Colon and Rectal Surgery

Colon and Rectal Surgery

MARVIN L. CORMAN, M.D.

Department of Colon and Rectal Surgery
Sansum Medical Clinic, Inc., Santa Barbara, California

Illustrated by Lois Barnes

J. B. Lippincott Company
PHILADELPHIA
London   Mexico City   New York   St. Louis   São Paulo   Sydney

Sponsoring Editor: Darlene D. Pedersen
Manuscript Editor: Rosanne Hallowell
Indexer: Julie Schwager
Art Director: Maria S. Karkucinski
Designer: Patrick Turner

Production Supervisor: J. Corey Gray
Production Assistant: Barney Fernandes
Compositor: Ruttle, Shaw & Wetherill, Inc.
Printer/Binder: The Murray Printing Company
Color Plate Printer: The Lehigh Press, Inc.

The author and publisher have exerted every effort to ensure that drug selection and dosage set forth in this text are in accord with current recommendations and practice at the time of publication. However, in view of ongoing research, changes in government regulations, and the constant flow of information relating to drug therapy and drug reactions, the reader is urged to check the package insert for each drug for any change in indications and dosage and for added warnings and precautions. This is particularly important when the recommended agent is a new or infrequently employed drug.

1 3 5 6 4 2

Library of Congress Cataloging in Publication Data

Corman, Marvin L.
    Colon and rectal surgery.

    Bibliography: p.
    Includes index.
        1. Colon (Anatomy)—Surgery.   2. Rectum—Surgery.
    I. Title. [DNLM: 1. Colon—Surgery.   2. Rectum—Surgery.
    WI 650 C811c]
    RD544.C67 1984   617'.5547   83-25598
    ISBN 0-397-50647-3

To my teachers

**John C. Goligher
Cornelius E. Sedgwick**

Master surgeons, inspiring leaders, treasured friends

PREFACE

In spite of its rather limited anatomical area, the colon and rectum commands a considerable proportion of a surgeon's attention. Developments in the field have proceeded apace so that many surgeons have elected to limit their area of interest to this specialty. Although it is true that some procedures are rather esoteric and should be undertaken only by those with special expertise, the majority of operations should be well within the purview of the well-trained general surgeon. It is my hope that *Colon and Rectal Surgery* is broad enough in scope to address the needs of both groups of surgical specialists, as well as those of surgical residents. If I have been able to demonstrate an organized approach to the diagnosis and treatment of the diverse conditions described, I will have succeeded in this venture.

I have tried to address what I believe are those disease processes in the anus, rectum, and colon for which surgical intervention may be considered. Where practical, I have included other conditions if they pose potential difficulty in differential diagnosis. Obviously, every physician and surgeon has areas of particular interest, but I have tried to avoid giving undue emphasis to one clinical entity or surgical procedure over another. I have particularly emphasized areas that have not been extensively discussed in most textbooks of surgery—for example, reconstructive anorectal surgery, incontinence, ostomy complications and their management, and dermatologic anal problems.

I think perhaps one of the unusual characteristics of this book is that it is a solitary endeavor. Many texts that are published today have multiple contributors or several coauthors. Some, as a result, may lack cohesiveness and uniformity. Conversely, an individually authored text has the potential deficiency of being restricted to its author's opinion, and consequently may be limited in perspective. In order to minimize this potential bias, I have tried to present diverse viewpoints, particularly in areas where there are controversies. I expect, however, that it will be abundantly clear to the reader where my opinion lies.

The text is supplemented with numerous artist's renditions depicting surgical technique, as well as extensive histologic, pathologic, and radiologic material. A comprehensive bibliography accompanies each chapter.

I think it is appropriate that the book be dedicated to two prominent men, John C. Goligher and Cornelius E. Sedgwick, who are part of a historic tradition of innovation and excellence in surgery.

It was my objective that *Colon and Rectal Surgery* effectively incorporate both the comprehension of a resource text and the pragmatism of a surgical atlas. The material is based on my experience in the clinical practice and teaching of colon and rectal surgery. I hope that the reader will find it of value.

Marvin L. Corman, M. D.

ACKNOWLEDGMENTS

Although this text is an individually authored effort, it could not have been prepared without the contributions and encouragement of many people.

I am very grateful to my fellows for their studies and writings during their year of training; their reviews have been incorporated within these pages. They have served as a source of learning for me.

The fine library of the Santa Barbara Cottage Hospital was indispensable. The director, Evelyn Fay, and her associate, Ann Campbell, enthusiastically furnished me with numerous references at my whim, and, I am certain, at great inconvenience to themselves. Elizabeth McChristie, whose outstanding work as a research assistant is evident to those familiar with the classic articles in the journal *Diseases of the Colon and Rectum,* must be recognized also for her contributions to this book. I am also very grateful to Rosalind Corman and Diane Schaefer for their assistance in searching the literature, abstracting data, and providing abundant material for this publication.

I must recognize the generous support of Paul Riemenschneider and his associates in the Department of Radiology at the Santa Barbara Cottage Hospital for making available their teaching collection for my use. Wayne Jakes, Sid Mauk, and Marshall Olson, my colleagues at the Sansum Clinic Department of Radiology, were also of great help.

The pathologic material is to a considerable extent based on the generosity of Rudolf Garret, Director of Pathology at the Sansum Medical Clinic, who spent many hours with me reviewing his voluminous personal collection. I am indeed fortunate to have benefited from his expertise. Rodger Haggitt, Director of the Section of Surgical Pathology at the Baptist Memorial Hospital, Memphis, Tennessee, provided further help in the field of intestinal pathology.

The book would not have been possible without the beautifully executed illustrations of Lois Barnes. Her artistic talent is matched by her scholarly diligence.

It is virtually impossible to include a comprehensive listing of the many individuals who provided their personal involvement, but I would be remiss if I did not mention Melissa Baughman, Estelle Light, Janet Layson, and Noel Hunt, enterostomal therapists, for their suggestions in the area of their special knowledge.

The influence of my colleagues John Libertino, John Clark, Arnold Medved, Albert Svoboda, George Scott, and Jerry Clark is felt throughout the book. I am particularly indebted to my associate, Elliot Prager, for his encouragement, endurance, and eternal optimism.

My publisher, the J. B. Lippincott Company, has been supportive, efficient, and highly professional. Special acknowledgment must be given to Darlene Pedersen, Rosanne Hallowell, Maria Karkucinski, John de Carville, and John Wehner. I would also like to mention Med-Photo Plus, who provided the excellent photographic reproductions. In addition, the dedication of Susan Lenkowec, who typed the manuscript, is most appreciated.

My nurses, Virginia Barone, Addé Donegan, Carol O'Brien, and Karin Ehde, were intimately involved throughout the writing. They were able to perform their clinical responsibilities as well as their extracurricular duties with grace and efficiency.

Finally, I wish to thank my wife, Bonnie, who read every page, reattached my dangling participles, and found my misplaced modifiers. In addition, I must apologize to her and to our sons, John and Alex, for my reclusion and for preempting our library and its writing desk.

CONTENTS

Color Figures/Chapter 1

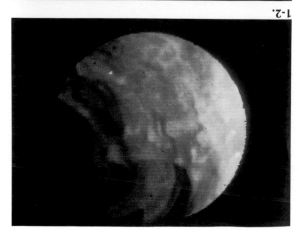

1-1.

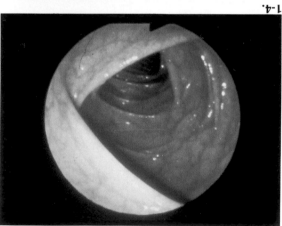

1-2.

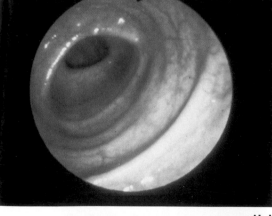

1-3.

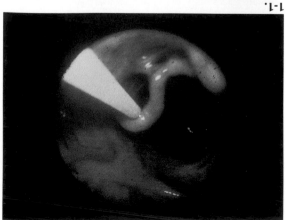

1-4.

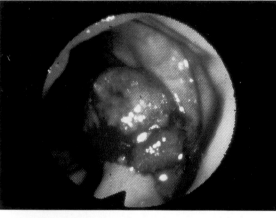

1-5.

1-1. Ulcerative colitis showing pseudopolyp.
1-2. Pseudomembranous colitis.
1-3. Normal descending colon.
1-4. Normal transverse colon.
Note the triangular folds.
1-5. Polyp of sigmoid on broad-based pedicle.

(Courtesy of Olympus Corporation of America)

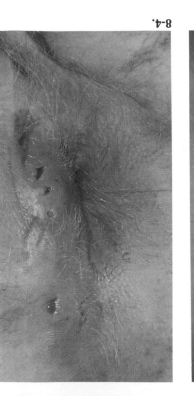

8-4.

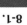

8-3.

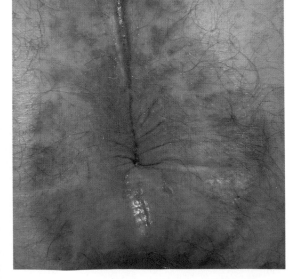

8-1.

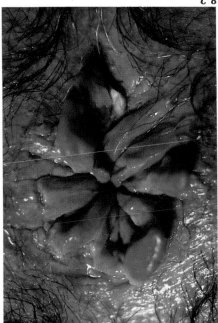

8-2.

8-1. Pruritus ani: Perianal neurodermatitis with lichenification and fissuring. (Courtesy of William G. Robertson, M.D.)

8-2. Pruritus ani: Marked edema with papillomatosis and nodularity, due to chronic abrading. (Courtesy of William G. Robertson, M.D.)

8-3. Psoriasis: Well-marginated erythematosquamous plaque with characteristic silvery scales. (Courtesy of Arnold Medved, M.D.)

8-4. Multiple external openings of fistula-in-ano.

Color Figures/Chapter 8

8-5. Mycosis fungoides: Violaceous tumor with adjacent reddish-brown, irregularly shaped plaques. (Corman ML, Veidenheimer MC, Swinton NW: Diseases of the Anus, Rectum and Colon. Part I: Neoplasms. New York, Medcom, 1972)

8-6. Leukemia cutis: Ulcerating, violaceous nodule. (Corman ML, Veidenheimer MC, Swinton NW: Diseases of the Anus, Rectum and Colon. Part I: Neoplasms. New York, Medcom, 1972)

8-7. Extramammary Paget's disease: Irregular but well-marginated, erythematous erosive patch. The edges are slightly indurated. (Courtesy of Arnold Medved, M.D.)

8-8. Extramammary Paget's disease: Recurrence after excision and skin grafting. (Courtesy of William G. Robertson, M.D.)

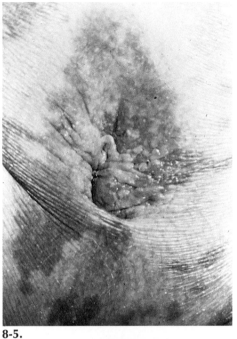

8-5.

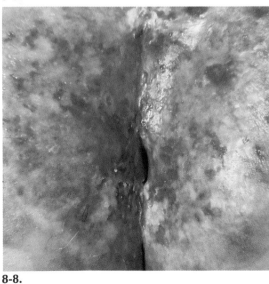

8-6.

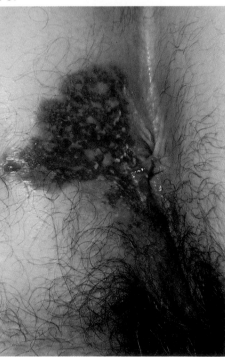

8-7.

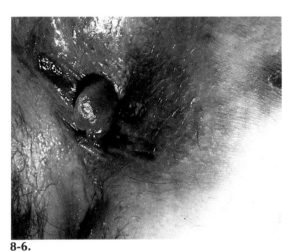

8-8.

9-1. Multiple (familial) polyposis.

10-1. Known polypoid carcinoma with surface ulceration; total colonoscopy is advised.

17-1. Melanosis coli.

(Courtesy of Olympus Corporation of America)

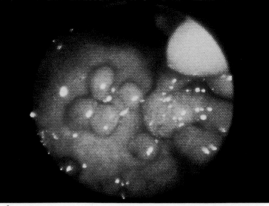

9-1.

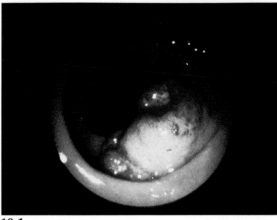

10-1.

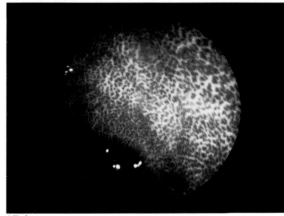

17-1.

CHAPTER 1

Evaluation and Diagnostic Techniques

This initial chapter addresses the evaluation of the symptoms frequently associated with diseases of the anus, rectum, and colon. In addition, the instrumentation and the studies available for the diagnosis of these condtions are presented.

HISTORY

As in all fields of medicine the assessment of the patient's history is the single most important piece of data that the physician can obtain. A carefully taken interview will in all probability either establish the diagnosis or at least suggest it. In the area of pathology of the anus, rectum, and colon there is a limited number of questions that are pertinent.

Bleeding

Bleeding from the rectum has long been established as an important warning sign of bowel cancer, yet cancer is not the most likely cause of hematochezia. Blood may be pink, bright red, mahogany, black, or inapparent (occult). It may be on the paper, in the toilet bowl, or both. None of the foregoing manifestations is diagnostic of the location or type of pathology with any degree of certainty. Blood on the paper alone is suggestive of a distal cause (e.g., hemorrhoids, fissure). Altered (dark) blood suggests a more proximal lesion

(e.g., carcinoma of the cecum). Blood in the bowl may or may not indicate greater blood loss. One drop of blood will turn the water pink, and a few drops will turn it red. Blood which is not observed by the patient but which is revealed through guaiac or orthotoluidine testing (see Occult Blood Determination) requires the same gastrointestinal evaluation that would be appropriate if it were perceived by the patient.

Bleeding usually is not an isolated symptom. When associated with a painful lump and unrelated to defecation it is usually due to a thrombosed hemorrhoid. When related to defecation it is often caused by an anal fissure, the most common cause of bleeding in the infant. When bleeding accompanies diarrhea, inflammatory bowel disease must be considered.

A reasonable index of suspicion must be present as well as competent clinical judgment before one embarks on additional studies to evaluate the cause of rectal bleeding. In exercising this judgment it is proper to withhold radiologic studies and defer esoteric procedures if the bleeding is due to a readily apparent cause. However, bleeding is an important symptom not to have. If it is felt to be due to hemorrhoids, appropriate treatment should be instituted to control the symptoms. If bleeding persists despite treatment, the responsibility falls on the physician to pursue the required studies necessary to establish a diagnosis, or to exclude within the limitations of the state of medical knowledge the presence of serious pathology.

2

Pain

Anorectal pain is a frequently heard complaint. It can be most disabling to the patient. If it is continuous, unrelated to defecation, and associated with a lump, a thrombosed hemorrhoid is the probable diagnosis. An anal abscess is another possibility. If the pain is worse during and following defecation, examination will usually reveal the presence of an anal fissure. If deep-seated, intermittent, and unrelated to defecation, the pain indicates that the patient is probably experiencing proctalgia fugax (levator spasm). If related to the coccyx and exacerbated by moving from a sitting to a standing position, it is coccygodynia. The diagnosis and management of these conditions are discussed in Chapter 17.

Anorectal pain is rarely associated with tumor unless the lesion invades the internal sphincter to produce tenesmus (a painful, ineffective desire to defecate).

Abdominal pain, if colicky in nature, may be caused by bowel obstruction, but most commonly is due to the irritable bowel syndrome. Physical examination and plain abdominal films readily distinguish the two entities. When abdominal pain is continuous, it may be due to peritoneal irritation from any of numerous causes. Here again physical examination and determination of the presence or absence of "peritoneal signs" will lead the physician to pursue the appropriate course.

Anal (Perianal) Mass

The differential diagnosis of an anal or perianal lump involves the spectrum of benign and malignant neoplastic lesions as well as a host of dermatologic conditions. However, the most common cause is a thrombosed hemorrhoid. Protrusion or prolapse of hemorrhoids that reduce spontaneously or require manual reduction may also be the etiology of the mass. Uncommonly, rectal prolapse (procidentia) may present as a rectal mass.

Other more frequently observed lumps include sebaceous cysts, lipomas, hypertrophied anal papillae, skin tags, and condylomata. With lesions of uncertain nature, biopsy is mandatory.

Rectal Discharge

Mucus discharge and soiling of the underclothes are not infrequent complaints. The patient may have had prior anal surgery with deformity and scarring, or he or she may have sphincter injury from surgical, accidental, or obstetric trauma. Hence, it is important to obtain an accurate history. Systemic disease (*e.g.,* diabetes mellitus) may be a factor. When purulent discharge is accompanied by a painful swelling, the patient usually has an anal or perianal abscess.

However, rectal discharge is usually not related to the presence of a specific pathologic entity. Most patients experience the difficulty because of dietary indiscretion or too vigorous attention to anal hygiene. Appropriate dietary and hygiene counseling may be all that is required. In patients with a lax anus, perineal strengthening exercises are advisable.

Incontinence

Fecal incontinence is usually due to fecal impaction, laxative abuse, or neurologic disease, but may also be the result of trauma. In the former situations medical management is usually the treatment of choice. The complaint of fecal incontinence requires at least a minimal neurologic examination (*e.g.,* sensory evaluation of the anal area). Repair or reconstruction is usually advocated for incontinence secondary to trauma or to congenital anomaly.

Change in Bowel Habits

The impression of the patient that the bowels have changed may have great significance. It is one of the symptoms suggestive of colonic neoplasm and almost always requires radiologic investigation for completeness.

Bowel habit change may be as obvious as diarrhea when the patient has had a long history of constipation, or as subtle as the development of normal, "easy" bowel movements in a patient after many years of a difficult or irregular pattern. The presence of bleeding with a bowel habit change increases the likelihood of the presence of a malignant neoplasm.

PHYSICAL EXAMINATION

A general physical examination of the patient with a colorectal complaint is usually an unrewarding experience. If one practices chief complaint medicine I see nothing improper in limiting the examination to the abdomen (also usually nonproductive) and to the rectum. Conversely, to embark upon radiologic investigation without performing a complete rectal examination is contraindicated.

The four basic approaches to colorectal evaluation

include inspection, palpation, anoscopy, and proctosigmoidoscopy. For the purpose of simplicity the term *proctosigmoidoscopy* is used interchangeably with the words *procto* and *sigmoidoscopy*. All three words imply the use of the 25-cm rigid instrument.

Positioning the Patient

The three commonly used patient positions for performing sigmoidoscopy are the prone, the left lateral, and the knee–chest (Fig. 1-1).

The prone (jackknife) position requires a special table that tilts the patient, head down (Fig. 1-2). The table is expensive, but this position provides the easiest access and the best view for the examiner. It is the least comfortable position, however, for patients.

The most comfortable position for patients is the left lateral (Sims') position. The patient lies on the left side on the examining table or bed with buttocks protruding over the edge, hips flexed, knees slightly extended, and right shoulder rotated anteriorly. The examiner may sit or stand depending on the height of the table or bed. Although this position is the easiest of the three for the patient, it is not as convenient for the examiner as is the prone position.

The knee–chest position is probably somewhat more comfortable for the patient than the prone position, but it is the least convenient for the examiner. In my opinion the knee–chest position should be abandoned.

Some physicians believe that the sigmoidoscope can be inserted farther when a patient is in one position rather than another, but there is no evidence to suggest that position either interferes with or expedites insertion of the instrument to its full length.

If one is to perform a satisfactory and reasonably comfortable examination, and to obtain all necessary information, it is essential to continually inform the patient what is to be expected and what is happening. Rectal examination may be a frustratingly unsuccessful experience for both the physician and the patient if proper concern is not demonstrated for the patient's understandable reluctance to submit to such an unpleasant intrusion of his intestinal tract. Warm hands and a reassuring demeanor are most helpful.

Inspection

Inspection of the anal area may reveal hemorrhoids, skin tags, dermatologic problems (including pruritic changes), abscess, fistula, scar, and deformity. Pain

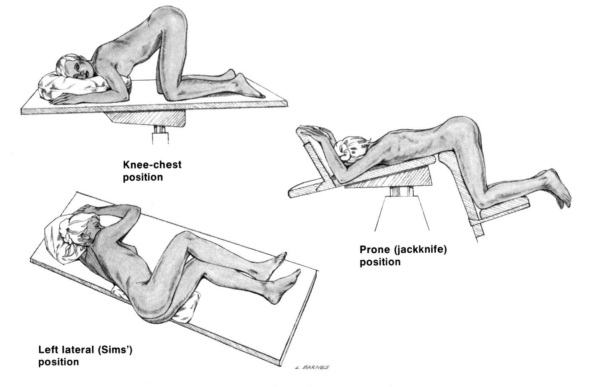

Knee-chest position

Prone (jackknife) position

Left lateral (Sims') position

L. BARNES

FIG. 1-1. Positions for performing sigmoidoscopy.

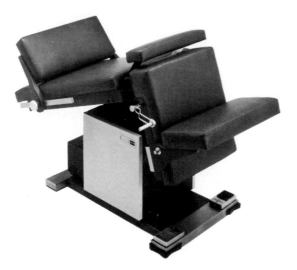

FIG. 1-2. Ritter table. (Courtesy of Sybron Corporation)

upon spreading the buttocks may indicate the presence of an anal fissure.

In addition to mere inspection of the perianal skin, evaluation of the resting state of the anal opening is important. A patulous anal opening may be seen with rectal prolapse, neurologic abnormality, sphincter injury, or the "gay bowel syndrome."[119]

By asking the patient to strain, further valuable information may be obtained. A rectal prolapse, hypertrophied anal papilla, or, most commonly, hemorrhoids may protrude. It should be remembered, however, that the prone (jackknife) position is least conducive to demonstrating conditions that tend to prolapse. If the physician suspects procidentia, then the patient should sit on the toilet for the examination.

Palpation

A water-soluble lubricant is applied to the gloved index finger. Although some physicians prefer the use of a finger cot, I prefer one of the disposable plastic gloves for rectal examination. The patient is informed that a finger will be passed into the rectum which will make him feel as if his bowels will move, but they won't. Again, it is imperative to inform continually and to reassure.

One should examine the rectum and its surrounding structures in an organized approach. In the man, first the prostate is felt anteriorly. Assessment of hypertrophy, nodularity, and firmness should be made. In the woman, the cervix is usually felt, unless it is surgically absent. The uterine body may be felt to be displaced posteriorly, and the presence of fibroid tumors may be noted. The uninitiated physician may misinterpret the nodularity as an intrarectal tumor. Another common error of rectal palpation in women is to misjudge a vaginal tampon for a rectal wall lesion. With experience, however, there should be no confusion. An enlarged prostate or a posteriorly displaced uterus may serve to warn the examiner tht rigid proctosigmoidoscopy will, in all probability, not be possible to the full length of the instrument.

One should then sweep the examining finger from anterior to posterior and back again, *consciously* thinking of a possible lesion that might be present. The conscious thought process is emphasized because all too often this phase of the examination is performed reflexively, with the assumption that any lesion will be identified by the instrument if it is not perceived by the examining finger. However, submucosal rectal nodules may not be visible and would otherwise be undiagnosed if direct visualization alone is employed. It is often possible to feel tumor in the sigmoid colon or a diverticular mass. Asking the patient to strain down (Valsalva's maneuver) will sometimes reveal a lesion in the upper rectum or rectosigmoid that otherwise might not be palpable.

Assessment of sphincter tone and contractility is an important part of the rectal examination and should be noted routinely whenever a patient complains of problems with fecal control or discharge.

Finally, as the finger is withdrawn, the presence of anal pathology is noted (*e.g.,* hypertrophied papilla, thrombosed hemorrhoid, stenosis, scarring, *etc.*). Digital examination of the anal canal is the most accurate means of diagnosing Crohn's disease in this area.

Anoscopy

Anoscopic examination unfortunately is employed too often as a substitue for proctosigmoidoscopy by physicians who do not have the sigmoidoscope in the office. A barium enema examination is then performed and a rectal lesion often overlooked. Conversely, when proctosigmoidoscopy is performed, anoscopy is usually omitted. The anoscope is not a substitute for the sigmoidoscope, and the proctoscopic examination is not an effective replacement for anoscopy. Anoscopy offers the best means to evaluate hemorrhoids, fissure, papillae, or other lesions of the anal canal. It is the requisite instrument if one is to perform an anal procedure or treat an anal canal condition.

There are a number of anoscopes available on the market (Fig. 1-3), but the one I prefer is the Hirschman. Fiberoptic modifications are available which have a light source that fits into the instrument (Fig. 1-4). These are preferred for convenience, but they are

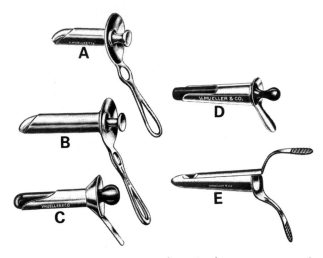

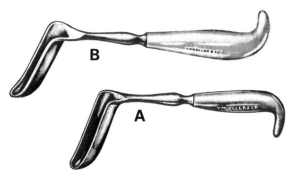

FIG. 1-5. A. The Hill-Ferguson rectal retractor, available in three depths and widths. **B.** The Ferguson-Moon rectal retractor, available in two depths and widths. (Courtesy of American V. Mueller)

FIG. 1-3. Anoscopes. **A.** The Hirschman anoscope is available in three diameters, ⅞ inches (2.2 cm), ¹¹/₁₆ inches (1.75 cm), and ⁹/₁₆ inches (1.43 cm). **B.** The Buie-Hirschman anoscope is similar to the Hirschman except it is 1 inch (2.5 cm) longer. **C.** The Ives anoscope has a hard rubber obturator and is available in one size (8.3 cm length). **D.** The Vernon-David anoscope is 3″ (7.6 cm) in length and 2 cm in diameter. **E.** The Brinkerhoff anoscope is a side-view instrument with a removable slide available in three sizes. (Courtesy of American V. Mueller)

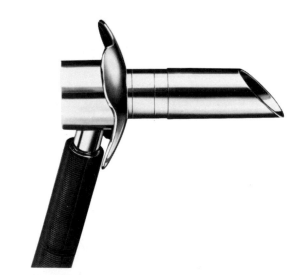

FIG. 1-4. The Welch Allyn fiberoptic anoscope (obturator not shown) is available in three diameters, 2.7 cm, 2.3 cm, and 1.9 cm. (Courtesy of Welch Allyn, Inc.)

relatively expensive. Alternatively, a hand-held light as an external light source (*e.g.*, a goose-neck lamp) is usually adequate but somewhat cumbersome. Side-view instruments in my hands fail to give adequate perspective of the anal canal and of anal pathology, so I avoid them. If a side view is required for performing an office procedure (*e.g.*, sphincterotomy) a narrow (2.2 cm) Hill-Ferguson retractor is preferred (Fig. 1-5). When rotating the anoscope around the anal cavity circumference it is helpful to reinsert the obturator in order to move the instrument. There is less tendency to drag or pinch the anal canal or perianal skin when one does this.

Finally, when noting or treating pathology, the site should be recorded as follows: right anterior, left lateral, and so forth. The use of the "o'clock" description should be abandoned, for it requires a known patient position, and this may differ from one examination to another.

Proctosigmoidoscopy

The sigmoidoscope is one of our most valuable diagnostic tools, perhaps even more useful than the stethoscope. The stethoscope is not likely to identify a cardiac, pulmonary, or abdominal abnormality that is not already evident from a carefully taken history. Also, stethoscopic findings almost always require confirmation by x-ray or electrocardiography. I do not expect physicians to discard their traditional auscultatory tool and begin carrying a sigmoidoscope in a hip holster to undertake the procedure on every patient they see. However, since the most common visceral malignancy in the United States today is colorectal cancer, it is a pity that more physicians do not do sigmoidoscopy.

Every patient should, at some time, undergo this procedure coincident with a complete medical examination. Ideally, an initial sigmoidoscopic examination should be performed when a patient is in his late teens in order to detect whether he has a tendency to form polyps. A number of investigators have confirmed a relatively high yield of asymptomatic polyps when proctosigmoidoscopic examination is performed as part of a complete physical examination. Swinton reported an incidence of 5% in a series of 3000 routine examination.[124] Portes and Majarakis reported almost an 8% incidence in 50,000 asymptomatic patients.[105] In our experience, approximately 9% of patients were found to have benign lesions.[26] After this initial examination sigmoidoscopy is not necessary as a routine diagnostic test for asymptomatic patients until age 50 and every 2 years thereafter. Of course, any patient who has such symptoms as rectal bleeding or a change in bowel habits should have this examination regardless of age.

The rigid sigmoidoscope is the best instrument available for evaluation of the rectum and rectosigmoid. Barium enema study is a poor technique for evaluating the rectum, and even fiberoptic sigmoidoscopy and colonscopy are not as satisfactory as sigmoidoscopy for evaluating ampullary lesions. Examination with the sigmoidoscope may reveal mucosal excrescences, polypoid lesions, cancer, inflammatory changes, stricture, vascular malformation, or anatomic distortion from extraluminal masses. It may also detect anal conditions, but, as mentioned, it is not an instrument to replace the anoscope for this purpose.

Equipment

There are numerous rigid sigmoidoscopes available, reusable and disposable, with proximal or with distal lighting, and with and without fiberoptics. The reusable instrument requires an initial expense that may exceed $300 (Fig. 1-6), whereas the disposable instruments (without the light source) are available for somewhat in excess of one dollar apiece (Fig. 1-7). The former obviously requires care and cleansing, whereas the latter is discarded. If only a few examinations a day are performed, the reusable instrument may be more appropriate. If many examinations are undertaken every day, unless one can afford the luxury of having a number of instruments and can justify the labor expense of cleansing them, the disposable instrument is usually preferred.

Reusable instruments are available in a number of diameters, ranging from 1.1 to 2.7 cm. The medium or 1.9-cm instrument is an excellent compromise that offers one the ability both to screen the patient and to perform procedures. The large bore instrument is less useful for screening because of greater patient discomfort but may be invaluable for removing a large polyp. The narrow sigmoidoscope (1.1 cm) is a good screening tool and is particularly useful if an anal stricture precludes the use of the larger-diameter instrument. It is very limiting, however, if one attempts to do procedures through it.

In addition to the speculum tube itself, the instrumentation includes a light source, a proximal magnifying lens, and an attachment for the insufflation of air.

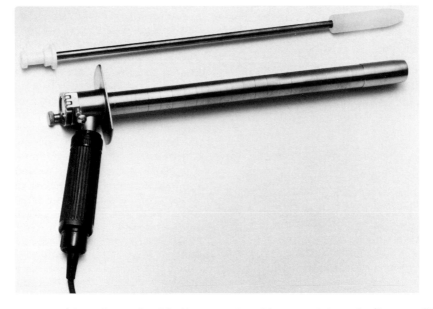

FIG. 1-6. Reusable and autoclavable fiberoptic sigmoidoscope, 1.9 cm in diameter, 25 cm in length. (Courtesy of Welch Allyn, Inc.)

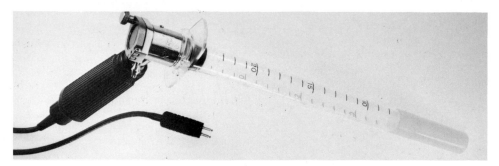

FIG. 1-7. Disposable fiberoptic sigmoidoscope. (Courtesy of Welch Allyn, Inc.)

There is the mistaken concept that the reservoir is an important piece of equipment, but its effect is to make the rigid sigmoidoscope an excessively long, cumbersome, and inconvenient apparatus. The first action one should take after purchasing new equipment is to remove the reservoir and attach the bulb to the eyepiece by the shortest length of tubing possible (Fig. 1-8).

Another important detail is adequate provision for suction. This can be accomplished by attachment to a vacuum pump or a water tap. Long swabs (chimney sweeps) are also helpful (Fig. 1-9).

Preparation

Adequate preparation of the distal bowel is a *sine qua non* for a complete and satisfactory examination. A small-volume enema (*e.g.,* Fleets) is administered just before examination unless the patient has a history suggesting inflammatory bowel disease. Vigorous catharsis the day before the examination and dietary restrictions are unnecessary.

Technique

There are five principles that should be adhered to if one is to conduct a safe, competent sigmoidoscopic examination:

Be expeditious.
Insufflate minimal air.
Have a nurse or assistant always available.
Keep talking: explain, reassure, distract.
Do no harm.

As mentioned earlier, a digital rectal examination should always precede instrumentation. Besides the information gleaned it permits the sphincter to relax sufficiently to accept the larger-diameter instrument. The well-lubricated, warmed sigmoidoscope is then inserted and passed to the maximum height as quickly as possible without causing significant discomfort.

Air insufflation is of value in demonstrating the lumen of the bowel and is of even greater benefit in visualizing the mucosa when the instrument is withdrawn. But air insufflation should be kept to a minimum because it tends to cause abdominal cramping that may persist for many hours after the examination. Although the novice should not pass the sigmoidoscope without clearly observing the lumen, as skill develops one can determine the amount of gentle pressure that can be safely exerted as long as the mucosa is seen to be sliding past. When an obstacle is reached, the instrument is withdrawn slightly and redirected to again view the lumen; it is then readvanced.

One should withdraw the sigmoidoscope in a rotating fashion, carefully viewing the entire circumference of the bowel wall and ironing out mucosal folds and the valves of Houston to be certain that no small lesion is missed. Particular care should be taken to view the posterior wall that sits in the hollow of the sacrum. This may necessitate the awkward placement of the examiner's head behind the patient's knees.

A key to success in inserting the sigmoidoscope is to be familiar with the anatomy of the rectum and the sigmoid colon. Knowing where the lumen probably is located without actually visualizing it permits the examiner considerable freedom in passing the instrument. When the instrument is inserted, the low and mid-rectal areas are midline structures. As the upper rectum is reached the bowel bends slightly to the left. At the rectosigmoid junction, the tendency is for the instrument to turn to the right and ventrally. Therefore, if difficulty is encountered at the level of 15 or 16 cm, a maneuver to the left might reveal the proximal bowel. At the level of 18 or 19 cm, a more vigorous maneuver to the right and ventrally might permit the proximal colon to be entered.

One must take care when passing the instrument without visualizing the lumen. However, perforation from rigid sigmoidoscopy is uncommon. Swinton reported 2 such occurrences in almost 100,000 examinations.[123] Gilbertsen reported 5 perforations in 103,000 examinations, and Nelson and associates noted 2 in over 16,000 proctosigmoidoscopies.[58, 95]

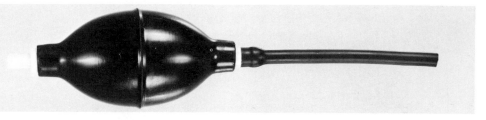

FIG. 1-8.   Insufflation bulb without reservoir. (Courtesy of Cameron-Miller, Inc.)

As of this writing I have not experienced this occurrence in over 50,000 examinations, but I have had one death from ventricular fibrillation. My own feeling is that perforation of the *normal* rectum or sigmoid colon should not occur from the instrument alone, but attempting to pass the instrument in a patient with inflammatory bowel disease, diverticulitis, radiation proctitis, or cancer can be a hazardous undertaking. Air insufflation can cause perforation of a diverticulum or of a walled-off abscess, and obviously such procedures as biopsy and electrocoagulation can result in perforation.

Bacteremia may be associated with lower gastrointestinal tract endoscopy.[3, 35, 77, 81] Even rectal examination may predispose to such a complication.[71] Although there is some difference of opinion about the incidence (0% to approximately 25%) and the significance of a transient nonfebrile episode, prophylactic antibiotic therapy should at least be considered in the patient at higher risk (*e.g.,* someone who has undergone heart valve replacement).

In my experience the average *length of instrument insertion* is 20 cm.[26] In a report from the Mayo Clinic, 25% of patients could not be examined beyond this point.[110] Nivatvongs and Fryd reported the average depth of insertion to be 19.5 cm.[97] The two structures that may preclude complete (25-cm) examination are the uterus and the prostate gland. An enlarged prostate, a uterus containing fibroid tumors, or a uterus that is displaced posteriorly may make it impossible to pass the instrument beyond the 15-cm level. Persistence in attempting to achieve a higher penetration is usually unrewarding and may be dangerous, and it is most uncomfortable for the patient. As mentioned, the potential for encountering this difficulty can often be predicted by careful digital examination.

Men are examined to the full length of the instrument much more often then women. Even when the uterus is surgically absent, fixation of the bowel in the pelvis may preclude passage of the instrument. A careful history will alert the examiner to expedite the procedure and to minimize further discomfort.

Younger patients are often more difficult to examine than older patients; because they usually have better sphincter tone, insertion of the instrument may cause

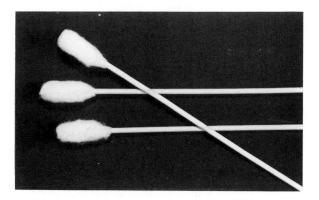

FIG. 1-9.   Chimney sweeps (long cotton-tip applicators for removing small amounts of stool).

more discomfort. The discomfort leads to apprehension and a tendency to "bear down," making the examination more tedious. Also, pelvic organs are less lax in younger than in older women, causing it to be somewhat more difficult to displace the uterus and to allow passage of the sigmoidoscope.

Procedures Through the Sigmoidoscope

There are three commonly employed procedures that one performs through the proctosigmoidoscope: biopsy, fulguration (electrocoagulation), and snare excision. Gear and Dobbins have published a comprehensive review on the diagnostic usefulness of rectal biopsy, to which is appended an extensive bibliography.[53] Biopsy forceps are available with various biting tips (Fig. 1-10). I prefer the Bouie instrument (Fig. 1-11), because in my hands it seems to cut what I wish it to, and I have had less success with the others. Some instruments are electrified for biopsy and coagulation, but the technique is cumbersome. Rarely is bleeding a problem when lesions for "disease" are biopsied. The occasional incident of bleeding usually occurs when biopsy is taken of a normal-appearing rectum, that is, when one is seeking a diagnosis (*e.g.,* Hirschsprung's disease, amyloidosis). Unless the bleeding is pulsatile at the site of the biopsy I rarely prolong the examina-

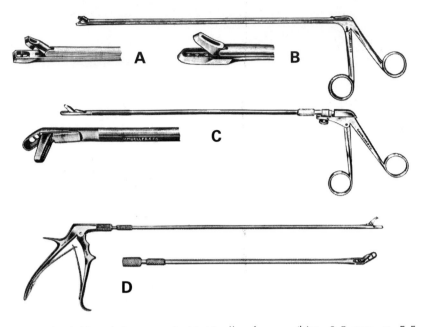

FIG. 1-10. Rectal biopsy forceps. **A.** V. Mueller forceps (bite, 3.5 mm × 5.5 mm). **B.** Yeomans forceps (bite, 4 mm × 10 mm). **C.** Turell angulated specimen forceps. **D.** Biopsy forceps; the curved upper jaw has a 360° rotation feature. (Courtesy of American V. Mueller)

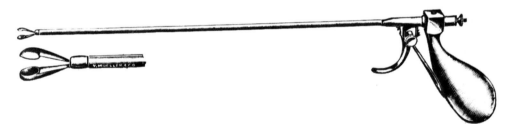

FIG. 1-11. Buie rectal biopsy forceps. (Courtesy of American V. Mueller)

tion to await complete hemostasis. If bleeding occurs it should be treated by applying pressure (tamponade) with an epineprhine-soaked, cotton-tipped stick (chimney sweep), rather than by electrocoagulation. Fulguration of a bleeding area when a biopsy has been taken of a grossly normal rectum may lead to perforation. Biopsy under such circumstances should always be performed on the posterior wall or at the valve of Houston.

Fulguration requires familiarity with electrosurgical equipment. Most surgeons find the instrument setting that works well for the procedure performed, but the same procedure carried out in the hospital with the same or different equipment may produce inadequate or too vigorous electrocoagulation. One is advised to test any unfamiliar equipment with a bar of soap, adjusting the setting for the appropriate conditions.

My own preference is for the suction-fulgurating unit made by Cameron-Miller (Figs. 1-12 and 1-13). This removes gas, smoke, liquid stool, and blood at the same time that the coagulation is being accomplished. Although it is helpful to know that a small lesion is a true polypoid adenoma rather than a hyperplastic polyp, biopsy of every mucosal excrescence is meddlesome and unnecessary. One can feel content to fulgurate (without biopsy) lesions under 5 mm. However, for larger tumors it is better to obtain pathologic confirmation through either a biopsy or a snare excision.

Use of the wire loop snare (Fig. 1-14) requires considerably more skill than fulguration alone. The technique usually permits complete excision with one application, although sometimes multiple snarings are required to remove larger growths. This is still an office procedure, however, if the surgeon has the appropriate equipment.

The snare is passed around the polyp and the wire

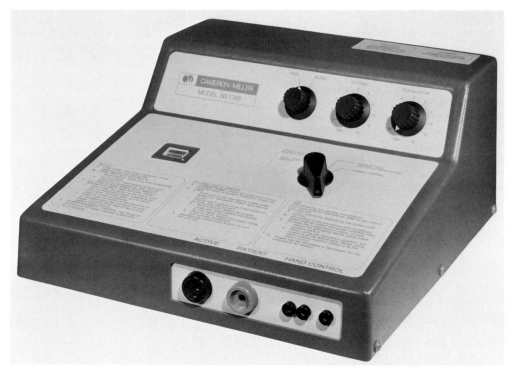

FIG. 1-12. Cameron-Miller electrosurgery unit. (Courtesy of Cameron-Miller, Inc.)

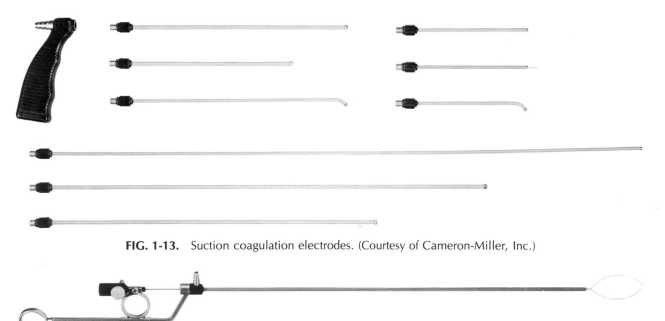

FIG. 1-13. Suction coagulation electrodes. (Courtesy of Cameron-Miller, Inc.)

FIG. 1-14. Wire loop snare and handle for polyp removal. (Courtesy of Cameron-Miller, Inc.)

loop slowly closed; the instrument is "jiggled" as the wire tightens the base. This maneuver permits adjacent mucosa to escape and minimizes the risk of burning the bowel wall. Coagulation rather than cutting current is preferred for snare excision because greater control of the speed of cutting through tissue can be exerted. If a thick pedicle is present, one may take several minutes to remove the specimen. After the polyp is removed it is helpful to have a long alligator or biopsy forceps to retrieve it.

If bleeding occurs from a pedicle, it may be secured by fulguration, application of pressure with an epinephrine-soaked chimney sweep, or the use of a long-armed (extended) rubber-ring ligator (see Chap. 2). By grabbing the pedicle with an alligator forceps, rubber-ring ligation can be performed to establish hemostasis. This technique, however, is not applicable to the sessile, bleeding area. Another method that has been recently advocated is the use of a "plumber's helper," or Frankfeldt forceps (Fig. 1-15), to grasp and twist the bleeding area.[5] The instrument is secured to the patient for up to 24 hours.

In contrast to closed-system fiberoptic endoscopy, electrocoagulation or snare excision with the open-ended sigmoidoscope does not require a full bowel preparation. Even in the situation in which an explosive gas mixture may be present, venting should be adequate enough to prevent proximal bowel injury. But bowel perforation under such circumstances is a potential hazard, albeit an uncommon one.

A patient may present with signs and symptoms of bowel perforation within a few minutes of electrocoagulation, polyp excision, or biopsy, or may develop septic problems as long as 10 days later. Anyone who complains of abdominal pain who underwent such a procedure in that interval requires urgent examination. The presence of free intra-abdominal or retro-peritoneal gas confirms the diagnosis, but in the absence of obvious peritonitis, treatment may consist of in-hospital observation, restriction of oral intake, intravenous fluid replacement, and broad-spectrum antibiotics. Fever or leukocytosis alone or in combination is not necessarily an indication for surgical intervention. Each clinical situation must be addressed individually. In the equivocal circumstance, one might consider a Gastrografin enema study (see Alternatives to the Use of Barium). But one can hardly be critical of the surgeon who performs a negative exploratory laparotomy in a patient whose abdominal signs and symptoms are increasing in severity or who continues to manifest fever and leukocytosis. If patients are to improve on "conservative" treatment, they almost always will do so within 24 hours.

FLEXIBLE FIBEROPTIC SIGMOIDOSCOPY

Flexible fiberoptic sigmoidoscopy (FFS) has developed more recently as an offshoot of colonoscopy (see Fiberoptic Colonoscopy) in order to simplify the former procedure and yet permit more bowel to be examined than is possible with a rigid instrument. Also, the examination has been touted to be more comfortable for the patient.

There is no doubt that FFS inspects more bowel surface area than is possible with the rigid proctosigmoidoscope. Marks and associates reached 50 cm or more in approximately two thirds of their patients.[86] The overall yield of pathology was more than three times greater with the flexible instrument. Others also report great satisfaction in this regard.[11, 20, 48, 138]

FFS is not, however, an easy examination to accomplish. Certainly the most difficult part of the procedure of colonoscopy is to negotiate the sigmoid, and this problem pertains equally to FFS; the only difference is that one does not usually have to employ various straightening maneuvers. The examination does require skill and patience. Experience is the best teacher. To paraphrase Hedberg, if only we could omit the first 100 endoscopies and begin with the 101st, a more comprehensive examination would be obtained, and we would experience very few complications indeed.[67]

In addressing the assertion that the procedure is more comfortable than rigid proctosigmoidoscopy, this may be more a reflection of patient position than of the examination itself. As mentioned earlier, the lateral Sims' position is preferred for patient comfort, and this is the recommended approach for FFS. But the examination does take longer; approximately half of the examinations took more than 5 minutes in Marks and associates' series, and my experience has been similar.[86] Furthermore, with air insufflation, gas cramping tends to persist for a much longer period of time following

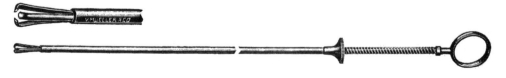

FIG. 1-15. Frankfeldt forceps. (Courtesy of American V. Mueller)

FFS. The list below illustrates a number of real and theoretic disadvantages of this examination.

Disadvantages of Flexible Fiberoptic Sigmoidoscopy

Cost
    Capital expense and repairs
    Personnel time (enema administration, cleaning)
    Duration
Communicable Disease
Complications
    Perforation
    Hemorrhage
    Explosion
Compromise of Adequate Colon Examination

The first and most often quoted criticism of the technique is the cost, which (excluding light source and accessories) approximates $4000. In addition to the outlay for the capital expense and repairs, there are the costs of personnel (longer time for examination, need for cleansing the instrument, patient preparation, *etc.*). And, of course, a critical consideration is the cost to the patient. In polling a number of medical centers and physicians, the cost of the examination ranged from a minimum of 25% more than for rigid proctosigmoidoscopy to as much as 150% more.

Another theoretical disadvantage of the procedure is that a more careful history must be obtained from the patient. With the difficulty in sterilizing the instrument, patients who have had a history of hepatitis, anal condylomata, and other infectious or communicable diseases should not be submitted to this examination routinely.[20]

Complications such as hemorrhage or perforation should not occur with any greater frequency with a flexible instrument than with the rigid. Care obviously is required whenever the procedure is undertaken in the presence of bowel disease, especially active inflammatory disease, diverticulitis, and ischemia. Minimal air should be used under these circumstances. Explosions should not occur, because electrocautery should not be employed for biopsy or snare excision with this instrument. The limited bowel preparation combined with a closed system presents a potential hazard for the presence of an explosive gas mixture. Biopsies should be carried out only with a ''cold'' forceps. Brush cytology may, of course, be safely employed.

One final point is that this examination is not a substitute for radiographic evaluation of the colon or total colonoscopy. It is an improvement over rigid proctosigmoidoscopy as a screening tool but is not the procedure of choice for evaluating the colon in a symptomatic patient.

FSS is indicated for the following reasons:

As a substitute for rigid proctosigmoidoscopy in screening, in evaluation of gastrointestinal complaints, and in polyp and cancer surveillance

Evaluation of questionable radiologic findings in the sigmoid colon

Confirmation of radiographic findings within range of the instrument

Diagnostic and follow-up evaluation of a patient with inflammatory bowel disease, especially if the disease is confined to the left or distal colon

Inspection of colon anastomosis when it is within range of the instrument

Therapeutically, FSS may be employed to reduce sigmoid volvulus and in combination with the snare to remove a foreign body.

Instrumentation

The flexible fiberoptic sigmoidoscope is available in the United States through a number of companies (American Cystoscope Makers, Inc. [ACMI], American Optical, Fuginon, and Olympus). Figure 1-16 illustrates the Olympus instrument. It has a working length of 68 cm and an outer diameter of 14 mm. It is forward viewing and has a wide-angle optical system (100°). The tip bends in four directions, 180° up and 180° down, 160° to the right and 160° to the left. It contains a 3.7-mm instrument channel for suction and for the passage of forceps, electrodes, or cytology brush (Fig. 1-17).

The flexible fiberoptic sigmoidoscope is quite similar from company to company. The tip of the instrument is deflected by rotation of the larger dial in each direction (Fig. 1-18). The smaller dial deflects the tip from

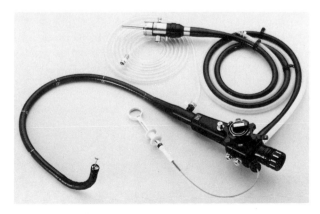

FIG. 1-16. Fiberoptic sigmoidoscope, CF-ITS2. (Courtesy of Olympus Corporation of America)

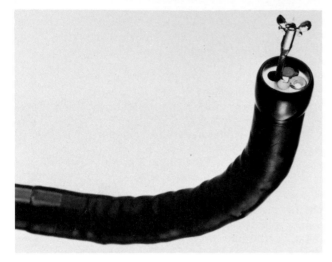

FIG. 1-17. Fiberoptic sigmoidoscope, CF-ITS2. Close-up of the bending section with biopsy forceps. (Courtesy of Olympus Corporation of America)

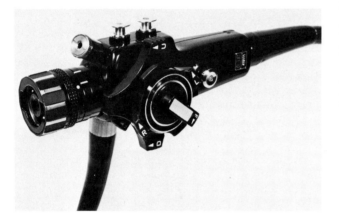

FIG. 1-18. Control unit of fiberoptic sigmoidoscope. (Courtesy of Olympus Corporation of America)

side to side. If both dials are turned maximally it produces a tight bend that causes the instrument to double back and impede further passage. When passing the instrument it is advantageous to keep the dials in the neutral position as much as possible.

Preparation

FFS requires only a limited bowel preparation Two small enemas (*e.g.,* Fleets) are given separately, the second approximately 10 minutes after the first has been eliminated. Dietary restrictions and oral laxatives are unnecessary.

Technique

The patient is placed in the left lateral (Sims') position on a relatively high examining table. The patient's right leg is flexed more than the left, and the right shoulder is rotated anteriorly. It is usually easier to stand than to sit. A two-person team approach is optimal, one person to handle the dials and the other to advance the instrument. Although one can do both, the procedure can be carried out much more expeditiously with two. This requires the addition of a fiberoptic teaching attachment (Fig. 1-19).

A well-lubricated finger is passed into the rectum, and then the instrument is inserted. Passing the blunt-ended FFS in without prior digital examination is difficult to accomplish and causes considerable apprehension and discomfort for the patient.

As with colonoscopy, what is usually encountered first is a dull pink or orange haze, perhaps with considerable fecal debris or retained enema fluid. While insufflating air rather than redirecting the tip, the instrument should be inserted further to 10 or 12 cm. This will usually permit visualization of the rectal ampulla. The person who advances the instrument has greater control of the course of the examination than the person handling the dials. In training an assistant or a resident to do FFS, I prefer to insert the instrument until the assistant has reached competence with the proximal end before reversing roles. In a surgical operation the assistant can either impede or expedite the procedure; he can make the surgeon appear either incompetent or highly experienced. Conversely, the skilled surgeon acting as a first assistant can orchestrate the procedure so effectively that the assistant can scarcely believe how ''talented'' he has become.

The instrument is passed with the lumen either under direct visualization or with the mucosa sliding past. Again, the person on the distal end can judge how firmly to push while watching the mucosa rush by.

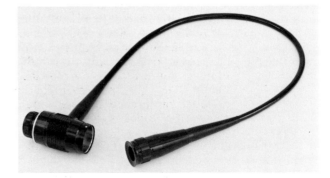

FIG. 1-19. Fiberoptic teaching attachment. (Courtesy of Olympus Corporation of America)

This approach is quite similar to that applicable to rigid proctosigmoidoscopy.

If further passage is impeded, the instrument is withdrawn slightly, the lumen is searched out by dial manipulation and rotation, and the instrument is advanced again. Coller describes in detail the various methods that are helpful in advancing the instrument; he calls them "torquing, dithering, and dither-torquing (accordianization)."[23] He also describes the familiar elongation and looping (alpha maneuver) techniques. I believe his article should be required reading for anyone who plans to employ FFS. By using the technique of "dithering" (the principle by which a person sitting on a chair with feet raised can move it across the floor by abrupt, jerking motions of the body), staccato movements of the instrument forward and back may permit the bowel virtually to intubate itself onto the 'scope.[23]

Negotiation of the sigmoid colon is the most difficult part of the procedure. With an intended limited examination, straightening the sigmoid colon is of less importance than it is with colonoscopy. But if all one accomplishes is to stretch the colon by attempts at advancement, another maneuver must be tried. Counterclockwise rotation of the instrument produces the so-called alpha loop (Fig. 1-20). Clockwise rotation results in relative straightening of the sigmoid colon and the opportunity to advance the instrument into the descending colon. Another means of proceeding up the descending colon when the sigmoid loop has already been traversed is to withdraw the instrument while rotating clockwise.

After the instrument has been passed to its full length or as far as is possible, it is carefully and slowly withdrawn. Suction, irrigation, and air insufflation are alternatively employed as indicated to obtain clear visualization of the entire mucosa. Biopsy (without electrocoagulation) or brush cytology is obtained if appropriate and the instrument removed. It is important to remember that FFS and colonoscopy are poor tools for evaluation of ampullary or distal rectal pathology. Particular care is required for examination of this area.

Finally, it is important not to forget why the patient is having the examination; if bleeding is the indication, it is not sufficient to reassure the patient that the FFS was normal. FFS does not diagnose pruritus ani, and it is not the appropriate instrument for evaluating the anal canal. Anoscopy and additional studies may be required.

BARIUM ENEMA

Since Cannon's original contrast studies of the gastrointestinal tract, the barium enema has been and continues to be the standard procedure for evaluation of the colon.[17, 18, 19]

Indications

Evaluation of the colon by barium roentgenogram is the most cost-effective means of identifying colon pathology (benign and malignant lesions, diverticular disease, inflammatory conditions, congenital anomalies), intrinsic as well as extrinsic abnormalities.[87] It can be usefully employed in urgent or emergency circumstances to differentiate between small and large bowel obstruction, acute appendicitis, and periappendiceal abscess. It has been successfully employed in the therapeutic setting to reduce volvulus and intussusception.

As a screening tool for neoplasm in an asymptomatic patient with no preexisting history of polypoid disease or cancer, it cannot be recommended. Benjamin and Todd performed barium enema examinations on 8420 asymptomatic patients and found that 45 had evidence suggestive of neoplasm, an incidence of 0.5%.[7] Gianturco and Miller reported a 2.3% incidence of polyps in 35,000 asymptomatic patients who underwent air-contrast barium enema studies.[57]

In patients with known asymptomatic rectal polyps, Drexler reported proximal lesions in 4.7%.[38] Our experience in 200 such patients revealed an incidence of only 2.5%.[27] However, if the rectal polyp that was initially identified was pedunculated, 13% of the patients had a proximal lesion as compared with approximately 1% with a sessile rectal polyp ($P = 0.01$).[27] One criticism of this study, however, is that not all rectal polyps have pathologic confirmation; some may have been hyperplastic and not true neoplasms.

Preparation

The procedure is essentially a meaningless exercise if the preparation has been inadequate. Without proper cleansing it may be difficult to distinguish tumor from stool and impossible to exclude the presence of small neoplasms (Fig. 1-21).

A number of bowel preparations have been recommended, but basically they consist of some dietary restriction the day prior to the procedure (usually a low-residue diet with a clear liquid supper), a vigorous laxative, and a suppository or enema the day of the examination. Sands was inspired to write the following ode to the subject:

O for a colon that's pure and untrammeled,
O for a colon that's clean.
You may have a heart that's as pure as the snow,
And still have a bowel that's obscene.[111]

There have been many studies concerning the optimal bowel preparation. Dodds and co-workers in a controlled evaluation demonstrated that regimens utiliz-

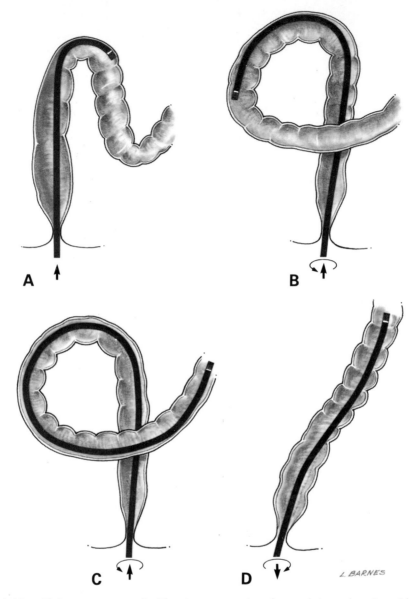

FIG. 1-20. Alpha maneuver. **A.** The instrument is advanced into the sigmoid colon. **B.** Counterclockwise rotation during advancement results in the loop. **C.** The colonoscope enters the descending colon. **D.** Clockwise torque during withdrawal permits straightening of the sigmoid colon.

ing magnesium citrate and bisacodyl were superior to those using castor oil, both in terms of effectiveness of cleansing and of patient complaints.[36] Other commercial preparations contain senna or cascara sagrada.

Another technique involves the oral administration (or more usually nasogastric tube installation) of Ringer's lactate or another saline solution.[70, 117] This preparation has also been advocated for colon cleansing prior to colonoscopy and bowel resection (Crapp prep).[29] Four to eight liters may be required, and evacuation may be complete in as little as two to as much as six hours.

It is important to maintain adequate hydration during laxative preparations. Many patients are elderly, and the barium enema study requires a considerable catharsis. This in turn can lead to renal, cardiac, and

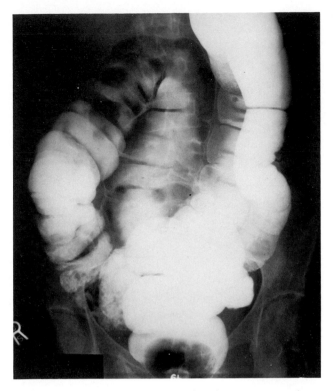

FIG. 1-21. A barium enema with a large amount of retained stool makes diagnosis of an intraluminal lesion virtually impossible.

Cannon first instilled contrast material into the gastrointestinal tract using bismuth subnitrate.[17] Shortly thereafter, barium began to be used because of its effective opacity, lack of absorption, ease of preparation, and low cost. Unfortunately, USP barium sulfate tends to settle and flocculate, and is composed of varying-sized particles. Newer preparations, however, are micronized with standard, small-sized particles in a suspending agent containing a measured amount of tannic acid. Barium is commercially available in a disposable bag, ready for the addition of a specified amount of water. High voltage (approximately 110 kv) is used in order to penetrate the barium column sufficiently.

It is important to realize that instillation of an opaque material within a hollow viscus does not fill the organ. What is being seen is the contrast material against one wall of the colon with the independent wall not identified and not filled. That is why most radiologists perform fluoroscopy with the patient in the supine position (evaluating the posterior wall of the bowel) and do the overhead films with the patient in the prone position (to evaluate the anterior wall). Questionable areas on the anterior wall then necessitate returning the patient to the x-ray table for fluoroscopy and respotting with the patient in the prone position.

Preliminary films of the abdomen, *i.e.*, kidney, ureter, and bladder (KUB), are obtained in order to identify areas of calcification, the presence of air or fluid-filled loops of intestine, residual fecal material, barium

electrolyte problems. By encouraging the patient to drink frequent glasses of water, in addition to clear juice and bouillon, these complications can be avoided. Cardiovascular and renal problems are more likely to occur with the gastric intubation technique. This method, therefore, is relatively contraindicated in elderly patients and in patients with renal or cardiovascular diseases. The morbidity can be reduced, however, by intravenous hydration. For my patients, however, I continue to favor magnesium citrate with supplemental enemas the morning of the study or the procedure.

Technique of Examination

The colon is not the easiest organ to examine. In order to evaluate all of the twists, turns, and redundancies, it is no longer appropriate to instill a measured amount of barium and "shoot" a film with the patient lying supine on the table. Most radiologists today believe that 90% of the information from the study is gleaned by means of fluoroscopy. The final films are really a modus for creating a permanent record for future reference and comparison.

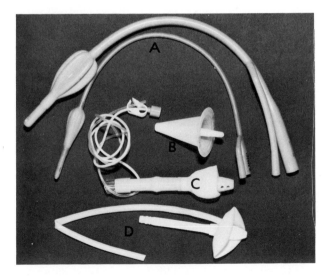

FIG. 1-22. Barium enema catheter tips. **A.** Bardex retention balloon catheters (pediatric and adult). **B.** Colostotip (Greer) for irrigating or performing contrast studies through a stoma. **C.** Catheter for air-contrast enema. **D.** Argyle retention cuff catheter.

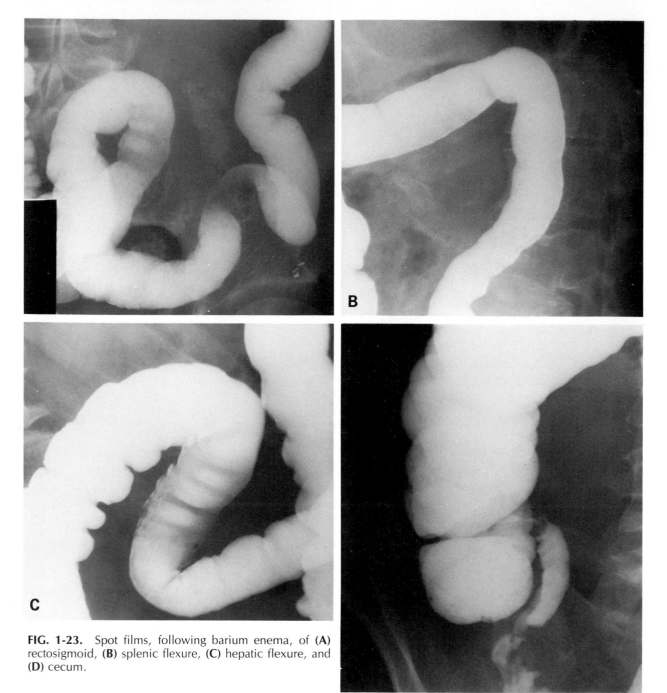

FIG. 1-23. Spot films, following barium enema, of **(A)** rectosigmoid, **(B)** splenic flexure, **(C)** hepatic flexure, and **(D)** cecum.

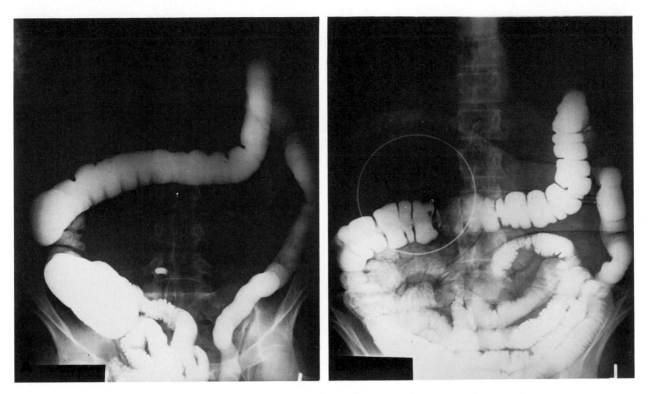

FIG. 1-24. Barium enema. **A.** Transverse colon polyp is poorly seen. **B.** Compression spot demonstrates small polyp.

from previous contrast studies, and any other soft tissue or bony abnormalities.

Using an appropriate catheter, the barium–water mixture is inserted into the colon with the patient in the prone position until the column of barium reaches the splenic flexure. The tubing and tip must be of sufficient caliber to allow free flow of the contrast medium. A smooth enema tip with both end and side hole openings is preferred. For those patients who have difficulty retaining an enema it is helpful to use a tip with an inflatable cuff (Fig. 1-22). It should be remembered, however, that an inflated balloon in the rectum may obscure the bowel wall. Endoscopic examination of the rectum should routinely be employed prior to this radiologic study.

As the barium flows the radiologist looks for distensibility and whether the flow is interrupted or deviated. Sometimes it is difficult to determine whether certain areas represent a fixed or anatomic narrowing or whether the narrowing is physiologic (*i.e.,* spasm). Anticholinergic agents have been employed to prevent spasm, but because of side-effects they are no longer recommended and have been abandoned by most physicians. Glucagon (2 mg) given by the intramusclar or intravenous route has been shown to be an effective smooth muscle relaxant when administered parenterally.[91] It is as effective as anticholinergic drugs and has fewer side-effects. Relaxation of the colon and reduction of discomfort allows the radiologist to perform a more satisfactory examination.

Spot films are usually taken of the rectosigmoid, hepatic flexure, splenic flexure, and cecum (Fig. 1-23). Compression spot films are useful to identify small polyps (Fig. 1-24). Angled views of the sigmoid colon (right anterior oblique [prone], and left posterior oblique [supine]) are most helpful in "opening up" this portion of the bowel to evaluate it (Fig. 1-25).[34] The Chassard-Lapiné view (Fig. 1-26) may be helpful in identifying sigmoid and rectosigmoid lesions but is hazardous in the reproductive years because of the increased radiation exposure.[39] On the other hand, spot films of the cecum are performed to prove that this area is indeed filled with barium, not necessarily because of difficulties with overlapping bowel. Peristalsis usually begins in the cecum so that it is frequently contracted or empty by the time the "overhead" films are taken.

How does one know that the cecum has been filled? Ideally, if the appendix fills or if reflux is seen in the terminal ileum, this would solve the issue, but the

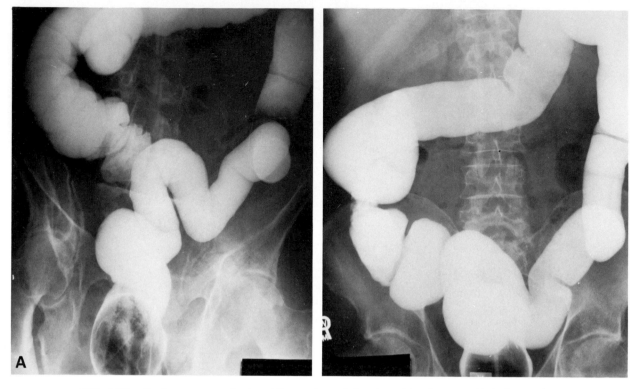

FIG. 1-25. Barium enema. **A.** An oblique view of the sigmoid colon permits better evaluation. **B.** In the posteroanterior projection the area would be obscured.

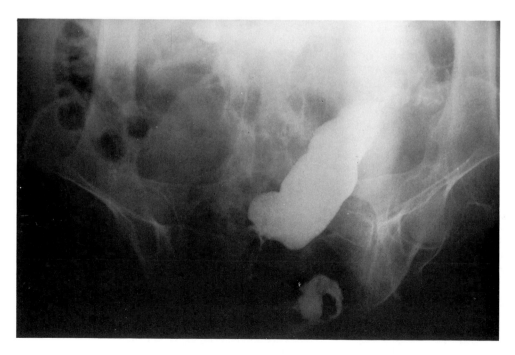

FIG. 1-26. Chassard-Lapiné view may be useful to demonstrate lesions in a redundant sigmoid colon. An annular carcinoma is seen.

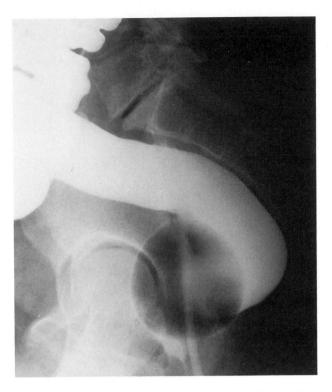

FIG. 1-27. Normal lateral view of rectum after barium enema.

the mucosa in spite of mucus secretion. Tannic acid is relatively contraindicated in patients with inflammatory bowel disease and in other ulcerative or inflammatory colon conditions because of the possibility of absorption and subsequent hepatic injury.

former is noted only 30% of the time, and the latter no more than half the time. However, there are certain characteristics of the cecum to look for: the largest haustral marking and the ileocecal valve.

The rectum also requires special radiologic views. The radiologist is constantly endeavoring to move and massage the colon, to empty it and to fill it. The rectum is the only area of the bowel that the radiologist cannot manipulate by abdominal pressure. A lateral view must be obtained to appreciate anterior and posterior wall lesions, and to be certain that the rectum lies well back in the hollow of the sacrum (Fig. 1-27) and is not displaced forward by retrorectal inflammation or by tumor (Fig. 1-28).

Probably the most important permanent film of the single-contrast barium enema is the post-evacuation study (Fig. 1-29). If there has been good evacuation it is the one time when all of the walls of the colon are demonstrated. With a completely collapsed bowel one can identify the mucosal pattern or lesions that disturb or destroy it.

In order to satisfactorily cover the colon a small amount of tannic acid is added to the barium. This substance stimulates the colon to empty more completely and effectively, and causes the barium to contact

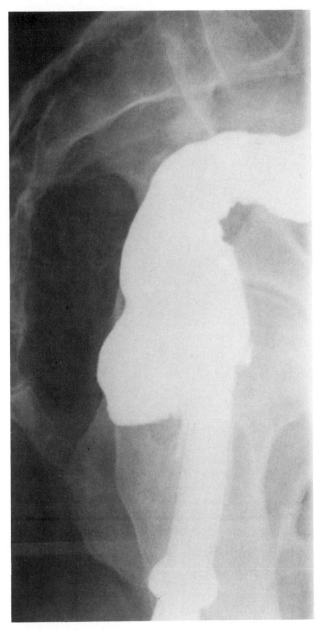

FIG. 1-28. On lateral projection after barium enema, anterior displacement of the rectum from recurrent tumor is evident. Note the increased distance from the sacrum when compared with the normal.

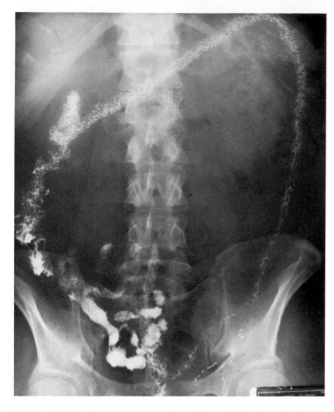

FIG. 1-29. A post-evacuation film following barium enema clearly demonstrates the normal mucosal pattern.

Alternatives to the Use of Barium

Barium is a substance that is potentially dangerous when it is used in a patient with suspected bowel perforation. Barium peritonitis is usually a lethal complication; that is why relative contraindications to barium enema include toxic megacolon, peritonitis, and recent biopsy or snare excision of a polyp (24 hours). However, if the biopsy was performed for an exophytic lesion, I believe the barium enema need not be deferred.

An alternative to barium is one of the water-soluble solutions of diatrizoate sodium (*e.g.,* Hypaque, Gastrografin). These solutions provide reasonable radiopacity and are nonirritating and relatively well tolerated if accidentally introduced into the peritoneal cavity. Since they are hypertonic with respect to plasma they can act as saline cathartics. The result is a rapid dilution of the opacity, but because of the cathartic effect they may be of benefit in the immediate preoperative situation.

There are, however, certain disadvantages of diatrizoate sodium. The major limitation is that, because of lesser opacification, visualization is sometimes less than

adequate. Also, in essence there is no post-evacuation residual. The problem of hypertonicity is a hazard in another respect; significant alteration in serum electrolytes can occur, especially in the pediatric patient and in the elderly patient. Patients with cardiac or renal disease are also at an increased risk when these agents are employed. Finally, the cost of the material is approximately $50 when compared with $4 for the barium preparation.

Double-Contrast (Air-Contrast) Barium Enema

The double-contrast barium enema study has been advocated as an improved means of evaluating the colon, of identifying small mucosal lesions, and of diagnosing inflammatory bowel disease.[79, 80, 135, 136] Others suggest that either study may be optimal under a given circumstance.[55, 84]

With the double-contrast examination an attempt is made to coat the colon with a thin layer of contrast material and to distend the bowel with air so that the entire mucosal circumference is visualized (Fig. 1-30).

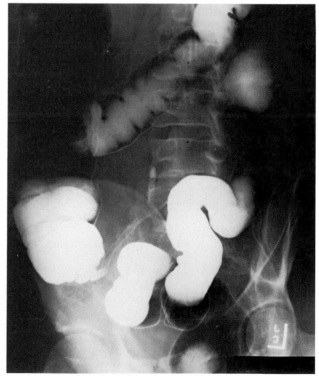

FIG. 1-30. Double-contrast (air-contrast) barium enema study demonstrating the normal colon.

The barium used is a heavy density, viscous material. In order to deliver this, a large caliber enema tube is required. This has a soft tip and an inflatable cuff, and uses a system that delivers air and barium separately (see Fig. 1-22, *C*).

There are a number of disadvantages to the air-contrast enema. First, the study inevitably results in considerably more radiation exposure: an adequate examination necessitates 10 or 12 overhead films plus several spot films. Second, it requires a cooperative patient who is able to roll around, support his own weight, and comprehend instructions. A third disadvantage is that fluoroscopy has very little role in the course of the examination. The radiologist endeavors to move the viscous barium around the colon as expeditiously as possible and then depends on the permanent films for diagnosis.

However, small lesions and ulcers *are* seen better with the double-contrast technique. There is a theoretical disadvantage of the study when a large lesion or a pedunculated polyp is present, but as with any other aspect of medicine, the skill and experience of the physician are the most important requisites.

Complications of Barium Enema Examination

Complications of barium enema examination are fortunately rare. When they occur they can be of catastrophic consequence. A number of complications have been reported, as listed below. Rectal perforation is usually due to trauma at the time the enema tip is inserted or from overinflation of a balloon catheter.[45, 115] The tip or balloon can also lacerate the rectal wall and produce rectal bleeding. The balloon technique for barium enema through colostomy has produced colonic perforation at and below the stoma. This technique should be abandoned and a colostotip or cone employed (see Fig. 1-22, *B*).

Complications of Barium Enema Examination

Rectal perforation (from enema tip or excessive balloon inflation)
Rectal tear or hemorrhage
Colonic perforation
Barium peritonitis
Barium submucosal granuloma
Toxic megacolon
Septicemia
Venous barium embolism
Retrograde gastrointestinal filling with vomiting and aspiration (in infants)

Colonic perforation and barium peritonitis carry at least a 50% mortality (see Fig. 17-9). Recognition of barium flowing into the peritoneal cavity is an indication for emergency surgical intervention. Although perforation at the site of tumor, diverticulitis, ischemic colitis, and nonspecific inflammatory bowel disease are the usual associated circumstances, perforation can occur in an otherwise normal bowel.[74, 142] It is said that idiopathic perforation occurs in 1 of 5000 barium enema studies, usually in the right colon. One might suspect that the term *idiopathic* might be a euphemism for overfilling the colon or employing a high hydrostatic pressure. Toxic megacolon and necrotizing enterocolitis are *absolute* contraindications to performing a barium enema study

Barium submucosal dissection, with its subsequent granuloma formation, is not common but is still a well-recognized clinical entity.[16, 83] The barium itself poses no threat, but the differential diagnosis of a submucosal, yellow rectal nodule includes carcinoid. It is, therefore, important to prevent this complication, which would otherwise necessitate a diagnostic biopsy. As previously mentioned, it is a wise idea to avoid mucosal biopsy and rectal polyp excision within the 24-hour period prior to a barium enema examination.

FIBEROPTIC COLONOSCOPY

In 1969 fiberoptic colonoscopy was introduced as a means of directly visualizing the colon and rectum, and even, in many instances, the terminal ileum. Within a few years Wolff and Shinya demonstrated that by using a wire loop snare and electrocautery, polyps could be removed through the instrument, thus ultimately relegating colotomy and polypectomy to near-historic interest.[139]

Instrumentation

The term *endoscope* is derived from two Greek words: *endon*, meaning within, and *skopein*, to view. As mentioned earlier, there are a number of suppliers of fiberscopes in the United States, most of which use similar optical structures that vary mainly in length, total diameter, and maneuverability, and which have a number of accessories. The diameters of the individual glass fibers in the image-conveying aligned bundles are similar, ranging from 9 to 12 µm.[43] In the flexible fiberoptic instruments the aligned individual fibers are bound together at their ends while the rest of the fibers remain loose and flexible. The fiberoptic endoscope can be made as long as necessary since light loss is negligible over several meters.[43]

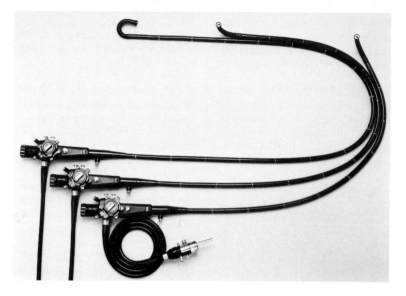

FIG. 1-31. Colonofiberscopes of the CF series, with total lengths of 2020 mm, 1670 mm, and 1270 mm respectively. (Courtesy of Olympus Corporation of America)

Several manufacturers make instruments of varying working lengths, from approximately 104 cm to almost 180 cm. They are forward viewing and may be of wide angle (*e.g.,* 120°) or of a narrower angle (*e.g.,* 85°). Figure 1-31 illustrates the three Olympus CF-type colonofiberscopes. A two-channel system is usually preferred in order to use two accessories for treatment, including polypectomy. Four-way angulation of the distal end is achieved from approximately 180° up or down and 160° right and left by manipulating the control knobs (see Fig. 1-18). Additional features include an air or water outlet and a suction/forceps channel. Air or carbon dioxide can be insufflated and liquid debris removed during the procedure. Accessories include a cold light supply and electrosurgical unit, as well as quite elegant photographic equipment. Requisite items for procedures include biopsy forceps, diathermy snare, and grasping forceps (Fig. 1-32).

Cost is a major factor, with a colonoscope itself now approximately $8000, and the entire unit over three times that amount. Repairs and the limited life expectancy of the instrument also must be considered in assessing the expense.[1] However, there is almost universal agreement that, with the plethora of colon pathology (especially neoplasms) in western countries, fiberoptic colonoscopy and colonoscopy–polypectomy are among the most valuable diagnostic and therapeutic modalities to become available in our armamentarium in the past 15 years.

Indications

It is generally agreed that colonoscopy supplements but does not replace the barium enema in the evaluation of colon disorders. The list on p. 25 summarizes the in-

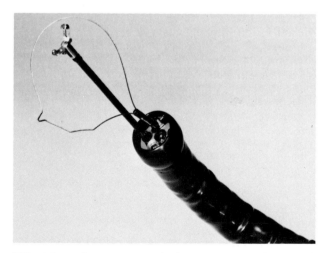

FIG. 1-32. Crescent type diathermy snare and rat-tooth grasping forceps. (Courtesy of Olympus Corporation of America)

dications for flexible colonoscopy. In most instances the procedure is employed either because the barium enema study has demonstrated a probable abnormality or because the barium enema has failed to indicate or identify the source when symptoms suggest colonic disease.[24]

Indications for Colonoscopy

Confirmation or refutation of suspected or equivocal radiologic abnormality (filling defects, narrowing [intrinsic versus extrinsic lesion], polyps)
Evaluation and follow-up of inflammatory bowel disease (e.g., dysplasia)
Differential diagnosis of diverticular disease or malignancy
Presence of a rectal polyp with or without barium enema abnormality (synchronous lesion)
Gastrointestinal symptoms (e.g., bleeding, abdominal pain, iron deficiency anemia) where radiologic investigation has failed to reveal the source
Follow-up evaluation of patient with prior solon surgery
Acute lower gastrointestinal bleeding
Endoscopic polypectomy
Reduction of sigmoid volvulus

Colonoscopy has been demonstrated to be of diagnostic usefulness in a number of clinical situations, for example, diverticular disease, inflammatory bowel disease (Color Fig. 1-1)*, ischemic colitis, pseudomembranous colitis (Color Fig. 1-2), tuberculosis affecting the bowel, and unexplained rectal bleeding.[10, 13, 14, 31, 33, 47, 49, 54, 66, 72, 76, 89, 93, 126, 128, 129, 132] In the two reports analyzing the results of unexplained rectal bleeding (Brand and co-workers, Tedesco and co-workers) 30% of the patients were found to have significant lesions in spite of a normal barium enema examination.[13, 129]

Other conditions in which diagnosis has been confirmed or expedited by colonoscopy include amebic colitis, the irritable bowel syndrome, pneumatosis cystoides intestinalis, and radiation colitis.[24, 32, 121]

Contraindications are essentially limited to those patients with an acute cardiovascular problem (e.g., myocardial infarction), and those with an acute abdominal inflammation (peritonitis, acute diverticulitis, bowel perforation, etc.).

Preparation of the Patient

As with barium enema examination the importance of an adequately cleansed colon cannot be overempha-

*Note: All color figures appear in the front of this volume.

sized. For most ambulatory patients a vigorous cathartic (e.g., 45 ml of castor oil) followed by colonic irrigation is generally satisfactory and can be commenced in the morning prior to an afternoon examination. Sedentary individuals may require several days to adequately prepare the bowel. Care must be taken to maintain adequate fluid intake and to avoid electrolyte abnormalities. Patients may lose as much as 7 pounds.[15, 136] This is of particular concern in those patients with cardiovascular or renal disease. A synthetic amino acid diet may facilitate bowel cleansing, and if hydration is maintained the osmotic catharsis will help in removing the fecal matter; however, it tends to be rather unpalatable and is quite expensive.[24]

In patients with ulcerative colitis there is a concern for exacerbating the condition following total colonoscopy when it is performed for dysplasia screening (see Chap. 15). Gould and Williams found that both castor oil (30 ml) and senna tablets (Senokot 75 mg sennosides) followed by two tap-water enemas produced equally good preparations in a prospective trial.[60] Neither group of patients developed a serious exacerbation of colitis. Certainly, acute ulcerative colitis and toxic megacolon are contraindications to this procedure.

Recently the nonabsorbed oligosaccharide, mannitol, has been advocated for colon preparation prior to barium enema examination and colonoscopy.[96] In Newstead and Morgan's study, during the afternoon of the day prior to the examination, 500 ml of a 10% or 20% solution were consumed; the mean number of bowel actions was 7. When using mannitol, additional oral fluid intake should be encouraged. Again, care must be taken with this technique in the elderly or the infirm. However, recent reports of fatal explosions after mannitol administration and colonoscopy–polypectomy have dampened most physician's ardor for this preparation.[9, 127] Hydrogen and methane produced by bacterial degradation of the mannitol have been suggested as causative factors.

The Crapp and associates preparation as described earlier in this chapter has been recommended as an effective, well-tolerated alternative to standard oral cathartics and enemata for colonoscopy as well as for barium enema examination.[29] Minervini and associates compared three methods of whole bowel irrigation: nasogastric saline solution alone, the solution with oral mannitol, and oral mannitol alone.[92] The best preparation was the combined approach, but patients and nursing staff preferred the oral mannitol alone.

Davis and co-workers[30] recently devised an electrolyte solution containing primarily sodium sulfate with polyethylene glycol (PEG) as an additional osmotic agent ("Golytely"). Approximately 1.5 liters per hour were administered orally. Goldman and Reichelderfer also have found this to be a good to excellent preparation, well-tolerated and without complication.[59]

Sedation is advised whenever total colonoscopy is contemplated. The insufflation of air or carbon dioxide (the latter is more rapidly absorbed) and traction on the bowel from the instrument may cause considerable discomfort and anxiety. Complete anesthesia, however, is contraindicated. It is important for the examiner to be aware of any excessive discomfort that the patient is experiencing in order to avoid possible injury to the bowel wall, mesentery, or adjoining structures.

Approximately 30 minutes prior to examination, the patient is given an intramuscular injection containing 50 mg each of sodium pentobarbital (Nembutal), meperidine hydrochloride (Demerol), and hydroxyzine hydrochloride (Vistaril). At the onset of the examination, diazepam (Valium) is given intravenously in an initial dose of about 1 mg per 8 kg of body weight.[24] Additional Valium is administered during the procedure if the patient requires it.

Technique of Examination

The examination can be performed by two persons or by one. The left lateral decubitus position is recommended by most endoscopists, although with fluoro-

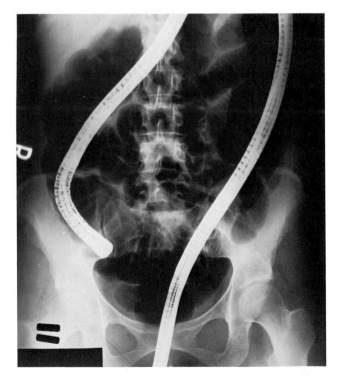

FIG. 1-33. Plain abdominal film demonstrating a colonoscope having achieved the cecum.

scopic control or the two-team approach, some physicians prefer the patient to be supine.[102, 131] Fluoroscopy is quite useful, but it is not mandatory. It obviously requires the availability of this expensive equipment and mandates protection from radiation exposure to personnel and to patient. Facilities should be available, however, for a plain abdominal x-ray should the need for accurate localization of the instrument be required (Fig. 1-33). Fluoroscopy, of course, not only accomplishes this end but aids in avoiding stretching of the colon and improper advancement of the instrument, as well as reducing patient discomfort. There are many articles and several books that describe in detail the techniques for passage of the colonoscope.[73]

After a careful digital examination of the rectum is performed, the instrument is inserted. Usually the examiner is confronted by a blurry pink haze. Air should be insufflated and the instrument advanced and rotated. At this point, the rectal lumen usually becomes apparent. If this is not the case, the instrument is slowly withdrawn and rotated. The valves of Houston may or may not be apparent in this area; advancement usually proceeds without difficulty to 16 or 18 cm.

The sigmoid colon presents the commonest location for difficulty in the passage of the instrument. Fixation of this area of the bowel in the pelvis by adhesions from prior surgery (*e.g.*, hysterectomy) may cause significant angulation and narrowing of the bowel lumen.

A frequently observed configuration of the colon is the so-called alpha loop (see Fig. 1-20). This is usually negotiated by withdrawing the instrument while applying clockwise rotation (Color Fig. 1-3). Additional sigmoid loops may present further problems. In some instances straightening may not be possible until the splenic flexure is achieved. Fluoroscopy may be necessary in order to resolve the problems of multiple loops. If these reform, a sigmoid stiffening device may be necessary. Air insufflation should be kept at a minimum because of the tendency for bowel distention to create more acute angulation.

At the level of the splenic flexure an acute angulation is encountered that after redirecting, permits visualization of the characteristic triangular transverse colon (Color Fig. 1-4). By withdrawing the instrument and straightening the tip, advancement further into the transverse colon is permitted (Fig. 1-34). Further negotiation of the transverse colon is achieved by hooking the tip against the wall of the colon, withdrawing, and reinserting (Fig. 1-34*D*). This maneuver can be repeated until the region of the hepatic flexure is reached. Gentle abdominal compression by the nurse or assistant will usually expedite the process.

The ascending colon is entered by angling the tip downward and withdrawing the instrument (Fig. 1-35). The use of suction and clockwise torque usually permits advancement of the instrument to the cecum.

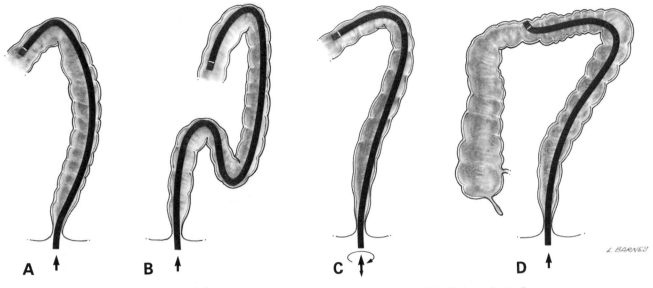

FIG. 1-34. Entering the transverse colon by colonoscopy. **A.** "Hooking" the splenic flexure. **B.** Advancing the instrument. **C.** Withdrawing and straightening the tip while maintaining clockwise torque. **D.** Negotiating the transverse colon by "hooking" the bowel wall.

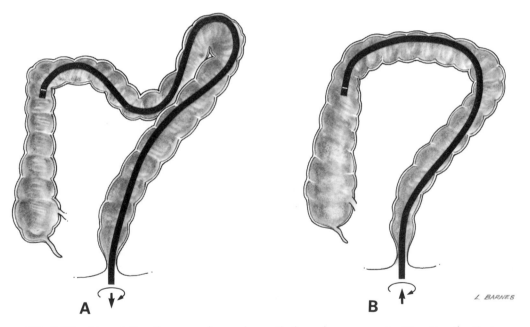

FIG. 1-35. Negotiating the ascending colon with the colonoscope. **A.** Directing the tip to visualize the ascending colon. **B.** Withdrawal produces advancement; this is expedited by the use of suction.

Waye suggests a number of possible steps that may be taken in order to advance the instrument:

1. Lubrication of the anal orifice to promote torquing
2. Withdrawal of air to deflate the bowel
3. Jiggling (dithering)
4. Withdrawal, clockwise rotation, and jiggling
5. Abdominal pressure
6. Locking the left–right control knob to stiffen the tip[133]

Obviously, anatomic variations are myriad, and only the skill developed through multiple endoscopic procedures permits consistent examination of the entire colon. Most experienced endoscopists now find that they can achieve the cecum more than 90% of the time. It should be remembered that the length of the instrument inserted does not accurately reflect the amount of colon examined. By straightening the redundant bowel one can in most instances reach the cecum using less than 90 cm of the instrument.

Withdrawal of the colonoscope should proceed slowly, and a careful search should be made for intraluminal lesions. Simultaneous maneuvering of the control knob as well as shaft rotation permit visualization of all walls of the bowel. By changing the position of the patient, difficult to see areas may be brought into view. Again, one should remember that the rectum may be inadequately visualized if care is not taken to ensure observation of the entire lumenal circumference.

Cleansing the Instrument

The concern for transmitting disease may be exaggerated, but the guidelines for cleaning and disinfecting as recommended by Hedrick are suggested.[68] The use of a chemical disinfectant (*e.g.,* glutaraldehyde or Betadine solution) followed by vigorous rinsing is the treatment of choice. The channels should be likewise cleansed and air dried.

Therapeutic Colonoscopy

Colonoscopy–Polypectomy

The advent of colonoscopy–polypectomy and its significance in the "prophylactic" treatment of colorectal cancer has received considerable attention in recent years. The concept of "following" a polyp observed on barium enema examination in order to avoid a laparotomy, colotomy, and polypectomy is no longer valid (see Color Fig. 1-5). Using colonoscopy, most polyps can be removed or at least biopsied. In patients who have demonstrated a colon or rectal polyp, I, as most others, have adopted an aggressive approach to the diagnosis and treatment of such lesions.[25] (See also Chap. 9.)

Equipment

As mentioned earlier, performance of polypectomy requires an electrical generating power source that for endoscopic use is transmitted by way of a wire loop snare or coagulating electrode. Polypectomy is undertaken through the accessory channel. Most commercially available high-frequency units permit tube or cutting current and a spark gap current, which produce coagulation or a blend of the two.[50]

Gas insufflation during polypectomy is a matter of particular concern because of the potential hazard of an explosive mixture being present. The necessity of adequate bowel preparation has been previously discussed. The use of an inert gas (most commonly carbon dioxide) has been recommended, but the requirements of tank storage and accessories have made this a rather impractical and, in the opinion of many, unnecessary alternative. Frühmorgen reported in over 2700 colonoscopy–polypectomy procedures no instance of gas explosion using standard methods of bowel preparation.[50]

In addition to the above, a large variety of cold and hot biopsy forceps, snares, and baskets and hooks for retrieval are commercially available.

Technique

The technique for removal of a polyp is not dissimilar to that employed for rigid proctosigmoidoscopy, but maintaining adequate visualization and holding instrument position obviously pose more of a problem. The two-team approach or the presence of an assistant is a requisite. Usually the polyp is visualized 2 or 3 cm distal to the endoscope. By maneuvering the tip of the colonoscope and sometimes the patient, the wire loop is advanced and the head of the polyp encircled (Fig. 1-36). The loop is drawn down to the pedicle until the latter is secured. The endoscope is then maneuvered to hold the polyp away from the bowel wall in order to avoid injury and possible perforation. The current is then applied and the polyp excised. It can then be removed using a forceps, hook, basket, or the suction itself. When other polyps are present, they may be removed individually or collected by straining the stool over the ensuing hours. Pathologic confirmation is, of course, required.

Large polyps (more than 2.5 cm) can be removed by the above technique if adequate visualization of the pedicle is possible, and the head can be ensnared. Failing this, however, it can be removed piecemeal, and the specimens collected as described. The expertise of the endoscopist determines the size and the degree of difficulty of lesion he is willing to approach. Even with the increased possibility of perforation, a properly informed patient may be well served by colonoscopy–polypectomy even if occasionally operative intervention is required for a complication (see Complications). The bowel is well prepared, and morbidity and mortality should be quite low indeed. But there still does remain a place for colotomy and polypectomy; it is a judgment that must rest with the endoscopist.

Sessile and even submucosal lesions can be removed by endoscopy but ulcerating tumors should not.[21, 22] Care must be taken to elevate the mucosa as the snare is tightened (Fig. 1-37). The result is to leave behind muscularis propria of the bowel. Obviously the risk of bowel perforation is increased when one attempts to remove such lesions.

Although in-hospital observation for 24 to 48 hours has been recommended strongly in the past, one may feel confident in outpatient treatment, providing the patient is well informed of the potential hazards and remains available in the immediate geographic vicinity for a day or so. At our institution virtually all patients are managed on an ambulatory basis.

Results and Complications

My associates and I performed colonoscopy on 146 patients with radiographically suspected polyps.[25] Of the 110 patients found to have a neoplastic lesion, 62 were found to have an additional neoplasm (19%). It is because of this association that total colonoscopy should be performed when a patient is found to harbor a colorectal polyp. Removing the lesion itself without such a complete evaluation is felt to be inadequate.

Shinya and Wolff reported their experience of 7000 polyps endoscopically removed.[116] There was no mortality. Most series report approximately two thirds of the lesions are adenomatous polyps (tubular adenomas), a few as villous adenomas, and the remainder as malignant tumors, other benign neoplasms, and nonneoplastic conditions. The significance of polyps, their distribution, and the follow-up of patients are discussed in Chapter 9.

The complications of colonoscopy and colonoscopy-polypectomy are listed on p. 30. Complications can be grouped in a number of categories: bowel preparation and medication, equipment misuse or malfunction, patient factors (communicable disease, underlying cardio-cerebral-pulmonary-renal disease), and factors related to trauma coincident with the procedure itself.[61, 85, 109, 114]

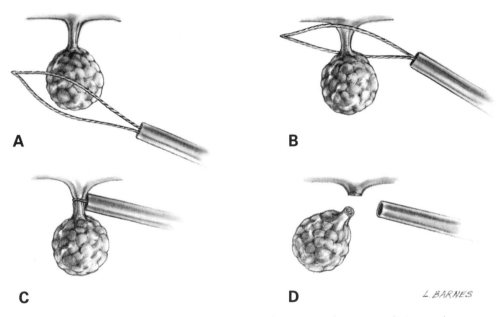

A   B

C   D   L. BARNES

FIG. 1-36. Technique of polypectomy. **A, B.** Polyp ensnared. **C.** Coagulation and strangulation. **D.** Polyp removed.

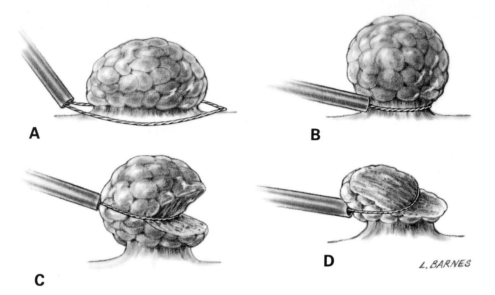

FIG. 1-37.   Technique for removal of sessile polyp. **A.** Polyp ensnared. **B.** Mucosa elevated. **C.** Piecemeal excision. **D.** Residual polyp removed.

Complications of Colonoscopy and Colonoscopy–Polypectomy

Hemorrhage (intraluminal, mesenteric injury,
    seromuscular tear, splenic trauma)
Perforation
Retroperitoneal and mediastinal emphysema
Pneumoscrotum
Explosion
Postcolonoscopy distention
Colonic obstruction
Volvulus
Bacteremia
Infections
Medical problems (pulmonary, cardiovascular, renal)
Mechanical failure

Smith polled members of the American Society of Colon and Rectal Surgeons.[118] He found from 162 respondents that over 20,000 colonoscopies were performed. The overall complication rate was 0.4% for diagnostic colonoscopy and 1.8% for polypectomy. In like manner, Berci and co-workers questioned members of the Southern California Society for Gastrointestinal Endoscopy.[8] The incidence of perforation following colonoscopy and polypectomy (901 procedures) was 0.33%, whereas that following colonoscopy alone (3850 procedures) was 0.25%. There was one death (0.02%). Bleeding occurred in 0.66% of polypectomized patients. In these and in other studies it becomes readily apparent that the incidence of complications decreases considerably as the examiner becomes more experienced. It is probably axiomatic that therapeutic colonoscopy not be performed by anyone until he has achieved at least 50 diagnostic studies.

Hemorrhage can be due to the polypectomy procedure, to biopsy, to laceration of the mucosa by the instrument, or to tearing of the mesentery or spleen. Familiarity with the electrical equipment, use of coagulating current, and the endoscopist's clinical experience reduce the incidence. Inevitably, if one performs sufficient examinations and procedures, the problem of bleeding will be encountered.

The decision of how to manage the problem depends on the magnitude of the hemorrhage. If bleeding is recognized at the time of polypectomy, the area should be resnared (if the pedicle is still apparent) and strangulated for at least 5 minutes. Electrocautery should not be used, particularly if no pedicle is present. If the area is within reach of the rigid proctosigmoidoscope, it may be controlled by one of the means suggested earlier in this chapter. In-hospital observation is mandatory if control has not been established with certainty, and operative intervention is occasionally necessary. This is particularly true if the bleeding is secondary to a mesenteric tear or splenic injury, both of which may not be readily apparent for a number of hours after the injury. Symptoms include the usual signs of hemorrhage (weakness, syncope, pallor, hypotension, and tachycardia), but peritoneal irritation and abdominal distention also may be observed. A falling hematocrit is obviously ominous.

Perforation of the colon with pneumoperitoneum usually becomes manifest almost immediately or within a few hours following the procedure. Usually this is due to the presence of disease in the colon (*e.g.*, diverticulitis) or to vigorous manipulation, rotation, or angulation of the instrument. Overdistention with air or gas can also precipitate a perforation. The disquieting observation of an appendix epiploica during colonoscopy establishes the diagnosis with certainty. Abdominal or pelvic pain and distention are observed. Again, in-hospital treatment is required. Occasionally the patient's symptoms may be minimal relative to the amount of gas that is apparent on abdominal roentgenogram. In selected cases, the bowel having been well prepared, cautious continued observation may be considered.[2] This is particularly true if the patient presents many hours or a day or two after the procedure. The patient should be kept from oral intake; intravenous fluid replacement and broad-spectrum antibiotics are advisable. A limited Gastrografin enema may also be considered in the equivocal situation (see Alternatives to the Use of Barium). The sigmoid is the commonest site of perforation. This may be due to its being the area of greatest difficulty to negotiate or the commonest location for pathology (*e.g.*, polyp, diverticulitis).

Laparotomy should be undertaken if the patient exhibits signs and symptoms of peritonitis. Fever and leukocytosis alone or in combination are not necessarily absolute indications for surgical intervention, but the burden of responsibility falls on the surgeon for unwarranted delay. A sealed perforation or negative laparotomy should not warrant criticism.

When a perforation is found, it usually can be closed primarily without the need for a diversionary procedure, the bowel having been well prepared. If a resection is required, it can also be safely undertaken without the need for proximal colostomy or ileostomy unless sepsis or gross contamination is observed.

Retroperitoneal and mediastinal emphysema have been reported as well as pneumoscrotum[46] after colonoscopy.[4, 82, 141] It is important to recognize these clinical entities because they do not of themselves constitute an indication for surgical exploration (*i.e.*, free perforation of the colon is not implied). It is, therefore, important to distinguish between retroperitoneal and intraperitoneal gas. In the former situation nonsurgical treatment should be at least the initial approach (see Fig. 15-89).

Explosion in a well-prepared colon should probably not occur, although as mentioned earlier the use of mannitol as a bowel preparation has been implicated as a causative factor. The use of an inert gas, such as carbon dioxide, has been advocated by some, but is probably an unnecessary caution. It should be remembered, however, that in an essentially closed system such as is present when colonoscopy–polypectomy is performed, there is no means for gas to escape once ignited. This is not true for the open-ended rigid proctosigmoidoscope. The examiner should be wary of using electrical current if he is dissatisfied with the adequacy of the bowel preparation.

Post-colonoscopy distention has been described as a syndrome manifested by abdominal distention, discomfort, and dilated loops of bowel on the roentenogram.[109, 122] Patients do not exhibit signs of peritonitis. Treatment consists of observation and medical management.

Colonic obstruction can be precipitated by colonoscopy, usually at the site of underlying sigmoid disease, and volvulus has been reported, possibly secondary to the alpha maneuver or to over-insufflation of air.

Bacteremia has been reported to be associated with colonoscopy, but other studies have failed to confirm this observation.[28, 35, 77, 99, 100] Routine antibiotic prophylaxis is probably not indicated except possibly in the high-risk patient, the person with valvular heart disease, or the patient in whom a prosthetic valve has been inserted.

Transmittal of bacterial, viral, and parasitic infections is possible. A carefully taken history prior to endoscopic examination, particularly with respect to hepatitis and to venereal disease, is necessary, although standard cleansing techniques should prevent communication.

A host of medical problems may be exacerbated by colonoscopy and its preparation. Respiratory depression and respiratory arrest can result from overdosage or too rapid administration of diazepam; this drug is also associated with a high incidence of phlebitis. Care in administration and the use of a dilute solution are helpful in preventing these complications.

Hypotension, bradycardia, tachycardia, and myocardial infarction have all been observed during and after colonoscopy. Electrocardiogram (EKG) monitoring with the addition of oxygen in patients at increased risk is worthy of consideration. Patients with pacemakers may require a fixed rate if electrocoagulation is employed, even though there may be proper grounding and adequate shielding of the pacemaker.

Numerous problems can develop from malfunction of the instruments and accessories; breakage of the colonoscope with entrapment of the instrument can occur. Defective electrical equipment and inexperience with its use are two of the commonest reasons for polypectomy hemorrhage and bowel wall necrosis. The snare wire can break or become fused with the polyp. Incomplete division of the pedicle can occur with the snare completely closed.

In spite of the long list of complications, colonoscopy and colonoscopy–polypectomy can be undertaken with a very low morbidity and a very rare mortality—certainly a lower mortality than can be expected after operative intervention.

Special Situations

Foreign Body Removal

The problem of removal of foreign bodies inserted into the rectum is addressed in Chapter 17). However, ingested foreign bodies have been reported by means of the colonoscope. Frühmorgen reported extraction of a dental prosthesis as well as intestinal tubes.[51]

Volvulus

Colonoscopy has been successfully applied in the treatment of sigmoid volvulus.[56, 122] Although rigid proctosigmoidoscopy is more readily available and easier to employ, there is the occasional situation when an attempt at reduction with a colonoscope may be indicated. The diagnosis and therapy of volvulus is discussed in Chapter 17.

Intraoperative Colonoscopy

Intraoperative colonoscopy may be considered when prior conventional colonoscopy has been unsuccessful, to evaluate the remainder of the colon when a partial resection is contemplated, to avoid contamination when an unsuspected polyp is found during a "clean" operation, and to complement arteriography in the diagnosis of the source of gastrointestinal hemorrhage.[42, 44, 88, 90] The patient is placed in the perineolithotomy position (see Fig. 11-4) as if for combined abdominoperineal resection of the rectum. The abdominal surgeon guides the instrument through the bowel, thus expediting the procedure.

Although the application of this technique is limited, it may become of greater value in the diagnosis and treatment of lower gastrointestinal hemorrhage with improved methods for clearing liquid and clotted blood through the colonoscope.

Pediatric Colonoscopy

Pediatric colonoscopy can be performed with a narrower caliber endoscope or with the standard instrument, depending on the age of the patient. A general anesthetic is usually recommended for infants and young children. Preparation in infants usually consists of a clear liquid diet for 24 hours, but a laxative is usually advised for older children. Evaluation of rectal

bleeding, suspicion of polyps, inflammatory bowel disease, and congenital anomalies are the commonest indications for the procedure.[52, 64, 104, 137]

Barium Enema Versus Colonoscopy

Generally speaking, there is little disagreement that colonoscopy is more likely to detect small excrescences than a barium enema examination, even with an optimal preparation and double-contrast technique.[37, 75, 130, 140] However, the difference in cost between the two studies is such that one must accept the reality that the procedures truly complement each other. One should put to rest the fallacious assumption that the radiologist can determine whether a polyp is benign or malignant. This is a diagnosis that must be made by histologic examination.

For screening purposes, barium enema is the procedure of choice. Once it has been determined that the patient is in a higher-risk group for the development of a neoplasm, colonoscopy should be the interval diagnostic study (see also Chap. 9).

Many physicians who discover and remove a polyp at the time of proctosigmoidoscopy now move directly to total colonoscopy rather than to barium enema or air-contrast enema. The need for a "road map" of the colon is felt no longer to be a requisite. On the other hand, the subject of cost must be addressed, and a normal, high-quality air-contrast enema should reassure the patient and the physican that a colonoscopy may be deferred. Perhaps colonoscopy might be considered as the screening technique the next time, 2 or 3 years later.

Although some physicians have developed protocols for follow-up evaluation of patients with rectal polyps, my own inclination is to start with the air-contrast enema and to use colonoscopy for follow-up. If the patient presents with more than one neoplasm, my tendency is to go directly to total colonoscopy. To date there is no justification for colonoscopy as a screening technique in the patient who is not at an increased risk for the development of a neoplasm.

EXFOLIATIVE CYTOLOGY

Exfoliative cytology has been recommended as a screening technique for evaluation of iron deficiency anemia, for early detection of colonic neoplasms, and to ascertain whether known lesions as determined by colonoscopy or roentgenography are benign or malignant.[107] The technique involves vigorous bowel cleansing.[6, 40, 101, 107] Raskin and Pleticka advocate in-

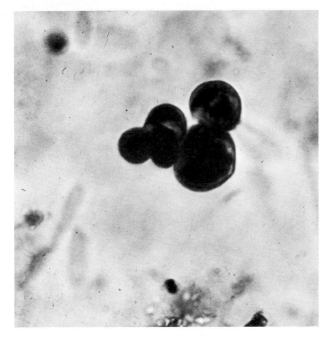

FIG. 1-38. Exfoliative cytology demonstrating cancer cells in colonic washings. (Original magnification × 600. Courtesy of Rudolf Garret, M.D.)

hospital evaluation in order to ensure such thoroughness.[108] Using a sigmoidoscope, a large-diameter red rubber catheter is inserted and the instrument withdrawn. Irrigation is then carried out, usually by a trained technician, and slides collected and reviewed by a pathologist (Fig. 1-38).

Exfoliative cytology has never gained much acceptance, primarily because of the cumbersome methodology and the fact that colonoscopy is far superior for evaluation of the entire bowel. Unless it can be simplified and the results interpreted with accuracy, the procedure will in all probability be relegated to that of historic interest only.

STOOL FOR OCCULT BLOOD DETERMINATION

Colorectal cancer is the commonest visceral malignancy. Probably the least expensive mass screening technique available for detection of gastrointestinal pathology is the occult blood determination. The value of this procedure is particularly enhanced because of recent evidence to suggest that colorectal cancer appears to be increasingly affecting the bowel in a more proximal location than has been previously appreciated (see Chap. 10).

Materials and Methods

The commercially available guaiac-impregnated slide (Hemoccult II) has come to be used as the primary resource for this screening study. But the test is essentially a meaningless exercise unless strict dietary instructions are adhered to.

For at least 48 hours prior to the collection of the first stool specimen, rare meat, turnips, horseradish, salmon, and sardines are to be avoided. A high-fiber diet is advised. Medications such as aspirin and vitamin preparations (especially vitamin C [ascorbic acid]) are excluded.

The test is commenced on the third day, with the patient taking a sample from the stool and smearing it on the card. Samples from three consecutive bowel movements are recommended. In interpreting results the American Cancer Society recommends that doubtful readings should be recorded as negative and trace readings as positive.[41] A single positive slide is treated as if all determinations are positive. With such a result, one is obligated to perform in sequential order a digital rectal examination, proctosigmoidoscopy, and barium enema examination (or air-contrast enema). If these studies are negative, colonoscopy should be considered; if normal, it should be followed by an upper gastrointestinal x-ray and small bowel series.

Recently a home-use occult blood detection kit has been marketed, the Fleet Detecatest. It will be interesting to ascertain how eagerly patients will purchase this product, and whether they will seek a physician's evaluation should a positive result be obtained.

Test Results

Numerous reports of the results of mass screening for colorectal cancer have been published (see also Chapter 10).[62, 63, 98, 120] Generally the studies have shown a high patient willingness to pursue further investigations when the test was positive. Those patients found to harbor a malignant lesion usually had a much earlier stage lesion. In the study of Sontag and associates, there was a 5% incidence of positive results.[120] Forty-eight percent of those who completed the gastrointestinal work-up were found to have neoplastic lesions, almost one third of which were malignant.

The occult blood determination of the stool should be an integral part of a complete physical examination.

FECES COLLECTION

The symptom of diarrhea and the frequency of infectious enteritis requires that the surgeon be familiar with at least the basic concepts of stool collection.

Stool for Culture

The stool collection should arrive in the laboratory within ½ hour of having been taken unless it is placed in a transport medium. Refrigeration is contraindicated. Swabs should not be used for collection.

Stool cultures are made by placing a sterile swab into the specimen and streaking a portion of several agar plates containing various inhibitory and noninhibitory agents to allow the recovery of both intestinal flora as well as pathogenic organisms (*e.g., Salmonella, Shigella, Campylobacter*). The plates are examined at 24 hours, and suspicious colonies are inoculated into identification media. If *Salmonella* or *Shigella* species are found, a subculture is sent for serologic typing or confirmation.

Certain organisms are somewhat unusual and are difficult to identify in a stool specimen. They are not routinely tested for, that is, a special request is usually necessary for their culture because they require special techniques. These organisms include fungi (the test is generally limited to screening for *Candida*), *Mycobacterium*, pathogenic *Vibrio* (cholera), *Campylobacter,* and *Yersinia*. The discovery of certain organisms mandates reporting to the local public health authority.

Stool for Ova and Parasites

The specimen must be less than 1 hour old when received by the laboratory. Three specimens are recommended for screening over a 5-day period. Collection can be made by using a warm saline or Fleet enema. Bismuth, mineral oil, castor oil, psyllium, and magnesium compounds used as laxatives produce specimens that are unsatisfactory for evaluation. Also, stools should not be collected if a barium study has been performed within 1 week.

Stool specimens for parasites are examined macroscopically for color and appearance (formed or liquid, with mucus or blood). They are also checked for adult worms or tapeworm proglottids.

A wet-mount preparation of stool on a glass slide with a drop each of saline and iodine is cover-slipped and examined microscopically for parasites (eggs, cysts, larvae) as well as for fecal leukocytes. A small portion of the specimen is also treated to concentrate the eggs and cysts, and later examined microscopically with wet mounts. Finally, a slide is streaked, stained (trichrome), and examined histologically with the oil emersion lens. For the diagnosis and treatment of the specific pathologic organism and disease, see the index.

INTRAVENOUS PYELOGRAPHY

The routine application of the intravenous pyelogram (IVP) in the preoperative assessment of patients undergoing bowel surgery is strongly encouraged. Prager and co-workers reviewed our experience with this study in 180 patients.[106] Seventy-eight (43%) were found to have abnormalities. Table 1-1 illustrates those that were felt related to the primary disease itself, and Table 1-2 summarizes the "unexpected" findings. Conditions such as inflammatory bowel disease, diverticulitis, and carcinoma of the rectum or rectosigmoid frequently are associated with urinary symptoms because of proximity to adjacent bladder or ureter.

Table 1-1. Abnormal IVP Findings Presumed Secondary to Primary Colon Disease

Abnormality	Number
Hydroureter	6
Bilateral hydroureter and hydronephrosis	2
Unilateral hydronephrosis	3
Ureteric deviation	3
Extrinsic pressure on bladder	7
Urinary tract calculi	8
Postvoiding residual	
Modest	22
Marked	5

(Prager E, Swinton NW, Corman ML, Veidenheimer MC: Intravenous pyelography in colorectal surgery. Dis Colon Rectum 1973; 16:479–481)

Table 1-2. Abnormal, Coincidental IVP Findings

Abnormality	Number
Ureteric duplication	4
Unilateral kidney	1
Ptotic kidney	1
Atrophic pyelonephritis	1
Bilateral sponge kidney	1
Bladder carcinoma	1
Neurogenic bladder	1
Poor visualization, both kidneys	1
Malrotated kidney	1
Renal carcinoma	1
Displaced kidney (secondary hypersplenism)	1
Caliectasis	4
Calyceal diverticulum	1
Renal pelvic cyst	1
Renal pelvic papilloma	2

(Prager E, Swinton NW, Corman ML, Veidenheimer MC: Intravenous pyelography in colorectal surgery. Dis Colon Rectum 1973; 16:479–481)

The concept of having a "road map" of the urinary tract prior to surgical intervention is supported by the high frequency of symptoms and of associated abnormalities. Tank and associates, for example, noted 30% of 150 patients who underwent abdominoperineal resection developed postoperative voiding difficulties.[125] Peel and associates, in a prospective series of 176 patients who underwent surgery for carcinoma or diverticular disease, noted urologic symptoms in almost one third.[103] As might be anticipated, the incidence of pyelogram abnormalities is much higher in symptomatic patients than in those without complaint, but the coincidental discovery of such conditions as ureteric duplication and unilateral kidney, as well as the risk of intraoperative injury to the urinary tract, strongly support the routine preoperative use of the IVP in all patients who are to undergo bowel surgery.

ANORECTAL PHYSIOLOGIC STUDIES

The physiology of the pelvic floor has been investigated primarily by means of electromyography (EMG) of the puborectalis and external sphincter muscles and by recording the manometric pressure in the anal canal and rectum.[34] These studies, however, are usually applied in a rather limited clinical setting, that is, in patients with anal incontinence due to congenital anomalies affecting the area (*e.g.,* myelomeningocele) or to trauma; following various surgical procedures; and coincident with certain diseases, such as rectal prolapse, neuropathy, and myopathy (see Chap. 5). In some centers patients with constipation are being evaluated using these techniques.[12, 65, 78]

Electrical activity is determined by inserting a fine needle electrode in the puborectalis muscle and the subcutaneous external sphincter.[78] On moving the exploring electrode from one part of the muscle to another a burst of electrical activity occurs, but when the needle is motionless there should normally be electrical silence.[134] The patient is then encouraged to maximally contract the sphincter, and the degree of response is evaluated. If the oscilloscope screen is filled with action potentials the sphincter is considered normal; this is called a Grade 4 response. A Grade 3 response would indicate some potentials missing; a Grade 2, many missing; a Grade 1, only a few present; and a Grade 0, no action potential.[134] With relaxation it is possible to identify such other electrical abnormalities as fibrillation.

Henry and co-workers recorded the latency of the anal reflex by EMG after electrical stimulation of the perianal skin.[69] In patients with fecal incontinence the latency period was considerably prolonged when compared with control subjects. They were able to conclude that denervation of the sphincter muscles was the primary cause of the incontinence in their patients.

Anorectal manometry reveals that the normal resting anal canal pressure is from 70 to 100 cm of water, which can be doubled during a contraction effort.[78] Patients who have undergone internal anal sphincterotomy or sphincter stretch may have a reduced pressure. It appears that the internal anal sphincter is the muscle responsible for the resting pressure in the anal canal.

The technique of anorectal manometry usually involves insertion of either a balloon-tipped catheter connected to a transducer or an open-tipped catheter. The calibration is determined at different levels of insertion with the patient in the resting state and while contracting the sphincter muscle.

The balloon can be inflated in the rectum to determine the rectosphincteric reflex and then distended further to the point at which the patient feels the urgency to defecate, and the results recorded.[94] Rapid balloon distention normally produces relaxation of the internal anal sphincter.[113] This response is felt to be due to an intramural reflex since it is preserved in the absence of any spinal pathway.[34] An intact rectosigmoid is required, and the response is absent in children with Hirschsprung's disease.

Borden and associates applied anal manometry to evaluate external sphincter activity.[12] They identified defects not previously described, which they postulated may be useful in determining the appropriate treatment for a given abnormality (*e.g.*, electrical stimulator, biofeedback, or bowel management).

This is the underlying question: Does physiologic evaluation of the anorectum aid in determining therapy? Because of the difficulty in obtaining these studies and the confusion in their interpretation, I have not found them useful in the usual clinical setting. In the vast majority of patients a carefully obtained history and physical examination (including sensory determination), and an appreciation for the sphincteric resting tone and contractility noted on digital examination, are the studies upon which one should rely.

REFERENCES

1. Abrams JS: A hard look at colonoscopy. Am J Surg 1977; 133:111–115
2. Adair HM, Hishon S: The management of colon-

oscopic and sigmoidoscopic perforation of the large bowel. Br J Surg 1981; 68:415–416

3. Adami B, Eckardt VF, Suermann RB, Karbach U, Ewe K: Bacteremia after proctoscopy and hemorrhoidal injection sclerotherapy. Dis Colon Rectum 1981; 24:373–374

4. Amshel AL, Shonberg IL, Gopal KA: Retroperitoneal and mediastinal emphysema as a complication of colonoscopy. Dis Colon Rectum 1982; 25:167–168

5. Anseline PF, Fazio VW: Management of massive postpolypectomy hemorrhage. Dis Colon Rectum 1982; 25:251–253

6. Bader, GM, Papanicolaou G: The application of cytology in the diagnosis of cancer of the rectum, sigmoid and descending colon. Cancer 1952; 5:307–314

7. Benjamin HG, Todd JD: Routine roentgenologic examination of the colon in patients with anorectal complaints. Dis Colon Rectum 1959; 2:196–199

8. Berci G, Panish JF, Schapiro M, Corlin R: Complications of colonoscopy and polypectomy. Gastroenterology 1974; 67:584–585

9. Bigard MA, Gaucher P, Lassalle C: Fatal colonic explosion during colonoscopic polypectomy. Gastroenterology 1979; 77:1307–1310

10. Blackstone MO, Riddell RH, Rogers BHG, Levin B: Dysplasia-associated lesion or mass (DALM) detected by colonoscopy in long-standing ulcerative colitis: An indication for colectomy. Gastroenterology 1981; 80:366–374

11. Bohlman TW, Katon RM, Lipshutz GR, McCool MF, Smith FW, Melnyk CS: Fiberoptic pansigmoidoscopy: An evaluation and comparison with rigid sigmoidoscopy. Gastroenterology 1977; 72:644–649

12. Borden EB, Sheran M, Sammartano RJ, Boley SJ: The complete anorectal function profile (abstr). Gastroenterology 1982; 82:1023

13. Brand EJ, Sullivan BH, Sivak MV, Rankin GB: Colonoscopy in the diagnosis of unexplained rectal bleeding. Ann Surg 1980; 192:111–113

14. Breiter JR, Hajjar JJ: Segmental tuberculosis of the colon diagnosed by colonoscopy. Am J Gastroenterol 1981; 76:369–373

15. Burbige E, Bourke E, Tarder G: Effect of preparation for colonoscopy on fluid and electrolyte balance. Gastrointest Endosc 1978; 24:286–287

16. Burnikel RH: Barium granuloma. Dis Colon Rectum 1962; 5:224–227

17. Cannon WB: The movements of the stomach studied by means of the Röntgen rays. Am J Physiol 1898; 1:360–362

18. Cannon WB: The movements of the intestines studied by means of the Röntgen rays. Am J Physiol 1901/1902; 6:251–277

19. Cannon WB, Moser A: The movements of the food in the esophagus. Am J Physiol 1898; 1:435–444

20. Carter HG: Short flexible fiberoptic colonoscopy in routine office examinations. Dis Colon Rectum 1981; 24:17–19

21. Christie JP: Colonoscopic excision of sessile polyps. Am J Gastroenterol 1976; 66:23-28

22. Christie JP: Colonoscopic excision of large sessile polyps. Am J Gastroenterol 1977; 67:430–438

23. Coller JA: Technique of flexible fiberoptic sigmoidoscopy. Surg Clin North Am 1980; 60:465–479

24. Coller JA, Corman ML, Veidenheimer MC: Diagnostic and therapeutic applications of fiberoptic colonoscopy. Geriatrics 1974; 29:67–73

25. Coller JA, Corman ML, Veidenheimer MC: Colonic polypoid disease: Need for total colonoscopy. Am J Surg 1976; 131:490–495

26. Corman ML, Coller JA, Veidenheimer MC: Proctosigmoidoscopy—age criteria for examination in the asymptomatic patient. CA 1975; 25:286–290

27. Corman ML, Veidenheimer MC, Coller JA: Barium-enema study findings in asymptomatic patients with rectal polyps. Dis Colon Rectum 1974; 17:325–330

28. Coughlin GP, Butler MHA, Grant AK: Colonoscopy and bacteraemia. Gut 1977; 18:678–679

29. Crapp AR, Powis SJA, Tillotson P, Cooke WT, Alexander-Williams J: Preparation of the bowel by whole-gut irrigation. Lancet 1975; 2:1239–1240

30. Davis GR, Santa Ana CA, Morawski SG, Fordtran JS: Development of a lavage solution associated with minimal water and electrolyte absorption or secretion. Gastroenterology 1980; 78:991–995

31. Dean ACB, Newell JP: Colonoscopy in the differential diagnosis of carcinoma from diverticulitis of the sigmoid colon. Br J Surg 1973; 60:633–635

32. Desbaillets LG, Mangla JC: Pneumatosis cystoides intestinalis diagnosed by colonoscopy. Gastrointest Endosc 1974; 20:126–127

33. Dickinson RJ, Dixon MF, Axon ATR: Colonoscopy and the detection of dysplasia in patients with longstanding ulcerative colitis. Lancet 1980; 2:620–622

34. Dickinson VA: Maintenance of anal continence: A review of pelvic floor physiology. Gut 1978; 19:1163–1174

35. Dickman MD, Farrell R, Higgs RH, Wright LE, Humphries TJ, Wojcik JD, Chappelka R: Colonoscopy associated bacteremia. Surg Gynecol Ob-

stet 1976; 142:173–176

36. Dodds WJ, Scanlon GT, Shaw DK, Stewart ET et al: An evaluation of colon cleansing regimens. Am J Roentgenol 1977; 128:57–59

37. Dodds WJ, Stewart ET, Hogan WJ: Role of colonoscopy and roentgenology in the detection of polypoid colonic lesions. Dig Dis Sci 1977; 22:646–649

38. Drexler J: Asymptomatic polyps of the colon and rectum. III. Proximal and distal polyp relationships. Arch Intern Med 1971; 127:466–469

39. Dysart DN: Angled sigmoid view. In Greenbaum EI (ed): Radiographic Atlas of Colon Disease, p. 31. Chicago, Year Book Medical Publishers, 1980

40. Ebeling CE, Little JW: The demonstration of malignant cells exfoliated from the proximal colon. Ann Intern Med 1957; 46:21–29

41. Eddy D: Cancer of the colon and rectum. CA 1980; 30:208–215

42. Eisenberg HW: Fiberoptic colonoscopy: Intraoperative colonoscopy. Dis Colon Rectum 1976; 19:405–406

43. Epstein M: Endoscopy: Developments in optical instrumentation. Science 1980; 210:280–285

44. Farinon AM, Vadora E: Endometriosis of the colon and rectum: An indication for preoperative coloscopy. Endoscopy 1980; 12:136–139

45. Fielding J, Lumsden K: Large-bowel perforations in patients undergoing sigmoidoscopy and barium enema. Br Med J 1973; 1:471–473

46. Fishman EK, Goldman SM: Pneumoscrotum after colonoscopy. Urology 1981; 18:171–172

47. Forde KA, Lebwohl O, Wolff M, Voorhees AB: Reversible ischemic colitis—correlation of colonoscopic and pathologic changes. Am J Gastroenterol 1979; 72:182–185

48. Foster GE, Vellacott KD, Balfour TW, Hardcastle JD: Outpatient flexible fiberoptic sigmoidoscopy, diagnostic yield and the value of glucagon. Br J Surg 1981; 68:463–464

49. Franklin GO, Mohapatra M, Perrillo RP: Colonic tuberculosis diagnosed by colonoscopic biopsy. Gastroenterology 1979; 76:362–364

50. Frühmorgen P: Therapeutic colonoscopy. In Hunt RH, Waye JD (eds): Colonoscopy: Techniques, Clinical Practice and Colour Atlas, pp 199–203. London, Chapman and Hall, 1981

51. Frühmorgen P: Therapeutic colonoscopy. In Hunt RH, Waye JD (eds): Colonoscopy: Techniques, Clinical Practice and Colour Atlas, p 222. London, Chapman and Hall, 1981

52. Gans SL: A new look at pediatric endoscopy. Postgrad Med 1977, 61:91–100

53. Gear EV, Dobbins WO: Rectal biopsy. Gastroenterology 1968; 55:522–544

54. Geboes K, Vantrappen G: The value of colonoscopy in the diagnosis of Crohn's disease. Gastrointest Endosc 1975; 22:18–23

55. Gelfand DW, Ott DJ: Single vs. double-contrast gastrointestinal studies: Critical analysis of reported statistics. Am J Roentgenol 1981; 137:523–528

56. Ghazi A, Shinya H, Wolff WI: Treatment of volvulus of the colon by colonoscopy. Ann Surg 1976; 183:263–265

57. Gianturco, C, Miller GA: Routine search for colonic polyps by high-voltage radiography. Radiology 1953; 60:496–499

58. Gilbertsen VA: Proctosigmoidoscopy and polypectomy in reducing the incidence of rectal cancer. Cancer (Suppl)1974; 34:936–939

59. Goldman J, Reichelderfer M: Evaluation of rapid colonoscopy preparation using a new gut lavage solution. Gastrointest Endosc 1982; 28:9–11

60. Gould SR, Williams CB: Castor oil or senna preparation before colonoscopy for inactive chronic ulcerative colitis. Gastrointest Endosc 1982; 28: 6–8

61. Graham J, Eusebio EB: Complications of colonoscopy. IMJ 1977; 152:39–42

62. Greegor DH: Occult blood testing for detection of asymptomatic colon cancer. Cancer 1971; 28:131–134

63. Greegor DH: Detection of colorectal cancer using guaiac slides. CA 1972; 22:361–363

64. Habr-Gama A, Alves PRA, Gama-Rodrigues JJ, Teixeira MG, Barbieri D: Pediatric colonoscopy. Dis Colon Rectum 1979; 22:530–535

65. Haddad H, Devroede-Bertrand G: Large bowel motility disorders. Med Clin North Am 1981; 65:1377–1396

66. Hagihara PF, Ernst CB, Griffen WO: Incidence of ischemic colitis following abdominal aortic reconstruction. Surg Gynecol Obstet 1979; 149:571–573

67. Hedberg SE: Personal communication.

68. Hedrick E: Guidelines for cleaning and disinfection of flexible fiberoptic endoscopes (FFE) used in GI endoscopy. Journal of American Practices in Infection Control 1978; 6:8–10

69. Henry MM, Parks AG, Swash M: The anal reflex in idiopathic faecal incontinence; an electrophysiological study. Br J Surg 1980; 67:781–783

70. Hewitt J, Reeve J et al: Whole-gut irrigation in preparation for large-bowel surgery. Lancet 1973; 2:337–340

71. Hoffman BI, Kobasa W, Kaye D: Bacteremia after rectal examination. Ann Intern Med 1978; 88:658–659

72. Hogan WJ, Hensley GT, Greenen JE: Endoscopic

evaluation of inflammatory bowel disease. Med Clin North Am 1980; 64:1083–1102

73. Hunt RH, Waye JD (eds): Colonoscopy: Techniques, Clinical Practice and Colour Atlas. London, Chapman and Hall, 1981

74. Kahn SP, Lindenauer SM, Wojtalik RS: Perforation of the normal colon during barium contrast examination. Am Surg 1976; 42:789–792

75. Knutson CO, Williams HC, Max MH: Detection of intracolonic lesion by barium contrast enema. JAMA 1979; 242:2206–2208

76. Koo J, Ho J, Ong GB: The value of colonoscopy in the diagnosis of ileo-caecal tuberculosis. Endoscopy 1982; 14:48–50

77. Kumar S, Abcarian H, Prasad ML, Lakshmanan S: Bacteremia associated with lower gastrointestinal endoscopy, fact or fiction? Dis Colon Rectum 1982; 25:131–134

78. Lane RH: Clinical application of anorectal physiology. Proc R Soc Med 1975; 68:28–30

79. Laufer I: The radiologic demonstration of early changes in ulcerative colitis by double contrast technique. J Can Assoc Radiol 1975; 26:116–121

80. Lanfer I, Mullens JE, Hamilton J: Correlation of endoscopy and double-contrast radiography in the early stages of ulcerative and granulomatous colitis. Radiology 1976; 118:1–5

81. LeFrock JL, Ellis CA, Turchik JB, Weinstein L: Transient bacteremia associated with sigmoidoscopy. N Engl J Med 1973; 289:467–469

82. Lezak MB, Goldhamer M: Retroperitoneal emphysema after colonoscopy. Gastroenterology 1974; 66:118–120

83. Lull GF Jr, Byrne JP, Sanowski RA: Barium sulfate granuloma of the rectum JAMA 1971; 217:1102–1103

84. Margulis AR: Is double-contrast examination of the colon the only acceptable radiographic examination? Radiology 1976; 119:741–742

85. Marino AWM: Complications of colonoscopy. Dis Colon Rectum 1979; 21:15–19

86. Marks G, Boggs HW, Castro AF, Gathright JB, Ray JE, Salvati E: Sigmoidoscopic examinations with rigid and flexible fiberoptic sigmoidoscopes in the surgeon's office. Dis Colon Rectum 1979; 22:162–168

87. Martel W, Robins JM: The barium enema: Technique, value and limitations. Cancer 1971; 28:137–143

88. Martin PJ, Forde KA: Intraoperative colonoscopy: Preliminary report. Dis Colon Rectum 1979; 22:234–237

89. Max MH, Knutson CO: Colonoscopy in patients with inflammatory colonic strictures. Surgery 1978; 84:551–556

90. Mendoza CB, Watne AL: Value of intraoperative colonoscopy in vascular ectasia of the colon. Am Surg 1982; 48:153–156

91. Miller RE, Chernish SM, Skucas J, Rosenak BD, Rodda BE: Hypotonic colon examination with glucagon. Radiology 1974; 113:555–562

92. Minervini S, Alexander-Williams J, Donovan IA, Bentley S, Keighley MRB: Comparison of three methods of whole bowel irrigation. Am J Surg 1980; 140:400–402

93. Myren J, Serck-Hanssen A, Solberg L: Routine and blind histological diagnoses on colonoscopic biopsies compared to clinical-colonoscopic observations in patients without and with colitis. Scand J Gastroenterol 1976; 11:135–140

94. Neill ME, Parks AG, Swash M: Physiological studies of the anal sphincter musculature in faecal incontinence and rectal prolapse. Br J Surg 1981; 68:531–536

95. Nelson RL, Abcarian H, Prasad ML: Iatrogenic perforation of the colon and rectum. Dis Colon Rectum 1982; 25:305–308

96. Newstead GL, Morgan BP: Bowel preparation with mannitol. Med J Australia 1979; 2:582–583

97. Nivatvongs S, Fryd DS: How far does the proctosigmoidoscope reach? N Engl J Med 1980; 303:380–382

98. Nivatvongs, S, Gilbertsen VA, Goldberg SM, Williams SE: Distribution of large-bowel cancers detected by occult blood test in asymptomatic patients. Dis Colon Rectum 1982; 25:420–421

99. Norfleet RG, Mitchell PD, Mulholland DD: Does bacteremia follow colonoscopy? II. Gastrointest Endoscopy 1976; 23:31–32

100. Norfleet RG, Mulholland DD, Mitchell PD, Philo J, Walters EW: Does bacteremia follow colonoscopy? Gastroenterology 1976; 70:20–21

101. Oakland DJ: The diagnosis of carcinoma of the colon by exfoliative cytology. Proc R Soc Med 1964; 57:279–282

102. Overholt BF: Colonoscopy: A review. Gastroenterology 1975; 68:1308–1320

103. Peel ALG, Benyon L, Grace RH: The value of routine preoperative urological assessment in patients undergoing elective surgery for diverticular disease or carcinoma of the large bowel. Br J Surg 1980; 67:42–45

104. Plucnar BJ: Colonoscopy in infancy and childhood with special regard to patient preparation and examination technique. Endoscopy 1981; 13:14–18

105. Portes C, Majarakis JD: Proctosigmoidoscopy–incidence of polyps in 50,000 examinations. JAMA 1957; 163:411–413

106. Prager E, Swinton NW, Corman ML, Veidenheimer MC: Intravenous pyelography in colorectal surgery. Dis Colon Rectum 1973; 16:479–481

107. Raskin HF, Palmer WL, Kirsner JB: Exfoliative cytology in diagnosis of cancer of the colon. Dis Colon Rectum 1959; 2:46–57

108. Raskin HF, Pleticka S: Exfoliative cytology of the colon. Cancer 1971; 28:127–130

109. Rogers BHG, Silvis SE, Nebel OT, Sugawa C, Mandelstam P: Complications of flexible fiberoptic colonoscopy and polypectomy. Gastrointest Endosc 1975; 22:73–77

110. Salazar M, Jackman RJ: Reasons for incomplete proctoscopy. Dis Colon Rectum 1969; 12:19–21

111. Sands J. Quoted by Masel H, Masel JP, Casey KV: A survey of colon examination techniques in Australia and New Zealand, with a review of complications. Australian Radiology 1971; 15:140–147

112. Sanner CJ, Saltzman DA: Detorsion of sigmoid volvulus by colonoscopy. Gastrointest Endosc 1977; 23:212–213

113. Schuster MM, Hendrix TR, Mendeloff AI: The internal anal sphincter response: Manometric studies on its normal physiology, neural pathways, and alteration in bowel disorders. J Clin Invest 1963; 42:196–207

114. Schwesinger WH, Levine BA, Ramos R: Complications of colonoscopy. Surg Gynecol Obstet 1979; 148:270–281

115. Seaman WB, Wells J: Complications of the barium enema. Gastroenterology 1965; 48:728–737

116. Shinya H, Wolff WI: Morphology, anatomic distribution and cancer potential of colonic polyps. Ann Surg 1979; 190:679–683

117. Skucas J, Cutcliff W, Fischer HW: Whole-gut irrigation as a means of cleaning the colon. Radiology 1976; 121:303–305

118. Smith LE: Fiberoptic colonoscopy: Complications of colonoscopy and polypectomy. Dis Colon Rectum 1976; 19:407–412

119. Sohn N, Robilotti JA: The gay bowel syndrome. Am J Gastroenterol 1977; 67:478–484

120. Sontag SJ, Durczak C, Aranha GV, Chejfec G et al: Fecal occult blood screening for colorectal cancer in a veterans administration hospital. Am J Surg 1983; 145:89–94

121. Stevens AF: Colonoscopy in the irritable bowel syndrome. Gut 1973; 14:432–433

122. Sugarbaker PH, Vineyard GC, Lewicki AM, Pinkus GS, Warhol MJ, Moore FD: Colonoscopy in the management of diseases of the colon and rectum. Surg Gynecol Obstet 1974; 139:341–349

123. Swinton NW: Personal communication.

124. Swinton NW: Polyps of rectum and colon. JAMA 1954; 154:658–662

125. Tank ES, Ernst CB, Woolston ST et al: Urinary tract complications of anorectal surgery. Am J Surg 1972; 123:118–122

126. Tawile NT, Priest RJ, Schuman BM: Colonoscopy in inflammatory bowel disease. Gastrointest Endosc 1975; 22:11–13

127. Taylor EW, Bentley S, Youngs S, Keighley MRB: Bowel preparation and the safety of colonoscopic polypectomy. Gastroenterology 1981; 81:1–4

128. Tedesco FJ: Antibiotic associated pseudomembranous colitis with negative proctosigmoidoscopy. Gastroenterology 1979; 77:295–297

129. Tedesco FJ, Pickens CA, Griffin JW, Sivak MV, Sullivan BH: Role of colonoscopy in patients with unexplained melena: Analysis of 53 patients. Gastrointest Endosc 1981; 27:221–223

130. Thoeni RF, Menuck L: Comparison of barium enema and colonoscopy in the detection of small colonic polyps. Radiology 1977; 124:631–635

131. Waye JD: Colonoscopy: A clinical view. Mt Sinai J Med (NY) 1975; 42:1–34

132. Waye JD: Colitis, cancer, and colonoscopy. Med Clin North Am 1978; 62:211–224

133. Waye JD: Colonoscopy intubation techniques without fluoroscopy. In Hunt RH, Waye JD (eds): Colonoscopy: Techniques, Clinical Practice and Colour Atlas, pp. 170–174. London, Chapman and Hall, 1981

134. Waylonis GW, Powers JJ: Clinical application of anal sphincter electromyography. Surg Clin North Am 1972; 52:807–815

135. Welin S: Results of the Malmö technique of colon examination. JAMA 1967; 199:119–120

136. Welin S: Newer diagnostic techniques: The superiority of double-contrast roentgenology. Dis Colon Rectum 1974; 17:13–15

137. Williams CB, Laage NJ, Campbell CA, Douglas JR, Walker-Smith JA, Booth IW, Harries JT: Total colonoscopy in children. Arch Dis Child 1982; 57:49–53

138. Winnan G, Berci G, Panish J, Talbot TM, Overholt BF, McCallum RW: Superiority of the flexible to the rigid sigmoidoscope in routine proctosigmoidoscopy. N Engl J Med 1980; 302:1011–1012

139. Wolff WI, Shinya H: Polypectomy via the fiberoptic colonoscope: Removal of neoplasms beyond the reach of the sigmoidoscope. N Engl J Med 1973; 288:329–332

140. Wolff WI, Shinya H, Geffen A, Ozoktay S, DeBeer R: Comparison of colonoscopy and the contrast enema in five hundred patients with colorectal disease. Am J Surg 1975; 129:181–186

141. Yassinger S, Midgley RC, Cantor DS, Poirier TJ, Imperator TJ: Retroperitoneal emphysema after colonoscopic polypectomy. West J Med 1978; 128:347–350

142. Yudis M, Cohen A, Pearce AE: Perforation of the transverse colon during barium enema and air-contrast studies. Am Surg 1968; 34:334–336

CHAPTER 2

Hemorrhoids

Hemorrhoids are dilated veins that lie beneath the anal canal lining and the perianal skin. External hemorrhoids occur below the pectinate line, internal hemorrhoids are found above it, and mixed hemorrhoids are located above and below the line.

The problem of hemorrhoids can occur at any age and affects both sexes. Women seem particularly prone to an exacerbation during pregnancy. Hemorrhoids are one of the commonest afflictions of Western civilization.

ANATOMY

The submucosa does not form a continuous ring of thickened tissue in the anal canal, but rather a discontinuous series of cushions; the three main ones are found in the left lateral, right anterior, and right posterior positions (Fig. 2-1).[14] The submucosal layer of each of these thicker regions is rich in blood vessels and muscle fibers known as the muscularis submucosa (Fig. 2-2).[60, 81] These fibers, arising from the internal sphincter and from the conjoined longitudinal muscle, are important in maintaining adherence of mucosal and submucosal tissue to the underlying internal sphincter and in supporting the blood vessels of the submucosa. The muscularis submucosa and its connective tissue fibers return the anal canal lining to its initial position after the temporary downward displacement that occurs during defecation.

The anal cushions receive their blood supply mainly from the terminal branches of the superior hemorrhoidal artery (superior rectal artery) and, to a lesser extent, from branches of the middle hemorrhoidal arteries.[11, 60] These branches communicate with one another and with branches of the inferior hemorrhoidal arteries, which supply the lower portion of the anal canal. The superior, middle, and inferior hemorrhoidal veins, which drain blood from the tissues of the anal canal, correspond to each of the hemorrhoidal arteries.[11, 35, 60]

ETIOLOGY

The three major theories of the cause of hemorrhoids are as follows:

1. Abnormal dilatation of the veins of the internal hemorrhoidal venous plexus, a network of the tributaries of the superior and middle hemorrhoidal veins[14, 59]
2. Abnormal distention of the arteriovenous anastomoses, which are in the same location as the anal cushions[35, 36]
3. Downward displacement or prolapse of the anal cushions[20, 72]

Other theories have been proposed to explain abnormal distention of hemorrhoidal vessels. Hemorrhoids might be caused by a backflow of venous blood from transient increases in intra-abdominal pressure. Pressure exerted on the hemorrhoidal veins by a fetus explains the occurrence of the condition in pregnant women.[48, 61] Engorgement of vessels might result from a defect in venous drainage, which, in turn, might be caused by failure of the internal sphincter to relax as it should during defecation. Vascular distention might be caused by augmented arterial flow, which would explain why people with hemorrhoids sometimes feel additional discomfort after a heavy meal; more blood is delivered to the digestive system through the mesenteric artery, of which the superior hemorrhoidal artery is a branch.[69]

The anal sphincters of many patients with hemorrhoids demonstrate an abnormal rhythm of contraction and exert a greater force of contraction than those of asymptomatic control subjects. Whether this sphincter abnormality is a cause or an effect of hemorrhoids is not known, but it might relate to any of the hypotheses outlined. An overactive sphincter might either contribute to venous congestion or expose the anal cushions to greater shear forces, or do both by constricting the anal canal.[5, 34]

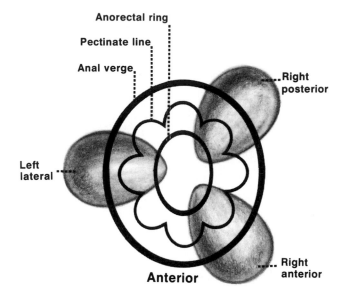

FIG. 2-1. Usual three primary hemorrhoidal groups.

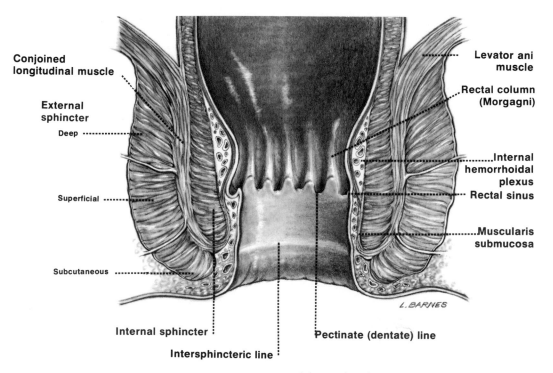

FIG. 2-2. Anatomy of the anal region.

Hemorrhoids may be caused by more than one factor. Although some evidence suggests that hemorrhoids are familial, it is not known whether they are caused by hereditary factors (weak-walled veins) or environmental factors (family members might have similar dietary or bowel habits). Excessive straining at defecation is believed to contribute to the formation of hemorrhoids, but this has not been proven.[22]

CLASSIFICATION

Hemorrhoids are classified by location (external, internal, or mixed) or by degree (first, second, third, and fourth). *External hemorrhoids* arise from the inferior hemorrhoidal plexus and are covered by modified squamous epithelium. They may thrombose and ulcerate. *Internal hemorrhoids* may prolapse and may be reducible or irreducible. They can ulcerate and bleed or thrombose. They arise from the superior hemorrhoidal plexus and are covered by mucosa. *Mixed hemorrhoids* (external–internal) may be prolapsed, irreducible, thrombosed, or ulcerated. They arise from the inferior and superior hemorrhoidal plexi and their anastomotic connections.

In *first-degree hemorrhoids* the veins of the anal canal are increased in number and size, and may bleed at the time of defecation. They are not prolapsed but project into the lumen. *Second-degree hemorrhoids* present to the outside during defecation but return spontaneously within the canal where they remain the rest of the time. *Third-degree hemorrhoids* (internal and mixed) prolapse outside the anal canal and require manual reduction. *Fourth-degree hemorrhoids* are irreducible and remain in a condition of prolapse all the time.

External Hemorrhoids

Two types of hemorrhoids are found at the external anal orifice. One occurs predominantly in the form of dilation and engorgement of the veins beneath the skin, and the other is manifested as thrombosis of these veins. When the clot forms, the patient becomes aware of its presence. The degree of pain depends on the size of the clot and the relationship it bears to the anal sphincters. A large clot will cause pain, but even if a clot is small, it can be painful if it lies within the anal musculature. Small, thrombosed hemorrhoids rarely rupture.

When infection spreads into external and internal tissues surrounding hemorrhoidal veins, excessive external swelling develops as edema fills the subcutaneous area of the perianal margins. The infection and swelling may result in acute external and internal hemorrhoids with associated thrombosis and prolapse.

External Tags or Skin Tabs

External tags or skin tabs are deformities of the skin of the external anal margin and occur as redundant folds. These tags may be found when an old thrombosed hemorrhoid has become organized into a fibrous appendage.

The practice of removing hemorrhoids in three primary groups usually leaves bridges of tissue between the sites of the hemorrhoidal masses. When hemorrhoidal disease is extensive, some of the diseased veins remain beneath these bridges of skin; these may become fibrous skin tags after the wounds have healed.

Internal Hemorrhoids

The ordinary internal hemorrhoid may not be evident on inspection, especially if the patient is relaxed. When the patient strains, a bulging mass may appear that involves all or part of the anal canal. The full extent of pressure is exerted on the anorectal outlet during defecation or straining, and therefore a reliable examination cannot be made while the patient is in either the recumbent or inverted (jackknife) position.

Thrombosed Hemorrhoids

Thrombosed hemorrhoids (clotted hemorrhoids) are seen most often in patients who strain while defecating, who have frequent bowel actions (in inflammatory bowel disease or malabsorption), or who maintain a library in the bathroom. Others include persons who sit for long periods of time—especially long-distance truck drivers, motorcycle policemen, and operators of heavy-duty construction equipment.

DIFFERENTIAL DIAGNOSIS

Polyps, Adenomas, and Carcinomas Versus Hemorrhoids

Sessile, polypoid (adenomatous) masses and true carcinomas, which are easily palpated or visualized, should be differentiated readily from hemorrhoidal tissue. Internal hemorrhoids uncomplicated by thrombosis, edema, prolapse, or other factors are usually easy to diagnose. Any anorectal abnormality that is readily palpable in the absence of a recent thrombosis or recent injection therapy is not likely to be hemorrhoidal tissue.

Biopsy and microscopic study of all suspicious lesions are essential to establish the correct diagnosis.

Hypertrophied Anal Papilla Versus Hemorrhoids

A firm mass that seems to arise from a pedicle attached in the region of the dentate line is most likely an hypertrophied anal papilla. Endoscopic study should establish the diagnosis by demonstrating that the pedicle arises from the dentate margin and that the entire lesion is invested by skin.

Rectal Prolapse Versus Hemorrhoids

Rectal prolapse may be either partial, involving only the mucosal layer of the rectal wall, or complete, involving the full thickness of the rectal wall. Partial prolapse may affect either a part or all of the circumference of the anal outlet. Differentiating prolapsed internal hemorrhoids from partial rectal prolapse may be somewhat difficult. Internal hemorrhoids are separated by sulci radiating peripherally from the center of the anal outlet. Partial rectal prolapse is unaccompanied by any evidence of inflammatory change. Usually there is some element of mucosal prolapse when a circumferential rosette of hemorrhoids becomes irreducible and thrombosed (Fig. 2-3). Complete rectal prolapse is distinguished by concentrically arranged mucosal folds that are strikingly different from the radiating sulci separating prolapsed internal hemorrhoids.

SIGNS AND SYMPTOMS

The commonest presenting complaint of patients with hemorrhoids is *bleeding.* This usually occurs during or after defecation and is exacerbated by straining and frequent defecation. Blood can be evident on the paper, in the toilet bowl, or both. Occasionally blood loss may be great enough to produce a profound anemia. *Pain* is usually *not* due to hemorrhoids, unless the hemorrhoidal vein is thrombosed, ulcerated, or gangrenous. The commonest cause of anal pain is fissure. *Prolapse* with spontaneous return, or requiring manual reduction, is a common presentation of hemorrhoids. The

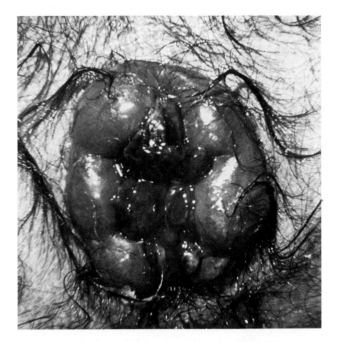

FIG. 2-3. Prolapsed, thrombosed hemorrhoids. These are irreducible and have an element of mucosal prolapse.

hemorrhoids may also be irreducible. *Pruritus ani* is often attributed to hemorrhoids, but frequently the examination fails to reveal significant hemorrhoidal disease. Unfortunately, many patients who undergo operative hemorrhoidectomy find that pruritus persists. Pruritus ani is a medical condition, the treatment of which includes diet, bowel management, anal hygiene, and occasionally medication (see Chap. 8).

Constipation is not a symptom of hemorrhoids, but defecation may be difficult when thrombosis or gangrene produces pain. Patients tend to avoid the toilet if hemorrhoidal symptoms are exacerbated by defecation, and this can lead to refusal of the call to stool with resulting obstipation.

EXAMINATION

Physical examination should include proctosigmoidoscopy and anoscopy. A barium enema examination should be performed in all patients who have rectal bleeding when the source is not obvious from these examinations. In the older age group (patients more than 50 years of age) a barium enema should be performed at some time, even if the hemorrhoids are the apparent cause of the patient's symptoms. A colonoscopic examination should also be considered.

GENERAL PRINCIPLES OF TREATMENT

Bleeding

Bleeding, if occasional and if related to straining or to diarrhea, should be managed medically. Treatment should be directed at the cause. Constipation can be controlled with appropriate dietary measures, bowel management programs, and laxatives. Diarrhea or frequent defecation may be managed with antidiarrheal medications and diet. Attention should also be given to improvement of anal hygiene.

Moesgaard and co-workers, in a prospective double-blind trial of a bulk agent (psyllium) versus a placebo in patients with bleeding and pain at defecation, noted a statistically significant difference in improvement of symptoms during a 6-week period (P<0.025).[52] They recommended the use of a high-fiber diet as the initial approach to management of patients with symptomatic hemorrhoids.

If bleeding persists, some form of treatment is advisable. If the patient believes that bleeding is caused by hemorrhoids and does not seek medical attention, a neoplasm could possibly supervene. Such a situation might jeopardize the opportunity for early diagnosis and treatment.

Prolapse

Prolapsed hemorrhoids that return spontaneously or are manually reducible can usually be treated by rubber ring ligation. The redundant mucosa and hemorrhoidal tissue are gathered in the drum of the ligator and can be removed effectively with minimal discomfort to the patient. If the prolapse is irreducible or if an external component is present, either excision using a local anesthetic or a surgical hemorrhoidectomy may be indicated.

Pain

If pain is due to gangrenous or ulcerated and thrombosed hemorrhoids, surgical hemorrhoidectomy is indicated. If hemorrhoids are associated with an anal fissure, hemorrhoidectomy should be considered and the fissure treated by internal anal sphincterotomy (see Chap. 3). A swollen, thrombosed external hemorrhoid that is producing pain should be treated by local excision.

AMBULATORY TREATMENT

Sclerotherapy: Injection Treatment of Hemorrhoids

In 1871, a unique form of treatment consisting of the injection of a chemical (phenol) into hemorrhoids was introduced in the United States and promised a "painless cure for piles without surgery."[4] Since specula were not available at that time, prolapsed hemorrhoids were selected for treatment. A single massive injection was intended to slough off the hemorrhoid. In 1879, Andrews reported on 3295 patients who were treated by injection, and estimated that at least 10,000 patients in the United States had been treated with this method.[4] Many complications, ranging from severe pain and slough to death, were reported. During this same period, Kelsey realized that the injection method was beneficial and substituted a weaker solution of carbolic acid, 5% to 7.5% in glycerine and water, which resulted in less sloughing.[39] Phenol (5%) in almond oil is still the primary sclerosing agent used in Great Britain today, 3 ml usually being injected into each hemorrhoidal site.

The combination of quinine and urea hydrochloride, widely used as a local anesthetic agent before the introduction of procaine, was associated with the development of fibrous tissue infiltration and sometimes slough at the site of injection.[71] Terrell, in 1913, first used this substance in the injection treatment of internal hemorrhoids with dramatic results. He concluded that a 5% solution was satisfactory from the standpoint of effectiveness and the patient's safety.[71]

Indications and Contraindications

The internal hemorrhoid, which does not prolapse, is the type most amenable to injection treatment. Sometimes a large, slightly protruding hemorrhoid can be treated in this manner. Injection usually affords only temporary relief of symptoms when hemorrhoids are extremely large, contain a great deal of fibrous tissue, or require digital replacement after defecation. External hemorrhoids should never be treated by injection. Internal hemorrhoids that are infected or that contain thrombi likewise should not be injected. Hemorrhoids with evidence of inflammation, such as ulceration and gangrene, are also unsuitable for injection treatment. External tags, fistulas, tumors, and anal fissures are complicating conditions that contraindicate use of the injection method. I believe injection treatment should be limited to those patients who have symptomatic hemorrhoids (especially bleeding) and who cannot tolerate rubber ring ligation.

Technique

With the patient in the semi-inverted (jackknife) position, the anoscope is inserted (Fig. 2-4). The scope should have an attachable light or an assistant should hold one. The entire region is inspected so that a diagram of the position of the hemorrhoids can be drawn on the patient's chart (see Fig. 2-1). This is important, especially when long intervals elapse between injections. The point at which each injection is made, the amount of solution used, and the date of injection should be recorded on the chart.

Figure 2-5 demonstrates the syringe and long-angled needle used for sclerotherapy. The needle is introduced through the mucous membrane into the center of the mass of varicose veins (Fig. 2-6). No antiseptic is necessary. Care must be taken to avoid bringing the point of the needle into contact with the sensitive margin of the pectinate line. Because of the remote possibility that the needle might enter the lumen of a vein and that the solution might be injected into the circulation, the injection should be preceded by partial withdrawal of the plunger of the syringe to see if blood appears. Unlike sclerotherapy for varicose veins, intraluminal injection must be avoided.

After the needle is in position, a solution of quinine and urea hydrochloride, 0.5 ml, is slowly injected submucosally into each pile site. No more than 3 ml should be used for each treatment. All sites should be treated initially.

If bleeding is not controlled by one complete injection treatment, alternative therapeutic approaches should be considered.

Complications

Sloughing

If sloughing follows the injection of a solution of quinine and urea hydrochloride, one or more of three errors are usually responsible; the injection was too superficial, too much solution was injected into one area, or a second injection was made into a hemorrhoid too soon after the first injection.

Thrombosis

Thrombosed hemorrhoids (internal or external, or both) are sometimes associated with sclerotherapy. With sloughing and thrombosis, treatment is conservative: sitz baths, analgesics, and topical anal creams.

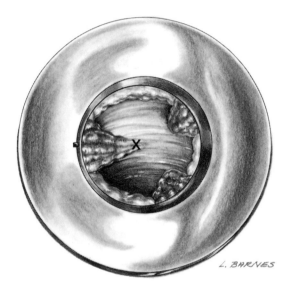

FIG. 2-4. Hemorrhoids in commonly seen locations in the anal canal as viewed through the anoscope. The X indicates the planned site for injection of the left lateral pile (in an insensitive area of the anal canal).

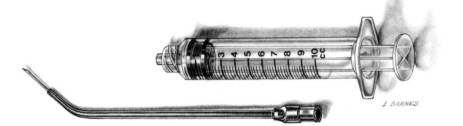

FIG. 2-5. Syringe and angled hemorrhoid needle. An angled needle permits better visualization than a straight needle.

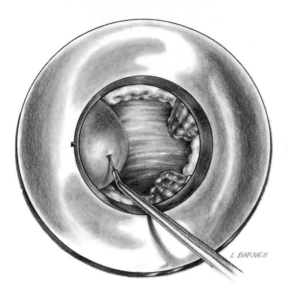

L. BARNES

FIG. 2-6.   Sclerotherapy. If a wheal is not produced, the injection is too deep, and the needle should be withdrawn. An injection that is too superficial will produce necrosis of the lining of the anal canal.

Burning

Burning in the anal canal is a late sequela of repeated sclerotherapy. I do not recommend repeated injections primarily for this reason.

Abscess and Paraffinoma

Submucous abscess and paraffinoma (oleogranuloma) can also occur, the latter after use of oil-based sclerosing agents.[26, 62]

Bacteremia

Bacteremia has been reported in 8% of patients following sclerotherapy.[2] Although none of the patients developed septicemia, antibiotic prophylaxis is probably a wise course for patients at an increased risk (*e.g.*, a patient with a prosthetic heart valve).

Results

Few reports of sclerotherapy have been published in the recent American and British literature. Dencker and associates reported on the comparative results obtained from three forms of treatment of internal hemorrhoids—ligation, operation according to Milligan, and injection—and concluded that the results obtained with

injection were poor.[21] Only 21% of patients were well at the review. Because other methods gave Dencker and co-workers much better results, they did not think that injection treatment should be used routinely for internal hemorrhoids.

Alexander-Williams and Crapp, in a report on conservative management of hemorrhoids, stated that they had used sclerotherapy extensively in the past and as part of clinical comparative trials, and found that it gave satisfactory short-term results, particularly in the treatment of patients with first-degree hemorrhoids.[3] I believe sclerotherapy should be limited to this group of patients.

Rubber-Ring Ligation

In 1954, Blaisdell described an instrument for ligation of internal hemorrhoids as an outpatient procedure.[12] In 1962, Barron modified this instrument and presented two series reporting excellent results.[8, 9] I am so satisfied with the ligation technique that it has replaced hemorrhoidectomy for approximately 80% of my patients.[17]

Any patient who has hemorrhoids manifested by bleeding or prolapse, or both, is a candidate for this procedure. The rubber rings must be placed on an insensitive area, usually at or just above the anorectal ring. If a patient has skin tags or hypertrophied anal papillae, these cannot be treated by ligation because of the pain that would result.

After a small cleansing enema has been given, complete proctosigmoidoscopy and anoscopy are performed. If the patient's history is suggestive of colonic disease, barium enema examination is completed before any treatment of the hemorrhoids is undertaken. The nature of the disease and the technique to be used are explained to the patient. Several treatments, spaced over 3-week to 4-week intervals, may be required, depending on how many pile sites must be eliminated to alleviate the symptoms. A moderate sense of discomfort or fullness in the rectum can be anticipated for a few days, but this discomfort is usually minimal and can be relieved by taking sitz baths and mild analgesics.

Technique

Figure 2-7 shows the McGivney ligator; I prefer this instrument to the Barron. It has a much more secure shaft, which may be rotated in a 360° arc to facilitate placement. A more recent modification is the suction hemorrhoidal ligator (Scanlan, Fig. 2-8). This latter instrument permits incorporation of the hemorrhoid without the need for a grasping forceps. It also seems

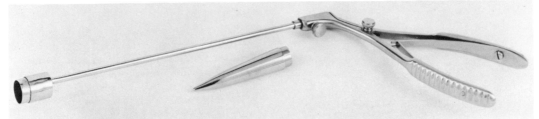

FIG. 2-7. McGivney ligator. (Courtesy of Miltex Instrument Co.)

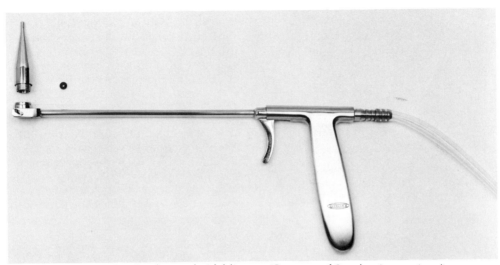

FIG. 2-8. Suction hemorrhoidal ligator. (Courtesy of Scanlan International).

to cause less discomfort to the patient, but this is perhaps because the drum incorporates a smaller volume of tissue; this is its one disadvantage.

Figure 2-9 demonstrates an anoscope in place through which the ligator and alligator forceps have been inserted. The most prominent hemorrhoid is treated first. It is grasped with the forceps (Fig. 2-10, *A*) and pulled up through the drum of the ligator (Fig. 2-10, *B*). If the patient experiences pain, a slightly more proximal point is selected, and this step is repeated. The tissue is drawn into the drum until it is taut, and the trigger is released, expelling two rubber rings (Fig. 2-10, *C*). Two rings are employed in case one breaks. When the rings are in place, the anoscope is withdrawn (Fig. 2-10, *D*). As mentioned, if one uses the suction ligator, no grasping instrument is required.

The patient rarely experiences pain necessitating removal of the rings, but this can be accomplished by interposing the end of a conventional disposable suture-removal scissors. Other methods for removing the rings tend to precipitate bleeding.

Post-Treatment Care

Stools should be kept relatively soft by diet, if this will suffice, or with the aid of a mild laxative. Some bleeding may occur when the rubber rings are dislodged. The patient is requested to return in 3 to 4 weeks for re-evaluation and further treatment. More than one hemorrhoidal site can be treated during an office visit, the number depending on the patient's tolerance.

One of the major advantages of rubber-ring ligation is the factor of timing. The patient need not return at fixed intervals for further ligation. Nothing is really lost if the patient chooses to return 3 months, 6 months, or even 1 year later. Other areas subsequently can be treated equally well despite such delays. However, the patient should realize that if symptoms are not completely relieved, it is probably because other areas need to be treated. If the patient experiences complete relief after the initial ligation, there is no reason for continuing therapy. Under these circumstances the patient is advised to return if and when symptoms recur.

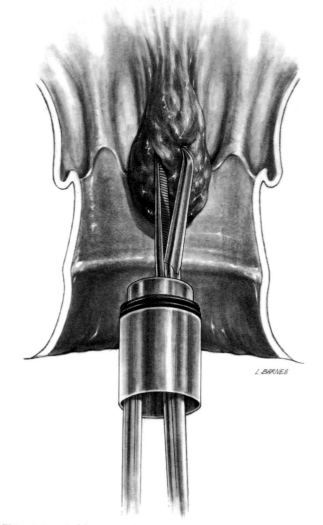

L.BARNES

FIG. 2-9. Rubber ring ligation. An alligator forceps is about to grasp the hemorrhoid. The forceps passes through the drum of the ligator.

Complications

Complications after rubber-ring ligation are occasionally seen and include delayed hemorrhage, severe pain, external hemorrhoidal thrombosis, ulceration, and slippage of the ligature.

Delayed Hemorrhage

Late hemorrhage (1 to 2 weeks) after rubber-ring ligation occurs in approximately 1% of patients. As in late hemorrhage after surgical hemorrhoidectomy, the reason is probably sepsis in the pedicle. This can be a major bleeding problem requiring hospitalization, suture ligation, and transfusion.

Pain

Pain requiring removal of the ring and measures to alleviate discomfort have been mentioned earlier. Tchirkow and associates recommend injection of a local anesthetic solution into the hemorrhoid bundle.[70] In my experience, however, most patients who complain of pain develop this symptom long after the anesthetic effect would have dissipated.

Thrombosis

With ligation of internal hemorrhoids, the risk of subsequent thrombosis of corresponding external hemorrhoids is 2 to 3%. If thrombosis occurs, sitz baths and stool softeners are recommended. Occasionally, excision of the thrombosed hemorrhoid is required.

Ulceration

Anal ulceration is a normal consequence of ligation. The rubber rings cause necrosis of tissue; they fall off in 2 to 5 days, leaving an ulcerated area. This is the principle that makes this treatment effective. On rare occasions a large ulcer, sometimes associated with a fissure, may be a troublesome complication.

Slippage

The rubber rings can slip or break at any time, but this usually happens after the first or second bowel movement. Breakage may be caused by a defective rubber band (hence, the use of two), but more commonly is caused by tension from a large bulk of tissue that has been ligated. The use of a mild laxative can help to prevent passage of hard stools, and thus one can avoid this problem.

Error in Diagnosis

The greatest disadvantage of rubber-ring ligation is that no pathologic specimen is obtained. Invasive epidermoid carcinoma or other tumor occasionally has been reported in the hemorrhoidal specimen, and in rare instances such a tumor will be missed. However, one should not condemn the procedure because of this concern.

Results

In 1977 Bartizal and Slosberg published a retrospective review of records of 670 patients who underwent 3208 rubber-band ligations for internal hemorrhoids.[10] The extent of post-banding discomfort and the presence and degree of rectal bleeding were assessed. All patients were followed for a minimum of 1 month after the completion of banding.

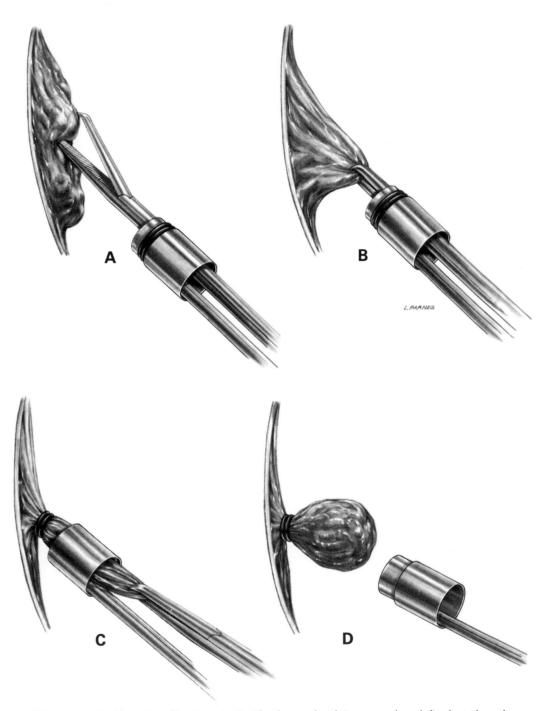

FIG. 2-10. Rubber ring ligation. **A, B.** The hemorrhoid is grasped and firmly tethered. **C, D.** The tissue is drawn into the drum, and two rubber rings are released. If the patient tolerates the maneuver, ligation can be performed with minimal or no discomfort.

Complications were confined to pain and bleeding. Only 21 patients (4%) had any pain. Mild pain was defined as pain that was reported but required no treatment, moderate pain required analgesics, and severe pain caused limitation of activities. No bleeding at all was reported by 642 (96%) of the patients. Bleeding to a slight degree was noted by 19 (3%) of the patients but required no treatment. Bleeding to a significant degree occurred in 9 patients (1%). Most were treated successfully with bed rest, but two required hospitalization. When those patients having moderate and severe pain were combined with those having severe bleeding only 13 (2% of all patients treated) had complications severe enough to interfere with daily activity.

Steinberg and co-workers by means of a questionnaire answered by 125 of 147 patients, conducted a long-term assessment (mean, 4.8 years) of the value of rubber-band ligation treatment for hemorrhoids.[68] The great majority (89%) of patients considered themselves cured or greatly improved by the treatment. However, only 44% were completely free of symptoms. Intermittent mild discomfort, occasional spotting of blood, and an awareness of lumps at the anus were the principal residual symptoms. Nevertheless, many patients were reportedly happier with this situation than with their state before treatment. Patients who suffered persistent or severe recurrent symptoms after rubber-band ligation were treated by further conservative measures. Fifteen patients (12%) had another rubber-band ligation, anal dilation, or lateral sphincterotomy.

Wrobleski, Veidenheimer, Coller, and I reported our long-term results of rubber-ring ligation.[83] Of 352 patients who were sent a questionnaire, 266 (76%) responded. Follow-up was for a mean of 60 months. Eight percent of the responders were improved by the procedure, although many continued to have some symptoms. The best results were obtained in patients who had Grade I hemorrhoids. Patients with Grade IV hemorrhoids were less likely to have had a good result (P<0.02).

The effectiveness of treatment did not depend on the number of hemorrhoids ligated. Patients who had a single pile treated were as likely to have had a good result as those in whom two or more bands were applied.

The Cleveland Clinic group reported 77% of their patients were asymptomatic following treatment.[29] Their technique differed in that approximately 90% were treated by multiple ligations in a single session. Although the long-term results indicate fewer symptoms, pain after treatment was more frequently observed and was more severe.

Lau and associates performed rubber-ring ligation on all three primary hemorrhoids at a single out-patient session.[42] Good to excellent results were noted in 91%, but moderate to severe pain was reported by 58 patients (29%). Although Lau and co-workers strongly endorsed this approach, their complication rate (hemorrhage, urinary retention, anal stenosis) was 3.5%.

Perhaps the most meaningful conclusion of our study was that a single treatment could achieve satisfactory results.[83] If more than three sessions are required to control symptoms, the procedure should probably be abandoned and hemorrhoidectomy performed.

Comment

Rubber-ring ligation is a reasonable alternative to surgical hemorrhoidectomy for most patients. But the patient must understand that the result may not equal that which can be achieved by surgery. Nevertheless, because of its decreased morbidity, adequate long-term effectiveness, convenience, and patient acceptability, I recommend this procedure as the primary outpatient therapy for hemorrhoidal complaints. However, in the presence of an external component, hypertrophied papilla, or associated fissure, surgical treatment is the most effective.

Cryosurgery

Cryosurgery is based on the concept of cellular destruction through rapid freezing followed by rapid thawing. The treatment of hemorrhoids by this technique has been advocated by Lewis, Williams and co-workers, and others as being painless, effective, and especially recommended for those patients who are medically unable to undergo general anesthesia.[15, 30, 45, 77, 79]

The tissue freezes around the tip of the cryoprobe. Thus, the distance between the tip and the outer border of the ice ball equals the depth of the ice ball. This allows the surgeon to determine visually how much tissue is being destroyed. Only that tissue encompassed within the ice ball will undergo irreversible cellular destruction. Changes at the boundary between the ice ball and normal tissue are reversible, and no true cellular destruction occurs. The principle of cryodestruction is well described in the articles cited above.

Technique

The following protocol is recommended by most authors:

The procedure is explained, and the patient is advised of the probability of profuse drainage and considerable swelling. If necessary, the patient is given an intravenous injection of 5 to 10 mg of diazepam (Valium). An injection of a local anesthetic is usually recommended, although the patient may experience more pain from the injection than from direct application of the cryoprobe to the external hemorrhoidal area.

The patient is placed in the left lateral or jackknife position. The fingers, a plastic vaginal speculum, or a modified plastic proctoscope are used to isolate one primary hemorrhoidal plexus at a time. Metal instruments are not used, as they would conduct cold. A water-soluble jelly is used to achieve good contact between the cryoprobe and the hemorrhoid. Both internal and external hemorrhoids can be treated in one operation. The tip of the cryoprobe is placed in the center of either the internal or the external hemorrhoidal plexus and remains there until the tissue to be destroyed is enveloped by the ice ball (Fig. 2-11). The period of freezing varies according to the cooling power of the probe. With a liquid nitrogen probe at $-196°C$ or a liquid nitrous oxide probe at $-89°C$, the application time is about 2 minutes per hemorrhoidal area. The greater the vascularity of the hemorrhoid, the greater the cooling power required to freeze it. Therefore, the liquid nitrogen probe is more effective for large hemorrhoids than the nitrous oxide probe. When an adequate amount of tissue has been frozen, the probe is switched off, rewarmed, and detached from the hemorrhoid; each plexus in turn is treated the same way.

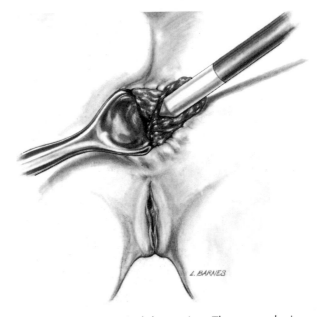

FIG. 2-11. Cryosurgical destruction. The cryoprobe is applied to a combined internal–external hemorrhoid.

Post-Treatment Care

Considerable swelling and edema occur within 24 hours but do not interfere with normal bowel function and elimination. Drainage, usually starting within several hours after the procedure, is fairly heavy for the first 3 to 4 days, but tapers off during the next 2 to 3 weeks. Patients are instructed to use some form of sterile pad and to change the pad several times a day during the first 3 to 4 days.

Two to three hours after freezing, the tissue becomes swollen and red. Within 72 hours pale spots appear on the surface, and these coalesce to form irregular patches by the fourth day. By the fifth or sixth day the whole hemorrhoidal area is pale, and black, gangrenous areas appear. Gangrene is usually complete between 7 and 9 days postoperatively. Thereafter, the hemorrhoid begins to disintegrate and comes away completely by the eighteenth day, leaving a normal-appearing anus.

Results

Wilson and Schofield reported 100 consecutive cases of hemorrhoids treated by cryosurgery.[80] All patients were treated as outpatients, usually without anesthesia, and the nitrous oxide cryoprobe was used.

Watery discharge has been said to occur in all patients, but in this study many patients did not notice the discharge at all, and only one complained that the discharge was a nuisance. Four patients experienced

immediate pain during the freezing process, and three needed a general anesthetic. An additional six patients underwent elective general anesthesia. Only one patient complained of pain during the first 5 days after treatment, and many patients returned to work the day after treatment. No major hemorrhage was encountered, although the watery discharge was sanguineous in some patients. The patients were assessed at 6 weeks and 3 months. Satisfactory results were obtained in 94%.

Savin reported on 444 operations performed with the nitrous oxide probe.[65] Excellent results were obtained in eliminating all hemorrhoids and symptoms in 431 of 434 patients. Ten patients were lost to follow-up study, and three patients had some residual hemorrhoidal tissue. Cryodestruction was successful in removing 97% of the concomitant pathologic conditions treated, such as anal fissure, anal fistula, hypertrophied anal papillae, condylomata acuminata, and mucosal prolapse. Of 155 patients evaluated 1 to 2 years after operation, 151 were graded as having excellent results, 3 had small asymptomatic internal varices, 1 had an external hemorrhoid, 3 were found to have hypertrophied anal papillae not present before, and 2 patients still had persistent hypertrophied anal papillae.

O'Connor reported results of nitrous oxide cryohemorrhoidectomy in 117 patients.[55] Skin tags larger than those the patients had before the procedure were found in four patients. Five had persistence of internal hemorrhoids. Three of the five patients complained of bleeding with bowel movements, and subsequently were treated by ligation. The major complications after cryosurgery were pain, bleeding, and fecal impaction. Six patients complained of pain lasting longer than 2 days, and two of these patients experienced pain for as long as 14 days. Bleeding necessitating hospitalization occurred in three patients. Fecal impaction also occurred in three patients. No urinary retention, ulceration, stenosis, or incontinence was reported. The average time lost from work was 2 days, with a range of 0 to 14 days. O'Connor concluded that internal hemorrhoids were easily treated by cryosurgery, and that thrombosed and edematous hemorrhoids should be treated by methods other than cryosurgery. He further advised that thick skin tags and large prolapsing hemorrhoids should be treated by excisional surgery.

Oh initially reviewed 100 patients who had undergone cryohemorrhoidectomy and subsequently reported on 1000.[56, 57] In his initial report, two thirds experienced pain, two suffered massive hemorrhage, and five encountered urinary difficulties. The effectiveness of 90% for cryotherapy noted by Oh[57] is similar to that for rubber-ring ligation, but the discomfort, prolonged drainage, and prolonged recovery were believed to be distinct disadvantages when compared with ligation. MacLeod, in his report on 528 patients treated by cryotherapy, recommended that this modality be used only on internal hemorrhoids and that the treatments be staged.[49]

Smith and co-workers reported a study in which closed hemorrhoidectomy and cryotherapy were performed on each of 26 patients.[67] One side of the anus was designated at random for surgery and the other for cryotherapy. Although pain was initially less after cryosurgery (only one patient reported severe pain on the cryotherapy side), 12 patients had pain for more than 2 weeks on the cryotherapy side, as compared with only three patients who experienced pain after 2 weeks on the surgical side. Interestingly, patients could determine which side was surgically treated and which side was "frozen." Of 24 patients examined 1 year after treatment, 13 had residual hemorrhoids (12 were at the cryosurgical site), six of whom requested further treatment. When preference was ascertained 1 year after treatment, 65% of patients said they preferred operative hemorrhoidectomy and 35% said they preferred cryodestruction.

Comment

When cryosurgical hemorrhoidectomy was first introduced, it was claimed to be painless, not requiring an anesthetic, and effective for external tags and hypertro-

phied papillae. Since that time more recent reports have affirmed that it is neither painless (local anesthetic is suggested by almost all observers) and that it is less effective, and in many ways ineffective, for treatment of hypertrophied anal papillae and skin tags. For internal hemorrhoids, rubber-ring ligation is superior to cryosurgery. It is quicker and cheaper, and requires no anesthetic. For the external component or hypertrophied papilla, excision after local infiltration rapidly removes the offending tissue, with complete healing in 7 to 10 days. Cryosurgical destruction requires the use of expensive equipment, is time-consuming to perform (some authors recommend hospitalization or an outpatient setting), and results in profuse drainage with delayed healing for many weeks. True, the initial postanesthetic pain may be somewhat less than with surgical hemorrhoidectomy, but this usually can be controlled with a mild analgesic.

In my opinion, cryosurgery adds nothing to the treatment of hemorrhoids that is not available by other means at lower cost, at greater efficiency, and with as good if not better results.

Infrared Coagulation

Recently, Neiger described a technique for the treatment of hemorrhoids using infrared coagulation.[53] Leicester and associates reported a prospective, randomized trial using this technique, and compared it with injection sclerotherapy or rubber-ring ligation.[44]

The apparatus, a German-made instrument, produces infrared radiation and is focused by a photoconductor. A 1-second pulse is used in the treatment of hemorrhoids, with the probe applied at the site where one would normally inject. The radiation causes protein coagulation 3 mm wide and 3 mm deep. The authors found the treatment to be more effective than sclerotherapy for nonprolapsing hemorrhoids; it offered no improvement, however, over rubber-ring ligation in hemorrhoids that prolapse.

I have had no experience with this new modality.

Lord's Dilatation

The three primary ambulatory methods of treatment of hemorrhoids—sclerotherapy, rubber-ring ligation, and cryosurgical destruction—have been discussed. Another procedure, dilatation, should be included in this category.

In 1968, Lord reported a method he had devised for the treatment of hemorrhoids.[46] He based his treatment on the hypothesis that increased anal canal pressure contributes to the hemorrhoid problem, and that dilatation reduces this pressure, thereby ameliorating the condition. Although this approach requires a general (or spinal) anesthetic, hospitalization can often be limited to a 1-day stay with discharge from an ambulatory care facility or similar surgicenter.

Technique

Lord states, "The procedure takes a little less time to perform than to describe."[47] The instruments are not sterile. The patient is placed on the left side and given an intravenous anesthetic. The constriction to the outlet, which Lord believes is present in all patients with third-degree hemorrhoids, is identified.

Two fingers of one hand are pulled upward, and the index finger of the other hand presses downward to feel the constriction. The aim is to dilate the lower part of the rectum and anal canal gently and firmly until no constrictions remain. It is an "ironing out" process that is carried out by a circular movement through all four quadrants. Tearing should be avoided. During the procedure, eight fingers are inserted as high as they will reach. Not all patients can be dilated safely to this extent, and Lord cautions that it is much better to do too little than to do too much.

As dilation is achieved, an assistant inserts a sponge, usually by means of a ring forceps. The sponge presses on the walls of the lower part of the rectum and anal canal to reduce postoperative hematoma formation. The sponge is left in place for 1 hour, and the patient is discharged when alert.

Postoperative Care

The patient is instructed on the insertion of a dilating cone (Fig. 2-12), which can be used as required for anal symptoms, but even Lord wonders whether it is vital to the success of the method. Vellacott and Hardcastle randomly allocated one group of patients to a bulk laxative, and the other group to a bulk laxative with a dilator.[74] Since there was no difference in results, they concluded that an anal dilator was not necessary. However, Greca and co-workers reported the opposite to be true.[33] Under normal circumstances the patient should take 2 or 3 days from work and is seen after 2 weeks, at which time, if free of symptoms, the patient is discharged.

Results

Lord claims less pain and less postoperative morbidity after dilatation than after hemorrhoidectomy. He states that his method does not cause urinary retention, deep vein thrombosis, postoperative bleeding, or fecal im-

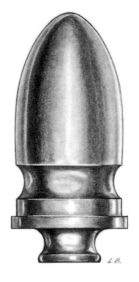

FIG. 2-12. Lord's dilator.

paction. The patients are free of pain during defecation, operating room time is saved, and the hospital stay is greatly shortened. In Lord's opinion, rubber-ring ligation is the treatment of choice for most hemorrhoid problems, and dilatation should be used as an alternative to hemorrhoidectomy. He suggests that hemorrhoidectomy should be considered when hypertrophied papillae and external tags are present.

Creve and Hubens noted the effect of the procedure on anal pressure.[18] They found a significant lowering following dilatation as compared with conventional hemorrhoidectomy.

A 5-year follow-up study of 100 patients who had Lord's dilatation for hemorrhoids was reported by Walls and Ruckley.[75] Hemorrhoids were first degree in 15, second degree in 48, and third degree in 37. Seventy-five patients were free of symptoms or greatly improved, but the treatment was unsuccessful in 22 patients, all except one of whom reported failure within 3 months. Nineteen of these patients were subsequently treated by hemorrhoidectomy.

A prospective study was carried out by McCaffrey on 50 patients with hemorrhoids treated by the Lord method; they were followed for at least 4 years.[50] Of 36 patients who were free of symptoms, 19 still had evidence of anal congestion but no distinct hemorrhoids, and 4 patients subsequently underwent a standard hemorrhoid operation for persistent prolapse and bleeding.

The complication that disturbs most surgeons is the possibility of causing incontinence by sphincter dilatation. Twenty (40%) of McCaffrey's patients had mild incontinence from 4 to 26 days after operation. The incontinence was for flatus and mucus, with relative control for feces.

Keighley and associates, in a prospective trial, compared dilatation, sphincterotomy, and a high-fiber diet in patients classified into two groups: those with a low and those with an elevated maximum resting anal pressure.[38] They concluded that since the Lord procedure significantly lowered the pressure, it was the treatment of choice in patients with preoperative elevation.

Comment

I do not employ the Lord dilatation for the treatment of hemorrhoids. Failure to deal with tags and papillae, and the risk of incontinence, especially in patients more than 60 years of age, preclude use of this technique in my opinion. However, if hospital time and cost savings are criteria, this method might be considered as an alternative to excisional surgery.

TREATMENT OF THROMBOSED HEMORRHOIDS

External

The patient with thrombosed external hemorrhoids usually presents with a painful, tender mass. If the problem has been present for more than 2 or 3 days, the discomfort usually has begun to improve. Under these circumstances, medical management should be considered. This consists of appropriate counseling (*e.g.,* removing the library from the toilet), sitz baths, and stool softeners. A mild analgesic may be recommended. With this regimen the mass will usually resolve in a week or 10 days.

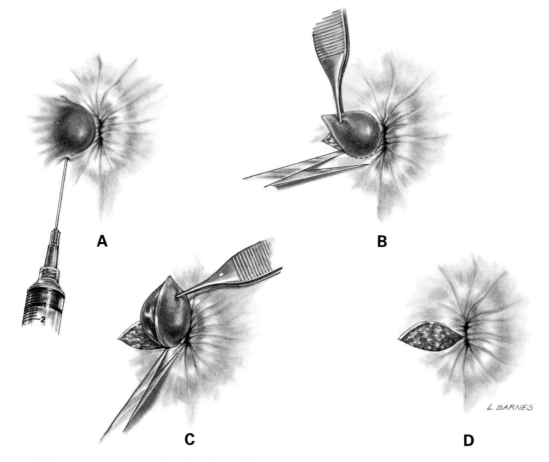

FIG. 2-13. Excision of a thrombosed hemorrhoid. **A.** The area is infiltrated with 0.5% bupivacaine in 1:200,000 epinephrine. **B, C.** The thrombosed hemorrhoid is excised along with a wedge of skin. **D.** Skin edges are sufficiently separate to permit adequate drainage, thereby preventing reaccumulation of a clot.

The patient may report that the lump appeared following a bout of constipation or diarrhea. If one or the other is a frequent occurrence, treatment of this needs to be discussed. If the area involved corresponds to the location where the patient reports a tendency for prolapse, rubber-ring ligation should be considered after the thrombosis resolves.

If ulceration or rupture has occurred, or if the patient is seen within 48 hours, it is usually advisable to excise the lesion. The hemorrhoid should be *excised*, not *incised*. Making a small incision and shelling the clot out like a pea from a pod all too often results in recurrent hemorrhage into the subcutaneous tissue and clot reaccumulation. Figure 2-13 demonstrates the proper technique for performing this procedure. The area is infiltrated with a solution of 0.5% bupivacaine (Marcaine) in 1:200,000 epinephrine. The underlying hemorrhoid is excised, as is a wedge of skin. Bleeding is controlled with pressure, topically applied epinephrine, or electrocautery. A pressure dressing is used.

The patient is instructed to keep the pressure dressing on if possible for 12 hours or until the morning after treatment. While sitting in the bath, the patient can remove the dressing without causing rebleeding, but if this occurs it can usually be controlled by the application of pressure on the wound with a cold cloth or compress. A small dressing can be used to avoid soiling. Daily sitz baths are recommended until the wound heals (7 to 10 days). A mild analgesic and a topical anesthetic cream may be of benefit.

Internal

In addition to the causes of thrombosed external hemorrhoids previously mentioned, thrombosed internal hemorrhoids may be due to prolapse with inadequate reduction. As a result, stasis develops within the vein and thrombosis occurs.

The treatment of thrombosed internal hemorrhoids is not as satisfactory as that for external hemorrhoids. Fortunately, however, pain is not as frequently observed. Excision of a thrombosed internal hemorrhoid requires instrumentation and a more extensive local infiltration. Suture is necessary for hemostasis, since the application of direct pressure is impossible (unless packing is undertaken).

Sitz baths are recommended, as well as a mild systemic analgesic and a topical anesthetic cream or suppository. A stool softener is also advisable. If the patient has extensive hemorrhoids, tags, hypertrophied papillae, or associated anal fissure, an urgent, in-hospital surgical approach is usually advocated.

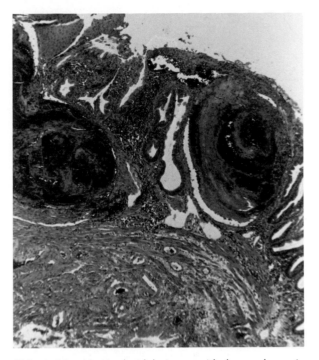

FIG. 2-14. Hemorrhoidal tissue with hemorrhage in a patient who underwent urgent hemorrhoidectomy. Note the dilated veins close to the surface containing recent blood clots. (Original magnification × 180)

TREATMENT OF GANGRENOUS (PROLAPSED, EDEMATOUS) HEMORRHOIDS

The patient who presents with severely disabling gangrenous hemorrhoids requires emergency medical measures and urgent (within 24 hours) surgical hemorrhoidectomy. Pain, swelling, bleeding, foul-smelling discharge, and difficulty with defecation are common presenting complaints. Of prior hemorrhoidal difficulties, prolapse is the most frequent. Proctosigmoidoscopic and anoscopic examination reveals edematous, thrombosed, irreducible hemorrhoids (Figs. 2-3 and 2-14).

In the office, a perianal field block is established using a solution of 40 ml of 0.5% bupivacaine (Marcaine) with 1:200,000 epinephrine, and adding to this two ampules (2 ml) of hyaluronidase (300 NF units of Wydase). A subcutaneous circumanal wheal is infiltrated in the edematous hemorrhoidal tissue (Fig. 2-15). Four deep injections are made in each quadrant to effect paralysis of the sphincter mechanism and total perianal anesthesia. The finger should be inserted into

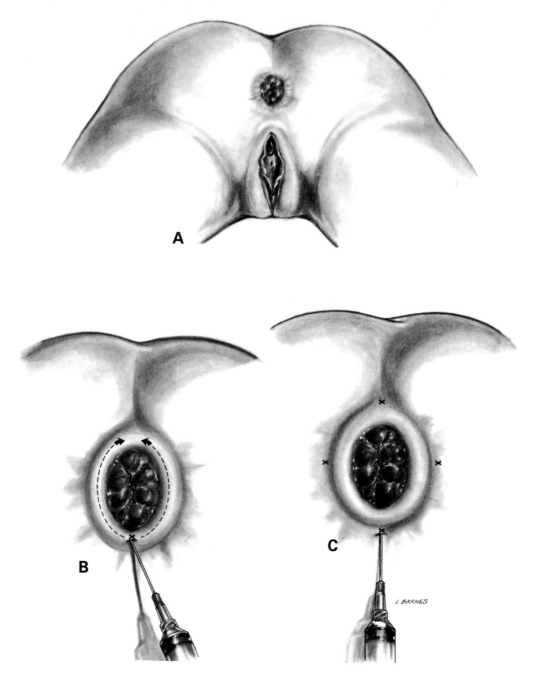

FIG. 2-15. Method of establishing perianal field block. **A.** The patient is placed in prone (jackknife) position. **B.** A subcutaneous perianal wheal is raised. **C.** Deep injections are made at four sites to effect further anesthesia and paralysis of sphincter muscles.

the rectum during introduction of the needle to avoid penetrating the lumen of the bowel. Care should also be taken to avoid entering the vagina, prostate, or urethra anteriorly. When the field block is completed, pressure is applied with a sterile pad as the hemorrhoidal mass is reduced. A pressure dressing is used, and the buttocks are taped.

The patient is admitted to the hospital on an emergency basis, and a hemorrhoidectomy is performed the following day. No enema is administered before the operation. With reduction maintained, the patient is comfortable, and an adequate, safe operation can be performed with less edema than would be present without reduction.

Eisenstat and co-workers used the above field block, and then performed multiple rubber-ring ligations and incised any thrombosis.[23] They reported gratifying results without significant complication.

Results of Emergency Surgery

Ackland reported results of 25 patients with prolapsed and strangulated hemorrhoids who underwent emergency operation.[1] The results were compared with those in a similar group having elective surgery for chronic hemorrhoids. According to this study, operation for prolapsed and strangulated hemorrhoids in the acute stage is safe and effective, comparable to that of elective operation. Secondary hemorrhage, ulceration, pylephlebitis, and stricture are no more common after emergency surgery for prolapsed and strangulated hemorrhoids than after elective operation for chronic hemorrhoids. Anal stenosis developed in one patient. Ackland concluded that emergency operation does not cause more postoperative pain than does elective surgery and that it is safe and effective.

Comment

Because conservative treatment of strangulated hemorrhoids (sitz baths, analgesics, and stool softeners) entails severe discomfort, prolonged disability, and financial hardship, urgent operation is advised for all such patients.

TREATMENT OF HEMORRHOIDS IN INFLAMMATORY BOWEL DISEASE

Jeffery and associates reported a retrospective review of 42 patients with ulcerative colitis and 20 patients with Crohn's disease who were treated for hemorrhoids and inflammatory bowel disease between 1935

and 1975.[37] Both surgical and conservative treatment of hemorrhoids in patients with ulcerative colitis had low complication rates: 4 complications after 50 courses of treatment. In Crohn's disease the complication rate was high: 11 complications after 26 courses of treatment. One of the 42 patients with ulcerative colitis and 6 of the 20 patients with Crohn's disease required rectal excision for complications apparently dating from the treatment of hemorrhoids. These results suggest that treatment of symptomatic hemorrhoids is relatively safe in patients with ulcerative colitis but is contraindicated in those with Crohn's disease.[37]

Comment

Any procedures on the anus or perianal skin in patients with inflammatory bowel disease should be limited to those minimal maneuvers that will effectively treat the patient's complaint. Definitive or extensive surgical treatment of any anorectal problem in such patients could result in delayed healing or nonhealing, with greater disability than before operation. Medical management of hemorrhoids should be practiced under these circumstances. In rare instances, when disease is quiescent and sepsis, fistula formation, and scarring are not present, hemorrhoids of severe degree might be treated by rubber-ring ligation.

SURGICAL HEMORRHOIDECTOMY

Surgical hemorrhoidectomy should be considered when the anorectal architecture has been severely and irreversibly compromised (in the presence of an external component, ulceration, thombosis, hypertrophied papillae, or associated fissure) and when the patient is not a candidate for outpatient hemorrhoidectomy. The goal of operation, which requires a hospital stay of 3 to 6 days, is complete excision of all hemorrhoidal tissue.

A hemorrhoidectomy should be planned at the operating table and should proceed according to the dictates of the individual case. Inserting a dry sponge into the rectum and withdrawing it is an excellent way to demonstrate hemorroidal tissue, tags, papillae, and the extent of redundant mucosa. Not every patient will have hemorrhoids in the three-quadrant distribution previously mentioned, but the surgeon should be prepared to excise all hemorrhoidal tissue and redundant mucosa. Whenever possible, a bridge of intact skin and mucosa should be left between excised hemorrhoidal sites to avoid subsequent stricture formation. This is particularly important when operating for acute, edematous, or gangrenous hemorrhoids.

Technique

Numerous approaches have been used for the surgical removal of hemorrhoids. Some eponymous operations include those of Buie, Fansler, Ferguson, Milligan-Morgan, Parks, Salmon, and Whitehead, to name a few.[13, 24, 25, 51, 59, 63, 78] The procedure that I favor is a modification of the Ferguson or closed hemorrhoidectomy.

Preoperative Preparation

The most important preoperative measure is a small enema (Fleets) the morning of operation. Vigorous mechanical cleansing by means of laxatives is counterproductive. The patient should be able to defecate as soon as possible after the operation, yet without the stool encumbering the surgeon during the procedure.

No antibiotics are indicated. Minimal intravenous fluids should be administered before induction of anesthesia, and the patient should be encouraged to void before entering the operating room.

Closed (Ferguson) Hemorrhoidectomy

The patient is placed in the prone (jackknife) position with the buttocks taped apart (Fig. 2-16). Having the patient in the lithotomy position is awkward for the assistant, since considerable suturing is required. Although the lateral decubitus position is recommended by the Ferguson group to avoid the need for spinal anesthesia or endotracheal intubation, this position is also awkward for the assistant.

The anus is infiltrated with a solution of approximately 15 ml of 0.5% bupivacaine in 1:200,000 epinephrine (Fig. 2-17). This low dose usually does not affect the pulse or blood pressure. The infiltration technique keeps bleeding to a minimum, and the anatomic plane between the hemorrhoidal mass and the underlying sphincter muscle is clearly delineated.

A Hill-Ferguson retractor placed in the anal canal reveals the extent of the hemorrhoids. For a right-handed surgeon, it is usually best to deal with the more difficult pile first, the one in the right posterior quadrant. Some surgeons prefer to place an anchoring suture in the rectum corresponding to the site of the hemorrhoid, but only a clamp need be placed, incorporating the skin tag and hemorrhoid to be excised (Fig. 2-18). The hemorrhoid is outlined with a scalpel and the incision is carried well outside the anal margin. The external hemorrhoidal plexus is removed by sharp dissection and the external sphincter muscle exposed (Fig. 2-19). The incision is carried into the anal canal; the internal sphincter muscle is carefully dropped away from the plane of dissection. Bleeding is avoided when

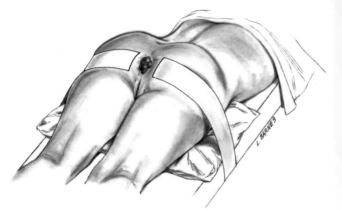

FIG. 2-16. Position of patient for hemorrhoidectomy. Spinal, caudal, or general endotracheal anesthesia is usually employed; the advantages of exposure and the surgeon's comfort outweigh inability to use a mask general anesthetic.

the dissection is outside the hemorrhoid and medial to the internal sphincter. When the entire hemorrhoid pedicle has been mobilized, a suture ligature is placed using a 5/8 circle hemorrhoidal needle with 2-0 or 3-0 chromic catgut. The pedicle is suture-ligated and the hemorrhoid is excised (Fig. 2-20). Any residual small internal or external hemorrhoids should be removed by means of a forceps and fine scissors. Hemostasis can be achieved with an electrocautery.

The wound is closed completely with a continuous suture, using the same suture that was used to ligate the hemorrhoid pedicle (Fig. 2-21). When the mucocutaneous junction is reached, the skin is closed in either a subcuticular fashion or by a continuous simple suture. In like manner, the remaining pile sites are excised, ligated, and primarily closed.

If a fissure is present (usually in the posterior position), an internal anal sphincterotomy is undertaken in the left lateral pile site by dividing the lower third of the internal anal sphincter. I do not employ sphincterotomy routinely, however.

The wounds are cleansed, and povidone-iodine (Betadine) ointment and a small dressing are applied. Minimal pressure is exerted; no packing is used.

Open Hemorrhoidectomy

Modifications of a closed or open hemorrhoidectomy are myriad. In the previous procedure, the wounds were completely closed. When hemorrhoids are gangrenous or thrombosed, or when closure is impossible because of narrowing of the anal lumen, an open procedure may be indicated.

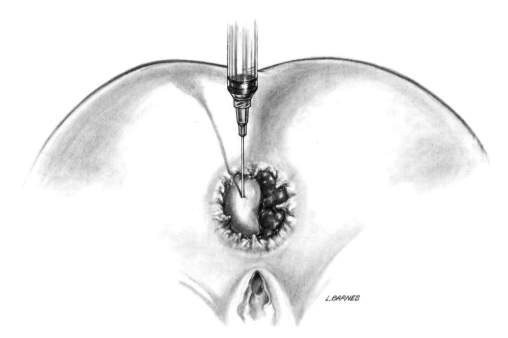

FIG. 2-17. Infiltration of the anus with a local anesthetic of bupivacaine in epinephrine, for hemorrhoidectomy.

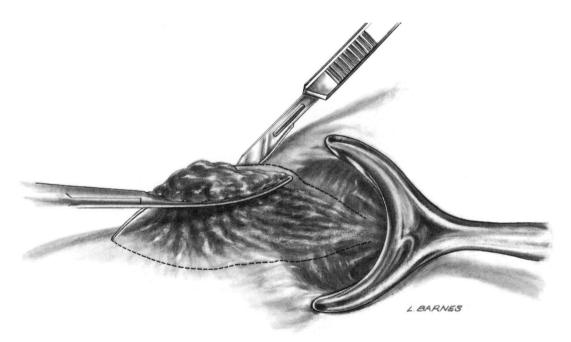

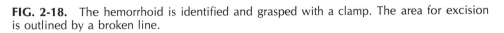

FIG. 2-18. The hemorrhoid is identified and grasped with a clamp. The area for excision is outlined by a broken line.

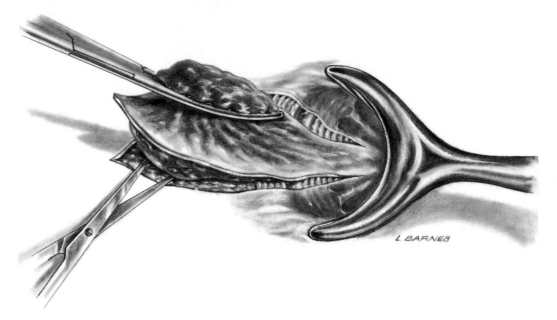

FIG. 2-19. After the area for excision is outlined, the hemorrhoidal plexus is removed from the underlying subcutaneous portion of the external sphincter and the internal sphincter.

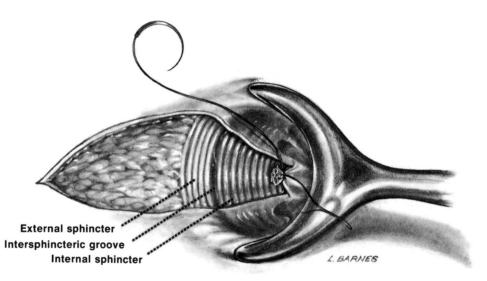

External sphincter
Intersphincteric groove
Internal sphincter

FIG. 2-20. Open wound after excision of the hemorrhoid. No external or internal veins remain.

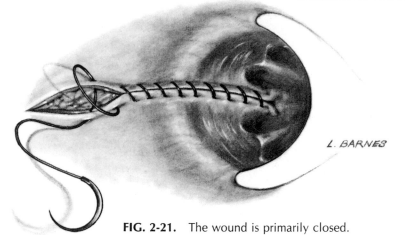

L. BARNES

FIG. 2-21. The wound is primarily closed.

In open hemorrhoidectomy, the procedure is identical to that described for the Ferguson operation, with ligation of the hemorrhoidal pedicle, except that the operation ends at this point (Figs. 2-22 and 2-23). Hemostasis is established with electrocautery. One or two sites may be left open, closed, or partially closed, depending on the individual circumstances. Good results are possible with a combination of techniques.

Submucosal (Parks) Hemorrhoidectomy

In the submucosal hemorrhoidectomy described by Parks, the mucosa of the anal canal and rectum is incised, and the hemorrhoidal tissue beneath is removed.[58] The mucosa is then reapproximated. The purpose of this method is to excise all the hemorrhoidal tissue without injuring the overlying squamous and columnar epithelium. The main potential advantage of this procedure is that the wounds allegedly heal more quickly, with less induration, scarring, and stricture formation.

A self-retaining anal (Parks) retractor is inserted to identify the pathologic condition, and a solution of 0.5% bupivacaine or lidocaine in 1:200,000 epinephrine is injected into the submucosa and the hemorrhoidal mass (Fig. 2-24). The skin incision starts outside the anus and is carried around the forceps holding the anal skin, removing minimal anal canal mucosa (Fig. 2-25). The anal canal is undermined by scissors dissection to expose the hemorrhoidal mass. The mucosa is elevated off the hemorrhoidal vessels (Fig. 2-26). The upper limit of the dissection should be about 4 cm above the mucocutaneous junction.

The external and internal sphincters are identified as the hemorrhoidal mass is elevated and stripped off the internal sphincter to an adequate level (Fig. 2-27). The hemorrhoidal mass is transfixed with a 2-0 chromic catgut suture (Fig. 2-28), and the hemorrhoid is excised. Hemostasis is maintained with an electrocautery. The flaps of the anal canal mucosa are reapproximated with 2-0 chromic catgut; the internal sphincter is incorporated in the sutures to prevent dislodgement (Fig. 2-29). Parks prefers to leave the skin open.

Postoperative Care: General Principles

The dressing is removed the evening after operation, and warm sitz baths are commenced for approximately 20 minutes, three or four times a day. A topical cream, such as Tucks, Balneol, Proctodon, or Americaine, is applied. The cream should be left at the bedside, and the patient instructed in its use. A small dressing (also kept at the bedside), such as a Tucks pad, prevents soiling of sheets and garments.

The patient is discharged if voiding is adequate in amount and if the bowels have moved. Discharge medications include an analgesic, a bulk laxative (and a stool softener or stimulant laxative, if necessary), and cream and pads for the dressing regimen.

The patient is not seen sooner than 3 or 4 weeks after discharge, at which time the wounds are usually healed. A properly performed operation is not likely to result in stricture formation; thus, weekly digital examinations are not necessary.

Complications

Pain

Although not a complication of the operation, pain is probably the single most important reason why patients avoid the procedure. It has been suggested that

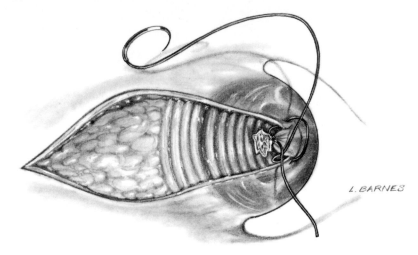

FIG. 2-22.   Open hemorrhoidectomy: technique of burying the hemorrhoidal pedicle.

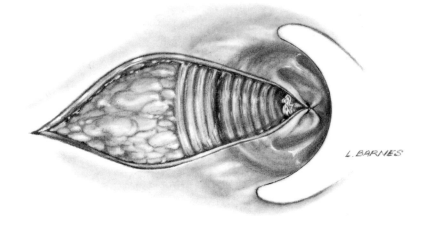

FIG. 2-23.   Completed open hemorrhoidectomy. Partial closure to the mucocutaneous junction is another option.

internal anal sphincterotomy or sphincter stretch ameliorates the problem, but I do not recommend either. They may subsequently be associated with incontinence for flatus and even for feces, particularly in older patients.

The appropriate prevention is narcotic analgesic medication administered in adequate doses and frequently (*e.g.*, Demerol, 75 to 125 mg every 3 hours).

Urinary Retention

Urinary complications after anorectal surgical procedures occur in a high percentage of patients, retention being the commonest complication. Bailey and Ferguson demonstrated the effectiveness of fluid restriction in a carefully controlled, prospective randomized study of 500 patients.[6] One group was given free access to oral fluids after operation; the other group was not permitted coffee or tea, and oral fluids were limited to 250 ml until voiding was spontaneous or until a catheter was inserted. Both groups were treated identically in all respects except for the postoperative fluid intake. Each patient was instructed to empty the bladder before going to the operating room. Anesthesiologists were asked to limit intravenous fluid to the amount they considered a safe minimum. Patients were not routinely catheterized; this was carried out only for bladder distention after examination by a physician.

Only 3.5% of the patients in the group having limited fluids required catheterization, as opposed to 14.9% of the patients in the group with unlimited fluids. No recognized postoperative complication was attributable to fluid restriction. The authors concluded that the postoperative catheterization rate was dramat-

hours thereafter as needed. Patients were told to take only sips of water until they voided. Nurses catheterized the patient only after approval of the physician and were instructed not to urge the patient to void. The morning after operation, the patient sat in a bathtub of hot water and was encouraged to void. Those who did not void immediately in the bath stood under a hot shower.

In the first group 52% of the patients were catheterized, and in the second group no patient was catheterized. Eighty-six percent of the patients voided before they took the hot bath, and the remaining voided in the bath or shower. None of the patients in this group was catheterized, and none complained of bladder fullness.

Factors commonly held responsible for postoperative urinary retention include spinal anesthesia, rectal pain and spasm, high ligation of the hemorrhoidal pedicle, rough handling of tissue, heavy suture material, numerous sutures, fluid overload, rectal packing, tight, bulky dressing, anticholinergics, and narcotics.[19, 40, 54, 64] Despite these possible contributing factors, dehydration

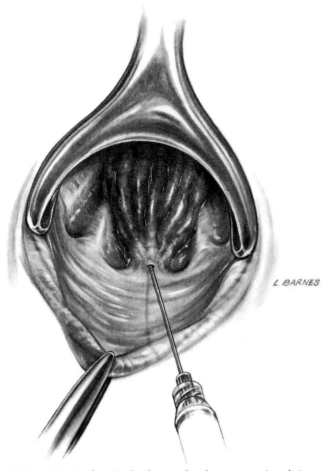

FIG. 2-24. Before Parks' hemorrhoidectomy, epinephrine is injected for hemostasis and clarification of planes of dissection.

ically reduced by restricting fluids and delaying catheterization until the bladder was distended.

Scoma reported a similar study that sought to abolish this common postoperative complication.[66] The charts of 100 patients who underwent hemorrhoidectomy before the study were reviewed. A second group consisted of 100 consecutive hemorrhoidectomies performed by the author using local anesthesia (bupivacaine hydrochloride with epinephrine and hyaluronidase). No patient received atropine or scopolamine. The anesthesiologist was asked to give diazepam (Valium) intravenously with small doses of Pentothal, if necessary, at the beginning of the local infiltration. Amounts of intraoperative fluids were limited at 200 ml, and the infusion was terminated as the dressings were being applied.

Postoperatively, meperidine hydrochloride (Demerol), 100 mg, was given intramuscularly 4 hours after hemorrhoidectomy was completed and every 2

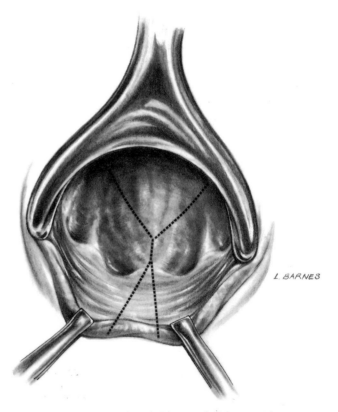

FIG. 2-25. Incision of Parks' hemorrhoidectomy is essentially cruciate. Two limbs of the V-shaped incision meet at the mucocutaneous junction and split again approximately 1 cm above this point.

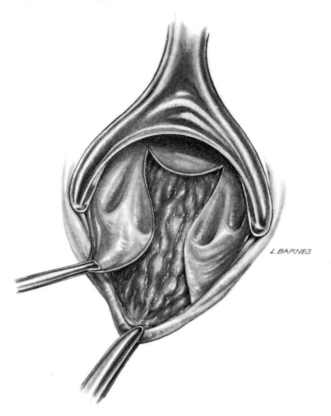

FIG. 2-26. Parks' hemorrhoidectomy. The mucosa is elevated from the underlying hemorrhoidal mass by scissors dissection.

sequelae. Here, again, the value of avoiding urinary retention cannot be overestimated.

Constipation

Patients having proctologic surgical procedures await their postoperative bowel evacuation less than enthusiastically and often view the enema intended to facilitate this function with apprehension. The enema is gladly forfeited by most patients if it can be replaced by some more acceptable method.

Constipation after anorectal surgery must be either relieved effectively or prevented, since, if untreated, it may lead to fecal impaction, a matter of special concern in this group of patients. Yet as long as 72 hours may elapse after operation before a laxative agent is first administered.[54, 73] Factors that contribute to this lag include the effects of analgesic medications administered before or after operation and of anesthesia, local physiologic dysfunction due to surgical manipulation, bed rest, and the patient's fear of painful defecation. A history of irregular bowel function and colonic hypomotility may complicate the problem further.

I evaluated the efficacy of senna (Senokot S) tablets in a prospective fashion on 50 patients who underwent anal operations.[16] Patients took two tablets with a full

of the patient and nursing education to delay catheterization appear to be the primary preventive measures required to reduce the incidence of postoperative urinary retention.

If catheterization is necessary, it should be performed with a balloon catheter. If the residual urine determination is greater than 500 ml, the catheter should be left in place for 24 hours, because it is unlikely that the patient will be able to void subsequently. Conversely, with a residual of less than 500 ml, the catheter can be removed with a reasonable expectation that spontaneous urination will occur.

Urinary Tract Infection

Urinary tract infection is usually a direct consequence of catheterization for urinary retention. The commonest offending organisms are coliform bacteria. Appropriate antibiotics and subsequent catheter removal usually result in rapid resolution, but chronic infection, chronic cystitis, and chronic pyelonephritis can be late

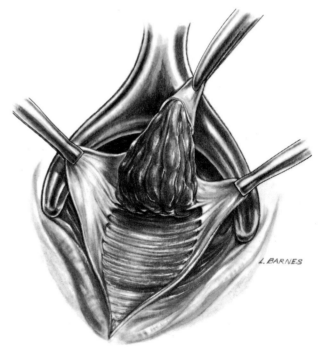

FIG. 2-27. Parks' hemorrhoidectomy. The hemorrhoid mass is elevated from the underlying internal anal sphincter.

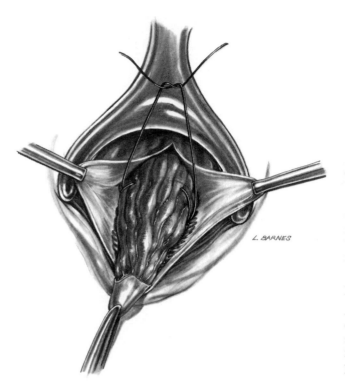

FIG. 2-28. Parks' hemorrhoidectomy: suture ligation of the hemorrhoid.

glass of water on the evening of the first day after operation. If evacuation occurred after this dose and the patient remained in the hospital, two tablets were taken on the following evening. If no bowel movement occurred by the evening of the second day, the dose was changed to two tablets at bedtime and two tablets the following morning. If no stool was passed by the evening of the third day of treatment, the dose at bedtime was increased to three tablets. Enemas or other suitable forms of treatment were administered if function of the bowel was not restored by the evening of the fourth day. One of the options was to increase the dose of the test medication to a maximum of four tablets. No other laxatives or stool modifiers were taken during the trial period. The test preparation was administered for a maximum of 4 days. All patients achieved bowel movements during the study, and none required enemas. None passed hard stools on the day of release from the hospital.

I believe that a stimulant laxative should be given on the evening of the operation and continued in a regimen similar to that described until defecation is achieved. After the fourth postoperative day, with no bowel action, a gentle tap water enema should be administered.

Hemorrhage

Massive hemorrhage that occurs in the recovery room is always the result of technical error. This hemorrhage is caused by inadequate ligation of the hemorrhoidal pedicle. Such a complication requires emergency surgical intervention, but should be quite rare with the Ferguson hemorrhoidectomy, because of the meticulous care taken in closing the wounds.

Delayed hemorrhage (7 to 14 days) is usually a result of sepsis in the pedicle. It occurs in 1% of hemorrhoidectomies. Patients may experience renewed bleeding that may involve clots or massive hemorrhage. Bleeding after 1 week when a patient has previously ceased bleeding warrants examination. Treatment varies from expectant management to in-hospital observation, transfusion, and reoperation. Delayed hemorrhage usually is not a preventable complication.

Infection

Although hemorrhoidectomy is viewed as a minor procedure by both patient and physician, it involves considerable dissection of an area with numerous and varied bacterial flora. Therefore, as Lal and Levitan have pointed out, it would not be surprising if hemorrhoi-

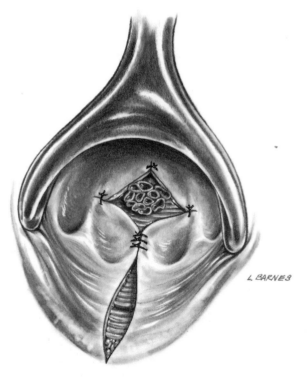

FIG. 2-29. Parks' hemorrhoidectomy. The anal mucosa is partially closed and the skin left open.

dectomy were followed by transient bacteremia and low-grade fever from relatively constant release of bacteria into the bloodstream from a feeding focus.[41] An 8.5% rate of transient bacteremia has been reported for proctoscopic examination of patients with no evidence of lower intestinal disease.[43]

It has been hypothesized that the major venous drainage of the rectum, by passing through the superior hemorrhoidal veins into the portal system, is cleared of organisms by the reticuloendothelial system of the liver.[43] This hepatic clearance, by effectively removing the bacteria released into the circulation, may be important in minimizing the impact of rectal colonic flora in the systemic circulation and may be the reason why infection is not a common complication after hemorrhoidectomy. Furthermore, since sitz baths are a routine part of the postoperative care, most skin problems (cellulitis, abscess) would be treated essentially in a prophylactic manner. In an experience of well over 1000 hemorrhoidectomies, I cannot recall ever having to drain an abscess in the postoperative period.

Anal Tags

The postoperative complication of skin tags is the accumulation of excess skin around the anus. Anal tags, which can interfere with proper cleansing of the anus and thus lead to skin irritation, can usually be avoided by excising redundant skin at the time of operation. Bothersome tags can be removed as an office procedure if symptoms warrant.

Mucosal Prolapse

Inadequate removal of rectal mucosa at the time of hemorrhoidectomy may result in mucosal prolapse. Patients' may complain of a lump that requires manual reduction. Problems with mucus discharge and pruritic symptoms are common.

Treatment usually consists of rubber-ring ligation of the prolapsed mucosa, but careful examination is suggested to look for procidentia.

Prevention of this complication requires that the surgeon remove any redundant mucosa at the time of hemorrhoidectomy.

Ectropion

If redundant mucosa above the site of the excised hemorrhoidal tissue is not properly fixed or excised, the mucosa can heal outside the anus. Ectropion can lead to mucus discharge, skin irritation, and pruritis ani.[9, 32] If the entire anal canal is removed and the cut edge of the rectum is sutured to the perianal skin, the characteristic Whitehead deformity may be produced. Since the mucosa is more mobile than the perianal skin, the

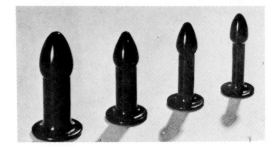

FIG. 2-30. Young Bakelite rectal dilators in a set of four adult sizes. (Courtesy of American V. Mueller)

tendency for mucosal descent is greater than the likelihood for the skin to reline the denuded anal canal. Excising redundant mucosa and suturing it to the underlying internal anal sphincter is the best way to avoid this complication. However, once an ectropion or Whitehead deformity develops, some form of anoplastic procedure is indicated (see Chap. 6).

Anal Stricture

Considerable portions of rectal mucosa and anoderm are removed to cure extensive, encircling hemorrhoids. Also, when multiple hemorrhoids are present, only minimal portions of intact, elastic anal tissue are left. With progressive healing, fibrous scar tissue may proliferate and contract the anorectal outlet.[76] When healing is complete, a narrow, foreshortened stenotic orifice may be left.

As with ectropion, anal stenosis is a preventable complication. If adequate skin bridges are preserved, the risk of reducing the circumference of the anal canal is minimized. However, in the presence of gangrenous hemorrhoids with extensive destruction of the anal canal, chronic fibrosis, chronic fissure, excess tags, and hypertrophied anal papillae, extensive removal of the anal canal is often necessary for an adequate hemorrhoidectomy. Under these circumstances, I recommend that anoplasty be performed at the time of hemorrhoidectomy (see Chap. 6). On the other hand, if because of sepsis, sloughing, or radical surgery (not treated by anoplasty), the potential for stricture formation becomes manifest, daily digital examination of the rectum is advisable while the patient is in the hospital. It is also often useful to advise the patient to insert a dilator twice daily after hospital discharge (Fig. 2-30). This, in my opinion, is the only indication for the use of a dilator. A bulk type of laxative is also prescribed. If the wound has healed without stricture formation, digital examination and the use of a dilator can be discontinued, usually within 6 to 8 weeks. However, if a healed, fixed stricture develops, I prefer to perform an anoplasty rather than to have the patient repeatedly use a dilator.

Fissure or Ulcer

An anal fissure may develop in the patient who has a contracted anorectal outlet after hemorrhoidectomy. Usually the fissure is situated posteriorly. Repeated trauma from defecation results in laceration of the scar, which may become a chronic, painful anal ulcer. Such postoperative fissures rarely respond to conservative management. Excision of the ulcer and associated scar tissue is required. The addition of internal anal sphincterotomy may further enlarge the anal canal lumen, although some form of anoplasty may ultimately be required.

Pseudopolyps

Hemorrhoidectomy usually requires ligation of the stump of the hemorrhoid. Tissue strangulation will take place at the site of ligation, and the stump will slough completely, leaving a defect that heals by granulation. Foreign body granulomas may result from the prolonged presence of suture material[28, 31] and may be manifest as an edematous, polypoid, or sessile tumor at the site of the suture. These can be excised locally or electrocoagulated.

Epidermal Cysts

In rare instances, some months after hemorrhoidectomy, asymptomatic inclusion cysts may appear in the anal canal or in the immediate perianal region. Their origin has been attributed to retention of keratin elements, hair particles, or exfoliated squamous epithelial cells in the wound.[28] If these cysts are bothersome, they should be removed by local excision.

Anal Fistula

Anal fistula is an unusual complication of hemorrhoidectomy. It may be more frequently observed following the closed operation, but the incidence is so low that I doubt whether the choice of operation is actually a factor. The fistula is always low and subcutaneous. Fistulotomy can often be accomplished in the office.

Pruritus Ani

Most causes of pruritus ani are diet related or due to overaggressive anal hygiene (see Chap. 8). However, pruritic symptoms following hemorrhoidectomy may have an anatomic basis. A mucosal ectropion, for example, can produce mucus discharge, which can contribute to the pruritus. With a specific anatomic abnormality, anoplasty may be advisable.

Fecal Incontinence

Fecal soilage or incontinence following hemorrhoidectomy is not as infrequent as one might expect. One possible etiology that has been suggested is the loss of anal canal sensation due to removal of sensory-bearing tissue and replacement by scar. I do not subscribe to such a theory.

Since most patients who have impairment of fecal control following hemorrhoidectomy are elderly, care should be taken when performing this operation in the older age group to avoid unnecessary sphincter stretch or sphincterotomy. Many surgeons are fond of sphincterotomy because they believe it ameliorates the postoperative pain problem. When performed at the posterior pile site, a "keyhole" deformity can result. It is a potentially hazardous maneuver in a patient without a concomitant fissure and should be avoided, especially in a patient over the age of 60.

Recurrence

Some patients have hemorrhoidal veins that become symptomatic within a few years after an assumed complete hemorrhoidectomy. However, varicosities that have been removed cannot recur. The "recurrence" consists of veins that, because of their normal appearance at the time of hemorrhoidectomy, were left undisturbed. With increased venous pressure over the years, dilatation of the venous walls occurs and symptomatic hemorrhoids result.

Because of this problem, all hemorrhoidal veins should be removed at the time of the surgical procedure. Tunneling out minute vessels from the underlying mucosa and debriding all veins over the external sphincter are useful prophylactic maneuvers. Ideally, internal hemorrhoidal veins that subsequently become symptomatic should be treated by an outpatient procedure, usually rubber-ring ligation.

Results

In 1971 Ganchrow and associates published results of a retrospective study of 2038 consecutive hemorrhoidectomies employing the Ferguson technique, together with 5-year follow-up results.[27] Eighty-two patients (4%) had postoperative complications. Forty patients (2%) had minimal bleeding, and 27 patients (1.3%) needed subsequent suture ligation. Two postoperative deaths occurred (0.1%). One patient died at home 10 days after operation following an uneventful course. Postmortem examination was not performed. Another patient died of gram-negative sepsis secondary to a urinary tract infection 37 days after operation.

Between the fifth and seventh postoperative days, 700 patients (34.3%) were discharged from the hospital; 524 patients (26%) were discharged on the eighth postoperative day, and 770 patients (38%) were discharged after the eighth day.

Questionnaires were returned by 1018 persons (50%). Of the responses, 970 patients (95%) answered that they had relief of symptoms, 892 patients (88%) answered that they had satisfactory bowel movements since the operation, 732 (72%) had no rectal complaints whatsoever during the 5 years, and 293 (28%) had some complaints, of which pruritus was the commonest.

Wolf and co-workers sent a questionnaire to members of the American Society of Colon and Rectal Surgeons.[82] There was no statistically significant difference with respect to pain, complications, and length of hospital stay. However, the open technique was felt to have a slightly more rapid healing time and was associated with a lower incidence of stenosis.

Barrios and Khubchandani reported their experience with a modified Whitehead operation.[7] Their modification involved removal of the entire anoderm, but the perianal skin was preserved, and the edges of the anal mucosa sutured to the subcutaneous tissue, not to the skin. Although reporting satisfactory results in 41 patients, they noted a 32% incidence of urinary retention, a 5% incidence of hemorrhage, and a 10% incidence of late complications (stenosis, ectropion, and incontinence).

Comment

Although I have not reviewed my experience with the Ferguson hemorrhoidectomy, rarely does a patient remain in the hospital more than 5 days after this operation. I have been very pleased with the technical aspects and the results of this operation and use this approach virtually exclusively in all patients submitted for the surgical removal of hemorrhoids. Usually the patient's only regret is that he procrastinated too long before permitting surgical intervention.

REFERENCES

1. Ackland TH: The treatment of prolapsed gangrenous hemorrhoids. Aust NZ J Surg 1961; 30:201–203
2. Adami B, Eckardt VF, Suermann RB, Karbach U, Ewe K: Bacteremia after proctoscopy and hemorrhoid injection sclerotherapy. Dis Colon Rectum 1981; 24:373–374
3. Alexander-Williams J, Crapp AR: Conservative management of haemorrhoids. Part I: Injection, freezing and ligation. Clin Gastroenterol 1975; 4:595–618
4. Andrews E: The treatment of hemorrhoids by injection. Medical Record 1879; 15:451
5. Arabi Y, Alexander-Williams J, Keighley MRB: Anal pressures in hemorrhoids and anal fissure. Am J Surg 1977; 134:608–610
6. Bailey HR, Ferguson JA: Prevention of urinary retention by fluid restriction following anorectal operations. Dis Colon Rectum 1976; 19:250–252
7. Barrios G, Khubchandani M: Whitehead operation revisited. Dis Colon Rectum 1979; 22:330–332
8. Barron J: Office ligation of internal hemorrhoids. Am J Surg 1963; 105:563–570
9. Barron J: Office ligation treatment of hemorrhoids. Dis Colon Rectum 1963; 6:109–113
10. Bartizal J, Slosberg P: An alterative to hemorrhoids. Dis Colon Rectum 1963; 6:109–113
11. Bernard A, Parnaud E, Guntz M et al: Radioanatomie normal du réseau vasculaire hémorrhoidel. (note préalable à propos d'une étude portant sur 15 cas). Ann Radiol (Paris) 1977; 20:483–489
12. Blaisdell PC: Prevention of massive hemorrhage secondary to hemorrhoidectomy. Surg Gynecol Obstet 1958; 106:485–488
13. Buie LA: Practical Proctology. Philadelphia, WB Saunders, 1937
14. Burkitt DP, Graham-Stewart CW: Haemorrhoids—postulated pathogenesis and proposed prevention. Postgrad Med J 1975; 51:631–636
15. Cooper IS, Lee AS: Cryostatic congelation: A system for producing a limited, controlled region of cooling or freezing of biologic tissues. J Nerve Ment Dis 1961; 133:259–263
16. Corman ML: Management of postoperative constipation in anorectal surgery. Dis Colon Rectum 1979; 22:149–151
17. Corman ML, Veidenheimer MC: The new hemorrhoidectomy. Surg Clin North Am 1973; 53:417–422
18. Creve U, Hubens A: The effect of Lord's procedure on anal pressure. Dis Colon Rectum 1979; 22:483–485
19. Crystal RF, Hopping RA: Early postoperative complications of anorectal surgery. Dis Colon Rectum 1974; 17:336–341
20. Davy A, Duval C: Modifications macroscopiques et microscopiques du réseau vasculaire hémorrhoidal dans la maladie hémorrhoidaire. Archives Françaises des Maladies de L'Appareil Digestif 1976; 65:515–521
21. Dencker H, Hjorth N, Norryd C et al: Comparison of results with different methods of treatment of internal haemorrhoids. Acta Chir Scand 1973; 139:742–745

22. Denis J: Étude numérique de quelques facteurs étiopathogéniques des troubles hémorrhoidaires de l'adulte. Archives Françaises des Maladies de l'Appareil Digestif 1976; 65:529–536

23. Eisenstat T, Salvati EP, Rubin RJ: The outpatient management of acute hemorrhoidal disease. Dis Colon Rectum 1979; 22:315–317

24. Fansler WA, Anderson JK: A plastic operation for certain types of hemorrhoids. JAMA 1933; 101:1064–1066

25. Ferguson JA, Heaton JR: Closed hemorrhoidectomy. Dis Colon Rectum 1959; 2:176–179

26. Gabriel WB: The Principles and Practice of Rectal Surgery, 4th ed. London, H K Lewis & Co, 1948

27. Ganchrow MI, Mazier WP, Friend WG et al: Hemorrhoidectomy revisited–a computer analysis of 2,038 cases. Dis Colon Rectum 1971; 14:128–133

28. Gaskin ER, Childer MD Jr: Increased granuloma formation from absorbable sutures. JAMA 1963; 185:212–214

29. Gehamy RA, Weakley FL: Internal hemorrhoidectomy by elastic ligation. Dis Colon Rectum 1974; 17:347–353

30. Gill W, Fraser J, Da Costa J et al: The cryosurgical lesion. Am Surg 1970; 36:437–445

31. Gillman T, Penn J et al: Reactions of healing wounds and granulation tissue in man to auto-Thiersch, autodermal, and homodermal grafts; with an analysis of implications of phenomena encountered for understanding of behavior of grafted tissue and genesis of scars, keloids, skin carcinomata, and other cutaneous lesions. Br J Plast Surg 1953; 6:153–223

32. Granet E: Hemorrhoidectomy failures: Causes, prevention and management. Dis Colon Rectum 1968; 11:45–48

33. Greca F, Hares M, Keighley MRB: Letter to the editor: Anal dilatation. Br J Surg 1981; 68:141

34. Hancock BD: Internal sphincter and the nature of hemorrhoids. Gut 1977; 18:651–655

35. Hansen HH: Neue Aspekte zur Pathogeneses und Therapie des Hämorrhoidalleidens. Deutsche Medizinische Wochenschrift 1977; 102:1244–1248

36. Hansen HH: Pathomorphologie und Therapie des Hämorrhoidalleidens. Hautartz 1977; 28:364–367

37. Jeffery PJ, Ritchie JK, Parks AG: Treatment of hemorrhoids in patients with inflammatory bowel disease. Lancet 1977; 1:1084–1085

38. Keighley MRB, Buchmann P, Minervini S, Arabi Y, Alexander-Williams J: Prospective trials of minor surgical procedures and high-fibre diet for hemorrhoids. Br Med J 1979; 2:967–969

39. Kelsey CB: Disease of the Rectum and Anus, p 178. New York, W Wood & Co, 1882

40. Kratzer GL: Local anesthesia in anorectal surgery. Dis Colon Rectum 1965; 8:441–445

41. Lal D, Levitan R: Bacteremia following proctoscopic biopsy of a rectal polyp. Arch Intern Med 1972; 130:127–128

42. Lau WY, Chow HP, Poon GP, Wong SH: Rubber band ligation of three primary hemorrhoids in a single session. Dis Colon Rectum 1982; 25:336–339

43. LeFrock JL, Ellis CA, Turchik JB et al: Transient bacteremia associated with sigmoidoscopy. N Engl J Med 1973; 289:467–469

44. Leicester RJ, Nicholls RJ, Mann CV: Infrared coagulation: A new treatment for hemorrhoids. Dis Colon Rectum 1981; 24:602–605

45. Lewis MI: Cryosurgical hemorrhoidectomy: A follow-up report. Dis Colon Rectum 1972; 15:128–134

46. Lord PH: A new regime for the treatment of hemorrhoids. Proc R Soc Med 1968; 61:935–936

47. Lord PH: Diverse methods of managing hemorrhoids: dilatation. Dis Colon Rectum 1973; 16:180–181

48. Lurz KH, Göltner E: Hämorrhoiden in Schwangerschaft und Wochenbett. Münchener Medizinigche Wochenschrift 1977; 119:1551–1552

49. MacLeod JH: In defense of cryotherapy for hemorrhoids: A modified method. Dis Colon Rectum 1982; 25:332–335

50. McCaffrey J: Lord treatment of haemorrhoids: Four-year follow-up of fifty patients. Lancet 1975; 1:133–134

51. Milligan ETC, Morgan CN, Jones LE et al: Surgical anatomy of the anal canal, and operative treatment of haemorrhoids. Lancet 1937; 2:1119–1124

52. Moesgaard F, Nielsen ML, Hansen JB, Knudsen JT: High-fiber diet reduces bleeding and pain in patients with hemorrhoids. Dis Colon Rectum 1982; 25:454–456

53. Neiger A: Hemorrhoids in everyday practice. Proctology 1979; 2:22–28

54. Nesselrod JP: Clinical Proctology, 3rd ed. Philadelphia, WB Saunders, 1964

55. O'Connor JJ: Cryohemorrhoidectomy: Indications and complications. Dis Colon Rectum 1976; 19:41–43

56. Oh C: The role of cryosurgery in management of anorectal disease: Cryohemorrhoidectomy evaluated. Dis Colon Rectum 1975; 18:289–291

57. Oh C: One thousand cryohemorrhoidectomies: An overview. Dis Colon Rectum 1981; 24:613–617

58. Parks AG: Surgical treatment of haemorrhoids. Br J Surg 1956; 43:337–351

59. Parks AG: Hemorrhoidectomy. Adv Surg 1971; 5:1–150

60. Parnaud E, Guntz M, Bernard A et al: Anatomie normal macroscopique et microscopique du réseau vasculaire hémorrhoidal. Archives Françaises des Maladies de l'Appareil Digestif 1976; 65:501–514

61. Parturier-Albot M, Rouzotte P, Elizalde N: Hémorrhoides et vie génitale de la femme. Archives Françaises des Maladies de l'Appareil Digestif 1976; 65:537–540

62. Rosser C: Chemical rectal stricture. JAMA 1931; 96:1762–1763

63. Salmon F: A Practical Essay on Stricture on the Rectum; Illustrated by Cases, Showing the Connexion of That Disease, with Affections of the Urinary Organs and the Uterus, With Piles and Various Constitutional Complaints, 3rd ed, pp 208–209. London, Whitaker, Treacher & Arnot, 1829

64. Salvati EP: Urinary retention in anorectal and colonic surgery. Am J Surg 1957; 94:114–117

65. Savin S: Hemorrhoidectomy—How I do it: Results of 444 cryorectal surgical operations. Dis Colon Rectum 1977; 20:189–196

66. Scoma JA: Hemorrhoidectomy without urinary retention and catheterization. Conn Med 1976; 40:751–752

67. Smith LE, Goodreau JJ, Fouty J: Management of hemorrhoids: Operative hemorrhoidectomy versus cryosurgery. Dis Colon Rectum 1979; 22:10–16

68. Steinberg DM, Liegois H, Alexander-Williams J: Long term review of the results of rubber band ligation of haemorrhoids. Br J Surg 1975; 62:144–146

69. Stelzner F, Staubesand J, Machleidt H: The corpus cavernosum recti—basis of internal hemorrhoids. Langebecks Arch Chir 1962; 299:302–312

70. Tchirkow G, Haas PA, Fox TA: Injection of a local anesthetic solution into hemorrhoidal bundles following rubber band ligation. Dis Colon Rectum 1982; 25:62–63

71. Terrell EH: The treatment of hemorrhoids by a new method. Transactions of the American Proctologic Society 1916; 65–73

72. Thomson H: A new look at hemorrhoids. Medical Times 1976; 104:116–123

73. Turell R: Preoperative and postoperative management in anorectal surgery. In Turell R (ed): Diseases of the Colon and Anorectum, Vol 2, 2nd ed, pp 883–894. Philadelphia, WB Saunders, 1969

74. Vellacott KD, Hardcastle JD: Is continued anal dilatation necessary after a Lord's procedure for hemorrhoids? Br J Surg 1980; 67:658–659

75. Walls ADF, Ruckley CV: A five-year follow-up of Lord's dilatation for haemorrhoids. Lancet 1976; 1:1212–1213

76. Watts JM, Bennett RC, Duthie HL et al: Healing and pain after hemorrhoidectomy. Br J Surg 1964; 51:808–817

77. White AC: Liquid air: Its application in medicine and surgery. Medical Record 1899; 56:109–112

78. Whitehead W: The surgical treatment of haemorrhoids. Br Med J 1882; 1:148–150

79. Williams KL, Haq IU, Elem B: Cryodestruction of haemorrhoids. Br Med J 1973; 1:666–668

80. Wilson MC, Schofield P: Cryosurgical haemorrhoidectomy. Br J Surg 1976; 63:497–498

81. Wilson PM: Anorectal closing mechanisms. S Afr Med J 1977; 51:802–808

82. Wolf JS, Munoz JJ, Rosin JD: Survey of hemorrhoidectomy practices: Open versus closed techniques. Dis Colon Rectum 1979; 22:536–538

83. Wrobleski DE, Corman ML, Veidenheimer MC, Coller JA: Long-term evaluation of rubber ring ligation in hemorrhoidal disease. Dis Colon Rectum 1980; 23:478–482

CHAPTER 3

Anal Fissure

Fissure is a common anorectal pathologic entity. It is of great significance because, if acute, the degree of patient discomfort and disability far exceeds that which might be expected for an otherwise rather trivial lesion.

An anal fissure is a "cut" or a "crack" that usually extends from the anal verge to the dentate line. It may be acute or chronic. It can occur at any age (it is the commonest cause of rectal bleeding in infants) but is usually a condition of young adults. Both sexes are affected equally, but women are much more likely to have an anterior fissure than men. However, 90% of fissures are located posteriorly in women; only 1% are anterior in men.[13]

ETIOLOGY AND PATHOGENESIS

Generally, anal fissure has been attributed to constipation or straining at stool. The theory is that the hard, fecal bolus "cracks" the anal canal. However, anal fissure can be a consequence of frequent defecation and diarrhea. It is also associated with nonspecific inflammatory bowel disease and must be considered in the differential diagnosis of several specific inflammatory conditions (*e.g.,* syphilis, tuberculosis). When anal fissure occurs in an aberrant location, especially laterally, one must entertain the possibility that the patient has ulcerative colitis or, more commonly, Crohn's disease.

Why the fissure is most commonly posterior is a subject of some controversy. Lockhart-Mummery felt that the explanation is found in the structure of the external sphincter.[19] The lower portion of this muscle is not truly circular, but consists of a band of muscle fibers that pass from posterior to anterior and split around the anus. He postulated that the anal mucosa is, therefore, best supported laterally and is weakest posteriorly. Because of the decreased support anteriorly in women, the condition occurs somewhat more readily in this location than it does in men. Further evidence to support Lockhart-Mummery's concept is apparent whenever one inserts an anal retractor too vigorously at the time of surgery for hemorrhoids. The split that may occur is almost invariably located posteriorly. If the sphincter is stretched in the cadaver, it will be found that tearing almost always occurs posteriorly.[20]

Why some fissures heal spontaneously and others develop chronicity is an unresolved question. Infection or lymphatic obstruction, secondary to the persistent inflammation, may be involved. What may develop distally is the characteristic skin tag or "sentinel pile," and proximally the hypertrophied anal papilla (Figs. 3-1 and 3-2). Another characteristic feature is that the internal anal sphincter muscle fibers are readily apparent at the base of the open wound (Fig. 3-3).

There is nothing in particular that is microscopically diagnostic of anal fissure (Fig. 3-4). Usually one observes only the typical inflammatory changes if the lesion is excised and sent for pathologic examination.

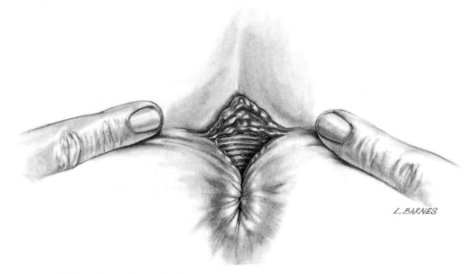

FIG. 3-1. ''Sentinel pile,'' or skin tab, at lower edge of anal fissure.

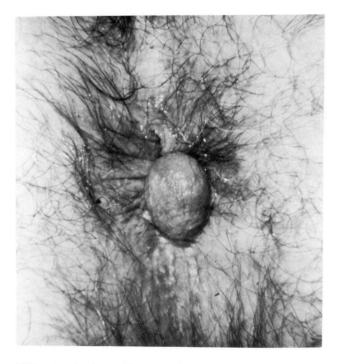

FIG. 3-2. Prolapsed hypertrophied anal papilla associated with anal fissure.

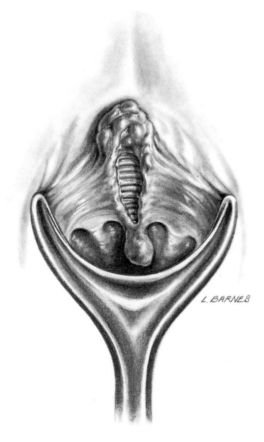

FIG. 3-3. Chronic posterior anal fissure with skin tag and hypertrophied anal papilla. Note fibers of the internal anal sphincter at the base of the wound.

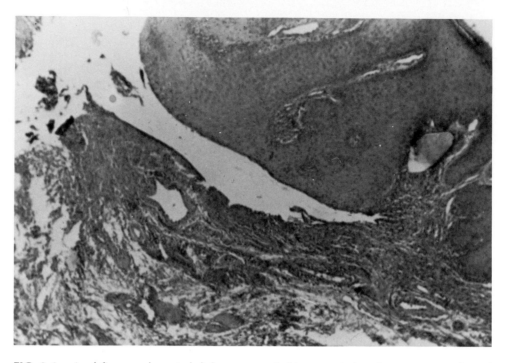

FIG. 3-4.   Anal fissure: elongated defect surrounded by granulation tissue on one side and acanthotic squamous epithelium on the other. (Original magnification × 180)

Duthie and Bennett measured sphincter pressures with an open-ended tube connected by a strain gauge to a recording device.[8] Although all patients had "spasm" of the sphincter on the basis of digital examination, no increase was found in the resting pressure over control subjects. Following sphincter stretch a moderate fall was noted, but it returned virtually to normal by the eighth postoperative day. It appeared to them that the therapeutic effect of sphincter stretch was not related so much to reduction in anal pressure as to prevention of the spasm.[8]

Nothmann and Schuster performed rectosphincteric manometry using balloons on patients with anal fissure.[27] "Resting" pressures were twice as high as in control subjects. It is important to recognize that resting pressures as measured with an open-tipped tube in patients with anal fissure are normal, whereas those measured by balloon catheter are elevated.[32] Others have observed a similar pattern, with reduction of the pressure to normal following internal anal sphincterotomy.[3, 6, 15] Following distension of the rectum there is the expected internal sphincter relaxation, but this is followed by a "marked and prolonged contraction above the initial baseline."[27] This has been termed the "overshoot" phenomenon. Nothmann and Schuster concluded that this reflexly stimulated sphincter spasm is involved in the etiology of the condition.[27]

Abcarian and associates in their manometric evaluation of patients with anal fissure concluded that the ameliorative effect of sphincterotomy really is due to an anatomic widening of the anal canal.[2]

SYMPTOMS

The characteristic complaints of the patient with an acute anal fissure are pain and bleeding. The pain usually occurs with defecation and right afterwards. Usually the pain ceases after a few minutes, but occasionally it may persist for hours. It can be differentiated from the pain of proctalgia fugax in that the latter condition produces discomfort that is usually not related to bowel action. Also, the patient feels the discomfort in the anus with a fissure, but it is higher and more deep-seated with proctalgia fugax. The other condition that commonly produces pain is a thrombosed hemorrhoid, but the patient also notes a lump, an observation that is not appreciated if an acute anal fissure is the cause.

Bleeding is usually minimal, frequently only on the paper, sometimes in the toilet bowl. Not uncommonly patients report no evidence of bleeding.

Patients with anal fissure of long standing (chronic) present with a different symptom complex. They complain of a lump (due to the sentinel tag), drainage or discharge (from the open wound), or pruritic symptoms. Bleeding may or may not be present and pain is usually mild or frequently absent. Problems with micturition and dyspareunia occasionally accompany the symptoms of both acute and chronic fissure.

The patient often relates that constipation is the antecedent event, but once pain develops, the fear of the act of defecation can exacerbate the problem. This can lead to fecal impaction, particularly in children and in the elderly.

EXAMINATION

Acute Fissure

As mentioned, the history is usually so characteristic that the diagnosis should be established easily. By mere inspection or gentle retraction of the perianal skin, the open wound often can be seen. If one is unable to pry the buttocks apart to view the area, the presence of an acute anal fissure is a virtual certainty. Under such circumstances, to attempt digital examination or to insert an instrument is an exercise in futility. Appropriate treatment should be initiated without this confirmation.

A topical anesthetic jelly may be useful if the physician is willing to wait a few minutes for it to take effect. Palpation will demonstrate spasm of the sphincter and exacerbate the patient's discomfort. The wound is usually not appreciated with the examining finger because there is usually no fibrosis and the cut is relatively superficial.

Anoscopic examination confirms the location of the fissure. The ability to perform the examination, however, may be a reflection of the chronicity of the problem. Proctosigmoidoscopic examination should be performed prior to any surgical procedure to establish that at least the rectum is not involved by inflammatory bowel disease. With both procedures it is suggested that one use narrow-caliber instruments.

Chronic Fissure

Examination of the patient with a chronic anal fissure usually reveals the characteristic sentinel pile. This can at times become rather large (3 or 4 cm). Digital examination readily reveals the presence of the fissure, the open wound, induration, and fibrosis. A hypertrophied anal papilla often can be appreciated at the apex of the ulcer.

Anoscopy frequently can be accomplished without difficulty since pain is not usually great. However, scarring may result in some narrowing of the anal canal, and it may be necessary to use a narrow diameter anoscope. Characteristically, the internal anal sphincter fibers are clearly seen at the base of a chronic anal fissure.

Proctosigmoidoscopy should be performed to rule out the possibility of a concurrent tumor or distal inflammatory bowel disease.

Occasionally a chronic anal fissure may be associated with a fistula (Fig. 3-5). When this occurs it is quite superficial, truly subcutaneous. Examination may reveal an external opening, virtually always in the midline, usually no more than 1 or 2 cm distal to the skin tag. Purulent material may be noted. A probe passed from the external opening emerges at the distal end of the fissure. The internal anal sphincter is frequently not traversed.

As suggested, chronic anal fissure may sometimes be associated with anal stenosis, particularly if the fissure is the result of prior anal surgery (e.g., hemorrhoidectomy; Fig. 3-6). Under this circumstance treatment may require an anoplasty (see Chap. 6).

If the fissure is ectopically located, extends proximal to the dentate line, is particularly broad-based, or is especially purulent, the presence of underlying inflammatory bowel disease must be considered. A history of diarrhea or abdominal pain is highly suggestive. When doubt exists about the etiology of the condition, biopsy should be performed before considering a definitive surgical procedure.

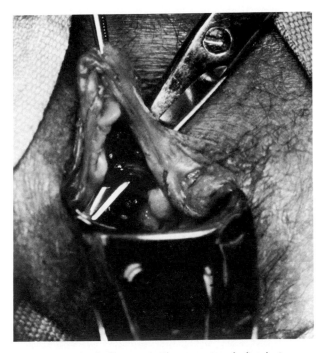

FIG. 3-5. Anal fissure with associated fistula-in-ano. (Courtesy of Daniel Rosenthal, M.D.)

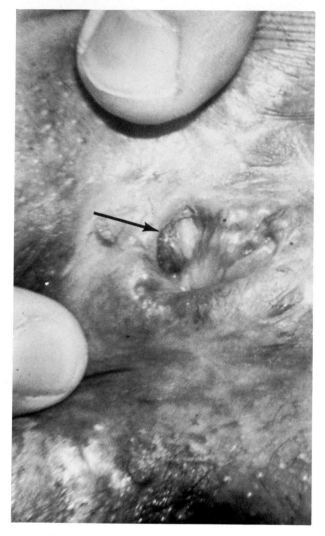

FIG. 3-6. Anal fissure *(arrow)* due to stenosis following hemorrhoidectomy. (Courtesy of Daniel Rosenthal, M.D.)

TREATMENT

Medical Management

Fissures of brief duration are usually successfully treated by conservative measures such as stool softeners (*e.g.*, dioctyl sodium sulfosuccinate, psyllium), encouragement of a high-fiber diet, and sitz baths. Preparations containing mineral oil are not advised because of difficulty in cleansing the area following defecation. Suppositories also are not recommended; they do not act effectively within the anal canal. Inserting any one of a number of proprietary creams and ointments to the area may offer some transient relief. The patient should be encouraged to continue with the diet even after symptoms have resolved, perhaps also with the addition of a bulk laxative agent, in order to prevent recurrence.

Injection of a long-acting local anesthetic offers only transient relief and permits examination, but its use on an ambulatory basis is impractical. Anal dilators should not be employed, and the application of silver nitrate will succeed only in clearing the physician's waiting room, so dramatic is the patient's response.

In some cases the history suggests a fissure of recent onset (2 weeks or less); almost all such fissures will heal by medical managment. However, if symptoms have been present for a longer period of time, resolution wihout surgery becomes increasingly less likely. My own attitude is to offer the patient a choice of continuing with medical measures or surgical intervention; the degree of disability, the degree of fear of the procedure, or both will determine the patient's course of action.

In the patient who complains of pruritus, the primary medical therapy is to cleanse the area with warm water following defecation. Many patients believe that the itching is due to lack of cleanliness and vigorously scrub the area with soap and water; this only serves to exacerbate the problem. The patient should be cautioned not to use soap in the perianal area. Avoiding coffee, alcoholic beverages, smoking, and spicy foods will also have an ameliorative effect (see Chap. 8).

If discharge is a problem and surgery is not appropriate, or the patient refuses, he can keep a ball of cotton at the anal opening, changing it as necessary, to avoid soiling underclothes and exacerbating pruritic symptoms.

Surgical Management

The choice of operative approach to the treatment of anal fissure depends on the duration of symptoms and on the physical findings. For an acute anal fissure, without a tag, hypertrophied papilla, or significant hemorrhoids, the two procedures advocated are *sphincter stretch* and *internal anal sphincterotomy*. For chronic anal fissure with external component, or when the condition is associated with symptomatic large hemorrhoids, excisional therapy is advised.

Sphincter Stretch

Sphincter stretch was originally described by Récamier in 1838 for the treatment of proctalgia fugax and anal fissure.[30] The procedure can be carried out with a local infiltration, but a brief general anesthetic is preferred.

If available, an ambulatory surgical facility is optimal. The patient is placed in the lithotomy position; sterile draping is unnecessary. The index finger of one hand is inserted into the rectum followed by the index finger of the opposite hand. Gentle lateral retraction with each finger commences for approximately 30 seconds. The long finger is inserted and then the other long finger. With four fingers in place, the anal canal is stretched cautiously for 4 minutes by the clock.

Results

Sphincter stretch is a reasonably effective procedure for the symptomatic relief of anal fissure. But there is a paucity of reports on the results of treatment, particularly within the past 15 years. This is probably because the procedure has been supplanted by internal anal sphincterotomy. Watts and associates performed sphincter stretch on 99 patients for anal fissure.[33] All were followed for at least 5 months. Three fourths of the patients achieved symptomatic relief within 48 hours; pain was resolved in 20% within 2 weeks. Six patients continued to have a fissure (two were free of pain), and five others developed recurrent discomfort without evidence of fissure. The troublesome complication in their series was related to control (usually for flatus alone, but occasionally for feces) or swelling. Twenty-eight percent were noted to have one of these complaints.

In my own experience, I have found sphincter stretch to be quite effective, but have abandoned the procedure in favor of lateral internal anal sphincterotomy. But if one is to use the former approach, it should be limited to younger patients and, in my opinion, is contraindicated over the age of 60, because of the high likelihood of incontinence problems.

Internal Anal Sphincterotomy

Goligher credits Miles as the surgeon who initially performed internal sphincterotomy for anal fissure, although Miles believed he was dividing what he called the "pecten band."[14, 22] In 1951 Eisenhammer became the first person to advocate internal anal sphincterotomy for this condition.[9]

The internal anal sphincter is the continuation of the distal portion of the circular muscle of the rectum (see Fig. 2-2). Its length is essentially equal to that of the anal canal itself. Distally, it can usually be easily felt medial to the intersphincteric groove outside the anal verge. The subcutaneous portion of the external sphincter is lateral to the groove.

The internal sphincter maintains the anal canal in the closed position; action is involuntary. The external sphincter is a striated muscle. The latter, with the levator ani muscle, are the muscles involved in voluntary control. Complete division of the internal anal sphincter is possible without creating significant impairment for fecal continence.[10]

The procedure has been performed in the posterior midline, but although usually curing the condition, it has been associated with the complication of the "keyhole" deformity (see Complications). Eisenhammer advocated the lateral position for sphincterotomy, dividing one half of the muscle in an open fashion.[10] Bennett and Goligher reported a high incidence of impairment for flatus with posterior internal anal sphincterotomy (34%) and a 15% incidence of difficulty with control of feces.[5] In time there was further improvement, but the fact remains that the operation has an appreciable morbidity, although the cure rate was 93%.

In 1969 Notaras reported a closed technique using a narrow-bladed scalpel, performing an internal anal sphincterotomy in a closed fashion in the lateral position.[24] In 66 patients so treated he reported a 6% incidence of fecal soiling. Notaras subsequently described his technique in detail, ultimately employing a scalpel used in cataract surgery.[25, 26] His method involves submucosal insertion of the knife, followed by an outward incision to the intersphincteric groove. I prefer inserting the knife into the groove and incising medially.

Technique

The procedure can be performed in the office using a local anesthetic (0.5% bupivacaine [Marcaine] in 1:200,000 epinephrine) or in an ambulatory surgical facility, using a short-acting general anesthetic. If the former method is used, the patient is placed either in the left lateral position or in the prone (jackknife) position. The fissure itself is infiltrated as well as the site for insertion of the knife, either the right lateral or left lateral position. No anal retractor is employed for the procedure if a local anesthetic is used. The index finger senses the knife blade beneath the anal mucosa, and the residual internal anal sphincter fibers are broken by the side of the finger (Fig. 3-7).

I prefer to perform the procedure with a general anesthetic in the outpatient surgical setting. The patient is placed in the lithotomy position on the operating table, and a Hill-Ferguson retractor is placed into the anal canal. The intersphincteric groove is usually easily felt, and the knife blade is inserted into the left lateral aspect (Fig. 3-8). Some surgeons use a No. 11 blade, but a 52-M Beaver blade is preferred (the type used for cataract surgery); it acts like a stiletto and creates a very small wound. For a left-handed surgeon the right lateral aspect is easier. There is a theoretical advantage of cutting on this side because the hemorrhoid

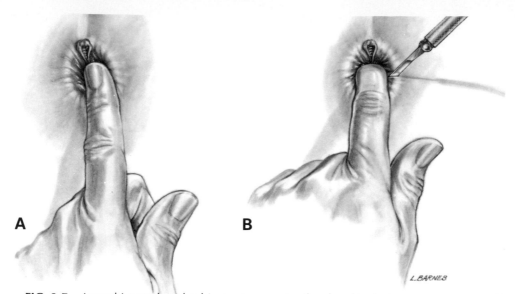

FIG. 3-7. Lateral internal anal sphincterotomy using the closed technique, no retractor, and a local anesthetic, with the patient in the prone position. **A.** A finger is inserted into the anal canal after anesthesia is established. **B.** Sphincterotomy is performed with the finger in place.

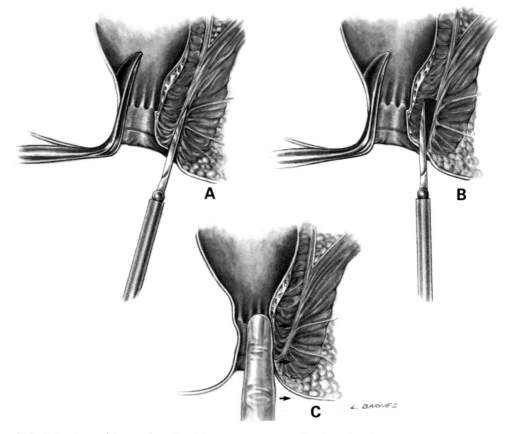

FIG. 3-8. Lateral internal anal sphincterotomy using the closed technique, a retractor, and a general anesthetic. The patient is in the lithotomy position. **A.** A knife is inserted into the intersphincteric groove. **B.** The lower one third to one half of the internal sphincter is divided. **C.** The residual fibers are broken with the finger.

sites are usually anteriorly and posteriorly located, but it requires that the right-handed surgeon operate backhanded; hence, I perform the sphincterotomy on the left.

The tip of the blade is angled medially (Fig. 3-8, *B*), pointing just above the dentate line, and the lower one third to one half of the internal anal sphincter is divided. When the knife is visualized beneath the intact anal mucosa, it is withdrawn. The side of the finger is then used to break any residual sphincter fibers (Fig. 3-8, *C*). If one pushes with the finger tip there is a tendency to tear the mucosa, which may then lead to bleeding and possibly the subsequent development of a fistula. If bleeding occurs at the wound puncture site it can be readily controlled by direct pressure for a few moments. If a tag or papilla is present it can be removed by excision with a scissors. No dressings are employed and the patient is discharged when alert.

Another variation of the lateral sphincterotomy is the open technique. This, too, can be performed in the office or in the hospital. It is more time consuming and usually requires suturing, so I do not recommend it, but for the sake of completeness, it is included in this discussion.

A small, radial incision is made laterally at the lower border of the internal sphincter into the intersphincteric groove (Fig. 3-9). Because of the open wound it is important to infiltrate the area with a local anesthetic containing epinephrine solution. The distal internal sphincter is grasped with an Allis forceps and bluntly freed. The lower one third to one half is divided with a scissors. The wound is closed with 2-0 chromic catgut or 5-0 Dexon. A small dressing is employed.

Postoperative Care

Sitz baths and a mild analgesic are the only measures advised postoperatively. Pain is usually less than what occurred preoperatively, and many patients resume their normal activity within 48 hours.

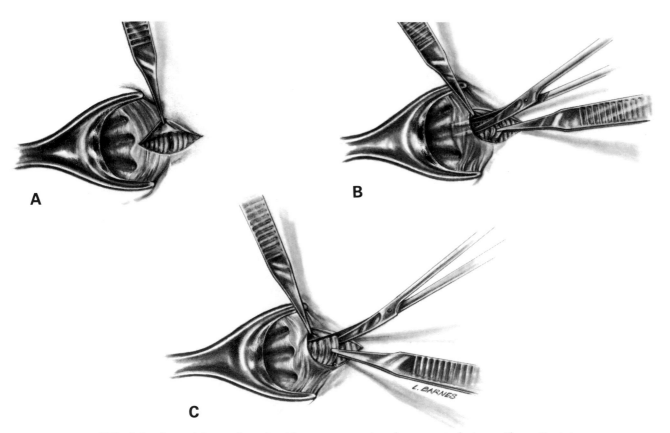

FIG. 3-9. Lateral internal anal sphincterotomy using the open technique. The patient is placed in the lateral or the prone (jackknife) position. **A.** A radial incision is made across the intersphincteric groove. A narrow Hill-Ferguson retractor is in place. **B.** The internal sphincter is separated from the anoderm by blunt dissection. **C.** The internal sphincter is divided. The wound may be closed or left open.

Complications

Ecchymosis is frequently noted around the site of the wound, but this is of no clinical significance. *Hemorrhage* is extremely rare, but is more likely to occur with the open procedure. Suture ligation may be required.

Perianal abscess occurs after 1% of closed internal anal sphincterotomies. It is virtually always associated with an *anal fistula*. This presumably is the result of penetration of the mucosa of the anal canal by the knife blade. It is surprising that this complication is not seen more frequently, because the anal canal mucosa must be breeched more often than is suspected. Treatment requires drainage of the abscess, identification of an internal opening (if present), and fistulotomy.

Fecal incontinence following sphincterotomy should not occur, because the internal and sphincter plays very little role in maintaining bowel control. Notaras reported on 73 patients who underwent this procedure and found 4 with soiling of the underclothes, 2 with imperfect control of flatus, and 1 with occasional fecal soilage.[25] This last patient was thought to have been a poor candidate for the procedure. Millar reported mucus or flatus control problems in 3 of 99 patients so treated; Hoffmann and Goligher noted 12 of 99 patients to have some minor defect of anal control.[17, 23] It is probably a wise idea to record the patient's preoperative bowel control status, especially if there is some degree of impairment noted from the history.

The incidence of *delayed healing* or *recurrence* is the standard of measurement for the success or failure of the operation. Millar reported 88% that were healed at 2 weeks, with 100% healed eventually.[23] Hoffman and Goligher reported 2% unhealed at 9 months.[17] Notaras, and Ray and co-workers, reported 100% healing.[25, 29] Marya and co-workers reported a 2% incidence of nonhealing.[21] Rudd reported on 200 patients and found only 1 unhealed, and that patient subsequently developed Crohn's disease.[31]

Keighley and associates compared a lateral sphincterotomy as performed with a local anesthetic versus a general anesthetic.[18] They found a 50% incidence of delayed healing with a local and a 3% incidence after a general anesthetic. They concluded that the operation should not be performed with local infiltration.

In my own experience I cannot claim a success rate of 100%. However, it is the rare patient indeed who complains of symptoms after the first postoperative month. I attribute a failure to inadequate partial sphincterotomy. All patients who were returned to surgery and on whom was performed a more generous sphincterotomy had their complaints alleviated and the fissure healed.

The statement should be reinforced about the inadvisability of performing internal anal sphincterotomy in the posterior midline, at the site of the open wound. Although the procedure is successful in alleviating pain and curing the fissure as frequently as is lateral sphincterotomy, it is associated with the troublesome consequence of "keyhole" deformity. This defect in the posterior midline may produce a mucus discharge, soiling of the underclothes, and pruritic symptoms. Correction requires an anoplasty (see Chap. 6). There is no reason to perform posterior sphincterotomy for anal fissure, and this approach should be abandoned.

Chronic Anal Fissure

The classical treatment of chronic anal fissure has been excision and internal anal sphincterotomy in the posterior position. This removes the eschar, skin tag, and papilla, but contributes to the problem of the previously mentioned "keyhole" deformity. Excision of the annoying tissue is useful, but the sphincterotomy should

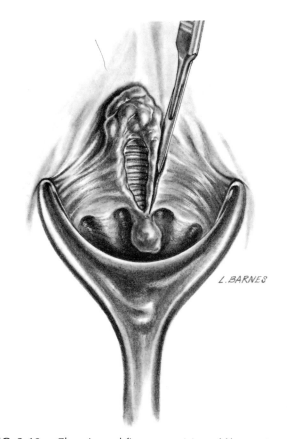

FIG. 3-10. Chronic anal fissure: excision of fibrous tissue, skin tag, and hypertrophied anal papilla. Sphincterotomy should *not* be performed at this site.

be performed in the lateral position. Unless the edges of the fissure are very fibrotic, removal of the tag and papilla by snipping with scissors should suffice. A more formal excision can be done if the surgeon prefers (Fig. 3-10). But the underlying internal anal sphincter should not be incorporated if this approach is utilized; the sphincterotomy should be performed at a lateral site by one of the methods described previously.

Reports of the treatment of chronic anal fissure by lateral internal anal sphincterotomy have been quite enthusiastic. Bell noted one failure in 56 patients.[4] Ravikumar and co-workers reported all fissures healed by 5 weeks, all but two within 3 weeks.[28]

Abcarian analyzed retrospectively 300 patients; one half underwent lateral internal anal sphincterotomy, and the other half underwent fissurectomy and midline sphincterotomy.[1] Although both groups had the same incidence of delayed healing (two patients), there was no patient who experienced fecal soilage in the former group; 5% noted this problem after the latter operation.

Hawley reported a prospective study of three methods of treatment of chronic anal fissure: sphincter stretch, posterior sphincterotomy, and lateral sphincterotomy.[16] He found that lateral internal anal sphincterotomy is the preferred operation because of earlier wound healing, less postoperative discomfort, and fewer problems with soiling.

Chronic Anal Fissure with Stenosis

Difficulty with defecation secondary to narrowing of the anal canal from chronic fissure can occasionally occur. The problem is more commonly seen when excess anal canal mucosa is removed at the time of hemorrhoidectomy. Stenosis and fissure may supervene. Conservative medical treatment with the use of a dilator has been recommended, but an anoplasty as has been recommended by Ferguson is the approach that I prefer (see Chap. 6).[7, 11]

Anal Fissure and Crohn's Disease

Fielding reported in a prospective study of 153 patients that over half had anal fissures, most of which were asymptomatic.[12] One must consider the possibility of underlying inflammatory bowel disease in any patient whose wound fails to heal. Lateral anal fissure or a history of frequent bowel actions should warn the surgeon to proceed with caution. Conservative (medical) treatment is advised. The wounds following surgery tend to be indolent, more symptomatic, and may actually precipitate the need for a diversionary procedure.

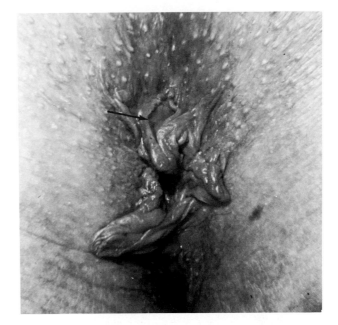

FIG. 3-11. Hemorrhoids with associated posterior anal fissure (arrow). This problem is optimally treated by hemorrhoidectomy and lateral internal anal sphincterotomy.

Anal Fissure and Hemorrhoids

When a patient has an anal fissure and a significant enough hemorrhoid problem to warrant surgical treatment, a hemorrhoidectomy and a sphincterotomy should be performed concurrently (Fig. 3-11). However, the sphincterotomy should be carried out laterally, usually at the site of the left lateral pile.

REFERENCES

1. Abcarian H: Surgical correction of chronic anal fissure: Results of lateral and internal sphincterotomy vs. fissurectomy—midline sphincterotomy. Dis Colon Rectum 1980; 23:31–36
2. Abcarian H, Lakshmanan S, Read DR, Roccaforte P: The role of internal sphincter in chronic anal fissures. Dis Colon Rectum 1982; 25:525–528
3. Arabi Y, Alexander-Williams J, Keighley MRB: Anal pressures in hemorrhoids and anal fissure. Am J Surg 1977; 134:608–610
4. Bell GA: Lateral internal sphincterotomy in chronic anal fissure—a surgical technique. Am Surg 1980; 46:572–575
5. Bennett RC, Goligher JC: Results of internal

sphincterotomy for anal fissure. Br Med J 1962; 2:1500–1503

6. Cerdán FJ, deLion AR, Azpiroz F, Martín J, Balibrea JL: Anal sphincteric pressure in fissure-in-ano before and after lateral internal sphincterotomy. Dis Colon Rectum 1982; 25:198–201

7. Crapp AR, Alexander-Williams J: Fissure-in-ano and anal stenosis. Part I: Conservative management. Clin Gastroenterol 1975; 4:619–628

8. Duthie HL, Bennett RC: Anal sphincteric pressure in fissure in ano. Surg Gynecol Obstet 1964; 119:19–21

9. Eisenhammer S: The surgical correction of chronic internal anal (sphincteric) contracture. South Afr Med J 1951; 25:486

10. Eisenhammer S: The evaluation of the internal anal sphincterotomy operation with special reference to anal fissure. Surg Gynecol Obstet 1959; 109:583–590

11. Ferguson JA: Fissure-in-ano and anal stenosis. Part II: Radical surgical managements. Clin Gastroenterol 1975; 4:629–634

12. Fielding JF: An enquiry into certain aspects of regional enteritis, p. 67. M.D. thesis, National University of Ireland (Quoted in Ref. 7)

13. Goligher JC: Surgery of the Anus, Rectum and Colon, p 136. New York, Macmillan, 1980

14. Goligher JC: Surgery of the Anus, Rectum and Colon, p 147. New York, Macmillan, 1980

15. Hancock BD: The internal sphincter and anal fissure. Br J Surg 1977; 64:92–95

16. Hawley PR: The treatment of chronic fissure-in-ano: A trial of methods. Br J Surg 1969; 56:915–918

17. Hoffmann DC, Goligher JC: Lateral subcutaneous internal sphincterotomy in treatment of anal fissure. Br Med J 1970; 3:673–675

18. Keighley MRB, Greca F, Nevah E, Hares M, Alexander-Williams J: Treatment of anal fissure by lateral subcutaneous sphincterotomy should be under general anesthesia. Br J Surg 1981; 68:400–401

19. Lockhart-Mummery P: Diseases of the Rectum and Anus. p 169–170. New York, Wm. Wood, 1914

20. Lockhart-Mummery P: Diseases of the Rectum and Anus, p 171. New York, Wm. Wood, 1914

21. Marya SK, Mittal SS, Singla S: Lateral subcutaneous internal sphincterotomy for acute fissure-in-ano. Br J Surg 1980; 67:299

22. Miles WE: Rectal surgery. London, Cassell & Co, 1939

23. Millar DM: Subcutaneous lateral internal anal sphincterotomy for anal fissure. Br J Surg 1971; 58:737–739

24. Notaras MJ: Lateral subcutaneous sphincterotomy for anal fissure—a new technique. Proc R Soc Med 1969; 62:713

25. Notaras MJ: The treatment of anal fissure by lateral subcutaneous internal sphincterotomy—a technique and results. Br J Surg 1971; 58:96–100

26. Notaras MJ: Fissure-in-ano. Lateral subcutaneous internal anal sphincterotomy. In Todd IP (ed): Colon, Rectum, and Anus, 3rd ed, pp 354–360 (Operative Surgery Series). London, Butterworth, 1977

27. Nothmann BJ, Schuster MM: Internal anal sphincter derangement with anal fissures. Gastroenterology 1974; 67:216–220

28. Ravikumar TS, Sridhar S, Rao RN: Subcutaneous lateral internal sphincterotomy for chronic fissure-in-ano. Dis Colon Rectum 1982; 25:798–801

29. Ray JE, Penfold JCB, Gathright JB, Roberson SH: Lateral subcutaneous internal anal sphincterotomy for anal fissure. Dis Colon Rectum 1974; 17:139–144

30. Récamier JCA: Extension, massage et percussion cadencée dans le traitement des contractures musculaires. Rev Medicale Franc 1838; 1:74–89 (Translated: Dis Colon Rectum 1980; 23:362–367)

31. Rudd WWH: Lateral subcutaneous internal sphincterotomy for chronic anal fissure, an outpatient procedure. Dis Colon Rectum 1975; 18:319–323

32. Schuster MM: The riddle of the sphincters. Gastroenterology 1975; 69:249–262

33. Watts J McK, Bennett RC, Goligher JC: Stretching of anal sphincters in treatment of fissure-in-ano. Br Med J 1964; 2:342–343

CHAPTER 4

Anorectal Abscess and Fistula

Anorectal abscess and fistula are frequently associated conditions. The former is an acute inflammatory process that may be caused by an underlying anal fistula. The latter represents a communication between two epithelial surfaces.

ANORECTAL ABSCESS

Etiology

Abscess may be the result of such specific causes as foreign body intrusion, trauma, malignancy, radiation, infectious dermatitides (*e.g.*, suppurative hydradenitis), tuberculosis, actinomycosis, Crohn's disease, hemorrhoids, and anal fissure.[38] It also may occur after anal operations (hemorrhoidectomy, sphincterotomy). The cause of nonspecific anorectal abscess and fistula is believed to be plugging of the anal ducts (the cryptoglandular theory). The anal glands and ducts (between 6 and 10 in number) are located around the anal canal, entering at the base of the crypts. Parks demonstrated by meticulous histologic review that half of all crypts are not entered by glands, that the ducts usually end blindly, and that the commonest direction of spread is downward into the submucosa.[54] Of greatest interest

is his observation that in two thirds of the specimens, one or more branches enter the sphincter, and in one half, the branches cross the sphincter completely to end in the longitudinal layer (Fig. 4-1). However, in his study, no branch crossed into the external sphincter. The implication is that infection of the duct can result in an abscess, which can spread in a number of directions and can lead to the subsequent development of anal fistula.

Age and Sex

Abscess and fistula occur more commonly in men than in women. McElwain and co-workers reported a ratio of three men to one woman, and Read and Abcarian reported a two-to-one ratio.[51, 61] McElwain and co-workers in their review of 1000 patients gave the average age at onset of 39 years for both sexes.[51] They also noted a seasonal occurrence for the disorder, with the highest incidence in the spring and summer.

Hill reported a personal experience of 626 patients.[36] The youngest was 2 months old, and the oldest was 79 years. There were almost twice the number of males as females. The vast majority of patients in his experience developed symptoms in the fourth, fifth, and sixth decades.

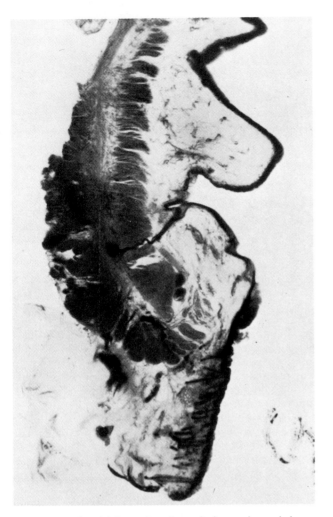

FIG. 4-1. This thick section through the anal canal shows an anal gland penetrating the internal sphincter, terminating in the longitudinal layer. (Parks AG: Fistula-in-ano. In Morson BC. [ed]: Diseases of the Colon, Rectum and Anus, p 277. New York, Appleton-Century-Crofts)

Types of Abscesses

The four presentations of anorectal abscess (perianal, ischiorectal, intersphincteric [submucosal], and supralevator) are depicted in Figure 4-2. It is important to distinguish among these presentations because the therapy and the implications for the subsequent development of anal fistula are different for each.

Perianal Abscess

Perianal (perirectal) abscess is a superficial, tender mass outside the anal verge. It is the commonest type of anorectal abscess (40% to 45% of cases). The patient usually presents with a relatively short history of painful swelling exacerbated by defecation and by sitting. Fever and leukocytosis are not common.

Physical examination reveals an area of erythema, induration, or fluctuance. Proctosigmoidoscopic examination may be difficult to perform because of pain, but even when it can be accomplished it is usually unrewarding. Occasionally, however, anoscopic examination demonstrates pus exuding from the base of a crypt.

When only erythema is present with no apparent mass, the surgeon may be misled into believing that incision and drainage will not be beneficial. Under such circumstances, the patient may be instructed to take sitz baths or may be given a broad-spectrum antibiotic and advised to return in 24 to 48 hours. Despite the absence of fluctuance or significant induration, an abscess is usually present. A patient who is dismissed without undergoing drainage may return a few hours later, distressed that spontaneous discharge has taken place, even though he may be more comfortable.

A hypodermic needle inserted into the region of induration is a simple diagnostic test. If purulence is present, a small incision is made using a local anesthetic. The pus is drained, an iodoform gauze wick is placed, and a dressing is applied. In 12 to 24 hours the patient, while taking a sitz bath, is instructed to remove the dressing and the drain. Baths three times daily are advised, and the patient is reexamined in 7 to 10 days. At this time proctosigmoidoscopic and anoscopic examinations are performed. If an external opening persists and a fistula is identified, a definitive procedure is indicated (see Anal Fistula, Principles of Surgical Treatment).

The value of antibiotics in the patient who has undergone incision and drainage is a matter of some controversy. In the patient who is at increased risk (*e.g.*, the patient with diabetes mellitus, valvular heart disease, or a compromised immune system), broad-spectrum antibiotics are suggested.

A fistula with an internal opening is occasionally seen concomitant with the abscess. The surgeon may elect to perform fistulotomy at the same time the abscess is drained if the internal opening is low-lying, in order to prevent recurrence; however, the literature is rather confusing on this point because it is not always clear what type of fistula–abscess the author is treating. A recurrence rate of a mere 3.4% has been reported by McElwain and associates following initial drainage and fistulotomy.[50] Their subsequent report demonstrated the rate of recurrence of abscess, fistula formation, or both to be 3.6%, which compared favorably with their own recurrence rate of 6% when the established fistula was excised.[51]

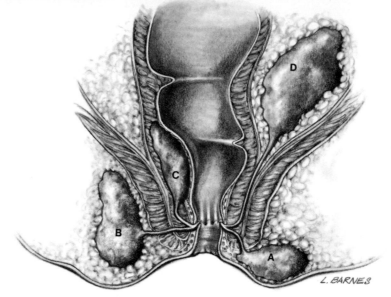

L. BARNES

FIG. 4-2. Infection of the anal duct can present as an abscess in a number of locations. **A.** Perianal. **B.** Ischiorectal. **C.** Intersphincteric. **D.** Supralevator.

Scoma and co-workers reported a retrospective review of 232 patients with anal abscess who underwent initial office drainage only.[66] Two thirds subsequently developed a fistula. Unfortunately, the authors failed to break down the incidence of fistula according to the type of abscess. They recommended that fistulotomy be delayed until the fistula becomes manifest. Waggener recommends the opposite approach.[73] In my own experience, anal fistula is usually not recognized at the time of drainage of a perianal abscess, and subsequently develops in approximately one third of the cases.

Ischiorectal Abscess

Ischiorectal abscess may present as a large, erythematous, indurated, tender mass of the buttock, or may be virtually inapparent, the patient complaining only of severe pain. This type of abscess is seen in 20% to 25% of patients. Pus is almost always present. Waiting for the abscess to "mature" causes the patient's suffering to persist needlessly. Needle aspiration will resolve the issue. Proctosigmoidoscopy and anoscopy are usually deferred because of considerable discomfort.

Drainage of ischiorectal abscess requires some planning because the condition is frequently the result of a transsphincteric fistula. Most patients with this type of abscess will require a subsequent fistula procedure. It is important, therefore, to drain the abscess by creating an external opening as close to the rectum as is possible (Fig. 4-3). If this is not properly performed, the subsequent fistulotomy will result in a large wound and

require a prolonged healing time (Fig. 4-4). The abscess cavity can be entered and adequate drainage established without attacking the point of presentation or the most fluctuant area.

The technique for drainage of a large ischiorectal abscess is little different from that for a small, perianal abscess. Neither necessarily requires a general anesthetic or vigorous operative manipulation. After installation of a local anesthetic, a small incision is made, and the pus is evacuated. The cavity is irrigated and an iodoform gauze wick inserted (not packed in). A dressing is applied, and the patient is instructed to remove it and the drain in 24 hours. This is best accomplished during a sitz bath. The patient is seen again in 7 to 10 days, and proctosigmoidoscopic and anoscopic examinations are performed for the probable fistula. As opposed to perianal abscess, an ischiorectal abscess is usually associated with the subsequent identification of a fistula.

Contraindications to Office Drainage

Several factors may contraindicate draining an ischiorectal abscess as an office procedure. First, a general, spinal, or caudal anesthetic may be required because of patient insistence or because the patient is unable to tolerate manipulation associated with a local procedure. In addition, ischiorectal abscesses should not be drained in the office when the patient is febrile. Systemic antibiotics and more vigorous irrigations than are possible with an office procedure may be advisable.

Finally, the surgeon may not have adequate office facilities; contamination of the examining room certainly limits its use for a time.

In-hospital drainage follows essentially the same procedure advocated for office treatment. The incision should be limited, minimal, and medial. Vigorous irrigation with saline or an antiseptic solution is followed by insertion of a small drain or wick. Administration of an anesthetic permits proctosigmoidoscopy and anoscopy, which may help to identify a specific cause for the abscess and localize an internal opening.

A simple way to determine the presence of an internal opening before drainage is to pass an anoscope while compressing the mass. Pus may be seen to exude from the crypt. If an opening is identified, its presence is noted for subsequent definitive treatment, usually in about 2 weeks. I do not advocate fistulotomy of a transsphincteric fistula synchronously with drainage of an ischiorectal abscess.

Antibiotics once started are continued for 48 hours. Although a culture of the pus is usually taken in the operating room, it is rarely of use in treatment. Drainage is the definitive therapy, and the patient almost invariably becomes afebrile within a few hours after the procedure.

Primary Closure

Ellis advocated incision, curettage, and primary suture with antibiotic coverage in the treatment of anorectal abscess.[17, 18] Although he reported excellent results (primary healing took place in the vast majority of cases), one wonders about the likelihood of subsequent fistula development. Wilson reported on 100 of 120 patients so treated and followed for an average of over 2 years.[75] Approximately two thirds of the patients initially had a perianal abscess; the remainder had an ischiorectal abscess. The overall recurrence rate was 22% (15.6% following perianal abscess and 33.3% following ischiorectal abscess). Wilson noted that recurrence was much more likely if the culture initially revealed predominantly *Escherichia coli* than if it yielded *Staphylococcus aureus*. The presence of the former organism might imply communication with the rectum.

Goligher reported a prospective trial of conventional laying open versus incision, curettage, and suture.[25] Patients identified as having an internal opening at the time of drainage were excluded from the study. Healing occurred in over 90% of those treated by primary suture. Because the follow-up period was less than 1 year, the rate of recurrence is difficult to judge.

I have had no experience with this technique, but I am reluctant to use it since I tend to advocate minimal manipulation in effecting drainage; hence, the wound is inevitably quite small.

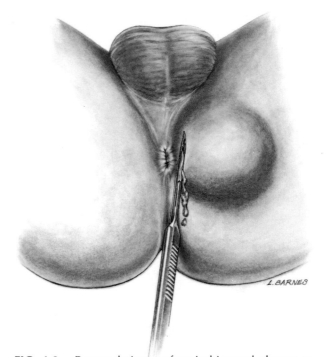

FIG. 4-3. Proper drainage of an ischiorectal abscess requires that the incision be made as medially as possible, not necessarily at the point of maximal fluctuance. This will enable one to avoid a subsequent long fistulotomy incision.

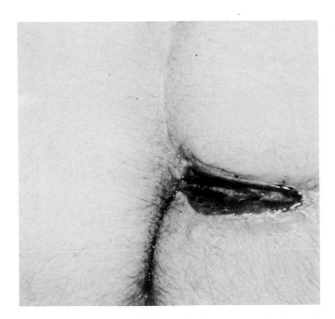

FIG. 4-4. Drainage of a buttock abscess too far laterally will result in a long fistula wound.

Deep Postanal Abscess

A transsphincteric fistula may present as an abscess in the deep postanal space (Fig. 4-5). This space is deep to the superficial external sphincter and inferior to the levator ani muscle. The patient will often complain of severe rectal discomfort. The pain may radiate to the sacrum, coccyx, or buttock, or display a sciatic distribution. It may be exacerbated by sitting. Defecation may be impaired, and a fecal impaction may be present. The symptoms may mimic proctalgia fugax, coccygodynia, or lumbosacral strain. The patient is frequently febrile.

Physical examination may be nonrevealing except for exquisite rectal tenderness posteriorly. A high degree of suspicion is required for early diagnosis and treatment. Very often, however, the diagnosis is missed, and the patient is sent home with instructions concerning sitz baths and perineal exercises and told to take an analgesic. Eventually the abscess presents at the skin or drains spontaneously, clearly establishing the diagnosis.

A patient with posterior rectal pain and tenderness that is of relatively short duration (less than 48 hours), that is continuous rather than intermittent, and that is not affected by position, must be suspected of having an abscess in the deep postanal space. An attempt at aspiration between the rectum and coccyx in the midline may prove diagnostic. If an extrarectal mass is felt, the differential diagnosis includes presacral cyst, teratoma, chordoma, and a host of rare inflammatory and neoplastic conditions.

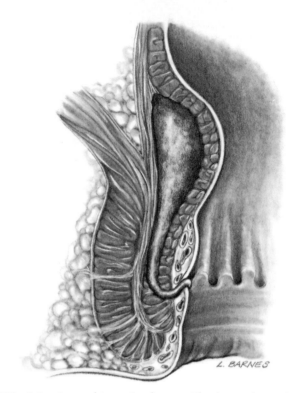

FIG. 4-6. Intersphincteric abscess. The internal opening is at the level of the crypt with cephalad extension in the intermuscular plane.

Treatment requires drainage of the deep postanal space, a procedure that cannot be accomplished adequately with a local anesthetic. Invariably at the time of drainage an internal opening in the posterior midline is identified. Since postanal infections can communicate with the ischiorectal fossa on either side, the patient may present with bilateral ischiorectal abscesses, the so-called horseshoe abscess.

The best access to the deep postanal space in order to effect drainage was initially described by Hanley.[33] He advocated placing a probe into the primary opening in the posterior midline and making an incision over the probe toward the tip of the coccyx. This incision bisects the superficial and subcutaneous external sphincter, and decompresses the cavity. Counterincisions can be made to drain the ischiorectal fossae if necessary. Packing is advised and should be left in place for 48 to 72 hours. I and others have found this to be the optimal method of treating this condition.[1, 31]

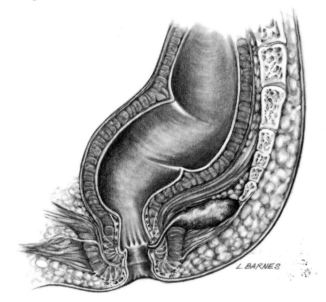

FIG. 4-5. Deep postanal abscess originating from a posterior crypt. Drainage is effected through an incision from the internal opening to the coccyx.

Intersphincteric Abscess

Intersphincteric abscess was initially described by Eisenhammer and subsequently subdivided by him into a high type and a low type.[15, 16] The condition arises from an infected crypt in the anal canal, and the infection burrows cephalad to present as a mass within the lower part of the rectum. It dissects in the intersphincteric and intramuscular plane, *not* under the mucosa, although it is frequently mistakenly called a "submucous" abscess (Fig. 4-6). Intersphincteric abscess is also sometimes classified as a submucous fistula, but this is an improper term because the condition does not fulfill the criterion for the definition of a fistula: a tract between two epithelial surfaces. Intersphincteric abscess represents 2% to 5% of perirectal abscesses.

The patient complains usually of rectal or anal discomfort, which may be exacerbated by defecation. A sense of fullness in the rectum is often felt. Pus or mucous discharge may be noted. The patient may or may not be febrile.

Rectal examination may reveal a tender submucosal mass, which may not be readily apparent by anoscopy or proctosigmoidoscopy. The condition can be confused with thrombosed internal hemorrhoids, but visual examination should distinguish the deep purple or black hemorrhoid from an abscess. The surface is edematous and indurated. An anal fissure is associated with the abscess in about 25% of patients.[58] Pus from the associated crypt leaves no doubt about the nature of the lesion (Fig. 4-7).

Treatment requires a general or spinal anesthetic. A Hill-Ferguson retractor or other appropriate anal retractor is inserted. The abscess is excised through the internal sphincter, removing the associated crypt-bearing area (Fig. 4-8). Finally, the cut edge of the rectum and the underlying internal sphincter are sutured for hemostasis, leaving the wound open for drainage (Fig. 4-9). No packing is required. The patient is discharged, and advised to take a stool softener and sitz baths. Healing usually takes place within 2 to 3 weeks; no further operation is required.

Supralevator Abscess

Supralevator abscess is relatively rare, less than 2.5% of abscesses in most series (see Fig. 4-2, *D*).[7, 11, 26, 36] However, Goldenberg, and Prasad and co-workers, reviewed the Cook County Hospital experience, and found the incidence to be 7.5% and 9.1%, respectively.[24, 59] It is difficult to understand this variation in incidence. The authors attribute their large experience to the low socio-economic status of the patients. Obesity and diabetes mellitus were considered important contributing factors (23%).

Perianal and buttock pain are the commonest presenting complaints. Most patients are febrile and demonstrate a leukocytosis.

In my experience, most patients have a pelvic inflammatory condition (Crohn's disease, diverticulitis, salpingitis) or have had recent abdominal or pelvic

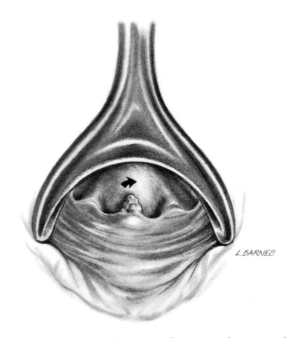

FIG. 4-7. Opening of an intersphincteric abscess at the level of the crypt. Induration *(arrow)* is usually present proximal to this point.

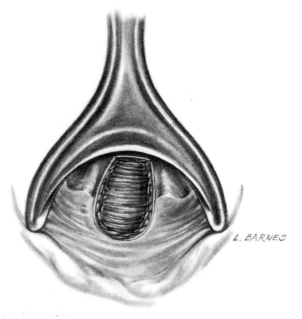

FIG. 4-8. Intersphincteric abscess. The mucosa and the underlying internal sphincter are excised.

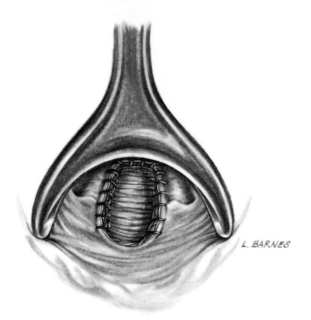

FIG. 4-9. Intersphincteric abscess. The cut mucosal edge with the internal anal sphincter is sutured for hemostasis.

surgery. Parks and Gordon reported a number of cases of perineal fistula that developed secondary to an intra-abdominal process.[56] Supralevator abscess may also occur as an extension of a transsphincteric anal fistula (Fig. 4-10).

The etiology of the abscess determines the therapy: transrectal drainage for abscess from pelvic sepsis and external drainage for abscess secondary to transphincteric fistula. Performing transrectal drainage when an internal opening is present at the level of the crypt is an invitation to disaster. Likewise, draining an abscess to the perineum when a communication is present in the rectum may result in a fecal fistula, and the need for bowel resection or a possible diversionary procedure.

How does one distinguish between the two situations? The history may be helpful (*e.g.*, knowledge that the patient has Crohn's disease, or has undergone recent abdominal surgery). More important, however, is evaluation under an anesthetic for the presence of an internal opening at the level of the crypt. If one is found, the drainage procedure should be external; if absent, drainage probably should be internal (see Fig. 4-10).

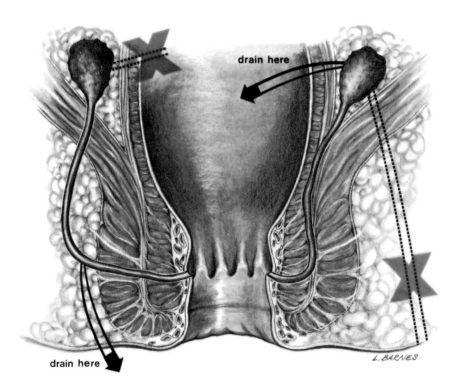

drain here

drain here

FIG. 4-10. Methods of drainage for supralevator abscess. **A.** Perineal drainage secondary to transsphincteric fistula. **B.** Transrectal drainage from pelvic sepsis.

Treatment

For internal drainage, the patient is placed in the prone position if the abscess is anterior, or in the lithotomy position if the abscess is posterior.

After aspiration, an incision is made either sharply with a knife or bluntly with a Kelly clamp into the cavity (Fig. 4-11). A Pezzer (mushroom) or Foley catheter is inserted into the cavity and delivered through the anal verge. The opening is made small enough for the catheter to remain without the need for suturing (Fig. 4-12). Other modifications of this technique are to place a cut piece of rubber catheter though the tip of another to hold it in place, or to use a T tube. The drain is removed in 48 hours.

In women, whenever possible an anterior abscess should be drained transvaginally through the posterior cul-de-sac. Drainage is technically easier to perform,

and the patient is more comfortable. If the intact anal sphincter is avoided, more adequate drainage can be accomplished.

If external drainage is deemed appropriate, the patient is placed in the prone (jackknife) position. A larger external wound is required than for other abscesses because it is imperative to drain the supralevator collection adequately. The location of the incision should be as medial as possible. The supralevator space should be packed or a Foley or mushroom catheter should be placed in the cavity, and should remain in place for 72 hours. Irrigation through the catheter is also advisable. In the series of Prasad and associates, primary fistulotomy was performed in two thirds of patients who were found to have concurrent fistulas.[59] In my opinion, however, definitive fistula surgery should be undertaken on a subsequent hospitalization.

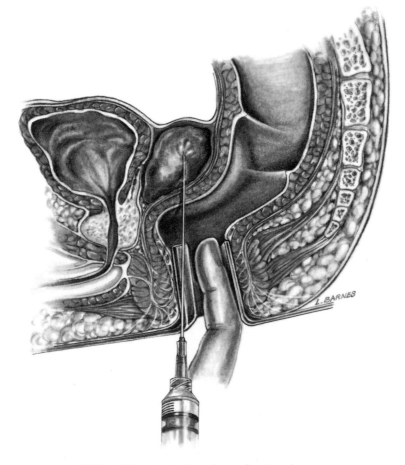

FIG. 4-11. Aspiration of supralevator abscess.

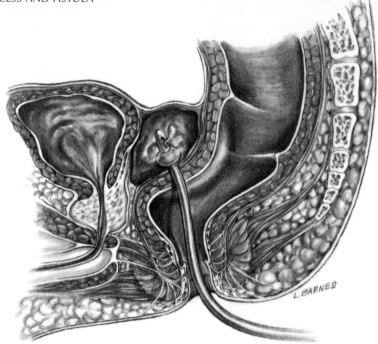

FIG. 4-12. A catheter is inserted into the supralevator abscess cavity to maintain adequate drainage.

Necrotizing Infections

Anorectal abscess can eventuate in severe necrotizing infection and death.[7, 9, 46] Perineal gas gangrene (Fournier's disease) can also develop.[43] Delay in diagnosis and treatment (a week or more in most cases) and associated diseases (diabetes, obesity, malignancy, tuberculosis) are causative factors (Fig. 4-13). Treatment requires antibiotics, nutritional support, wide debridement, adequate drainage, and frequently colostomy.

Anal Infections in Hematologic Diseases

Abscess and fistula are not uncommonly seen in patients with hematologic abnormalities (leukemia, granulocytopenia, lymphoma).[40, 65, 67, 72] The incidence in granulocytopenia has been reported to be 11%.[72] Half of the patients died within 1 month of diagnosis, most from septic complications.

Patients present with fever and pain. Conservative treatment (antibiotics, sitz baths, and radiotherapy) is advocated for patients with leukemia if the disease is under poor control. Surgical drainage under such circumstances may result in fulminant sepsis and death. Drainage should be performed, however, if the patient is in remission.

ANAL FISTULA

More surgeons' reputations have been impugned because of problems with fistula operations than from any other operative procedure. Complications of fistulectomy are myriad, and include fecal soilage, mucous discharge, anal incontinence, and recurrent abscess and fistula. The surgeon who initially has the opportunity to treat the patient is the one most likely to effect cure without creating subsequent difficulties.

Symptoms

The commonest presenting complaints of anal fistula are swelling, pain, and discharge. The former two symptoms usually are associated with abscess when the external or secondary opening has closed. Discharge may be from the external opening or may be reported by the patient as mucus or pus mixed with the stool. The majority of patients have an antecedent history of abscess.

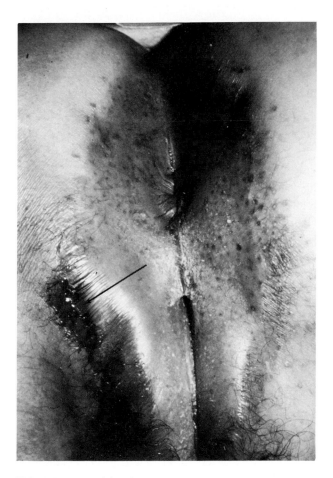

FIG. 4-13. Anal fistula *(arrow)* in a patient with diabetes. Note the severe pruritic changes. (Courtesy of Daniel Rosenthal, M.D.)

Anal fistula may be confused with suppurative hydradenitis and pilonidal sinus, which are discussed in Chapter 8 (Dermatologic Anal Conditions).

Classification

Four types of fistulas are described by most authors: submucous (see Fig. 4-6), intersphincteric (Fig. 4-14), transsphincteric (Fig. 4-15), and extrasphincteric (Fig. 4-16). The submucous fistula is a misnomer and has been described in the section on abscess.

How does one identify the type of fistula, the course of the tract, and the location of the internal opening? The two basic procedures used in the office are the application of Goodsall's rule[28] and careful physical examination, including probing of the tract.

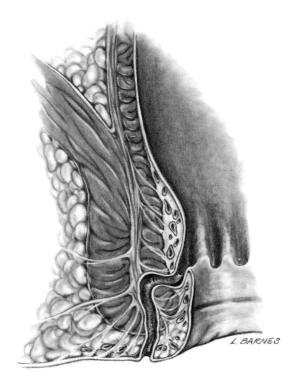

FIG. 4-14. Intersphincteric fistula. The tract passes through the internal sphincter and in the intersphincteric plane.

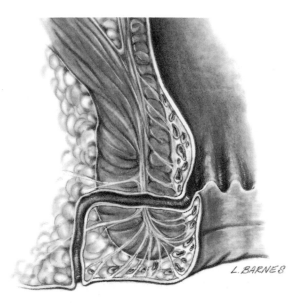

FIG. 4-15. Transsphincteric fistula. The tract passes through both the internal and external sphincters, into the ischiorectal fossa, and thence to the skin.

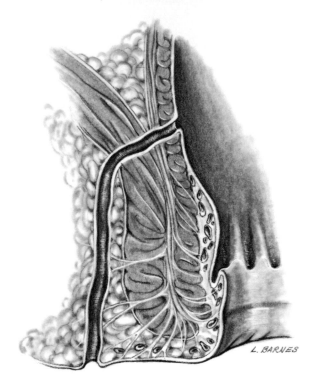

FIG. 4-16. Extrasphincteric fistula. The internal opening is above the level of the levator ani muscle, and the tract passes to the skin deep to the external sphincter.

Goodsall's Rule

When the external opening lies anterior to the transverse plane, the internal opening tends to be located radially. Conversely, when the external opening lies posterior to the plane, the internal opening is usually located in the posterior midline (Fig. 4-17). There is some controversy over the reason for this, but it may result from a defect in fusion of the longitudinal muscle and the external sphincter in the posterior midline. A transsphincteric fistula is, therefore, more likely to occur here; the tract can then dissect into one or both ischiorectal fossae.

Although the rule is relatively consistent, exceptions are occasionally seen. Accordingly, it should be used as a guide to help the surgeon find the tract when it may not be apparent. It is not a substitute for meticulous technique, and clear identification of the direction of the tract and the location of the internal opening.

Most commonly, fistulas pass in the intersphincteric plane, but with transsphincteric fistulas, multiple openings can develop from the deep postanal space and from the ischiorectal fossa; this is the etiology of the so-called horseshoe fistula.

Physical Examination

Careful palpation may reveal the thickened tract proceeding into the anal canal if it is in a relatively superficial location. This finding is most characteristic of an intersphincteric fistula. Failure to identify the tract by palpation implies that it may be deep and more likely to be a transsphincteric fistula. Anoscopic examination may reveal purulent material exuding from the base of the crypt. By gentle probing with a crypt hook or malleable probe (Fig. 4-18), the presence of the tract may be confirmed. This maneuver is easier to accomplish for a radially located fistula than for one that opens in the posterior midline. Occasionally, the tract will pass subcutaneously for a considerable distance: into the perineum, scrotum, labia, and thigh (Fig. 4-19). Failure to identify the internal opening does not mean that it has closed, however. Angulation or narrowing of the tract may make it impossible to follow it into the anal canal without causing considerable discomfort to the patient. Under these circumstances examination under an anesthetic is required.

Principles of Surgical Treatment

The surgeon who first treats the patient has the best opportunity to identify the tract, find the opening, and cure the patient. When this is not accomplished in the first instance, further surgery may be more complex, and the patient will be exposed to potentially serious complications.

Failure to cure the patient is usually the result of timorousness or temerity. If the surgeon traces the tract

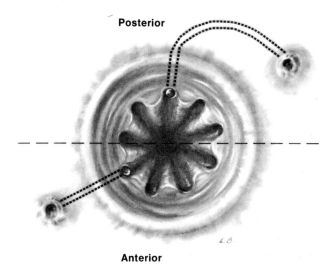

FIG. 4-17. Typical course of fistula tracts according to Goodsall's rule.

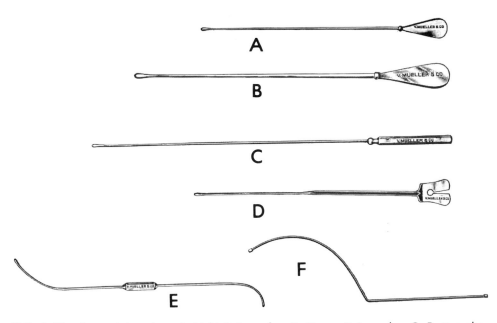

FIG. 4-18. Anorectal probes. **A.** Light Buie probe. **B.** Heavy Buie probe. **C.** Pratt probe. **D.** Larry Probe. **E.** Barr probe. **F.** Earle probe. (Courtesy of American V. Mueller)

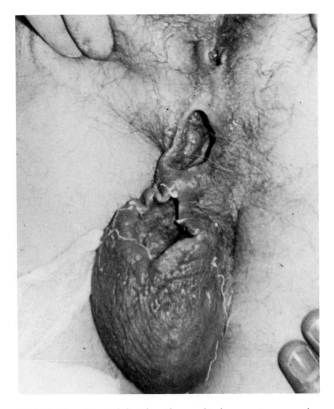

FIG. 4-19. Scrotal fistula. The multiple openings are due to extensive subcutaneous tracking. Although on cursory examination the fistula may appear to be difficult to treat, the tract is usually quite superficial.

from the external opening to the level of the crypt, but cannot pass the probe into the anal canal and subsequently desists from excising the crypt-bearing area, he is being too timid. In this situation it is reasonable to assume that the crypt opening has sealed and that it was the source of the fistula. Alternatively, if the surgeon identified the internal opening, but is reluctant to lay it open because of the fear that it is ''too high,'' he jeopardizes the opportunity to alleviate the condition and to cure the patient. The fistula will recur, and the subsequent procedure will be performed without the security of knowing that the internal opening occurred naturally. With rare exception, in the initial operation, if the patient does not have Crohn's disease or some other specific cause for the fistula (trauma, for example), the surgeon should be able to open the tract without fear of causing incontinence. If question exists about the level of the internal opening, a seton can be employed (see Extrasphincteric Fistula, Seton Division).

Conversely, if the tract has not been identified to the level of the crypt, and the surgeon elects to guess where the opening should be and creates an artificial internal opening, he is being too aggressive. The opening and the tract may have been missed completely. When operating for recurrence after such a procedure, both the natural and the artificial internal openings must be considered.

Identification of Fistula Tract

Several methods can be employed to identify a fistula tract.

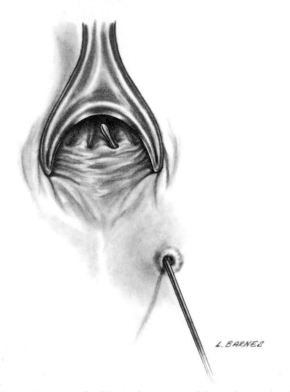

Passing a Probe

Passage of a probe should be attempted from both the external and the internal aspects. Sometimes it is easier to identify the tract from the internal opening, but usually probing the external one will reveal the course. Simultaneous passage of two probes (from the internal and the external openings) may confirm the tract's location when the tips of the probes touch. A stenotic area within the tract may preclude complete passage from either end. The probe should never be forced, only gently maneuvered (Fig. 4-20).

Injection of Dye

If a substance such as methylene blue or indigo carmine is injected through the tract, the dye may appear in the rectum and confirm the patency of the tract and its communication with an internal opening. The problem with this technique is that the surgeon may have only one opportunity to visualize the internal opening before the material stains every bit of tissue. Therefore, I do not recommend this approach.

Injection of Milk

Milk can be used to identify the tract and the internal opening. Sterility is not required. A Marx needle is used to inject the milk while an anoscope is in position in the rectum (Fig. 4-21). The milk can be wiped away

FIG. 4-20. A malleable probe is passed from the external to the internal openings, confirming the course of the tract.

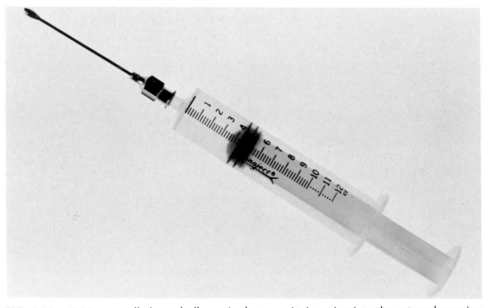

FIG. 4-21. A Marx needle has a bulbous tip that permits insertion into the external opening without penetrating the wall of the tract.

without staining the tissue, and the internal opening can be identified. Failure to demonstrate communication with the internal opening implies stenosis of the tract, but if the milk is seen in the submucosa of the anal canal, even without escape into the lumen, the associated crypt-bearing area can be safely excised.

Injection of Hydrogen Peroxide

Hydrogen peroxide injection is probably the best means for identifying the internal opening. The liberated oxygen can be seen bubbling through the internal opening. The pressure created by the oxygen may be sufficient to penetrate even a stenotic tract and pass into the anal canal. Obviously, staining of the tissue does not occur.

Comment

The aforementioned injection techniques confirm the presence of the fistula and the internal opening. They do not, however, identify the course of the tract itself. If a probe can be passed it is only necessary to incise down onto it. However, if this cannot be accomplished, the dissection must be carried out slowly and meticulously, following the epithelialized tract until it communicates with the anal canal.

A fistula operation should always be performed using an electrocautery. Identification of the tract requires a dry operative field. In such a vascular area no better means can be found for maintaining hemostasis than by this technique.

Fistulotomy Versus Fistulectomy

Whether to perform fistulectomy or fistulotomy is a commonly asked question. I do not believe that the tract should be excised completely, because this often creates a large, gaping wound that requires a prolonged healing time (Fig. 4-22). A fistulotomy is usually adequate, but a small portion of the tract should be removed for pathologic examination, especially to rule out Crohn's disease.

Office Fistulotomy

Office fistulotomy may be undertaken synchronously with drainage of an abscess if the internal opening is low-lying or of the intersphincteric type. It may also be performed in the office as an interval procedure after abscess drainage. For the vast majority of patients, however, definitive fistula surgery should be performed in the operating room under general, spinal, or caudal anesthesia.

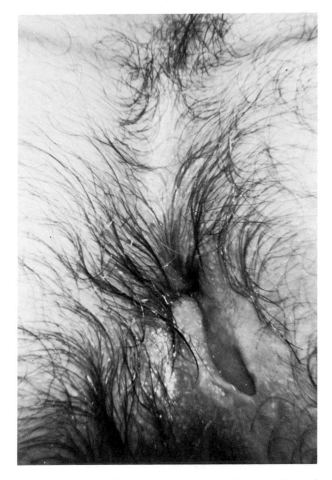

FIG. 4-22. Anal fistulectomy may require a prolonged healing time. This wound is still open 6 weeks following the operation.

Surgical Techniques

Conventional Fistula. After the external and internal openings have been identified by one of the means mentioned, the tract is incised (Fig. 4-23). Continuity of the epithelial lining confirms the completeness of the operation. Granulation tissue is removed by curettage. A portion of the tract is excised and sent for pathologic examination. The external portion of the incision is widened relative to the size of the opening in the anal canal, because skin tends to heal more rapidly than does the anal mucosa. If this is not performed properly, delayed healing of the anal canal may result. The cut edges of the anal mucosa and the underlying internal anal sphincter are oversewn for

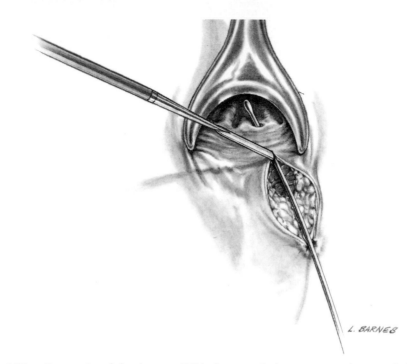

FIG. 4-23. Conventional fistulotomy. With the use of electrocautery the tract is laid open between the internal and external openings.

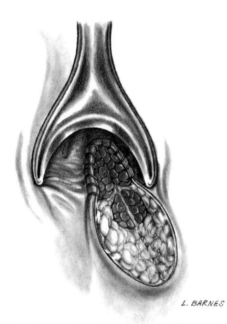

FIG. 4-24. Conventional fistulotomy. The anal opening with the underlying internal sphincter is sutured for hemostasis.

hemostasis (Fig. 4-24). The wound is otherwise left open and gently packed. A vaseline gauze is preferred because subsequent removal is less likely to induce bleeding.

To reiterate, the principles of operative treatment are to identify the tract, incise the tract, excise the specimen for biopsy material, widen the external wound, and suture the cut edge of the anal canal. The dressing is removed that evening or the next day, and sitz baths are commenced. An office visit is recommended approximately 10 days later, and then every 2 weeks until healing has taken place.

This technique is applicable to virtually all intersphincteric fistulas and most transsphincteric fistulas. Occasionally, however, supralevator extension of a transsphincteric fistula is found (Fig. 4-25). Treatment requires recognition of this entity, curettage, irrigation, and packing of the supralevator extension. Under no circumstances should the extension be drained into the rectum.

Horseshoe Fistula. Horseshoe fistula is a type of transsphincteric fistula. It is so called because it is composed of multiple external openings joined by a subcutaneous communication in a U or horseshoe shape. The arms of the U are directed anteriorly, and the internal opening is in the posterior midline. Rarely, a horseshoe fistula may present with the opposite con-

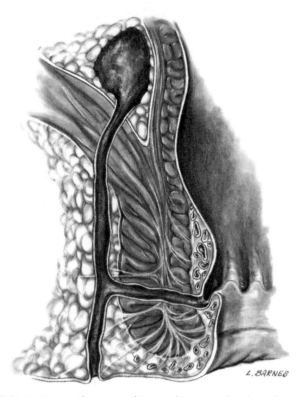

FIG. 4-25. In the case of transsphincteric fistula with su-pralevator extension, drainage of the extension into the rectum is contraindicated.

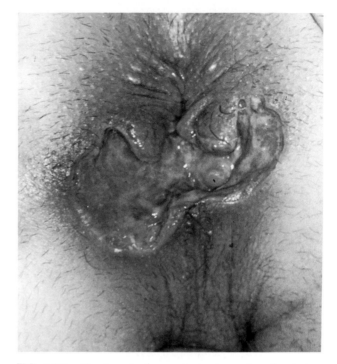

FIG. 4-26. Treatment of an anterior horseshoe fistula by the classical technique leaves a large, gaping wound that requires a prolonged time to heal.

figuration, that is, the internal opening is in the anterior midline, and the arms of the U are directed posteriorly.

Treatment of this condition has evolved to be much less radical than had often been described. The classic procedure required identification of the tracts and internal opening, and unroofing or excision of each of them. This resulted in a huge, gaping wound, which required a prolonged healing time (Fig. 4-26). Disability after this operation can last for many months.

I no longer advocate this method for treating horseshoe fistula. Friend and Hanley observed that the most important aspect of any fistula operation is to excise the internal opening into the deep postanal space and to establish adequate drainage.[21, 33] If the internal opening has been removed, the external openings will heal when adequate drainage has been established.

The tracts and openings of a horseshoe anal fistula are illustrated in Figure 4-27. The deep postanal space must be entered, curetted, and irrigated. It is then only necessary to unroof the external openings, curette out the tracts, and drain (Fig. 4-28). The cut edges of the anal canal and underlying internal sphincter are sutured for hemostasis. The deep postanal space is packed with iodoform gauze and a dressing is applied.

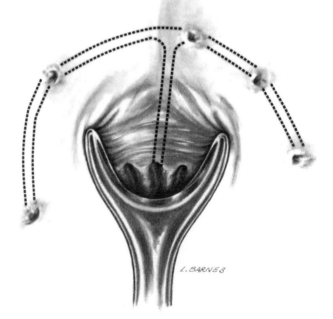

FIG. 4–27. Diagrammatic representation of a horseshoe anal fistula. The internal opening is in the posterior midline.

When the fistula is approached in this way, healing is rapid, and the risk of functional impairment to the anus from scarring and deformity is lessened considerably. Length of disability is markedly reduced.

Extrasphincteric Fistula.   When the internal opening is thought to lie above the levators (Figs. 4-16 and 4-29), division of the tract may result in fecal incontinence. If the puborectalis sling is completely divided, anal incontinence will certainly ensue. When diagnosis is in doubt, a seton can be employed. This involves placing a heavy suture through the tract and out the anal canal. The thread may be passed through the eye of the probe to permit insertion. The suture is loosely tied, and no further procedure is undertaken at this time.

When the patient is alert, rectal examination is performed. While the patient alternately tightens and relaxes the sphincter, the seton can be felt to be above or below the levators. If it is below, a fistulotomy can be performed safely. Conversely, if the internal opening is above the levators an alternative procedure must be undertaken. A number of possible operative approaches exist for the treatment of extrasphincteric fistula.

Seton Division.   The principle involved in the use of the seton as a *therapeutic* tool is analogous to that of a wire cutting through a block of ice. The ice is still adherent after division by the wire. Theoretically, by

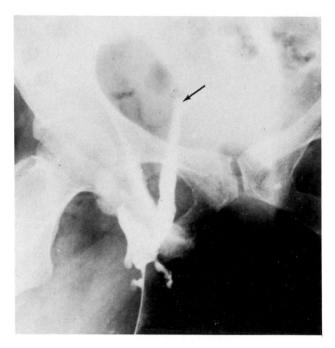

FIG. 4-29.   Fistulogram of an extrasphincteric fistula. The tract enters the rectum at the level of the arrow.

tightening the suture and permitting it to cut through over a number of days, the resultant inflammatory response keeps the sphincter muscle from retracting and separating.

If a seton is employed, the skin and anal canal mucosa between the openings must be excised and the suture then passed (Fig. 4-30, *A*). I prefer doubled number 2 silk, but another alternative is to use elastic bands. The seton is securely tied, usually with maximum tension (Fig. 4-30, *B*).

The patient is discharged after bowel function has been restored, and he is re-examined 1 week later. By this time the suture has either loosened or has passed by necrosing through the tissue (usually the former). It is then a relatively simple matter to change the seton by injecting a local anesthetic into the sphincter and securely tying it again. If an elastic band has been used, it can be twisted or stretched and tied. Two weeks later the seton has usually eroded out. If not, the fistulotomy can be completed in the office, because little tissue usually remains to be divided. If the surgeon prefers, a third insertion can be performed. This technique was described by Hippocrates but is still applicable for the difficult fistula problem. It is certainly the simplest of the methods available for the treatment of extrasphincteric fistula.

Fistulotomy with Sphincter Repair.   Complete excision of an extrasphincteric fistula is a hazardous undertaking. Although direct repair is performed imme-

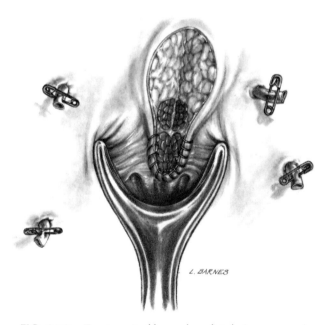

FIG. 4-28.   Treatment of horseshoe fistula-in-ano requires unroofing in the posterior midline to adequately drain the deep postanal space. The external openings are individually drained with curettage only of the underlying tracts.

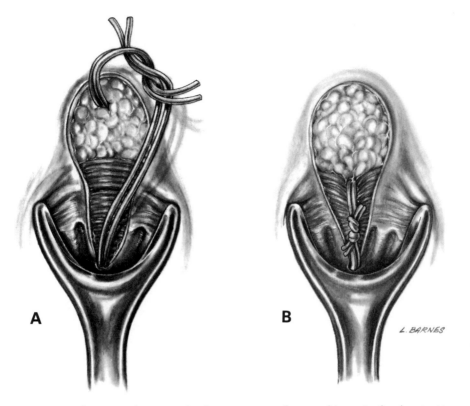

FIG. 4-30.   Application of a seton in the treatment of extrasphincteric fistula. **A.** Heavy sutures (silk is preferred) are passed through the external and internal openings. **B.** The sutures are firmly secured.

diately, breakdown is common. It should be considered, however, as an alternative technique for the treatment of high-level fistulas.

The entire tract between the external and the internal openings is divided. The epithelial lining is excised and the wound irrigated. A layered closure is performed using polyglycolic acid sutures, closing the rectal wall and reconstructing the sphincter muscles. The ischiorectal fossa is widely drained externally. A colostomy is advisable.

This operation is usually reserved for patients who have had multiple failed attempts at repair. It is a difficult procedure and should be performed by someone with specialized knowledge of anorectal anatomy and with experience in complex fistula surgery.

Closure of Internal Opening and Drainage of Extrasphincteric Tract.   Closure of the internal opening and drainage of the extrasphincteric tract is less destructive of tissue than the former repair, but it too is technically difficult to perform. The procedure involves debridement and closure of the internal opening through a transanal approach. External drainage is widely established and the supralevator area vigorously

curetted, irrigated, and packed (Fig. 4-31). A concurrent colostomy is indicated. This procedure is less likely to cause further harm, and, therefore, theoretically is preferred to the potentially destructive operation previously mentioned.

Other Techniques.   Other approaches that can be used to treat an extrasphincteric fistula include low anterior resection, abdominosacral resection, and transsacral excision. Sometimes a diverting colostomy alone will permit spontaneous healing. When the patient has minimal symptoms, expectant management (using a small dressing and sitz baths), draining an abscess when it occurs, and perhaps even inserting a small drain in the tract (suturing it into place for a prolonged time) may offer adequate palliation.

Results

It is difficult to evaluate the results of treatment for anal fistula because so much depends on the individual surgeon's technique and the type of fistula encountered. The three primary criteria for determining success or failure in fistula surgery are recurrence, delayed healing, and incontinence.

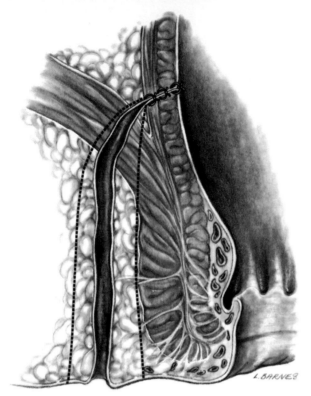

FIG. 4-31. Treatment of extrasphincteric fistula by closure of the internal opening, and wide drainage of the supra-levator space and ischiorectal fossa, as indicated by the broken line.

Parks and Stitz reviewed 158 patients treated by the senior author over a 15-year period.[57] Follow-up was available in 142 patients for over 1 year. There were 12 recurrences (9%) and 10 fistulas that were unhealed (7%). The recurrences were noted with all types of fistulas, all but two of which healed with reoperation. The authors also evaluated bowel control in their patients and found that 17% who had an intersphincteric fistula had difficulty with flatus or occasional soiling. One third of those with transsphincteric fistulas reported one or the other complaint. No patient in either group was truly incontinent. However, 2 of 13 patients who had extrasphincteric fistulas were incontinent. Kuypers reported an overall recurrence rate of 4%, and a 10% incidence of some control difficulty.[41] Bennett noted in 114 patients that 12% had inadequate control for feces, 16% had poor flatus control, and 24% had frequent soiling of their underclothes.[6] Thirty-six percent of patients complained of one or more of the above problems. Adams and Kovalcik reported an overall recurrence rate of 4% in 133 patients.[2]

Hill followed 476 patients for up to 20 years.[36] Delayed wound healing occurred in only 7; 4 experienced recurrence and 19 experienced varying degrees of control difficulties.

Hanley and co-workers reported their results in 41 patients with horseshoe fistula.[34] There was no problem with healing, recurrence, or incontinence using the technique previously described. Hamilton, using the same approach, reported 4 recurrences in 57 patients.[31]

Treatment of defects in the skin following fistula operations by means of skin grafting was described rather unenthusiastically by Wilson.[76] I prefer to employ advancement or rotation flaps when scarring produces sufficient symptoms to warrant anoplasty (see Chap. 6). The methods of sphincter reconstruction to correct problems with fecal incontinence are discussed in Chapter 5.

Dual Anal Fistulas

A patient may rarely present with two anal fistulas, each with separate external and internal openings. Mazier noted an incidence of approximately 2% of 1000 patients who presented with anal fistulas, and Hill reported 27 patients with more than one fistula in a total of 626 patients (4%).[36, 49]

The treatment of simultaneous low-lying fistulas consists of identifying the external and internal openings and performing a fistulotomy in the standard fashion. This condition should be distinguished from horseshoe fistula; the latter becomes obvious by careful delineation of the tracts and the internal openings.[53]

Anal Fistula in Crohn's Disease

In our experience anal fissures, fistulas, and abscesses occurred as complications in 22% of 1098 patients with Crohn's disease.[74] Alexander-Williams found that half of his patients with anal fistula and Crohn's disease had no symptom.[3] When anal fistula occurs as a complication of this condition, it is important to distinguish between anal Crohn's disease with fistula, and Crohn's disease of the intestinal tract with no anal disease and a coincidental fistula-in-ano. This distinction is important because the fistula procedure can be performed with relative safety in a patient who has Crohn's disease and in whom the disease does not involve the anus or anal canal, provided that the abdominal condition is quiescent. Any fistula procedure that is performed in the presence of active inflammatory bowel disease, however, is a hazardous undertaking, because the resultant wound may be a greater management problem than was the original condition (Fig. 4-32).

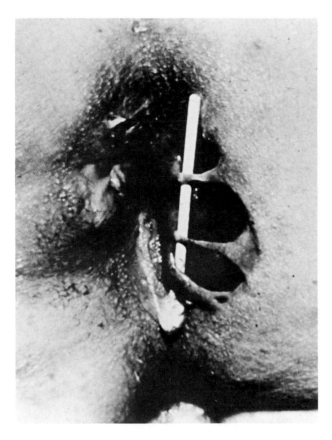

FIG. 4-32. Indolent, ulcerating wound resulting from an ill-conceived fistulectomy in a patient with Crohn's disease. (Corman ML et al: Diseases of the Anus, Rectum and Colon. Part II: Inflammatory Bowel Disease. New York, Medcom, 1976)

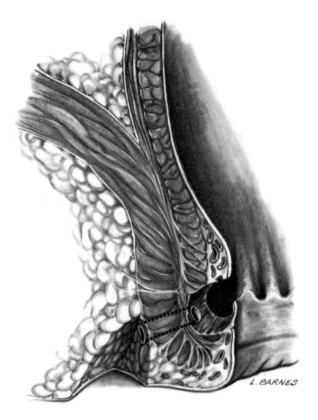

FIG. 4-33. Treatment of a fistula in the presence of anal Crohn's disease. The internal opening and a portion of the internal sphincter are excised *(arrow)*. The external opening has been adequately drained. The dotted lines indicate a fistula tract through the external sphincter; this is *not* incised.

In the presence of known anal Crohn's, however, it may be possible to ameliorate the patient's condition and relieve the discomfort associated with anal abscess and fistula.

One of the most effective ways, albeit aggressive, of treating patients with this complication is to establish adequate drainage of the internal opening. This is best accomplished by excising the internal opening and the underlying internal anal sphincter in the same manner described for the treatment of intersphincteric abscess. The external opening can then be unroofed, and drainage can be established between the external sphincter and the external opening (Fig. 4-33). This is not a conventional fistulotomy but is a complete drainage of the fistula on either side of the external sphincter. However, since this lesion frequently heralds the onset of intestinal manifestations, the most prudent course of action is usually to merely incise and drain the abscess when it becomes symptomatic.

Anal Fistula and Carcinoma

Rarely, carcinoma can develop in a chronic anal fistula (Figs. 4-34 and 4-35). Getz and associates reported 2 cases and noted less than 150 in the literature.[14, 22, 39, 60] Millar reported three cases of villous tumors arising in anal fistulas.[52] Long-standing, chronic inflammation is felt to lead to the malignant degeneration.

Differential diagnosis includes anal canal carcinoma with fistula (epidermoid, cloacogenic), carcinoma of the rectum with fistula, and carcinoma arising in an anal duct.[20, 22]

Treatment usually requires abdominoperineal resection.

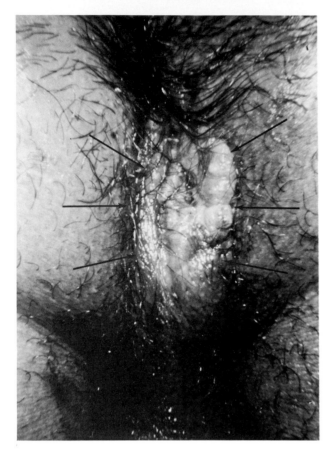

FIG. 4-34. Adenocarcinoma arising in an anal fistula. (Courtesy of Daniel Rosenthal, M.D.)

RECTOVAGINAL FISTULA

Rectovaginal fistula is not a manifestation of fistula-in-ano because it is not a result of cryptoglandular infection. The condition occurs most commonly following trauma, especialy obstetric injury. Other etiologic factors are inflammatory bowel disease (Fig. 4-36), carcinoma, radiation, diverticulitis, hysterectomy (especially vaginal), and perineal septic processes.

Symptoms and Signs

Patients complain of passage of flatus, feces, or pus from the vagina. Depending on the etiology, location, and extent of the problem, the woman may also have difficulty with the control of flatus and feces.

Physical examination should include both rectal and vaginal evaluation. I prefer to categorize the fistula on the basis of three locations: anal, low rectal, and high rectal. If one is a gynecologist, the equivalent classification would be low, mid-, and high vaginal. The location of the fistula is important because it will determine the operative approach necessary.

A low fistula is usually readily apparent on inspection or anoscopy. One usually has little difficulty in identifying the tract and passing a probe. A mid-rectal (mid-vaginal) fistula is also relatively easily identified, particularly in passing the probe from vagina to rectum. A high fistula may be quite difficult to visualize, especially if the opening is small. This type of fistula is usually a complication of diverticulitis or hysterectomy. Proctosigmoidoscopic examination rarely will demonstrate the opening, but gentle probing at the apex of the vagina will often identify the defect. Barium enema examination will frequently show opacification of the vagina (Fig. 4-37).

If the patient's symptoms are characteristic, but the surgeon is unable to confirm a fistula by one of the above means, there are two other approaches worth

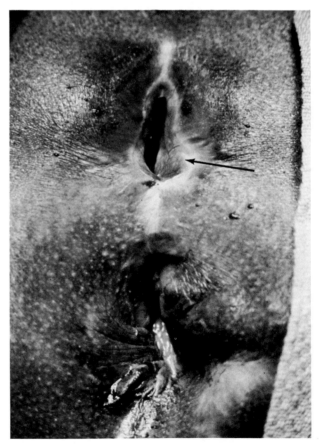

FIG. 4-35. Squamous cell carcinoma *(arrow)* in a 4-year-old fistula. (Courtesy of Daniel Rosenthal, M.D.)

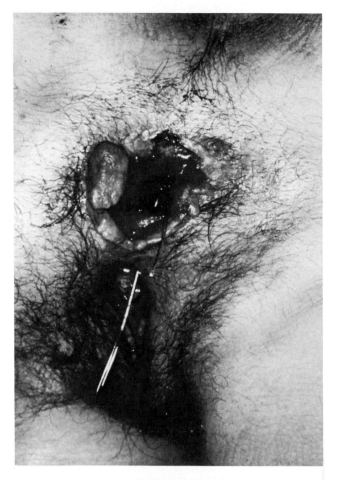

FIG. 4-36. Rectovaginal fistula secondary to Crohn's disease.

attempting. One procedure is to place the patient in the lithotomy position and insert a proctoscope in the rectum. With the patient in a slight Trendelenberg position, the vagina is filled with warm water. Air is then insufflated through the proctoscope; if bubbles are seen in the vagina, the diagnosis is confirmed. Another alternative is to give the patient a methylene blue small retention enema, and leave a tampon in the vagina. The tampon is removed after an hour to see if the blue color appears on it.

Treatment

General Principles

As suggested, the treatment of rectovaginal fistula depends on the location and the etiology. High rectovaginal fistulas are approached transabdominally and involve a bowel resection if colon or rectal disease precipitated the communication. If secondary to hysterectomy, it may suffice to separate the bowel from the vagina, close the opening, and interpose omentum, a peritoneal flap, or fascia. For mid- and low rectovaginal fistulas, a number of operative approaches have been advocated: transvaginal, perineal, transanal, transsphincteric, and transsacral (transcoccygeal). One operation that should not be done, even for anovaginal fistulas, is simple fistulotomy. Dividing the perineum, even for relatively superficial fistulas, will usually cause some degree of impairment of fecal control.[63]

All patients should be placed on a bowel preparation as if for colon resection; this includes a vigorous laxative 1 day before and a tap water enema the morning of surgery until the returns are clear. Neomycin and

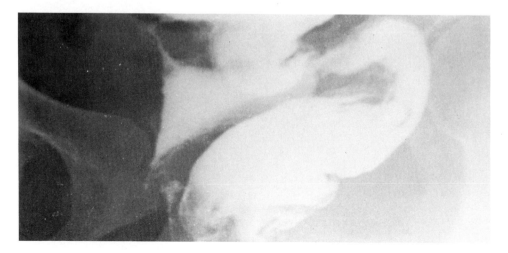

FIG. 4-37. Rectovaginal fistula following hysterectomy. A barium enema demonstrates contrast material in the vagina.

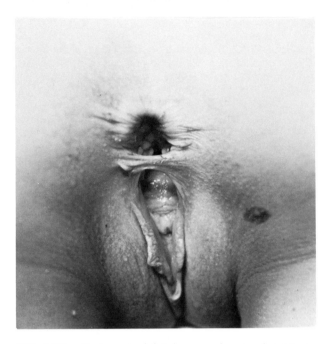

FIG. 4-38. Rectovaginal fistula secondary to obstetric injury. Note the ectopic (anterior) displacement of the rectum.

erythromycin, 1 g each, are given at 1:00 P.M., 2:00 P.M., and 10:00 P.M. the day before the operation. A broad-spectrum perioperative antibiotic is also advisable. A Foley catheter should be inserted before surgery and kept in place until the perineum is reasonably comfortable.

Technique

Any attempt at repair must primarily address the rectal opening, even though the fistula may have arisen from a vaginal source (*e.g.*, from obstetric trauma). Many surgeons prefer to repair a rectovaginal fistula by the transvaginal approach. This is not recommended, since the high-pressure zone is in the rectum. If the repair of the rectal opening is satisfactorily accomplished, it is not even necessary to deal with the vagina. Conversely, no matter how meticulous the technique is when performed through the vagina, if the rectal closure does not remain secure, failure will result.

In the low or mid-vaginal fistula secondary to trauma my own preference is to perform a perineal operation with a concomitant anoplasty and sphincteroplasty. The reason why I believe this is necessary is that the condition is usually the result of an ectopic location (anterior displacement of the rectum); that is, the rectum is too close to the vagina (Fig. 4-38). Many

of these patients have significant impairment for the control of feces even if they do not have a rectovaginal fistula. In order to effect a satisfactory repair, it is necessary to reconstruct the perineal body, and to accomplish this an anoplasty is required.

The patient is placed in the prone (jackknife) position. A cruciate incision is made across the perineal body (Fig. 4-39), and full-thickness flaps of skin are developed. A Hill-Ferguson retractor is kept in place in the anal canal for the entire operation in order to maintain adequacy of the lumen while the muscle repair is completed. The rectovaginal septum is infiltrated with 0.5% lidocaine in 1:200,000 epinephrine. This aids in hemostasis and facilitates the dissection. The rectum is separated from the vagina, and the fistula tract is divided. The cephalad limit is reached, and a plication of the levator ani muscle is carried out anterior to the rectum. This reefing usually requires three or four 0-Dexon sutures. The redundant mucosa is excised from the vagina and the rectum (Fig. 4-40). The external sphincter muscle is reapproximated using the same suture material. Sometimes it is rather difficult to identify residual external sphincter, but there is usually fibrous tissue that can be used to build up the perineal body. The final step in the operation is to advance and interdigitate the two triangular flaps of skin (Fig. 4-41). The skin is mobile enough so that the suture line will ac-

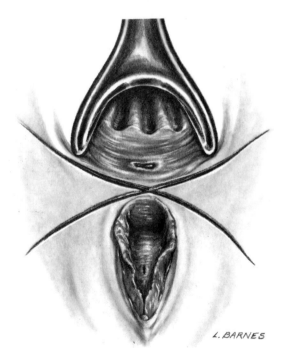

L. BARNES

FIG. 4-39. Rectovaginal fistula repair. A cruciate incision is made across the perineum.

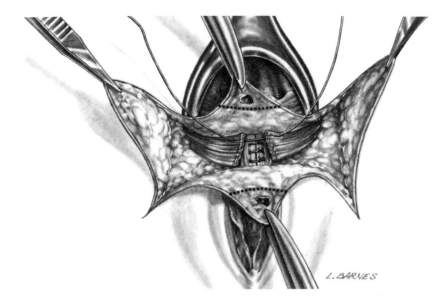

FIG. 4-40. Rectovaginal fistula repair. The levator ani muscle has been plicated. The redundant mucosa and fistula are excised.

tually be within the anal canal and within the vagina in the midline (Fig. 4-42). A Jackson-Pratt drain is placed under the skin and brought out through a stab wound in the buttock. The drain is removed in 48 to 72 hours.

Postoperatively, the patient is placed on a bowel-confining regimen; this consists of a clear liquid diet and codeine (60 mg), Lomotil (2 tablets), and deodorized tincture of opium (15 drops), each four times daily. The wounds are cleansed thrice daily with a topical antiseptic solution. After 5 days, the medications are discontinued, and a regular diet is instituted.

Results

I reported 21 women who underwent rectovaginal reconstruction (sphincteroplasty and anoplasty) after sustaining obstetric injury.[13] All patients had varying degrees of incontinence for flatus or for feces. Most wore a pad. Five patients had an associated rectovaginal fistula. All had the deformity consistent with anterior or ectopic displacement of the anus.

Following reconstruction, all patients had their incontinence problems considerably ameliorated. All were continent for feces and all the fistulas remained healed.

Although rectovaginal fistula is an uncommon complication of vaginal delivery, the obstetrician should be wary of performing episiotomy in the midline if the woman is recognized to have the rectum close to the vagina.

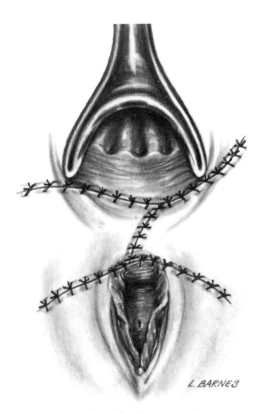

FIG. 4-41. Rectovaginal fistula repair. The two triangular flaps are transposed. The effect is to displace the rectum farther from the vagina.

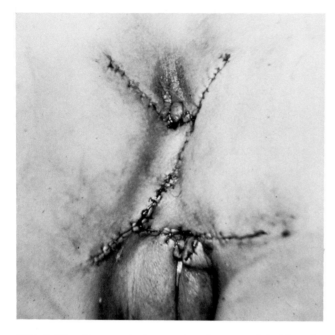

FIG. 4-42.   Rectovaginal reconstruction completed by advancement of the skin flaps. The distance between the anus and the vagina is normal. Compare this with preoperative Fig. 4-38.

Other Techniques and Results

Many other approaches to the treatment of rectovaginal fistula have been described.[5, 8, 23, 30, 35, 37, 42, 62, 64] In general, gynecologists tend to prefer a transvaginal repair, either excising the fistula, closing the defects in the rectal and vaginal walls, or performing a fistulotomy and repairing the perineum.

Given incised the perineal body, converting the fistula into a laceration.[23] A layered closure was effected. He reported primary healing in all ten cases.

Lawson described a transvaginal approach to high rectovaginal fistulas that developed following obstetric injury.[42] This involved incising the vagina and sometimes dividing the cervix, and opening the pouch of Douglas. As previously mentioned, it would seem that such a fistula could be more easily treated by an abdominal approach.

Belt and Belt reported good results in all ten patients treated by dissecting out and interposing the internal sphincter muscle.[5] Greenwald and Hoexter excised the fistula by a transanal approach and performed a layered closure.[30] They reported 100% success in 20 patients.

Others advocate a transanal approach with advancement of the rectum.[37, 62] Rothenberger and co-workers reported 91% success in 35 patients.[62]

Rectovaginal Fistula in Crohn's Disease

Rectovaginal fistula as a complication of inflammatory bowel disease almost inevitably will require a diversionary procedure or proctectomy. Although attempted repair has been suggested for the occasional patient,[4, 19, 71] in my experience the results are horrendous and are likely to precipitate an early requirement for colostomy or ileostomy.

Rectovaginal Fistula Following Radiotherapy

Rectovaginal fistula following radiation therapy presents a particularly difficult problem in management. However, there are some patients for whom repair may produce quite satisfactory results.

Patients with this complaint often give a history of having undergone radiotherapy many years previously, usually for carcinoma of the cervix. In more recent years, such a complication may be the result of radiation treatment for cancer of the anal canal, rectum, or bladder. The vast majority of these patients present with a fistula above the sphincters, usually in the mid- or upper rectum.

With a history of previous malignancy, it is imperative to establish whether the patient has any evidence of recurrent disease. Obviously, reconstruction is contraindicated under such circumstances. Complete evaluation by means of multiple biopsies, radiologic investigation (including CT scan), and hematologic studies is required. The genitourinary tract should also be investigated, using intravenous pyelography and cystoscopy.

Techniques

A number of operative approaches to the repair of radiation-induced rectovaginal fistula have been described.[10, 12, 29, 45, 47, 55, 68] The difference between the handling of this etiology of fistula and the treatment of other etiologies is that layered closure, fistulotomy, and rectal advancement are contraindicated. Normal (non-radiated) tissue must be brought to the area.

Sartorius muscle interposition has been used successfully, as has gracilis.[12, 29] Resective procedures have also been employed. These include the pull-through operation, coloanal anastomosis, vascular pedicle graft of bowel, and the abdominotranssacral resection.[10, 45, 47, 55, 68]

In order to have a reasonable chance of success and to avoid the risks inherent in these very low anastomoses, a colostomy at the time of the repair–resection should be performed (see Chap. 17). Of course, if the patient is not a candidate for one of the above operations, some form of diversionary procedure is indicated.

RECTOURETHRAL FISTULA

Rectourethral fistula is, fortunately, a rare condition. It is most frequently encountered as a complication of prostatectomy, especially when performed by way of the perineal route. It is also occasionally seen as a sequela of radiation therapy for carcinoma of the bladder or prostate. Trauma and infection are more unusual causes. Even in the adult, a congenital anomaly may be the cause.[32] Looser and co-workers reported the experience of colorectal–urinary tract fistulas at the Memorial Hospital in New York and found only two cases of rectourethral communication during a 17-year period.[44] One followed a low anterior rectal resection and the other a radical perineal prostatectomy.

Thompson reported the Mayo Clinic experience over a 30-year period.[69] There were 36 rectourethral fistulas. Fourteen followed prostatectomy, six occurred after trauma, three with Crohn's disease, and four from "other causes." Nine patients had malignant fistulas. Although the authors did not distinguish between the symptoms of rectovesicle and rectourethral fistulas, 90% of the patients had urinary tract infections, and 83% reported urine from the rectum. Over half of the patients noted pneumaturia and fecaluria. Bleeding through the rectum implied a malignant process. Cystoscopy established the diagnosis in 84% of patients; proctoscopy was of value in 70%.

Treatment

Many approaches have been used to treat the condition. Hampton and Bacon favor the abdomino-anal pull-through with perineal repair.[32] Turner-Warwick prefers an abdominal operation with interposition of appropriately tailored omentum.[70] Mason exposed the area by dividing the rectum and sphincters posteriorly; the fistula is repaired in layers and the rectum reconstructed.[48] The perineal approach with advancement of the rectal mucosa has also been used.[27]

In patients with unresectable malignant disease, a diversionary procedure is the treatment of choice. If the tumor is resectable, a pelvic exenteration is the optimal course of action. For benign conditions, successful repair requires long-term catheter or suprapubic drainage of the urinary tract.

In Goligher's hands, either the Mason approach or that of Turner-Warwick offers the best results.[27] The former technique is described in Chapter 11. My own preference is to use the services of a urologist who has a particular proficiency in performing reconstructive urologic procedures.

REFERENCES

1. Abcarian H: Surgical management of recurrent anorectal abscesses. Contemp Surg 1982; 21:85–91
2. Adams D, Kovalcik PJ: Fistula in ano. Surg Gynecol Obstet 1981; 153:731–732
3. Alexander-Williams J: Fistula-in-ano: Management of Crohn's fistula. Dis Colon Rectum 1976; 19:518–519
4. Beecham CT: Recurring rectovaginal fistula. Obstet Gynecol 1972; 40:323–326
5. Belt RL Jr, Belt RL: Repair of anorectal vaginal fistula utilizing segmental advancement of the internal sphincter muscle. Dis Colon Rectum 1969; 12:99–104
6. Bennett RC: A review of the results of orthodox treatment for anal fistulae. Proc R Soc Med 1962; 55:756–757
7. Bevans DW Jr, Westbrook KC, Thompson BW, Caldwell FT: Peri-rectal abscess: A potentially fatal illness. Am J Surg 1973; 126:765–768
8. Block IR, Rodriguez S, Olivares AL: The Warren operation for anal incontinence caused by disruption of the anterior segment of the anal sphincter, perineal body, and rectovaginal septum. Dis Colon Rectum 1975; 18:28–34
9. Bode WE, Ramos R, Page CP: Invasive necrotizing infection secondary to anorectal abscess. Dis Colon Rectum 1982; 25:416–419
10. Bricker EM, Johnston WD: Repair of post irradiation rectovaginal fistula and stricture. Surg Gynecol Obstet 1979; 148:499–506
11. Buchan R, Grace RH: Anorectal suppuration: The results of treatment and the factors influencing the recurrence rate. Br J Surg 1973; 60:537–540
12. Byron RL Jr, Ostergard DR: Sartorius muscle interposition for the treatment of the radiation-induced vaginal fistula. Am J Obstet Gynecol 1969; 104:104–107
13. Corman ML: Rectovaginal reconstruction. Dis Colon Rectum (in press)
14. Dukes CE, Galvin C: Colloid carcinoma arising within fistulas in the ano-rectal region. Ann R Coll Surg Engl 1956; 18:246–261
15. Eisenhammer S: The internal anal sphincter; its surgical importance. S Afr Med J 1953; 27:266–270
16. Eisenhammer S: The internal anal sphincter and the anorectal abscess. Surg Gynecol Obstet 1956; 103:501–505
17. Ellis M: The use of penicillin and sulphonamides in the treatment of suppuration. Lancet 1951; 1:774–775
18. Ellis M: Recurrence of infection following treat-

ment of anorectal abscesses by primary suture. Proc R Soc Med 1962; 55:757–758

19. Faulcolon HT, Muldoon JP: Rectovaginal fistula in patients with colitis. Dis Colon Rectum 1975; 18:413–415

20. Fincato M, Corsi C, Perrone A, Gargiulo M, Familiari G: Perianal fistulous abscesses and cloacogenic cancer. Proctology 1980; 2:105–109

21. Friend WG: Anorectal problems: Surgical incisions for complicated anal fistulas. Dis Colon Rectum 1975; 18:652–656

22. Getz SB, Ough YD, Patterson RB, Kovalcik PJ: Mucinous adenocarcinoma developing in chronic anal fistula: Report of two cases and review of the literature. Dis Colon Rectum 1981; 24:562–566

23. Given FT Jr: Rectovaginal fistula: A review of 20 years' experience in a community hopital. Am J Obst Gynecol 1970; 108:41–46

24. Goldenberg HS: Supralevator abscess diagnosis and treatment. Surgery 1982; 91:164–167

25. Goligher JC: Fistula-in-ano: Management of perianal suppuration. Dis Colon Rectum 1976; 19:516–517

26. Goligher JC: Surgery of the Anus, Rectum and Colon, 4th ed, p 156. New York, Macmillan, 1980

27. Goligher JC: Surgery of the Anus, Rectum and Colon, 4th ed, pp 193–194. New York, Macmillan, 1980

28. Goodsall DH: Anorectal fistula. In Goodsall DH, Miles WE (eds): Diseases of the Anus and Rectum, Part I, pp 92–173. London, Longmans, Green & Co, 1900

29. Graham JB: Vaginal fistulas following radiotherapy. Surg Gynecol Obstet 1965; 120:1019–1030

30. Greenwald JC, Hoexter B: Repair of rectovaginal fistulas. Surg Gynecol Obstet 1973; 146:443–445

31. Hamilton CH: Anorectal problems: The deep post-anal space—surgical significance in horseshoe fistula and abscess. Dis Colon Rectum 1975; 18:642–645

32. Hampton JM, Bacon HE: Diagnosis and surgical management of rectourethral fistulas. Dis Colon Rectum 1961; 4:177–180

33. Hanley PH: Conservative surgical correction of horseshoe abscess and fistula. Dis Colon Rectum 1965; 8:364–368

34. Hanley PH, Ray JE, Pennington EE, Grablowsky OM: Fistula-in-ano: A ten-year follow-up study of horseshoe-abscess fistula-in-ano. Dis Colon Rectum 1976; 19:507–515

35. Hibbard LT: Surgical management of rectovaginal fistulas and complete perineal tears. Am J Obst Gynecol 1978; 130:139–141

36. Hill JR: Fistulas and fistulous abscesses in the anorectal region: Personal experience in management. Dis Colon Rectum 1967; 10:421–434

37. Hilsabeck JR: Transanal advancement of the anterior rectal wall for vaginal fistulas involving the lower rectum. Dis Colon Rectum 1980; 23:236–241

38. Jackman RJ, Buie LA: Tuberculosis and anal fistula. JAMA 1946; 130:630–632

39. Kline RJ, Spencer RJ, Harrison EG Jr: Carcinoma associated with fistula-in-ano. Arch Surg 1964; 89:989–994

40. Kott I, Urca I: Perianal abscess as a presenting sign of leukemia. Dis Colon Rectum 1969; 12:338–339

41. Kuypers JHC: Diagnosis and treatment of fistula-in-ano. Neth J Surg 1982; 34:147–152

42. Lawson J: Rectovaginal fistulae following difficult labour. Proc R Soc Med 1972; 65:283–286

43. Lichtenstein D, Stavorovsky M, Irge D: Fournier's gangrene complicating perianal abscess: Report of two cases. Dis Colon Rectum 1978; 21:377–379

44. Looser KG, Quan SHQ, Clark DGC: Colo-urinary tract fistula in the cancer patient. Dis Colon Rectum 1979; 22:143–148

45. Marks G: Combined abdominotranssacral reconstruction of the radiation-injured rectum. Am J Surg 1976; 131:54–59

46. Marks G, Chase WV, Mervine TB: The fatal potential of fistula-in-ano with abscess: Analysis of 11 deaths. Dis Colon Rectum 1973; 16:224–230

47. Marks G, Mohiudden M: The surgical management of the radiation-injured intestine. Surg Clin North Am 1983; 63:81–96

48. Mason AY: The place of local resection in the treatment of rectal carcinoma. Proc R Soc Med 1970; 63:1259–1262

49. Mazier WP: The treatment and care of anal fistulas: A study of 1,000 patients. Dis Colon Rectum 1971; 14:134–144

50. McElwain JW, Alexander RM, MacLean MD: Primary fistulectomy for anorectal abscesses, clinical study of 500 cases. Dis Colon Rectum 1966; 9:181–185

51. McElwain JW, MacLean MD, Alexander RM et al: Anorectal problems: Experience with primary fistulectomy for anorectal abscess, a report of 1,000 cases. Dis Colon Rectum 1975; 18:646–649

52. Millar DM: Villous neoplasms in anorectal fistulas. Proctology 1979; 2:50–53

53. Mirelman D, Corman ML: Dual anal fistulas—an uncommon manifestation of fistula-in-ano. Dis Colon Rectum 1978; 21:54–55

54. Parks AG: Pathogenesis and treatment of fistula-in-ano. Br Med J 1961; 1:463–469

55. Parks AG, Allen CLO, Frank JD, McPartlin JF: A

method of treating post-irradiation rectovaginal fistulas. Br J Surg 1978; 65:417–421

56. Parks AG, Gordon PH: Perineal fistula of intra-abdominal or intrapelvic origin simulating fistula-in-ano—Report of seven cases. Dis Colon Rectum 1976; 19:500–506

57. Parks AG, Stitz RW: The treatment of high fistula-in-ano. Dis Colon Rectum 1976; 19:487–499

58. Parks AG, Thomson JP: Intersphincteric abscess. Br Med J 1973; 2:537–539

59. Prasad ML, Read DR, Abcarian H: Supralevator abscess: Diagnosis and treatment. Dis Colon Rectum 1981; 24:456–461

60. Prioleau PG, Allen MS Jr, Roberts T: Perianal mucinous adenocarinoma. Cancer 1977; 39:1295–1299

61. Read DR, Abcarian H: A prospective survey of 474 patients with anorectal abscess. Dis Colon Rectum 1979; 22:566–568

62. Rothenberger DA, Christenson CE, Balcos EG, Schottler JL, Nemer FD, Nivatvongs S, Goldberg SM: Endorectal advancement flap for treatment of simple rectovaginal fistula. Dis Colon Rectum 1982; 25:297–300

63. Rothenberger DA, Goldberg SM: The management of rectovaginal fistulae. Surg Clin North Am 1983; 63:61–79

64. Russell TR, Gallagher DM: Low rectovaginal fistulas. Am J Surg 1977; 134:13–18

65. Schimpff SC, Wiernik PH, Block JB: Rectal abscesses in cancer patients. Lancet 1972; 2:844–847

66. Scoma JA, Salvati EP, Rubin RJ: Incidence of fistulas subsequent to anal abscesses. Dis Colon Rectum 1974; 17:357–359

67. Sehdev MK, Dowling MD, Seal SH, Stearns MW: Perianal and anorectal complications in leukemia. Cancer 1973; 31:149–152

68. Thomford NR, Smith DE, Wilson WH; Pull-through operation for radiation-induced rectovaginal fistula. Dis Colon Rectum 1970; 13:451–453

69. Thompson JS, Engen DE, Beart RW Jr, Culp CE: The management of acquired rectourinary fistula. Dis Colon Rectum 1982; 25:689–692

70. Turner-Warwick R: The use of pedicle grafts in the repair of urinary tract fistulae. Br J Urol 1972; 44:644–656

71. Tuxen PA, Castro AF: Rectovaginal fistula in Crohn's disease. Dis Colon Rectum 1979; 22:58–62

72. Vanheuverzwyn R, Delannoy A, Michaux JL, Dive C: Anal lesions in hematologic diseases. Dis Colon Rectum 1980; 23:310–312

73. Waggener HU: Immediate fistulotomy in the treatment of perianal abscess. Surg Clin North Am 1969; 49:1227–1233

74. Williams DR, Coller JA, Corman ML, Nugent FW, Veidenheimer MC: Anal complications in Crohn's disease. Dis Colon Rectum 1981; 24:22–24

75. Wilson DH: The late results of anorectal abscess treated by incision, curettage, and primary suture under antibiotic cover. Br J Surg 1964; 51:828–831

76. Wilson E: Skin grafts in surgery for anal fistula. Dis Colon Rectum 1969; 12:327–331

CHAPTER 5

Anal Incontinence

115

Anal incontinence is not a life-threatening disease, but it is a traumatizing and disabling condition. The psychological effects can be as severe as any physical disability.

Anal incontinence can result from a disturbance of any one or more of the mechanisms that normally ensure continence: central nervous system or spinal cord injuries and disease, loss of the afferent sensory component of the rectosphincteric reflex, diseases that impair smooth muscle (scleroderma) or striated muscle (polymyositis), or direct muscle damage occurring with perianal disease or surgical trauma.[1, 49, 51, 63]

Before discussing the physiology of continence and defecation, and the treatment of patients with control difficulties, it is important to define what is meant by incontinence. I am attracted to the classification of Lane.[33] He separates anal incontinence into three categories:

True incontinence: Passage of feces without the patient's knowledge, or without voluntary contraction, or both

Partial incontinence: Passage of flatus or mucus under the above circumstances

"Overflow" incontinence: Result of rectal distention with relaxation of the anal sphincters (*e.g.*, fecal impaction)

PHYSIOLOGIC BASIS OF CONTINENCE

The neuromuscular control for fecal continence has been a subject of considerable investigation and debate.[15, 41, 42, 49, 50–53, 55] Schuster has been one of the leaders in the evaluation and treatment of incontinent patients in this country. Much of the following represents his thoughts on the subject.

Continence is maintained partly under voluntary control and partly through the autonomic nervous system. Parks and co-workers have suggested that the anorectal angle is a very important factor.

Mechanical and physiologic retentive forces in the rectosigmoid normally maintain the distal rectum empty and in a collapsed state.[50, 52] The bends and folds of the rectosigmoid as well as the valves of Houston are believed to retard the material from entry into the rectum.[51] As feces accumulates in the rectum, the bowel wall muscle relaxes, allowing for distention and accommodation of the enlarging fecal mass. Threshold stimulation of the afferent nerve endings* is reached, and involuntary precipitation of the anal reflex occurs, enabling the rectum to empty. Successive functional segments of colon coordinate their activity to produce a mass peristaltic wave above the fecal mass. Concomitantly, the distal part of the intestine and the internal sphincter relax, and the external sphincter contracts. If elimination is to proceed, voluntary inhibition of the external sphincter contraction occurs.

The *internal sphincter* is maintained in a state of near maximal contraction at all times; its major reflex response to rectal distention is relaxation. The *external sphincter* is also in a state of contraction; its major reflex response to stimuli, however, is contraction.[50] The degree of external sphincter contraction varies with alteration of intra-abdominal pressure and posture. As

---

* Preganglionic, parasympathetic, afferent fibers originating in the second, third, and fourth sacral segments.

116

intra-abdominal pressure is increased or as the patient rises to a more upright posture, electrical activity and tone increase gradually. Resting activity may be supplemented by voluntary contraction, which is accompanied by a marked rise in electrical action potentials and a substantial increase in recorded intrasphincteric pressure. Because of fatigure, maximal voluntary contraction can be maintained only for approximately 50 seconds. The internal sphincter plays no major role in maintenance of continence, but if elimination is to be suppressed, continued voluntary contraction of the external sphincter must be maintained.

The *external anal sphincter* is part of a composite muscle that enables voluntary control of continence. It is a striated muscle encircling the anal canal; contraction closes off the anal aperture. The *levator ani,* arising from the bony pelvis and the obturator fascia, spreads out to form a muscular pelvic floor (Fig. 5-1). The *puborectalis muscle* is the anteromedial portion of this diaphragm and, arising from the back of the symphysis, passes posteriorly around the lower part of the rectum, meeting fibers from the opposite side in a loop or U-shaped girdle. The puborectalis blends with the deep portion of the external sphincter, the longitudinal muscle, and the adjacent part of the internal sphincter to form the *anorectal ring.* Contraction of the levator ani and the puborectalis sling pulls the anorectal junction forward and upward, elongating the anal canal and increasing angulation between the anal canal and the rectum. Contraction of the levator ani coordinated with that of the external anal sphincter results in effective closure of the anal canal.[18]

A relatively recent theory of pelvic muscle anatomy and function has been described by Shafik.[55] This involves a three-loop system with two U-shaped loops directed anteriorly and one posteriorly (Fig. 5-2)

The practical importance of these two muscles in maintaining continence is that if the external anal sphincter is divided completely, satisfactory continence will be provided by the intact puborectalis muscle. If both the external sphincter and the puborectalis muscle are divided, the patient will be incontinent. Division of the puborectalis without division of the external sphincter may occur in infants during operation for

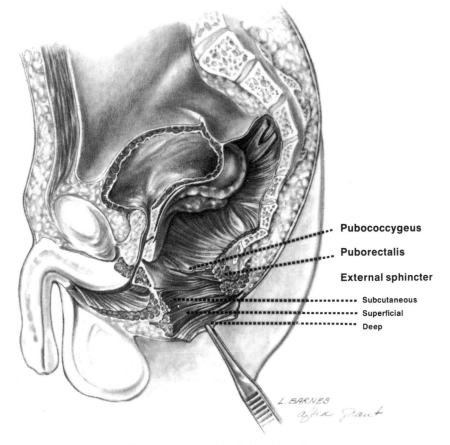

Pubococcygeus

Puborectalis

External sphincter

Subcutaneous
Superficial
Deep

L. BARNES
after Grant

FIG. 5-1. Muscles of the pelvic floor.

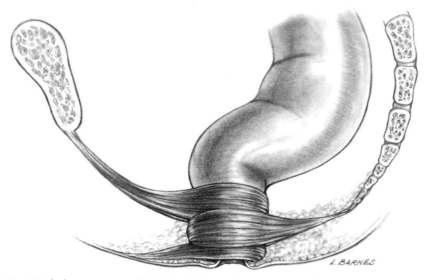

L. BARNES

FIG. 5-2. Triple-loop system of Shafik.[55] The top loop arises and inserts on the pubis, and is made up of the deep external sphincter and puborectalis. The middle loop attaches to the coccyx (superficial external sphincter). The lower loop inserts in the anterior perianal skin (subcutaneous external sphincter).

high imperforate anus. These children are rendered incontinent despite having a normal functioning external sphincter.[31]

The internal sphincter reflex is mainly initiated by rectal distention. Response of the external sphincter can be initiated by voluntary effort, postural change, rectal distention, increased intra-abdominal pressure, and anal dilation. These responses involve several different neural pathways. Therefore, neurologic impairment can be differentiated from muscle disease if the sphincter responds to any one of these stimuli.[54] Failure to respond to all stimuli is indicative either of muscle disease or of diffuse neurologic disorder.

The neural pathway for response of the internal sphincter is not known. The internal sphincter is supplied by a dual innervation and contains a motor supply that travels through the hypogastric nerves from the sympathetic outflow tract as well as an inhibitory supply from the parasympathetic outflow tract (Fig. 5-3).[23, 34] The internal sphincter is also continuously active, with strips of the muscle demonstrating spontaneous contraction *in vitro.*[15]

Receptors for the external sphincter response lie either in or near the rectal mucosa, since the reflex disappears after application of a topical anesthetic. The external sphincter is supplied only by somatic pudendal nerves, arising from the second, third, and fourth sacral nerves. Therefore, its relaxation can be caused only by reduction in frequency of existing motor impulses in

the pudendal nerves. Since lesions of the cauda equina abolish the external sphincter reflex, it is evident that it is mediated through the spinal cord.[3, 45] This is not true of the internal sphincter response, which can persist after transection of the lower spinal cord.[14, 53]

DEFECATION

Distention of the rectum is the stimulus for defecation. As the stool enters the rectum the internal sphincter relaxes and the external sphincter contracts. If one is to voluntarily inhibit external sphincter contraction during a mass peristaltic propulsion, defecation will be achieved without a voluntary effort. With contraction of the external sphincter, accomodation occurs by relaxation of the rectal wall muscle. This, in a matter of seconds, will remove the urgency to defecate unless the volume is large, or the individual has impairment of the sphincter mechanism.

If a voluntary effort is required to defecate, intra-abdominal pressure is increased by closure of the glottis and by contraction of the muscles of the pelvic floor (resisting the forward movement of stool and closing the lumen distally).[46] The diaphragm descends, and the voluntary muscles of the abdominal wall are contracted, creating a closed system.[46] Relaxation of the pelvic muscles produces descent of the pelvic floor and straightening of the previously angulated rectum.[24,25]

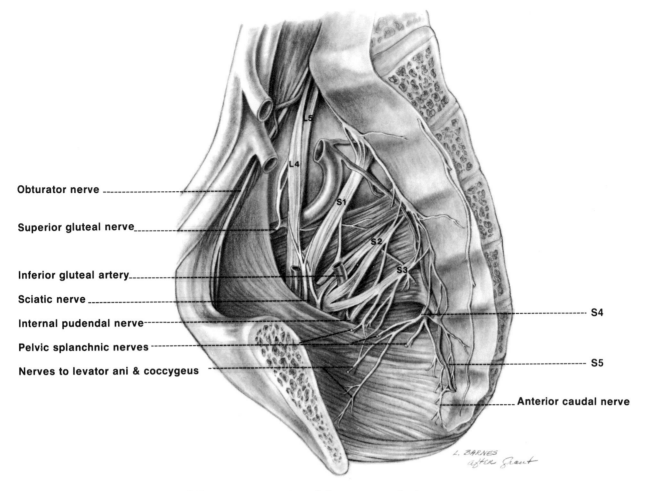

FIG. 5-3.   Innervation of the rectum and sphincters.

Closure of the anal canal by the sphincters allows increase of pressure within the rectum so that subsequent sphincteric inhibition results in expulsion of stool.[46] The point at which complete inhibition of the external sphincter occurs can be demonstrated experimentally with an intrarectal balloon. When the volume reaches 150 to 200 cc of air, the intrarectal pressure reaches 45 to 55 mm Hg.[44] At the end of defecation, when straining is discontinued, the pelvic floor rises to its normal position and again obliterates the lumen. A rebound contraction of the anal sphincter occurs; this has been termed the "closing reflex."[45, 46]

ETIOLOGY OF INCONTINENCE

The causes of fecal incontinence are summarized in the list on this page.

Causes of Fecal Incontinence

Trauma
  Surgical (fistulectomy, hemorrhoidectomy,
    sphincterotomy, sphincter stretch)
  Obstetric
  Accidental
Congenital anomalies (spina bifida, myelomeningocele,
  imperforate anus, Hirschsprung's disease)
Neurogenic diseases (multiple sclerosis, arteriosclerosis,
  diabetes)
Colorectal diseases (hemorrhoids, rectal prolapse,
  inflammatory bowel disease)
Miscellaneous
  Laxative abuse
  Chronic diarrhea
  Fecal impaction
  Encopresis

Surgical Trauma

The development of incontinence after anorectal surgery is usually the result of inappropriate division of the anorectal ring. This is most likely to occur when a high-level fistula is laid open or an artificial opening created. This is probably the commonest cause of fecal incontinence.[4, 5] Familiarity with anorectal anatomy and the extent of disease present is imperative (see Chap. 4).

Internal anal sphincterotomy when performed for anal fissure may produce partial anal incontinence (see Chap. 3). Since the internal sphincter is not involved in voluntary control, fecal incontinence should not occur. However, if the surgeon injudiciously divides the external sphincter, incontinence may ensue.

Sphincter stretch for anal fissure or manual dilatation as a treatment for hemorrhoids (Lord procedure) may be associated with fecal incontinence. This should not be done on patients over the age of 60; it is because of this complication, in fact, that I no longer employ manual dilatation (see Chap. 2)

Partial incontinence may be a late complication of *hemorrhoidectomy.* Removal of excess mucosa of the anal canal, such as is performed during the Whitehead operation, may produce this distressing complication. Eschar may interfere with sphincter contraction, and rectal mucosa may prolapse through the cicatrix at the site of the excision. This may further impair closure of the canal and allow for continuous discharge of mucus (see Chaps. 2 and 6).[24]

Bowel resections designed to preserve the anal sphincter (low anterior resection, the various pull-through procedures, colo-anal anastomosis, abdominosacral resection) frequently result in discharge of mucus or incontinence for flatus, probably by interrupting the neural reflex.[22]

Several *misconceptions* concerning sphincteric surgery should be mentioned if only to be refuted:

Complete division of the muscle does not impair its power of control provided that its nerve supply is not interfered with.

Dividing the sphincter in the posterior midline is safe.

Dividing the sphincter transversely at right angles to the direction of the fibers but not obliquely is safe.

Division of the muscle at several places instead of one will not lead to permanent loss of control.

Although some surgeons continue to believe some of these misconceptions, the fact remains that if the sphincter muscle is divided through the puborectalis sling, the patient will be incontinent.

Obstetric Trauma

Fecal incontinence may result from birth-canal injury during vaginal delivery. Although not common, this may result from median episiotomy. The condition may also be associated with rectovaginal fistula. The obstetrician should be wary of the patient who has an ectopic (anterior displacement) location of the rectum (see Chap. 4).

Accidental Trauma

Trauma to the perineum can impair the sphincter mechanism. Impalement on a spike or pole may result in division of the sphincter and contamination of the extrarectal spaces. Sepsis can supervene and lead to excessive scar formation with a resultant patulous anal canal and an incompetent sphincter. Initial treatment usually consists of debridement of nonviable tissue, removal of foreign material, open drainage, and often proximal colostomy. Reconstructive sphincteric surgery is deferred for a later time (see also Chap. 17).

Congenital Anomalies

Congenital incontinence may be due to spina bifida, meningocele, myelomeningocele, anorectal malformations, and congenital megacolon (Hirschsprung's disease). Involvement of sensory or motor nerves may produce urinary and fecal incontinence and, ultimately, rectal prolapse.

Neurogenic Diseases

Any neurologic disease may affect bowel control. Perhaps the most common condition that produces a neuropathy is diabetes mellitus. Patients with this disease may be particularly troubled because diarrhea (from autonomic neuropathy) and fecal incontinence often are seen together. Schiller and associates, in their study on 16 such patients, concluded that incontinence in this group was due to abnormal internal anal sphincter dysfunction, and that diabetics with no diarrhea do not have impairment for fecal control.[48]

Colorectal Disease

Incontinence for flatus or feces is often associated with local anorectal disease in the absence of antecedent surgery or trauma. Prolapse of rectal musoca or hemorrhoids and complete rectal prolapse interfere with closure of the anal canal. With time, the protruding mass stretches the sphincter and attenuates it, thus leading to further symptoms of incontinence. Other conditions that may be associated with incontinence include nonspecific inflammatory bowel disease (ulcerative colitis and Crohn's disease), malignant conditions, and infectious and parasitic diseases.

Other Causes

Probably the commonest cause of nonsurgical fecal incontinence is *laxative abuse.* A common offender is mineral oil. The greasy stool that results from mineral oil abuse slides past the sphincter without producing any significant dilatation. Over the years, because the sphincter is not stretched by a normal stool, the muscle atrophies. Any attempt to repair the sphincter in a patient with such a history will be futile.

Fecal impaction frequently is associated with incontinence, probably on an overflow basis. Patients with this problem are usually elderly and often suffer from systemic disorders for which they may be taking constipating medications. For example, the medications frequently employed for treating Parkinsonism are quite constipating; impaction is very common in these patients.

Fecal impaction is also a troubling problem for the senile and psychiatrically disturbed patient. Treatment may require manual disimpaction, enemas, and laxatives. After the impaction is cleared, prevention consists of the establishment of a proper bowel managment program. This may be supplemented by colonic irrigations and perineal strengthening exercises.

Chronic diarrhea may be associated with fecal incontinence. Read and co-workers evaluated 29 patients with this symptom complex, determining the severity of the diarrhea by 72-hour stool collections.[46] They also studied anal manometry and continence for liquid, the latter by the patient's ability to retain a saline enema. Most, but not all, patients had low sphincter pressures and an impaired ability to retain the enema. This would suggest a defect in sphincteric function. However, a group of patients exhibited a normal sphincter mechanism. Theoretically, with a large volume of stool, the normal sphincter was overwhelmed.

Encopresis, or psychogenic soiling, was first recognized by Weissenberg, who realized that this form of fecal incontinence was based on emotional disturbances and analogous to enuresis as it pertains to urinary soiling.[62] Encopresis is an involuntary evacuation of the bowel not caused by organic factors. The condition is commoner in men. Treatment is usually directed toward psychotherapy, which can be performed by a family physician or psychiatrist, depending on the patient's needs.[2, 16, 56] Recently, uridine-5-triphosphate has been advocated, and its use has shown some success.[36] Although the mechanism of action of this drug is not certain, it is believed to stimulate the cortical substance of the brain to make the person more aware of the need to defecate.

EVALUATION OF THE PATIENT

History

In order to determine the appropriate therapy for the patient with anal incontinence, probably the single most important criterion is the etiology of the problem. Patients who have sustained loss of sphincter function through injury (surgical, obstetric, accidental) are the most amenable to reconstructive efforts. However, those who are incontinent because of disease are generally poor candidates for reconstruction. In this group of patients appropriate counseling (dietary, exercise, bowel management) may be the most efficacious mode of therapy.

Physical Examination

Although proctosigmoidoscopy and barium enema examination are important studies in the evaluation of any patient with a colorectal problem, they are usually unrewarding in someone with anal incontinence. Inspection and palpation reveal the information that will dictate the therapy. By spreading the buttocks the physician will be able to determine whether there is a patulous anus, implying a loss of sphincter muscle or poor resting tone (Figs. 5-4, 5-5, and 5-6). A mucosal ectropion (Fig. 5-7) or rectal prolapse may be noted (see Chap. 7).

By palpation, the resting tone of the sphincter can be assessed, and by asking the patient to "tighten up," the contractility can be evaluated. Any defect in the sphincter muscle can also be perceived. In neurologic lesions (including spinal cord and cauda equina) normal tone may be apparent; however, if gentle traction is applied to any segment of the anorectal ring, it is followed by gaping of the anal canal.[26] Even though this evaluation is relatively subjective, the information obtained, in my opinion, is more valuable than so-called objective, investigative studies.

Sensory determination is also useful in examining a patient with anal incontinence. Reconstructive surgery in someone with impairment of sensation to touch or

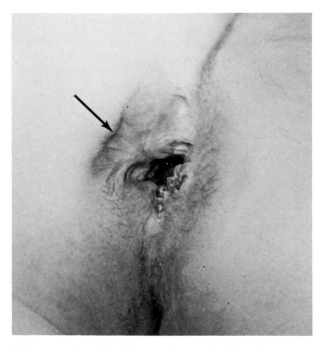

FIG. 5-4.   Considerable scarring and deformity *(arrow)* from perineal trauma (avulsion injury) with a patulous anus.

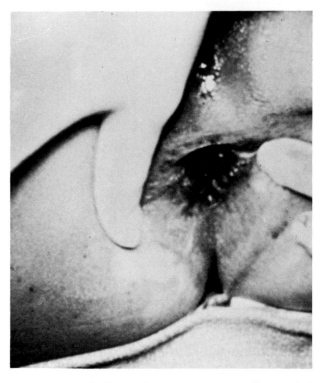

FIG. 5-6.   Markedly patulous anus in a mentally retarded young woman with congenital absence of the external sphincter. The patient was incontinent from birth.

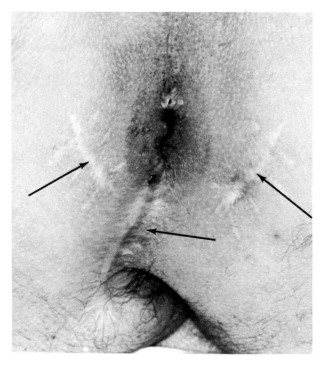

FIG. 5-5.   Patulous anus following multiple operations for anal fistula. Note scars *(arrows)*.

pinprick implies that any repair effort will be compromised.

The ability to retain a small-volume enema has been suggested as a means for evaluating incontinence. Although retaining liquid implies good sphincter function, I have never found an incontinent patient able to perform this feat. Hence, I do not rely upon this test.

Physiologic Studies

The two investigations for evaluating pelvic floor physiology are electromyography (EMG) and anorectal pressure. Cineradiography and bowel transit time have also been employed, the former particularly for rectal prolapse patients, and the latter in patients with constipation and fecal impaction.[7, 15] If incontinence is secondary to a neurologic cause, evaluation by a neurologist and appropriate studies are suggested.

Neill and associates, in evaluation of patients with fecal incontinence and rectal prolapse by means of EMG and anorectal manometry, demonstrated abnormal results in this group of patients.[37] This indicated

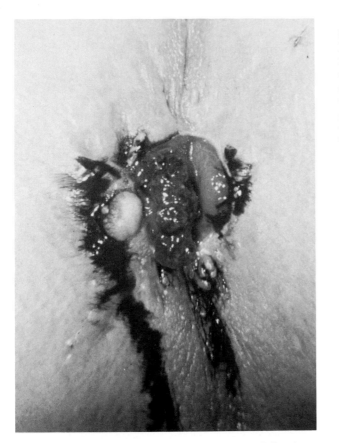

FIG. 5-7. Mucosal ectropion in a young man following a pull-through operation for an imperforate anus. Note the ready bleeding.

damage to the innervation of the pelvic floor muscles. Henry and associates recorded the latency of the anal reflex in patients with fecal incontinence by means of EMG.[27] In 22 patients with idiopathic fecal incontinence (no prior history of trauma), they concluded that a major cause was denervation of the sphincter musculature.

Waylonis and Powers analyzed 184 pediatric and 81 adult patients, the former with suspected bowel and bladder dysfunction and the latter following abnormal EMG determinations.[61] Forty-nine of 54 children with myelomeningocele had reduced or absent external sphincter function. This implied the need for frequent urologic follow-up. Nineteen of 26 children who were incontinent following surgery for Hirschsprung's disease or imperforate anus had abnormal findings. They felt that the EMG was particularly useful in determining the presence or absence (and location) of sphincter tissue in cases of imperforate anus. In the adults with abnormal EMGs, 36% had abnormal spinal x-rays.

Borden and co-workers developed an anorectal function profile by using pressure studies and the EMG.[6] They identified discrete defects in anorectal function, including high sensory threshold levels, discomfort with minimal rectal distension, persistence of external sphincter activity with maximum tolerable volume, and increasing rather than decreasing external sphincter activity with rectal distension. They suggested that on the basis of these studies specific therapy can be selected (*e.g.,* electrical stimulator for absent tonic external sphincter activity, biofeedback for abnormal external sphincter contraction reflex, rectal distension for high resting sphincter pressure, and bowel management for patients with high rectal volume and sensation thresholds).

Comment

While in my opinion the history and physical examination are the most useful studies for determining the treatment in a patient with fecal incontinence, selective application of physiologic studies should be considered. For example, EMG may be very helpful in determining the presence of muscle in patients with congenital anomalies.

NONSURGICAL TREATMENT

The treatment of anal incontinence should be directed to the cause. However, despite the potential appeal of surgical intervention, initial treatment should be medical and include the bowel management program outlined here.

*Bowel Management Program**

The aim of a bowel management program is to develop and establish for the patient a routine for defecation that is safe, convenient, and dependable. Eventually, the bowel can be "reeducated" to empty regularly and at predictable times. Through maintaining proper fecal consistency, stimulating peristalsis, and controlling the time of evacuation, a conditioned reflex can be developed to ensure adequate fecal elimination. Individual patterns differ. Not all patients need to have a bowel movement every day; two or three times a week may be sufficient.

* After Sylvia Nott, RN, BSN, MSN, Clinical Nurse Specialist, Rehabilitation, New England Deaconess Hospital, Boston, Massachusetts

1. Make certain that the patient has a well-balanced diet with sufficient fiber and adequate fluid intake (2500 to 3000 ml a day).
2. Establish a workable time for defecation. Find the patient's previous bowel habits and his or her future plans for a daily schedule. Take advantage of the gastrocolic reflex, that is, the time when peristalsis is most stimulated by eating: 20 to 30 minutes after meals.
3. Start with a clean bowel. Disimpact if necessary and give enemas until clear if required.
4. Position the patient on a toilet or commode. Squatting is the optimal position because it both compresses the abdomen and allows gravity to facilitate defecation. The patient may take a cup of coffee or any similar stimulus that has been found helpful in the past.
5. Insert a suppository, such as glycerine or bisacodyl (Dulcolax). For patients with a spinal cord injury a carbon dioxide suppository may be of greater benefit. The suppository should be inserted at the same hour every day (night) during the first week of the program, and then every other day thereafter.
6. Instruct the patient to massage the abdomen from right to left and down several times, beginning 15 to 20 minutes after insertion of the suppository; having the patient bend forward and "strain" may also be helpful.
7. Stool softeners or bulk laxative preparations can be added as required.

Perineal Exercises

The following perineal strengthening exercises also may be of benefit.

- Lying on back with knees bent, raise head and reach hands toward knees. (1) Raise head and reach right hand toward left knee. Relax. Raise head and reach left hand toward right knee. Relax. (2) Flatten back. Pull abdomen in and squeeze buttocks together.
- Take a deep breath in. Squeeze buttocks together and close anal passage. *Sitting:* Squeeze buttocks together. Relax. *Standing:* Pull abdomen in and squeeze buttocks together (knees should be relaxed).

Although it probably is not possible to increase internal anal sphincter tone by perineal strengthening exercises, muscle bulk and voluntary contractility of the external anal sphincter, puborectalis sling, and levatores can be improved significantly by such exercises. Another simple strengthening exercise is to pretend to hold in a bowel movement and count to 20. This can be done 15 or 20 times a day, while walking down the street, riding in a car, or sitting in a chair—whenever the patient thinks of it. Bulging muscles should not be expected overnight, but given sufficient time (several weeks to several months), the patient should note an improvement in voluntary control.

Operant Conditioning

An interesting observation on the value of exercise was made by Engel and associates in a report of six patients who had severe fecal incontinence of diverse etiologies.[17] These authors used a Miller-Abbott balloon with a 50-ml capacity inserted into the rectum to record on a polygraph a measurable response to sphincter contractility. By positive or negative verbal reinforcement, each patient was able to sense the rectal distension, and knew that this stimulus was the cue to initiate sphincteric control. During follow-up periods ranging from 6 months to 5 years, four patients remained completely continent, and the other two were improved. One patient was able to relax the internal sphincter as well as to contract the external sphincter. It appears, therefore, that autonomic regulation may be brought under voluntary control with such techniques as operant conditioning. However, the success of this particular approach needs further substantiation.

Whitehead and co-workers employed behavioral modification in incontinent patients with spina bifida.[63] Using a bowel management program in addition to biofeedback, they reported improvement in 65% of patients and complete control in 30%.

Exercises, in combination with a bowel management program, can in most instances ameliorate difficulties with control. However, if these methods fail, and if the patient has a condition amenable to reconstruction, a surgical approach is indicated.

Electrical Treatment

Caldwell, Hopkinson and Lightwood, and Glen have reported success with electrical stimulation of the anal sphincter by means of an anal canal electrode.[9, 20, 28, 29] The device applies a tetanizing stimulus to the anal sphincter and pelvic floor through a plug-shaped electrode (Fig. 5-8). After the plug is inserted, the current is slowly increased until the patient is aware of a tingling sensation. This causes contraction of the anal musculature with gradual buildup in sphincter tone and contractility. Although perineal strengthening exercises would undoubtedly accomplish the same goal, the use of electrical stimulation, particularly in a patient who is unable to perform such exercises, seems to offer encouraging results in selected patients.

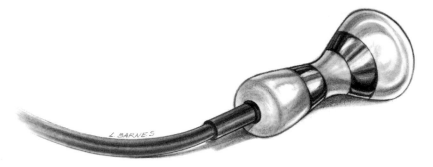

FIG. 5-8. The anal canal electrode, used for stimulating the sphincter mechanism, is available in several diameters.

MacLeod reported the use of the intra-anal plug which adapts to an electromyometer and not to a generator.[35] The sphincter muscle contractions were converted to an audible sound to guide the patient in sphincter contraction. Weekly 20-minute sessions were carried out, and the patients were advised to perform frequent exercises in the interim. Ten of 17 patients studied subjectively reported good to excellent results, but only 3 of these were shown to have measurable improvement.

SURGICAL TREATMENT

Successful surgical repair of incontinence requires an understanding of the underlying pathophysiology, and only those patients who have lesions amenable to reconstruction should be selected. Knowledge of the patient's history of previous injury, childbirth, or anorectal surgery is essential. Inspection of the anal area and palpation, if one asks the patient to "tighten-up" and to "relax," will permit an accurate definition of the condition. Although a thorough examination may require an anesthetic, it is imperative to obtain as much information as possible with the patient fully awake to assess the voluntary and resting tone of the sphincter as well as any defect in the sphincter muscle. This information cannot be obtained if the patient is anesthetized.

The two primary methods of surgical treatment of anal incontinence are direct repair of a localized sphincter defect, and repair designed to supplement the sphincter mechanism. A modified classification of the various methods of surgical treatment, which was proposed by Hagihara and Griffen, is presented in the list on this page.[25]

Direct repair of local sphincter conditions may produce excellent results, but anatomic structures may be distorted or obliterated by scar. It may not be possible to effect accurate dissection or identification of individual muscles, and even if possible, the dissection might

Types of Anal Surgical Repair

Anorectal muscle repairs
  Apposition of sphincter muscles
  Overlapping of sphincter muscles
  Reefing of sphincter muscles
  Narrowing the anal canal
  Use of perineal muscles other than the sphincter
    muscle
  Puborectalis repair (postanal perineorrhapy)
  Pubococcygeus repair
Use of other muscles
  Gluteus
  Vastus internus
  Adductor longus
  Gracilis
Anal procedures
  Fascia lata
  Thiersch procedures (wire, Teflon, Marlex, catgut,
    Dacron-impregnated Silastic mesh)

compromise viability of the tissue. Definitive treatment, therefore, includes excision of the scar, definition of the ends of the sphincter muscle, and suture of the ends together.

The three basic operative approaches to repairing the injured sphincter are apposition. overlapping, and reefing. All have their advocates, but no one method can consistently be employed with success. In principle, the surgeon usually attempts to repair the external sphincter muscle or puborectalis sling, or both. The internal sphincter is usually not identifiable or substantial enough to contribute meaningfully to the result. Repair of the sphincter in patients with incontinence is most successfully undertaken after operative or nonoperative trauma and is best accomplished as soon as possible after the incident. The considerable success that gynecologists have in repairing the torn perineal musculature after childbirth is a testament to this fact. However, repair can be carried out many months after the original injury with a good result. A point comes, however, when disuse takes its toll, with ultimate loss of muscle tissue. An attenuated muscle lacks holding power; sutures tend to cause necrosis and pull out easily.

A discussion of the three common types of sphincter repair follows. In addition, a detailed description of gracilis muscle transposition is included; this is a procedure that I have utilized with some success. The Thiersch repair, described in Chapter 7, is not recommended as a specific treatment for anal incontinence. However, by incorporating Silastic-impregnated Dacron mesh, this approach for the treatment of anal incontinence has proved most useful. Colostomy is a last resort and should rarely be used to treat anal incontinence.

Skin incisions for sphincter repair are described in Chapter 6. A curvilinear incision has the advantage of exposure but is best used in men since it does not readily lend itself to a closure that can displace the vagina away from the rectum. In women, an important step in any sphincter repair is to increase the distance between the rectum and vagina. A cruciate incision with bilateral flap advancement is an effective way to accomplish this (see Figs. 4–39 through 4–42).

Preoperative Preparation

All patients undergoing reconstructive anorectal surgical procedures should be prepared as if for colonic resection. The morning of operation, tap water enemas are given until the returns are clear. The orally administered antibiotic regimen of erythromycin base and neomycin, as popularized by Nichols and co-workers, is advised.[38] In addition, systemic antibiotics, such as a cephalosporin, clindamycin (Cleocin) or metronidazole (Flagyl), should be administered just before operation and in the immediate postoperative period. An indwelling urinary catheter is suggested for women. Any operation to repair the sphincter should be performed in the prone (jackknife) position.

Direct Sphincter Repair

Apposition

Figure 5-9, *A* demonstrates the typical appearance of a deformed anus after trauma, secondary to fistulectomy, impalement injury, or avulsion (see Fig. 5-4). The dashed line represents residual normal muscle. In Figure 5-9, *B*, the skin eschar is excised, and the divided muscle ends are identified.

For simplicity, the Hill-Ferguson retractor is not il-

lustrated, but it should be used and kept in place for the entire operation in order to maintain the lumenal diameter. Repair of the sphincter muscle is then undertaken. It is preferable to permit scar to remain on the sphincter to hold the sutures when the ends are apposed, but as illustrated here, all such tissue has been debrided. The commonly employed apposition technique is shown in Figure 5-9, *C*. The sutures can be nonabsorbable, pull-out-wires, or long-term absorbable material. I use this last suture material (either 0 or 2-0), inserted either as simple or preferably horizontal mattress sutures.

Overlapping

When sufficient sphincter muscle remains, an overlapping technique is preferred (Fig. 5-9, *D*). Further length can be achieved by undermining the skin and by freeing the muscle for 1 or 2 cm at each end. With this technique, breakdown of the repair is less likely. Unfortunately, the clearly illustrated problem shown in Figure 5-9 is not always the typical appearance found at the operating table. All too often merely eschar and insufficient viable muscle tissue are found. Under these circumstances the surgeon ultimately may resort to suturing "stuff to stuff" in the hope of incorporating some tissue that will permit better voluntary control or that will at least narrow the anal orifice. Such a frustrating operative session, however, rarely produces significant improvement in bowel control. When everything surgically possible has been done to ensure a good result, external sphincter repair is frequently combined with puborectalis plication (Figs. 5-10 and 5-11).

An important consideration at the completion of the repair is to determine the means to establish proper skin coverage over the defect. If loss of skin has been minimal, primary closure is the most convenient method; with considerable loss of skin, a new covering must be found. A split-thickness graft may be employed, but I prefer sensory-bearing full-thickness skin, either advanced or rotated into position, as illustrated in Figure 5-12 and in Chapter 6 (Anoplasty). Usually drains are not necessary, but occasionally, with the potential of dead space, a small, appropriately tailored Jackson-Pratt drain brought out through a counterincision may be useful.

Reefing

Reefing, a procedure involving plication of the deep portion of the external sphincter and puborectalis sling, is the procedure commonly employed transvaginally for posterior repairs (rectocele). As illustrated in Figure 5-10, reefing may be performed anteriorly or, as shown in Figure 5-11, it may be done posteriorly. In the anterior repair, the approach commonly employed in

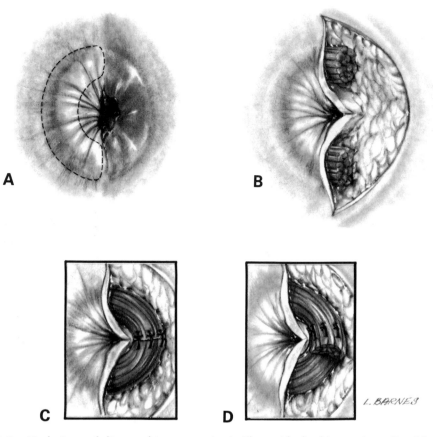

FIG. 5-9. Technique of direct sphincter repair. **A.** The residual sphincter is outlined by a dashed line; tissue loss is demonstrated on the opposite side. **B.** The ends of the divided sphincter are identified. Eschar has been debrided. **C.** Technique of apposition. **D.** Technique of overlapping.

women, the vagina is mobilized and the external sphincter is divided. The first suture is placed in the external sphincter, and the plication proceeds in a cephalad direction until the puborectalis muscle is likewise plicated. Care must be taken to avoid narrowing the anal orifice; a finger or retractor should be placed into the rectum during the tying of the sutures. The vagina is reapproximated with interrupted fine Dexon sutures.

In the posterior plication (Fig. 5-11) the external sphincter is identified and sutured medially to narrow the anal orifice. Here, again, care must be taken to avoid too tight a closure. If it is not necessary to excise skin, the incision for this approach is often curvilinear. It should be made approximatley 1 cm from the mucocutaneous junction, and offers excellent exposure of the sphincter muscle.

Parks emphasized the importance of levator plication in the procedure he calls the deep postanal repair.[39] A posterior incision is made and the dissection carried out in the intersphincteric plane. By retracting the external sphincter the levatores are identified and plicated. The external sphincter is also plicated.

Postoperative Care

All patients who undergo reconstructive anorectal procedures that involve repair of the sphincter or replacement of skin, or both, should have a bowel-confining regimen in the immediate postoperative period. This consists of a clear liquid diet with the addition of "slowing" medications—Lomotil, up to 8 tablets a day; codeine, up to 240 mg a day; and deodorized tincture of opium, up to 60 drops a day. With such a regimen it is rare indeed for a patient to have a bowel movement. The duration of this program depends on the amount of surgical trauma and may vary from 3 to 7 days. In women, an indwelling catheter is useful until

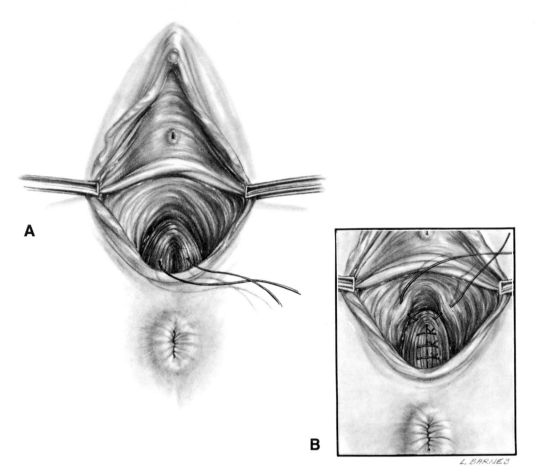

FIG. 5-10. The reefing procedure as performed anteriorly in women. **A.** The vaginal mucosa has been elevated and the sphincter identified. **B.** The sphincter is reefed, and the perivaginal fascia is used to complete the repair.

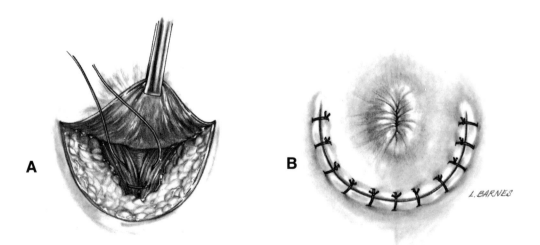

FIG. 5-11. Posterior reefing procedure. **A.** A curvilinear incision exposes the sphincter posteriorly. The sphincter is plicated posteriorly. **B.** Closure.

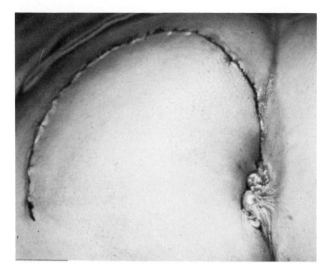

FIG. 5-12.   Rotation flap to cover the defect in the patient shown in Fig. 5-4

defecation is permitted. Systemic antibiotics may be useful for from 2 to 7 days, depending on the amount of surgical manipulation and degree of contamination.

Local care includes gentle cleansing of the wounds with antiseptic solution three times daily and application of a topical antiseptic ointment, such as povidone-iodine (Betadine). Sitz baths are not advised for at least 5 days. Patients are encouraged to perform perineal strengthening exercises immediately after operation. When the patient is able to take a regular diet, a stool softener, such as dioctyl sodium sulfosuccinate (Colace), and a bulk laxative preparation containing psyllium (Metamucil, Konsyl-D, Konsyl) are often advisable.

Operation for Supplementing the Sphincter Mechanism (Gracilis Muscle Transposition)

When there is sufficient residual sphincter, direct repair usually produces satisfactory results. However, if muscle tissue has been lost either as a result of trauma or disuse, such an approach is usually unsuccessful. In such instances surgical reconstruction designed to create an artificial sphincter may have some merit.

In 1936, Stone reported the use of preserved fascia as a pursestring suture about the anus.[58] Although this did not permit voluntary control, it narrowed the anal outlet so that the patient had some degree of continence. The operation was subsequently extended and revised to encircle the fascia around the anus and to

anchor the free ends to the gluteus maximus muscle on each side.[59, 64] The anal canal was thus enclosed in a fascial ring, which could theoretically be tightened by contraction of the gluteal muscle. Satisfactory results were reported in 30 patients.[60] Other operations have been developed to supplement the sphincter muscle, but very little experience has been reported.[8, 11]

In 1952, Pickrell and associates developed a procedure using the gracilis muscle as a substitute anal sphincter.[43] I have used this operation when a supplementary sphincter was required,[12, 13] and when multiple attempts at direct repair have been unsuccessful. This operation is not for elderly patients who complain of soiling their underclothes. It is an esoteric sphincter-repairing approach to be used only in limited circumstances. It is beneficial in young patients, in patients who have sustained trauma, and in those with congenital abnormalities.

The gracilis muscle, the most superficial muscle in the medial aspect of the thigh, is broad in the upper thigh, becomes narrow, and tapers to a tendon which inserts below the tibial tuberosity. The major blood supply enters proximally so that division at the insertion and mobilization of the muscle to the proximal neurovascular bundle do not compromise viability.

Technique

The method of preoperative preparation has been described. Patients are placed in the perineolithotomy position to expose the thighs and the anus. The side selected for transposition is draped so that it can be removed easily from the stirrup.

The three medial incisions required to mobilize the gracilis muscle are in the upper thigh, in the mid-thigh, and across the knee joint. The muscle is identified initially through the proximal incision. A quarter-inch Penrose drain is passed under the muscle (Fig. 5-13), and the dissection is carried cephalad to the neurovascular bundle *(inset)*, which is the upper limit of the dissection. The muscle is mobilized to the tendinous insertion (Fig. 5-14) by incising the investing fascia and by blunt dissection beneath the skin bridges. The tendon of the gracilis muscle passes under the sartorius muscle so that the latter muscle must be retracted anteriorly to identify the gracilis tendon. The dissection proceeds distally as far as possible, and the tendon is divided. The two distal incisions are closed in two layers (subcutaneous tissue and skin) and the muscle delivered through the proximal incision (Fig. 5-15).

Attention is then turned to the anal dissection. A curvilinear incision is made approximately 1.5 cm from the anal verge anteriorly and posteriorly. If possible an attempt should be made to preserve the raphes (as illustrated) so that the muscle can be pulled around

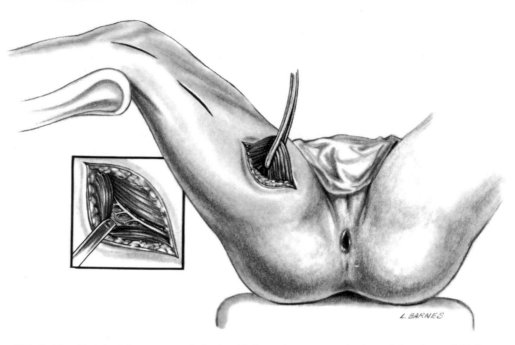

FIG. 5-13. Two incisions are made in the thigh, and one across the knee joint, for mobilizing the gracilis muscle. A Penrose drain is placed around the muscle proximally; this tethers the muscle and facilitates identification of the neurovascular bundle *(inset)*.

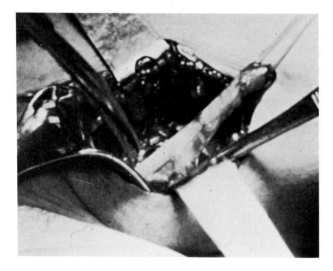

FIG. 5-14. The gracilis muscle is fully mobilized to the tendinous insertion.

them as a pulley (Fig. 5-16). A tunnel is developed between the proximal thigh incision and the anterior perianal incision, and the muscle is pulled through (Fig. 5-17). The thigh incision is then closed.

A tunnel is developed in the extrasphincteric space on either side of the anal canal. The tendon is passed clockwise if the right gracilis muscle is being transposed, or counterclockwise if the left gracilis muscle is used (Fig. 5-18).

After the tendon is passed 360° and *behind* the muscle, an incision is made over the contralateral ischial tuberosity. Three monofilament nonabsorbable sutures (Prolene) are placed in the gluteal fascia and held in place (Fig. 5-19). The tendon is pulled through a tunnel developed between the ischial incision and the anterior perianal incision (Fig. 5-20). At this point the leg from which the gracilis muscle was taken is removed from the stirrup and adducted (Fig. 5-21). This is an extremely important maneuver because it releases some tension on the muscle. If the tendon were to be anchored without adduction, the substitute sphincter would be too loose, and the results would be unsatisfactory. With maximal adduction the surgeon pulls the tendon taut. It should be quite snug when the finger is inserted in the rectum. Too tight an anal orifice may be corrected by dilation. The sutures are placed into the tendon and secured. All incisions are closed, and

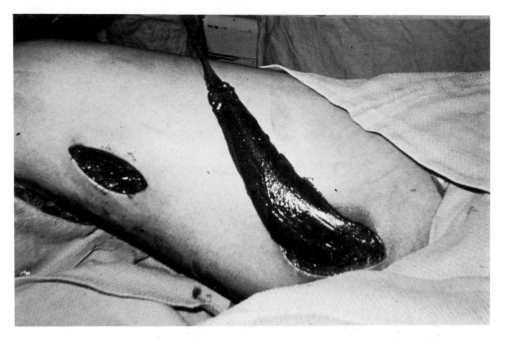

FIG. 5-15. The gracilis muscle is delivered through the proximal incision.

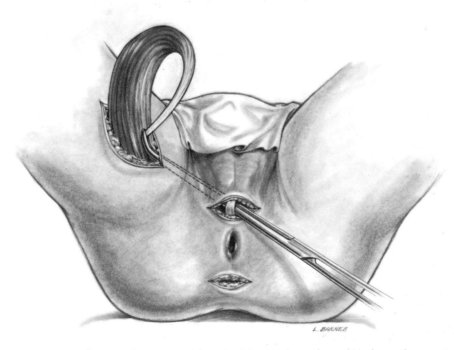

FIG. 5-16. Gracilis muscle transposition. Incisions are made anteriorly and posteriorly outside the anus, preserving the raphes. The placental forceps serves to deliver the tendon through the thigh tunnel.

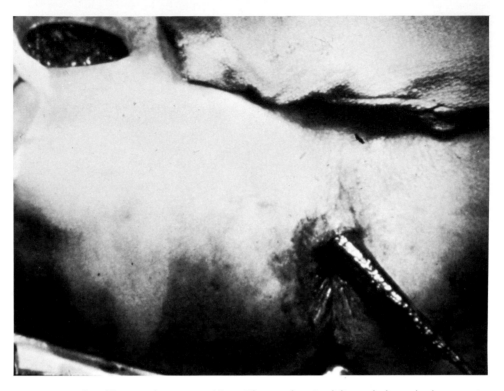

FIG. 5-17. Gracilis muscle transposition. The tendon is delivered through the anterior perianal incision.

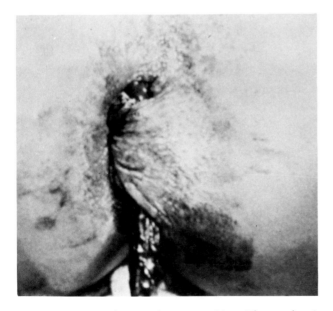

FIG. 5-18. Gracilis muscle transposition. The tendon is brought out through the posterior incision.

no drains are employed (Fig. 5-22). A protective colostomy is unnecessary.

Postoperative Care

Postoperatively the bowels are confined for 1 week. The patient is kept at bed rest for 48 hours, after which ambulation is permitted. The wounds are gently cleansed three times daily, and a topical antiseptic ointment is applied. The postoperative management of these patients must be vigorous. Lack of success in the past with this procedure may have been the result of insufficient attention to this aspect of treatment. This repair is much like the Thiersch operation in narrowing the anal orifice except that this "pursestring" is dynamic. The anal orifice can be stretched open, and then it passively closes.

The goal in the postoperative period is establishment of a workable time for defecation. For most patients this is in the morning. When the patient is eating a regular diet, a suppository, such as bisacodyl, is inserted immediately after breakfast. Ideally the patient will defecate and remain clean until the next morning when the procedure is repeated. Ultimately the patient will

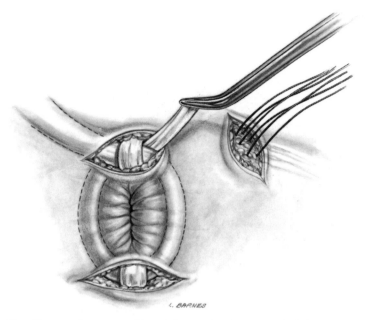

FIG. 5-19. Gracilis muscle transposition. The tendon has encircled the anus. An incision is made over the contralateral ischial tuberosity, and sutures are placed in the gluteal fascia.

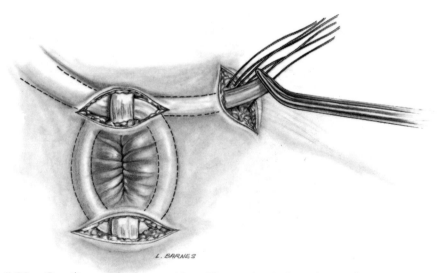

FIG. 5-20. Gracilis muscle transposition. The tendon is brought out through the ischial tuberosity incision.

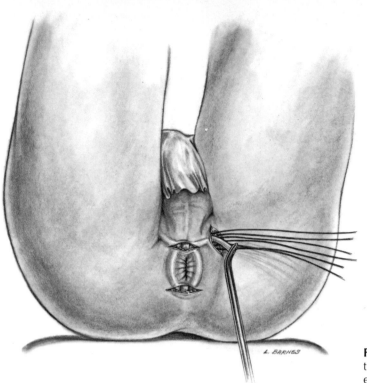

FIG. 5-21. Gracilis muscle transposition. Adduction of the thigh before the tendon is secured is an extremely important maneuver.

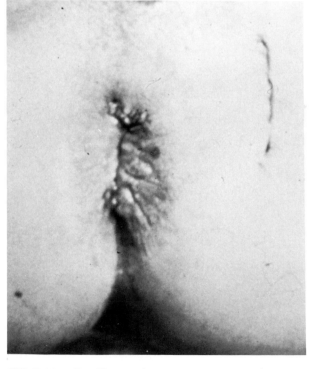

FIG. 5-22. Gracilis muscle transposition: immediate postoperative appearance of the perianal area.

establish a pattern that would avoid the need for a suppository. Obviously each patient must be treated individually; some may require laxatives, others "slowing" medications.

Anal Encircling (Thiersch) Procedure

Gabriel recommended encircling the anus using silver wire.[19] He reported good results in 11 patients for anal incontinence. Generally this procedure has been advocated for the treatment of rectal prolapse, but because of complications and difficulty in handling, most surgeons prefer another type of suture. My own preference is Mersilene (5 mm). However, I have not found it useful for the treatment of anal incontinence (see Chap. 7).

A simple and quite effective alternative to the transposition of the gracilis muscle for supplementing the sphincter mechanism is implanting a Dacron-impregnated Silastic sheet as a prosthesis encircling the anus (See Fig. 7-10). Although Labow and co-workers described the use of this material as an alternative to wire in the treatment of rectal prolapse, I have found it quite useful as a substitute anal sphincter in patients with fecal incontinence.[32]

A strip is cut to 1.5 cm wide; it should be prepared by the surgeon in such a way that it is elastic along its longitudinal axis (Fig. 5-23, *A*). An overlap of 1 cm is created, and a TA stapler is used to secure the edges (Fig. 5-23, *B*). The diameter can be checked before applying the stapler by holding the material in place with a hemostat and returning the sheet to the proper position in the wound. Digital examination confirms the adequacy of the narrowing. The suture line is reinforced with interrupted Prolene sutures (Fig. 5-23, *C*). All wounds are closed. Figures 5-24 and 5-25 show the preoperative and immediate postoperative appearance of the anus in a young man who suffered sphincter injury following a motorcycle accident.

Because of the risk of infection, the patient should be placed on a bowel preparation and systemic perioperative antibiotics. The patient is discharged in 3 to 5 days, when bowel function has occurred.

I have used this procedure on 19 patients with anal incontinence. One patient developed sepsis, necessitating removal of the sling. In spite of this complication the patient reported some improvement, presumed secondary to scarring. The other patients reported good to excellent control for feces.

The particular advantage of this material is that it can stretch, and on rectal examination it is difficult to distinguish the sensation of the sheet from that of the normal, intact anal sphincter.

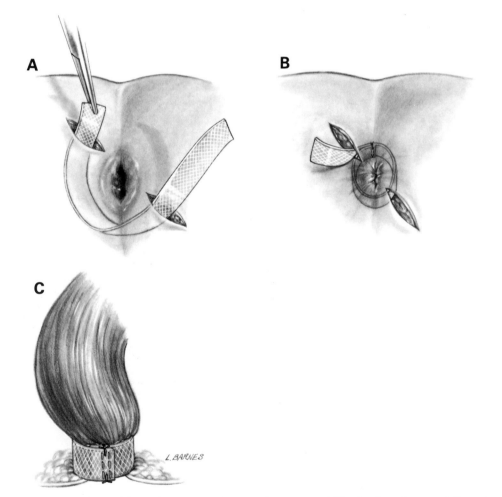

FIG. 5-23. Elastic fabric sling. **A.** The Dacron-impregnated Silastic sheet is passed through the two incisions. **B.** The sheet is passed circumferentially around the anus and sutured into place. **C.** Final position of the sheet.

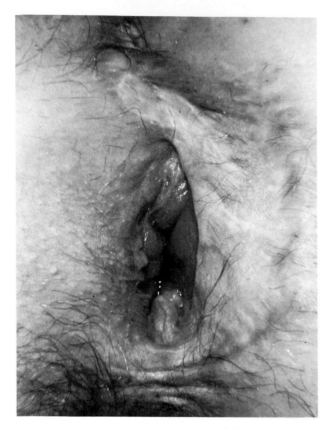

FIG. 5-24. Patulous anus and scarring following accidental trauma.

Results

It is very difficult to evaluate the relative merits of different operations in the treatment of fecal incontinence. Generally, the best results are obtained if direct sphincter repair is possible. [10, 21, 47, 57] If there is little or no sphincter remaining, obviously an attempt at resuture will be of little avail, whereas a gracilis muscle transposition, for example, may be quite ameliorating. Much, therefore, depends on the judgment of the surgeon and the type of surgical problem that the patient presents. Unfortunately, neither of these variables is readily apparent in a literature search on the subject.

Goldberg and associates reviewed 47 cases treated by sphincteroplasty.[21] Almost half of the patients sustained obstetric or gynecologic trauma. The total complication rate was 8.5%. An independent examiner found that 52% had excellent results, 37% good results, and 11% fair or poor results.

Rudd reported the treatment of 136 patients with anal incontinence.[47] Approximately one third were treated with exercises and bowel management, and another third by operant conditioning. Twenty-one patients had direct external sphincter repair, all but one of whom had good or excellent results. Of six patients requiring a puborectalis–external sphincter repair, five had good results.

Parks reported 75 patients who underwent the deep postanal repair; approximately two thirds had a rectal prolapse.[39] The best results were in the group without prolapse. The overall success rate was 83%. Keighley and Matheson found that rectopexy alone resulted in restoration of continence in 80% of 20 procidentia patients with this symptom.[30] Those with incontinence (4 patients) were submitted to postanal repair. Three became completely continent and one noted some improvement.

I reported 13 patients who underwent gracilis muscle transposition.[13] Patients were followed for a mean of 22 months. Good or excellent results were achieved in those who sustained prior trauma or had a congenital anomaly, providing they did not have a neurologic problem or underlying bowel disorder.

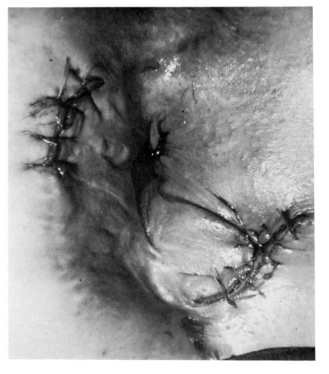

FIG. 5-25. Postoperative appearance following elastic fabric sling.

It was felt that gracilis muscle transposition could be advised when sphincter muscle had been lost or other sphincteroplastic approaches had failed. Relative contraindications included neurologic deficit, diarrhea, and severe constipation.

SUMMARY

Anal incontinence following trauma should be treated by direct sphincter repair or puborectalis plication, if possible. If this fails or if there is inadequate residual muscle, a gracilis muscle transposition or insertion of Silastic-impregnated Dacron should be considered.

Perineal strengthening exercises with or without "biofeedback" and bowel management should supplement the above, and should be the primary treatment in those patients deemed inappropriate for reconstruction.

Colostomy should rarely be necessary in the treatment of this condition.

REFERENCES

1. Ala J, Mendeloff AI, Hendrix TR et al: Studies of fecal incontinence by combined manometric-electromyographic techniques (abstr). Gastroenterology 1965; 48:863
2. Bellman M: Studies on encopresis. Acta Paediatr Scand Suppl 1966; 170:1–151
3. Bishop B, Garry RC, Roberts TDM et al: Control of the external sphincter of the anus in the cat. J Physiol 1956; 134:229–240
4. Blaisdell PC: Repair of the incontinent sphincter ani. Surg Gynecol Obstet 1940; 70:692–697
5. Block IR: Repair of the incontinent sphincter ani following operative injury. Surg Gynecol Obstet 1959; 109:111–116
6. Borden EB, Sheran M, Sammartano RJ, Boley SJ: The complete anorectal function profile (abstr). Gastroenterology 1982; 82:1023
7. Brocklehurst JC: Management of Anal Incontinence. Clin Gastroenterol 1975; 4:479–487
8. Bruining HA, Bos KE, Colthoff EG, Tolhurst DE: Creation of an anal sphincter mechanism by bilateral proximally based gluteal muscle transposition. Plast Reconstr Surg 1981; 67:70–73
9. Caldwell KPS: The electrical control of sphincter incompetence. Lancet 1963; 2:174–175
10. Castro AF, Pittman RE: Repair of the incontinent sphincter. Dis Colon Rectum 1978; 21:183–187
11. Chittenden AS: Sphincter muscle and reconstruction. Ann Surg 1930; 92:152–154
12. Corman ML: Gracilis muscle transposition. Contemp Surg 1978; 13:9–16
13. Corman ML: Follow-up evaluation of gracilis muscle transposition for fecal incontinence. Dis Colon Rectum 1980; 23:552–555
14. Denny-Brown D, Robertson EG: An investigation of the nervous control of defaecation. Brain 1935; 58:256–310
15. Dickinson VA: Maintenance of anal continence: A review of pelvic floor physiology. Gut 1978; 19:1163–1174
16. Easson WM: Encopresis—psychogenic soiling. Can Med Assoc J 1960; 82:624–628
17. Engel BT, Nikoomanesh P, Schuster MM: Operant conditioning of rectosphincteric responses in the treatment of fecal incontinence. N Engl J Med 1974; 290:646–649
18. Gabriel WB: The Principles and Practice of Rectal Surgery, 5th ed, p 18. London, HK Lewis and Co, 1963
19. Gabriel WB: The Principles and Practice of Rectal Surgery, 5th ed, pp 106–132. London, HK Lewis and Co, 1963
20. Glen ES: Effective and safe control of incontinence by the intra-anal plug electrode. Br J Surg 1971; 58:249–252
21. Goldberg SM, Gordon PH, Nivatvongs S: Essentials of anorectal surgery, pp 286–287. Philadelphia, JB Lippincott, 1980
22. Goligher JC, Duthie HL, DeDombal FT et al: Abdominoanal pull-through excision for tumours of the mid-third of the rectum: A comparison with low anterior resection. Br J Surg 1965; 52:323–335
23. Gorsch RV: Proctologic Anatomy. Baltimore, Williams & Wilkins, 1955
24. Granet E: Hemorrhoidectomy failures: Causes, prevention and management. Dis Colon Rectum 1968; 11:45–48
25. Hagihara PF, Griffen WO Jr: Delayed correction of anorectal incontinence due to anal sphincteral injury. Arch Surg 1976; 111:63–66
26. Hardcastle JD, Porter NH: Anal continence. In Morson BC (ed): Diseases of the Colon, Rectum and Anus, pp 251-260. New York, Appleton-Century-Crofts, 1969
27. Henry MM, Parks AG, Swash M: The anal reflex in idiopathic faecal incontinence: An electrophysiologic study. Br J Surg 1980; 67:781–783
28. Hopkinson BR, Lightwood R: Electrical treatment of anal incontinence. Lancet 1966; 1:297–298
29. Hopkinson BR, Lightwood R: Electrical treatment of incontinence. Br J Surg 1967; 54:802–805
30. Keighley MRB, Matheson DM: Results of treatment for rectal prolapse and fecal incontinence. Dis Colon Rectum 1981; 24:449–453
31. Kiesewetter WB, Turner CR: Continence after surgery for imperforate anus: A critical analysis and

preliminary experience with the sacroperineal pull-through. Ann Surg 1963; 158:498–512

32. Labow S, Rubin RJ, Hoexter B, Salvati EP: Perineal repair of rectal procidentia with an elastic fabric sling. Dis Colon Rectum 1980; 23:467–469

33. Lane RH: Clinical application of anorectal physiology. Proc R Soc Med 1975; 68:28–30

34. Louw JH: Congenital abnormalities of the rectum and anus. Curr Probl Surg 1965; May:1–64

35. MacLeod JH: Biofeedback in the management of partial anal incontinence: A preliminary report. Dis Colon Rectum 1979; 22:169–171

36. Musicco N: Encopresis: A good result in a boy with UTP (uridine-5-triphosphate). Am J Proctol 1977; 28:43–46

37. Neill ME, Parks AG, Swash M: Physiological studies of the anal sphincter musculature in faecal incontinence and rectal prolapse. Br J Surg 1981; 68:531–536

38. Nichols RL, Broido P, Condon RE et al: Effect of preoperative neomycin-erythromycin intestinal preparation on the incidence of infectious complications following colon surgery. Ann Surg 1973; 178:453–462

39. Parks AG: Anorectal incontinence. Proc R Soc Med 1975; 68:681–690

40. Parks AG, Porter NH, Hardcastle JD: The syndrome of the descending perineum. Proc R Soc Med 1966; 59:477–482

41. Parks AG, Porter NH, Melzak J: Experimental study of the reflex mechanism controlling the muscles of the pelvic floor. Dis Colon Rectum 1962; 5:407–414

42. Phillips SF, Edwards DAW: Some aspects of anal continence and defaecation. Gut 1965; 6:396–406

43. Pickrell KL, Broadbent TR, Masters FW et al: Construction of a rectal sphincter and restoration of anal continence by transplanting gracilis muscle: Report of four cases in children. Ann Surg 1952; 135:853–862

44. Porter NH: Megacolon: A physiological study. Proc R Soc Med 1961; 54:1043–1047

45. Porter NH: A physiological study of the pelvic floor in rectal prolapse. Ann R Coll Surg Engl 1962; 31:379–404

46. Read NW, Harford WV, Schmulen AC et al: A clinical study of patients with fecal incontinence and diarrhea. Gastroenterol 1979; 76:747–756

47. Rudd WWH: Anal incontinence (Symposium). Dis Colon Rectum 1982; 25:97–102

48. Schiller LR, Santa Ana CA, Schmulen AC et al: Pathogenesis of fecal incontinence in diabetes mellitus: Evidence for internal-anal sphincter dysfunction. N Engl J Med 1982; 307:1666–1671

49. Schuster MM: Clinical significance of motor disturbances of the enterocolonic segment. Am J Dig Dis 1966; 11:320–335

50. Schuster MM: Motor action of rectum and anal sphincters in continence and defecation. In Code CR (ed): Handbook of Physiology: A Critical, Comprehensive Presentation of Physiological Knowledge and Concepts. Section 6, Alimentary Canal; Vol 4: Motility, pp 2121-2140. Baltimore, Williams & Wilkins, 1968

51. Schuster MM: The riddle of the sphincters. Gastroenterology 1975: 69:249–262

52. Schuster MM, Mendeloff AI: Characteristics of rectosigmoid motor function: Their relationship to continence, defecation and disease. In Glass GBJ (ed): Progress in Gastroenterology, Vol 2, pp 200-220. New York, Grune & Stratton, 1970

53. Schuster MM, Hendrix TR, Mendeloff AI: The internal anal sphincter response: Manometric studies on its normal physiology, neural pathways, and alteration in bowel disorders. J Clin Invest 1963; 42:196–207

54. Schuster MM, Hookman P, Hendrix TR et al: Simultaneous manometric recording of internal and external anal sphincteric reflexes. Bull John Hopkins Hosp 1965; 116:9–88

55. Shafik A: A new concept of the anatomy of the anal sphincter mechanism and the physiology of defecation— The external anal sphincter: A triple-loop system. Invest Urol 1975; 12:412–419

56. Silber DL: Encopresis: Discussion of etiology and management. Clin Pediatr (Phila) 1969; 8:225–231

57. Slade MS, Goldberg SM, Schottler JL et al: Sphincteroplasty for acquired anal incontinence. Dis Colon Rectum 1977; 20:33–35

58. Stone HB: Plastic operation for anal incontinence. Trans South Surg Assoc 1928; 41:235–240

59. Stone HB: Plastic operation for anal incontinence. Arch Surg 1929; 18:845–851

60. Stone HB, McLanahan S: Results with the fascia plastic operation for anal incontinence. Ann Surg 1941; 114:73–77

61. Waylonis GW, Powers JJ: Clinical application of anal sphincter electromyography. Surg Clin North Am 1972; 52:807–815

62. Weissenberg S: Encopresis. Ztschr f Kinderh 1926; 40:674–677

63. Whitehead WE, Parker L, Bosmajian LS et al: Behavioral treatment of fecal incontinence secondary to spina bifida (abstr). Gastroenterology 1982; 82:1209

64. Wreden RR: A method of reconstructing a voluntary sphincter ani. Arch Surg 1929; 18:841–844

CHAPTER 6

Anal Stenosis and Anoplasty

Anal stricture can be one of the most disabling complications of anal surgery or of anal disease. Anal stenosis can occur as a consequence of a number of conditions: benign and malignant tumors, inflammations (especially Crohn's disease), congenital anomalies (ectopic and imperforate anus), laxative abuse, and trauma (particularly surgical). This last cause is by far the commonest reason for performing an anoplasty.

SYMPTOMS AND FINDINGS

The most troublesome complaint of patients with anal stenosis is difficulty defecating. Constipation, obstipation, painful bowel movements, narrow caliber of the stool, abdominal cramping, and bleeding are frequently associated symptoms. The fear of fecal impaction or pain usually causes the patient to rely on daily laxatives or enemas.

Physical examination will readily reveal the problem. It may be impossible to perform digital examination, or only the little finger alone may be tolerated. Since there is a tendency to confuse anal stenosis with anal spasm, especially in the presence of anal fissure, the correct diagnosis can sometimes be made only by employing an anesthetic. This abolishes the spasm associated with an acute fissure but will not produce an increased luminal diameter in a patient with a stenosis.[14] Proctosigmoidoscopy and anoscopy will require narrow caliber instruments. Examination of the proximal bowel, however, must be undertaken prior to any reconstructive approach in order to rule out the presence of colon disease.

It is important to ascertain the etiology of the stricture in order to determine the proper therapy. Inflammatory bowel disease is an absolute contraindication to anoplasty, and obviously a malignant process must be treated by extirpation. Perhaps the most useful diagnostic tool is obtaining an accurate history. If the patient associates the onset of the problem with prior hemorrhoidectomy or electrocoagulation of anal condylomata, the condition will be appropriately treated by anoplasty. Conversely, with no such history, in a patient with long-term laxative abuse, correction of the stricture may lead to anal incontinence. This occurs when sphincter muscle wasting accompanies the anal stricture, a consequence of passing small, narrow stools over many years. Mineral oil is particularly notorious for lubricating the stool so that it fails to dilate the anal canal, thereby precipitating stenosis.

Symptoms from birth imply a congenital etiology. Commonest is an anteriorly situated *ectopic anus*, usually at the orifice of the vagina.[1] The *hooded anus* (Fig. 6-1) and *anorectal atresia* are also congenital lesions that may produce stenosis in spite of treatment early in life.

TREATMENT

Medical

The conservative treatment of anal stenosis includes laxatives, suppositories, and enemas. These permit easier defecation but do not treat the defect itself, narrowed anal canal diameter. The patient may be given an anal dilator (see Fig. 2-30) in order to widen the anal canal, but all too often the stricture is too severe

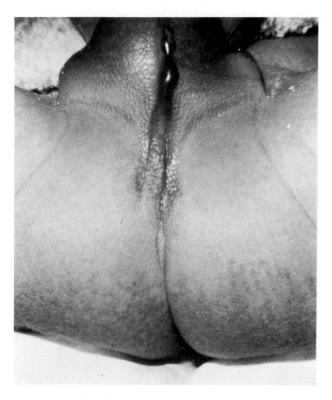

FIG. 6-1. A hooded anus predisposes to anal stenosis later in life. Tracking of meconium can be seen along the median raphe. Initial management often involves the use of a dilator.

and precludes insertion of any instrument. Furthermore, even if it is possible to use such a device, its application does not replace the loss of anal canal tissue. Hence, dilation is usually required indefinitely. The procedure itself is quite traumatic and may tear the canal; the subsequent complications may require surgical intervention.[13]

Surgical

Excision of the Eschar and Sphincterotomy

The classic surgical treatment of anal stricture is lysis and excision of the eschar, transverse suture of the rectal mucosa to the underlying internal anal sphincter, and sphincterotomy: the same procedure as described for the treatment by excision of chronic anal fissure (see Fig. 3-10). Although the results have been reported as excellent ("several hundred" patients of Pope, over 200 patients of Turell, 17 patients of Shropshear, and 224 patients of Malgieri),[6, 9, 12, 15] it is difficult to interpret whether the patients had significant narrowing or merely spasm associated with an anal

fissure. Furthermore, the term *anoplasty* should be limited to the procedures that actually replace the anal canal with skin.

The procedure is performed as follows:

A deformed anal orifice is present (Fig. 6-2, *A*) that does not admit the index finger (Fig. 6-2, *B*). When the stricture is excised or lysed (Fig. 6-3, *A*) and when a 29-mm Hill-Ferguson retractor is inserted, the cut edge of the rectum can be sutured to the underlying internal anal sphincter in a transverse fashion, thereby widening the anal canal (Fig. 6-3, *B*). If the lumen is still inadequate, the same maneuver can be performed on the opposite side (Fig. 6-3, *C*).

This is a perfectly acceptable technique and will yield satisfactory results if sufficient skin bridges remain. If this is not the case, frequent digital examinations must be performed or dilators employed to prevent restricture. As with sphincterotomy or sphincter stretch, this operation does not create a new anal canal lining with sensory-bearing mucosa. However, this procedure, or even the simpler approach of sphincterotomy, is satisfactory for most patients. For more profound narrowing, anoplasty should be performed in order to treat the basic problem: loss of anal canal tissue.

Anoplasty

Anoplasty is a procedure whereby perianal skin is moved to cover a defect in the anal canal. This defect is usually the result of an operative procedure, such as excision of a portion or all of the anal canal, hemorrhoidectomy, excision of an anal fissure, or excision of a lesion of the anal canal. Anoplasty is performed to correct anal stenosis or is employed coincident with sphincteroplasty for sphincteric injury or for repair of a rectovaginal fistula.[2–8, 10, 11] The list below summarizes the indications for this procedure.

Indications for Anoplasty

Anal stenosis
  Congenital
  Inflammatory (fistula, abscess)
  Trauma
    Accident
    Operative (hemorrhoidectomy, fissurectomy, pull-through procedure, excisional procedures)
    Disuse (laxatives, enemas, chronic diarrhea)
Coincident with excision of anal lesions
  Ulcer
  Tumor
Coincident with reconstructive anorectal operations
  Rectovaginal fistula repair
  Sphincteroplasty
  Congenital anomaly (imperforate anus, ectopic anus)

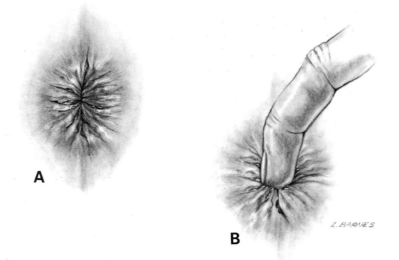

FIG. 6-2.   Anal deformity (**A**) with stricture that does not permit digital examination (**B**).

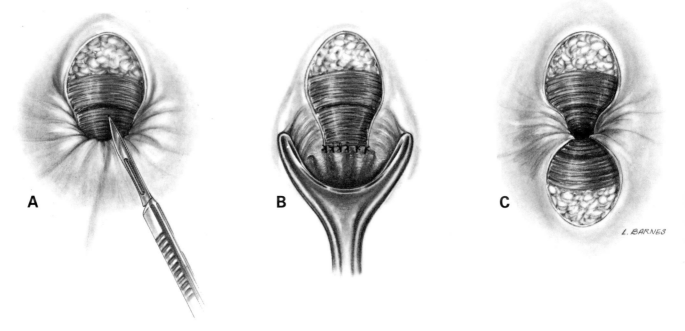

FIG. 6-3.   **A, B.** Lysis of the stricture, permitting insertion of a Hill-Ferguson retractor (29 mm). The rectum is sutured to the underlying internal anal sphincter. **C.** When further widening is required, this can be done on the opposite side.

Preoperative Preparation

Vigorous mechanical cleansing of the colon is a requisite for all anal procedures if skin grafting to the anus is planned. Patients should be given a cathartic on the day before operation (300 ml of magnesium citrate or 60 ml of castor oil) followed by colonic irrigations until the returns are clear. It is not certain whether nonabsorbable, orally administered antibiotics are useful, but a systemic antibiotic given before the operative procedure, intraoperatively, and for one or two doses postoperatively is of benefit in reducing the incidence of subsequent wound infection.

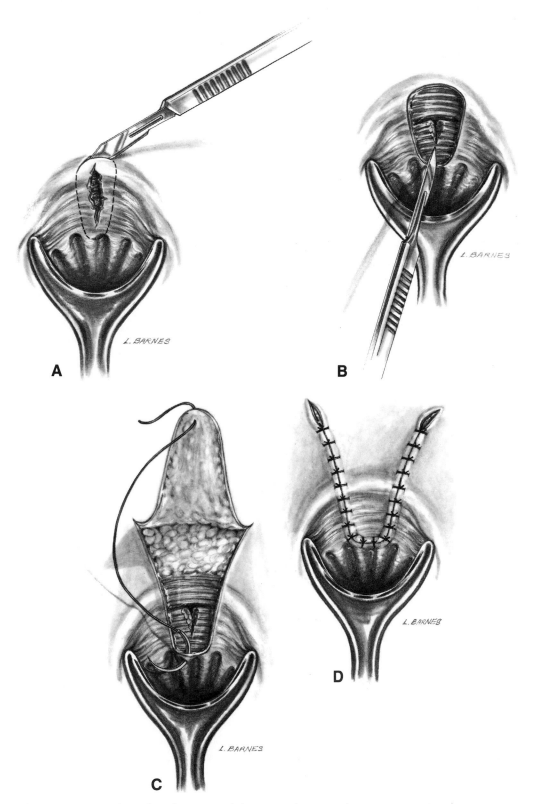

FIG. 6-4. Anoplasty for chronic anal fissure with minimal stenosis. **A.** The excision is outlined with a dashed line. **B.** An internal anal sphincterotomy is performed. **C.** The skin flap is elevated. **D.** The flap is advanced and sutured to the rectum.

Anoplasty for Chronic Anal Fissure with Minimal Stenosis

Esoteric anoplastic maneuvers should be reserved for loss of anal canal tissue, but even mild anal stenosis can be treated by skin replacement. A small advancement flap may be useful for stenosis accompanying chronic posterior anal fissure.

Operative Technique.   The patient is placed in the prone (jackknife) position on the operating table with the buttocks taped apart. Spinal, caudal, general endotracheal, or local anesthesia is employed. The fissure or stricture is excised (Fig. 6-4, *A*), and an internal anal sphincterotomy is performed (Fig. 6-4, *B*). A flap of skin is elevated in the posterior midline (Fig. 6-4, *C*). A Hill-Ferguson retractor is kept in place for the entire operation to determine the adequacy of the opening of the anal canal. If the anal canal can be reconstructed with the retractor in place, the opening will be adequate.

Incisions are carried proximally for 5 to 8 cm. Care must be taken to avoid creating a narrow pedicle that might compromise blood supply at the apex of the flap. Mobilization over the sacrum is unnecessary for this degree of anal canal defect. The full thickness of the skin is sutured to the rectal mucosa and to the underlying internal anal sphincter with interrupted 3-0 polyglycolic acid (synthetic absorbable) sutures. The completed repair is shown in Figure 6-4, *D*. The external aspect may be left open if tension is produced by closure, or the entire wound may be closed primarily.

This technique is simple and useful for stricture associated with anal fissure. However, if more than 25% of the circumference of the anal canal needs to be covered, another anoplastic approach is indicated (see the following).

Postoperative Management.   In all anoplastic operations, an antibiotic, usually a cephalosporin, is given parenterally for 3 to 5 days. In the previously described procedure no attempt is made to prevent

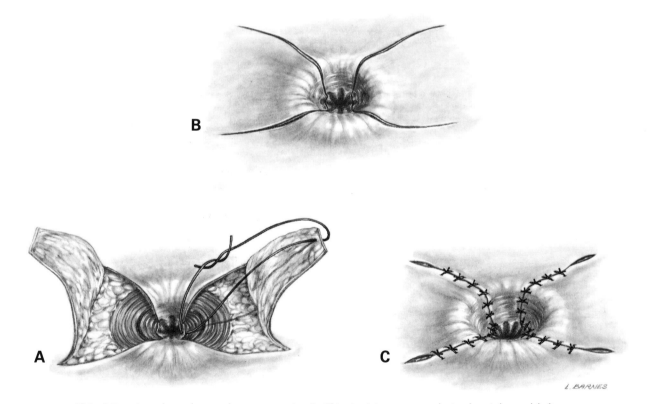

FIG. 6-5.   Anoplasty for moderate stenosis. **A.** Skin incisions are made in the right and left lateral positions. **B.** The skin flaps are elevated. **C.** Skin is advanced and sutured to the cut edge of the rectum and underlying sphincter. (Hill-Ferguson retractor is not shown.)

bowel movements after operation, and the patient is allowed a regular diet supplemented by a bulk laxative containing psyllium. On the first day after operation, sitz baths are begun, and if no bowel movement occurs by the second postoperative day, a laxative is given. Erythema of the skin flap is common, but purulent drainage is unusual. Probing under the pedicle may express a hematoma or purulent collection, but the skin graft is rarely compromised. The patient is discharged when a bowel movement is achieved, and he is seen weekly until the wounds heal, usually in 3 to 6 weeks.

Anoplasty for Moderate Stenosis

When more skin coverage is required than is offered by the single advancement flap described previously, sufficient skin can often be obtained by performing a double advancement flap in the right lateral and left lateral positions. This will permit coverage of up to approximately 50% of the anal canal.

Operative Technique. The patient is placed in the prone (jackknife) position with the buttocks taped apart. A local anesthetic is not advisable because of the extensive amount of infiltration that would be required. Figure 6-5, *A*, demonstrates the incisions before mobilization of the pedicle of the skin. In Figure 6-5, *B*, the full thickness of skin has been elevated in the two positions, and a suture is placed through the full thickness of the skin to the cut edge of rectum, incorporating a small portion of the underlying internal anal sphincter. Interrupted sutures of 4-0 Dexon are placed. Closure is effected as seen in Figure 6-5, *C*. The diameter of the anal canal has clearly been increased.

Postoperative Management. It is usually advisable to confine the bowel movements after this procedure. Sitz baths are withheld; the wound is cleaned, and a topical antiseptic, such as povidone-iodine, is applied 4 times a day.

After 5 days, medications are discontinued, and a regular diet supplemented with a laxative containing psyllium is commenced. Sitz baths are begun at this time. Some separation of the wound may occur, but satisfactory results can be expected. The patient is discharged when bowel function is adequate and is seen weekly until the wounds heal.

Anoplasty for Severe Anal Stenosis or for Significant Loss of Anal Canal Tissue

The plastic maneuvers previously described are useful for minimal or moderate problems of skin coverage.

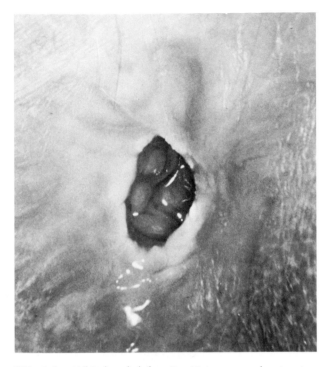

FIG. 6-6. Whitehead deformity. Note mucosal ectropion following excision of all of the anal canal: the characteristic "wet anus."

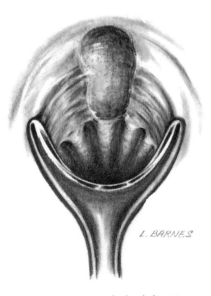

FIG. 6-7. Keyhole deformity.

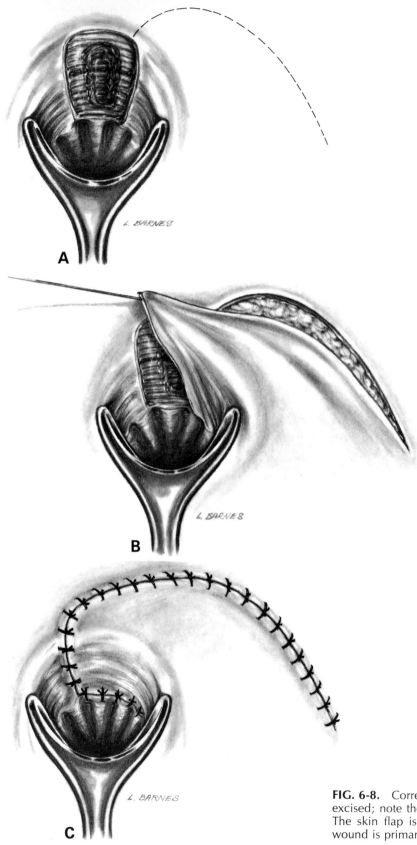

FIG. 6-8. Correction of keyhole deformity. **A.** The scar is excised; note the outline of the skin flap *(dashed line)*. **B.** The skin flap is mobilized and rotated medially. **C.** The wound is primarily closed.

However, if 50% or more of the anal canal needs to be reconstructed, an S-plasty should be considered. The conditions that may necessitate this maneuver to effect an optimal result include strictures secondary to radical hemorrhoidectomy, recurrent fissure, and laxative (especially mineral oil) abuse. Other instances in which S-plasty should be considered are when excision of lesions of the anal canal create tissue loss, and in correcting the characteristic Whitehead deformity (Fig. 6-6), the "keyhole" deformity (see Fig. 6-7), and the mucosal ectropion after abdomino-anal pull-through (see Fig. 5-7).

Operative Technique. The patient is placed in the prone (jackknife) position, and the buttocks are taped apart. In most instances a single rotation flap will more than suffice for adequate skin coverage (see Fig. 5-12). In such patients the left side may be taped farther laterally to permit a wider incision. Figure 6-7 illustrates a keyhole deformity in the posterior midline, a

consequence of excisional fissure surgery. After excision of the scar, an outline for the incision is made (Fig. 6-8, A). The flap is rotated medially (Fig. 6-8, B) and the wound closed primarily with interrupted 4-0 Dexon (Fig. 6-8, C).

In the correction of a Whitehead deformity or when the entire anal canal must be replaced, a bilateral rotation flap (S-plasty) must be performed. Spinal, caudal, or general endotracheal anesthesia is employed. A locally administered anesthetic is not advised. The anal canal is incised posteriorly, and the lower portion of the internal sphincter is divided. The anal canal is incised farther to permit insertion of a Hill-Ferguson retractor.

A full-thickness flap of skin is elevated, with the incision begun in the midline and carried laterally in a curvilinear fashion for approximately 8 to 10 cm (Fig. 6-9, A). A longer length can be obtained by incising farther laterally and, eventually, somewhat medially. Care must be taken to avoid necrosis of the flap. As

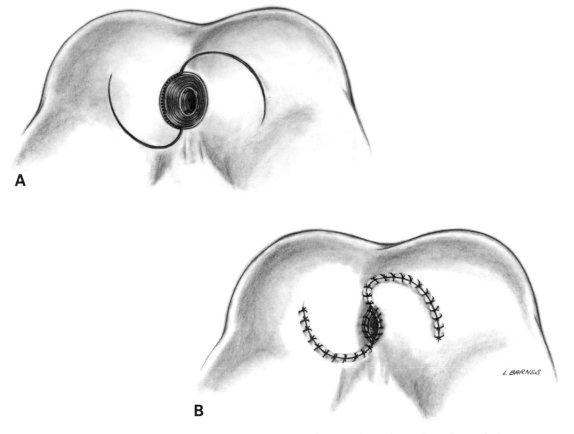

FIG. 6-9. Anoplasty for severe anal stenosis or for significant loss of anal canal tissue. **A.** The skin flaps are outlined; the eschar has been excised. **B.** The flaps are rotated and sutured to the rectum and underlying internal sphincter. (Hill-Ferguson retractor is not shown.)

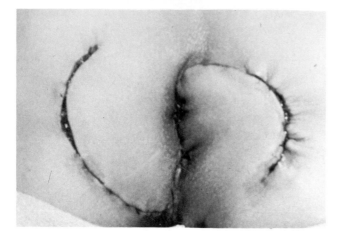

FIG. 6-10. S-plasty: immediate postoperative appearance following correction of Whitehead deformity.

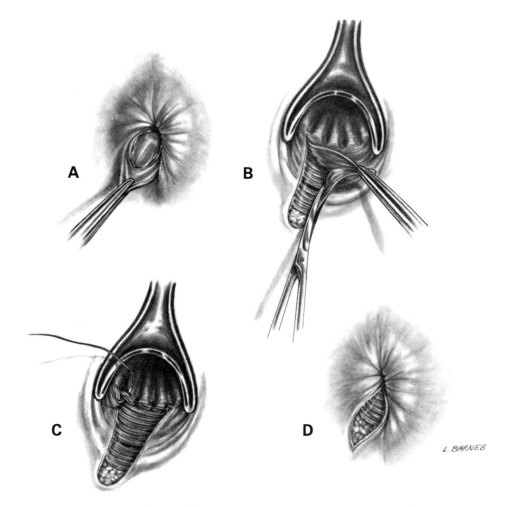

FIG. 6-11. Treatment of mucosal ectropion. **A.** Mucosa projects in one quadrant. **B.** Mucosa is excised. **C.** The edge of the rectum is sutured to the underlying internal sphincter. **D.** The wound is left open to granulate.

mentioned, more than one flap is rarely required since a new anal canal along half of the circumference is more than adequate. However, if the entire anal canal must be reconstructed, such as becomes necessary with the Whitehead deformity (in which all the mucosa must be excised completely, denuding the anal canal), a similar incision is performed on the opposite side. Hemostasis is effected with an electrocautery. Saline irrigation is carried out, and the skin is rotated medially and sutured to the rectum and to the underlying internal sphincter with interrupted Dexon sutures (Fig. 6-9, *B*). After the new mucocutaneous junction has been completed, subcuticular sutures of similar material are used, and the wound is closed completely by mobilizing a full-thickness flap of skin cephalad and laterally (Fig. 6-10). If this produces tension, the lateral aspect is left open to granulate (the usual method) or is grafted using split-thickness skin from the thigh (rarely indicated).

Postoperative Management.　No bowel movements are permitted for 5 days after operation. The regimen is identical to that described for double advancement flaps. Preoperative systemic antibiotic coverage is continued through the postoperative period for 5 days.

Rarely, a hematoma or an abscess will develop underneath the flap. By insertion of a hemostat between the sutures, evacuation of the collection usually can be achieved without compromising the graft.

Prolonged anal stenosis or a Whitehead deformity usually results in an attenuated sphincter mechanism. With a widely patent anal orifice, discharge of mucus and incontinence for flatus or even for feces may occur during the initial few weeks after operation. It is, therefore, advisable to start a regimen of perineal strengthening exercises, 10 to 15 times a day. Significant improvement may take many weeks, but normal continence should be achieved. An exception to this is in the patient who has anal stenosis and a virtually nonexistent sphincter mechanism caused by prolonged laxative abuse. These patients should be carefully selected for anoplastic restorative procedures, and a less than generous opening should be created.

Although the previous operation described the treatment of the classic Whitehead deformity, the mucosal ectropion producing the wet anus can be less than circumferential. In the patient illustrated in Figure 6-11, the mucosa projects in only one quadrant (Fig. 6-11, *A*). As long as no stricture is present, a simple excision (Fig. 6-11, *B*) and transverse suture of the rectum to the underlying internal anal sphincter (Fig. 6-11, *C*) will suffice. The open wound, as shown in Figure 6-11, *D*, will heal without the mucosal extrusion.

Anoplasty Concomitant with Sphincteroplasty, Ectopic Anus, or Perineal Body Reconstruction

In restorative procedures of the anal sphincter mechanism, as described in Chapter 5, the skin must often be mobilized concomitantly to effect adequate repair.

The anoplasty described in Chapter 4 (see Figs. 4-39 to 4-42) is most useful, especially in women with ectopic anus, rectovaginal fistula, or sphincter injury. A cruciate incision is made, the dissection and repair are completed, and the triangular flaps are advanced.

Postoperative Care.　Postoperative care must be directed not only to the skin but also to the underlying reconstruction or sphincter repair. The bowels are usually confined, as has been described, for a period of approximately 5 days, after which the previously mentioned regimen is begun.

Results

Sarner reported 21 patients who underwent from one to four advancement flaps for symptomatic anal stenosis.[11] He stated, "Adequate relief was achieved in all cases." Others have reported uniform satisfaction with advancement flaps.[7, 10] Ferguson and others have had equally gratifying results with rotation of the skin.[4, 8] Although there are no controlled studies, and individual observers may be biased in their interpretations, the fact remains that anoplasty is a simple and generally effective technique. In almost 100 anoplastic operations, regardless of the method, I have been pleased that every patient has had his or her symptoms ameliorated.

Comment

The methods for plastic reconstruction of the anal canal and perianal skin described are very useful procedures but should be performed only in carefully selected patients. They should not be employed routinely for uncomplicated fissurectomy, hemorrhoidectomy, or fistula repair. However, in certain disabling conditions, such as anal stenosis, Whitehead deformity, incontinence, sphincter injury, and rectovaginal fistula, one of these operations can be extremely effective in ensuring a successful result.

REFERENCES

1. Bentley JFR: Developmental anomalies and other diseases in children. In Morson BC: Diseases of the Colon, Rectum and Anus, p 64. New York, Appleton-Century-Crofts, 1969

2. Corman ML: Anoplasty. In Maingot R. (ed): Abdominal Operations, 7th ed, pp 2367-2374. New York, Appleton-Century-Crofts, 1980

3. Corman ML, Veidenheimer MC, Coller JA: Anoplasty for anal stricture. Surg Clin North Am 1976; 56:727–731

4. Ferguson JA: Repair of "Whitehead deformity" of the anus. Surg Gynecol Obstet 1959; 108:115–116

5. Hudson AT: S-plasty repair of Whitehead deformity of the anus. Dis Colon Rectum 1967; 10:57–60

6. Malgieri JA: Anoplasty to correct anal stricture. Dis Colon Rectum 1961; 4:289–291

7. Nickell WB, Woodward ER: Advancement flaps for treatment of anal stricture. Arch Surg 1972; 104:223–224

8. Oh C, Zinberg J: Anoplasty for anal stricture. Dis Colon Rectum 1982; 25:809–810

9. Pope CE: An anorectal plastic operation for fissure and stenosis and its surgical principles. Surg Gynecol Obstet 1959; 108:249–252

10. Rand AA: The sliding skin-flap graft operation for hemorrhoids: a modification of the Whitehead procedure. Dis Colon Rectum 1969; 12:265–276

11. Sarner JB: Plastic relief of anal stenosis. Dis Colon Rectum 1969; 12:277–280

12. Shropshear G: Posterior and anterior anal proctotomy: A simplified technic for postoperative anal stenosis. Dis Colon Rectum 1971; 14:62–66

13. Turell R: Postoperative anal stenosis. Surg Gynecol Obstet 1950; 90:231–233

14. Turell R, Gelernt IM: Anal stenosis. In Turell R (ed): Diseases of the Colon and Anorectum, 2nd ed, p 1046. Philadelphia, WB Saunders, 1969

15. Turell R, Gelernt IM: Anal stenosis. In Turell R (ed): Diseases of the Colon and Anorectum, 2nd ed, p 1051. Philadelphia, WB Saunders, 1969

CHAPTER 7

Rectal Prolapse

Rectal prolapse or procidentia is an uncommon clinical entity that has long fascinated surgeons. It is a condition that was recognized in antiquity, having been described in the Ebers Papyrus of 1500 B.C.[34] It often occurs in persons in the extremes of life. The two types of presentation are a complete or full-thickness involvement of the bowel and a partial or incomplete type involving prolapse of the mucosa only. The latter may be circumferential or may involve only part of the rectal mucosa.

ETIOLOGY

The precise cause of rectal prolapse is not thoroughly understood, but a number of factors seem to be implicated in the development of the condition.[62] To understand the cause, it is helpful to review the anatomy. The normal spine with its vertebral curves and the tilt of the pelvis shift the weight of the abdominal organs forward, away from the pelvic floor, and cause the rectum to follow a serpentine course through the pelvis. The stability of the rectum is greatly aided by the support of the levator ani muscle. An extensive interweaving of the longitudinal fibers of the rectum with the levator fibers creates a stable attachment between the rectum and this muscle. This provides a firm attachment to the pelvic floor and is an important element in rectal fixation, because without it the rectum would slip down through the muscle during defecation.[45, 46, 47]

The puborectalis sling functions by elevating the lower end of the rectum upward and forward toward the pubis, creating an acute anorectal angle and compressing the structures in front of it to decrease the opening of the pelvic floor. Relaxation of the puborectalis sling results in descent of the pelvic floor, obliterating the anorectal angle so that the rectum becomes more vertical.

During the act of defecation, intra-abdominal pressure is increased by contraction of the abdominal wall musculature and the diaphragm. Contraction of the levator ani muscle is inhibited, the puborectalis sling lengthens, and the pelvic floor descends, thereby obliterating the anorectal angle. The external sphincter muscle, which functionally forms a single unit with the puborectalis sling, relaxes at the same time. The rectum now occupies a vertical position, and the fecal mass is expelled by the contraction of the circular muscle of the rectum combined with the pressure from above. The rectum is held in place by fixation of the levator muscle anteriorly and by the various ligamentous structures laterally when the rectum is in a vertical position. The levator sling returns to its usual support position after defecation.

Etiologic factors believed to produce rectal prolapse may be congenital or acquired. The list on p 153 summarizes the predisposing influences. The unique pelvic anatomy, especially as observed at the time of laparotomy, is thought to play an important role in the cause of prolapse. A redundant rectosigmoid is often seen, as is a deep pouch of Douglas (a deep rectovaginal or rectovesical pouch of peritoneum).[37] Whether these are causative factors or associated anatomic conditions has been a subject of considerable debate.

Predisposing Factors for Rectal Prolapse

Poor bowel habits (esp. constipation)
Obesity
Chronic cough
Neurologic disease (e.g., congenital anomaly, cauda equina lesion)
Female sex
Nulliparity
Redundant rectosigmoid
Deep pouch of Douglas
Patulous anus (weak internal sphincter)
Diastasis of levator ani (defect in pelvic floor)
Lack of fixation of rectum to sacrum
Intussusception (secondary to colonic lesion)
Operative procedure (e.g., hemorrhoidectomy, fistulectomy, abdomino-anal pull-through)

Similarly, the patulous or weak sphincteric mechanism with diastasis of the levator ani muscle that causes a defect in the pelvic floor is more the result of prolapse than a causative factor (Fig. 7-1).

In infants, prolapse may be caused by a lack of skeletal support and by excessive pressures from above. In adults, prolapse may result from incomplete skeletal development. A free mesentery to the entire colon and rectum is a congenital anomaly that may undermine the support mechanism. Because of the complicated development of the levator ani muscle and its fixation to the rectum, anomalies of this muscle (including tenuous fixation to the rectum) may occur more often than is realized and may also contribute to instability of the rectum.

After many years of debate concerning the nature of the pathologic condition, Ripstein and Lanter and others described intussusception.[11–13, 54, 57, 60, 62] What initiates the intussusception is not clear, but, as demonstrated cineradiographically, over a period of time the intussusception pulls the rectum farther from the sacrum as it descends, eventually presenting at the anal verge.[6, 55, 60] Lack of fixation of the rectum to the sacrum can be observed at the time of laparotomy. When the act of defecation is viewed cineradiographically, the sequence of events is confirmed.

Rectal prolapse may be a consequence of a number of anorectal surgical procedures. An ectropion, sometimes referred to as a mucosal prolapse, is a frequent complication of the radical hemorrhoidectomy of Whitehead (see Fig. 6-6). It is important to differentiate this condition from procidentia. Surgical injury to the puborectalis muscle, such as might occur after anal fistula procedures and pull-through operations, also may be a predisposing factor (Fig. 7-2). If considerable sphincter has been divided, mucosal prolapse may be seen on the side of the injury.

Diseases of the nervous system and lesions of the cauda equina may contribute to rectal prolapse. Patients in psychiatric hospitals and nursing homes are not uncommonly afflicted with this otherwise rare condition. Goligher believes that one third of his patients were "rather odd," and approximately 3% were "definitely psychotic."[16] When it could be determined, nearly half of our patients demonstrated somewhat aberrant behavior.[26] The cause of the problem in these patients is not clearly understood, but it may have something to do with a systemic degenerative process. Excessive pressure on the pelvic floor, particularly when related to attenuated muscle, is another etiologic factor.[62]

In adults, the overwhelming majority with rectal prolapse (90% in our experience) are women.[26] The peak incidence occurs in the sixth decade. Multiparity

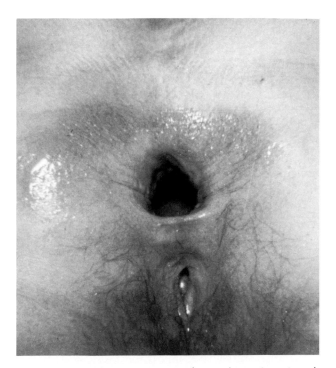

FIG. 7-1. Patulous anus seen after prolapse is reduced. (Corman ML, Veidenheimer MC, Coller JA: Managing rectal prolapse. Geriatrics 29:87–93, 1974)

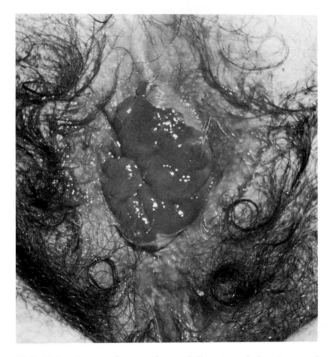

FIG. 7-2. Incomplete prolapse following abdomino-anal pull-through for imperforate anus.

has sometimes been mentioned as a possible etiologic factor, but in our experience 40% of patients were *nulliparous.*[26] Boutsis and Ellis reported that 58% of their patients with prolapse were childless, and Hughes reported an incidence of 39%.[5, 24] Such rates of nulliparity are much higher than would be expected from the general population. With the frequent occurrence of bowel management problems in this disease, the most likely candidate for rectal prolapse is a neurotic, constipated, single woman.

CLINICAL FEATURES AND EVALUATION

The most frequent primary complaint is referable to the prolapse itself: three fourths of patients complain of the protrusion. Problems with bowel regulation and incontinence are also presenting features. Almost half of our patients had a history of constipation.[26] Significant bleeding is rarely seen unless the prolapse is massive or irreducible.

Fecal incontinence associated with prolapse is not an uncommon symptom. Parks and associates suggested that because of stretch injury to pudendal and perineal nerves, loss of continence in patients with

rectal prolapse is secondary to prolonged protrusion.[50] They cite studies that demonstrate histologic abnormalities of small nerves supplying the anorectal musculature. Neill and associates reported EMG studies that showed reduced amplitude of action potentials in the external sphincter and puborectalis muscles in patients with fecal incontinence but not in those with rectal prolapse without incontinence.[39] Their findings indicated that denervation caused pelvic floor weakness, with prolapse and incontinence in some patients; in others, prolapse occurred without detectable abnormality of the pelvic musculature.

Incontinence becomes more severe as the protrusion increases in degree. Dilatation of the canal by the mass results in further relaxation of the sphincter muscles and further prolapse.[58] Mucous discharge may also become a problem. Protrusion may occur from lifting or coughing even without defecation. Manual replacement eventually becomes necessary, and ultimately the mass may be outside most of the time. Infrequently, the prolapse may become incarcerated or even strangulated if it has occurred after excessive straining.

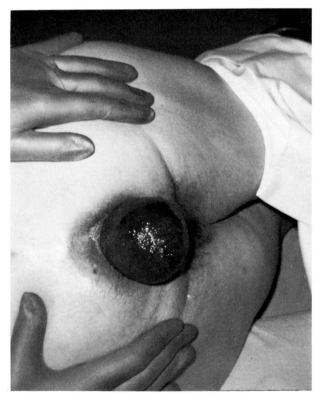

FIG. 7-3. Rectal prolapse, or procidentia. (Corman ML, Veidenheimer MC, Coller JA: Managing rectal prolapse. Geriatrics 29:87–93, 1974)

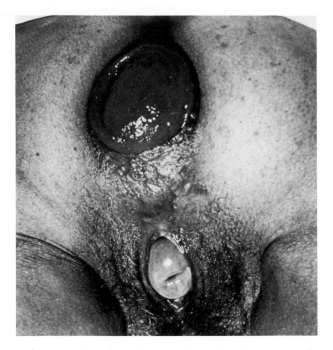

FIG. 7-4. Rectal prolapse with uterine descensus. The cervical os appears at the introitus. (Corman ML, Veidenheimer MC, Coller JA: Managing rectal prolapse. Geriatrics 29:87–93, 1974)

The duration of symptoms may be prolonged. This may be a reflection of the patient's psyche, but all too often it represents failure of the physician to recognize the entity and to recommend treatment. Usually the diagnosis of a full-thickness prolapse presents no problem (Fig. 7-3); it can be associated with uterine descensus (Fig. 7-4), uterine prolapse (Fig. 7-5), or cystocele (Fig. 7-6).[8]

When a patient's symptoms are suggestive of rectal prolapse, having the patient sit on the toilet and bear down may not be a particularly aesthetic experience for the patient or the surgeon, but it may be the only means by which rectal prolapse can be visualized. The least effective way of seeing the lesion is to place the patient in the jackknife position on the examining table.

A thorough proctosigmoidoscopic examination is required of patients with any anorectal complaint and particularly of patients with rectal prolapse. It is important to specify the degree of prolapse and whether it is full thickness or mucosal. Occasionally, carcinoma of the rectum or rectosigmoid may be the cause of intussusception, especially in a man with no associated neurologic disease.

An important part of the examination of the patient with rectal prolapse is determination of the tone and contractility of the sphincter mechanism. If the sphincter tone is poor and the anus patulous, and if the patient is unable to contract the puborectalis sling voluntarily, functional results after repair of the prolapse may not be satisfactory. On the other hand, if the patient has relatively good sphincter tone and contractility, a good functional result can be expected.

A barium enema examination is usually required for completeness but is all too often unrewarding. Patients with rectal prolapse have considerable difficulty retaining the contrast material, and abundant fecal residue is the rule rather than the exception. Colonoscopy is not usually indicated, but flexible fiberoptic sigmoidoscopy may reveal the intussusception if the examination is performed with the patient straining and in a sitting position. Ripstein believes that on colonoscopic examination the straightened rectal segment of prolapse is almost always present, and the intussusception can easily be seen and recognized.[56] Likewise, cinefluorography may be helpful if the diagnosis is questionable.

The Preprolapse Situation

Occasionally a patient complains of a feeling of a lump inside the rectum and perception of an obstruction when attempting to pass flatus or to have a bowel

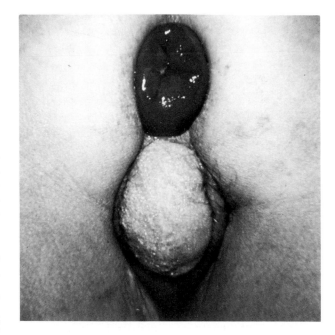

FIG. 7-5. Rectal prolapse with uterine prolapse. (Corman ML, Veidenheimer MC, Coller JA: Managing rectal prolapse. Geriatrics 29:87–93, 1974)

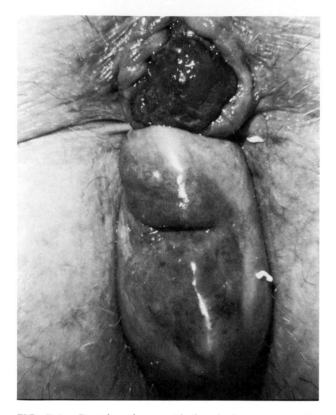

FIG. 7-6. Rectal prolapse with fourth-degree cystocele. (Corman ML, Veidenheimer MC, Coller JA: Managing rectal prolapse. Geriatrics 29:87–93, 1974)

movement. There may be a sensation of incomplete evacuation. Pain may be present in the perineal area with sciatic or obturator radiation.

Proctosigmoidoscopic examination by the inexperienced examiner may be singularly unrewarding. However, careful inspection of the mucosa may reveal an area of hyperemia and edema from 8 to 15 cm, and the bowel wall may appear thickened. Occasionally, one may perceive intussusception of the rectosigmoid. This history and the proctoscopic findings are suggestive of preprolapse. All the manifestations of procidentia will usually develop within 1 year.

Syndrome of the Descending Perineum

When a healthy person increases intra-abdominal pressure and relaxes the pelvic musculature, no significant change can be observed in the concavity of the peri-

neum. However, in patients with chronic illness, malnutrition, and preprolapse, the syndrome of the descending perineum may be observed.[49] The normal concavity may be obliterated with straining. In patients with this syndrome, either the anal canal is situated several centimeters below a line drawn between the pubis and coccyx or it descends 3 or 4 cm during straining.[49] The perineal area can even descend 5 or 6 cm in some persons (Fig. 7-7). Relaxation of the pelvic floor is a result of injury to the pelvic muscles, particularly the levatores.

Patients usually complain of tenesmus and difficulty evacuating. Treatment is directed to bowel management (diet, laxatives, suppositories) and to education; the patient is cautioned to avoid straining. Many, however, will ultimately develop further problems such as incontinence and rectal prolapse.

DIFFERENTIAL DIAGNOSIS

The condition that most often misleads the examiner into believing he is dealing with procidentia is prolapsed hemorrhoids (see Fig. 2-3). A protruding mass of hemorrhoidal tissue tends to be lobular; a definite sulcus or groove is present between the masses of tissue down to the level of the anal skin. With very large hemorrhoids that have become edematous and thrombosed, the enlarged size frequently gives the incorrect impression that the entire rectal wall is protruding. However, with rectal prolapse, concentric rings of intact tissue are evident throughout the entire circumference.

Sometimes the differential diagnosis may include a large rectal or sigmoidal polypoid lesion prolapsing through the anus. The physician should replace the mass and examine the rectum digitally and endoscopically. A polypoid lesion is usually mobile and can be separated from the lower part of the rectum and anal canal by digital examination. A polypoid tumor feels quite different from the rectal mucosa. Proctosigmoidoscopic examination should clarify any differential diagnostic problem

As already mentioned, the anal deformities associated with radical hemorrhoidectomy, fistula surgery, and pull-through procedures may produce an ectropion or mucosal prolapse, but again this should pose no difficulty in differential diagnosis. It is extremely important to distinguish full-thickness prolapse from mucosal prolapse because treatment of the two conditions is decidedly different. Therefore, it is helpful to examine the patient sitting or squatting and straining. Many patients have been submitted to multiple anal procedures because rectal prolapse has been mistaken for hemorrhoids.

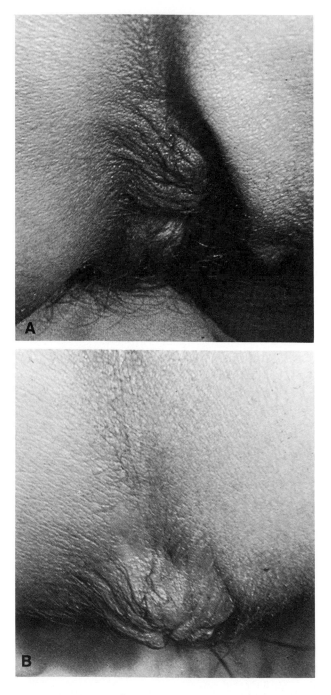

FIG. 7-7. Descending perineum (perineal descensus). **A.** At rest. **B.** During straining. (De los Rios Margrina E: Color Atlas of Anorectal Diseases, p 199. Philadelphia, W B Saunders, 1980)

RECTAL PROLAPSE IN CHILDREN

Rectal prolapse in children is a self-limited condition usually seen in infancy or early childhood, and disappears in a few months or years. Usually the mother notices a lump protruding from the anus, which may or may not reduce spontaneously. The commonest differential diagnostic condition is that of a juvenile polyp. Distinction between the two conditions should not be difficult, however.

Occasionally a child is seen in whom rectal prolapse develops in the early teen years. Often a history of chronic constipation and poor bowel habits is elicited. These children usually have been instructed on the importance of daily evacuation, and they sit on the toilet for an hour or more trying to defecate.

TREATMENT

Children. The most important aspect of treatment in a child is to reassure the parents and child that this is a self-limited condition. Treatment consists of reduction of the prolapse and support of the rectum with a pad or taping of the buttocks; both should be reserved for prolapse that does not reduce spontaneously. When constipation is a problem in the infant or young child, the use of stool softeners and the provision of ample liquid in the diet will tend to ameliorate the condition. In the older child, supporting the rectum during defecation and manual reduction of the prolapse immediately after it appears are important therapeutic measures.

The child should be reeducated and given an appropriate diet. The injection of a sclerosing agent may be considered for minor degrees of prolapse (see Chap. 2). Irreducibility or even gangrene of the prolapsed segment may occur and require emergency resection. In the nonurgent situation, when repeated prolapse necessitates some form of surgical intervention, a Thiersch type of repair is the recommended approach. The material can be subsequently removed.

Adults. Partial or incomplete (mucosal) prolapse should be treated by an *anal* operation in adults. If only one quadrant is involved, excision, with the wound left open, may be all that is required (see Fig. 6-11). If the lesion is circumferential, excision with S-plasty is the preferred procedure (see Figs. 6-9 and 6-10).

If surgical treatment for incomplete or complete prolapse is contraindicated, or if the patient refuses operative intervention, a number of noninvasive approaches and limited office procedures may be employed for palliation (see the list on p 158). Although instructing the patient on proper bowel management and perineal exercises may be salutary, these measures cannot be expected to cure the condition.

Nonoperative Treatment for Rectal Prolapse

Adhesive strapping of buttocks
Manual anal support during defecation
Correction of constipation
Proper habit of defecation
Perineal strengthening exercises
Electronic stimulation (see Fig. 5-8)
Injection of sclerosing agent
Rubber ring ligation

More than 100 operations have been designed for the treatment of complete rectal prolapse. Most operative procedures are a variation of a few basic modes of surgical therapy and depend on the surgeon's concept of the anatomic defect. The options for treatment include narrowing of the anal orifice, obliteration of the peritoneal pouch of Douglas,[37] restoration of the pelvic floor, resection of the bowel (either by an abdominal or a perineal approach), and suspension or fixation of the rectum to the sacrum or other structures. Additional operations combine one or more of these approaches (see the list below).

Modes of Surgical Therapy

Narrowing of anal orifice
Obliteration of peritoneal pouch of Douglas
Restoration of pelvic floor
Resection of bowel
   Peritoneal (abdominal) approach
   Perineal approach
Suspension or fixation of rectum
   To sacrum
   To other structures
Combination of two or more of the above

(Modified from Boutsis C, Ellis H: Ivalon-sponge-wrap operation for rectal prolapse: An experience with 26 patients. Dis Colon Rectum 1974; 17:21–37)

General Principles

All patients undergoing surgery for rectal prolapse should have thorough mechanical cleansing of the bowel with an orally administered laxative and colonic irrigation the night before and the morning of the operation. A preoperative intravenous pyelogram is recommended if a laparotomy is planned. Nonabsorbable, orally administered antibiotics should be ordered routinely whenever resection is contemplated or intrusion into the bowel is a possibility. Systemic broad-spectrum antibiotics are advised during the perioperative period, especially when foreign material is to be implanted.

Postoperative care for abdominal repairs is essentially the same as for bowel resection (see Chap. 10). Intravenous fluid replacement is continued until flatus is passed. Progressive diet is initiated, and the patient is discharged when the bowels have functioned.

Narrowing of the Anal Orifice

Thiersch Repair

In the older, poor-risk patient, many surgeons prefer the Thiersch operation for rectal prolapse.[21] The procedure can be performed with a local anesthetic, making it a satisfactory technique in these patients. In this procedure, silver wire is placed into the perianal space to encircle and narrow the anus. Today, most surgeons have abandoned the silver wire because of the complications of breakage and ulceration. Other materials, such as nylon, Mersilene, polypropylene mesh (Marlex), Teflon, fascia lata, silicone rubber, and Dacron-impregnated Silastic have been used for the same purpose.[20, 23, 29, 32, 42, 52]

Operative Technique

The patient is placed in the lithotomy position on the operating table, and the perianal area is vigorously prepared with an antiseptic solution. A local anesthetic can be used to infiltrate the area, but for convenience, a general or spinal anesthetic is optimal. I prefer to use the double-armed Mersilene (5 mm) suture (Fig. 7-8).

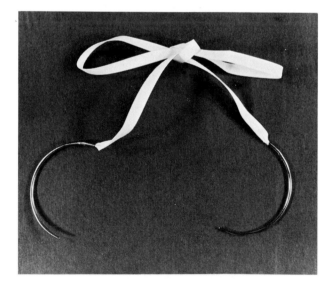

FIG. 7-8. Double-armed, 5-mm Mersilene for Thiersch repair.

A small incision is made in the anterior and posterior positions 1 cm outside the anal verge (Fig. 7-9, *A*). The suture is passed anterior to posterior on either side of the anus in the ischiorectal fossa (Fig. 7-9, *B*). The knot should be buried *posteriorly.* The recommendation that the diameter be the proximal interphalangeal joint of the operating surgeon is problematical (Fig. 7-9, *C*). The proximal interphalangeal joint is not a standard size, with the result that one patient's anal canal orifice

may be created relatively large, and another is made relatively narrow. A No. 16 or No. 18 Hegar dilator (see Fig. 11-59) is a better standard for determining lumenal size. Suturing is required for Mersilene tape to avoid a bulky knot; alternatively, a stapling device may be used to secure the tape. I prefer the modification suggested by Thorlakson whereby an "eye" is cut near one end of the tape, and the other end brought through like a noose, doubled-back, and secured

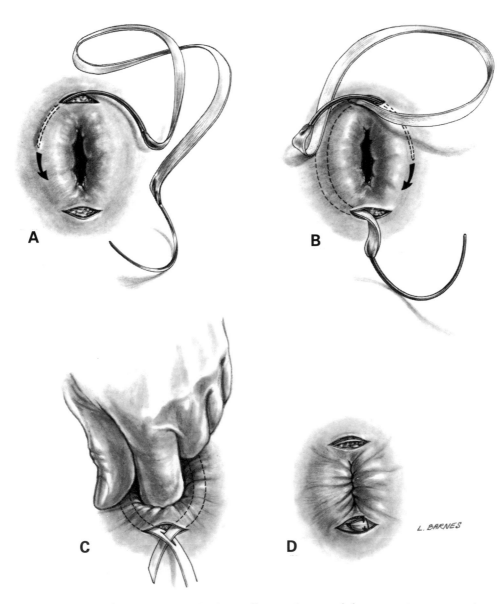

FIG. 7-9. Thiersch repair. **A, B.** Each needle arm is passed from anterior to posterior. **C.** The tape is secured after tightening to the level of the proximal interphalangeal joint. (A Hegar dilator is the preferred measuring device.) **D.** The tape is sutured to itself rather than knotted.

(Fig. 7-9, *D*).[61] The two wounds are primarily closed with 4-0 Dexon.

Postoperative Care

Frequent examinations are necessary to be certain that fecal impaction does not develop. Stool softeners, laxatives, suppositories, or enemas may be required. A topical antiseptic ointment, such as povidone-iodine (Betadine), is advised. The patient is discharged when bowel function has been established.

Complications

Complications are frequently seen with Thiersch and Thiersch-type repairs. The material may be too tight, necessitating removal because of repeated impaction or incontinence. Wound infection is a common problem, and when this occurs, the suture must be removed. Finally, if the prolapse recurs, it may become incarcerated and even strangulated. Recurrent prolapse following a Thiersch repair requires immediate evaluation.

Other Thiersch-Type Repairs

Other approaches have been advocated as alternatives to the Thiersch operation. Marlex mesh has been employed by Lomas and Cooperman.[32] Despite their wound infection rate of 33%, they believe this is a rapid, safe procedure to use in the elderly patient who is not a candidate for a more extensive surgical operation.

Mersilene mesh, a synthetic, polyester, woven fiber, has been advocated for Thiersch-type operations. Notaras employs a ribbon of Mersilene (approximately 4 cm wide) and passes it around the anus, as has been described with the other material except that a more extensive mobilization is required.[42] The mesh is sutured together so that the opening permits two fingers. Notaras reported an experience with 18 patients with no infection, breakage, or erosion.

Elastic Fabric Sling

Recently Labow and co-workers described the use of an elastic fabric sling, a Dacron-impregnated Silastic sheet.[29] I have used this technique in the treatment of fecal incontinence in order to supplement the sphincter mechanism (see Fig. 5-23). The operative technique is similar to that of any Thiersch approach except that the authors recommend the jackknife position. The strip is cut to 1.5 cm wide, with care taken to prepare it in such a way that it is elastic along its longitudinal axis (Fig. 7-10). An overlap of 1 cm is created, and a TA stapler is used to secure the edges, which are then

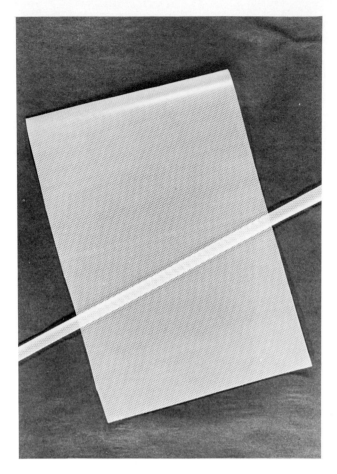

FIG. 7-10.   Elasticity of the 1.5-cm-wide strip can be readily appreciated. Care must be taken to trim the sheet along the proper axis.

reinforced with interrupted nonabsorbable sutures. All wounds are primarily closed.

The authors noted no problems with infection, erosion, or impaction in nine patients. In my experience, removal of the material was required in one patient because of erosion and sepsis. The particular appeal of this material is that it can stretch; on rectal examination it simulates the normal sphincter.

Comment

Evaluation of the long-term results of the classical Thiersch procedure (using wire) is absent from contemporary writings, and even the newer materials are described with little more than "case report" experience. The Thiersch-type operations in my opinion should rarely be employed. Under most circumstances the complication rate is prohibitively high. Furthermore, the procedure does not cure the prolapse; it most certainly would recur if the material were removed.

There are certain limited situations in which the use of the Thiersch operation is indicated. For example, in a moribund patient it is a simple and reasonably safe operation. If an individual cannot tolerate the anesthetic required for a major operation, it is appropriate to consider this procedure.

Obliteration of the Pouch of Douglas

The Moschcowitz procedure was designed on the theory that the cause of rectal prolapse is a sliding hernia.[29, 37] The technique involves serial pursestring sutures placed in the floor of the pelvis (Fig. 7-11). The recurrence rate, however, as reviewed by Theuerkauf and associates was close to 50%.[60] Although I have had no experience with this technique, the lack of success of others and the theoretical premise on which it is based

would seem to imply that the procedure should be abandoned.

Restoration of the Pelvic Floor

Plication of the levatores has been advocated either alone or in combination with other modes of surgical therapy to restore the pelvic floor.[2, 14, 15, 18, 25, 44] The procedure can be performed through the abdomen or the perineum (see Chap. 5), or after removing the coccyx or lower sacrum.[25] Reefing the levatores transabdominally can be performed anterior or posterior to the rectum, although the latter may be technically difficult to accomplish (Fig. 7-12). When it is employed with sacral fixation or resection, I believe it is an unnecessary and often tedious maneuver that does not improve the chance of cure. With plication of the levatores alone for the treatment of rectal prolapse, the incidence of recurrence is so great as to preclude its use.

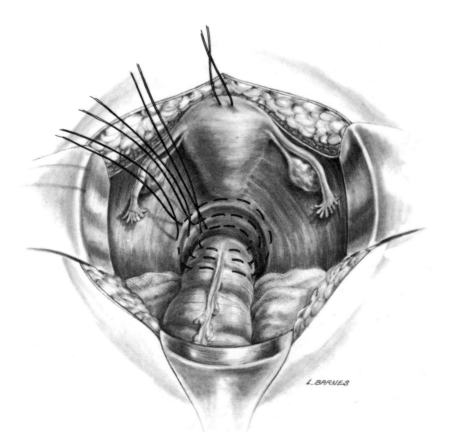

FIG. 7-11. The Moschcowitz procedure involves the obliteration of the pouch of Douglas by serial pursestring sutures.

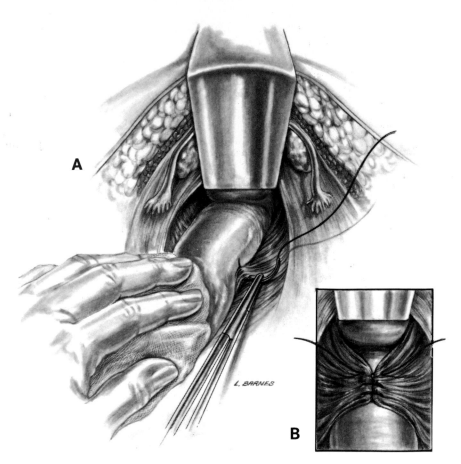

FIG. 7-12. **A.** Reefing of the levator ani muscle performed transabdominally. A suture is placed into the muscle adjacent to the right lateral aspect of the rectum. **B.** Reefing or plication accomplished anterior to the rectum.

Resection of the Bowel

Anterior Resection

High Anterior Resection

High anterior resection for the treatment of rectal prolapse has many advantages over other techniques but also has some disadvantages. One major advantage is the removal of the redundant sigmoid colon; this excess colon can pose a problem in some patients who are to undergo suspension or fixation procedures. A mobile sigmoid colon may predispose to torsion or to volvulus. Patients who undergo resection may have some of their bowel symptoms (especially constipation) improved by removal of the redundant segment. Patients who have a long history of bowel management problems will not have this complaint ameliorated by a sling procedure; in fact, they may be made worse.

The major disadvantage of resection is the inherent risk of an anastomotic leak, but this risk should be minimal. The technique for performing anterior resection is described in Chapter 11. It is important to remember that when this operation is performed for prolapse, the rectum must be mobilized completely to the levatores.

Beahrs and co-workers reported on the treatment of rectal prolapse at the Mayo Clinic.[3] Of 118 patients, 28 underwent anterior resection. One operative death occurred, and in one patient prolapse recurred. The cause of this was thought to be failure to free the rectum down to the level of the levator ani muscle. The authors concluded that anterior resection is the operation of choice for rectal prolapse.

Despite the success of this approach, dependence on adhesions to fix the rectum posteriorly may be unpredictable. Therefore, some authors advise some form of rectal fixation when high anterior resection is performed.

Anterior Resection with Sacral Fixation

A modification of anterior resection to include fixation of the distal rectal segment to the sacrum can be performed. The posterior rectal wall or intact lateral ligaments are secured to the sacrum with three or four heavy nonabsorbable sutures; the redundant sigmoid colon is then removed (Fig. 7-13). Goldberg reported 125 cases using this technique with no recurrence.[53]

Comment

Despite a considerable experience with the Teflon sling repair (see Teflon Sling Repair [Ripstein Opera-

tion]), I have become in recent years much more enthusiastic about anterior resection as the optimal operation for rectal prolapse. I have not found it necessary to suture the rectum or lateral ligaments to the sacrum and have had no recurrence in 21 patients. Since so many patients are constipated and have a redundant sigmoid colon, this procedure should yield a better functional result.

Perineal Resection

Perineal resection of the prolapsed segment appears to be a relatively simple means of addressing the problem, but unfortunately the high rate of recurrence has prevented most contemporary surgeons from adopting this approach. It might, however, still be employed usefully in the rare instance of gangrene of the prolapsed bowel. Altemeier and Culbertson developed a modification of the perineal resection, which is described below.[1]

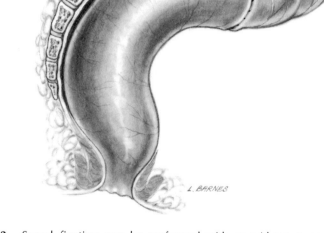

FIG. 7-13. Sacral fixation can be performed with or without concomitant rectosigmoid resection. Sutures are placed directly into the muscularis of the rectum and through the periosteum of the sacrum.

Altemeier Operation

With the patient in the lithotomy position and an indwelling Foley catheter in place, the perianal area is prepared and draped. The prolapse is exteriorized, and its apex is grasped with clamps. A circumferential incision is made through all layers of the outer bowel wall just proximal to the mucocutaneous junction (Fig. 7-14, *A*). When the circumferential incision is completed, clamps are reapplied to the distal edge of rectum, and the prolapse is delivered as a single loop of exteriorized bowel. Any hernial sac (located on the anterior surface of the bowel) is identifed and the peritoneal cavity entered. A continuous suture obliterates the sac. The levator ani muscles are identified and interposed anterior to the bowel by interrupted long-term absorbable sutures (Fig. 7-14, *B*). This eliminates the large defect in the pelvic diaphragm. The redundant intestine is then divided in half by anterior and posterior incisions carried to the point of the proposed resection (Fig. 7-14, *C*). The intestine is transected obliquely and progressively in quadrants, completing the anastomosis of the intestinal wall to the anal ring in each quadrant (Fig. 7-14, *D*). Anastomosis is effected

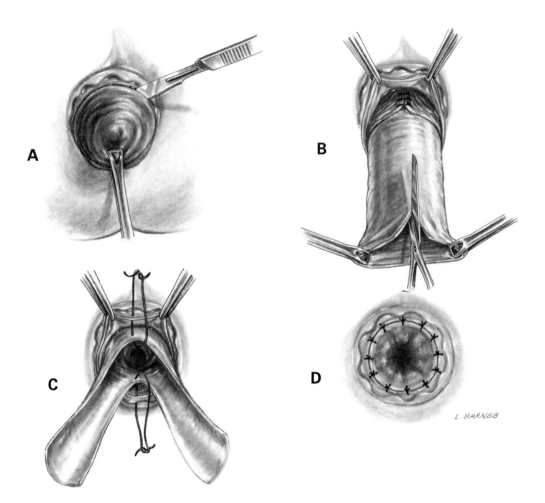

FIG. 7-14. Altemeier procedure. **A.** An incision is made circumferentially at the level of the mucocutaneous junction. **B.** The levator ani muscle is reefed anteriorly after the rectum has been delivered. **C.** The redundant bowel is incised longitudinally and sutured in the anterior and posterior midline to the residual cuff of the rectal mucosa. **D.** After the redundant bowel is trimmed, interrupted sutures are placed between the anal canal and the underlying internal sphincter to the full thickness of the rectum.

with interrupted, fine polyglycolic acid sutures; no drains are used. In principle, the operation obliterates the pelvic pouch, plicates the levators, and resects the redundant bowel. The rectum is not fixed to the sacrum, however.

Despite the successful experience of some authors, the complex technique and the unfamiliar approach dissuades most surgeons from attempting this operation. Altemeier and associates reported on their results with 106 patients; three developed recurrences.[2]

Vermeulen and associates recently reported a simplified approach to perineal rectosigmoidectomy without levator plication, using the end to end autosuture device (see Chapter 11).[64] In nine women (mean age, 79 years) they noted no significant complications and no recurrences. They felt that this approach is the procedure of choice in the elderly, poor-risk patient.

Delorme Procedure

The Delorme operation, uncommonly employed today, is basically a perineal procedure.[10] It is performed with the patient in the lithotomy position, and a circumferential incision is made similar to that for the Altemeier procedure. Dissection, however, is hemorrhagic because it is a mucosal stripping (Fig. 7-15, *A*).

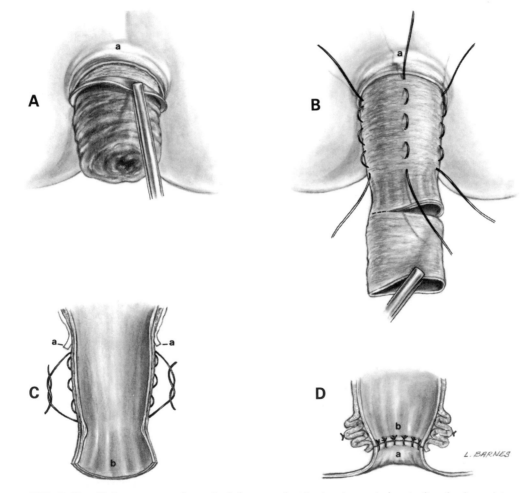

FIG. 7-15. Delorme procedure. **A.** Submucosal stripping is carried out after the bowel is circumferentially incised. **B.** Multiple sutures are placed into the submucosa and muscularis, and the redundant mucosa is excised. **C.** The sutures are secured and the bowel pleated. **D.** The final position is established and the mucosa is sutured.

The denuded muscularis is pleated longitudinally, collapsing the bowel like an accordion (Fig. 7-15, B–D).

In 30 patients treated by Nay and Blair, a 10% incidence of poor results was noted.[38] This was defined as incontinence or development of a recurrent, complete prolapse. Uhlig and Sullivan were quite enthusiastic, reporting only three failures in 44 patients, an incidence of less than 7%.[63] McCaffrey recommended this approach after a failed "Ripstein" operation.[35] He reported good results in three patients. But most surgeons report cumbersome dissection and a relatively high recurrence rate, implying that the procedure has limited usefulness.

Combined Abdominal and Perineal Operation

Dunphy has advocated a combined abdominal and perineal operation for rectal prolapse.[14] The perineal operation is essentially the same as that described by Altemeier and co-workers.[1, 2] The abdominal operation, however, is done several days later. Full mobilization of the rectum is carried out, and a plication of the ligamentous structures lateral to the rectum is performed. The pouch of Douglas is obliterated in the manner of Moschowitz. Dunphy described this technique and results of treatment in four patients; no recurrence was noted.

This is an extensive operative approach requiring two major procedures. Although the belt-and-suspenders approach may be useful under some circumstances, there are simpler and at least as reliable alternatives.

Transsacral Resection

The transsacral operation uses the approach to the rectum described by Kraske for resection of rectal cancer.[28] This operation has been advocated by Davidian and Thomas and by Jenkins and Thomas.[9, 25]

An incision is made overlying the sacrum and coccyx, and the latter is disarticulated and removed. The levator ani muscles are divided to expose the rectum. The peritoneum is incised anteriorly and the rectum fully mobilized. The redundant colon is liberated and delivered through the sacral wound (Fig. 7-16, A). The levator ani muscles are approximated anterior to the rectum (Fig. 7-16, B), the peritoneum is closed, and resection of the redundant bowel is carried out. After anastomosis all wounds are primarily closed.

Theoretical advantages of this procedure are that the operation does not require a laparotomy and that the levator ani muscles are reconstituted, narrowing the defect in the pelvic floor. The pouch of Douglas is obliterated, and the rectum is secured posteriorly. The major disadvantage is that the patient has an extremely painful sacrococcygeal wound that is subject to infection. The possibility of a fecal fistula, although not noted by Davidian and Thomas, is still real.[9, 25] The authors reported 30 patients who underwent this operative approach; there was no mortality or recurrence.[9] As with other procedures for the treatment of this condition, the extensive operation described would contraindicate it for most surgeons, particularly in light of the simpler alternatives available for cure.

Suspension or Fixation of the Rectum

Teflon Sling Repair (Ripstein Operation)

The commonest surgical approach for the treatment of rectal prolapse in the United States is the Teflon sling repair, first described by Ripstein in 1965.[55] The patient is placed in the Trendelenburg position on the operating table, and a midline hypogastric incision is made. Exploration of the abdomen usually reveals the characteristic defect of redundant sigmoid colon, lack of fixation of the rectum to the sacrum, and a deep pouch of Douglas. The rectosigmoid is mobilized, usually without difficulty, with care taken to avoid injury to the ureters. The presacral space is entered and the *inferior mesenteric vessels carefully preserved.* Mobilization of the rectum to the level of the levator ani muscle can be accomplished without effort, but this is usually not necessary.

Fixation of the Teflon mesh to the sacrum can be performed in one of two ways. Sutures are placed into the periosteum of the sacrum approximately 1 cm to the right of the midline using a one-half circle Mayo trocar-point needle. Three or four nonabsorbable sutures are used (Fig. 7-17, A). If a presacral vein is entered the ligature can be tied. All too often, however, the vein exits directly from the bone, and only application of pressure to the area will stop the bleeding.

The Teflon mesh is trimmed to approximately 4 cm wide and secured into place along the right side of the sacrum (Fig. 7-17, B). At this point in the operation it is important for the assistant to maintain proximal traction while the mesh is anchored to the muscularis propria of the rectum. If the rectum is not maintained under tension in a cephalad direction and redundant rectum is left below the mesh, prolapse will recur. Nonabsorbable sutures are placed from the mesh into the rectal wall (Fig. 7-17, C). After the mesh has been laid around two thirds of the bowel, the redundant material is trimmed so that it can be placed around the rectum without tension (Fig. 7-17, D). Sutures are placed into the sacrum on the left side and secured into the mesh. An approximately 1-cm defect is present posteriorly (Fig. 7-17, E). The remaining sutures on the

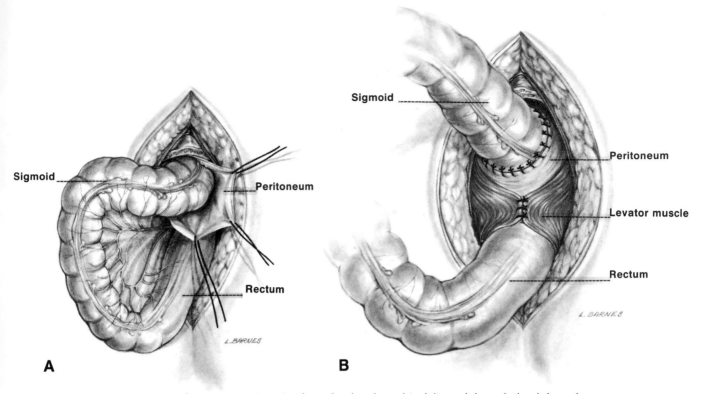

A

B

FIG. 7-16. Thomas operation. **A.** The redundant bowel is delivered through the defect after the levatores are incised. The hernial sac is identified anteriorly, the sac is opened, and the redundant sigmoid is delivered. **B.** The hernial sac is excised and the floor of the pelvis reconstituted by suturing the seromuscular layer of the proximal bowel to the peritoneum. The levator ani muscle is plicated anterior to the rectum. The bowel is resected and an anastomosis performed (not shown.)

left side are placed through the mesh into the muscularis of the bowel (Fig. 7-17, *F*).

Another method of securing the mesh is to place a single row of sutures into the midline of the sacrum. The middle of the mesh is sutured into place and the material brought onto either side of the rectum (Fig. 7-18). With proximal traction maintained on the rectum the mesh is anchored, leaving a 1-cm defect anteriorly (Fig. 7-18, *inset*). This is a simpler technique than the former but has the potential disadvantage of having only a solitary row of sutures posteriorly.

It is not necessary to reperitonealize the floor of the pelvis, but it can be done at the surgeon's discretion. If hemostasis is secure, no pelvic drains are employed. However, when sacral venous bleeding has been encountered or hemostasis is a concern, a Jackson-Pratt drain is placed into the pelvis and brought out through a stab wound in the left lower quadrant. This is usually maintained for 2 or 3 days.

Postoperative management of the Teflon sling repair is essentially the same as that for bowel resection. An indwelling urinary catheter is recommended for several days. Patients are given intravenous fluids until bowel sounds develop and the patient passes flatus, at which time a progressive diet is instituted. The patient is discharged when the bowel has functioned, usually by the seventh or eighth postoperative day.

Results

Until my recent adoption of anterior resection, the Teflon sling repair had been my primary method of treatment of rectal prolapse. Half of the patients in our reported experience had prior colorectal operations.[26] Most had undergone anorectal procedures; 20% underwent multiple operative procedures.[26] In excess of 100 such operations, the success rate was over 95%.[31] Four patients early in our experience required reoperation, two because of recurrent rectal prolapse and two because of postoperative rectal stricture. One patient with recurrent rectal prolapse was a young

(Text continues on p 170)

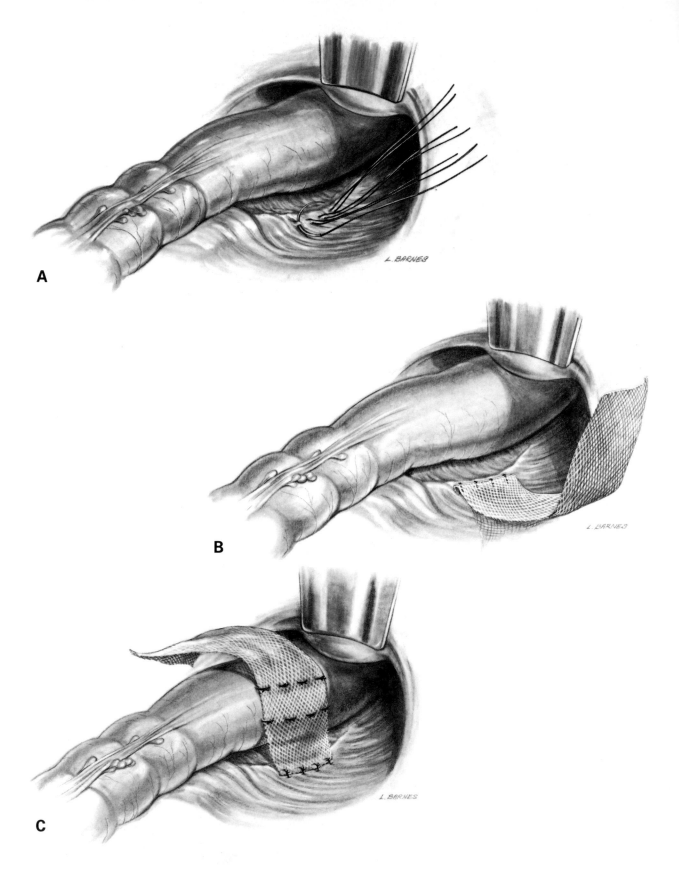

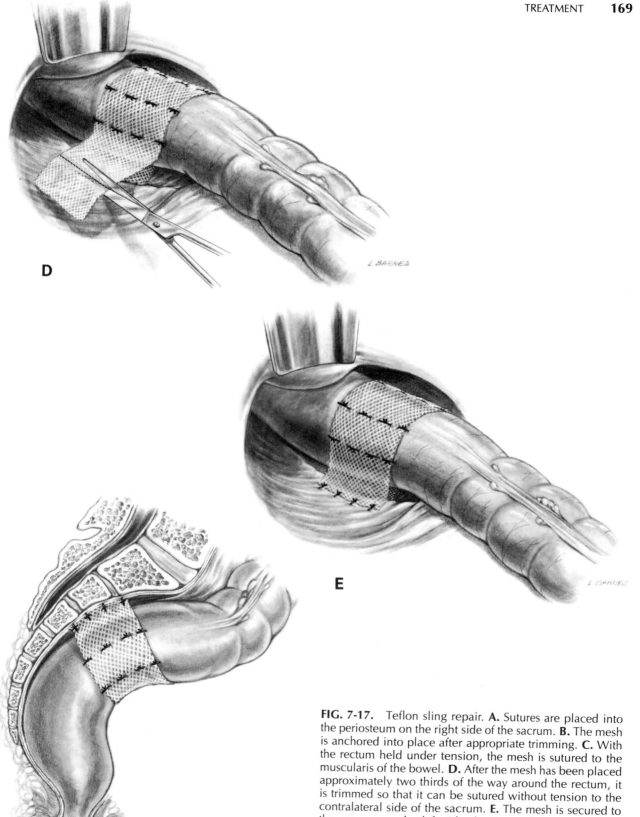

FIG. 7-17. Teflon sling repair. **A.** Sutures are placed into the periosteum on the right side of the sacrum. **B.** The mesh is anchored into place after appropriate trimming. **C.** With the rectum held under tension, the mesh is sutured to the muscularis of the bowel. **D.** After the mesh has been placed approximately two thirds of the way around the rectum, it is trimmed so that it can be sutured without tension to the contralateral side of the sacrum. **E.** The mesh is secured to the sacrum on the left side, leaving a defect of approximately 1 cm posteriorly. **F.** Lateral view showing the position of the mesh as secured to the sacrum.

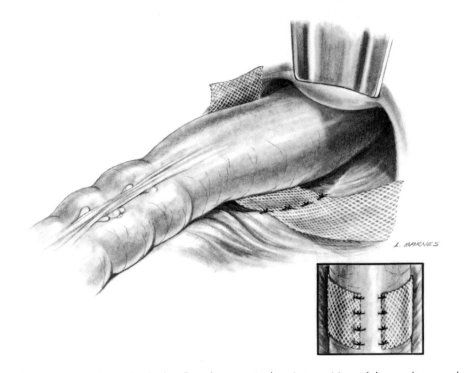

FIG. 7-18. Alternate method of Teflon sling repair showing position of the mesh sutured in the midline. The mesh is brought around either side of the rectum and sutured to the anterior wall, leaving a defect of approximately 1 cm anteriorly *(inset)*.

woman in whom recurrent prolapse developed with the vaginal delivery of a child; subsequent repair was performed without incident. The second patient was 80 years old and quite active. The prolapse recurred within 6 weeks after the operation while the patient was building a stone wall and lifting an 80-pound bag of cement.

There were no operative deaths in our experience. On the basis or our initial report on 55 patients, 48 (87%) had an uneventful postopertive course (Table 7-1).[26] The average hospital stay was 16 days, with 80% of the patients discharged in less than 3 weeks. Long-term follow-up information was obtained on all but one patient. The mean follow-up period was 46 months with 35 patients having been followed up for more than 5 years. Bowel management and incontinence remained persistent problems after the prolapse was corrected. In our experience approximately one third of our patients complained of difficulty in regulating bowel function after the repair, and approximately 11% complained of incontinence or soiling. Of course, bowel function and incontinence problems are commonly expressed before surgical intervention. The habits of excessive straining at stool and dependence on laxatives are often long standing and not remedied by anatomic correction of the prolapse. This is the

primary reason why I have become more enthusiastic about resection.

The success of the repair and patient satisfaction depend on the ability to improve bowel habits. Dietary measures, stool softeners, and periodic enemas may be advised. Although laxative use may be discouraged, many patients tend to return to cathartic abuse. Certainly the operation does nothing for the patulous, dilated anus, or diminished anal sphincter tone. To improve continence, a physiotherapy program of perineal strengthening exercises has been successful in many patients (see Chap. 5).

Gordon and Hoexter, in a study of members of the American Society of Colon and Rectal Surgeons based on a questionnaire, were able to gain information on 1111 Teflon sling repairs performed by 129 surgeons.[17] The overall complication rate was 16.5% with a recurrence rate of 2.3%. Fecal impaction was seen in 6.7% of patients. It was the opinion of the authors that the complications seem to be related primarily to too tight an application of the mesh around the rectum. The complication rate seems to decrease with increased experience.

Holmström and associates reported their experience with the Teflon sling repair in 59 patients.[22] The operative mortality was high (5%). However, in two of

Table 7-1. Operative Morbidity

Complication	Frequency	Percent
None	48	87.3
Wound sepsis	4	7.3
Urinary tract infection	2	3.6
Wound separation	1	1.8
Pulmonary problems	1	1.8
Total	56*	

* One patient had both a urinary tract infection and wound sepsis.
(Jurgeleit HC, Corman ML, Coller JA et al: Procidentia of the rectum: Teflon sling repair of rectal prolapse, Lahey Clinic experience. Dis Colon Rectum 1975; 18:464–467)

the three patients the cause of death was coronary disease. Their recurrence rate was 5.4% with a mean observation period of 5 years. At the Ochsner Clinic, the Ripstein procedure has been used exclusively since 1970. Biehl and co-workers reported on their experience and compared it with the Altemeier, sigmoidectomy, and Thiersch procedures formerly used.[4] The Ripstein operation was associated with a lower recurrence rate and a lower morbidity rate.

Launer and co-workers reported the Cleveland Clinic experience with the Teflon sling repair.[30] Although there was no operative mortality in 57 patients there was a rather high morbidity (26%). Seven patients (14%) developed recurrent mucosal prolapse, and six patients (12%) had a complete recurrence. Despite the disappointing results the authors still believe that the Ripstein procedure remains the treatment of choice for rectal prolapse.

Late Complications

We have reported the late complications of Teflon sling repair including our experience when the original procedure was performed elsewhere.[31] Rectal stricture developed in five patients postoperatively. These patients had in common a troublesome history of bowel management problems, specifically severe constipation that antedated insertion of the Teflon sling. Patients with rectal stricture also had a longer history of prolapse (79 months versus 37 months). Barium enema examination showed stenosis in all these patients (Fig. 7-19), ranging from a diameter of 3 mm to 19 mm. The presence of narrowing was also confirmed by proctosigmoidoscopy.

The problem of constipation is not altered by the Teflon sling repair. On the contrary, constipation became more severe in three patients, and early obstructive signs soon evolved. In some patients who presented with obstructive symptoms relatively soon after the operation, faulty technique must be assumed. However, fibrotic reaction secondary to the mesh must be considered a possible factor. In any patient with a history of chronic constipation, particularly with a history of long-standing rectal prolapse, consideration should be given to performing an anterior resection.

Recurrent rectal prolapse after Teflon sling repair usually is related to faulty surgical technique. The mesh may not be secured adequately to the presacral fascia or bone. Furthermore, when traction on the rectosigmoid is insufficiently maintained while the sling is inserted, the mesh will not be anchored low enough on the rectum. The error is more likely in a man whose pelvis is narrow and in whom mobilization and suture placement are more difficult. In our experience a higher ratio of men to women is observed in the group of patients with this complication. I believe that one should abandon the Teflon sling repair for anterior resection in men.

Ivalon Sponge Implant

The use of Ivalon sponge as a wrapping about the rectum has been advocated by the British.[5, 36, 51, 59, 65] The operation basically consists of the implantation of a synthetic polymer around the rectum. After full mobilization of the rectum the appropriately tailored sponge is sutured to the sacrum in the posterior midline. It is then wrapped around the rectum, leaving a defect in the anterior midline.

Results of this procedure on 26 patients were reported by Boutsis and Ellis.[5] One operative death occurred, but no instance of pelvic sepsis or wound complication was reported. Follow-up study revealed nine mucosal recurrences (an incidence of 35%). Complete rectal prolapse developed in 11.5%. Stewart reported 41 patients: no operative deaths occurred, complete recurrence developed in three patients (7%), and a mucosal recurrence developed in 10 patients (24%).[59] One apparent advantage of this technique is that fecal impaction has not been a problem.[36, 51] The incidence of recurrence appears to be higher than that reported for the Teflon sling repair. This operation has not been used in the United States.

Teflon Sling Suspension

A unique approach to rectal suspension has been devised by Nigro, who believes the most effective way to correct prolapse is to perform a method that most closely simulates the normal anatomic arrangement.[41] It is his contention that the most important factor is the angulation and fixation provided by the pelvic floor musculature and that maximum support comes with contraction of the muscle that lifts and angulates the

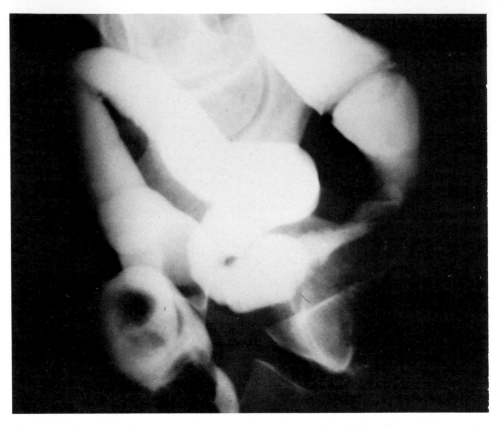

FIG. 7-19. Barium enema study showing rectal stricture after Teflon sling repair. (Lescher TJ, Corman ML, Coller JA et al: Management of late complications of Teflon sling repair for rectal prolapse. Dis Colon Rectum 22:445–447, 1979)

lower rectum upward and forward toward the pubis.[40] Accordingly, he designed an intra-abdominal sling approach that suspends the rectum from the pubis. He has had six successful results. Since I have had no experience with this technique, it is difficult to comment on its advisability. The concept is presented here because it is unique and new.

The patient is placed in the Trendelenburg position on the operating table. A midline incision is made in the lower part of the abdomen, and the rectum is mobilized in the same manner as for a Teflon sling repair. Care is taken to avoid injury to the inferior mesenteric vessels. The dissection is carried posteriorly down to the coccyx. The mesh is tailored approximately 4 cm wide by 20 cm long. The central portion is secured to the rectum with interrupted nonabsorbable sutures. It is then sutured to the posterior and lateral walls of the rectum as low as possible to the rectal wall.

The space of Retzius, in front of the bladder and close to the pubic rami, is opened. A long curved clamp is placed into this space and directed downward and posteriorly to the presacral space. The mesh is then grasped and pulled forward to lie on the pubic bone. The same is accomplished on the contralateral side. Each end is then secured to the pubic ramus with interrupted nonabsorbable sutures. The length of graft is determined by holding it to the pubic bone with just enough tension to prevent slack (Fig. 7-20). The presacral space is left open, and the abdomen is closed without drainage. Postoperative care is essentially the same as for Teflon sling repair.

Greene reported 15 patients who underwent this operation. There was no mortality, no operative morbidity, and no recurrences with a minimum follow-up of 6 months.[19] Severe incontinence was corrected in all but one patient, and this person was improved. There were no problems with sexual function or the urinary tract.

Greene feels that the particular advantage of this

operation is in patients who experience incontinence problems.

This unique operation is rather problematical. Dissection along the anterior pelvis is more likely to injure vital urinary or genital structures, and if carried out in a woman of childbearing age, a subsequent pregnancy requires a caesarian section. Impotence seems more likely to result than with the Ripstein when this procedure is performed in men.

Rectopexy

Perhaps the simplest abdominal approach to the treatment of rectal prolapse is rectopexy. The operation consists of mobilizing the rectum down to the levator ani muscle and securing the mesentery of the rectum and muscularis to the sacral fascia or bone. This is usually performed with interrupted nonabsorbable sutures or strips of fascia lata. The operation was originally described by Orr, but Loygue and associates modified the procedure to include full rectal mobilization.[33, 43] They reported their experience with 140 patients; two operative deaths were noted, and the incidence of recurrent prolapse was 3.6%. Christiansen and Kirkegaard reported two recurrences (8%) in 24 patients who underwent this procedure.[7]

It is evident that fixation of the rectum to the sacrum by whatever means has a high success rate with low morbidity and mortality. Although I have had no experience with this technique as the sole treatment, its simplicity makes it appealing.

RECTAL PROLAPSE AND FECAL INCONTINENCE

The great majority of patients will have their incontinence difficulties alleviated with resolution of the procidentia. There is, however a small group of patients in whom anal incontinence may be quite disabling. Parks advocated the deep postanal repair of the pelvic floor muscles in these patients (see Chapter 5).[48] Although his overall failure rate for patients with incontinence was 17%, many of these individuals did not have a prolapse initially. He suggested that the more severe the prolapse, the worse the result.

Keighley and Matheson reported 20 patients with prolapse and anal incontinence.[27] Rectopexy alone controlled the incontinence in all but four patients (20%). Following postanal repair all but one became continent.

I have never found it necessary to perform an operative procedure for fecal incontinence following successful treatment of the rectal prolapse. Bowel management in the rare patient who complains usually suffices. If such a problem persisted I believe I would recommend a Dacron–Silastic implant (see Chap. 5).

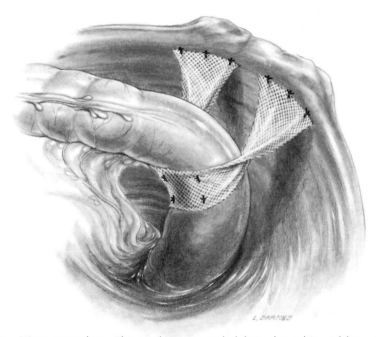

FIG. 7-20. Nigro procedure. The mesh is suspended from the pubis and brought around the posterior wall of the rectum as a halter.

SUMMARY

The varied operative procedures available for rectal prolapse can be confusing. Most of the maneuvers are relatively esoteric and can be performed successfully only by the few surgeons who have developed the specialized technique. It is recommended, therefore, that the less experienced surgeon adopt one of the standard procedures. A rectopexy or suspension procedure without resection can be performed safely with good results, a low morbidity, and low mortality. Anterior resection with or without sacral fixation, an operation familiar to most surgeons, also offers an excellent cure rate.

The Thiersch-type approach should probably be reserved for those patients who cannot tolerate laparotomy. The material chosen should be one of the commercially available synthetic products. Wire should not be used. The Dacron-impregnated Silastic prosthesis for this operation has potential, especially for the incontinent patient. Results of further study are awaited.

REFERENCES

1. Altemeier WA, Culbertson WR: Technique for perineal repair of rectal prolapse. Surgery 1965; 58:758–764
2. Altemeier WA, Culbertson WR, Schowengerdt C et al: Nineteen years' experience with the one-stage perineal repair of rectal prolapse. Ann Surg 1971; 173:993–1006
3. Beahrs OH, Theuerkauf FJ Jr, Hill JR: Procidentia: Surgical treatment. Dis Colon Rectum 1972; 15:337–346
4. Biehl AG, Ray JE, Gathright JB Jr: Repair of rectal prolapse: Experience with the Ripstein sling. South Med J 1978; 71:923–925
5. Boutsis C, Ellis H: The Ivalon-sponge-wrap operation for rectal prolapse: An experience with 26 patients. Dis Colon Rectum 1974; 17:21–37
6. Brodén B, Snellman B: Procidentia of the rectum studied with cineradiography: A contribution to the discussion of causative mechanism. Dis Colon Rectum 1968; 11:330–347
7. Christiansen J, Kirkegaard P: Complete prolapse of the rectum treated by modified Orr operation. Dis Colon Rectum 1981; 24:90–92
8. Corman ML, Veidenheimer MC, Coller JA: Managing rectal prolapse. Geriatrics 1974; 29:87–93
9. Davidian VA, Thomas CG Jr: Trans-sacral repair of rectal prolapse: Efficacy of treatment in thirty consecutive patients. Am J Surg 1972; 123:231–235
10. Delorme R: Sur le traitement des prolapsus du rectum totaux part 1' excision de la muquese rectale au rectal-colique. Bull Soc Chir Paris 1900; 26:498–518
11. Devadhar DS: A new operative treatment for complete prolapse of the rectum. J Christ Med Assoc India 1961; 36:18–23
12. Devadhar DS: New thoughts on the mechanism and treatment of rectal procidentia. J Int Coll Surg 1964; 42:672–681
13. Devadhar DS: A new concept of mechanism and treatment of rectal procidentia. Dis Colon Rectum 1965; 8:75–77
14. Dunphy JE: A combined perineal and abdominal operation for the repair of rectal prolapse. Surg Gynecol Obstet 1948; 86:493–498
15. Dunphy JE, Botsford TW, Savlov E: Surgical treatment of procidentia of the rectum: An evaluation of combined abdominal and perineal repair. Am J Surg 1953; 86:605–607
16. Goligher JC: Surgery of the Anus, Rectum and Colon, 3 ed, p 293. London, Bailliere Tindall, 1975
17. Gordon PH, Hoexter B: Complications of the Ripstein procedure. Dis Colon Rectum 1978; 21:277–280
18. Graham RR: The operative repair of massive rectal prolapse. Ann Surg 1942; 115:1007–1014
19. Greene FL: Repair of rectal prolapse using a puborectal sling procedure. Arch Surg 1983; 118:398–401
20. Haskell B, Rovner H: A modified Thiersch operation for complete rectal prolapse using a Teflon prosthesis. Dis Colon Rectum 1963; 6:192–195
21. Henschen C: Ueber den Ersatz des Thierschschen Drahtringes bei der Operation des Mastdarmvorfalls durch geflochtene Seidenriemen, frei überpflanzte Gefäss-Sehnen-Periost-oder Faszien stücke. München Med Schnschr 1912; 59:128
22. Holmström B, Ahlberg J, Bergstrand O et al: Results of the treatment of rectal prolapse operated according to Ripstein. Acta Chir Scand (Suppl) 1978; 482:51–52
23. Hopkinson BR, Hardman J: Silicone rubber perianal suture for rectal prolapse. Proc R Soc Med 1973; 66:1095–1098
24. Hughes ESR: Discussion on rectal prolapse of the rectum. Proc R Soc Med 1949; 421:1007–1011
25. Jenkins SG Jr, Thomas CG Jr: An operation for the repair of rectal prolapse. Surg Gynecol Obstet 1962; 114:381–383
26. Jurgeleit HC, Corman ML, Coller JA et al: Procidentia of the rectum: Teflon sling repair of rectal prolapse, Lahey Clinic experience. Dis Colon Rectum 1975; 18:464–467
27. Keighley MRB, Matheson DM: Results of treatment for rectal prolapse and fecal incontinence.

Dis Colon Rectum 1981; 24:449–453

28. Kraske P: Zur Exstirpation hochsitzender Mastdarmkrebse. Verh Dtsch Ges Chir 1885; 14:464–474

29. Labow S, Rubin RJ, Hoexter B et al: Perineal repair of rectal procidentia with an elastic fabric sling. Dis Colon Rectum 1980; 23:467–469

30. Launer DP, Fazio VW, Weakley FL et al: The Ripstein procedure: a 16-year experience. Dis Colon Rectum 1982; 25:41–45

31. Lescher TJ, Corman ML, Coller JA et al: Management of late complications of Teflon sling repair for rectal prolapse. Dis Colon Rectum 1979; 22:445–447

32. Lomas MI, Cooperman H: Correction of rectal procidentia by use of polypropylene mesh (Marlex). Dis Colon Rectum 1972; 15:416–419

33. Loygue J, Huguier M, Malafosse M et al: Complete prolapse of the rectum: A report on 140 cases treated by rectopexy. Br J Surg 1971; 58:847–848

34. Mann CV: Rectal prolapse. In Morson BC: Diseases of the Colon, Rectum and Anus, pp 238-250. New York, Appleton-Century-Crofts, 1969

35. McCaffrey JF: Delorme repair for prolapse of the rectum following "failed" Ripstein opertion. Am J Proctol Gastroenterol Colon Rectal Surg 1983; 34:5–6

36. Morgan CN, Porter NH, Klugman DJ: Ivalon (polyvinyl alcohol) sponge in the repair of complete rectal prolapse. Br J Surg 1972; 59:841–846

37. Moschowitz AV: The pathogenesis, anatomy and cure of prolapse of the rectum. Surg Gynecol Obstet 1912; 15:7–21

38. Nay HR, Blair CR: Perineal surgical repair of rectal prolapse. Am J Surg 1972; 123:577–579

39. Neill ME, Parks AG, Swash M: Physiological studies of the anal sphincter musculature in faecal incontinence and rectal prolapse. Br J Surg 1981; 68:531–536

40. Nigro ND: An evaluation of the cause and mechanism of complete rectal prolapse. Dis Colon Rectum 1966; 9:391–398

41. Nigro ND: A sling operation for rectal prolapse. Proc R Soc Med (Suppl) 1970; 63:106–107

42. Notaras MJ: The use of Mersilene mesh in rectal prolapse repair. Proc R Soc Med 1973; 66:684–686

43. Orr TG: A suspension operation for prolapse of the rectum. Ann Surg 1947; 126:833–840

44. Palmer JA: Prolapse of the rectum: Treatment by the Moschowitz-Graham operation. Can J Surg 1969; 12:116–123

45. Paramore RH: The supports-in-chief of the female pelvic viscera. J Obstet Gynaecol 1908; 13:391–409

46. Paramore RH: The pelvic floor aperture: With an appendix. J Obstet Gynaecol 1910; 18:95–121

47. Paramore RH: The Hunterian lecture on the intra-abdomino-pelvic pressure in man. Lancet 1911; 2:1677–1683

48. Parks AG: Anorectal incontinence. Proc R Soc Med 1975; 68:681–690

49. Parks AG, Porter NH, Hardcastle J: The syndrome of the descending perineum. Proc R Soc Med 1966; 59:477–482

50. Parks AG, Swash M, Urich H: Sphincter denervation in anorectal incontinence and rectal prolapse. Gut 1977; 18:656–665

51. Penfold JC, Hawley PR: Experience of Ivalon-sponge implant for complete rectal prolapse at St. Mark's Hospital, 1960-1970. Br J Surg 1972; 59:846–848

52. Plumley P: A modification to Thiersch's operation for rectal prolapse. Br J Surg 1966; 53:624–625

53. Rectal prolapse (Symposium). Contemp Surg 1980; 17:54–88

54. Ripstein CB: The repair of massive rectal prolapse. Surg Proc 1965; 2:2

55. Ripstein CB: Surgical care of massive rectal prolapse. Dis Colon Rectum 1965; 8:34–38

56. Ripstein CB: Procidentia of the rectum: Internal intussusception of the rectum (stage I rectal prolapse). Dis Colon Rectum 1975; 18:458–460

57. Ripstein CB, Lanter B: Etiology and surgical therapy of massive prolapse of the rectum. Ann Surg 1963; 157:259–264

58. Schuster MM: The riddle of the sphincters. Gastroenterology 1975; 69:249–262

59. Stewart R: Long-term results of Ivalon wrap operation for complete rectal prolapse. Proc R Soc Med 1972; 65:777–778

60. Theuerkauf FJ Jr, Beahrs OH, Hill JR: Rectal prolapse: Causation and surgical treatment. Ann Surg 1970; 171:819–835

61. Thorlakson RH: A modification of the Thiersch procedure for rectal prolapse using polyester tape. Dis Colon Rectum 1982; 25:57–58

62. Todd IP: Etiological factors in the production of complete rectal prolapse. Postgrad Med J 1959; 35:97–100

63. Uhlig BE, Sullivan ES: The modified Delorme operation: Its place in surgical treatment for massive rectal prolapse. Dis Colon Rectum 1979; 22:513–521

64. Vermeulen FD, Nivatvongs S, Fang DT et al: A technique for perineal rectosigmoidectomy using autosuture devices. Surg Gynecol Obstet 1983; 156:85–86

65. Wells C: New operation for rectal prolpase. Proc R Soc Med 1959; 52:602–603

CHAPTER 8

Dermatologic Anal Conditions

Dermatologic anal problems are usually rather trivialized by the surgeon, who often categorizes them as complaints of a psychoneurotic or anal obsessive personality. The patient may be referred directly to a dermatologist, or he may be given any one of a number of proprietary creams or the ubiquitous topical steroid, without benefit of a physical examination. Dermatologists are understandably more adept at establishing the diagnosis of skin problems and usually will perform a biopsy for confirmation in questionable cases. But the dermatologist is loath to perform rectal examination and does not have endoscopic equipment available. In my opinion, therefore, patients with anal complaints, including dermatologic problems, should be seen by a physician or surgeon who has the knowledge and the equipment to perform a complete rectal evaluation. If the problem appears to be limited to the skin and of uncertain diagnosis, consultation with a dermatologist is certainly appropriate.

The purpose of this chapter is to describe the skin conditions that affect the perianal area, emphasizing the differential diagnosis, the indications for biopsy, and the treatment of the more important diseases. Those conditions that may be found in the anal area only incidental to the systemic cutaneous process are mentioned *en passant* if recognition of the disease in the area is felt to be unique or of particular interest. This chapter is *not* meant to be a précis of a textbook of dermatology.

CLASSIFICATION

Dermatologic diseases may be categorized in a number of ways: on the basis of the type of lesion (flat, elevated, depressed), whether primary or secondary, histopathologically, or by the commonly employed classification: inflammation, infection, neoplasm. A modification using this last method is illustrated on p. 179.

In addition, a glossary of dermatologic terms may aid the reader in interpreting the description of the lesions; this is presented on p. 180.

INFLAMMATORY CONDITIONS

Pruritus Ani

By far the commonest symptom of anorectal disease presenting to the dermatologist is pruritus ani.[6] Although the condition may be due to specific disease (hemorrhoids,[74] anal fissure, previous anal surgery, constipation, or diarrhea), most patients are not found to have significant anorectal pathology except for the obvious skin changes. The rich nerve supply to the perianal area is thought to be the primary reason for the sensitivity to potential irritants.[73]

Itching is usually noted in the anal or occasionally the genital areas, but the condition is not generalized. Although the anus is frequently the site for autoeroticism, most patients do not appear to fall into this category. The condition tends to be worse at night, awakening the patient from sleep. This leads to scratching, which exacerbates the complaint even further. Pruritus ani is more common in men.

Besides anorectal pathology as a specific etiology for the condition, allergic (contact) dermatitis, mycoses, seborrhea, diabetes, and *Oxyuris* (pinworm) have all been implicated as causative factors. Anal neurodermatitis may cause violent itching, which may lead to tearing of the perianal area (Color Fig. 8-1). With chronicity the skin can become atrophic or hypertrophic with nodularity and scarring (Color Fig. 8-2).

Physiologic studies have demonstrated that in patients with idiopathic pruritus ani the anal sphincter relaxes in response to rectal distention more readily than in patients with no anal disease.[44] It is postulated that soiling may occur as a result of this factor and lead to the genesis of the condition.

Physical examination should include anoscopy and proctosigmoidoscopy to look for specific cause of the symptoms. Usually, however, the procedures are unrewarding. Examination with a magnifying lens may be helpful.[27] Evaluation with a Wood's lamp may reveal fluorescence,[91] but this equipment is usually not readily available in the office practice of most physicians and surgeons. Skin scrapings of the perianal area examined with a potassium hydroxide slide preparation and cultured on Sabouraud's medium for yeast and fungi should be performed if suspicion warrants (see Fungal Infections).

Treatment

An accurate history will usually dictate the appropriate treatment. Attention in recent years has been drawn to the role of diet in the cause of the condition. Items that have been implicated include coffee, tea, carbonated beverages (especially colas), milk products, alcohol (particularly wine and beer), tomatoes and tomato products (like ketchup), cheese, chocolate, and

Dermatologic Anal Conditions

Inflammatory Diseases

  Pruritus ani
  Psoriasis
  Lichen planus
  Lichen sclerosis et atrophicus
  Atrophoderma
  Contact (allergic) dermatitis
  Seborrheic dermatitis
  Atopic dermatitis
  Radiodermatitis
  Behçet's syndrome
  Lupus erythematosus
  Dermatomyositis
  Scleroderma
  Erythema multiforme
  Familial benign chronic pemphingus (Hailey-Hailey)
  Pemphigus vulgaris
  Cicatricial pemphigoid

Infectious Diseases

  Nonvenereal
    Pilonidal sinus
    Suppurative hidradenitis
    Fistula-in-ano
    Crohn's disease
    Tuberculosis
    Actinomycosis
    Herpes zoster
    Vaccinia
    Fournier's gangrene
    Tinea cruris
    Candidiasis (moniliasis)

    "Deep" mycoses
    Amebiasis cutis
    Trichomoniasis
    Schistosomiasis cutis
    Bilharziasis
    Oxyuriasis (pinworm, enterobiasis)
    Creeping eruption (larva migrans)
    Larva currens
    Cimicosis (bedbug bites)
    Pediculosis
    Scabies

  Venereal
    Gonorrhea
    Syphilis
    Chancroid
    Granuloma inguinale
    Lymphogranuloma venereum
    Molluscum contagiosum
    Herpes genitalis
    Condylomata acuminata

Premalignant and Malignant Diseases

  Acanthosis nigricans
  Leukoplakia
  Mycosis fungoides
  Leukemia cutis
  Basal cell carcinoma
  Squamous cell carcinoma
  Malignant melanoma
  Bowen's disease
  Extramammary Paget's disease

Glossary of Dermatologic Terms

Elevated Lesions

Abscess
Bulla (bullae): bleb; blisters containing serous or sero-purulent fluid
Crusts: dried masses of serum, pus, or blood, with epithelial and bacterial debris
Cysts: sac containing liquid or semi-solid material
Desquamation: scales; result from abnormal keratinization and exfoliation of cornified epithelial cells
Exfoliation: scales; laminated masses of keratin; desquamated epidermis
Exudate: crusts; dried blood or pus
Furuncle: necrotizing form of folliculitis; many may coalesce to form a *carbuncle*
Hyperkeratosis: increased thickening of the stratum corneum
Keratosis (keratotic): horny growth
Lichenification (lichenoid): thickened, leathery; exaggerated, mosaic-appearing skin markings
Nodule (nodular): larger papule
Papule (papular, papilloma, papillomatosis): circumscribed solid elevations with no fluid
Plaque: minimal height, relatively large surface area

Pustule: "pimple"; elevation of the skin containing pus
Urticaria: wheals
Vegetation (vegetative): luxuriant, fungal-like growth
Vesicle: blister; circumscribed epidermal elevation
Wheal: evenescent, edematous, variable-sized flat elevation

Flat Lesions

Infarct: coagulation necrosis due to ischemia
Macule (macular); circumscribed change in skin color
Sclerosis (sclerotic): induration or hardening
Telangiectasia: condition caused by dilatation of capillary vessels and minute arteries

Depressed Lesions

Atrophy (atrophic): thin, almost transparent epidermis
Erosion
Excoriation: mechanical abrasion
Gangrene
Scar: cicatrix secondary to injury or disease
Sclerosis: circumscribed or diffuse hardening in the surface of the skin
Sinus: tract from a suppurative cavity to skin surface
Ulcer: excavation involving loss of dermis as well as epidermis (variable depth)

(Modified from Domonkos AN, Arnold HL Jr, Odom RB: Cutaneous symptoms, signs and diagnosis. In Andrew's Diseases of the Skin, 7th ed, pp 15–19. Philadelphia, WB Saunders, 1982; Fitzpatrick TB: Fundamentals of dermatologic diagnosis. In Fitzpatrick TB, Eisen AZ, Wolff K et al (eds): Dermatology in General Medicine, 2nd ed, pp 10–37. St Louis, McGraw-Hill, 1979; and Rook A, Wilkinson DS: The principles of diagnosis. In Rook A, Wilkinson DS, Ebling FJG (eds): Textbook of Dermatology, 3rd ed, pp 57–67. Oxford, Blackwell Scientific Publications, 1979)

nuts.[48,96] Cigarette smoking is another factor. It is postulated that these products induce mucous discharge, probably through a systemic route, or possibly in some instances by changing the *p*H of the stool.

Since most patients indulge in one or more of the above, it is probable that the surgeon will receive an affirmative response when he inquires about the dietary history. By recognizing the association of one of these agents with pruritus ani, the patient will ally himself with the surgeon. The patient may have been previously told that the problem is psychoneurotic; the physician's reassurance and sympathy are one of the most important factors contributing to the resolution of the problem.

Removing or changing the dietary factor (*e.g.*, by using decaffeinated coffee) may cause the symptoms to disappear. But the most important advice that can be given is on the management of anal hygiene. Many patients perceive their problem to be one of lack of cleanliness; the opposite is more likely. Vigorously scrubbing the area with soap and water will cause the skin to be defatted, and a contact dermatitis may supervene. Rarely have I identified a patient with pruritus

who was not scrupulous with respect to anal cleanliness; the difficulty is to convince the patient that the anal orifice need not be sterilized.

Advise the patient to remove the soap from the area! He should cleanse the perineum with plain water, particularly when bathing or showering, and ideally following defecation. Some patients may actually be allergic to toilet paper, so that in stubborn cases a moist cloth should be used for cleansing. Even in a public toilet a moistened paper towel is preferable to the irritative effects of continued rubbing with toilet paper. For patients with copious discharge, a cotton ball placed at the anal verge, changed as necessary, may be helpful.

A wealth of topical creams and ointments, over-the-counter and prescription, are available for the pruritus ani sufferer. The use of anesthetic ointments and creams (*e.g.*, Nupercaine, Americaine) is not advised. Symptoms are only temporarily masked, the underlying problem is not addressed, and allergic dermatitis can develop. Soothing creams are generally preferred to ointments; many are quite satisfactory (*e.g.* Balneol, Tucks, Proctodon). However, when the proprietary

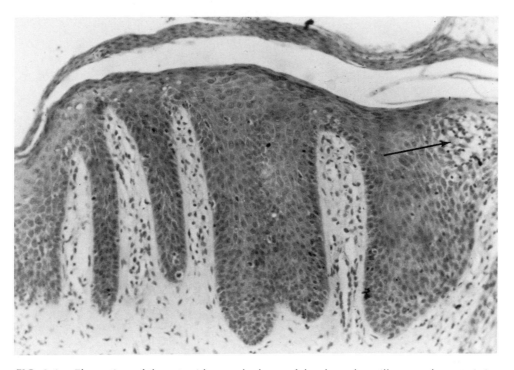

FIG. 8-1. Elongation of the rete ridges and edema of the dermal papillae are characteristic features of psoriasis. Note parakeratosis, "Munro abscess" *(arrow),* and the absence of a granular cell layer. (Original magnification × 180. Courtesy of Rudolf Garret, M.D.)

preparation fails, one must consider using a topical steroid; this almost inevitably will bring immediate relief. My own preference is for Proctocort (1% hydrocortisone cream) because it is nicely packaged with a plastic applicator and finger cots. It is applied at bedtime and once or twice more during the day. It should be discontinued, however, as soon as symptoms resolve, in order to avoid problems of skin atrophy (see Atrophoderma).

In the rare intractable case, sedation and tranquilization must be considered. In addition, biofeedback and self-hypnosis have been of demonstrable benefit. Consultation with a professional familiar with these techniques may be advisable.

Psoriasis

Psoriasis is a common, chronic inflammatory disease of the skin, characterized by rounded, circumscribed, erythematous, dry, scaling patches covered by grayish-white or silvery-white scales. The lesions have a predilection for the scalp, nails, extensor surfaces of the limbs, elbows, knees, and the sacral region.[35] When the condition occurs in the anal area it may cause severe pruritic symptoms. The perianal lesions are usually sharply marginated; psoriatic lesions may be present on other sites in the body. There may be a characteristic butterfly distribution with an extension over the coccyx and sacrum (Color Fig. 8-3).

Histologically, characteristic features include epidermal thickening (acanthosis), elongation of the rete ridges, and elongation of the dermal papillae (Fig. 8-1). There may be increased mitotic activity in the epidermis. Cells of the stratum corneum usually have retained nuclei (parakeratosis). Focal collections of inflammatory cells in the subcorneum are known as Munro microabscesses.

Treatment usually consists of topical corticosteroids, tars, or both. In addition, the use of ultraviolet (UV) light has been found to be beneficial. More recently the so-called PUVA treatment has been advocated. This consists of a combined systemic–external therapy, using a potent photoactive agent (psoralen) followed by administration of a special light system emitting long-wave UV-A. Cancer chemotherapeutic drugs, such as methotrexate, have also been used.

I am reluctant to treat psoriasis without dermatologic consultation unless the condition is quite localized to the perianal area.

Lichen Planus

Lichen planus is a skin condition that consists of an eruption of papules that are distinct in color and configuration. The lesion is characteristically found on the flexor surfaces, mucous membranes, genitalia, and occasionally the perianal area. It may appear as a small, flat, glistening papule, frequently with central umbilication.

Histologically the papule shows thickening of the granular layer, degeneration of the basement membrane and basal cells, and a lymphocytic and histiocytic infiltrate in the upper dermis (Fig. 8-2). Biopsy of the skin establishes the diagnosis.

Treatment often has less than satisfactory results. Corticosteroids appear to be the most useful for this condition. Topical preparations with occlusive dressings are quite helpful; systemic administration as well as intralesional injection have also been used. In mild cases, antipruritic lotions and antihistamines are employed. Rest is also helpful.

Lichen Sclerosis et Atrophicus (LSA)

Lichen sclerosis et atrophicus (LSA) is an uncommon condition of unknown cause. It occurs much more frequently in women than in men. The genital area appears to be the most commonly involved site.

Physical examination may reveal the characteristic "inverted keyhole" distribution. In this situation the disease extends beyond the mucocutaneous border to involve the skin of the vulva, perineum, and the perianal area. In the vulva, the condition affects the labia, the vestibule, and the entroitus (Fig. 8-3). Discomfort, pruritus, dysuria, and dyspareunia are common.

The characteristic histologic change in LSA is hyalinization of the collagen below the epidermis (Fig. 8-4). The epidermis also shows variable hyperkeratosis and follicular plugging. LSA is associated with squamous cell carcinoma of the vulva. In a recent report, an association between the condition and squamous cell carcinoma of the perianal region was noted.[90]

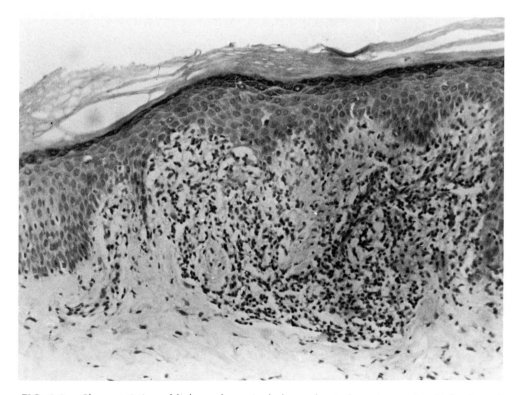

FIG. 8-2. Characteristics of lichen planus include moderate hyperkeratosis, thickening of the stratum granulosum, sawtooth configuration of the rete ridges, and lymphocytic infiltration of the dermis and basal cell layer. Note the sharp demarcation of the lymphocytic infiltrate. (Original magnification × 120. Courtesy of Rudolf Garret, M.D.)

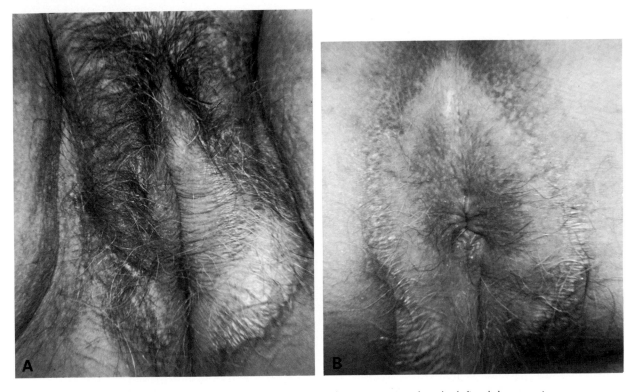

FIG. 8-3. Characteristic of lichen sclerosis et atrophicus (LSA) is a sharply defined dermatosis in the vulvar area **(A)** and perianum **(B)** with hypopigmentation centrally and hyperpigmentation peripherally. Note the lichenoid papules about the periphery. (Courtesy of John A. Clark, M.D.).

Treatment consists primarily of the relief of the pruritic symptoms in the hope of lessening the risk of leukoplakia and carcinoma. A mild topical steroid sufficient to control the symptoms is advocated. Secondary infection should be treated with appropriate antibiotics.

Atrophoderma (Atrophy of the Skin)

Atrophy of the skin is a reaction to the repeated and prolonged application of topical corticosteroids or following local injection of these products.[51] Telangiectasia, indicating loss of dermal collagen, occurs, and the patient who originally complained of pruritus now reports discomfort and burning.[92] The friction of walking rubs the already atrophic and thinned epidermis.

Patients usually report a history of self-application of topical corticosteroids for many years. Attempting to remove the medication is frequently unsuccessful. Biopsy may reveal atrophy and hyperkeratosis. Because

of the possibility of subsequent development of this condition it is important to discontinue the use of cortisone treatment when the pruritic symptoms have abated.

Contact (Allergic) Dermatitis

There are two types of dermatitis caused by substances coming in contact with the skin: irritant dermatitis (due to a nonallergic reaction from exposure to an irritating substance) and allergic (contact) dermatitis (due to allergic sensitization to a number of substances).[33] Irritants include alkalis, acids, metal salts, dusts, gases, and hydrocarbons.

Allergic contact dermatitis results from a hypersensitivity of the delayed type, also known as cell-mediated hypersensitivity or immunity.[33] A person may be exposed to an allergen for many years befor developing hypersensitivity. The allergens are numerous and varied: substances such as dyes, oils, resins, chemicals used for fabrics, cosmetics, and insecticides, as well as the products or the substances of bacteria, fungi, and parasites.[33] The most common causes of contact dermatitis are, in order of frequency, poison ivy, oak and sumac, paraphenylenediamine, nickel, common rubber compounds, and the dichromates.[46]

The patch test is used to detect hypersensitivity to a substance that is in contact with the skin. A nonirritating concentration of substances suspected to be the cause of the contact dermatitis is applied. The patches remain in place for 48 hours or less if burning or itching occurs. A positive reaction will produce severe pruritus and erythema or vesicles.

Therapy obviously is directed toward removing the underlying cause of the skin problem or the allergen. Iodine and adhesive tape are common dermatitis-inducing products in patients who undergo anal surgery. Soothing compresses such as Aveeno colloidal oatmeal, in addition to corticosteroids and possibly antipruritics, may be advisable.

Seborrheic Dermatitis

Seborrheic dermatitis is a chronic, superficial, inflammatory disease of the skin, with a predilection for the scalp, eyebrows, nasolabial crease, ears, axillae, submammary folds, umbilicus, groin, and gluteal crease. The disease is characterized by dry, moist, or greasy scales, and by crusted, pink-yellow patches of diverse size and shape.[35] The condition is believed to be due to hypersecretion of sebum and is apparently exacerbated by increased perspiration and by emotional stress. The presence of a high fat intake is frequently noted in patients with this condition.

Histologically the picture is not dissimilar to that of psoriasis, but Munro abscesses are not seen. There is a school of thought that the two conditions are so similar that there is some justification for thinking that their etiology must be the same. Likewise, treatment is similar to that of psoriasis, but the application of corticosteroids is the primary therapy.

Atopic Dermatitis (Atopic Eczema)

The term *atopy* is derived from the Greek word meaning "out of place" or "strange," and it is defined as the tendency to develop allergies to various substances manifested by systemic symptoms such as asthma, hay fever, and eczema.[32] The condition is believed to be either a form of immunologic deficiency or possibly a blockade of beta-adrenergic receptors in the skin.

Atopic dermatitis can occur as localized, erythematous, scaly, papular, or vesicular patches, or in the form of pruritic, lichenified lesions.[35] Pruritus is commonly the symptom causing additional skin changes; it occurs in paroxysms. Emotional upset may exacerbate an attack. Other factors initiating the problem may be clothing, some foods, and dryness of the skin. Superimposed infections such as intertrigo and dermatophytosis may produce further exacerbations.

Histologically, hyperkeratosis and parakeratosis with acanthosis is noted (Fig. 8-5). When there is lichenification, the acanthosis is increased and there is papillomatosis, with long papillary bodies reaching to the stratum corneum. These changes may resemble somewhat those seen in psoriasis.

Treatment consists of avoiding, if possible, emotional stress, avoiding extremes of cold and heat, limiting the use of stimulant beverages, and using antihistamines and corticosteroids. Oral prednisone is the commonly used preparation, 30 to 60 mg given every 4 to 6 weeks (possibly longer).

Radiodermatitis

Radiodermatitis is a particular problem in the anal area because current therapy for carcinoma of the rectum and anus often involves ionizing radiation. In some patients, unfortunately, the cure of the cancer may be actually worse than the disease (see also Chap. 17).

Many changes are found in the cell as the result of radiation therapy. Mitoses are temporarily arrested, chromosomal abnormalities occur, and there is at least a temporary halt in the normal cell cycle. The amount of skin change resulting from radiotherapy is dependent on the dose. Changes may be manifested as erythema, edema, and ulceration, and symptoms may include burning, itching, or severe pain. After a period of time, telangiectasis, atrophy, and freckling may appear. The skin becomes dry, thin, smooth, and shiny. Radiation injury may result in the subsequent development of malignancy, in most cases following a rather prolonged latent period. The incidence of this complication increases with the passage of time (Fig. 8-6).

Results of treatment are often less than satisfactory. If there is no evidence of malignant change, little or no specific therapy is advisable. Cleansing the area with a mild soap and water, in addition to the use of an emollient, a corticosteroid preparation, or both, may be of help. Any suspicious lesions should be biopsied.

Behçet's Syndrome

Behçet's syndrome is characterized by four main symptoms: recurrent aphthous ulcers in the mouth, skin lesions, eye lesions, and genital ulcerations.[60] Genital

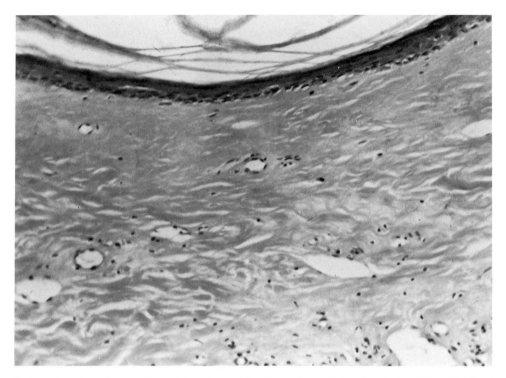

FIG. 8-4. Atrophy of the epidermis and hyalinization of the dermis in LSA. (Original magnification × 120. Courtesy of Rudolf Garret, M.D.)

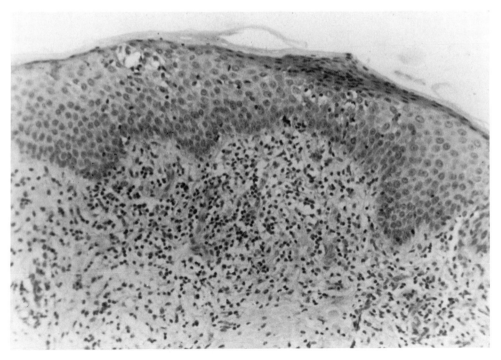

FIG. 8-5. Histologic characteristics of atopic dermatitis include mild acanthosis, spongiosis, focal parakeratosis, and dermal mononuclear cell infiltrate. (Original magnification × 180. Courtesy of Rudolf Garret, M.D.)

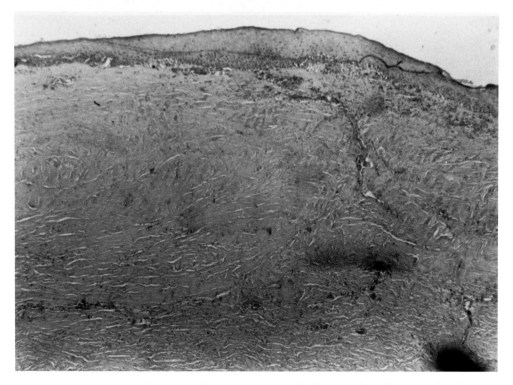

FIG. 8-6.   Histologic findings of radiodermatitis include fibrosis of the dermis with sclerosis, atrophy of the epidermis, and absence of skin appendages. (Original magnification × 120. Courtesy of Rudolf Garret, M.D.)

ulcerations may be found in both sexes on the genitocrural fold, on the anus, on the perineum, or in the rectum. Ulcerations are similar to those seen in the mouth. Although the cause of the condition is unknown, there is some evidence to suggest that it is of viral etiology, or possibly an autoimmune disease. Histologically the lesions usually show a vasculitis.

The anal condition may be misdiagnosed as hemorrhoids, fissure, Crohn's disease, condylomata, or veneral disease.[60] Surgery is contraindicated. Corticosteroid treatment systemically or topically is the treatment of choice.

Lupus Erythematosus

Lupus erythematosus, like other connective tissue diseases, only rarely occurs in the anal area, and still more rarely occurs as an isolated finding in this location. The cutaneous finding is called discoid lupus erythematosus (DLE). It may begin with single or multiple lesions involving entire regions of the body, especially the head and neck, the sternum, the vulva, and the perineum. The typical plaque is approximately 1 cm or more in diameter with characteristic scales. Removal of the scales reveals patulous follicular orifices with dry, horny keratinous plugs.[34] Occasionally a basal cell or squamous cell carcinoma may develop in long-standing DLE lesions.

In laboratory investigation, the LE cell test usually yields a negative result in DLE. The direct immunofluorescence test result is usually positive, however, as is the result of the antinuclear antibody test.

Treatment consists of avoidance of strong sunlight, extremes in temperature, and localized trauma. Corticosteroid creams and ointments are particularly beneficial. Intralesional steroid therapy is helpful. Systemic therapy with antimalarials also has been advised.

Dermatomyositis

Dermatomyositis (polymyositis) is an inflammatory condition that produces angiopathy in the skin, subcutaneous tissue, and muscles. The disease usually starts in the face and eyelids, and may spread to other areas. It is associated with a number of other disturbances including Raynaud's phenomenon, alopecia, urticaria, and erythema multiforme. Of particular interest to the surgeon is the fact that a visceral cancer is frequently associated with the condition. Histologic changes are similar to those of lupus erythematosus.

Treatment consists of rest, salicylates, steroids, methotrexate, and azathioprine.

Scleroderma (Systemic Sclerosis)

Scleroderma is characterized by the appearance of circumscribed or diffuse, smooth, hard, ivory-colored areas that are immobile and give the skin the appearance of being "hide-bound."[34] The skin becomes smooth, yellowish, and firm, and it shrinks, so that the underlying structures are bound down. Although the condition frequently involves the face and hands, leading to an expressionless appearance on the former and a claw-like appearance of the latter, it can progress to involve most of the internal organs. Involvement of the small intestine may cause constipation, diarrhea, and abdominal distention. Although the colon is only rarely involved, it can produce the signs and symptoms of Ogilvie's syndrome (see Chap. 17). Treatment consists of general supportive measures, baths, a high-protein diet, corticosteroids, and a number of other medications including immunosuppressives.

Erythema Multiforme

Erythema multiforme is a clinically and histologically distinctive condition precipitated by a number of agents: virus infections, bacterial infections, radiotherapy, carcinomatosis, pregnancy, connective tissue disease, drug reactions, and many others. The mechanism for this particular reaction is unknown. The lesions present as dull red, flat, maculopapules which may be rather small or which may increase to 1 or 2 cm in 48 hours. The periphery may remain red, whereas the center is cyanotic. The lesions appear almost like *targets*. Lesions in the oral mucous membrane are common, but genital lesions are also frequent.

Histologically, the abnormality is confined to the upper dermis and lower epidermis. In more severe cases there is necrosis of the whole epidermis. Bullae usually are subepidermal. Treatment consists of symptomatic relief in the mild case, but in severe cases the use of corticosteroids has been suggested. Antibiotics are advised to prevent secondary infection.

Familial Benign Chronic Pemphigus (Hailey-Hailey)

Familial benign chronic pemphigus is a hereditary disease characterized by a recurrent bullous and vesicular dermatitis of the neck, axillae, flexors, and surfaces that oppose. The disease is transmitted as an autosomal dominant trait. The histologic pattern is rather unique, with prominent intraepidermal vesicles and bullae (Fig. 8-7). The condition has been found localized to the perianal area and may pose confusion in differential diagnosis.[103]

Treatment consists of antibiotics (local or systemic) and the use of topical corticosteroids. Additionally, low-dose radiation treatment has been recommended. Localized areas have been treated by excision and skin grafting.

Pemphigus Vulgaris

Pemphigus vulgaris is characterized by bullae appearing on apparently normal skin and mucous membranes.[38] The lesions usually begin first in the mouth and next in the groin, scalp, face, neck, axillae, and genitals. It appears that an autoimmune mechanism is the etiology. The condition occurs equally in both sexes, usually in adults in their fifth and sixth decades. Circulating intercellular antibodies may be demonstrated in these patients.

The pathologic changes are acantholysis, cleft and blister formation in the intraepidermal areas just above the basal cell layer, and the formation of acantholytic cells (Fig. 8-8).[38] Characteristic of the separation of keratinocytes is the presence of the Tzanck cell lining the bulla, as well as lying free in the cavity.

Because of the pain associated with advanced cases, prolonged daily baths with permanganate solution are advised. Silvadene, which is effective in the treatment of burn patients, is also useful in this condition. Corticosteroids remain the primary therapy, 160 mg of prednisone daily. Cancer chemotherapeutic agents have also been advised.

Cicatricial Pemphigoid (Benign Mucosal Pemphigoid)

Cicatricial pemphigoid is characterized by the presence of transient vesicles that heal by scarring to mucous membranes. The condition most commonly occurs in the mouth and conjunctiva. Other areas of involvement include the pharynx, esophagus, genitalia, and anus. In rare cases the lesion has been confined to the genital

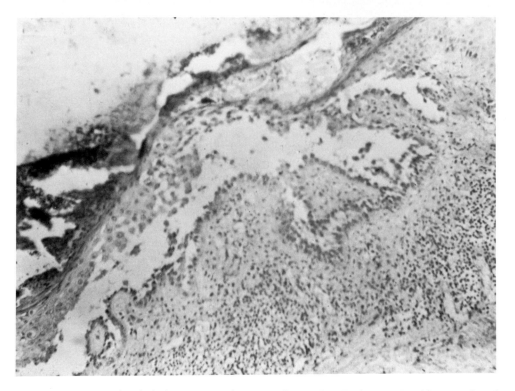

FIG. 8-7. Benign familial chronic pemphigus (Hailey-Hailey) is characterized by suprabasal bullae, such as the one shown here, containing detached prickle cells, and good preservation of acantholytic cells. Note the moderate inflammatory reaction in the underlying dermis. (Original magnification × 180. Courtesy of Rudolf Garret, M.D.)

and anal area.[64] Direct immunofluorescence of the lesional area reveals the presence of antibodies at the basement membrane. The absence of acantholysis differentiates the condition from pemphigus vulgaris.

There is no effective medication for the condition. Obstructing areas in the larynx and esophagus may require tracheostomy or gastrostomy.

INFECTIOUS CONDITIONS

For the purposes of discussion I have taken the liberty of classifying the infectious processes according to those that are nonvenereal and those that are usually attributable to venereal causes.

Nonvenereal Infections

Pilonidal Sinus

Pilonidal sinus is a common infective process that occurs in the natal cleft and sacrococcygeal region in young adults and teenagers. There is a 3:1 male predominance. In 1973, over 70,000 patients were admitted to nongovernmental hospitals in the United States with the primary diagnosis of pilonidal sinus disease.[71] A total of over 77,000 soldiers were admitted to army hospitals for pilonidal sinus problems during 1942 through 1945, remaining an average of 44 days.[83] The condition was originally described by Anderson, and was subsequently named "pilonidal sinus" by Hodges in 1880.[7, 59] The term literaly means "nest of hair"; usually the epithelium-lined sinus is found to contain hair.

When the sinus becomes infected, usually after puberty, it drains from an opening or openings overlying the coccyx and sacrum (Fig. 8-9). The infected abscess may extend to the perianal area in a presentation that may be mistaken for anal fistula. The disease can also be confused with suppurative hydradenitis. Although the condition is by no means life threatening, it does cause considerable disability for many patients. Time lost from school or from work can amount to a number of months.

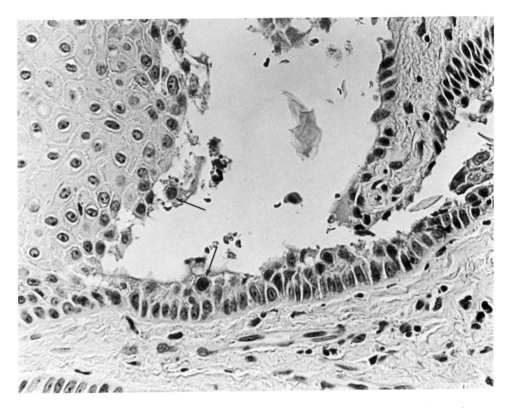

FIG. 8-8. Intraepithelial vesicles such as this one are characteristic of pemphigus vulgaris. The arrows indicate cells with large hyperchromatic nuclei (Tzanck cells). There is an absence of inflammatory reaction in the dermis. (Original magnification × 600)

The etiology of the condition has recently been the subject of some controversy and discussion. One possible theory that has been espoused is the failure of fusion in the embryo, with resultant entrapment of hair follicles in the sacrococcygeal region. Proponents of this theory are quick to point out the frequent incidence of eyebrow hair meeting in the midline in such patients. Another theory attributes the problem to the result of trauma, introducing hair shafts into the subdermal areas. Lord observed a number of interesting features of the condition.[70] He felt that there was a constant relationship between the lateral sinus openings and the midline pits; the openings are always cephalad to the pits. Lord observed in a patient the presence of 23 hairs of exact same length, diameter, color, and orientation. He postulated that it would be impossible for this number of hairs to follow each other into a pilonidal sinus and be identical in every respect. Lord applied this observation by suggesting that the treatment of pilonidal sinus can be made, therefore, quite simple. He suggested that all that is required is the removal of the offending hair follicle and the hairs that have been shed. These observations were subsequently confirmed by Bascom.[10]

The patient usually presents with pain, swelling, and purulent drainage. Fever and leukocytosis may also accompany the symptoms. As with other septic processes in the perianal area, antibiotics have no place in the therapy, except to augment the surgical procedure.

Treatment

For acute pilonidal abscess, incision and drainage will relieve the patient's symptoms. Regardless of the size of the septic process, this can usually be done in a physician's office, or in an outpatient surgicenter or ambulatory care facility. Whenever possible it is advisable to simultaneously drain the abscess and curette or excise the infected sinus.

Definitive elective treatment of pilonidal disease includes excision and primary closure, excision and grafting, excision leaving the wound open to close secondarily, incision and curettage, follicle excision (Lord), and cryosurgical destruction.

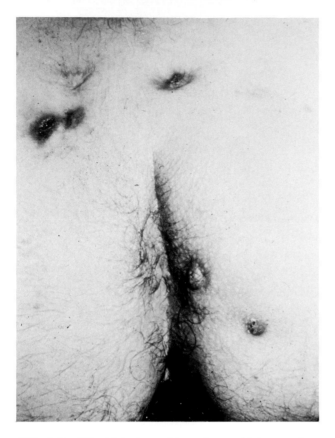

FIG. 8-9. Pilonidal sinus. Note the multiple openings overlying the sacrum and buttocks.

Excision and packing is rather simple to accomplish, requires minimal hospital stay, and in fact usually can be accomplished with a local anesthetic in the office. A probe is passed from opening to opening and the sinus is unroofed (Fig. 8-10, *A*). Alternatively, the multiple openings can be excised en bloc, curetting out any further extensions or side tracts (Fig. 8-10, *B*). If the procedure is undertaken on an outpatient basis, the patient is instructed to remove the packing the following morning, usually while taking a bath. With this approach, an expeditious surgical procedure and shortened hospital stay (or no hospital stay) are substituted for a prolonged postoperative convalescence. All too often such wounds require frequent treatments, necessitating cauterization, shaving, cleansing, and packing. It is not uncommon for pilonidal sinus wounds that extend toward the anal verge to take 6 months or longer to heal (Fig. 8-11). Delayed healing may persist to the point when re-excision is advised. Multiple operative procedures are not uncommon sequelae under these circumstances. It is for this reason that I am reluctant to advise this particular approach except for rather small lesions.

Excision with marsupialization is a compromise between a completely open wound and a completely closed one. This approach permits a somewhat smaller opening than does an approach in which the wound is left totally open (Fig. 8-12). If the suture material (a long-term absorbable substance) succeeds in holding the edges together, more rapid healing should occur. Unfortunately, the sutures frequently pull out, and the patient is left with as wide a wound as he would have

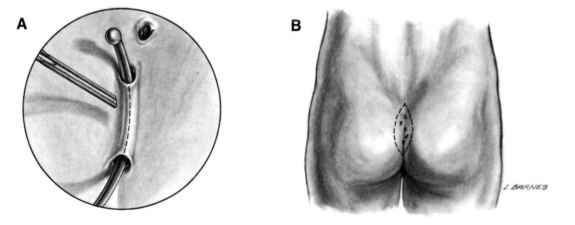

FIG. 8-10. Excision and packing for the treatment of pilonidal sinus can be accomplished by unroofing the individual tract **(A)** or by an all-encompassing excision **(B)**.

had with excision and packing. Even without this development, the wound still requires careful attention, including packing, shaving, and cleansing.

Excision and primary closure can be performed in an ambulatory surgical facility if the sinus is relatively small. However for more extensive lesions, inpatient therapy is recommended. This has the disadvantage of a relatively prolonged hospital stay, but provides the potential benefit of a healed wound within perhaps 10 to 14 days. For large, complex pilonidal sinus problems, particularly when multiple procedures have been performed (see Fig. 8-11), the excision and primary closure technique may be very effective. The pilonidal sinus is excised to the gluteal fascia (Fig. 8-13, *A*). The fascia is incised and a periosteal elevator is used to lift the fascia off the sacrum (Fig. 8-13, *B*). This maneuver permits the placement of heavy retention sutures through all layers. These are laid into position, and the fascia is reapproximated with absorbable suture material (Fig. 8-14, *A*). The wound is copiously irrigated, and the skin is closed (Fig. 8-14, *B*); the retention sutures are secured over a stent dressing (Fig. 8-14, *C*). The dressing is left in place for approximately 10 days. When the pilonidal sinus extends near the anal opening, the bowels are confined for this period. This requires a clear liquid diet and the use of "slowing" medications (deodorized tincture of opium, Lomotil, and codeine). With considerable skin loss it is sometimes useful to rotate skin flaps to cover the defect.[55, 71] This can be performed using one of the techniques described in Chapter 6 (Anoplasty).

Other operations have been advocated that require excision of less tissue. The Lord modification has been mentioned earlier. This consists of drainage of the abscess, removal of the hair, and excision of the hair follicle (if present). The cavity is cleansed through incisions adjacent to but not inside the pilonidal sinus. The cavity walls are not excised but are permitted to collapse.

The use of cryosurgical destruction has been advocated.[50, 78] The technique consists of surgery, opening of the tracts and side branches, curettage, and electrocoagulation of bleeding points. The open wound is then sprayed with liquid nitrogen for approximately 5 minutes.

I have had no experience with this technique, but O'Connor states that there is less deformity and scarring when compared with a wider excision.[78] However, since it has been generally recognized that a wide excision is not a necessary part of the treatment, the comparison may be inappropriate.

Results. Hanley is an advocate of emergency surgery of acute pilonidal abscess by excision and open

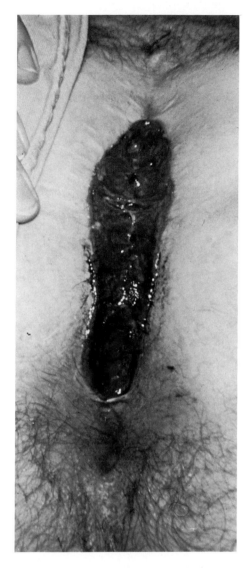

FIG. 8-11. Indolent, granulating, nonhealing wound of recurrent (persistent) pilonidal sinus.

treatment.[56] With this technique he reports uniform healing with no evidence of recurrence in a small group of patients. Bascom and Edwards reported their experience with the Lord treatment: removal only of the follicles and hairs.[10, 41] In the former report, 50 patients were treated in the office under local anesthesia. Acute abscesses received drainage only, whereas chronic abscesses were treated by excision of the enlarged follicles from the midline skin. One to ten follicles were removed, individually if possible. The specimens weighed under 1 g per patient. Incisions were kept smaller than

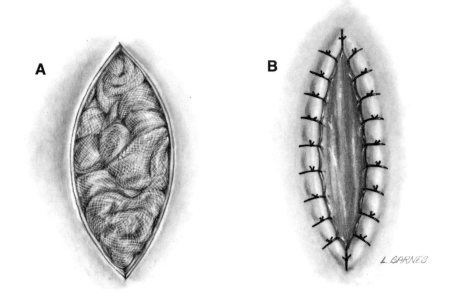

FIG. 8-12. Appearance of the pilonidal sinus after two different approaches: open and packed, usually with iodoform gauze **(A),** and marsupialized, suturing the full thickness of the skin to the underlying epithelialized tract or fascia **(B).**

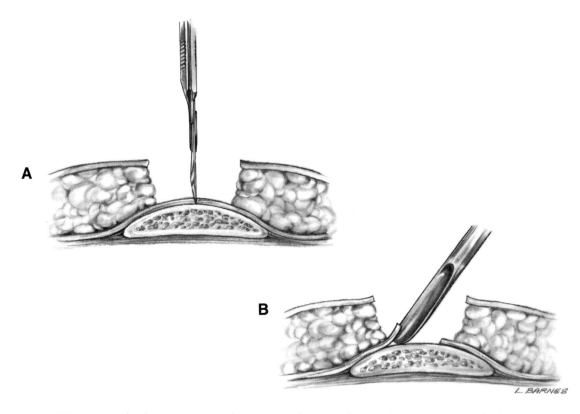

FIG. 8-13. The first two steps in the primary closure technique for the treatment of pilonidal sinus infection. **A.** The fascia is incised. **B.** The fascia is elevated.

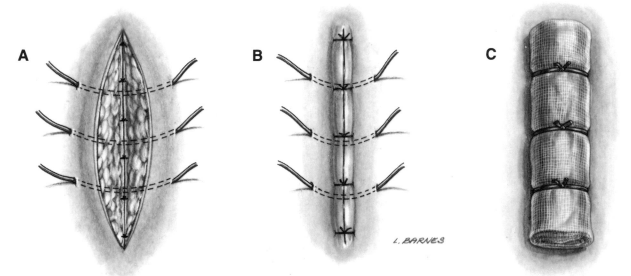

L. BARNES

FIG. 8-14.   The last three steps in the primary closure technique for treating pilonidal sinus infection. **A.** With retention sutures in place, the fascia is closed. **B.** The skin is closed. **C.** Stent dressing is secured.

7 mm. Follow-up averaged 24 months. The mean disability was 1 day, and the mean wound-healing time was 3 weeks. Recurrences appeared in four patients (8%); all were healed 3 weeks following reoperation. There was no incident of a second recurrence.

In Edwards' report, 102 patients were treated by this technique.[41] The median number of days off work was 10, and the median number of days requiring healing was 39. Eighty-nine percent were free of recurrent disease, provided they attended the follow-up clinic. Since a number of patients failed to attend it is difficult to interpret the results of this study. It appears, however, that the author was not as successful as Bascom.

Zimmerman reported outpatient excision and primary closure on 32 patients.[105] Follow-up was for a mean of 24 months. In all cases primary healing was obtained, a result that is not dissimilar to my own experience.

Reports of the success of excision and grafting are somewhat difficult to interpret in light of the lack of a control in these studies.[55, 71] In the report from the Cleveland Clinic, 58 patients were reviewed who underwent extensive or recurrent pilonidal disease surgery with primary skin grafting.[55] More than 72% had recurrent disease when initially seen at the clinic. The average hospital stay was 10 days. The time off from work averaged 28 days; the recurrence rate was 1.7%, and the failure rate, 3.4%. Using the Z-plasty technique, 120 patients were treated by Mansoory and Dickson.[71] There were two recurrences, a very favorable experience. When skin loss is present in association with pilonidal sinus disease (particularly in the recurrent situation), mobilizing skin to cover the defect will more reliably lead to a satisfactory result.

Comment.   It is now generally agreed that minimal surgery should be applied to the treatment of pilonidal disease whenever possible. The concept of Lord and of others in removing the hair follicles and the hairs themselves without extensive excision and debridement is an excellent one. Every attempt should be made to keep the patient out of the hospital and to limit the morbidity of the procedure. However, there are some patients who benefit from a more extensive excision, particularly those who have had multiple procedures. Under these circumstances, inpatient hospital treatment with excision and primary closure may offer a lower morbidity.

Suppurative Hidradenitis (Hidradenitis Suppurativa)

Suppurative hidradenitis is a chronic, recurrent, indolent infection involving the skin and subcutaneous tissue arising in the apocrine glands (axillary, inguinal, genital, perineal, and mammary). The condition was originally described in 1839 by Velpeau.[99] Sexes are equally susceptible, and most cases occur between the ages of 16 and 40. The most frequent area of involvement is the axilla, but the perianal area is not uncommonly affected. The etiology is unknown. Acne appears to be a predisposing etiologic factor, although poor skin hygiene, hyperhidrosis, and chemical depilatories may play a role.[22] The condition can be confused with anal fistula, Crohn's disease, tuberculosis, pilonidal sinus, and other infections in the anal area. Examination reveals tender, erythematous, purulent lesions, which may be associated with adenopathy and systemic signs (fever, malaise, and leukocytosis; Fig. 8-15). The condition frequently produces burrowing sinuses that can extend for many inches around the anus, into the scrotum, buttock, labia, and sacrum. Although the tracts are usually relatively superficial, they can actually invade deeply and extend to involve the area around the femoral vessels.

Histologically, the earliest inflammatory changes are seen within and around the apocrine glands, the ducts of which may be distended with leukocytes. In the chronic stage, multiple abscesses, intercommunicating sinus tracts, and irregular hypertrophied scars form.[20] The scars, ulceration, and infection extend within the subcutaneous tissue to the fascia (Fig. 8-16).

Treatment

It is generally felt that early antibiotic therapy is of considerable value in the treatment of this condition. Local and systemic broad-spectrum antibiotics are advised; this includes penicillin, erythromycin, and tetracycline in some cases, especially where acne is noted in other areas. The antibiotics should be used until resolution of the process is complete. Unfortunately, there is a group of patients who do not respond to this regimen, and disability is such that surgical intervention is required to treat the extensive sinus tracts and abscesses.

With minimal involvement and inadequate palliation by medical means, incision and drainage of an abscess may result in cure. When the condition progresses to extensive sinus formation, excision is the only means by which the condition can be effectively ameliorated.

The four methods of surgical treatment are excision with primary closure, excision with grafting, excision with marsupialization, and excision with packing (Fig. 8-17, A–D). All four methods can be applied usefully even in the same patient. Primary closure usually requires a relatively narrow wound, but often by elevating the full thickness of skin on either side of the excision site, the wound may be approximated without tension. Wide excision, leaving the wound open to heal by second intention, is probably the commonest method of surgical treatment. This has the obvious disadvantage of a prolonged healing time.

Methods to close the wound include the application of a split-thickness graft or some form of plastic procedure (e.g., Z-plasty). It would certainly be preferable to close the wound by some means if this were possible. Occasionally it is necessary to perform a diverting colostomy if extensive surgery and grafting is required in the perianal area. Rarely does the disease progress to the point where such significant deformity of the anal canal develops to necessitate a permanent colostomy. In patients who have both anterior and posterior disease in the perineal area it is usually wise to perform surgery on one side only and treat the opposite side only after healing has taken place.

Results. Culp reported the Mayo Clinic experience with 132 patients observed with anogenital hidradenitis suppurativa during a 6-year period.[26] Of the 30 patients whose disease was limited to the anal canal and adjacent areas, two thirds were men. Most of the patients had previous multiple attempts at surgical drainage or extirpation. The author commented that although excision with grafting had been used extensively in the past, such a program had not been necessary in recent years. Although extensive exteriorization was the method employed in 17 of the 30 patients, the wounds were healed within 8 weeks in all cases. A diverting colostomy was not felt to be necessary. Although there was no recurrence in the patients (follow-up more than 1 year), the length of time for healing is still in my opinion rather considerable.

Thornton and Abcarian reviewed 104 patients who underwent surgery for the condition at the Cook County Hospital in Chicago.[98] Approximately two thirds of the patients were men. A sample of the drained pus sent for culture and antibiotic sensitivity revealed no growth in approximately half of the patients. The operative procedure for all patients consisted of wide excision down to normal fat or fascia using electrocautery. The wounds were then packed with iodoform gauze; patients were followed on a biweekly basis. The average hospital stay was approximately 1 week. However, patients over the age of 40 years had an average hospital stay of approximately 19 days. Healing times ranged from approximately 1 month for relatively small wounds to 2 months for larger ones. Four patients developed a recurrence.

Broadwater and co-workers reviewed their experience of 23 patients treated between 1967 and 1981.[16] Sixty-one percent were male; the average age was 30 years. The mean duration of symptoms was in excess of 5 years. The authors' primary treatment included wide and deep excision with selective (individualized) closure. Although it is difficult to evaluate the reason for selection of the procedure, the overall recurrence rate in those patients undergoing primary closure was 30%. Those patients who underwent excision with application of a split-thickness graft had a 13% incidence

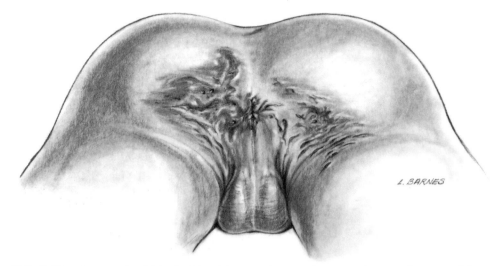

FIG. 8-15. Suppurative hidradenitis with extensive involvement of perianal area and buttocks.

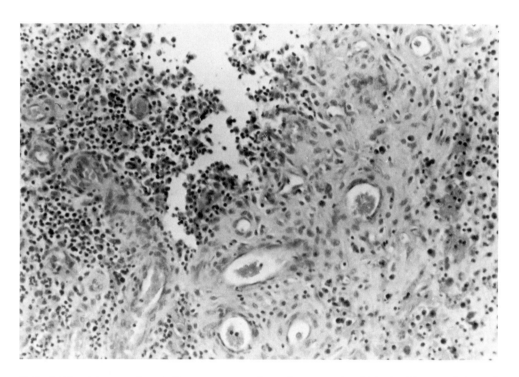

FIG. 8-16. Mononuclear inflammatory exudate of suppurative hidradenitis, consisting of monocytes, lymphocytes, and plasma cells. (Original magnification × 280. Courtesy of Rudolf Garret, M.D.)

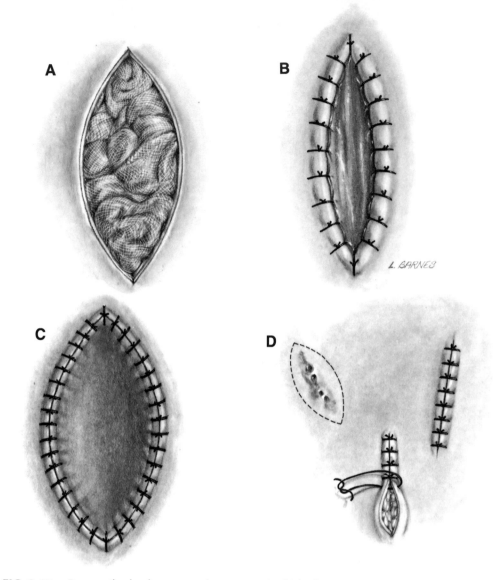

FIG. 8-17.   Four methods of treatment for suppurative hidradenitis. **A.** Excision with packing. **B.** Excision with marsupialization. **C.** Excision with grafting. **D.** Excision and primary closures.

of recurrence. Half of the patients treated by excision, with the wound left open to heal by secondary intention, developed recurrences. However, only four lesions were so treated.

Comment   Suppurative hidradenitis is a complicated condition to treat; the approach to each case must be individualized. My own inclination is to excise relatively small lesions and perform primary closure wherever possible. I am reluctant to embark on various plastic procedures because of my discomfort with opening up extensive planes of dissection in the presence of possible sepsis. For large lesions I prefer to widely excise and leave the area to granulate for 4 or 5 days. Application of a split-thickness graft at that time affords an excellent opportunity for primary healing.

Fistula-in-ano (Anal Fistula)

Anal fistula (Color Fig. 8-4) is another perianal infective process that may be confused with pilonidal sinus and suppurative hidradenitis. Chapter 4 is dedicated to the diagnosis and management of this condition.

Crohn's Disease

Anal and perianal Crohn's disease present a difficult mangement problem (see Figs. 4-32, 4-33, 4-36, and 15-1). This condition is discussed in Chapter 4, and the diagnosis and management of inflammatory bowel disease is presented in Chapter 15.

Tuberculosis

Tuberculosis distal to the ileocecal valve is uncommon; it is seldom considered in the differential diagnosis when the disease process is located in the large intestine.[54] It can be confused with Crohn's disease, actinomycosis, anal fistula, and the other cutaneous conditions affecting the perianal area. Most reported cases occur in developing countries. The disease is seen most commonly in men and is usually associated with pulmonary tuberculosis. However, there have been case reports of the lesion occurring in the absence of pulmonary infection.[102] Primary inoculation of the microbacterium may result from trauma to the skin or mucosa. The lesion may appear as a brownish-red papule that can progress into an ulcerating plaque; this is known as a *tuberculous chancre*. Regional lymphadenopathy is common. A high index of suspicion is necessary if one is to establish the diagnosis early and to initiate appropriate therapy. An anal fissure in an unusual location that is slow to heal should be pathologically confirmed with appropriate staining and cultures to rule out the presence of the bacterium.[102]

The ulcers are usually painful and indolent, with blue, irregular edges. The diagnosis can be established by means of demonstration of the acid-fast bacilli in the biopsy specimen, positive guinea pig culture, and the presence of caseating granulomas in the histologic examination of skin lesions. Demonstration of active disease in the lungs and the presence of a positive tuberculin skin test are helpful in confirming the nature of the lesion (see Chap. 17).

In western countries, tuberculosis is not likely to be considered in the differential diagnosis of a perianal ulcer.[4] In the absence of a pulmonary lesion it would be very difficult for me not to treat the patient, initially at least, for Crohn's disease. Obviously, antituberculous drugs are the treatment of choice. Therapy with isoniazid (INH), rifampin, and ethambutol will usually resolve the anal condition in a matter of 2 or 3 weeks. However, treatment should be continued for many months following resolution of the local or systemic manifestations.

Actinomycosis

Actinomycosis is a chronic infectious disease involving the cervicofacial area, thorax, or abdomen. It is caused by an anaerobic, gram-positive bacterium, *Actinomyces israelii*. It produces a suppurative, fibrosing inflammation that forms sinus tracts, discharging granules (Fig. 8-18). In the abdominal form, a mass is usually present, and a psoas abscess occasionally occurs (see Chap. 17)

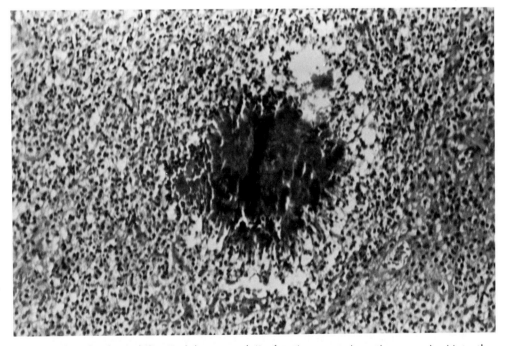

FIG. 8-18. The basophilic "sulphur granule" of actinomyces in actinomycosis. Note the homogeneous center and the club-shaped filaments at the periphery. (Original magnification × 120. Courtesy of Rudolf Garret, M.D.)

The diagnosis is established by identification of the microorganism in cultures of tissue or from the exudate of the lesion. The diagnosis is absolutely established if sulfur granules are seen. In the anal area, sinus tracts and fistulas may resemble Crohn's disease, anal fistula, suppurative hydradenitis, and tuberculosis. The presence of the disease elsewhere (particularly in the abdomen) is helpful in alerting the surgeon to the nature of the problem.

Treatment consists of surgical excision and drainage of the abscess as well as antibiotics (usually penicillin). A 4-week period of treatment is recommended.

Viral Infections

A number of viral infections can affect the anal area. Those that are presumed nonvenereal in origin follow.

Herpes Zoster

Herpes zoster (presumed reactivation of varicella) may affect the anal area. The condition, also known as "shingles," affects both sexes equally. Jellinek and Tulloch described 7 patients with retention, loss of sensation, or incontinence.[63] The lesion is characterized by groups of vesicles on an erythematous base along the distribution of a spinal nerve leading to a posterior ganglion. Itching, tenderness, and pain are characteristically located along the region supplied by the nerve.

Diagnosis can be established by means of tissue culture and by demonstration of antibiodies in the serum by immunofluorescent techniques. Histologically, vesicles are seen to be intraepidermal; within these vesicles are found large, swollen cells called "balloon cells" (Fig. 8-19).

Treatment consists of medical measures, including rest and the application of heat. Analgesics are advisable for acute neuralgia. For older patients with severe pain, systemic corticosteroid therapy is advisable. The condition may be particularly troublesome in patients who have been immunosuppressed by the treatment for malignancy.

Vaccinia

Vaccinia virus is an attenuated cowpox virus that has been propagated in laboratories for immunization against smallpox. Perianal vaccinia is a rare complication of vaccination, and usually occurs in young children.[24] It has also been reported as a complication of diarrhea with probable transmission to the excoriated area by the fingers.[25] In adults the condition may be confused with syphilis or with herpes simplex infection. The history is helpful if the patient underwent a recent vaccination or was exposed to someone who had.

Treatment is generally supportive because complete resolution usually occurs spontaneously. However, vaccinia immune globulin (VIG) has been recommended in severe cases or to expedite resolution of the process.

Bacterial Infections

Infective processes associated with bacterial organisms such as pilonidal sinus and suppurative hydradenitis

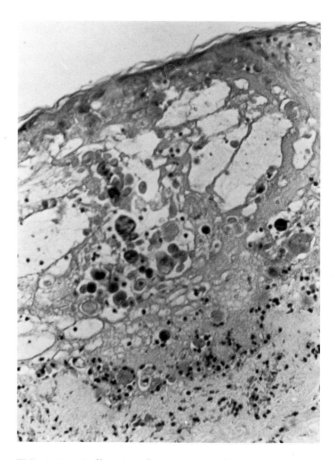

FIG. 8-19. Ballooning degeneration of prickle cells with the formation of multilocular vesicles in herpes zoster. Note cells with large inclusion bodies. (Original magnification × 240. Courtesy of Rudolf Garret, M.D.)

have already been discussed. There is, however, a unique infective condition in the perianal area that is worthy of discussion, *Fournier's gangrene.*

Fournier's Gangrene

Fournier's syndrome is a gangrenous infection that may involve the genital area, groin, and perineum. A number of organisms have been identified, both aerobic and anaerobic, including *Clostridium welchii.*[58]

Because of the prevalence of two or more species of bacteria in the infection, the term "synergistic gangrene" has been employed. *Necrotizing fasciitis* is another descriptive term that has been employed for the condition. It is important to distinguish the entity from clostridial myonecrosis, because the treatment is so obviously different.[12] Many patients have a history of prior anorectal surgery or pelvic surgery for infective processes (*e.g.,* perforated diverticulitis). Broad specimen (appropriate) antibiotic therapy is recommended, but vigorous surgical debridement must be undertaken. This includes unroofing of all of the tracts and excision of devitalized tissue. The wounds are left open and packed. Vigorous irrigation with antiseptic solution is recommended.

Fungal Infections

The primary site of involvement of recognized fungal infections is the skin. Those that cause superficial involvement are called *dermatophytes,* and include *Microsporum, Trichophyton,* and *Epidermophyton.*[36] Fungi digest and live on keratin.

Tinea Cruris (Jock Itch, Crotch Itch)

Tinea cruris occurs most commonly in the intertriginous areas; the condition is exacerbated by heat and humidity. It is also known as ringworm of the groin and is caused by a species of *Trichophyton.* The differential diagnosis includes seborrheic dermatitis, psoriasis, and vegetative pemphigus. Demonstration of the fungus by potassium hydroxide microscopic examination and culture confirms the diagnosis (Fig. 8-20).

Treatment consists of reduction of perspiration and enhancement of evaporation from the crural area. Loose-fitting clothes are suggested. Griseofulvin is considered the most effective drug in the treatment of all ringworm fungi.[101] Its action is believed to be a modification of the keratin so that the fungus will not invade. Three to four weeks of treatment is advised. Topical fungicides are not very satisfactory, so an oral route

is suggested. Other medications include tolnaftate, clotrimazole, and miconazole.[101]

Candidiasis (Monoliasis)

Candidiasis is caused by the yeast-like fungus, *Candida albicans.* The fungus is a frequent commensal in humans and is present in the alimentary tract and vagina of many healthy people.[101] Intertriginous areas are frequently affected, the perianal and inguinal folds and the axillae.

The organism is usually found outside the epidermis and behaves primarily as an opportunistic infection, especially in patients who have impaired resistance. The condition may be somewhat difficult to recognize. Pustules without surrounding inflammation may leave a "collarette" of scale; satellite lesions can be often seen in adjacent skin. Some eruptions in the inguinal area may resemble tinea cruris, but usually there is less scaling and a greater tendency to fissuring.[36] When the condition occurs in children it is called diaper or napkin dermatitis.

The diagnosis of candidiasis is made by demonstrating the yeast, spores, or pseudomycelium under the microscope with potassium hydroxide. Culture on Sabouraud's glucose agar shows a growth of creamy, grayish, moist colonies in about 4 days.[36]

Treatment consists of topical nystatin, clotrimazole, or miconazole. For very severe cases, usually in patients with immunologic deficiency, amphotericin B can be administered intravenously.

Sporotrichosis, Coccidioidomycosis, Histoplasmosis, North American Blastomycosis, Chromomycosis, Cryptococcosis, Nocardiosis, and Mycetoma

The above fungal infections are generally known as the "deep mycoses." These usually come from inhalation of dust contaminated with the fungus, from droppings of animals infected by it, or from contamination from other sources.[36] All have associated skin lesions, which have generally a good prognosis if it is a primary cutaneous infection. However, when the skin lesion is a result of dissemination from a visceral focus, the prognosis can be very serious indeed. Generally, skin biopsy will reveal the presence of the fungi. The treatment varies with the type of fungus and with the extent of disease, either localized or systemic. The reader is referred to a textbook of medicine for the clinical features, diagnosis, and management of the conditions.

Parasitic Diseases

There are numerous parasitic diseases that have cutaneous manifestations, many of which also affect the

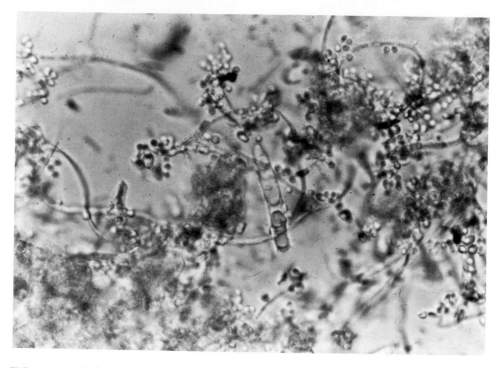

FIG. 8-20. *Trichophyton mentagrophytes* in potassium hydroxide preparation, a species of Trichophyton that can cause tinea cruris (ringworm of the groin). (Original magnification × 600. Courtesy of Rudolf Garret, M.D.)

alimentary tract. Included are infections due to protozoa (single-cell organisms), nematodes (roundworms), arthropods, trematodes (flukes), cestodes (flatworms), annelids (leeches), and chordates. A number of these conditions are discussed in some detail in Chapter 17. The discussion that follows is limited to those important cutaneous manifestations which would be of value to the surgeon.

Amebiasis Cutis

Entamoeba histolytica is an organism that causes disease most commonly in the tropics. Cutaneous amebiasis occurs less frequently than the intestinal disease except for the cutaneous manifestations in the genitalia and perianal area. It is believed that the reason for this is direct extension from the involved bowel. Lesions begin as deep abscesses that rupture and form distinct ulcerations. Characteristically, skin lesions spread rapidly and may terminate fatally. There is an erythematous halo around the ulcer. Histologically there are areas of necrotic ulcertion with many lymphocytes, neutrophils, plasma cells, and eosinophils. The organism is frequently demonstrated in the fresh material from the base (see Chap. 17). Although abscesses may require surgical drainage, the cutaneous manifestation will usually respond to either metronidazole or emetine.

Trichomoniasis

Trichomonas vulvovaginitis causes vaginal pruritus, burning, and leukorrhea. The condition is caused by the protozoan *Trichomonas vaginalis*. Because of the discharge and pruritic symptoms, the anal area may be secondarily involved by the irritation. Eliciting a history of the vaginal discharge will alert the physician to the source of the problem. Treatment is metronidazole (Flagyl), 250 mg for 10 days.

Flatworms: Schistosomal Dermatitis (Schistosomiasis Cutis, Swimmer's Itch)

Schistosomal dermatitis is a severe pruritic, papular dermatitis caused by cercarial species of *Schistosoma*, a genus of trematodes. Exposure to the cercaria (Fig. 17-55) occurs by swimming or wading in water containing them. They attach by burrowing into the skin. Clinically there is severe itching at the time of the exposure secondary to an urticarial reaction. A papular, pruritic lesion results which spontaneously regresses after a few days, disappearing by 2 weeks. Antipruritic measures are used for treatment.

Visceral schistosomiasis (bilharziasis) may produce cutaneous manifestations as a result of deposition of eggs in the dermis. Fistulous tracts may develop in the perineum and buttocks, with hard masses, sinus tracts, and seropurulent discharge with a foul, characteristic odor. In the severe vegetating form, malignant change in the granulomas has been noted. Treatment consists of trivalent antimony compounds (tartar emetic, stibophen, triostam, or Astiban).

Nematode Infections

Oxyuriasis (Pinworm, Enterobiasis). *Enterobius (Oxyuris) vermicularis* is the helminth that most commonly infects humans. Children are more frequently affected than adults. It is more common in temperate climates than in the tropics. The worm lives in the proximal colon and is commonly found in the appendix (Fig. 8-21), but the disease is not truly related to the bowel itself. The worms migrate to the rectum at night and emerge on the perianal skin to deposit thousands of ova (Figs. 8-22 and 8-23). The ova are

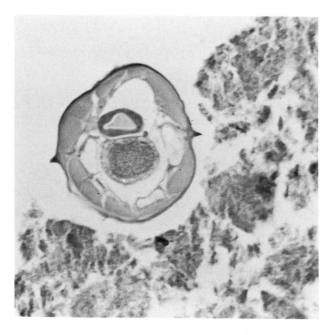

FIG. 8-22. Pinworm ovum *(Enterobius vermicularis)*. Note the lateral spines. (Original magnification × 170)

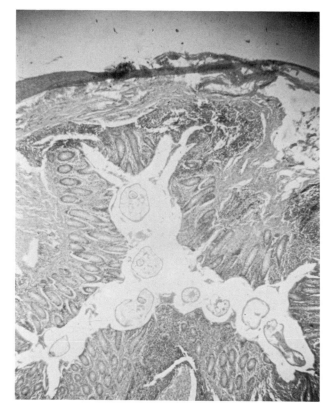

FIG. 8-21. *Enterobius vermicularis* infection: pinworms in the appendix, cross-section. (Original magnification × 80. Courtesy of Rudolf Garret, M.D.)

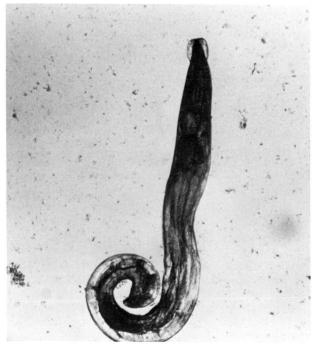

FIG. 8-23. *Enterobius vermicularis,* the adult pinworm (female). (Courtesy of Rudolf Garret, M.D.)

returned to the mouth by the patient; the larvae hatch in the duodenum, and migrate to the small and large intestine. Fertilization occurs in the cecum, completing the life cycle.

The diagnosis is usually established by demonstration of the ova in smears taken from the anal region early in the morning. Applying cellophane tape against the perianal region, adding a drop of iodine, and examining the tape under a microscope slide may facilitate detection of the ova. Demonstration of the pinworm in the stool is rarely successful. Because of the high likelihood of communication it is appropriate to study members of the patient's family.

Piperazine (Antepar) and pyrvinium pamoate (Povan) are effective medications for the treatment of the condition. The former is given in single daily doses of 65 mg per kg (not to exceed 2500 mg) taken 1 hour before breakfast for 8 consecutive days, and the latter is given in a single dose of 5 mg per kg; a second dose may be given 1 week after the first treatment.[37] Undergarments, towels, sheets, pajamas, and other clothing should be thoroughly laundered separately from those of other members of the family.

Creeping Eruption (Larva Migrans). Larva migrans is a cutaneous eruption caused by larvae of several nematodes, most commonly the cat or dog hookworm, *Ancylostoma braziliense* or *Ancylostoma caninum*. The ova of these hookworms are deposited in the soil and hatch into infected larvae which penetrate the skin. People who go barefoot at the beach, children playing in sandboxes, carpenters and plumbers working under homes, and gardeners are the most common victims.[37] The feet, buttocks, hands, and genitals are most frequently involved by the process. Raised, pruritic, thin, linear, tunnel-like lesions are noted which contain serous fluid.

The disease is usually self-limited, but freezing of the larvae with ethyl chloride or liquid nitrogen has been effective. An alternative internal treatment is thiabendazole (Mintezol).

Larva Currens. Larva currens is a form of cutaneous larva migrans that is caused by *Strongyloides stercoralis*. The condition is so called because of the speed of larval migration. It is caused in essence by an autoinfection, penetration of the perianal skin by larvae excreted in the feces. The eruption is usually associated with intestinal strongylodiasis, beginning in the skin round the anus, and may involve the buttocks, thighs, and back. The itching is quite severe. As the larvae leave the skin to enter the bloodstream (settling in the intestinal mucosa), the rash disappears. The skin demonstrates a papular eruption with edema and urticaria.

Treatment consists of thiabendazole, 25 to 50 mg per kg for 2 to 4 days.

Insect Diseases

Cimicosis (Bedbug Bites). The bedbug (*Cimex lectularius*) hides in crevices during the daytime and feeds on human blood at night.[37] The bedbug usually produces a linear series of bites on the ankles and buttocks. Since the bites are painless the patient may not be aware of what has happened until finding the bedclothes stained with blood. Some patients may react with severe urticaria and pain. Treatment consists of soothing antipruritic lotions. The pests are eliminated by means of fumigation (*e.g.*, with malathion).

Pediculosis (Phthiriasis). There are several varieties of *Pediculus* that affect man, but the one that concerns us for the purpose of this discussion is Pediculus pubis *(Phthirus pubis)*, the pubic or crab louse. The condition is usually transmitted by sexual intercourse or from contaminated bedding. The lice are found on the hair or skin, appearing as yellowish brown or gray specks.[37] The so-called nits are attached to the hair shaft. Symptoms include pruritus and the secondary effects of persistent excoriation. The condition frequently coexists with other sexually transmitted diseases. Treatment consists of Kwell lotion or shampoo, or crotamiton (Eurax).

Arachnid Infection: Scabies

Scabies is a skin condition resulting from infestation by the mite *Sarcoptes scabiei* (Fig. 8-24). The female burrows into the stratum corneum and there deposits her eggs (Fig. 8-25). Patients complain primarily of itching that is worse at night. Areas commonly involved include the interdigital folds, flexor aspects of the wrist, nipples, navel, genitals, buttocks, and outer aspects of the feet. The lesion appears as a whitish burrow, which is rather tortuous and threadlike. Papules and pustules are frequently seen. The condition is usually contracted by close contact with a person harboring the mite. Treatment consists of lindane (gamma benzene), crotamiton (Eurax), or thiabendazole.

Venereal Diseases

Sexually transmitted diseases are the commonest communicable conditions in industrialized countries; a recent estimate by the World Health Organization (1974) indicated that 250 million people are infected annually with gonorrhea and about 50 million people with sy-

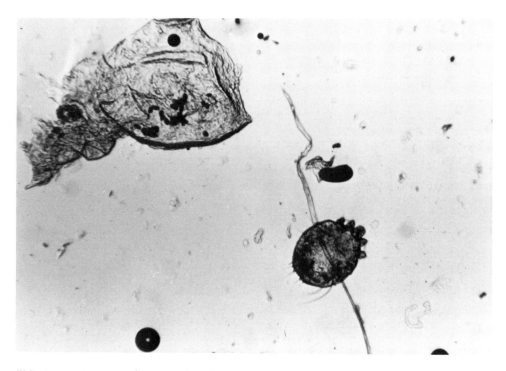

FIG. 8-24.   Scrapings from a scabies lesion showing the female mite. (Original magnification × 240. Courtesy of Rudolf Garret, M.D.)

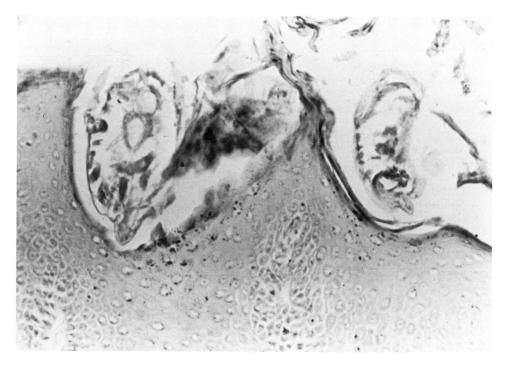

FIG. 8-25.   Scabies. A biopsy specimen showing the female mite burrowing into the epidermis. (Original magnification × 280. Courtesy of Rudolf Garret, M.D.)

philis.[18] Sohn and Robilotti coined the phrase "The Gay Bowel Syndrome" to indicate a constellation of diseases and conditions to which male homosexuals fall victim.[93] Although the classical venereal diseases such as syphilis, gonorrhea, chancroid, lymphogranuloma venereum, and granuloma inguinale are of interest, they represent only a minority of the sexually transmitted infections in the United States. The epidemic venereal conditions today are anogenital herpes and condylomata acuminata. With the changes in mores and attitude to sexual matters, it is incumbent upon the physician to be knowledgeable about the manifestations, differential diagnosis, and treatment of sexually transmitted disease.

Gonorrhea

Gonorrhea is a bacterial infection caused by *Neisseria gonorrhoeae*, a gram-negative diplococcus. The only known reservoir is man. The disease affects mucous membranes of the urethra, cervix, rectum, and oropharynx. Gonococcal dermatitis is a rare infection that may develop in a wound that has come in contact with the bacterium. It can also develop in the genital area. The complication of gonorrheal proctitis is of particular interest to the surgeon. This usually results from infection from anal intercourse in the gay population, but in women the condition is frequently the result of spread to the rectum from the genital tract. Gonococcal proctitis is discussed in Chapter 17.

Syphilis (Lues)

Syphilis is caused by the spirochete *Treponema pallidum*. The organism enters the skin or mucous membrane, producing a chancre approximately 3 weeks following the infection. This is the primary stage of the disease. The lesion is usually single and is most commonly found on the penis. In women, it may be inapparent because of its location within the vagina or cervix. A chancre is usually painless, but not always so. In the homosexual population the chancre is usually situated at the anal margin or in the anal canal (Fig. 8-26). As mentioned, the lesion may be painless, but there may be severe discomfort, tenesmus, and difficulty with defecation and discharge. Unless there is an index of suspicion, the condition may be confused with an anal fissure; inguinal adenopathy, however, is often present. The aberrant location of the fissure (*e.g.*, lateral) should alert the examiner, but this also could be a finding consistent with anal Crohn's disease.

Although most writings on the subject state that the diagnosis is established on the basis of identification of the organism by means of dark-field examination (Fig. 8-27), the test is of limited value. Since the absence of a positive test does not exclude the diagnosis, it is

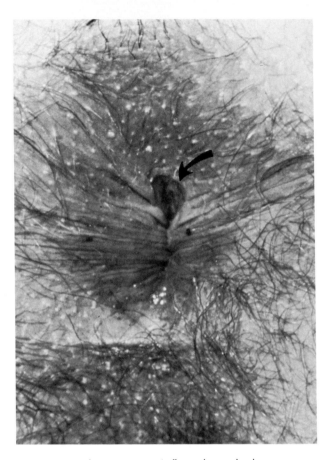

FIG. 8-26. Chancre, a noninflamed punched-out-appearing ulcer that was dark-field positive for *Treponema pallidum*.

probably better to treat the patient and to await the results of serologic tests. However, serologic tests for syphilis do not become positive until the primary chancre has been present for several weeks.

Although excision of the lesion is not recommended, there are characteristic histopathologic changes (Fig. 8-28). There is dense infiltration of round cells, plasma cells, and fibroblasts. Proliferation of endothelial cells results in a progressive arteritis.

Penicillin is the treatment of choice in nonallergic patients, whereas in those who are allergic to penicillin, tetracycline, 500 mg orally four times daily for 15 days, is recommended.[39]

The other cutaneous manifestation of lues is the secondary stage of syphilis, *condylomata lata*. The signs and symptoms of secondary syphilis may develop 2 to 6 months after infection and usually 6 to 8 weeks after the appearance of the primary chancre. Both lesions may exist synchronously. A maculopapular rash de-

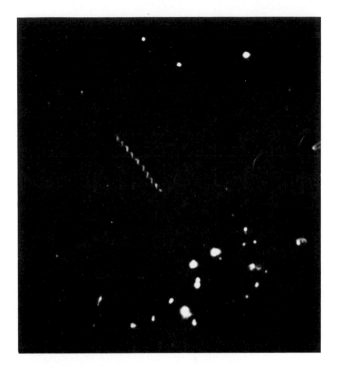

FIG. 8-27. *Treponema pallidum*, the causative agent of syphilis, appears as a corkscrew-shaped organism on dark-field examination. (Original magnification × 600. Courtesy of Rudolf Garret, M.D.)

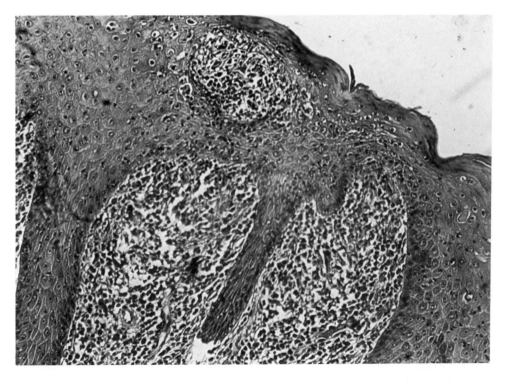

FIG. 8-28. Syphilitic chancre demonstrating pseudoepitheliomatous hyperplasia and plasma cell infiltration of the dermis with dilated lymphatics. (Original magnification × 250. Courtesy of Rudolf Garret, M.D.)

velops, which gives rise to a proliferating, weeping mass containing the spirochetes. The lesions may appear rather flat, scaling, red, and indurated; in the anal area particularly they may become papillomatous and vegetative, with an associated foul odor (Fig. 8-29). Although most literature suggests that the lesions are nonpruritic, other authors suggest that this may be the primary complaint.[21] The diagnosis may be established by demonstrating the organism using dark-field microscopic examination, but serologic tests are virtually always positive. The histopathology of secondary syphilis varies depending on the clinical presentation. Condylomata lata show acanthosis and edema in the epidermis with broadening of the rete ridges (Fig. 8-30). Some lesions may show a nonspecific chronic inflammatory reaction (Fig. 8-31).

Treatment with penicillin, erythromycin, or tetracycline is effective. An important part of the management of the patient includes the tracing of all sexual contacts, which in the case of secondary syphilis necessitates a 1-year retrospective review.[18]

Chancroid

Chancroid is a rare sexually transmitted disease caused by the gram-negative bacillus *Hemophilus ducreyi*. The condition is more common in tropical and subtropical areas and in the poorer populations. The disease begins on the genitals as an inflammatory macule or pustule; the latter ruptures, forming a punched-out ulcer with irregular edges. Within a few days to 2 weeks, inguinal adenitis frequently develops, which may lead to perforation of the lymphatics. The inguinal node is called a *bubo*. The diagnosis is established by demonstrating the bacterium in smears from the ulcer. In addition to the involvement of the anal area, extragenital involvement may be noted in the hands, eyelids, and elsewhere.

Treatment is usually given with sulphonamides (sulfisoxazole) or tetracycline.

Granuloma Inguinale (Granuloma Venereum)

Granuloma inguinale is a chronic, granulomatous, ulcerative skin disease caused by *Calymmatobacterium granulomatis,* formerly known as *Donovania granulomatis.* There is some question whether it may be transmitted nonvenereally as well as venereally. The lesions appear as cauliflower-like proliferations from which develop pustules and papules (Fig. 8-32). Sinuses and scars are characteristic. The lesions are usually not painful, and adenopathy is not necessarily present. Squamous cell carcinoma may develop in the lesions.

The diagnosis is usually established by the appearance and the history, and the preparation by staining of a punch biopsy specimen. Donovan bodies appear as deeply staining, bipolar, safety-pin-shaped rods in the cytoplasm of macrophages (Fig. 8-33). Biopsy usually reveals a massive inflammatory reaction (predominantly polymorphonuclear), thickening of the epidermis at the periphery, and pale-staining macrophages usually in the upper parts of the granuloma (Fig. 8-34).

A host of antibiotics have been successful in the treatment, tetracycline being preferred. When irreversible tissue destruction has developed, resective surgery may be necessary.

Lymphogranuloma Venereum (Lymphogranuloma Inguinale, Lymphopathia Venereum)

Lymphogranuloma venereum (LGV) is a suppurative venereal disease caused by *Chlamydia trachomatis.* It is not a common condition, and it is most frequently seen

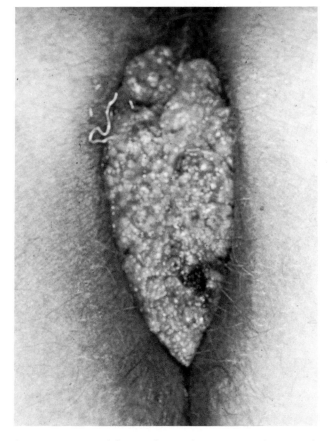

FIG. 8-29. Condylomata lata, a large, perianal, mucoid, warty mass composed of smooth-surfaced lobules. (Courtesy of Rudolf Garret, M.D.)

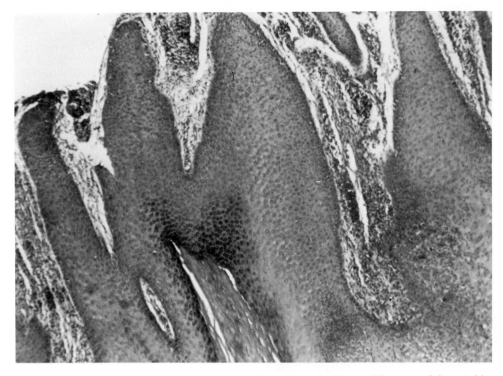

FIG. 8-30. Condylomata lata demonstrating dilated lymphatics, proliferation of the prickle-cell layer (acanthosis), and an inflammatory exudate. (Original magnification × 250. Courtesy of Rudolf Garret, M.D.)

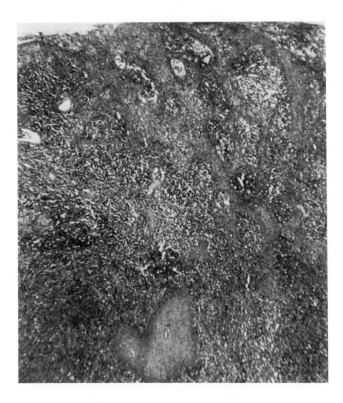

FIG. 8-31. Condylomata lata showing pseudoepitheliomatous hyperplasia of the squamous epithelium. A heavy plasma cell infiltrate is evident in the dermis, with dilated lymphatics. (Original magnification × 250. Courtesy of Rudolf Garret, M.D.)

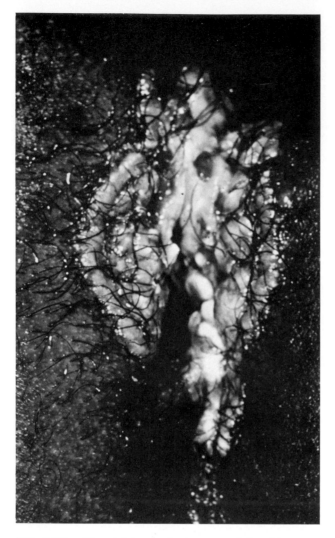

FIG. 8-32. Cicatricial granulomatous nodule with a surrounding erythematous border, characteristic of granuloma inguinale. (Courtesy of Rudolf Garret, M.D.)

in the homosexual population, with a particularly high incidence among blacks. The lesion initially appears as a herpetiform vesicle on the genitalia or anal area. LGV may start in the rectum as a proctitis, which may then progress to stricture formation. Clinical symptoms under these circumstances are rectal discharge, bleeding, and tenesmus. An associated anal fissure is not uncommon. Perianal fistulas may develop and in late cases severe rectal stricture. Approximately 2 weeks following the appearance of the primary lesion, regional lymphadenopathy occurs. Characteristically, in men,

the nodes fuse together in a large mass. Histologically, the changes consist of an infectious granuloma with the formation of stellate abscesses (Fig. 8-35).

Laboratory studies reveal characteristic abnormalities. There is often an inverted albumin–globulin ratio. The so-called Frei test has been classically employed to establish the diagnosis of LGV; this is an intradermal test similar to the tuberculin test. The procedure has fallen into disrepute and in many places is no longer available. The complement fixation test is now considered to be the most accurate for detecting antibodies and establishing the diagnosis. Elevated titers are noted approximately 1 month after the onset of the illness. Tetracycline is the recommended treatment,[28] although sulfonamides have been usefully employed in the early stage. Rectal stenosis may require a resective procedure (Fig. 8-36).

Molluscum Contagiosum

Molluscum contagiosum is a communicable skin disease caused by a poxvirus. It can involve the skin of the abdomen, thighs, groin, genitalia, buttocks, and, in homosexual men, the perianal area.[18] The lesions begin as papules, often develop central umbilication, and may be widely disseminated. They are often asymptomatic but may exhibit pruritic symptoms. Molluscum contagiosum has a characteristic histopathology. There is a downward proliferation of the rete ridges and envelopment by the connective tissue to form a deep crater. So-called molluscum bodies are found in the cytoplasm of the cells of the stratum malpighii (Fig. 8-37).

Treatment may not be required because the lesions usually heal without scarring unless secondarily infected. Curettage can be employed using ethyl chloride spray for freezing. Liquid nitrogen and electrocoagulation also have been effective.

Herpes Genitalis

Herpes simplex is a virus that has been associated with a number of acute, limited, vesicular eruptions near mucocutaneous junctions. Synonyms include fever blister, cold sore, herpes febrilis, herpes labialis, and genital herpes. In the genital area the lesions may appear on the prepuce, glans, shaft of the penis, labia, vulva, clitoris, and cervix. The anal area is also commonly involved.

Cutaneous lesions associated with herpes simplex infections are usually characteristic. A direct fluorescent antibody technique with the fluid from the vesicle is a rapid means for confirmation. The Tzanck preparation will reveal intranuclear inclusion bodies upon smearing. But basically the clinical picture of grouped vesicles

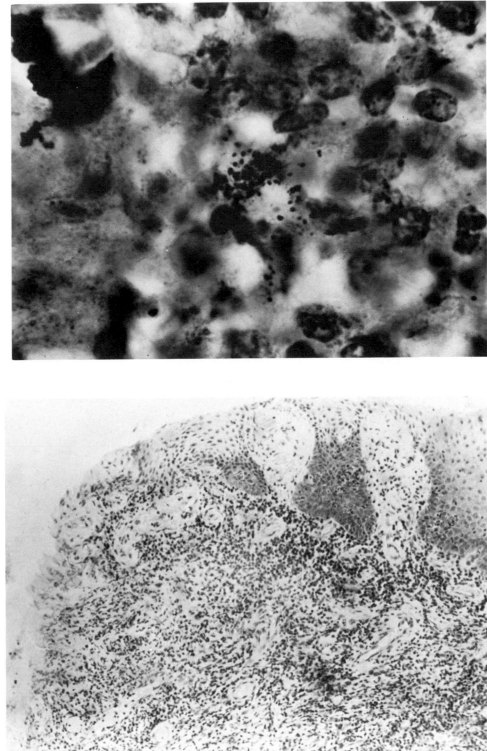

FIG. 8-33. Granuloma inguinale. Donovan bodies in macrophages, demonstrated by Leischman's stain. (Original magnification × 600. Courtesy of Rudolf Garret, M.D.)

FIG. 8-34. Granuloma inguinale. Mononuclear cell infiltrate in the dermis with ulcer on the left. (Original magnification × 120. Courtesy of Rudolf Garret, M.D.)

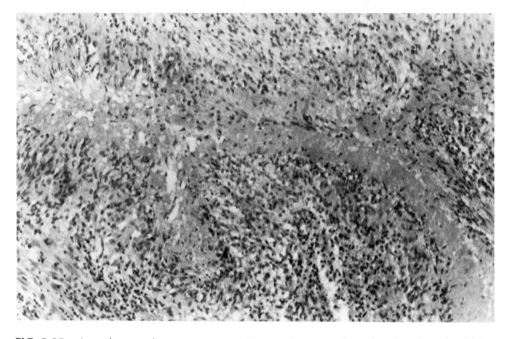

FIG. 8-35.   Lymphogranuloma venereum (LGV): Stellate granuloma in a lymph node. (Original magnification × 280. Courtesy of Rudolf Garret, M.D.)

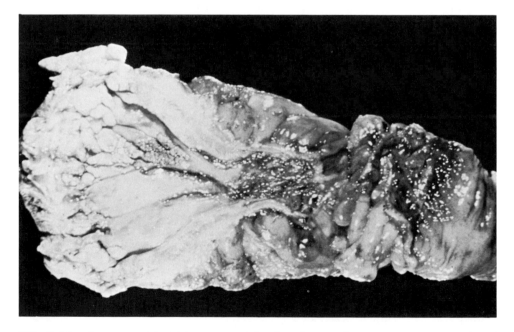

FIG. 8-36.   Severe rectal stricture caused by lymphogranuloma venereum necessitated proctectomy. If resection is necessary, reestablishment of intestinal continuity should be attempted if possible. (Corman ML, Veidenheimer MC, Swinton NW: Diseases of the Anus, Rectum, and Colon. Part I: Neoplasms. New York, Medcom, 1972)

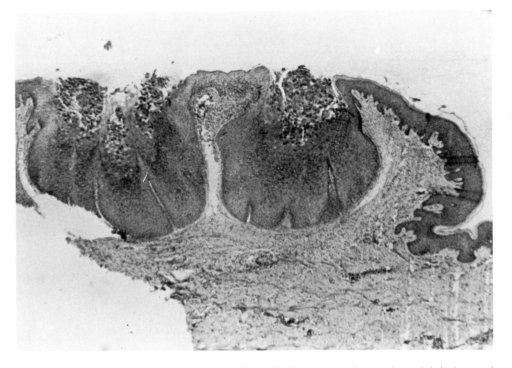

FIG. 8-37. Proliferation of squamous cells with formation of pear-shaped lobules and molluscum bodies in the central, crater-like area, characteristic of molluscum contagiosum. (Original magnification × 120. Courtesy of Rudolf Garret, M.D.)

on an erythematous base anywhere in the body suggests herpes infection.

Jacobs reported 16 patients with herpes simplex infection of the perianal skin and anal canal over a 2-year period.[62] There were 14 men and 2 women; all were either homosexual or bisexual.

Of great concern are the recent reports of the acquired immunodeficiency syndrome and its association with viral infections. Siegal and associates reported four homosexual men who presented with enlarging perianal ulcers from which herpes simplex virus was cultured.[88] Three patients died, and Kaposi's sarcoma developed in the fourth. The most prominent observation was the presence of a profound lymphopenia in all patients. The authors suggest that their findings were part of a national epidemic of immunodeficiency among male homosexuals.

Anal herpes infections usually are self-limiting, however. The application of soothing compresses and the use of mild analgesics are helpful; steroids should not be employed. The most recent therapy for the condition is the use of an antiviral ointment, acyclovir (Zovirax). This is a synthetic acyclic purine nucleoside analog that exhibits *in vitro* inhibitory activity against the virus. As of this writing the management of herpes genitalis and its disturbing associated conditions is rapidly changing.

Condylomata Acuminata (Venereal Warts)

Condylomata acuminata represents the commonest venereal disease in the practice of most surgeons. It is also one of the most troublesome conditions to eliminate. The disease is caused by a papilloma DNA virus, a member of the papovavirus group.[11] Recent evidence suggests that the virus is antigenically, biochemically, and immunologically distinct from the virus of the common wart, verruca vulgaris.[11] Although the condition may occur in heterosexual men and women, it is most commonly seen in homosexual males. It may be found in association with other conditions, such as gonorrhea, lymphogranuloma venereum, and syphilis, especially in patients who have had homosexual contact.[72]

The appearance of the wart usually makes the diagnosis quite obvious. These warts are usually small, discrete, elevated, pink vegetative excrescences in the anal canal, perianal skin, and urogenital region (Fig. 8-38). They may be single or multiple, or coalesce to

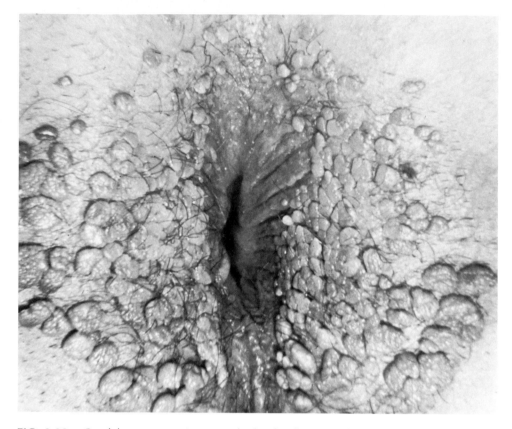

FIG. 8-38. Condylomata acuminata. Multiple closely grouped papillomas creating a cauliflower-like appearance. (Corman ML, Veidenheimer MC, Swinton NW: Diseases of the Anus, Rectum, and Colon. Part I: Neoplasms. New York, Medcom, 1972)

form polypoid masses. Lesions in the anal canal rarely extend into the rectum but are confined to the squamous epithelium and transitional zones. The wart itself is a hyperplastic epithelial lesion with irregular acanthosis and marked hyperkeratotis (Fig. 8-39).

Patients usually complain of the lump or lumps and often think that the problem is due to hemorrhoids. Other symptoms include discharge, pruritus, difficulty with defecation, anal pain, tenesmus, and rectal bleeding. A characteristic scenario is that the patient reports having received some form of topical external therapy over many weeks or months. The fact that the treatment has failed precipitates the second opinion or referral. Treatment of the external component should not be considered unless the patient has undergone a complete proctosigmoidoscopy. External application of various medicaments is doomed to failure if there is disease present in the anal canal.

Treatment and Results

Numerous methods of treating anal condylomata have been proposed: surgical excision, bichloracetic acid, podophyllin, cryotherapy, electrocoagulation, immunotherapy, antitumor therapy, laser beam, and many other caustic agents. Simmons performed a randomly allocated double-blind study of 10% and 25% podophyllin in 140 men with anogenital warts.[89] There was no significant difference in the effect of the two preparations; only 22% of the patients were free of warts following 3 months of therapy. Bichloracetic acid, an extremely powerful keratolytic and cauterant, has been employed. Swerdlow and Salvati treated 34 patients by bichloracetic acid only, in an uncontrolled study comparing a number of patients who had undergone other forms of therapy. [97] The authors concluded that the recurrence rate was lower and discomfort was less.

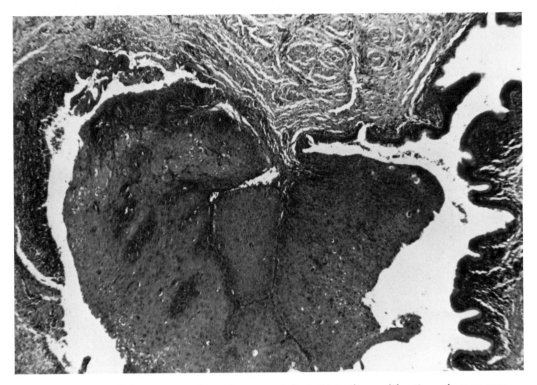

FIG. 8-39. Condylomata acuminata in an anal duct. Note the proliferation of squamous cells, vacuolated squamous cells, hyperchromatic nuclei, and and the absence of a cornified layer. Note also the columnar epithelium lining the anal duct. (Original magnification × 120. Courtesy of Rudolf Garret, M.D.)

Cryotherapy has been advocated in the treatment of this condition.[75, 85] Savin reported one failure in six patients so treated.[85]

Billingham and Lewis reported a controlled study on 38 patients.[11] Surgical therapy was performed on the left half of the anus (electrocoagulation), while the right half was treated with the carbon dioxide laser. The authors concluded that the laser was associated with at least as much pain as electrocoagulation. Furthermore, recurrences were seen more often on the laser side. These factors along with the high cost of the equipment implied no advantage to this new form of treatment.

Various chemotherapeutic agents have been advocated in the treatment of this condition, including 5-fluorouracil,[77] thiotepa,[19] and bleomycin.[45] This last drug was injected directly into the body of the wart in 10 patients at intervals of every 2 to 3 weeks. An overall success rate of 70% was achieved. Three patients experienced total resolution of the condylomata after the first treatment, but three patients failed to respond after

several sessions. With the exception of discomfort there were no systemic effects following the treatment.

Abcarian and Sharon evaluated the efficacy of immunotherapy in the treatment of anal condylomata acuminata.[2] Two hundred consecutive patients were studied over an 8-year period. A vaccine was prepared by excising and washing the condyloma tissue. A 10% suspension was prepared in Medium 199 supplemented with antibiotics. Following homogenization and freezing, it was then centrifuged, and the supernatant was heated. The inactivated material was then centrifuged again, and the supernatant was collected and tested for bacterial sterility. The patient was vaccinated with six consecutive weekly injections of 0.5 ml, subcutaneously administered in the deltoid area. The vaccine was frozen between injections.[1-3] Excellent results were seen in 84% of patients, and fair results in 11%; no improvement was noted in 5% of patients. There was no adverse reaction or complication. The authors concluded that immunotherapy was the recommended method of treatment for extensive, recurrent, or persistent anal condyloma acuminatum. Eftaiha and co-workers reported their experience with immunotherapy and compared it to other, more conventional forms of treatment.[42] Condylomata were successfully eradicated in approximately 94% of patients by this means. It was the authors' opinion that this modality of treatment should be reserved for recurrent and giant anal condylomata.

For those interested in employing the technique, there is a laboratory that will provide this service.*

Comment

External lesions in the absence of any internal warts can usually be effectively treated by chemical means (*e.g.*, podophyllin, bichloracetic acid). If the lesions do not respond to treatment, then physical destruction by electrocoagulation is the recommended approach. If there are only a few warts, the use of a local anesthetic in the office will permit adequate outpatient treatment. For more extensive lesions I prefer a general anesthetic, preferably administered on an outpatient basis.

Anal canal lesions do not respond to topical treatment. Here again, if there are few in number, a local anesthetic and electrocoagulation are appropriate. For more extensive lesions, a general anesthetic is preferred.

Close follow-up examination is required to treat recurrent lesions. Less than half of my patients have resolution of the process after only one treatment. It is important for the patient to understand, therefore, that the therapy may be rather prolonged. For some reason, once the warts have been removed and the wounds have healed, the condition does not usually recur.

At the time of electrocoagulation it is important for the surgeon to create a first- or second-degree burn, not a third-degree burn. The condylomata are literally exploded on the surface of the skin with the needle-tip electrocautery. Any residual tissue is wiped off with a dry sponge. This leaves an erythematous, smooth base. An antiseptic dressing is applied and the patient is discharged. If the "burn" is not undertaken too deeply, pain is not very severe; it can usually be controlled with a nonnarcotic prescription. The patient is advised to take sitz baths and is seen every 2 weeks for evaluation and possible office treatment. Occasionally there is profound recurrence of the warts on the first postoperative visit, and the patient must be returned to the operating room to undergo another surgical session.

---

* Madison Clinical Laboratory, Ltd., 330 N. Madison St., Suite 200, Joliet, Illinois 60435 (815-741-8100)

Giant Condyloma Acuminatum (Buschke-Löwenstein Tumor) and Malignant Degeneration

The Buschke-Löwenstein tumor, also known as giant condyloma acuminatum, is a variant of anal condylomata that tends to behave in a locally malignant fashion, burrowing deeply into adjacent structures (see Fig. 12-15).[5, 43] Wide local excision is the recommended treatment. Occasionally malignant transformation of anal condyloma can occur;[67, 80] squamous cell carcinoma has arisen in a number of these rare cases. Although abdominoperineal resection is probably the treatment of choice, some consideration should be given to multimodality therapy (see Chap. 12).

PREMALIGNANT AND MALIGNANT DERMATOSES

Malignant neoplasms of the anal margin and perianal skin include basal cell carcinoma, extramammary Paget's disease, Bowen's disease, malignant melanoma, and epidermoid carcinoma. The last two conditions are discussed in Chapter 12. Leukemia and lymphoma also commonly involve the anal area. In addition to the above, there are two cutaneous lesions that may be premalignant or associated with cancer elsewhere: acanthosis nigricans and leukoplakia.

Acanthosis Nigricans

Acanthosis nigricans is known chiefly for its ominous association with abdominal cancer in adults.[15] Regions affected include the face, neck, axillae, external genitalia, groin, inner thighs, umbilicus, and anus. The condition may present as a grayish, velvety thickening or roughening of the skin. The pathologic changes are epidermal, with papillomatosis, hyperkeratosis, and hyperpigmentation (Fig. 8-40). Pruritus is the most frequent symptom.

The malignant form of acanthosis nigricans may antedate, accompany, or follow the onset of the internal cancer. Most abdominal malignancies are adenocarcinomas, usually of gastric origin (60%). The tumor itself usually is advanced at the time of discovery and has a rapid progression. Treatment is directed to the malignant condition.

Leukoplakia

Leukoplakia is a whitish thickening of the mucous membrane epithelium occurring in patches of diverse size and shape. In the anal canal it is seen mostly in

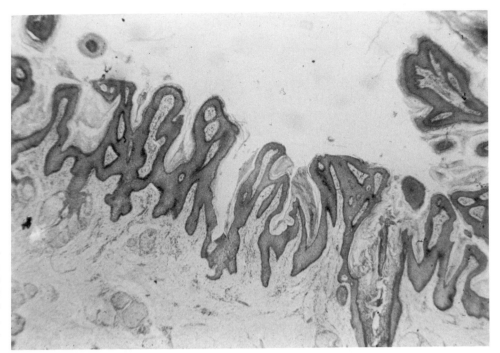

FIG. 8-40. Acanthosis nigricans. Epithelium in a papillary configuration with pigmented cells in the basal cell layer. (Original magnification × 260. Courtesy of Rudolf Garret, M.D.)

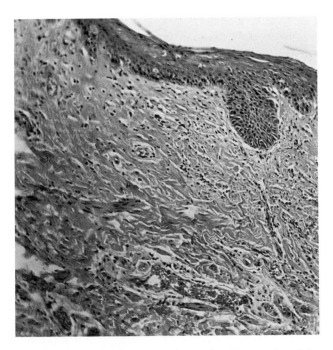

FIG. 8-41. Leukoplakia. Parakeratosis with atrophy of the epidermis and fibrosis of the dermis. Note the few cells with hyperchromatic nuclei close to the basal cell layer. (Original magnification × 240. Courtesy of Rudolf Garret, M.D.)

men and is occasionally associated with delayed wound healing (*e.g.,* following excision of fissure, hemorrhoids, and condylomata). Bleeding, discharge, and pruritic symptoms are the commonest complaints. Microscopically, hyperkeratosis and squamous metaplasia are seen (Fig. 8-41). Although the anal condition itself does not represent a malignancy, when it occurs in the gingival and buccal mucosa there is a high risk of the development of epidermoid carcinoma.

Excision of the lesion has been unsuccessful in my experience; the condition simply recurs. Because of the questionable malignant potential, annual proctosigmoidoscopy (anoscopy) with biopsy of any suspicious area is advised.

Mycosis Fungoides

Mycosis fungoides is an uncommon, pruritic, usually fatal cutaneous malignant neoplasm of the lymphoreticular system, specifically the thymus-derived (T-) lymphocytes. Subsequent involvement of lymph nodes and internal organs develops as the disease progresses.

The cutaneous lesion can occur anywhere; the overlying skin may have only telangiectasia or be violaceous (Color Fig. 8-5). The lesions are often of varied vivid color. As the lesions advance ulcerations occur (Fig. 8-42), and pain is a predominant symptom. Microscopic changes include perivascular accumulation

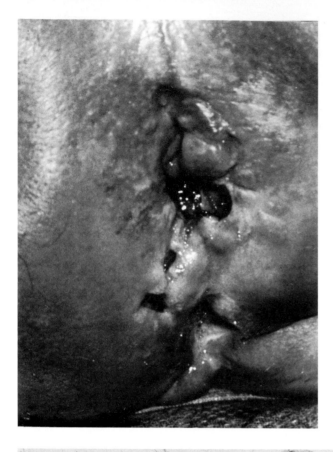

of lymphocytic cells; as the disease progresses increased numbers of abnormal, malignant cells are demonstrated (Fig. 8-43). Treatment is directed toward management of the systemic disease.

Leukemia Cutis

Perianal complications of the leukemias are not commonly seen, but they are a well-recognized clinical entity.[13, 87, 100] Occasionally they may be the first manifestation of the malignancy. Leukemic infiltrations may consist of diffuse infiltrations, erythema, and ulceration (Color Fig. 8-6). Lymphocytic leukemia characteristically may have a discrete nodular appearance (Fig. 8-44). It may present as a fistula, an abscess, or a tender, erythematous area. Cellulitis may be quite marked.

Histologically, masses of cells may be seen in the upper dermis or as nodules in the dermis (Fig. 8-45). The type of cells and immature forms are those of the systemic process; mitoses are infrequently seen in the skin lesions.

Sehdev and co-workers reported 22 cases of perianal complications in leukemic patients.[87] Conservative,

FIG. 8-42. Lymphoma. Perianal ulceration, nodules, and skin infiltration by biopsy-proved lymphomatous infiltrate. (Courtesy of Daniel Rosenthal, M.D.)

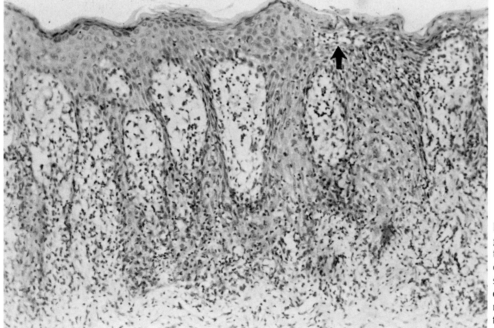

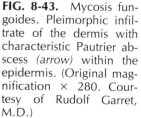

FIG. 8-43. Mycosis fungoides. Pleimorphic infiltrate of the dermis with characteristic Pautrier abscess *(arrow)* within the epidermis. (Original magnification × 280. Courtesy of Rudolf Garret, M.D.)

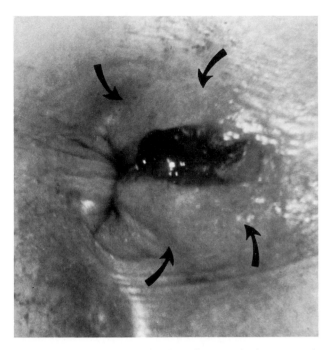

FIG. 8-44. Leukemia cutis (lymphocytic leukemia). Diffuse swelling and infiltration (outlined by arrows) with ulceration. (Courtesy of Daniel Rosenthal, M.D.)

symptomatic treatment with the addition of radiotherapy is advised in patients with leukopenia who are moribund, or in whom the lesions have spontaneously drained.

Any leukemic patient who complains of pain in the perianal area is presumed to have this serious complication and is started on precautionary measures; this includes interdiction of rectal examinations, instrumentation, or enemas.[87] Antibiotics are advised. Surgical treatment should be withheld if the leukemia is not under control or in remission. Operative intervention under these circumstances may result in rapid progression of the septic process, necrosis of the perineum, and death. Radiation therapy to the anal area is preferred. If surgical drainage or excision is performed (in patients with remission), bleeding may be a difficult management problem.

Basal Cell Carcinoma

Basal cell carcinoma of the anus is an extremely rare tumor. Only one case was reported in Gabriel's experience of 1700 malignant tumors of the anus and rectum.[49] Most published reports involve one or two patients.[9, 17, 65, 84] Nielsen and Jensen reported the largest single series of basal cell carcinoma of the anus.[76]

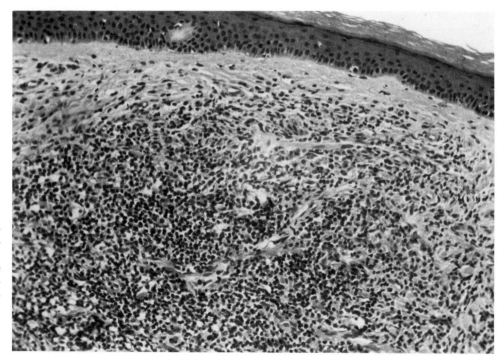

FIG. 8-45. Leukemia cutis. Infiltration of the dermis by leukemic cells. Note the collagen bundle separating the mass of tumor cells from the underlying epidermis. (Original magnification × 240. Courtesy of Rudolf Garret, M.D.)

Thirty-four patients were treated over a 30-year period. There was no sex predominance. Tumors were usually between 1 and 2 cm and localized to the anal margin. Symptoms included the sensation of a lump or of an ulcer in two thirds of patients. Bleeding, pain, pruritus, and discharge were other noted complaints.

The characteristic appearance of the lesion is that of a chronic indurated growth with rolled edges (pearly border) and a central depression or ulceration (Fig. 8-46). Histologically, the tumor arises from the basal cells of the malpighian layer of the skin (Fig. 8-47). Sheets of basophilic-staining cells are seen to contain large blue-staining nuclei with minimal cytoplasm.

Local excision with adequate margins is the treatment of choice. Radical (abdominoperineal) resection is performed for neglected, extensive, infiltrating tumors. There were no deaths due to the basal cell carcinoma in the series of Nielsen and Jensen.[76] Those

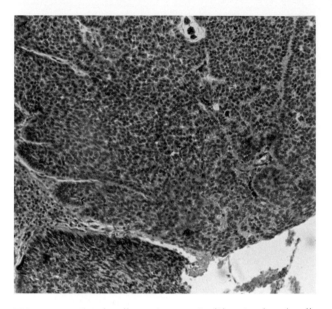

FIG. 8-47. Basal cell carcinoma. Proliferating basal cells infiltrate the dermis. Note the peripheral palisading. (Original magnification × 240. Courtesy of Rudolf Garret, M.D.)

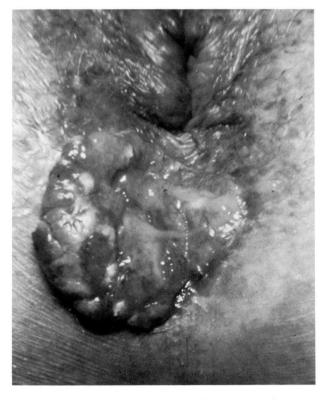

FIG. 8-46. Basal cell carcinoma (rodent ulcer). Ulcerating tumor with a pearly border. (Rosenthal D: Basal cell carcinoma of the anus: Report of two cases. Dis Colon Rectum 1967; 10:397–400)

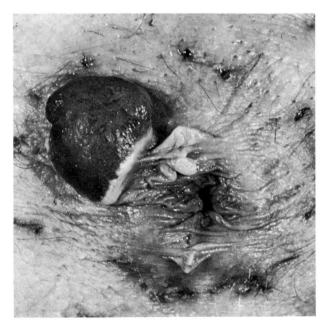

FIG. 8-48. Squamous cell carcinoma. Ulcerating, friable tumor. (Courtesy of Rudolf Garret, M.D.)

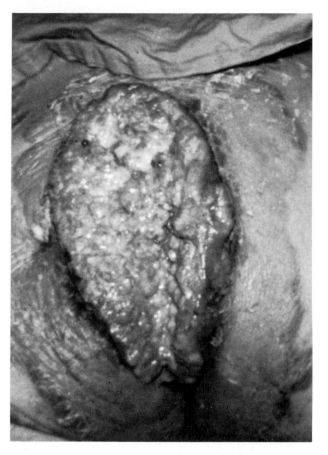

FIG. 8-49. Squamous cell carcinoma. Fungating, cauliflower-like mass. (Courtesy of Daniel Rosenthal, M.D.)

tumors in other series that were reported to have metastasized were probably basaloid (cloacogenic) carcinomas with both squamous and basal cell histologic features.

Squamous Cell (Epidermoid) Carcinoma

Squamous cell carcinoma of the perianal skin is manifested and treated in a similar manner to the lesion elsewhere on the body. The tumor may appear superficial, discrete, and hard. With progression it may ulcerate (Fig. 8-48) or become papillomatous or cauliflower-like (Fig. 8-49). Although this tumor is relatively slow growing, metastases to regional lymph nodes occur. Wide local excision is the treatment of choice for most lesions.[30, 81] If there is question about

the site of origin (anal versus perianal), treatment in accordance with the protocol described in Chapter 12 is suggested.

Malignant Melanoma

Malignant melanoma is described in Chapter 12.

Bowen's Disease

Bowen's disease is an intraepidermal squamous cell carcinoma that tends to spread intraepidermally, but it may invade. The condition is eponymously associated with the author of the paper of 1912.[14] Approximately 100 cases involving the anus have been reported. The condition is more commonly seen on the face, hands,

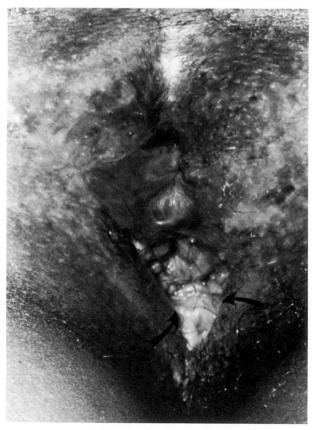

FIG. 8-50. Bowen's disease. Indurated erythematosquamous patch involving the perianal area. (Courtesy of Daniel Rosenthal, M.D.)

and trunk.[81] Graham and Helwig reported a relationship of this condition to malignant tumors elsewhere (thymoma, bronchogenic carcinoma, hypernephroma, gastrointestinal cancer, *etc.*).[52, 53] One third of their patients developed neoplasms within 10 years of the original diagnosis. They suggested that Bowen's disease may represent a cutaneous manifestation of a predisposition to the development of cancer.

The disease usually presents with itching and burning, although pain and bleeding may be noted.[86] Strauss and Fazio, in their report from the Cleveland Clinic of 12 patients, noted that the diagnosis was usually made as an incidental finding after anorectal surgery.[94]

The lesion appears as an erythematous, slightly crusted, placque-like area with well-defined margins (Fig. 8-50). The condition may be confused with psoriasis and with Paget's disease. Microscopically the epidermis is thickened by hyperkeratosis; there may be parakeratosis and acanthosis (Fig. 8-51). In contrast to Paget's disease, a Bowenoid cell does not pick up aldehyde–fuchsin stain (Fig. 8-52).[81]

Treatment requires wide local excision with frozen section examination to ensure adequate margins, although radical surgical extirpation has been used when this procedure fails.[40] The condition has been also reported to respond to topical dinitrochlorobenzene and 5-fluorouracil.[82]

In the 12 patients reviewed by the Cleveland Clinic group, there was no recurrence or metastasis when adequate excision with or without grafting was employed.[94] Seven of the patients previously had or subsequently developed a systemic or cutaneous cancer. Of the 11 patients treated at the Memorial Sloan Kettering Cancer Center, 5 were free of disease after 5 years and 1 died of colon cancer; the remainder had a limited follow-up.[81]

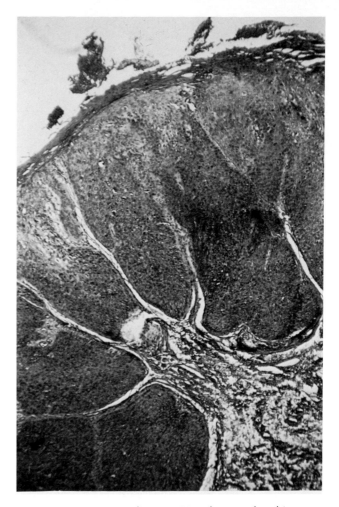

FIG. 8-51. Bowen's disease. Disturbance of architecture of the squamous epithelium. (Original magnification × 250. Courtesy of Rudolf Garret, M.D.)

Extramammary Paget's Disease

In 1874 Sir James Paget described a cutaneous lesion of the breast that histologically demonstrated the presence of large, round, clear-staining cells with large nuclei.[79] Darier and Couillaud subsequently described the condition in the perineal area.[29] The lesions of extramammary Paget's disease are not unlike those seen in the breast.

Helwig and Graham reviewed material from the Armed Forces Institute of Pathology; a total of 40 patients were identified with lesions in this area.[57] They found that the lesion usually appeared erythematous to whitish gray, elevated, crusty, scaly, eczematoid, and occasionally papillary (Color Fig. 8-7). Microscopically, hyperkeratosis, parakeratosis, acanthosis, and pale,

vacuolated cells are seen within the epidermis (Fig. 8-53). Sialomucin may be identified by periodic acid–Schiff (PAS) stain; Bowen's disease does not show this positive staining (Fig. 8-54).

Most patients complain of ulceration, discharge, pruritus, and occasionally bleeding and pain. The mean age of onset has been reported to be 59 years.[57]

Carcinoma is found in a high percentage of patients in adjacent areas. Thirteen of the 40 patients in Helwig and Graham's series had an immediate underlying cutaneous carcinoma.[57] Another seven had primary internal or extracutaneous cancer. Lock and associates reported four patients, three of whom developed car-

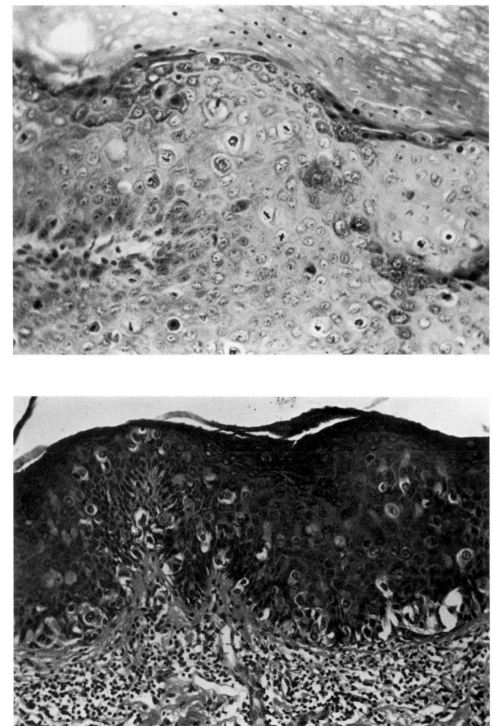

FIG. 8-52. Bowen's disease. Note cells with hyperchromatic nuclei (Bowenoid cells) scattered throughout the epithelium. Many mitotic figures are seen. (Original magnification × 600. Corman ML, Veidenheimer MC, Swinton NW: Diseases of the Anus, Rectum, and Colon. Part I: Neoplasms. New York, Medcom, 1972)

FIG. 8-53 Extramammary Paget's disease. Note the large, pagetoid cells within the epithelium. These were mucicarmine positive, thus ruling out Bowen's disease. (Original magnification × 240. Courtesy of Rudolf Garret, M.D.)

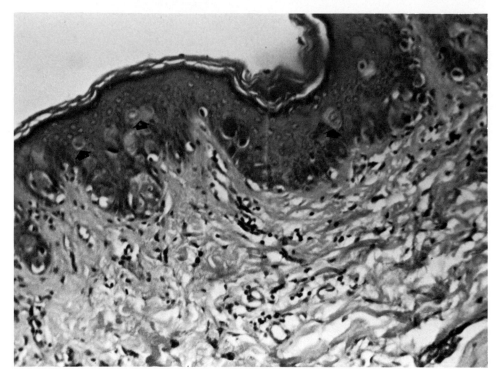

FIG. 8-54 Extramammary Paget's disease. Mucicarmine positive cells *(arrows)* within the epithelium. (Original magnification × 240. Courtesy of Rudolf Garret, M.D.)

cinoma.[69] Others report a similar association: for example, with cloacogenic carcinoma, and with villous adenoma of the rectum.[8, 61, 81, 95, 104] In addition, a familial occurrence has been reported.[66]

Treatment depends on the presence or absence of an underlying invasive carcinoma. Linder and Myers suggest that a distinction be made between an *in situ* carcinoma and that of an infiltrating growth.[68] In the latter situation abdominoperineal resection may be required or consideration may be given to multimodality therapy (see Chap. 12). Wide local excision with or without grafting should be adequate for noninvasive disease. Careful follow-up is essential, with recurrence probably dictating a more radical approach (Color Fig. 8-8).

REFERENCES

1. Abcarian H, Sharon N: The effectiveness of immunotherapy in the treatment of anal condylomata acuminata. J Surg Res 1977; 22:231–236
2. Abcarian H, Sharon N: Long-term effectiveness of immunotherapy of anal condyloma acuminatum. Dis Colon Rectum 1982; 25:648–651
3. Abcarian H, Smith D, Sharon N: The immunotherapy of anal condyloma acuminatum. Dis Colon Rectum 1976; 19:237–244
4. Ahlberg J, Bergstrand O, Holmström B et al: Anal tuberculosis: A report of two cases. Acta Chir Scand 1980; (suppl) 500:45–47
5. Alexander RM, Kaminsky DB: Giant condyloma acuminatum (Buschke-Lowenstein tumor) of the anus: Case report and review of the literature. Dis Colon Rectum 1979; 21:561–565
6. Alexander S: Dermatological aspects of anorectal disease. Clin Gastroenterol 1975; 4:651–657
7. Anderson AW: Hair extracted from ulcer. Boston Med Surg J 1847; 36:74
8. Arminski TC, Pollard RJ: Paget's disease of the anus secondary to a malignant papillary adenoma of the rectum. Dis Colon Rectum 1973; 16:46–55
9. Armitage G, Smith I: Rodent ulcer of the anus. Br J Surg 1955; 42:395–398
10. Bascom J: Pilonidal disease: origin from follicles of hairs and results of follicle removal as treatment. Surgery 1980; 87:257–272
11. Billingham RP, Lewis FG: Laser versus electrical cautery in the treatment of condylomata acuminata of the anus. Surg Gynecol Obstet 1982; 155:865–867
12. Blanchard RJ: Fulminating nonclostridial gas-

forming infection: A case of necrotizing fasciitis. Can J Surg 1975; 18:339–344

13. Blank WA: Anorectal complications in leukemia. Am J Surg 1955; 90:738–744

14. Bowen JT: Precancerous dermatoses: A study of two cases of chronic atypical epithelial proliferation. J Cutan Dis 1912; 30:241–255

15. Braverman IM: Skin Signs of Systemic Disease, pp 669-671. Philadelphia, WB Saunders, 1981

16. Broadwater JR, Bryant RL, Petrino RA et al: Advanced hidradenitis suppurativa: Review of surgical treatment in 23 patients. Am J Surg 1982; 144:668–670

17. Bunstock WH: Basal cell carcinoma of the anus. Am J Surg 1958; 95:822–825

18. Catterall RD: Sexually transmitted diseases of the anus and rectum. Clin Gastroenterol 1975; 4:659–669

19. Cheng SF, Veenema RJ: Topical application of thio-tepa to penile and urethral tumors. J Urol 1965; 94:259–262

20. Ching CC, Stahlgren LH: Clinical review of hidradenitis suppurativa: Management of cases with severe perianal involvement. Dis Colon Rectum 1965; 8:349–352

21. Cole GW, Amon RB, Russell PS: Secondary syphilis presenting as a pruritic dermatosis. Arch Dermatol 1977; 113:489–490

22. Conway H, Stark RB, Climo S et al: The surgical treatment of chronic hidradenitis suppurativa. Surg Gynecol Obstet 1952; 95:455–464

23. Corman ML, Veidenheimer MC, Swinton NW: Diseases of the Anus, Rectum, and Colon. Part I: Neoplasms. New York, Medcom, 1972

24. Crapp AR, Macbeth WAAG: Perianal vaccinia: A case report. Aust NZ J Surg 1976; 46:83–85

25. Crighton JL: Diarrhoea and perianal vaccinia. Br Med J 1976; 2:732–733

26. Culp CE: Chronic hidradenitis suppurative of the anal canal—a surgical skin disease. Dis Colon Rectum 1983; 26:669–676

27. Dailey TH: Pruritus ani. Practical Gastroenterol 1980; 4(7)

28. Dan M, Rotmensch HH, Eylan E et al: A case of lymphogranuloma venereum of 20 years' duration: Isolation of Chlamydia trachomatis from perianal lesions. Br J Vener Dis 1980; 56:344–346

29. Darier J, Couillaud P: Sur un cas de maladie de Paget de la région périnéo-anale et scrotale. Société Française de Dermatologie et de Syphiligraphie 1983; 4:25–31

30. Dillard BM, Spratt JS Jr, Ackerman LV, Butcher HR Jr: Epidermoid cancer of anal margin and canal. Arch Surg 1963; 86: 772–777

31. Domonkos AN, Arnold HL Jr, Odom RB: Cutaneous symptoms, signs and diagnosis. In Andrew's Diseases of the Skin, 7th ed, pp 15–19. Philadelphia, WB Saunders, 1982

32. Domonkos AN, Arnold HL Jr, Odom RB: Cutaneous symptoms, signs, and diagnosis. In Andrew's Diseases of the Skin, 7th ed, pp 75–96. Philadelphia, WB Saunders, 1982

33. Domonkos AN, Arnold HL Jr, Odom RB: Cutaneous symptoms, signs, and diagnosis. In Andrew's Diseases of the Skin, 7th ed, pp 97–143. Philadelphia, WB Saunders, 1982

34. Domonkos AN, Arnold HL Jr, Odom RB: Cutaneous symptoms, signs, and diagnosis. In Andrew's Diseases of the Skin, 7th ed, pp 175–205. Philadelphia, WB Saunders, 1982

35. Domonkos AN, Arnold HL Jr, Odom RB: Cutaneous symptoms, signs, and diagnosis. In Andrew's Diseases of the Skin, 7th ed, pp 218–247. Philadelphia, WB Saunders, 1982

36. Domonkos AN, Arnold HL Jr, Odom RB: Cutaneous symptoms, signs, and diagnosis. In Andrew's Diseases of the Skin, 7th ed, pp 341–403. Philadelphia, WB Saunders, 1982

37. Domonkos AN, Arnold HL Jr, Odom RB: Cutaneous symptoms, signs, and diagnosis. In Andrew's Diseases of the Skin, 7th ed, pp 526–580. Philadelphia, WB Saunders, 1982

38. Domonkos AN, Arnold HL Jr, Odom RB: Cutaneous symptoms, signs, and diagnosis. In Andrew's Diseases of the Skin, 7th ed, pp 581–606. Philadelphia, WB Saunders, 1982

39. Drusin LM, Homan WP, Dineen P: The role of surgery in primary syphilis of the anus. Ann Surg 1976; 184:65–67

40. Edwards M: Bowen's disease: A case report. Dis Colon Rectum 1965; 8:297–299

41. Edwards MH: Pilonidal sinus: a 5-year appraisal of the Millar-Lord treatment. Br J Surg 1977; 64:867–868

42. Eftaiha MS, Amshel AL, Shonberg IL, Batshon B: Giant and recurrent condyloma acuminatum: Appraisal of immunotherapy. Dis Colon Rectum 1982; 25:136–138

43. Elliot MS, Werner ID, Immelman EJ, Harrison AC: Giant condyloma (Buschke-Loewenstein tumor) of the anorectum. Dis Colon Rectum 1979; 22:497–500

44. Eyers AA, Thomson JPS: Pruritus ani: Is anal sphincter dysfunction important in aetiology? Br Med J 1979; 2:1549–1551

45. Figueroa S, Gennaro AR: Intralesional bleomycin injection in treatment of condyloma acuminatum. Dis Colon Rectum 1980; 23:550–551

46. Fisher AA: New advances in contact dermatitis. Int J Dermatol 1977; 16:552–568

47. Fitzpatrick TB: Fundamentals of dermatologic diagnosis. In Fitzpatrick TB, Eisen AZ, Wolff K et al (eds): Dermatology in General Medicine, 2nd ed, pp 10-37. St. Louis, McGraw-Hill, 1979

48. Friend WG: The cause and treatment of idiopathic pruritus ani. Dis Colon Rectum 1977; 20:40–42

49. Gabriel WB: Principles and Practice of Rectal Surgery, 4th ed, p 469. London, HK Lewis & Co, 1948

50. Gage AA, Dutta P: Cryosurgery for pilonidal disease. Am J Surg 1977; 133:249–254

51. Goldman L, Kitzmiller KW: Perianal atrophoderma from topical corticosteroids. Arch Dermatol 1973; 107:611–612

52. Graham JH, Helwig EB: Bowen's disease and its relationship to systemic cancer. Arch Dermatol 1959; 80:133–159

53. Graham JH, Helwig EB: Bowen's disease and its relationship to systemic cancer. Arch Dermatol 1961; 83:738–758

54. Gupta AS, Sharma VP, Rathi GL: Ano-rectal tuberculosis simulating carcinoma. Am J Proctol 1976; 27:33–38

55. Guyuron B, Dinner MI, Dowden RV: Excision and grafting in treatment of recurrent pilonidal sinus disease. Surg Gynecol Obstet 1983; 156:201–204

56. Hanley PH: Acute pilonidal abscess. Surg Gynecol Obstet 1980; 150:9–11

57. Helwig EB, Graham JH: Anogenital (extramammary) Paget's disease. Cancer 1963; 16:387–403

58. Himal H, McLean AP, Duff JH: Gas gangrene of scrotum and perineum. Surg Gynecol Obstet 1974; 139:176–178

59. Hodges RM: Pilo-nidal sinus. Boston Med Surg J 1880; 103:485–486

60. Iwama T, Utzunomiya J: Anal complication in Behçet's syndrome. Jpn J Surg 1977; 7:114–117

61. Jackson BR: Extramammary Paget's disease and anaplastic basaloid small-cell carcinoma of the anus: Report of a case. Dis Colon Rectum 1975; 18:339–345

62. Jacobs E: Anal infections caused by Herpes Simplex virus. Dis Colon Rectum 1976; 19:151–157

63. Jellinek EH, Tulloch WS: Herpes zoster with dysfunction of bladder and anus. Lancet 1976; 2:1219–1222

64. Joost Th v, Faber WR, Manuel HR: Drug-induced anogenital cicatricial pemphigoid. Br J Dermatol 1980; 102:715–718

65. Krause EW: Perianal basal cell carcinoma. Arch Dermatol 1978; 114:460–461

66. Kuehn PG, Tennant R, Brenneman AR: Familial occurrence of extramammary Paget's disease. Cancer 1973; 32:145–148

67. Lee SH, McGregor DH, Kuziez MN: Malignant transformation of perianal condyloma acuminatum: A case report with review of the literature. Dis Colon Rectum 1981; 24:462–467

68. Linder JH, Myers RT: Perianal Paget's disease. Am Surg 1970; 36:342–345

69. Lock MR, Katz DR, Parks A, Thomson JPS: Perianal Paget's disease. Postgrad Med J 1977; 53:768–772

70. Lord PH: Etiology of pilonidal sinus. Dis Colon Rectum 1975; 18:661–664

71. Mansoory A, Dickson D: Z-plasty for treatment of disease of the pilonidal sinus. Surg Gynecol Obstet 1982; 155:409–411

72. Marino AW Jr: Proctologic lesions observed in male homosexuals. Dis Colon Rectum 1964; 7:121–128

73. Marks MM: The influence of the intestinal pH on pruritus ani. South Med J 1968; 61:1005–1006

74. Murie JA, Sim AJW, Mackenzie I: The importance of pain, pruritus and soiling as symptoms of haemorrhoids and their response to haemorrhoidectomy or rubber band ligation. Br J Surg 1981; 68:247–249

75. Nahra KS, Moschella SL, Swinton NW Sr: Condyloma acuminatum treated with liquid nitrogen: Report of five cases. Dis Colon Rectum 1969; 12:125–128

76. Nielsen OV, Jensen SL: Basal cell carcinoma of the anus—a clinical study of 34 cases. Br J Surg 1981; 68:856–857

77. Nel WS, Fourie ED: Immunotherapy and 5% topical 5-fluorouracil ointment in the treatment of condylomata acuminata. S Afr Med J 1973; 47:45–49

78. O'Connor JJ: Surgery plus freezing as a technique for treating pilonidal disease. Dis Colon Rectum 1979; 22:306–307

79. Paget J: On disease of the mammary areola preceding cancer of the mammary gland. St Bartholomew's Hosp Rep 1874; 10:87–89

80. Prasad ML, Abcarian H: Malignant potential of perianal condyloma acuminatum. Dis Colon Rectum 1980; 23:191–197

81. Quan SHQ: Anal and para-anal tumors. Surg Clin North Am 1978; 58:591–603

82. Raaf JH, Krown SE, Pinsky CM et al: Treatment of Bowen's disease with topical dinitrochlorobenzene and 5-fluorouracil. Cancer 1976; 37:1633–1642

83. Rook A, Wilkinson DS: The principles of diagnosis. In Rook A, Wilkinson DS, Ebling FJG (eds): Textbook of Dermatology, 3rd ed, pp 57–67. Oxford, Blackwell Scientific Publications, 1979

84. Rosenthal D: Basal cell carcinoma of the anus:

Report of two cases. Dis Colon Rectum 1967; 10:397–400

85. Savin S: The role of cryosurgery in management of anorectal disease: Preliminary report on results. Dis Colon Rectum 1975; 18:292–297

86. Scoma JA, Levy EI: Bowen's disease of the anus. Dis Colon Rectum 1975; 18:137–140

87. Sehdev MK, Dowling MD Jr, Seal SH, Stearns MW Jr: Perianal and anorectal complications in leukemia. Cancer 1973; 31:149–152

88. Siegal FP, Lopez C, Hammer GS et al: Severe acquired immunodeficiency in male homosexuals, manifested by chronic perianal ulcerative herpes simplex lesions. N Engl J Med 1981; 305:1439–1444

89. Simmons PD: Podophyllin 10% and 25% in the treatment of ano-genital warts. Br J Vener Dis 1981; 57:208–209

90. Sloan PJM, Goepel J: Lichen sclerosus et atrophicus and perianal carcinoma: A case report. Clin Exp Derm 1981; 6:399–402

91. Smith LE, Henrichs D, McCullah RD: Prospective studies on the etiology and treatment of pruritis ani. Dis Colon Rectum 1982; 25:358–363

92. Sneddon IB: Atrophy of the skin: The clinical problems. Br J Dermatol, 1976; 94:121–122

93. Sohn N, Robilotti JG Jr: The gay bowel syndrome: A review of colonic and rectal conditions in 200 male homosexuals. Am J Gastroenterology 1977; 67:478–484

94. Strauss RJ, Fazio VW: Bowen's disease of the anal and perianal area: A report and analysis of twelve cases. Am J Surg 1979; 137:231–234

95. Subbuswamy SG, Ribeiro BF: Perianal Paget's disease associated with cloacogenic carcinoma: Report of a case. Dis Colon Rectum 1981; 24:535–538

96. Sullivan ES, Garnjobst WM: Pruritus ani: A practical approach. Surg Clin North Am 1978; 58:505–512

97. Swerdlow DB, Salvati EP: Condyloma acuminatum. Dis Colon Rectum 1971; 14:226–231

98. Thornton JP, Abcarian H: Surgical treatment of perianal and perineal hidradenitis suppurativa. Dis Colon Rectum 1978; 21:573–577

99. Velpeau A: Dictionnaire en 30 volumes. Articles: Aiselle, II, p 91; Anus, III, p 304; Mamelles, XIX, 1939; Clinique cirug, II, p 133. Quoted by Conway H, Stark RB, Climo S et al: The surgical treatment of chronic hidradenitis suppurativa. Surg Gynecol Obstet 1952; 95:455–464

100. Walsh G, Stickley CS: Acute leukemia with primary symptoms in the rectum: A rapid increase in the white cells and fatal outcome. South Med J 1934; 96:684–689

101. Warin RP: Antifungal agents. Practitioner 1974; 213:494–507

102. Whalen TV Jr, Kovalcik PJ, Old WL Jr: Tuberculous anal ulcer. Dis Colon Rectum 1980; 23:54–55

103. Wilkin JK: Chronic benign familial pemphigus: Minimal involvement mimicking chronic perianal candidiasis. Arch Dermatol 1978; 114–136

104. Williams SL, Rogers LW, Quan SHQ: Perianal Paget's disease: report of seven cases. Dis Colon Rectum 1976; 19:30–40

105. Zimmerman CE: Outpatient excision and primary closure of pilonidal cysts and sinuses. Am J Surg 1978; 136:640–642

CHAPTER 9

Polypoid Diseases

A polyp is a well-circumscribed projection above the surface epithelium. It may be pedunculated or sessile. It can vary in size from 1 or 2 mm to more than 10 cm. It is not a histologic diagnosis; *polyp* is merely a descriptive term. Three types of polyps are discussed in this chapter: hyperplastic (metaplastic) polyps, hamartomas, and adenomas.

HYPERPLASTIC (METAPLASTIC) POLYP

In 1934 Westhues described a nonneoplastic mucosal lesion that has come to be known in the United States as a hyperplastic polyp; in England the tumor is called *metaplastic*, the term having been introduced by Morson.[107, 155] He prefers the latter terminology because the former has a connotation suggestive of neoplasm. In truth, the lesion is often associated with a cancer in the resected specimen, as frequently as 50% of the time (see Fig. 10-18). It is, however, generally felt that the tumor bears no relationship to benign or malignant neoplastic lesions of the colon and rectum. Hayashi and co-workers suggested that the cells forming the hyperplastic polyp grow more slowly and have a longer life span than adjacent normal mucosal cells.[72] The retained epithelium fails to detach, becoming "hypermature."[72]

Hyperplastic polyps are usually found in the rectum and sigmoid, often at the summit of mucosal folds and on the apex of the valves of Houston. They are nearly always multiple and can present in such large numbers that on both endoscopic examination and barium enema they may simulate familial (multiple) polyposis.[57] Their usual size is from 2 to 5 mm. They appear approximately the same color as the rectal mucosa, or slightly paler; often they are overlooked. Microscopically, crypts are seen to be lined by a hyperplastic epithelium that gives the crypt lumen a scalloped appearance (Fig. 9-1). The structure is quite different from that of an adenomatous polyp. The lining epithelium loses its regular columnar and goblet cell pattern and appears serrated because of flattening of the cells (Fig. 9-2).[107] Goblet cells are diminished and the lamina propria may demonstrate increased inflammatory reaction: plasma cells and lymphocytes (Fig. 9-3).

Since it is accepted that hyperplastic polyps are not neoplasms and do not connote increased risk for the development of tumors, either benign or malignant, the question of how to treat them must be addressed. The fact that a patient harbors hyperplastic polyps is of no clinical significance; hence, therapy is unnecessary. The problem arises, however, in establishing with certainty the nature of the lesion. This can be accomplished only by submitting the lesion for pathologic confirmation. This is an important step, because if it is discovered that the tumor is a neoplasm (*e.g.*, polypoid adenoma), the procedure for total colonic evaluation and follow-up is quite different. My own philosophy is to effect a compromise between an aggressive "search and destroy" attitude with every identifiable mucosal excrescence and a laissez-faire approach. The following protocol is recommended.

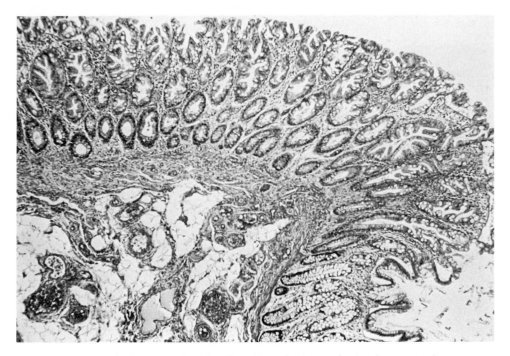

FIG. 9-1. Hyperplastic (metaplastic) polyp. Note the hyperplastic changes in the mucosa, and the serrated glands near the surface with papillary projections. (Original magnification X 240. Corman ML, Veidenheimer MC, Swinton NW: Diseases of the Anus, Rectum, and Colon. Part I: Neoplasms. New York, Medcom, 1972)

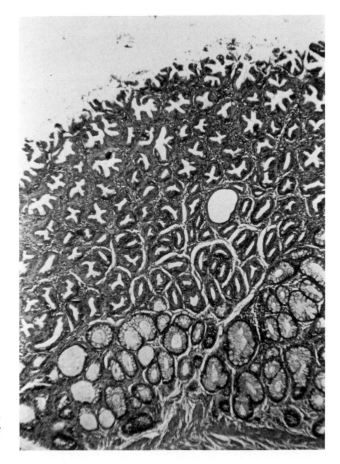

FIG. 9-2. Hyperplastic (metaplastic) polyp: A polypoid lesion with serrated glands, some of which are cystically dilated. (Original magnification × 280. Courtesy of Rudolf Garret, M.D.)

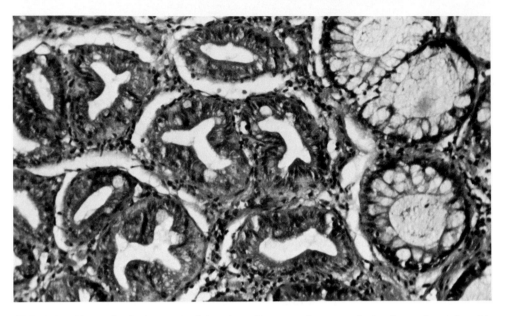

FIG. 9-3. Hyperplastic (metaplastic) polyp. Compare the normal glands on the right with the serrated glands on the left. (Original magnification × 600. Courtesy of Rudolf Garret, M.D.)

Excise the lesion initially to confirm the diagnosis. No follow-up other than the routine colorectal cancer screening appropriate for any patient with no previous history is suggested if the polyp is nonneoplastic. If the patient on subsequent proctosigmoidoscopic examination is found to harbor additional lesions, no treatment is advised, except possibly fulguration of the relatively larger ones. There are four reasons why I suggest ignoring them. First, they tend to spontaneously disappear and recur elsewhere; some patients simply are hyperplastic polyp makers. Second, I am reluctant to create further anxiety by reinforcing the phobia most people have about cancer. Third, there are complications associated with excision of lesions; bleeding and perforation are encountered more frequently when small lesions are removed than when large tumors are biopsied. This occurs because normal bowel must be injured in order to completely extirpate the growth. If the surgeon performs procedures through the endoscope frequently enough, sooner or later, he will encounter a complication. Finally, it adds considerably to the cost of the patient's care.

Despite my impression that I am able to determine on clinical inspection alone the likelihood of a lesion being hyperplastic, there are times when I am certainly mistaken. The surgeon must establish his own criteria and his own philosophical approach to the removal, fulguration, or nonintervention of presumed hyperplastic polyps.

HAMARTOMAS

A hamartoma is defined as a nonneoplastic growth that is composed of an abnormal mixture of normal tissue, which in the colon includes juvenile and Peutz-Jeghers polyps.[152]

Juvenile Polyps

The juvenile polyp (congenital polyp, retention polyp, juvenile adenoma) is usually found in children under 10 years of age, but it is also seen in older children and may occur in adults at any age.[107] It is an uncommon condition, occurring in approximately 1% of asymptomatic children.[56] The age distribution has been reported to have a bimodal pattern.[126] According to Roth and Helwig, the childhood group has a modal age of 4 years, whereas the adult group was found to have a modal age of 18 years.[126] The incidence is twice as frequent in boys, and there is a 13-to-1 ratio of men to women in adults.[126]

The commonest presenting complaint is rectal bleeding, followed by prolapse or protrusion of the mass, passing of tissue, and abdominal pain.[50, 79, 103, 126] Autoamputation is noted in up to 10% of patients. Diarrhea, mucus, proctalgia, tenesmus, and rectal prolapse are also reported complaints.[14]

Mazier and associates reported 258 patients with juvenile polyps.[103] Sixty percent of the polyps were located within 10 cm of the anal verge; only 10% were located farther away than 20 cm, but these were scattered throughout the colon. Approximately three fourths were larger than 1 cm in diameter.

Macroscopically, the lesions are usually round or oval, with a smooth, continuous surface, in contrast to the papillary surface that characterizes the adenomatous polyp.[91] They usually have a short stalk. The cut surface demonstrates numerous cystic spaces filled with mucus (Fig. 9-4). Microscopic examination reveals that juvenile polyps are composed of an epithelial and a connective tissue element, with the latter contributing the bulk of the tumor mass (Fig. 9-5).[107] Acute and chronic inflammatory cells are frequently seen. Alexander and co-workers noted that a frequent microscopic finding is infiltration by eosinophils.[1] They postulated that since eosinophils usually connote an allergic response, the polyps are probably the result of allergy. In support of this theory was the observation that there is a statistically significant increased incidence of allergy in the children with polyps and in the families of those children.

Despite the suggestion by some that juvenile polyps may be neoplastic, most pathologists today agree with Morson that the lesion is a hamartoma.[107] He bases his conclusion on the observations that there is an abnormality of the mucosal connective tissue or lamina propria and that this connective tissue stroma bears a resemblance to primitive mesenchyme. This lends support to the contention that the lesion is a malformation rather than a neoplasm.

The diagnosis is usually confirmed by means of proctosigmoidoscopy, and the lesion is removed transanally. In those polyps beyond the reach of the instrument, the barium enema has identified the lesion. In the not too distant past, prior to the advent of colonoscopy, many of these patients were observed, because the alternative meant colotomy and polypectomy. With the advent of flexible fiberoptic colonoscopy, today there is no reason to adopt such an approach. In many centers colonoscopy is the initial means employed for investigating children with undiagnosed rectal bleeding.[40, 139]

Although the majority of patients present with a single polyp (70%), approximately 30% are found to have multiple polyps (Fig. 9-6). Rarely, a patient presents with so-called juvenile polyposis, a condition in-

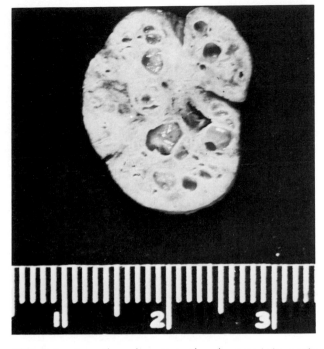

FIG. 9-4. Juvenile polyp. Note the characteristic cystic spaces in cross section. (Courtesy of Rudolf Garret, M.D.)

itially described by McColl and associates in a number of children.[105] Many of these patients have a family history of adenomatous polyposis and of carcinoma of the colon.[66, 135] Reed and Vose recently reported simultaneous diffuse juvenile polyposis and adenomatous polyps in a 17-year-old girl.[122] The authors theorize that the two histologically different lesions may represent phases in a spectrum of diffuse colonic polyposis that may be initiated or exacerbated by a yet undetermined stimulus. The recurrence rate for solitary juvenile polyps is less than 20%, whereas the rate approaches 90% in familial cases.[66]

Since juvenile polyposis should be considered a potentially premalignant condition, an aggressive approach is indicated. Unless one is satisfied that the colon has been "cleared" (usually by means of colonoscopy and polypectomies), total abdominal colectomy is the recommended procedure. Consideration should be given to ileoanal anastomosis with intervening pouch if the rectum is densely involved (see Chap. 15). Proctocolectomy and ileostomy may have to be performed in some cases. Finally, family members should undergo colorectal evaluation.

Although juvenile polyps are the most common colorectal tumors in children, benign and malignant neo-

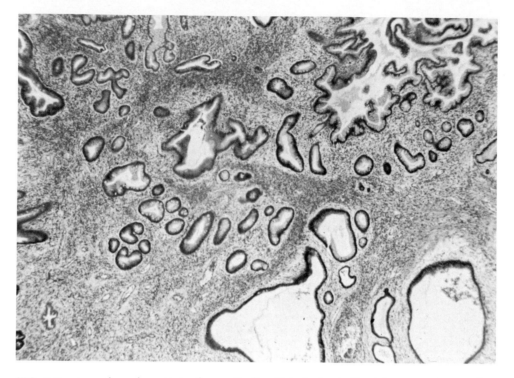

FIG. 9-5. Juvenile polyp. Note the cystically dilated glands lined by normal-appearing epithelium. (Original magnification × 170. Courtesy of Rudolf Garret, M.D.)

plasms can present at virtually any age.[9, 93] Billingham and co-workers observed that solitary adenomas accounted for 7.4% of all polyps found in patients under 20 years of age.[9] Despite the likelihood that a lesion proximal to a juvenile polyp in the rectum is most probably another juvenile polyp, an aggressive attitude should be taken to confirm the true histologic nature of the lesion. With the availability of colonoscopy and colonoscopy–polypectomy there is no justification for continued observation. It is, however, generally agreed that a juvenile polyp itself is neither a neoplasm nor a premalignant condition. Once the polyp is removed, no further follow-up is required.

Peutz-Jeghers Polyps

In 1921, Peutz described a familial syndrome that included pigmentation of the mouth and other parts of the body and polyps of the gastrointestinal tract.[118] Later Jeghers and his colleagues established the syndrome by describing a number of cases.[86, 87] The disease appears to be transmitted as an autosomal dominant,

but *de novo* cases have been reported without any suggestive family history.

The polyps are found most freuently in the small bowel, particularly the jejunum, but they also can involve the stomach, colon, and rectum.[107] Well over 300 patients with the syndrome have now been described.

Cutaneous pigmentation usually is noted at birth or in infancy; the skin changes may actually disappear after puberty.[153] They consist of clusters of black or dark brown freckle-like spots, 1 to 2 mm in diameter, on and around the lips and buccal mucosa, fingers, and toes.[12] The commonest symptom and the one most difficult to manage is abdominal pain, often due to intestinal obstruction. The obstruction is usually the result of a polyp or of intussusception. The other frequent complaint is rectal bleeding. Other signs and symptoms include prolapse of the polyp, passage of the polyp, hematemesis, and anemia.

Macroscopically, the polyps vary in size; they can be as large as several centimeters in diameter. When large, they are usually pedunculated. Grossly, they look very much like adenomatous polyps (see Polypoid Adenoma).

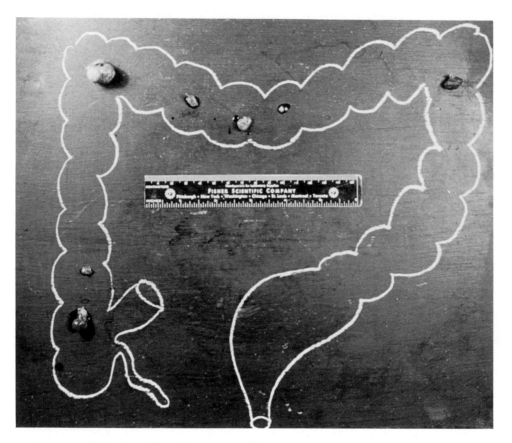

FIG. 9-6. Multiple juvenile polyps removed from one patient. (Courtesy of Rudolf Garret, M.D.)

Microscopically, the polyps appear to originate from intestinal glandular epithelium along with a muscular branching framework that arises from the muscularis mucosa (Fig. 9-7).[57] The tubules of epithelium rest on the branching bands of smooth muscle in a relationship similar to that which the glandular epithelium has to the muscularis mucosa in the normal bowel.[107] Since there is no evidence of hyperplasia, cytologic variation, or loss of differentiation, Morson suggests that the lesion represents a hamartomatous process or malfunction, rather than a neoplasm.[107]

Diagnosis of the syndrome can usually be made on the basis of family history, skin pigmentation, and gastrointestinal symptoms. Contrast studies confirm the extent of the polypoid disease. The major problem lies with the treatment, particularly for the most frequent manifestation, small bowel disease. Many of these young patients undergo multiple laparotomies because of small bowel obstruction and bleeding.[5] Holt reported

the application, on a prophylactic basis, of small bowel plication in a patient who had undergone multiple prior bowel resections because of complications of the disease.[80] With frequent episodes of obstruction or bleeding, a massive small bowel resection may be necessary, thus relegating the patient to the fate of a gastrointestinal cripple, surviving on intravenous hyperalimentation.

Another concern that has been expressed is the suggestion that there may be an association between Peutz-Jeghers syndrome and gastrointestinal cancer.[22, 81, 102, 123, 130] However, Linos and co-workers reported the considerable Mayo Clinic experience (48 patients) and failed to document one definite case; the median follow-up period was 33 years.[97] The authors, furthermore, found that survival was similar to that of the population at large. They recommended that every effort should be made to conserve intestine in the management of this condition.

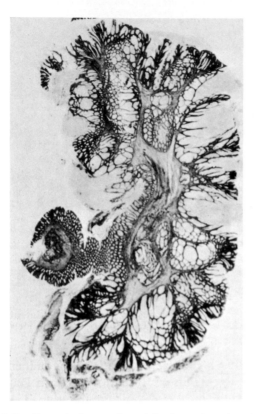

FIG. 9-7. Peutz-Jeghers polyp of the large intestine. Note the tree-like muscular framework. (Morson BC: Some peculiarities in the histology of intestinal polyps. Dis Colon Rectum 1962; 5:337–344)

Williams and associates, of St. Mark's Hospital, reported the management of 10 patients with Peutz-Jeghers syndrome by means of upper and lower gastrointestinal endoscopy.[158] As many as 17 polypectomies were performed in one patient. They recommend upper and lower gastrointestinal endoscopy every other year, the same evaluation if the patient develops symptoms, and laparotomy for any small bowel polyp 1.5 cm in diameter or greater. There is evidence to suggest that an aggressive approach is justified because the frequency of recurrent tumors decreases as the patient becomes older.

Of course, it is of paramount importance to distinguish and identify those lesions that represent true (adenomatous) polyps from the hamartomatous tumors. The malignant potential of the former is not a subject for debate.

ADENOMAS

Whereas hyperplastic polyps are the commonest "tumors" of the colon and rectum, adenomas are by far the most frequently observed neoplasm. They are classified into three categories: polypoid, villous, and mixed. The lesions are by definition benign, but their relationship to the subsequent development of cancer is important (see The Polyp–Cancer Sequence).

Polypoid Adenoma (Adenomatous Polyp, Tubular Adenoma)

Probably the most comprehensive study of polyps was published in 1975 by Muto, Bussey, and Morson.[110] Over 3000 patients were evaluated at St. Mark's Hospital during a period of almost 12 years. Approximately 4500 benign and malignant neoplasms were interpreted pathologically in these patients. Seventy-five percent of the benign tumors were classified as adenomatous polyps and 10% as villous adenomas.

The lesions may be as small as 1 mm or larger than 5 cm. They may be pedunculated (Fig. 9-8) or sessile (Fig. 9-9), with a relatively smooth surface broken by clefts into multiple nodules. The smaller tumors are more likely to have a regular outline and the larger adenomas a lobulated pattern.[75]

Microscopically, polypoid adenomas consist of closely packed epithelial tubules separated by normal lamina propria, which grow and branch horizontally to the muscularis mucosae.[37] There is, however, no consistent appearance of the tubules; they may be quite regular or irregular, with or without inflammatory reaction (Fig. 9-10). The epithelial cells may become distorted, the nuclei may be hyperchromic (stain more deeply) with increased number, and mucus is reduced (Fig. 9-11). Mitoses can be quite frequently observed, but there is no invasion of the muscularis mucosae. Whereas some authors describe certain changes as representative of *in situ* carcinoma, others may call the same phenomenon "atypical" or "dysplastic." I prefer not to use the expression *carcinoma-in-situ* because it is confusing. If there is no invasion of the muscularis mucosae the lesion is benign (Figs. 9-12 and 9-13).

Minute adenomas can actually be detected microscopically as single-gland structures. Oohara and coworkers studied their histogenesis and concluded that they originate from basal cells of the deep layer of mucosa, with those on the lymphoid follicles most likely to undergo neoplastic change.[114] The glands then grow by branching.

(Text continues on p. 238)

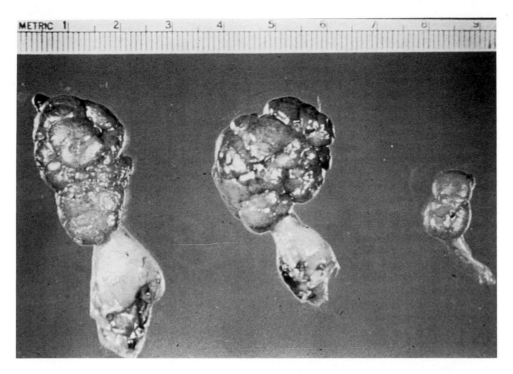

FIG. 9-8. Adenomatous polyps. These three pedunculated tumors were removed from the same patient. (Corman ML, Veidenheimer MC, Swinton NW: Diseases of the Anus, Rectum, and Colon. Part I: Neoplasms. New York, Medcom, 1972)

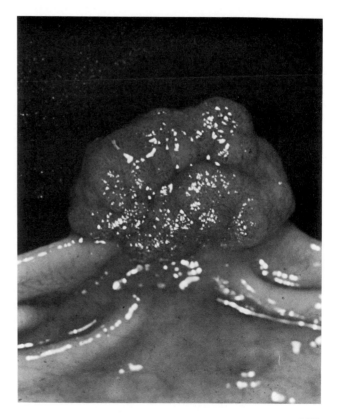

FIG. 9-9. Sessile adenomatous polyp. (Courtesy of Rudolf Garret, M.D.)

235

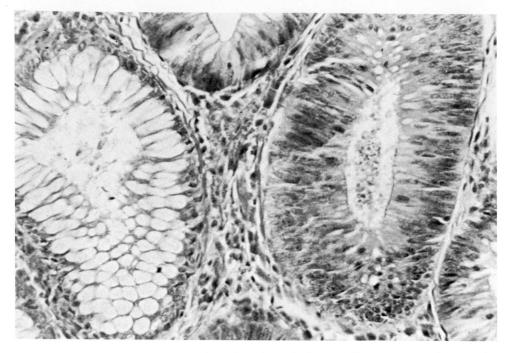

FIG. 9-10. This section from the edge of a polypoid adenoma illustrates a neoplastic and a normal gland side by side. Note the crowding of cells, the piling up of nuclei, and the loss of ability to produce mucus in the neoplastic gland on the right. (Corman ML, Veidenheimer MC, Swinton NW: Diseases of the Anus, Rectum, and Colon. Part I: Neoplasms. New York, Medcom, 1972)

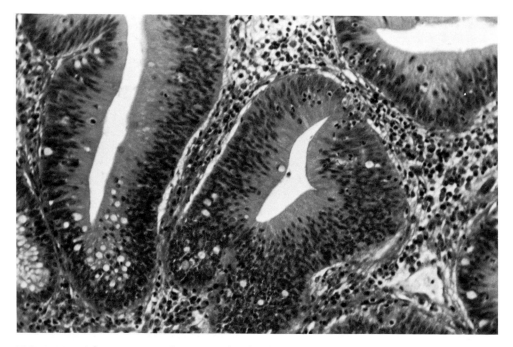

FIG. 9-11. Adenomatous polyp. Note the dysplasia, characterized by loss of polarity with some mitotic figures. (Original magnification × 600. Courtesy of Rudolf Garret, M.D.)

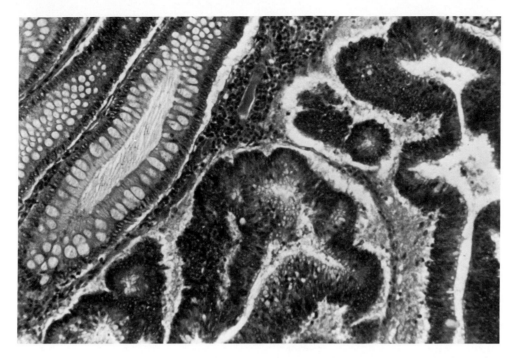

FIG. 9-12. Adenomatous polyp with severe dysplasia on the right, normal glands on the left. (Original magnification × 600. Courtesy of Rudolf Garret, M.D.)

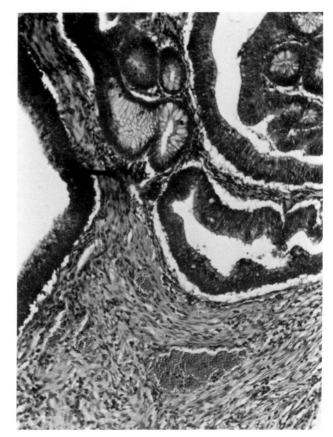

FIG. 9-13. Adenomatous polyp with severe dysplasia: the whole thickness of the glandular epithelium shows total loss of polarity. (Original magnification × 600. Courtesy of Rudolf Garret, M.D.)

Normal surface epithelial cells of the colonic mucosa are replaced every 4 to 8 days.[37] Exfoliation of the cells is balanced by cell division and migration. Elias and associates, using stereologic methods, determined that epithelial surfaces were increased up to 226 times in adenomatous polyps when compared with the normal mucosa.[45] They demonstrated, furthermore, that the number of cells was increased up to 370 times. The authors concluded that the increased number was not primarily dependent on mitotic activity but upon amitotic nuclear fragmentation.

Villous Adenoma (Villous Papilloma)

The villous adenoma generally appears larger than a polypoid adenoma and is more frequently sessile (Fig. 9-14). The margins are usually less well defined than in adenomatous polyps. Despite its size, however, its velvety soft texture may cause it to be missed on digital examination of the rectum (Fig. 9-15). However, sigmoidoscopy will readily demonstrate the presence of a lesion.

Although rectal bleeding is the commonest presenting complaint for both adenomatous conditions, change in bowel habits and mucous discharge are not uncommonly observed, especially in a patient with a large villous adenoma. There is a unique symptom complex associated with villous adenoma that is now infrequently seen: hypokalemia and dehydration. The syndrome was originally reported by McKittrick and Wheelock in 1954 (Fig. 9-16).[106] Others have noted severe fluid and electrolyte depletion in some patients.[36, 63, 84, 121, 129] Jeanneret-Grosjean and Thompson reported that *sodium* loss is as frequently seen and may be the dominant feature of this syndrome in some cases.[85]

Chiu and Spencer reported the Mayo Clinic experience with villous lesions of the colon.[20] During the decade 1964 through 1973, 331 such patients without an associated carcinoma were identified. The median age was 64 years (range, 36 to 82 years); one third of the patients were asymptomatic. Whereas others have reported a more distal location for the lesions, in the Mayo Clinic experience they were evenly distributed throughout the colon. Seven percent were smaller than 1 cm, and 61% were smaller than 3 cm.

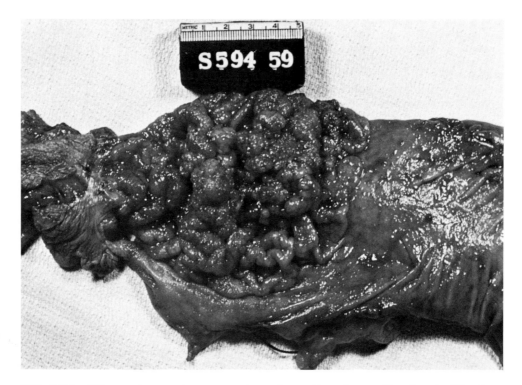

FIG. 9-14. Villous adenoma in a resected specimen. Note the papillary fronds. (Courtesy of Rudolf Garret, M.D.)

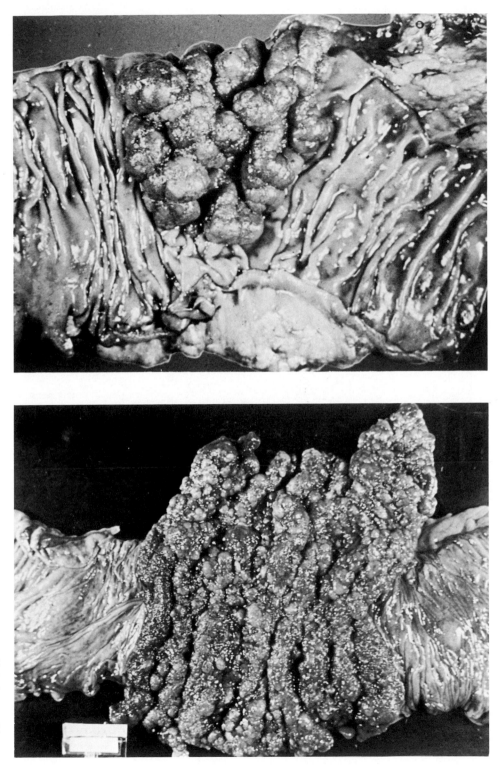

FIG. 9-15. A villous adenoma in a resected specimen demonstrates the soft, velvety appearance of this lesion. (Corman ML, Veidenheimer MC, Swinton NW: Diseases of the Anus, Rectum, and Colon. Part I: Neoplasms. New York, Medcom, 1972)

FIG. 9-16. Villous adenoma: A huge lesion that produced electrolyte depletion. (Corman ML, Veidenheimer MC, Swinton NW: Diseases of the Anus, Rectum, and Colon. Part I: Neoplasms. New York, Medcom, 1972)

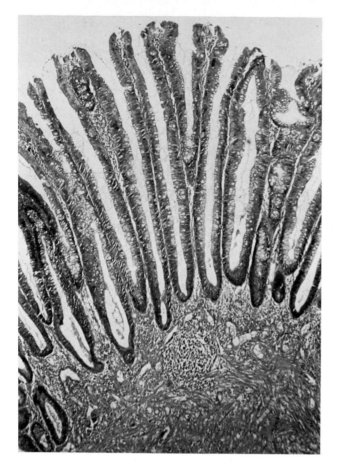

FIG. 9-17. Villous adenoma. Papillary fronds extend from the mucosa. (Original magnification × 280. Corman ML, Veidenheimer MC, Swinton NW: Diseases of the Anus, Rectum, and Colon. Part I: Neoplasms. New York, Medcom, 1972)

Microscopically, the villous adenoma consists of finger-like processes, each made up of a core of lamina propria covered by epithelial cells growing vertically toward the bowel lumen (Fig. 9-17).[37] The epithelium sits on the muscularis mucosae, and in the benign lesion there is no evidence of invasion (Fig. 9-18). Whereas there is decreased mucus in polypoid adenomas, some villous adenomas may actually demonstrate an increase (Fig. 9-19). Atypia or dysplasia is commonly observed (Figs. 9-20 and 9-21).

Tubulovillous Adenoma (Villoglandular Adenoma, Papillary Adenoma, Villoglandular Polyp, Mixed Adenoma, Polypoid–Villous Adenoma)

The combination of polypoid and villous elements is frequently seen in benign neoplasms of the colon and rectum (Fig. 9-22). Histologically, the changes are intermediate between a villous and a polypoid adenoma (Fig. 9-23). The distinction, however, between this presentation and that of a "pure" polypoid adenoma is academic. The patient's symptoms, the methods of diagnosis, and the therapy for the benign lesion are identical.

Evaluation and Diagnosis

Adenomas are commonly observed in countries where there is a high incidence of colorectal cancer; their frequency increases with the age of the patient.[38] Depending on the mean age of the patients in the various reported series, benign neoplasms in the colon and rectum have been observed in from 12% to 60%. Radiographic studies generally identify fewer polyps than do postmortem examinations.[38, 43, 51, 124]

The three methods for diagnosing polypoid disease are proctosigmoidoscopy, barium enema, and fiberoptic colonoscopy. The techniques are discussed in Chapter 1.

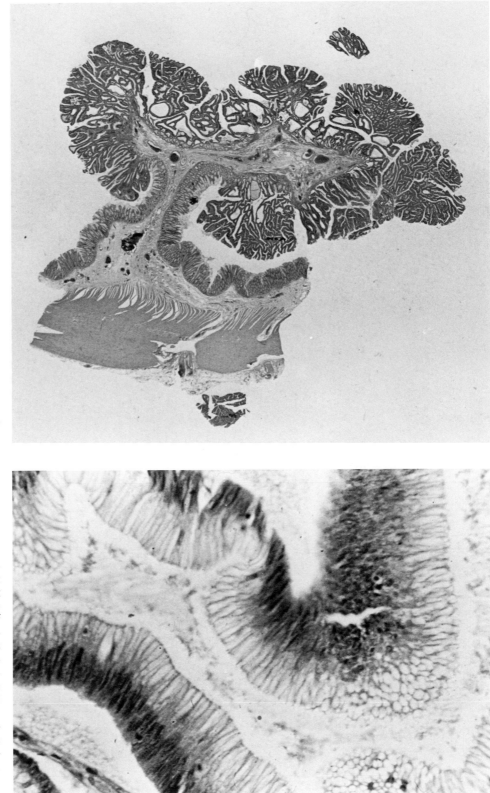

FIG. 9-18. Villous adenoma (whole mount specimen). Note the papillary projections with transition between the normal large bowel mucosa and the polyp. (Courtesy of Rudolf Garret, M.D.)

FIG. 9-19. Villous adenoma. The neoplastic gland is lined by cells that have retained their capacity for the production of mucus. Rich in electrolytes, this mucus accounts for the occasionally observed abnormalities occurring in patients with large lesions. (Original magnification × 600. Corman ML, Veidenheimer MC, Swinton NW: Diseases of the Anus, Rectum, and Colon. Part I: Neoplasms. New York, Medcom, 1972)

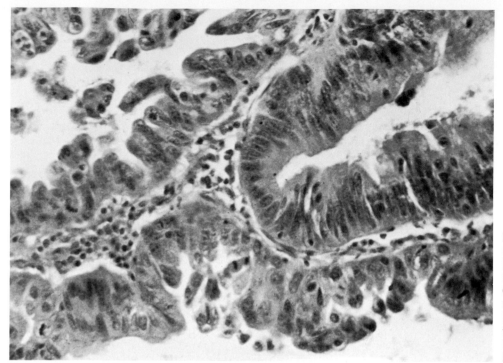

FIG. 9-20. Villous adenoma: Foci of atypical epithelial hyperplasia. (Original magnification × 600. Corman ML, Veidenheimer MC, Swinton NW: Diseases of the Anus, Rectum, and Colon. Part I: Neoplasms. New York, Medcom, 1972)

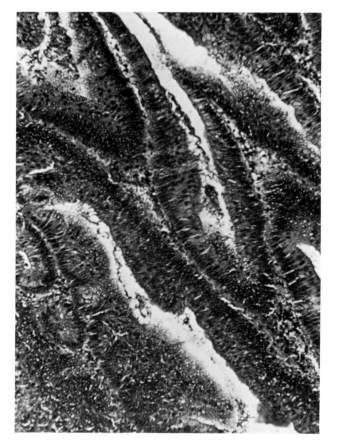

FIG. 9-21. Villous adenoma. The lining cells of the glandular epithelium show a loss of polarity; this represents a mild dysplastic change. (Original magnification × 600. Courtesy of Rudolf Garret, M.D.)

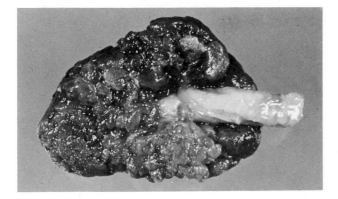

FIG. 9-22. Villoglandular polyp. This pedunculated lesion has areas of varied coloration that on microscopic examination showed both villous and adenomatous changes. (Corman ML, Veidenheimer MC, Swinton NW: Diseases of the Anus, Rectum, and Colon. Part I: Neoplasms. New York, Medcom, 1972)

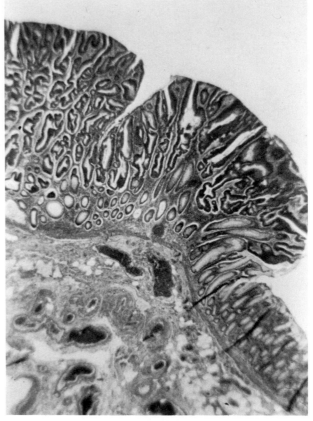

FIG. 9-23. Villoglandular polyp. (Original magnification × 280. Courtesy of Rudolf Garret, M.D.)

We reported the results of proctosigmoidoscopy as performed on an asymptomatic population.[26] Three quarters were men (mean age, 51 years) and one quarter were women (mean age, 55 years). Benign lesions were found in 220 patients (9%). Gilbertsen's ongoing studies from the University of Minnesota Medical Center have demonstrated a marked reduction in the incidence of lower bowel cancers by a program of follow-up proctosigmoidoscopy after polypectomy.[58] Only 15% of the statistically anticipated carcinomas developed, and each of these was an early lesion. Prager and associates traced approximately 300 patients 15 years following sigmoidoscopy–polypectomy for a benign neoplasm.[120] Twelve patients were found to have developed a carcinoma in the interval. The number of malignancies was twice the expected number and their distribution was more proximal. The authors concluded as follows: first, patients with colorectal polyps have a greater tendency to develop colorectal cancer than do unaffected persons; second, carcinomas develop in areas not previously the site of polyps; third, proctosigmoidoscopy is inadequate as the only modality of surveillance; and finally, without the prior polypectomy the incidence of cancer would in all probability have been higher.

Depending on the technique employed, polyps of the colon can be identified in from 1% to 13% of patients; the double contrast (air contrast) approach gives a higher yield (see Chap. 1).[2, 8, 94, 115] An air contrast enema is probably the preferred radiologic approach to evaluating the colon under all circumstances, but especially when the patient has a prior history of polyps or carcinoma; lesions as small as 2 or 3 mm may be identifiable by this technique. We determined, in 200 asymptomatic patients who were found to have one or more rectal polyps, that a barium enema demonstrated a synchronous, proximal neoplasm in 2.5%.[28]

The radiologist cannot ascertain the histologic diagnosis of a polyp, although certain characteristic features may be identified. Of particular importance is to note the presence or absence of a pedicle or stalk (Figs. 9-24 through 9-26); although a pedicle does not connote benignity, it implies that one should attempt to remove the lesion by way of the colonoscope, and that an adequate margin will probably be obtained (see Fig. 1-36). Sessile lesions are more likely to be malignant and are more difficult to remove by means of colonoscopy (Fig. 9-27; see also Fig. 1-37). Again, the ra-

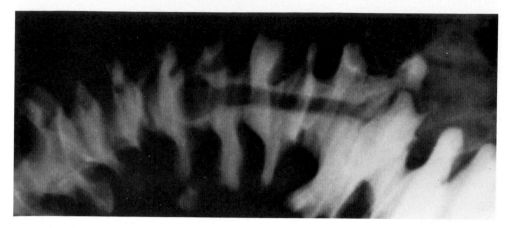

FIG. 9-24. Adenomatous polyp. Barium enema demonstrates a 1.5-cm lesion on a very long pedicle.

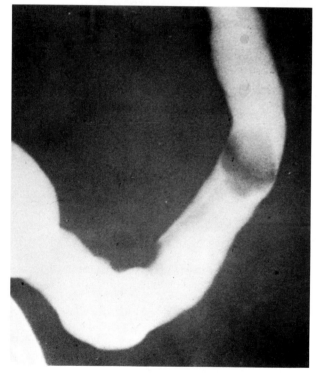

FIG. 9-25. Villoglandular polyp. Note the slightly lobulated filling defect on a long pedicle, demonstrated by barium enema. (Corman ML, Veidenheimer MC, Swinton NW: Diseases of the Anus, Rectum, and Colon. Part I: Neoplasms. New York, Medcom, 1972)

diologist should not be the arbiter of the pathologic diagnosis.

Villous adenomas have a characteristic radiologic appearance. They have an irregular surface because of the frond-like growths; barium in the interstices of the tumor surface produces striated or lace-like radiographic features (Fig. 9-28).[8]

Colonoscopy and colonoscopy–polypectomy are the diagnostic and therapeutic modalities that have been responsible for the quantum advance in our knowledge of polypoid disease in the past 15 years (see Color Fig. 1-5). The indications, equipment, methodology, and complications have been discussed in Chapter 1. Although the procedure of polypectomy has usually required hospitalization in the recent past, outpatient management is now considered safe if the patient is without serious illness, is reliable, and is near adequate medical facilities should the need for medical care arise.[113] The following is a brief summary of the results in a number of selected studies.

Knutson and Max reported their experience of 662 patients.[92] A total of 421 polypoid lesions were seen in 281 patients, three quarters of which were benign. In their report, the comparative overall inaccuracy rate for air-contrast barium enema (false positive and false negative) was 30%. The major morbidity was the "lost polyp." Cowen and associates reported 741 polyps removed during 300 examinations.[31] Thirty-six were excised in one patient, and a 7-cm villous adenoma was removed in another. Forty percent were not identified by barium enema. Others, in a comparison of two techniques, demonstrated 90% accuracy of air contrast enema and 91% accuracy of colonoscopy.[49]

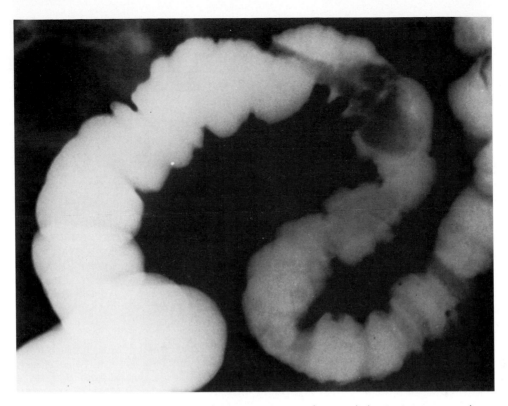

FIG. 9-26. Villous adenoma: Large lesion (3.5 cm) on long pedicle. Barium enema demonstrates irregularity of the surface due to a frond-like growth.

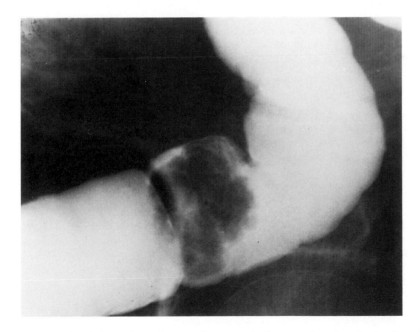

FIG. 9-27. Villoglandular polyp. This sessile, 3-cm lesion was found to be benign; it was removed by colonoscopy–polypectomy.

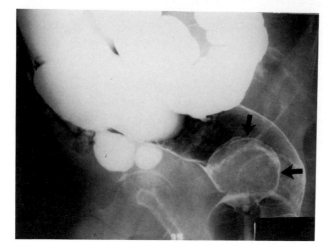

FIG. 9-28. Villous adenoma of the rectum. Barium enema shows a slightly lobulated, broad-based filling defect on the anterior wall. The frond-like appearance is suggestive of a villous adenoma.

A colonoscopic survey of adenomas was reported from the St. Mark's Hospital.[60] Over 1000 polyps were removed, three quarters of which were left sided. With increasing polyp size there was a greater tendency to villous involvement; this was associated with a higher incidence of malignant change. Shinya and Wolff, in an analysis of 7000 polyps endoscopically removed, found that polyp size was related to malignant change, but they noted that invasive cancer *was* found in polyps less than 1 cm in diameter.[133]

Determining the neoplastic or nonneoplastic, benign or malignant natures of polyps is often an unsuccessful exercise. Despite the generalizations about size, color, and presence or absence of a pedicle, the only certain means for establishing the diagnosis is histologic confirmation. Tedesco and co-workers, in a study of small polyps (less than 5 mm), reported that approximately half were neoplastic and half metaplastic (hyperplastic).[142] Nishizawa and colleagues used the magnifying fiberoptic colonoscope and dissecting microscope.[112] They could detect a characteristic "pit pattern" of abnormality in apparently normal colonic mucosa (as small as 1 mm) with the frequent presence of an "incipient" adenoma. Chapuis and associates, using the flexible fiberoptic sigmoidoscope, attempted to diagnose the nature of the lesion by inspection; the diagnosis was correct in 82 percent of the cases.[17] Although the size of the polyp prejudiced the examiner, this was not a reliable indicator of the diagnosis.

The problem of the management of the sessile lesion has been the subject of debate. Most people today, depending on the "aggressiveness" and experience of the endoscopist, would recommend at least an attempt at colonoscopic removal of a benign-appearing lesion. Christie reported the removal of 47 sessile lesions, from 2 to 6 cm in size.[21] There was one incident of complication requiring operative intervention. The author recommends that the appearance at endoscopy determines the advisability of resection by this approach. Smooth, soft, lobulated, non-ulcerated tumors are excisable, provided one has good instrument tip control at the level of the lesion.[21] For those patients at high risk for an anesthetic and for laparotomy, the endoscopist should attempt removal of even very large tumors.[35]

Total colonoscopy is a requisite for patients found to harbor a neoplasm of the colon. We reported colonoscopic examination of the entire colon performed in 146 patients for radiographically suspected benign polypoid disease.[25] Of 36 patients who did not have a neoplastic lesion at the suspected site, 7 (19%) had unsuspected small benign polypoid adenomas elsewhere in the colon. Sixty-two of 110 patients (56%) who were found to have a lesion at the radiographically demonstrated location, harbored a total of 128 additional, unsuspected polyps. Whereas the radiographically demonstrated polyps were predominantly on the left side, two thirds of the unsuspected neoplasms were found proximal to the splenic flexure, resulting in a more uniform distribution of neoplastic colonic polypoid disease (Fig. 9-29).[25] There *has* been a change in the distribution of colon and rectal cancer to a more proximal location, an observation originally reported by Cady and co-workers (see also Chap. 10).[15] Others, in analyzing *benign* polypoid disease, have shown a similar left-to-right shift.[65]

How to follow patients who have undergone colonoscopy–polypectomy is a subject of some controversy. As mentioned, if the patient has had only a polypectomy, complete endoscopic evaluation of the entire colon should be accomplished as early as possible. Unfortunately, there has been little objective evidence upon which to decide the correct intervals for follow-up examination.[157]

Waye and Braunfeld reported over 200 patients with a "cleared" colon who underwent repeat colonoscopy within 1 year of endoscopic polypectomy.[151] Further adenomas were found in 56%. Patients with single adenomas had as much likelihood of having further lesions as did those with multiple tumors. Of the remaining patients in whom no adenomas were found at 1 year, 35% developed new growths within 4 years; those with a single tumor initially had half the rate of a subsequent neoplasm when compared with patients who had multiple adenomas. The authors recommend colonoscopy every 2 years if more than one adenoma was removed and every 3 years in patients with only one index lesion.

Kronborg and colleagues reported the results of 629 colonoscopies and 130 double-contrast examinations performed during the first 2 years of a prospective program.[94] Three months following polypectomy 13 patients required additional polypectomy. The yield was highest with patients who had sessile villous adenomas, those with dysplasia, and those with carcinoma. Wiliams and co-workers reported a prospective study from St. Mark's Hospital.[159] Recall of 300 patients who had previously undergone colonoscopic polypectomy was conducted using multiple diagnostic tests (occult blood testing, proctosigmoidoscopy, double contrast barium enema, flexible fiberoptic sigmoidoscopy, and total colonoscopy). The mean follow-up interval since polypectomy was 3.6 years. Since double contrast enema missed 71% of adenomas, the authors suggested that colonoscopy is the preferred method for follow-up.

If one is to carry out a vigorous effective polyp–cancer surveillance program in a patient who underwent prior polypectomy for neoplastic disease (benign or malignant), I advocate *no* radiologic investigation and limiting the procedure to colonoscopy every 3 years. In order to help ensure maximum patient commitment to follow-up, a flexible fiberoptic sigmoidoscopy is advised for the other yearly visits.

The Polyp–Cancer Sequence

The significance of neoplastic polyps would be of academic interest only, were it not for the relationship between these lesions and the subsequent development of carcinoma. I have already alluded to this relationship, but it is important to document the evidence for this conclusion. Some documentation is indeed circumstantial, but it is not without impact.

Synchronous Cancer

Morson and Dawson demonstrated that about one third of resected specimens for colon and rectal cancer harbor one or more adenomas.[109] Greene reported an incidence of 13%.[65] In a postmortem study Helwig demonstrated adenomas in half the patients found to have a large bowel carcinoma (Fig. 9-30).[75] In ten others who were found to have "an adenoma with carcinomatous transition," eight harbored additional adenomas. In those patients found to have two or more synchronous *carcinomas*, Heald and Bussey found that

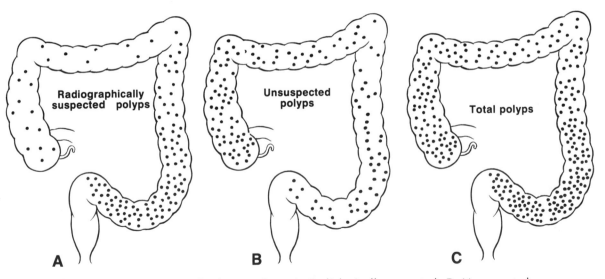

FIG. 9-29. Distribution of colonic polyps. **A.** Radiologically suspected. **B.** Unsuspected. **C.** Total distribution. (Illustration by F. E. Steckel, based on data from Coller JA, Corman ML, Veidenheimer MC: Colonic polypoid disease: Need for total colonoscopy. Am J Surg 1976; 131:490–494)

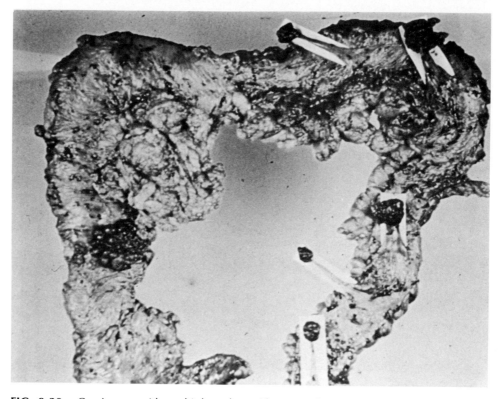

FIG. 9-30. Carcinoma with multiple polyps. There are five pedunculated, adenomatous polyps in the left and transverse colon, and a carcinoma in the ascending colon. (Corman ML, Veidenheimer MC, Swinton NW: Diseases of the Anus, Rectum, and Colon. Part I: Neoplasms. New York, Medcom, 1972)

75% had an associated adenoma.[74] Numerous colonoscopy studies have confirmed this frequent association.

Metachronous Cancer

It has long been known that patients who underwent colon resection for carcinoma are at an increased risk for the subsequent development of a malignancy.[13] Morson reported that the metachronous cancer rate at St. Mark's Hospital was approximately 4%.[108] The average time interval was about 10 years, implying that the polyp–cancer development period is that length of time. The frequency of identifying benign neoplasms in such patients is also high. Henry and colleagues reported 154 patients who had previously undergone polypectomy and were followed for a mean of 7 years.[76] Thirty percent developed recurrent polyps; the rate was 16 times that expected in a population of similar age and sex during the first year. Furthermore, in patients who developed a recurrent polyp, one third developed another recurrence.

Geographic Distribution

Carcinoma of the colon and rectum is a disease of western civilization (the epidemiology is discussed in Chap. 10). Adenomatous polyps parallel the geographic distribution, with a high incidence in Europe and the United States, in other meat-consuming countries, and in urban populations.

Anatomic Distribution

The distribution of benign tumors of the colon is similar to that of cancers: more frequent in the distal bowel, with a relatively high incidence in the cecum. Ekelund, in an autopsy study, found over one half of patients to have adenomas of the rectum and sigmoid colon, slightly less than those who were found to have a carcinoma.[44] Nineteen percent of the benign lesions were in the right colon, virtually the same as the distribution for cancer. In Helwig's series, the sigmoid colon was the most common site of adenomas, adenomas with malignant transformation, and carcinomas.[75] Other sites were correspondingly involved. Additional studies demonstrated a more even distribution for adenomas than for carcinomas; this may be in anticipation of a further trend to more proximal cancers. Greene observed that a left-to-right shift was noticeable in the decade from 1971 to 1980 in comparison with the prior 10-year period.[65] Thirty-two percent of adenomas were found in the rectum in the former decade and 13% in the latter.

Age

It would be expected that adenomatous polyps antedate cancer by several years, but until recently this could not be well documented. The reason for this probably is that cancer patients are usually symptomatic and the date of onset can be quite accurately reported. Polyps, especially when small, may be asymptomatic for a considerable period of time. Morson estimates that evolution of the polyp–cancer sequence is approximately 10 years.[108] In my own experience, patients who underwent colonoscopy–polypectomy had a mean age of 55, compared with colorectal cancer patients whose mean age was 62.

Sex

Men and women have an approximately equal frequency of colorectal cancer; the same observation is true for adenomas. Women have a slightly greater number of right-sided lesions (both benign and malignant).

Evolution

There are two situations in which the life history of the adenoma–carcinoma sequence can be demonstrated: first, in the unusual situation in which a patient with a benign polyp refuses removal of the lesion and subsequently develops a carcinoma at the same site; and second, in familial polyposis, a condition that always results in a bowel cancer if the colon is not resected (see Familial Polyposis).[38] In the latter situation, the histologic nature of the neoplasm is identical to the solitary polypoid adenoma.

Muto and co-workers reported four patients who had untreated adenomatous polyps.[110] In one, cancer

was diagnosed at the same site over 5 years later; in the second, a cancer was found after 6 years. The third patient had a cancer of the rectum develop 13 years after the original observation of a benign polyp. In the fourth case, after 11 years the tumor was still benign. The authors concluded that the life history of the polyp–cancer sequence is probably at least 5 years and may in some cases be more than 10 years.

Patients with large, sessile villous adenomas represent a special situation, because the lesions are frequently removed locally by a transanal approach and have a tendency to recur. Muto and associates observed the long-term follow-up in 10 such patients (5 to 30 years).[110] All patients had periodic evaluation and further treatment as necessary for recurrence. Two patients subsequently developed cancers: one after 10 years and one at 28 years.

In patients with familial polyposis, the onset of the cancer is on average approximately 15 years following establishment of the initial diagnosis. In the St. Mark's series the average age at diagnosis of polyposis without cancer was 27 years, and polyposis with cancer, 39 years, a 12-year time interval.[110]

Histologic Change

The most direct evidence for the polyp–cancer sequence is the demonstration of all stages in the development of malignancy within the same specimen: normal epithelium, adenomatous tissue, atypia, and frank invasion (Fig. 9-31). Occasionally, from macroscopic examination alone, an otherwise benign lesion may appear to have undergone malignant change (Fig. 9-32). In large series of colonoscopy–polypectomies, 4% to 5% of polyps demonstrate some element of invasive carcinoma.[46, 60, 162] Generally, the larger the lesion the greater the likelihood of malignant degeneration. Polypoid adenomas under 1 cm have been shown to have a 1% incidence of malignant change; those from 1 to 2 cm have a 10% incidence, and those over 2 cm, a 35% incidence.[110] In patients with villous adenomas, the incidence was reported as follows: under 1 cm, 10%; 1 to 2 cm, 10%; and over 2 cm, 53%.[10] If carcinomas of the large bowel arose *de novo* from normal mucosa, without passing through the stage of benignity, it would not be uncommon to observe a cancer of 0.5 cm in diameter.[38] Since this is not the case, one must assume that the vast majority of colorectal cancers arise from benign polyps. Figure 9-33 demonstrates schematically how the various presentations may evolve. It has been said that if one seeks vigorously enough and performs sufficient serial sections of the pathologic specimen, an element of benign

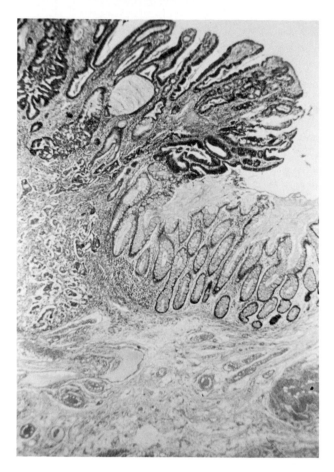

FIG. 9-31. Villous adenoma. Note the marked dysplasia of the lining cells on the left, with infiltrating well-differentiated adenocarcinoma penetrating the muscularis mucosae. (Original magnification × 260. Courtesy of Rudolf Garret, M.D.)

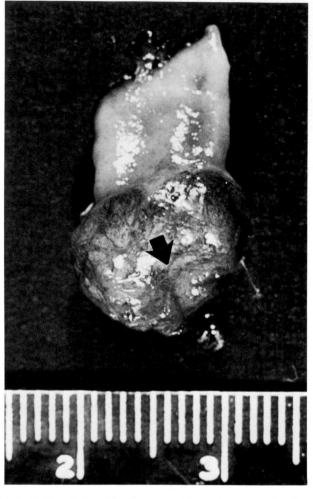

FIG. 9-32. Polypoid adenoma with carcinoma at the tip. Ulcer is indicated by the arrow. (Courtesy of Rudolf Garret, M.D.)

polyp can virtually always be found in a cancer, particularly if the tumor is relatively small. Although some cancers of the colon and rectum probably arise *de novo* from otherwise normal mucosa, the majority originate from adenomas.

Pseudocarcinomatous Invasion

Benign-appearing glandular tissue has been described deep to the muscularis mucosae; this condition has been termed pseudocarcinomatous invasion.[110] It is believed to be associated with larger tumors, those with a long pedicle, and lesions of the sigmoid colon.[37] Day and Morson suggest the histologic appearance is due to trauma, possibly secondary to repeated twisting of the stalk.[37]

Histologic features reveal gland-like or cyst-like structures in the submucosa that show a cytologic appearance similar to that of the overlying benign tumor (Fig. 9-34).

Differentiation of pseudocarcinomatous invasion from invasive cancer is important; in the St. Mark's Hospital series of 56 patients, no one developed a recurrence or metastasis following excision.[37]

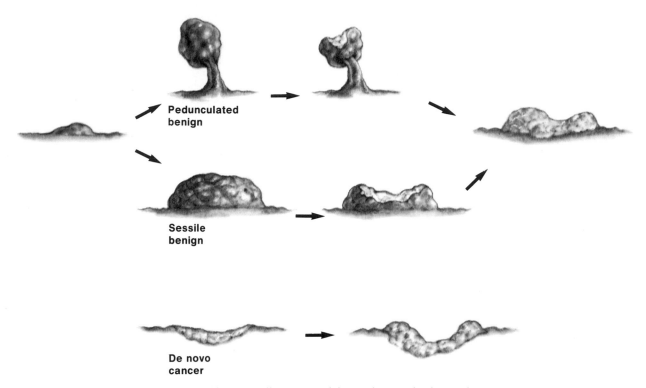

FIG. 9-33.   Schematic illustration of the evolution of colorectal cancer.

Treatment and Results

With the advent of colonoscopy, the presence of a polypoid lesion virtually dictates endoscopic evaluation and, in most cases, polypectomy. There is no justification today for observation to determine the lesion's change in appearance or size with the passage of time, except in the rare situation when the risk of endoscopy is great. Colotomy and polypectomy for pedunculated lesions is a procedure that has been relegated almost completely to the realm of historic interest (Fig. 9-35). If colonoscopy is not available, if removal of the lesion is felt to be outside the limits of the endoscopist's ability, if the instrument cannot be passed to the level of the lesion, or if adequate control cannot be obtained during an attempt at polypectomy, abdominal operation is justified. Figure 9-36 illustrates the technique of colotomy and polypectomy for a pedunculated lesion; the tumor shown in Figure 9-35 is illustrated after removal in Figure 9-37.

The major concern with the requirement for laparotomy as the means to remove the lesion is the operative risk. Prior to the advent of colonoscopy, the generally quoted operative mortality was from 1% to 2%. There is reason to defer surgery in the occasional high-risk patient who harbors a relatively small lesion, since there is little risk of cancer (less than 1% for a tumor less than 1 cm in size). Unfortunately, this information is not terribly helpful in such patients, because lesions of this diameter can usually be removed by way of the colonoscope. Those that cannot are larger, and hence the likelihood of the presence of a cancer is that much greater. For pedunculated polyps, when laparotomy is required, a colotomy and polypectomy is acceptable. Sessile lesions are usually best treated by a resection. Frozen section examination is indicated for sessile lesions (if resection is not performed) and for pedunculated tumors with a short pedicle or in which there is indication of possible cancerous change; it is more than embarrassing to return the patient to surgery for a second laparotomy because the resection margin is deemed inadequate. The techniques of bowel resection are described in the following chapter and the indications, technique, and complications of colonoscopy are discussed in Chapter 1.

The most controversial issue of management is the

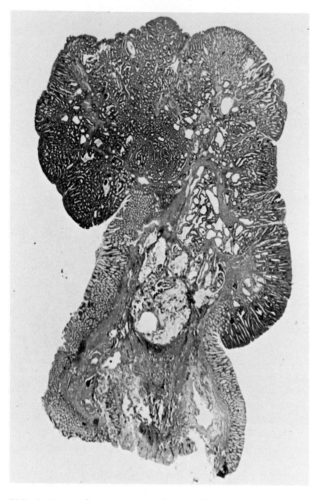

FIG. 9-34. Adenomatous polyp with pseudoinvasion of the pedicle. The glands are cystically dilated and look identical to those in the polyp itself. The glands in the stalk are lined by normal-appearing epithelium. (Original magnification × 80. Corman ML, Veidenheimer MC, Swinton NW: Diseases of the Anus, Rectum, and Colon. Part I: Neoplasms. New York, Medcom, 1972)

problem of what to do if invasive carcinoma is found.[6, 7, 30, 131, 134, 161] Most series have relatively few cases; some authors advocate resection whereas others do not. Some selectively advise resection (*e.g.,* in patients with poorly differentiated lesions, or simply in young patients). Wolff and Shinya recommend resection if the cancer is close to the plane of resection, if there is tumor in the lymphatics, or if the lesion is poorly differentiated.[161] Interestingly, however, in five patients with small polypoid cancers (no benign element identified), no residual cancer was identified by the authors. How-

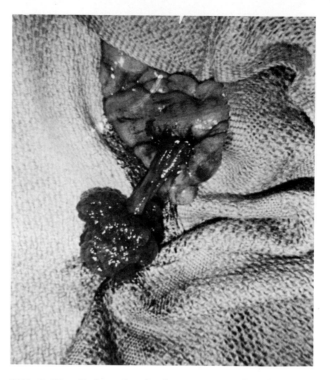

FIG. 9-35. Pedunculated adenomatous polyp delivered through colotomy. (Corman ML, Veidenheimer MC, Swinton NW: Diseases of the Anus, Rectum, and Colon. Part I: Neoplasms. New York, Medcom, 1972)

ever, Colacchio and associates, in analyzing size, depth of invasion of the pedicle, degree of differentiation, and involvement of lymphatics with the stalk, could not accurately predict the likelihood of tumor spread to regional lymph nodes.[23] They recommend conventional colonic resection in all patients who harbor polyps with invasive carcinoma.

It must be remembered that the polyp must be totally removed. Biopsy alone is worthless. If the cancer invades the pedicle it is theoretically possible for it to metastasize. The likelihood, however, is extremely remote if the margin is free. In this situation my preference is to inform the patient that in all probability cure has been achieved, but there is the remote possibility (perhaps 1% or 2%) that residual tumor may still be present. The decision for resection is left to the patient. Conversely, if the margin is not clear, resection is advised. Parenthetically, if laparotomy is performed, it is important for the surgeon to know exactly where the lesion originally was located. If the specimen is opened it is usually possible to identify the site of the polypectomy up to 5 weeks later.[68]

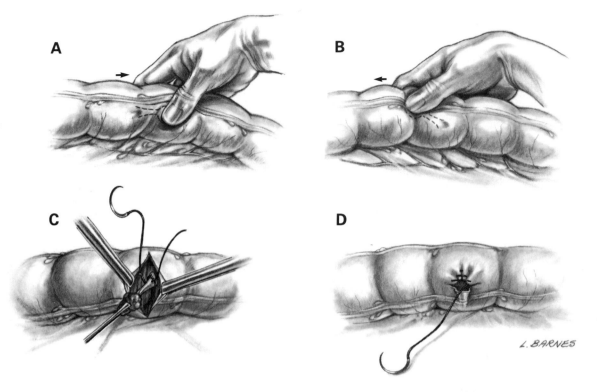

FIG. 9-36. Colotomy and polypectomy. The base of the pedicle is determined by traction to create dimpling **(A),** or the polyp is moved in both directions with site for colotomy determined by splitting the difference **(B).** Transverse colotomy is preferred, and the base is suture-ligated **(C).** Longitudinal enterotomy with transverse closure (to avoid lumenal narrowing) is also acceptable **(D).**

An alternative to colotomy and polypectomy when colonoscopy has been unsuccessfully employed is the procedure of *operative colonoscopy:* laparotomy and transanal polypectomy. Wilson and associates[160] describe the technique as follows:

The patient is placed in the perineolithotomy position as if for combined abdominoperineal resection (see Fig. 11-4). Following laparotomy, the colonoscope is inserted into the rectum; a noncrushing clamp is placed proximal to the tumor to avoid air insufflation beyond the area for polyp excision. With the guidance of the abdominal surgeon the endoscope is expeditiously passed, and the polyp is removed by the endoscopist.

Others have been pleased with the technique in the rare instance when it has been advised.[101] Besides cases of unsuccessful colonoscopy, the procedure can be usefully employed in combination with laparotomy for other conditions (*e.g.,* cholelithiasis), in order to avoid opening the colon, and for localization of nonpalpable colonic lesions. Although the advantages of the approach are limited, consideration should be given to its application in the occasional difficult polypectomy problem.

Large benign neoplasms of the rectum, especially villous adenomas, are tumor management problems that present a challenge to all surgeons (see Figs. 9-14 through 9-16). It is generally agreed that these lesions have an increased likelihood of malignant degeneration as compared with polypoid adenomas. This may be in some measure due to the usually larger size of villous lesions; however, even when comparing the two histologic types size for size an increased frequency of cancerous change is noted.

Biopsy results of any grossly benign polyp are notoriously inaccurate, but with villous adenoma this dictum is especially true. The tumor should be inspected carefully, and pale or white areas that may be suggestive of malignant change should be noted. These are the areas that should be biopsied. Palpation is often very helpful in identifying firm or hard sites for biopsy;

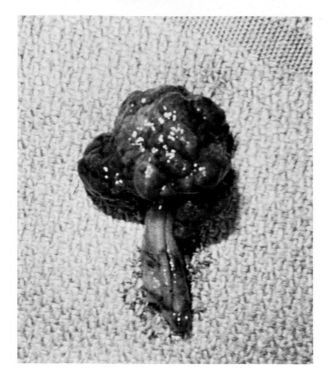

FIG. 9-37. Pedunculated polyp, shown in Fig. 9-35, after removal. (Corman ML, Veidenheimer MC, Swinton NW: Diseases of the Anus, Rectum, and Colon. Part I: Neoplasms. New York, Medcom, 1972)

the presence of ulcer implies cancerous change. Taylor and co-workers reported their experience with preoperative assessment of villous adenomas.[141] Forty-four percent of the biopsy reports were misleading when compared with the report of the excised specimen. Most disturbing was a 10% false-positive incidence. The most important criterion for determining the type of operative approach in my opinion is the clinical impression gained by palpation and inspection. If one is not convinced that the lesion harbors invasive cancer, every effort should be made initially to perform a sphincter-saving approach.

There are basically four methods of removing rectal tumors: transanal excision, transcoccygeal excision (Kraske), transsphincteric excision (Mason), and rectal resection with or without restoration of intestinal continuity. All of these methods are discussed in Chapter 11.

Transanal excision is the preferred operation if resection precludes restoration of continuity. The procedure can be performed by snare electrocoagulation or by excision; I prefer to use the former approach for large lesions and the latter for small ones. The reason for this apparent contradiction is that it is helpful to have the specimen removed intact and submitted for pathologic evaluation. With a small lesion, this can usually be achieved by excision; however, excision of large or circumferential tumors requires a tedious, often bloody dissection. A compromise is suggested, wherein a wire-loop snare is used to remove the bulk of the mass, and the base is electrocoagulated.

A sphincter stretch is necessary for both procedures, and a plastic anoscope of appropriate size is inserted (see Fig. 11-82). The tumor is visualized and an anchoring suture is placed distally (Fig. 9-38). It is often helpful to infiltrate the submucosa with a dilute adrenaline solution to facilitate dissection and limit blood loss. The full thickness of the bowel is incised with an adequate margin around the tumor, and the rectum is reapproximated as the dissection proceeds. Each suture is held for traction.

The procedure is performed with the patient in the prone position for an anterior lesion and in the lithotomy position for a posterior lesion. Only a small-volume enema is given preoperatively; usually, for relatively small tumors, the operation is performed as an outpatient procedure.

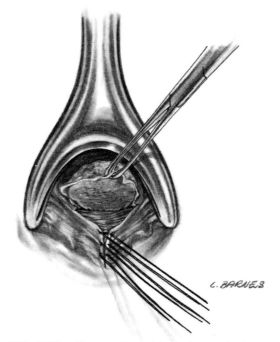

FIG. 9-38. Transanal excision. An anchoring suture is placed distal to the tumor; the lesion is excised in a stepwise fashion, and the bowel is reapproximated as the polypectomy proceeds.

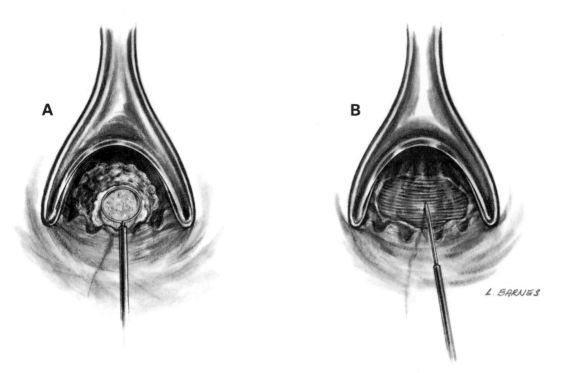

FIG. 9-39.   Transanal snare electrocoagulation. **A.** A wire loop snare cautery pares the tumor mass down. **B.** A needle electrode is employed for electrocoagulation of residual tumor.

With snare electrocoagulation of a large tumor, inpatient surgery is necessary. A bowel preparation as if for colectomy is advisable, as is a perioperative antibiotic. The tumor is pared down with the wire loop until only minimal tumor remains (Fig. 9-39, *A*). Using the needle-tip electrode the remainder is coagulated with an adequate margin (Fig. 9-39, *B*).

Chiu and Spencer reported the Mayo Clinic experience of 331 villous adenomas treated over a 10-year period.[20] Excluded were patients with synchronous carcinomas. Numerous methods were employed, depending on the location and size of the tumors. Only three patients underwent abdominoperineal resection. Sixty-nine electrocoagulations were associated with four recurrences, whereas 26 transanal excisions yielded 7 patients who developed recurrences. The authors reiterate the importance of nonradical resection for lesions without invasive carcinoma.

In the Memorial Hospital (New York) experience, 72 patients underwent local excision, and 9 developed recurrences.[121] The authors advocate local excision by means of cautery snare for all benign-appearing villous adenomas. Because of the 12% recurrence rate, frequent follow-up examination is recommended. The recurrence rate in 24 patients who underwent transanal excision as reported by Jahadi and Bailey was also 12%.[84]

Westbrook and colleagues reported 19 patients who underwent transsacral (transcoccygeal) or transsphincteric operations; 9 patients had villous adenomas.[154] Despite four fecal fistulas, two wound dehiscences, one rectal stricture, and one sacrococcygeal hernia, the authors stated that "the posterior approach to the rectum is safe and effective. . . ." I cannot agree; the procedure may be effective (there were no recurrences), but in the authors' experience as well as in my experience and that of others,[19] the morbidity rate is excessively high. Transanal snare electrocoagulation or local excision are the approaches recommended for villous adenomas of the rectum.

FAMILIAL POLYPOSIS

Familial (multiple) polyposis is an heritable (autosomally dominant) disease in which the colon is involved with numerous adenomatous polyps. The condition becomes apparent during youth, and if colectomy is not performed, it is associated with a high incidence of colorectal cancer, usually by the age of 40. The largest

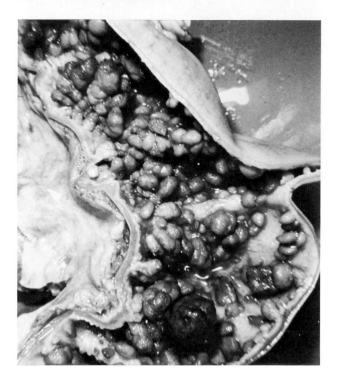

FIG. 9-40. Multiple (familial) polyposis. This portion of a sigmoid colon demonstrates numerous, variable-sized polypoid excrescences throughout the bowel. (Corman ML, Veidenheimer MC, Swinton NW: Diseases of the Anus, Rectum, and Colon. Part I: Neoplasms. New York, Medcom, 1972)

experience with familial polyposis has been published by Bussey in a monograph based upon approximately 300 families contained in the St. Mark's Hospital Polyposis Register.[11] Much of the following data is derived from that publication. Bussey stresses that distinction should be made between multiple polyposis and the condition of multiple adenomas. In the former, colon polyps number as many as several thousand (Fig. 9-40). The author suggests that the number 100 be the cutting-off point to distinguish between the two conditions.[11]

A number of individual case reports of patients with multiple polyps were described in the 18th and 19th centuries, but Cripps is generally credited with being the first to note the condition in two members of the same family.[18, 29, 33] Handford described the association of cancer in 1890.[70] The establishment of the St. Mark's Hospital register was the result of the initial observations of Lockhart-Mummery; this was succeeded by other reports from the same institution.[41, 42, 99] Following these publications, a number of families were identified by other authors as harboring this genetic defect. Gardner and his co-workers, although not the first to identify extracolonic manifestations, accumulated sufficient data to isolate a group of patients who were subsequently determined to have Gardner's syndrome (see below).[52, 54, 55]

Signs and Symptoms

Polyps may be present for a number of years before the onset of symptoms. Family members who are routinely screened for polyps are often identified as polyposis patients while still asymptomatic. Bussey theorized that polyps exist for at least a decade before causing symptoms of sufficient import to the patient to cause him to seek medical attention.[11] The mean age of the appearance of polyps in the St. Mark's Hospital series was 22.[11]

Bleeding is the most common complaint (80%), followed by diarrhea (70%), abdominal pain, and mucous discharge. Weight loss, anemia, and intestinal obstruction are ominous signs, implying the presence of a cancer.

In addition to the symptoms and findings indicating intestinal polyploid disease, patients may manifest other pathologic entities of an extracolonic nature.

Gardner's Syndrome

Gardner's syndrome is characterized by the presence of multiple osteomata (usually skull and mandible), cysts, and soft-tissue tumors. Other conditions associated with the syndrome include desmoid tumors of the abdominal wall, mesentery, and retroperitoneum; dental abnormalities; thyroid carcinoma; periampullary carcinoma; and gastrointestinal adenomatosis and carcinoma.

Osteomata were originally described in the skull and mandible, but more recently they have been shown to involve other areas and may be the only extracolonic manifestations.[147, 149] The boney tumors may be present for many years before the onset of intestinal symptoms.[11]

Epidermoid cysts are a frequent finding in patients with Gardner's syndrome. Because of the common occurrence in the general population of the cutaneous lesion, however, little thought is usually given to the possibility of its being associated with the condition. But because they are uncommon before the age of puberty, the presence of epidermoid cysts in this age group should alert the physician to pursue colorectal investigation.[11, 96]

Desmoid tumors are usually benign fibromata that tend to infiltrate locally into adjacent tissue. Although the lesion appears occasionally to emulate fibrosarcoma, metastasis does not occur. Local recurrence is the rule rather than the exception. The mass tends to develop in abdominal incisions, in the abdominal cavity (particularly the small bowel mesentery), and the retroperitoneum.[64, 104] The condition may antedate the appearance of the polyposis by developing in an abdominal incision performed for another purpose (*e.g.,* appendectomy). Usually, however, desmoid tumors become manifest from 1 to 3 years following surgery for polyposis.[11]

In my experience, desmoid tumors are by far the most troublesome, indeed disabling, consequence of Gardner's syndrome. Complete extirpation in some patients may not be possible. Involvement of retroperitoneal structures may cause urinary obstruction, which in turn may require a diversionary procedure. Attempting to remove a large tumor from the small bowel mesentery may compromise the viability of a large portion of the intestine; prior to the advent of hyperalimentation this was usually a fatal complication.

Desmoid tumors are reported to arise in from 3.5% to 5.7% of patients who have Gardner's syndrome.[11, 136] Surgical removal should be performed only if the tumors are symptomatic, and one should recognize that the likelihood of recurrence is great. Intestinal bypass rather than resection should be considered for large mesenteric lesions.

Dental abnormalities have more recently been recognized as part of the syndrome complex,[53] including impacted supernumerary teeth, unerupted teeth, early cavities, edentulousness, dentigerous cysts, and abnormal mandibular bone structure.[11]

Thyroid carcinoma has been reported to be associated with Gardner's syndrome.[16, 32, 90, 95, 137, 138] Unique about this observation is the fact that the proliferative abnormalities of the syndrome as listed above are of mesenchymal origin, whereas thyroid tumors are not; this suggests a broader potential for the genetic defect.[16] It is known, for example, that pheochromocytoma is associated with medullary carcinoma of the thyroid.

Periampullary carcinoma is a well-recognized disease that is associated with Gardner's syndrome. Twelve percent of patients in the St. Mark's Hospital series who survived for 5 years after colectomy developed a carcinoma of the duodenum, ampulla of Vater, or pancreas.[11] Sugihara and associates reviewed the literature and identified 29 such cases.[140] The mean age of the patient was 45. Eleven patients developed colorectal cancer, all of them having presented with symptoms before the periampullary malignancy. Fundamental advice would be to recommend periodic upper gastrointestinal radiologic investigation (preferably with double contrast technique) and endoscopy at intervals in all patients found to have Gardner's syndrome.[39, 71]

Gastrointestinal polyps have been frequently reported with the syndrome (Fig. 9-41). Japanese studies reveal the incidence of gastric polyps to be as high as 70% in patients with Gardner's syndrome, and the incidence of duodenal polyps approaches 100%.[140] Numerous case reports indicate the association of gastrointestinal polyps with this syndrome, as well as an association of the syndrome with small bowel carcinoma.[10, 67, 78, 90, 119, 125]

Other conditions that are believed to represent manifestations of this syndrome include *carcinoid of the small bowel, adrenal cancer, skin pigmentation,* and *lymphoid polyposis.*[73, 100, 144, 148, 156] There is, however, the possibility that the observations may merely be coincidental.

Turcot's Syndrome

Turcot's syndrome is the eponym given to familial polyposis in association with malignant tumors of the central nervous system; the condition was originally described by Turcot and co-workers in 1959.[145] Others have also reported a relationship between the two diseases.[3, 16] Rothman and associates noted the development of a medulloblastoma before the colonic condition was recognized.[128] Turcot's syndrome is thought to be distinct from Gardner's syndrome because of the pattern of inheritance; a generation is frequently missed. Smith and Kern attributed this observation to variable gene penetrance.[138] Others suggest that the disease is transmitted as an autosomal recessive trait.[47, 83]

Cronkhite-Canada Syndrome

In 1955, Cronkhite and Canada described a syndrome of gastrointestinal polyposis, pigmentation, alopecia, and nail dystrophy.[34] Other cases have been reported.[59, 88] Diarrhea and malabsorption produce severe vitamin deficiency, hypoproteinemia, and fluid and electrolyte abnormalities. The polyps may not always be neoplastic, and the condition perhaps should not be considered as one of the polyposis syndromes.

Evaluation

Traditionally, proctosigmoidoscopy has been the procedure employed for identification of familial polyposis in relatives of a family member known to harbor the condition. Unfortunately, the rectum may be relatively or even totally spared, and patients may be given false reassurance. In addition to considering the means of evaluation, the age at which screening should begin must be addressed. Naylor and Lebenthal reported three children (all asymptomatic) who were related to

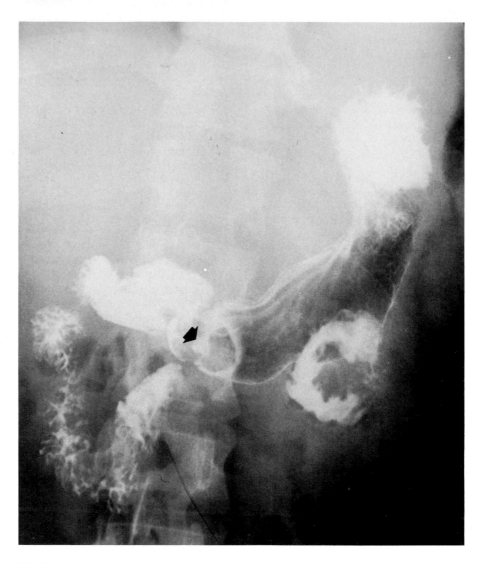

FIG. 9-41. Antral polypoid lesion with central ulceration *(arrow)* on an upper GI series in a patient with multiple (familial) polyposis.

a patient with Gardner's syndrome to have evidence of polyps.[111] The children were 18 months, 6 years, and 9 years old; barium enema was not always diagnostic. The authors recommend colonoscopy and biospy in at-risk children; in their opinion, by deferring colonic examination until adolescence, the opportunity to diagnose polyposis and possibly prevent a cancer might be jeopardized (see Color Fig. 9-1).

Pavlides and colleagues assessed colonoscopy, barium enema, and occult blood determination in families of patients with a hereditary polyposis.[117] Colonoscopy was demonstrated to be superior to barium enema; results of occult blood determination were positive in 30% of patients with polyposis, more than five times as frequently as in those patients without polyposis. Although barium enema or double contrast study will demonstrate the disease in most patients (Fig. 9-42), small lesions such as those illustrated in Figure 9-43 may be missed. My own preference is to proceed directly to colonoscopy as the screening tool in the at-risk family member. In children especially, I prefer to avoid radiation exposure.

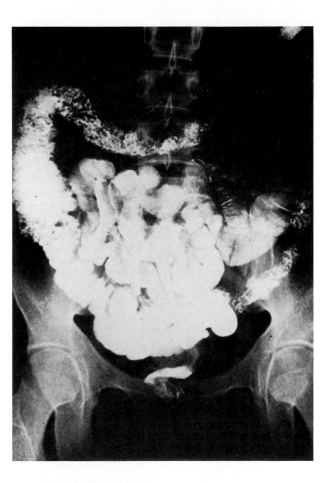

FIG. 9-42. Multiple (familial) polyposis. Barium enema reveals multiple filling defects throughout the colon and rectum. The air contrast technique is preferred. (Corman ML, Veidenheimer MC, Swinton NW: Diseases of the Anus, Rectum, and Colon. Part I: Neoplasms. New York, Medcom, 1972)

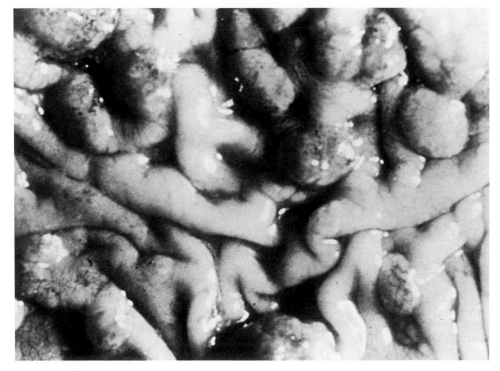

FIG. 9-43. Multiple (familial) polyposis. These multiple small mucosal excrescences may be inapparent upon barium enema study. (Corman ML, Veidenheimer MC, Swinton NW: Diseases of the Anus, Rectum, and Colon. Part I: Neoplasms. New York, Medcom, 1972)

Treatment and Results

There are four operations that are employed for the treatment of familial polyposis: proctocolectomy and ileostomy; total colectomy with ileorectal anastomosis (periodically fulgurating residual or recurrent rectal polyps); total colectomy, mucosal proctectomy, and ileoanal anastomosis; and, finally, the same as the last procedure, except with an intervening pouch. The technical aspects of total colectomy and ileorectal anastomosis are discussed in Chapter 10; the other procedures are detailed in Chapter 15.

The Cleveland Clinic group recommends total abdominal colectomy and ileorectal anastomosis for this condition.[61, 62] The protocol includes early surgical intervention (before age 20), with anastomosis at approximately 12 cm from the dentate line, and close follow-up (every 6 months).[61] The authors point out that polyps may spontaneously regress following total colectomy.[24, 82, 98, 132] A lowered pH of the stool has been stated to be a factor. The administration of vitamin C has also been felt to increase the tendency to regression.[150] Although the regression may be only temporary, the avoidance of an esoteric operation or an ileostomy in the patient who is likely to comply with the follow-up regimen makes this the most useful procedure for surgeons.

Total colectomy and ileorectal anastomosis has also been the procedure of choice at St. Mark's Hospital.[11] Total proctocolectomy was performed on 22 patients, 19 of whom had rectal cancer. In 91, the former procedure was employed; there were two operative deaths. Regression of the polyps seemed to take place in the first decade after surgery, but this trend was reversed in the second decade. Of the 89 patients surviving this operation, two subsequently developed a carcinoma of the rectum. Since the patients had been closely followed, at the time of proctectomy all were found to have Dukes' A lesions (see Chap. 10). Only one other required proctectomy; this patient originally had over 5000 polyps. The numerous recurrences finally made further surgery necessary. Bussey computes the cumulative risk of development of cancer in the retained rectum at 3.6%.[11]

Beart and co-workers reported the results of total colectomy, mucosal proctectomy, and ileoanal anastomosis in 50 patients, 7 of whom had polyposis.[4] Three quarters of the patients preferred the operation to the alternative of ileostomy. Each patient obviously serves as his own control.

In the same series, Heppell and co-workers analyzed continence in three polyposis patients; nine others with ulcerative colitis were also evaluated.[77] The patients were generally continent during the day; however, all but one reported leakage at night. Although the procedure did preserve the sphincter, it decreased the capacity and compliance of the distal bowel and impaired fecal control.

Parks and associates reported four patients with polyposis coli who underwent proctocolectomy with an ileal reservoir and ileoanal anastomosis.[116] Seventeen patients with ulcerative colitis were also treated. There was no disturbance of urinary or sexual function. Every patient was continent during the day; one was incontinent at night. The average frequency of evacuation was approximately four times in 24 hours. The authors felt that this operation was a reasonable alternative to proctocolectomy and ileostomy. Others have also felt that the pelvic reservoir procedure is desirable.[48, 69, 89, 127, 143] Utsunomiya and colleagues reported the use of multiple operative variations to effect ileoanal anastomosis in 11 polyposis patients.[146] The side-to-end ileoanal anastomosis with J-loop reservoir provided the best functional results in their experience.

Comment

Conventional proctocolectomy and ileostomy achieves complete extirpation of the polyp-bearing intestine but at the expense of the loss of intestinal continuity. The fear of having a permanent stoma may dissuade some patients from having needed surgery or members of polyposis families from undergoing screening evaluation. But if one is to consider retaining the rectum, a considerable burden of responsibility falls upon the surgeon and the patient. The confidence of being asymptomatic lulls patients into a false sense of security; rationalization and denial are frequently employed defense mechanisms. Under such circumstances, when rectal bleeding or a change in bowel habits develops, the cancer is often far advanced. Of the four patients upon whom I operated for rectal cancer, who did not undergo periodic evaluation and who became symptomatic following total colectomy, all had metastatic disease. The patient must be informed of the risk and be willing to undergo proctosigmoidoscopy every 6 months for an indefinite period. It is easier to justify this position if the rectum is relatively spared, but even with extensive involvement I prefer this approach, at least in the first instance. If rectal polyposis cannot be adequately treated by a local procedure, an esoteric sphincter-saving operation should be considered.

I do not believe that ileoendoanal anastomosis without intervening pouch is a functionally satisfactory alternative. If the patient has only the choice between this procedure and an ileostomy, many will opt to avoid a stoma. Although the anastomosis with pouch is the preferred alternative to conventional ileostomy, the procedure has a very high morbidity, and the functional results are certainly less than perfect. The patient should not be "convinced" by the surgeon to undergo this complicated operation; rather, he must be well motivated to avoid an ileostomy. In my opinion all pouch anastomotic operations require a diversionary procedure temporarily; the patient must understand the necessity for at least two operations.

In summary, total abdominal colectomy is the recommended approach, with a pouch anastomotic procedure available for possible subsequent use. Proctocolectomy is advised for patients with rectal cancer or for those who wish the best operation for cure. This operation is also suggested for those who will not adhere to the required follow-up regimen.

REFERENCES

1. Alexander RH, Beckwith JB, Morgan A, Bill AH: Juvenile polyps of the colon and their relation to allergy. Am J Surg 1970; 120:222–225
2. Andren L, Frieberg S, Welin S: Roentgen diagnosis of small polyps in colon and rectum. Acta Radiol (Stockh) 1955; 43:201–208
3. Baughman FA Jr, List CF, Williams JR et al: The glioma-polyposis syndrome. N Engl J Med 1969; 281:1345–1346
4. Beart RW Jr, Dozois RR, Kelly KA: Ileoanal anastomosis in the adult. Surg Gynecol Obstet 1982; 154:826–828
5. Beck AR, Jewett TC Jr: Surgical implications of the Peutz-Jeghers syndrome. Ann Surg 1967; 165:299–302
6. Behringer GE: Polypoid lesions of the colon. Which should be removed? Surg Clin North Am 1974; 54:699–712
7. Berci G, Panish J Morgenstern L: Diagnostic colonoscopy and colonoscopic polypectomy. Arch Surg 1973; 106:818–819
8. Berk RN: Polypoid lesions of the colon. In Greenbaum EI: Radiographic Atlas of Colon Disease, pp 401–411. Chicago, Year Book Medical Publishers, 1980
9. Billingham RP, Bowman HE, MacKeigan JM: Solitary adenomas in juvenile patients. Dis Colon Rectum 1980; 23:26–30
10. Boley SJ, McKinnon WM, Marzulli VF: The management of familial gastrointestinal polyposis involving stomach and colon. Surgery 1961; 50:691–696
11. Bussey HJR: Familial Polyposis Coli. Baltimore, Johns Hopkins University Press, 1975
12. Bussey HJR: Polyposis syndromes. In Morson BC: The Pathogenesis of Colorectal Cancer, pp 81–94, Philadelphia, WB Saunders, 1978
13. Bussey HJR, Wallace MH, Morson BC: Meta-chronous carcinoma of the large intestine and intestinal polyps. Proc R Soc Med 1967; 60:208–210
14. Cabrera A, Lega J: Polyps of the colon and rectum in children. Am J Surg 1960; 110:551–556
15. Cady B, Persson AV, Monson DO, Maunz DL: Changing patterns of colorectal carcinoma. Cancer 1974; 33:422–426
16. Camiel MR, Mulé JE, Alexander LL, Benninghoff DL: Association of thyroid carcinoma with Gardner's syndrome in siblings. N Engl J Med 1968; 278:1056–1058
17. Chapuis PH, Dent OF, Goulston KJ: Clinical accuracy in the diagnosis of small polyps using the flexible fiberoptic sigmoidoscope. Dis Colon Rectum 1982; 25:669–672
18. Chargelaigue A: Des polypes du rectum. Paris, Thesis, 1859
19. Christiansen J: Excision of mid-rectal lesions by the Kraske sacral approach. Br J Surg 1980; 67:651–652
20. Chiu YS, Spencer RJ: Villous lesions of the colon. Dis Colon Rectum 1978; 21:493–495
21. Christie JP: Colonoscopic excision of large sessile polyps. Am J Gastroenterol 1977; 67:430–438
22. Cochet B, Carrel J, Desbaillets L et al: Peutz-Jeghers syndrome associated with gastrointestinal carcinoma: report of two cases in a family. Gut 1979; 20:169–175
23. Colacchio TA, Forde KA, Scantlebury VP: Endoscopic polypectomy: Inadequate treatment for invasive colorectal carcinoma. Ann Surg 1981; 194:704–707
24. Cole JW, Holden WD: Postcolectomy regression of adenomatous polyps of the rectum. Arch Surg 1959; 79:385–392
25. Coller JA, Corman ML, Veidenheimer MC: Colonic polypoid disease: Need for total colonoscopy. Am J Surg 1976; 131:490–494
26. Corman ML, Coller JA, Veidenheimer MC: Proctosigmoidoscopy—age criteria for examination in the asymptomatic patient. CA 1975; 25:286–290
27. Corman ML, Veidenheimer MC, Swinton NW: Diseases of the Anus, Rectum, and Colon. Part I: Neoplasms. New York, Medcom, 1972
28. Corman ML, Veidenheimer MC, Coller JA: Barium enema study findings in asymptomatic patients with rectal polyps. Dis Colon Rectum 1974; 17:325–330
29. Corvisart L: Hypertrophie partielle de la muqueuse intestinale. Bull Soc Anat 1847; 22:400
30. Coutsoftides T, Sivak MV Jr, Benjamin SP, Jagelman D: Colonoscopy and the management of polyps containing invasive carcinoma. Ann Surg 1978; 188:638–641

31. Cowen AE, Stitz RW, Ward M: Colonoscopic polypectomy. Med J Aust 1981; 1:627–628

32. Crail HW: Multiple primary malignancies arising in the rectum, brain and the thyroid. US Nav Med Bull 1949; 49:123–128

33. Cripps WH: Two cases of disseminated polypus of the rectum. Trans Path Soc Lond 1882; 33:165–168

34. Cronkhite LW, Canada WJ: Generalized gastrointestinal polyposis. Unusual syndrome of polyposis, pigmentation, alopecia and onychotrophia. N Engl J Med 1955; 252:1011–1015

35. Dagradi AE, Riff DS, Ford EA: Colonoscopic polypectomy excision of a huge villous adenoma. Am J Gastroenterol 1976; 66:464–466

36. Davis JE, Seavey PW, Sessions JT Jr: Villous adenomas of the rectum and sigmoid colon with severe fluid and electrolyte depletion. Ann Surg 1962; 155:806–816

37. Day, DW, Morson BC: Pathology of adenomas. In Morson BC: The Pathogenesis of Colorectal Cancer, pp 43–57. Philadelphia, WB Saunders, 1978

38. Day DW, Morson BC: The polyp problem. In Hunt RH, Waye JD (eds): Colonoscopy—Techniques, Clinical Practice and Colour Atlas, pp 301–326. London, Chapman and Hall, 1981

39. Denzler TB, Harned PK, Pergam CJ: Gastric polyps in familial polyposis coli. Radiology 1979; 130:63–66

40. Douglas JR, Campbell CA, Salisbury DM et al: Colonoscopic polypectomy in children. Br Med J 1980; 281:1386–1387

41. Dukes CE: The hereditary factor in polyposis intestine or multiple adenomata. Cancer Rev 1930; 5:241–256

42. Dukes CE: Familial intestinal polyposis. Ann Eugen Lond 1952; 17:1–29

43. Eide TJ, Stalsberg H: Polyps of the large intestine in northern Norway. Cancer 1978; 42:2839–2848

44. Ekelund G: On cancer and polyps of colon and rectum. Acta Pathol Microbiol Scand 1963; 59:165–170

45. Elias H, Hyde DM, Mullens RS, Lambert FC: Colonic adenomas: stereology and growth mechanisms. Dis Colon Rectum 1981; 24:331–342

46. Enterline HT, Evans GW, Mercado-Lugo R et al: Malignant potential of adenomas of colon and rectum. JAMA 1962; 179:322–330

47. Erbe RW: Inherited gastrointestinal polyposis syndromes. N Engl J Med 1976; 294:1101–1104

48. Fonkalsrud EW: Endorectal ileal pullthrough with ileal reservoir for ulcerative colitis and polyposis. Am J Surg 1982; 144:81–87

49. Fork F-T: Double contrast enema and colonoscopy in polyp detection. GUT 1981; 22:971–977

50. Franklin R, McSwain B: Juvenile polyps of the colon and rectum. Ann Surg 1972; 175:887–891

51. Gabrielsson N, Granqvist S, Ohlsén H, Sundelin P: Malignancy of colonic polyps: Diagnosis and management. Acta Radiol [Diagn] (Stockh)1978; 19 (Fasc 3): 479–495

52. Gardner EJ: A genetic and clinical study of intestinal polyposis, a predisposing factor for carcinoma of the colon and rectum. Amer J Hum Genet 1951; 3:167–176

53. Gardner EJ: Gardner's syndrome re-evaluated after twenty years. Proc Utah Acad 1969; 46:1–11

54. Gardner EJ, Plenk HP: Hereditary pattern for multiple osteomas in a family group. Amer J Hum Genet 1952; 4:31–36

55. Gardner EJ, Richards RC: Multiple cutaneous and sub-cutaneous lesions occurring simultaneously with hereditary polyposis and osteomatosis. Am J Hum Genet 1953; 5:139–147

56. Gelb AM, Minkowitz S, Tresser M: Rectal and colonic polyps occurring in young people. NY State J Med 1962; 62:513–518

57. Gibbs NM, Katz D: Hyperplastic polyps. In Morson BC (ed): The Pathogenesis of Colorectal Cancer, pp 14–32. Philadelphia, WB Saunders, 1978

58. Gilbertsen VA: Proctosigmoidoscopy and polypectomy in reducing the incidence of rectal cancer. Cancer 1974; 34:936–939

59. Gill W, Wilkin BJ: Diffuse gastrointestinal polyposis associated with hypoproteinaemia. J R Coll Surg Edinb 1967; 12:149–156

60. Gillespie PE, Chambers TJ, Chan KW et al: Colonic adenomas—a colonoscopy survery. GUT 1979; 20:240–245

61. Gingold BS, Jagelman DG: Sparing the rectum in familial polyposis: Causes for failure. Surgery 1981; 89:314–318

62. Gingold BS, Jagelman DG, Turnbull RB Jr: Surgical management of familial polyposis and Gardner's syndrome. Am J Surg 1979; 137:54–56

63. Gjöres JE, Örndahl B: Villous adenoma with severe fluid imbalance. Acta Chir Scand 1974; 140:82–84

64. Gorlin RJ, Chaudhry AP: Multiple osteomatosis, fibromas, lipomas and fibrosarcomas of the skin and mesentery, epidermoid inclusion cysts of the skin, leiomyomas and multiple intestinal polyposis. N Engl J Med 1960; 263:1151–1158

65. Greene FL: Distribution of colorectal neoplasms: A left to right shift of polyps and cancer. Am Surg 1983; 49:62–65

66. Haggitt RC, Pitcock JA: Familial juvenile polyposis of the colon. Cancer 1970; 26:1232–1238

67. Halstead JA, Harris EJ, Bartlett MK: Involvement of the stomach in familial polyposis of the gastrointestinal tract: report of a family. Gastroenterology 1950; 15:763–770

68. Hambrick E: Fiberoptic colonoscopy: The fate of colonoscopic polypectomy sites. Dis Colon Rectum 1976; 19:400–404

69. Handelsman JC, Fishbein RH, Hoover HC Jr et al: Endorectal pull-through operation in adults after colectomy and excision of rectal mucosa. Surgery 1983; 93:247–253

70. Handford H: Disseminated polypi of the large intestine becoming malignant. Trans Path Soc Lond 1890; 41:133

71. Harned RK, Williams SM: Familial polyposis coli and periampullary malignancy. Dis Colon Rectum 1982; 25:227–229

72. Hayashi T, Yatani R, Apostol J, Stemmerman GN: Pathogenesis of hyperplastic polyps of the colon: A hypothesis based on ultrastructure and in-vitro kinetics. Gastroenterology 1974; 66:347–356

73. Heald RJ: Gardner's syndrome in association with two tumours in the ileum. Proc R Soc Med 1967; 60:914–915

74. Heald RJ, Bussey HJR: Clincial experiences at St. Mark's Hospital with multiple synchronous cancers of the colon and rectum. Dis Colon Rectum 1975; 18:6–10

75. Helwig EB: Adenomas and the pathogenesis of cancer of the colon and rectum. Dis Colon Rectum 1959; 2:5–17

76. Henry LG, Condon RE, Schulte WJ et al: Risk of recurrence of colon polyps. Ann Surg 1975; 182:511–514

77. Heppell J, Kelly KA, Phillips SF et al: Physiologic aspects of continence after colectomy, mucosal proctectomy, and endorectal ileo-anal anastomosis. Ann Surg 1982; 195:435–443

78. Hoffmann DC, Goligher JC: Polyposis of the stomach and small intestine in association with familial polyposis coli. Br J Surg 1971; 58:126–128

79. Holgersen LO, Miller RE, Zintel HA: Juvenile polyps of the colon. Surgery 1971; 69:288–293

80. Holt RW: Prevention of intussusception in Peutz-Jeghers syndrome. Dis Colon Rectum 1979; 22:274–275

81. Hsu S-D, Zaharopoulos P, May JT et al: Peutz-Jeghers syndrome with intestinal carcinoma: Report of the association in one family. Cancer 1979; 44:1527–1532

82. Hubbard TB Jr: Familial polyposis of the colon: The fate of the retained rectum after colectomy in children. Am Surg 1957; 23:577–580

83. Itoh H, Ohsato K, Yao T et al: Turcot's syndrome and its mode of inheritance. Gut 1979; 20:414–419

84. Jahadi MR, Bailey W: Papillary adenomas of the colon and rectum: A twelve year review. Dis Colon Rectum 1975; 18:249–253

85. Jeanneret-Grosjean AJ, Thompson WG: Villous adenoma with hyponatremia and syncope: Report of a case. Dis Colon Rectum 1978; 21:118–119

86. Jeghers H: Pigmentation of skin. N Engl J Med 1944; 231:88–100

87. Jeghers H, McKusick VA, Katz KH: Generalized intestinal polyposis and melanin spots of the oral mucosa, lips and digits. A syndrome of diagnostic significance. N Engl J Med 1949; 241:993–1005

88. Johnson MM, Vosburgh JW, Wiens AT, Walsh GC: Gastrointestinal polyposis associated with alopecia, pigmentation, and atrophy of the fingernails and toenails. Ann Intern Med 1962; 56:935–940

89. Johnston D, Williams NS, Neal DE, Axon ATR: The value of preserving the anal sphincter in operations for ulcerative colitis and polyposis: A review of 22 mucosal proctectomies. Br J Surg 1981; 68:874–878

90. Keshgegian AA, Enterline HT: Gardner's syndrome with duodenal adenomas, gastric adenomyoma and thyroid papillary—follicular adenoma. Dis Colon Rectum 1978; 21:255–260

91. Knox WG, Miller RE, Begg CF et al: Juvenile polyps of the colon: A clinicopathologic analysis of 75 polyps in 43 patients. Surgery 1960; 48:201–210

92. Knutson CO, Max MH: Diagnostic and therapeutic colonoscopy. Arch Surg 1979; 114:430–435

93. Kottmeir PK, Clatworthy HW Jr: Intestinal polyps and associated carcinoma in childhood. Am J Surg 1965; 110:709–716

94. Kronberg O, Hage E, Deichgraeber E: The clean colon: A prospective, partly randomized study of the effectiveness of repeated examinations of the colon after polypectomy and radical surgery for cancer. Scand J Gastroenterol 1981; 16:879–884

95. Lee FI, MacKinnon MD: Papillary thyroid carcinoma associated with polyposis coli. Am J Gastroenterol 1981; 76:138–140

96. Leppard B: Epidermoid cysts and polyposis coli. Proc R Soc Med 1974; 67:1036–1037

97. Linos DA, Dozois RR, Dahlin DC, Bartholomew LG: Does Peutz-Jeghers syndrome predispose to gastrointestinal malignancy? Arch Surg 1981; 116:1182–1184

98. Localio SA: Spontaneous disappearance of rectal

polyps following subtotal colectomy and ileoproctostomy for polypsis of the colon. Am J Surg 1962; 103:81–82

99. Lockhart-Mummery JP: Cancer and heredity. Lancet 1925; 1:427–429

100. Marshall WH, Martin FIR, Mackay IR: Gardner's syndrome with adrenal carcinoma. Aust Ann Med 1967; 16:242–244

101. Martin PJ, Forde KA: Intraoperative colonoscopy: Preliminary report. Dis Colon Rectum 1979; 22:234–237

102. Matuchansky C, Babin P, Coutrot S et al: Peutz-Jeghers syndrome with metastasizing carcinoma arising from a jejunal hamartoma. Gastroenterology 1979; 77:1311–1315

103. Mazier WP, MacKeigan JM, Billingham RP, Dignan RD: Juvenile polyps of the colon and rectum. Surg Gynecol Obstet 1982; 154:829–832

104. McAdam WAF, Goligher JC: The occurrence of desmoids in patients with familial polyposis coli. Br J Surg 1970; 57:618–631

105. McColl I, Bussey HJ, Veale AMO, Morson BC: Juvenile polyposis coli. Proc R Soc Med 1964; 57:896–897

106. McKittrick LS, Wheelock FC Jr: Carcinoma of the Colon, pp 61–63. Springfield, Charles C Thomas, 1954

107. Morson BC: Some peculiarities in the histology of intestinal polyps. Dis Colon Rectum 1962; 5:337–344

108. Morson BC: Evolution of cancer of the colon and rectum. Cancer 1974; 34:845–849

109. Morson BC, Dawson IMP: Gastrointestinal Pathology. Blackwell Scientific, Oxford, 1972

110. Muto T, Bussey HJR, Morson BC: The evolution of cancer of the colon and rectum. Cancer 1975; 36:2251–2270

111. Naylor WE, Lebenthal E: Early detection of adenomatous polyposis coli in Gardner's syndrome. Pediatrics 1979; 63:222–226

112. Nishizawa M, Okada T, Satō F et al: A clinicopathological study of minute polypoid lesions of the colon based on magnifying fiber-colonoscopy and dissecting microscopy. Endoscopy 1980; 12:124–129

113. Norfleet RG: Colonoscopy and polypectomy in nonhospitalized patients. Gastrointest Endosc 1982; 28:15–16

114. Oohara T, Ogino A, Tohma H: Histogenesis of microscopic adenoma and hyperplastic (metaplastic) gland in nonpolyposis coli. Dis Colon Rectum 1981; 24:375–384

115. Ott DJ, Gelfand DW: Colorectal tumors: Pathology and detection. AJR 1978; 131:691–695

116. Parks AG, Nicholls RJ, Belliveau P: Proctocolectomy with ileal reservoir and anal anastomosis. Br J Surg 1980; 67:533–538

117. Pavlides GP, Milligan FD, Clarke DN et al: Hereditary polyposis coli I: The diagnostic value of colonoscopy, barium enema, and fecal occult blood. Cancer 1977; 40:2632–2639

118. Peutz JLA: Very remarkable case of familial polyposis of mucous membrane of intestinal tract and nasopharynx accompanied by peculiar pigmentations of skin and mucous membrane. Nederl Maandschr V Geneesk 1921; 10:134–146

119. Phillips LG Jr: Polyposis and carcinoma of the small bowel and familial colonic polyposis. Dis Colon Rectum 1981; 24:478–481

120. Prager ED, Swinton NW, Young JL et al: Follow-up study of patients with benign mucosal polyps discovered by proctosigmoidoscopy. Dis Colon Rectum 1974; 17:322–324

121. Quan SHQ, Castro EB: Papillary adenomas (villous tumors): A review of 215 cases. Dis Colon Rectum 1971; 14:267–280

122. Reed K, Vose PC: Diffuse juvenile polyposis of the colon: A premalignant condition. Dis Colon Rectum 1981; 24:205–210

123. Reid JD: Intestinal carcinoma in the Peutz-Jeghers syndrome. JAMA 1974; 229:833–834

124. Rickert RR, Auerbach O, Garfinkel L et al: Adenomatous lesions of the large bowel: An autopsy study. Cancer 1979; 43:1847–1857

125. Ross JE, Mara JE: Small bowel polyps and carcinoma in multiple intestinal polyposis. Arch Surg 1974; 108:736–738

126. Roth SI, Helwig EB: Juvenile polyps of the colon and rectum. Cancer 1963; 16:468–479

127. Rothenberger DA, Vermeulen FD, Christenson CE et al: Restorative proctocolectomy with ileal reservoir and ileoanal anastomosis. Am J Surg 1983; 145:82–88

128. Rothman D, Su CP, Kendall AB: Dilemma in a case of Turcot's (glioma-polyposis) syndrome: Report of a case. Dis Colon Rectum 1975; 18:514–515

129. Roy AD, Ellis H: Potassium-secreting tumours of the large intestine. Lancet 1959; 1:759–760

130. Ryo UY, Roh SK, Balkin RB et al: Extensive metastases in Peutz-Jeghers syndrome. JAMA 1978; 239:2268–2269

131. Shatney CH, Lober PH, Gilbertsen VA, Sosin H: The treatment of pedunculated adenomatous colorectal polyps with focal cancer. Surg Gynecol Obstet 1974; 139:845–850

132. Shepard JA: Familial polyposis of the colon with special reference to regression of rectal polyposis after subtotal colectomy. Br J Surg 1971; 58:85–91

133. Shinya H, Wolff WI: Morphology, anatomic distribution and cancer potential of colonic polyps: An analysis of 7,000 polyps endoscopically removed. Ann Surg 1979; 190:679–683

134. Silverberg SG: Focally malignant adenomatous polyps of the colon and rectum. Surg Gynecol Obstet 1970; 131:103–114

135. Smilow PC, Pryor CA, Swinton NW: Juvenile polyposis coli: A report of three patients in three generations of one family. Dis Colon Rectum 1966; 9:248–254

136. Smith WG: Desmoid tumors in familial multiple polyposis. Mayo Clin Proc 1959; 34:31–38

137. Smith WG: Familial multiple polyposis: Research tool for investigating the etiology of carcinoma of the colon? Dis Colon Rectum 1968; 11:17–31

138. Smith WG, Kern BB: The nature of the mutation in familial multiple polyposis: Papillary carcinoma of the thyroid, brain tumors, and familial multiple polyposis. Dis Colon Rectum 1973; 16:264–271

139. Sokhi GS, Hashemi K: Colonoscopic polypectomy in children. Br Med J 1981; 282:145

140. Sugihara K, Tetsuichiro M, Kamiya J et al: Gardner's syndrome associated with periampullary carcinoma, duodenal and gastric adenomatosis: Report of a case. Dis Colon Rectum 1982; 25:766–771

141. Taylor EW, Thompson H, Oates GD et al: Limitations of biopsy in preoperative assessment of villous papilloma. Dis Colon Rectum 1981; 24:259–262

142. Tedesco FJ, Hendrix JC, Pickens CA et al: Diminutive polyps: Histopathology, spatial distribution, and clinical significance. Gastrointest Endosc 1982; 28:1–5

143. Telander RL, Perrault J: Colectomy with rectal mucosectomy and ileoanal anastomosis in young patients: Its use for ulcerative colitis and familial polyposis. Arch Surg 1981; 116:623–629

144. Thomford NR, Greenberger NJ: Lymphoid polyps of the ileum associated with Gardner's syndrome. Arch Surg 1968; 96:289–291

145. Turcot J, Despres JP, St Pierre F: Malignant tumors of the central nervous system associated with familial polyposis of the colon. Dis Colon Rectum 1959; 2:465–468

146. Utsunomiya J, Iwama T, Imajo M et al: Total colectomy, mucosal proctectomy and ileoanal anastomosis. Dis Colon Rectum 1980; 23:459–466

147. Utsunomiya J, Nakamura T: The occult osteomatous changes in the mandible in patients with familial polyposis coli. Br J Surg 1975; 62:45–51

148. Venkitachalam PS, Hirsch E, Elguezabal A, Littman L: Multiple lymphoid polyposis and familial polyposis of the colon: A genetic relationship. Dis Colon Rectum 1978; 21:336–341

149. Watne AL, Core SK, Carrier JM: Gardner's syndrome. Surg Gynecol Obstet 1975; 141:53–56

150. Watne AL, Lai HY, Carrier J, Coppula W: The diagnosis and surgical treatment of patients with Gardner's syndrome. Surgery 1977; 82:327–333

151. Waye JD, Braunfeld S: Surveillance intervals after colonoscopic polypectomy. Endoscopy 1982; 14:79–81

152. Welch CE, Hedberg SE: Polypoid lesions of the gastrointestinal tract, 2nd ed, p 131. Philadelphia, WB Saunders, 1975

153. Welch CE, Hedberg SE: Polypoid lesions of the gastrointestinal tract, 2nd ed, pp 186–199. Philadelphia, WB Saunders, 1975

154. Westbrook KC, Lang NP, Broadwater JR, Thompson BW: Posterior surgical approaches to the rectum. Ann Surg 1982; 195:677–685

155. Westhues M: Die pathologisch-anatomischen Grundlagen der Chirurgie des Rektumkarzinoms. Leipzig, Georg Thieme Verilg, 1934

156. Weston SD, Weiner M: Familial polyposis associated with a new type of soft-tissue lesion (skin pigmentation): Report of three cases and a review of the literature. Dis Colon Rectum 1967; 10:311–321

157. Williams CB: Editorial: Follow-up after polypectomy. Endoscopy 1982; 14:73

158. Williams CB, Goldblatt M, Delaney PV: "Top and tail endoscopy" and follow-up in Peutz-Jeghers syndrome. Endoscopy 1982; 14:82–84

159. Williams CB, Macrae FA, Bartram CI: A prospective study of diagnostic methods in adenoma follow-up. Endoscopy 1982; 14:74–78

160. Wilson SM, Poisson J, Gamache A et al: Intraoperative fiberoptic colonscopy—"The difficult polypectomy." Dis Colon Rectum 1976; 19:136–138

161. Wolff WI, Shinya H: Definitive treatment of "malignant" polyps of the colon. Ann Surg 1975; 182:516–525

162. Wolff WI, Shinya H: Endoscopic polypectomy: Therapeutic and clinicopathologic aspects. Cancer 1975; 36:683–690

CHAPTER 10

Carcinoma of the Colon

Colorectal carcinoma is the commonest visceral malignancy found in most western countries. It was estimated that in 1983, in the United States alone, 126,000 new cases would be diagnosed, and 58,000 deaths would occur.[246] An infant born in the United States today has a 5% chance of developing colorectal carcinoma during his lifetime.

EPIDEMIOLOGY

In recent years the epidemiology of large bowel cancer has become a major concern of investigators. Interpopulation and nationality differences were the inspiration for Burkitt's hypothesis on the causal role of a low-residue, high-carbohydrate diet in colorectal cancer.[28, 30] Burkitt's observations have generated interest about the incidence and mortality of large bowel cancer, and other hypotheses have been suggested.[19, 118, 122, 123, 202]

The mortality data for colorectal cancer in most Western European countries is high.[68, 277] Scotland has the world's highest rate of bowel cancer, much higher even than that of England.[240] Spain and Portugal on the other hand have a relatively low rate, more consistent with that of Eastern Europe.[68] The two populations with risks similar to Western Europe are the people of Israel and the Chinese in Singapore. With the exception of Singapore, people in Asia have a low incidence of colorectal cancer. In Israel, a considerable difference exists between Israelis born in Europe and those born in North Africa or Asia. The incidence in the former is 2.5 times that of the latter. African countries generally have a very low frequency of colorectal cancer; in Latin American countries the incidence rate varies.[53, 142]

In addition to the variation in the incidence of colorectal cancer from one population to another, observations have been made concerning the variations in the distribution within the colon and rectum. It has been postulated that low-risk populations have a relatively increased incidence of right-sided cancers, whereas relatively high-risk communities have an increased risk of left-sided malignancies.[22, 28, 30, 120]

A difference in incidence of cancer has been observed from country to country when comparing an urban population to a rural population.[18, 42, 61, 162, 197, 254, 261] The nature of the *urban–rural gradient* in risk has been extensively investigated in the United States. By comparing metropolitan and nonmetropolitan countries, Haenszel and Dawson showed that in the United States increased risk for large bowel cancer is found in urban populations in each major region of the country.[121]

With respect to *immigration*, colorectal cancer is less common among Japanese Americans than American whites.[247] However, the rates for Japanese Americans is higher than for Japanese living in Japan. The children of these immigrants have an incidence approximating native American Caucasians.[122] A similar phenomenon has been seen in other populations.[253]

With respect to *race*, there is very little difference between blacks and whites within each community and region of the country.[55, 289] However, the risk of large bowel cancer in American Indians is less than half that for whites.[54, 248]

Some studies have shown a higher death rate for colorectal cancer in more affluent people.[43, 206] Colombia, a country with a low incidence, reported a higher rate in this group of people.[124]

Occupation has been investigated as a possible causative factor.[186, 206] The relative affluence associated with some occupations appears to be the reason why certain professionals have a higher incidence of colorectal cancer.

In studies of the *religion* of patients, Jews have a higher incidence than people of other religions.[118, 119, 199, 241] Members of the Church of Jesus Christ of Latter-Day Saints (Mormons) have a low incidence.[26, 72, 171] Their religion prohibits use of tobacco, alcohol, tea, and coffee. Seventh-Day Adventists have a significantly lower rate of colorectal cancer; their church proscribes tobacco and alcohol.[160, 161, 213]

A number of studies have been published evaluating the association of *tobacco* and cancer.[38, 60, 128, 140, 152, 238] There appears to be no causative relationship between smoking and malignancy in this organ.

Diet is the epidemiologic area that has been receiving the most attention during the past decade, especially since Burkitt's observations.[27-30] He and Painter postulated that high fiber content was the primary factor responsible for the low incidence of colorectal cancer in African natives.[209] Theoretically, whatever carcinogen was ingested or produced would be present in a diluted form, and because of the decreased transit time, would be excreted rapidly. Fleiszer and co-workers, and Chen and co-workers, found that rats were greatly protected when they were given dimethylhydrazine (a known colon carcinogen) parenterally if the dietary fiber were increased.[40, 76]

Other studies have demonstrated correlations between colorectal cancer and additional dietary factors. For example, Nigro and colleagues demonstrated that cancer in the animal model can be inhibited by an increased fiber intake only when the fat content is relatively low.[202, 203] They presented a program for possible prevention of colorectal cancer: a 10% reduction in fat consumption, the addition of 25 g of a dietary fiber per day, and the addition of chemical inhibitors: selenium, retinoids, and plant steroids.[202] These substances have been shown to inhibit cancer that can be induced by carcinogens. The results of ongoing, controlled clinical trials are awaited.

Hill and associates determined that feces from people in the West exhibited a high concentration of bile acids when compared with that of African and Eastern countries.[143] Others have demonstrated strong correlations between high intake of animal fat and protein, and colorectal cancer.[7, 144, 145] Populations with high beef consumption generally have the highest incidence of bowel cancer.[59, 61]

Bacteria are thought to play a role in the causation of colorectal cancer; presumably it is their action on ingested fat or metabolites that is critical. Hill and associates demonstrated that people in the Unites States and Great Britain have a higher colony count of anaerobic flora and a lower count of aerobic bacteria.[143] Others have confirmed this observation.[6] The similarity between the chemical structure of bile salts and the carcinogen methylcholanthrene has been observed. It is not unreasonable to hypothesize that the action of bacteria on bile salts might produce a substance capable of inducing malignant degeneration. Burkitt, in fact, postulated that one of the reasons for the preponderance of carcinoma in the distal bowel is the higher concentration of bacteria in this location.[28]

Patients with *inflammatory bowel disease*, especially *ulcerative colitis*, are at increased risk for the development of a malignancy; perhaps this risk is as high as 60 percent with 30 years of active, total bowel disease.[163, 172, 185] With respect to *Crohn's disease*, a number of reports have been published implicating an association between regional enteritis and small bowel carcinoma.[193, 231, 245] The relationship between granulomatous colitis and large bowel cancer is less well established (see Chap. 15).

There has been considerable difference of opinion about the risk of development of colorectal cancer following pelvic irradiation. A recent report demonstrated an increased risk for women who were radiated for gynecologic cancer.[235] Additional studies are required for confirmation and for accurate assessment of this possibility.

Because of the clinical evidence for an increased quantity of secondary bile acids in the feces of patients with bowel cancer, and experimental studies which demonstrate that secondary bile acids promote chemical carcinogenesis, *cholecystectomy* has been implicated as a possible precipitating factor.[270, 273] This operation increases secondary bile acids in the enterohepatic circulation.[270] A more recent report by Abrams and colleagues failed to confirm a relationship between gall bladder removal and the subsequent development of colorectal cancer.[2]

McVay reported an appreciably increased incidence of colorectal carcinoma in patients who had undergone *appendectomy*.[184] He suggested that the relationship might be explained by immunologic factors. Other reports, however, have failed to substantiate this relationship.[113, 146, 148]

A number of authors have recognized the relationship between *ureterosigmoidostomy* and carcinoma of the colon at the site of the ureteral implant into the colon.[129, 156, 174, 272, 279] The frequency of this complication may be several hundred times greater than that expected in the general population. The etiology of this complication is not clearly understood; it might be related to the urine bathing the colonic mucosa, the presence of a carcinogen in the urine, or the effects of the ureter implanted into the colon. It is suggested that this type of diversion of the urinary tract be abandoned, especially in young patients with benign disease.[244] Periodic evaluation of the bowel is required; consideration should be given to resecting that area of the colon, and another procedure should be employed.[73, 158]

Excluding the polyposis syndromes (see Chap. 9), carcinoma of the colon has been reported in *cancer families*.[168, 169] These studies have demonstrated an increased incidence of cancer in siblings and parents of probands. There also appears to be an increased association of proximal colonic involvement.[170] There is, however, no evidence of greater frequency of bowel tumors in spouses of colorectal cancer victims.

AGE AND SEX

The incidence of carcinoma of the colon and rectum increases with *age*, but the progression also varies by anatomic site, population, and *sex*. In our experience the mean age at diagnosis for men was 63 years, and for women, 62 years.[49] Cook and associates computed the slopes of the logarithm of the incidence against the logarithm of the age from a number of cancer registries and demonstrated that the slopes of the curves for colon and rectal cancer for men were consistently higher than the slopes of the curves for women in almost every population.[47] They noted, furthermore, that this variation in male/female difference was greater for colon than for rectal carcinoma.

In women, colorectal cancer ranks second in the United States both in number of deaths from cancer and new cases (breast cancer is number one in both categories). In the past 25 years there has been a noticeable decrease in age-adjusted death rate for women (22%), whereas no such decrease has been noted for men.

In men, colorectal cancer ranks second for deaths by cancer and third for new cases. Lung cancer is number one in deaths and new cases, with prostatic cancer recently moving into the second position in number of new male cancer cases in the United States.

Colorectal cancer accounts for 14% of cancers in men and 15% in women. Men have a preponderance of rectal cancer and a slight excess of cancer of the descending and transverse colon. The incidence of cancer of the ascending colon and cecum is essentially the same for both sexes.[55] Of cancer deaths in men, 12% are attributable to cancer of the colon and rectum, and in women, 15%.

SYMPTOMS AND SIGNS

Change in bowel habits is the commonest presenting symptom of colorectal cancer. The change may be as insignificant as that from a bowel movement every other day to one daily. All too often, patients place little emphasis on this symptom until a profound alteration occurs. Generally, a more distal lesion creates more obvious symptoms than a proximal one. The reasons for this are threefold: first, formed stool in the distal colon has greater difficulty passing though an area of narrowing than liquid stool present in the proximal bowel; second, the lumen of the bowel itself is larger proximally than it is distally; and third, because of other symptoms (bleeding, pain, discharge), the distal tumor producing a change in bowel habits is often of greater importance in the patient.

Bleeding is the second commonest symptom of colorectal cancer. It may be overt or occult. The blood may be bright red, purple, mahogany, black, or inapparent. The more distal the location of the lesion, the less altered the blood will be, and the redder it will appear. Although bleeding can represent a relatively early sign of cancer of the bowel, it is often a neglected symptom. Patients frequently attribute bleeding to hemorrhoids, particularly if they have had prior hemorrhoid difficulties. For this reason it is important to treat bleeding hemorrhoids, so that the presence of this symptom alerts the patient to seek medical attention.

Conversely, the physician himself may attribute bleeding to hemorrhoids. Nothing is more tragic than the misdiagnosis of a potentially curable cancer because of inadequate examination or investigation. Too often, patients are treated with suppositories, creams, and laxatives, and only when symptoms become severe enough is proper investigation undertaken.

Mucus, either as a discharge (implying a distal lesion) or mixed with the stool, is a symptom which often accompanies bleeding. The presence of mucus and bleeding should be considered a highly suggestive combination that necessitates bowel investigation.

Rectal pain is an unlikely presenting symptom of cancer. The commonest reasons for anorectal pain are thrombosed hemorrhoids, anal fissure, and proctalgia fugax. When rectal cancer produces pain, the lesion usually is very distal or very large. Pain may result from infiltration of the sensitive anal canal or from sphincteric invasion. Such invasion may produce tenesmus, a painful urgency to defecate.

Abdominal pain resulting from tumor implies an obstructing or partially obstructing lesion. This pain is usually colicky in nature and may be associated with abdominal distention, nausea, or vomiting. Intestinal obstruction is a presenting complaint in 5% to 15% of patients. *Weight loss* frequently accompanies these symptoms. *Back pain* from retroperitoneal extension of a tumor of the ascending or descending colon is unusual and a late sign.

A palpable or visible *abdominal mass* in the absence of other signs and symptoms implies a slow-growing, infiltrative process that may be much more amenable to surgical extirpation than might otherwise be anticipated. Such tumors often metastasize quite late in the course of the disease.

Weight loss in the absence of other symptoms is a poor prognostic sign. Inanition and loss of strength and appetite suggest metastatic disease, most commonly to the liver. Presentation with symptoms of *metastatic disease* occurs in approximately 5% of patients with colorectal cancer. Hepatomegaly is a frequent observation, but even pulmonary, cerebral, and osseous metastases as isolated findings may reveal an occult colorectal primary on investigation.

Perforation with peritonitis is an unusual presentation today (except in certain hospitals that serve an indigent population). Differentiating carcinoma from perforated diverticulitis, particularly for a sigmoid lesion, may be extremely difficult (see Surgical Treatment).

Rarely, a carcinoma of the cecum can obstruct the lumen of the appendix and cause signs and symptoms of *acute appendicitis*. Nitschke and co-workers reported on 12 patients who presented in such a manner and who were found to have carcinoma of either the appendix or the cecum.[204] The development of a fecal fistula after appendectomy should lead the physician to suspect an underlying malignancy. Although such presentations are rare, any patient over the age of 50 years in whom acute appendicitis develops should be evaluated carefully at the time of surgery for an underlying carcinoma.

It has been thought that *inguinal hernia* present on admission in older men is associated with colorectal carcinoma.[56, 180, 262] Because of this observation, routine barium enema examination has been advocated in all patients before herniorrhaphy. Brendel and Kirsh reported no such association.[23] I have not been impressed with the yield of such screening studies and do not advocate routine barium enema examination in patients before inguinal herniorrhaphy.

Nonmetastatic *cutaneous presentations* of colorectal cancer have been reviewed by Rosato and associates.[228] They noted a number of conditions associated with gastrointestinal malignancy, including acanthosis nigricans, dermatomyositis, pemphigoid, and others. Such manifestations are rare, but any disseminated skin condition that is unresponsive to conventional therapy should encourage the physician to consider gastrointestinal investigation.

Duration of Symptoms

I continue to be impressed by the long history of symptoms presented by many patients who come for surgical treatment of colorectal cancer. Symptoms have been present for longer than 6 months in one third of our surgically treated patients. Some patients have sought early medical advice because of symptoms, but lack of suspicion of carcinoma or inadequate examination of the patient at the time of the evaluation delayed operative intervention. However, patients with a short history of symptoms do not have a better prognosis. Patients with symptoms of less than 5 months' duration have a higher incidence of resection for cure, but the long-term survival is not noticeably related to the duration of symptoms.[149]

EVALUATION

Digital Rectal Examination

Mayo stated, "The physician often hesitates to make the necessary examination because it involves soiling the finger."[181] The efficacy of digital examination in identifying rectal cancer has been a subject of considerable debate. Only 10% of colorectal cancers are potentially within reach of the examiner's finger. Even when the cancer is within reach, the physician may not be diligent enough or thorough enough in palpation to discover the presence of a lesion. The risks, however, are nonexistent, and no one would argue the cost versus the benefit.

Digital examination will identify the location of the lesion, whether anterior or posterior; the lesion can be judged to occupy the whole of the circumference or part of it. The tumor may be fixed or movable, ulcerated or scirrhous, exophytic or invasive. Careful palpation of the presacral space may reveal hard lymph nodes suggestive of tumor metastases; this may be a valuable prognostic sign. The fact that the tumor is palpable will often dictate the type of operation possible or whether the lesion is resectable. Fixity may indicate a need for supplemental treatment, such as radiotherapy. Therefore, despite the numerous, often esoteric studies available to evaluate today's patient, digital examination of the rectum is still a very important adjunct.

Proctosigmoidoscopy

The sigmoidoscope is one of the most valuable diagnostic tools used. Examination with this instrument may reveal mucosal excrescences, polyps, polypoid lesions, cancer, inflammatory changes, strictures, vascular malformation, and anatomic distortion from extraluminal masses. It may also detect numerous anal conditions, such as fistulas, hemorrhoids, fissures, and abscesses. When the instrument is passed to its full length of 25 cm, about two thirds of all cancers of the colon and rectum can be identified. Unfortunately, with the rigid instrument, insertion to its full length is possible in only about 50% of patients, the average penetration being approximately 20 cm.

Many investigators have advocated routine proctosigmoidoscopy for early diagnosis,[35, 41, 87, 139, 151, 215, 243, 257] but others have questioned the need for this procedure on an annual basis.[62, 63, 189] The American Cancer Society encourages physicians to search for colorectal cancer before the onset of symptoms. Optimally, an annual proctosigmoidoscopic examination for all patients 40 years of age and older would be recommended. With over 80 million such persons in the United States, this is indeed an awesome task. It was estimated in 1980 that annual sigmoidoscopic examination on all people over age 40 in the Unted States would cost approximately $2.75 billion.[37]

We examined 2500 consecutive asymptomatic patients with the rigid sigmoidoscope as part of a general examination. Excluded from the study were symptomatic patients and those with a prior history of colorectal disorders. The proctoscope was inserted to a mean length of 20 cm. Adenocarcinoma was found in eight patients, and in two of these patients carcinoma developed in a polypoid adenoma. A total of 432 benign polypoid lesions was found in 228 patients (9.1%).[48]

In this study all lesions found in patients less than 50 years old were benign; no cancers were detected in patients before the sixth decade of life. This is not surprising because only 5% of colorectal cancer occurs in patients less than 45 years old.[12] Although colorectal cancer can develop in a person of any age, because of the limitations of time, space, and manpower we suggested that routine proctosigmoidoscopic examination be performed in those age groups most likely to benefit from the procedure: patients aged 50 and older. If this criterion is met, 30% fewer examinations would need to be performed.

Obviously, when a patient has symptoms a proctosigmoidoscopic examination is mandatory. When a tumor is identified a biopsy of the lesion should be performed. This is usually a simple office procedure requiring no anesthetic and minimal special tools (see Fig. 1-10). For polypoid, exophytic lesions, appreciable

bleeding is rarely a problem after biopsy. If electrocoagulation equipment is not readily available and bleeding is encountered, pressure with a long, cotton-tipped applicator soaked in a topical solution of adrenalin will usually suffice.

The sample for biopsy should be taken from the edge of the lesion at the junction of the tumor and normal-appearing bowel, and placed in a fixative solution. Notation should be made of the distance from the anal verge to the lower level of the lesion. Also, the size, the macroscopic appearance (whether ulcerated or polypoid), and which wall the lesion occupies should be recorded.

Flexible Fiberoptic Sigmoidoscopy and Colonoscopy

The flexible fiberoptic sigmoidoscope has recently been introduced to supplement the rigid instrument as a screening tool for colorectal cancer. It has one primary advantage: more proximal evaluation of the bowel. It must be remembered, however, that the rectal ampulla is better evaluated by the rigid sigmoidoscope than by the fiberoptic instrument. Also, the examiner must be wary of performing such procedures as biopsy-cautery and snare excision with the fiberoptic instrument with an inadequately prepared colon. With the limited preparation required for fiberoptic sigmoidoscopy, the risk of explosion with the use of electrical equipment for tumor biopsy or removal is very real.

Total *colonoscopy* as a screening technique cannot be justified in the asymptomatic patient who is not in a high-risk group. It usually requires sedation and is not without complication (*e.g.*, a perforation rate of 0.1% to 0.5%).

Colonoscopy has been of demonstrated value in the patient with a known neoplasm in identifying the presence of a synchronous tumor (see Color Fig. 10-1). Barium enema, of course, serves the same purpose. Herbst and associates, in a retrospective study of 55 patients, found that nine (16%) harbored another lesion.[136] This discovery caused the operation to be modified.

Since most symptomatic patients undergo proctosigmoidoscopy and barium enema sequentially, Winawer suggests that the colonoscope may be used if small to moderate tumors are present, because it can usually pass the lesion.[284] He also believes that the procedure is more valuable for right colon, known primary lesions; the yield is higher and the distal bowel can be more easily examined. Two to eight percent of patients will have a synchronous carcinoma elsewhere in the colon.[208, 225] Furthermore, when polyps are present, the risk is even higher. Perhaps as many as 50% of colon cancer patients will harbor one or more colon polyps.[208] In the report of Reilly and associates, 7.6 percent of 92 patients had a synchronous cancer.[225] All were missed on barium enema examination, and none was more advanced than the index lesion. These studies confirm what has long been suspected: often the metachronous tumor really represents the missed synchronous one.

Gilbertsen and co-workers believe that *barium enema examination* is not sufficiently reliable in evaluating pa-

tients for suspected colorectal cancer and have abandoned the routine use of this modality in favor of colonoscopy in patients in whom a colorectal lesion is suspected.[89] They hold that often barium enema examination need not be performed if colonoscopy is diagnostic. I believe, however, that the studies are complementary and would rarely perform colonoscopy without the "road map" of a barium enema or air contrast enema.

Barium Enema and Air Contrast Enema Examination

The barium enema is the most commonly employed investigative study for evaluation of carcinoma of the large bowel. When it is performed in the presence of a known rectal carcinoma it should be done with great care (Fig. 10-1). After the procedure, the rectum must be cleansed vigorously by multiple enemas to avoid the possibility of obstruction from inspissated barium.

Figure 10-2 demonstrates a typical apple-core lesion at the rectosigmoid juncture. This segment is fairly long; loss of the normal mucosal pattern occurs in the involved bowel, and characteristically the mucosa over-

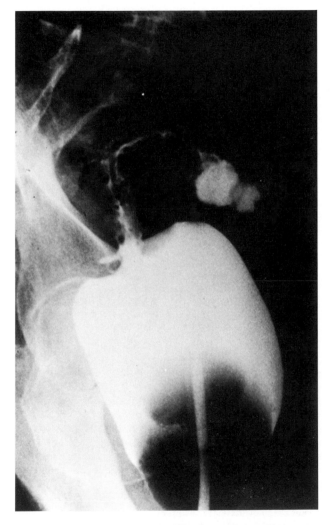

FIG. 10-1. Barium enema study of a patient with known rectal carcinoma invites the hazard of inspissated barium precipitating colonic obstruction. The physician must weigh the value of screening the proximal bowel against this risk. (Corman ML, Veidenheimer MC, Swinton NW: Diseases of the Anus, Rectum and Colon. Part I: Neoplasms. New York, Medcom, 1972)

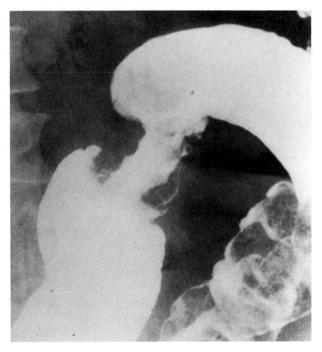

FIG. 10-2. Apple-core carcinoma at the rectosigmoid juncture. (Corman ML, Veidenheimer MC, Swinton NW: Diseases of the Anus, Rectum and Colon. Part I: Neoplasms. New York, Medcom, 1972)

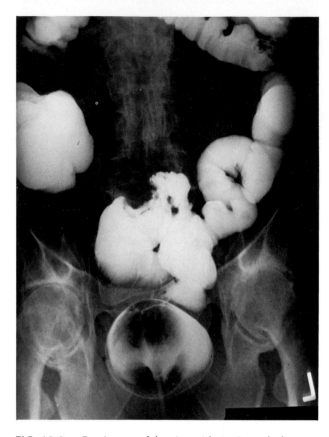

FIG. 10-3. Carcinoma of the sigmoid. An irregularly marginated mass projecting into the lumen of the colon shows the characteristic shoulders of a malignancy.

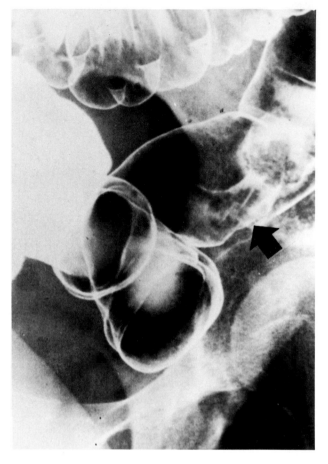

FIG. 10-4. The presence of a pedicle *(arrow)* does not exclude carcinoma. This lesion was entirely malignant. (Corman ML, Veidenheimer MC, Swinton NW: Diseases of the Anus, Rectum and Colon. Part I: Neoplasms. New York, Medcom, 1972)

hangs the lesion. Another frequently seen appearance of carcinoma of the sigmoid is shown in Figure 10-3.

The presence of a pedicle (as seen in Fig. 10-4) does not rule out the diagnosis of carcinoma. In fact, the illustration shows a polypoid carcinoma on a stalk measuring more than 2 cm in length. The radiologist is not in a position to recommend whether a polyp is benign or malignant.

Barium enema study (Fig. 10-5) reveals complete retrograde obstruction at the level of the midsigmoid colon. Retrograde obstruction, although an impressive radiologic finding, is not necessarily indicative of antegrade obstruction. Occasionally, patients will report little change in bowel habits, even with this radiologic picture. The resected specimen is shown in Figure 10-6.

The barium enema study shown in Figure 10-7 demonstrates a carcinoma of the sigmoid colon with associated diverticular disease. Differentiating between these two conditions is often difficult. It is sometimes said that the presence of diverticula as seen in this patient excludes the diagnosis of carcinoma. This is certainly not true. A normal mucosal pattern usually is maintained in diverticular disease, whereas in carcinoma the mucosa is destroyed or the mucosal pattern lost. In some patients, however, it is impossible to distinguish between the two conditions, and resection must be performed to rule out malignancy.

Carcinoma of the sigmoid colon with perforation is shown in Figure 10-8. Under such circumstances differentiation between carcinoma and diverticular disease is extremely difficult. However, the mucosal destruction and the overhanging edges of the neoplasm indicate the presence of carcinoma. Another compli-

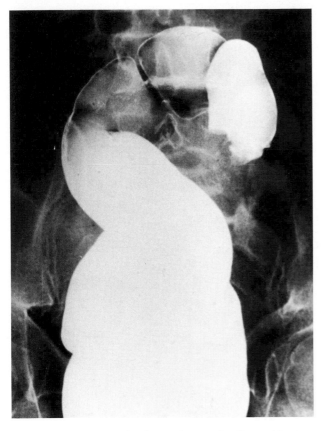

FIG. 10-5. Retrograde obstruction to the flow of barium from a carcinoma may or may not be associated with significant obstructive symptoms clinically. (Corman ML, Veidenheimer MC, Swinton NW: Diseases of the Anus, Rectum and Colon. Part I: Neoplasms. New York, Medcom, 1972)

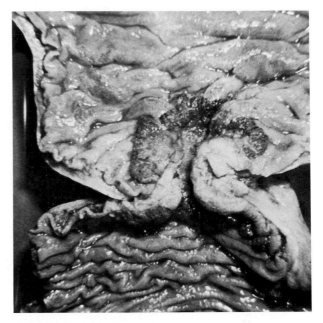

FIG. 10-6. String stricture: resected specimen of the carcinoma causing obstruction shown in Fig. 10-5. (Corman ML, Veidenheimer MC, Swinton NW: Diseases of the Anus, Rectum and Colon. Part I: Neoplasms. New York, Medcom, 1972)

cation of colon cancer is fistulization. Figure 10-9 demonstrates reflux of barium into the upper intestinal tract from a carcinoma near the hepatic flexure.

Figure 10-10 demonstrates a carcinoma involving one wall of the cecum in a patient who presented with anemia. Careful bowel preparation is necessary for evaluation of cecal tumors, because fecal matter frequently obscures this area.

Occult Blood Determination

The stool guaiac or orthotoluidine test has been the subject of a number of reports (see Chap. 1). Greegor studied patients with known asymptomatic colorectal cancers and found the presence of blood in at least one of three stool specimens.[106] Because of the relatively high false-positive rate, he recommended a diet that reduced this rate to approximately 1%. This diet is free of meat, fish, and chicken and relatively high in roughage (fiber) to stimulate bleeding from an existing lesion. Ostrow and associates studied healthy volunteers and found that the test slide preparation gave consistently positive results after the administration of 25 ml of blood and usually gave positive results with only 10 ml.[207]

In Gilbertsen's study guaiac testing revealed that cancer was responsible for positive test results in 5.1% of patients, and benign tumors in 24%, with no evidence of gastrointestinal neoplasm in 68%.[88] A more recent report from that center evaluated 48,000 asymptomatic patients over a period of approximately 4 years.[205] Invasive carcinoma was found in 113; over half of the tumors had not breached the bowel wall.

Although evaluation of a patient with a positive guaiac determination can be expensive (perhaps in excess of $1000), other pathologic entities, which may be of significance, are worth identifying.[37] While the cost versus the benefit of a massive screening program using occult blood testing is debatable, no one doubts the value of early diagnosis.[88, 283, 286] Scudamore

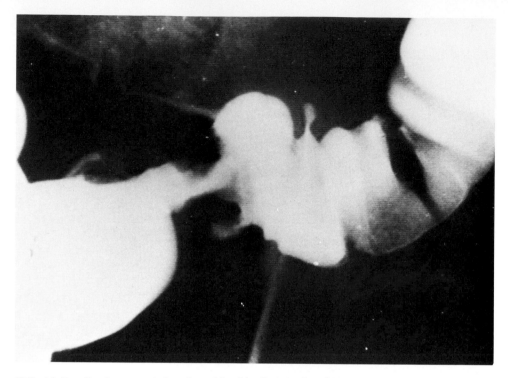

FIG. 10-7. Carcinoma of the sigmoid with diverticular disease. Because of the relative frequency of both conditions, this is not an uncommon picture. (Corman ML, Veidenheimer MC, Swinton NW: Diseases of the Anus, Rectum and Colon. Part I: Neoplasms. New York, Medcom, 1972)

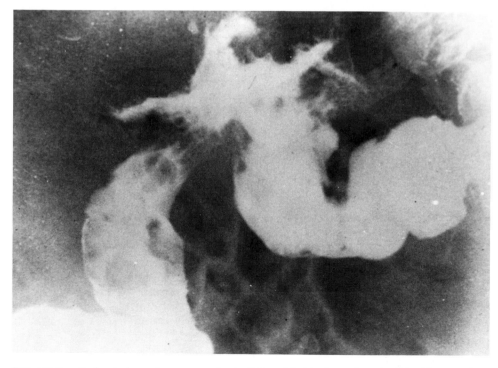

FIG. 10-8. Perforated carcinoma may be indistinguishable from diverticulitis. (Corman ML, Veidenheimer MC, Swinton NW: Diseases of the Anus, Rectum and Colon. Part I: Neoplasms. New York, Medcom, 1972)

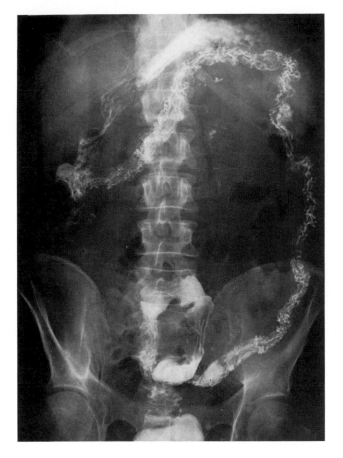

FIG. 10-9. Carcinoma with fistula. Note the reflux of barium into the duodenum and stomach through a fistula from an hepatic flexure lesion.

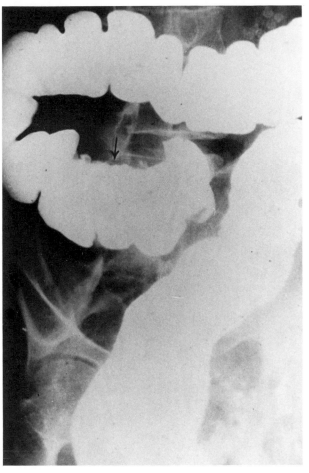

FIG. 10-10. Carcinoma of the cecum occupying one wall of the bowel *(arrow)*. (Corman ML, Veidenheimer MC, Swinton NW: Diseases of the Anus, Rectum and Colon. Part I: Neoplasms. New York, Medcom, 1972)

showed that when a patient has no gastrointestinal symptoms, a 100% possibility of curative resection can be expected with an 88% 5-year survival.[239]

Cytology

Establishing the diagnosis of carcinoma of the colon by means of cytologic evaluation, lavaging the colon with saline solution, has been advocated (see Chap. 1).[218] Winawer and colleagues performed brush cytology and lavage on selected patients with colonic neoplasms.[285] They believed that brush cytology improved the yield of tissue diagnosis when combined with biopsy, but lavage cytology alone did not seem to be as useful.

Although I have had only limited experience with this technique, the addition of brushing or lavage ap-

pears relatively academic. When the lesion cannot be excised by the colonoscope, exploratory laparotomy and resection are advisable.

Carcinoembryonic Antigen

Attention to the immunologic aspects of bowel cancer has been stimulated by the findings of Gold and Freedman; they identified an antigen in extracts from colon cancer tissue.[94, 95] This antigen, a glycoprotein absent from normal adult intestinal mucosa but present in primitive endoderm, was therefore called carcinoembryonic antigen (CEA). Thomson and associates described a radioimmunoassay for CEA in the serum.[263]

They reported positive results in 97% of patients with colon cancer in their series. However, the high accuracy of CEA as a diagnostic test for bowel cancer that was reported in earlier papers apparently resulted from the fact that most of the patients studied had advanced disease with extensive metastases. In such patients CEA was not only frequently detected but was present at very high levels in the blood, especially when the liver was involved. However, in cancer localized to the mucosa and submucosa, without invasion into the muscularis propria, the percentage of positive tests falls to between 30% and 40%. Even when recurrence is confined to the bowel wall, the results of the test are usually negative. Therefore, the use of CEA as a screening technique for the asymptomatic population is not justified.[93, 135, 226]

However, levels of CEA can be applied usefully in the prognosis of patients with colorectal cancer. If the tumor has been completely excised, the elevated level of the antigen should return to normal within a few days. A limited fall to an intermediate, albeit elevated, level is indicative of incomplete excision. Subsequent elevation after return to normal implies recurrence of tumor.

The preoperative CEA level in and of itself has some prognostic significance. Patients with localized disease (as evaluated by clinical methods) have a higher recurrence rate when a high preoperative CEA level is noted than when the preoperative level is low. Such an elevation may be suggestive of inapparent spread of the tumor.

Carcinoembryonic antigen is of limited value in the search for a primary site if metastatic carcinoma is noted. The antigen is detected in about 50% of tumors of the breast, stomach, and lung and other solid tumors. Levels above normal have also been found in heavy smokers and in patients with cirrhosis, pancreatitis, uremia, peptic ulcer, intestinal metaplasia of the stomach, and ulcerative colitis. The antigen has been reported in tissue of intestinal polyps, colonic inflammatory mucosa, and normal intestinal mucosa of children. Carcinoembryonic antigen has also been found in cancerous tissue from the breast, liver, and lung, as well as in body fluids exposed to cancer. In colonic washings, high levels of CEA were found in patients with colon cancer and colon polyps, intermediate levels in those with ulcerative colitis, and lower levels in normal subjects.[282]

A more recent modification of the CEA assay involves the use of radiolabeled antibodies to the antigen followed by an external photoscan.[96–98] Goldenberg and co-workers evaluated 50 patients by injecting ^{131}I-labeled antibody against CEA and performing total-body scans.[97] In this study 83% of the patients evaluated preoperatively and approximately 90% postoperatively were found to have the tumors correctly localized. The authors conclude that among other potential benefits this technique can help to stage the tumor preoperatively and complement other methods used to assess tumor response to therapy.

Although I use the CEA determination preoperatively in all patients diagnosed as having carcinoma of the colon or rectum, I have found it of limited value. At the present time the primary application of the determination is in the postoperative patient, when increasing values suggest recurrence and persistently normal values suggest absence of recurrence (see Follow-Up Evaluation).

Leukocyte Adherence Inhibition

The leukocyte adherence inhibition (LAI) assay is an *in vitro* test that is based on the observation that leukocytes from cancer patients following incubation with tumor extracts from the same organ lose their ability to adhere to glass surfaces.[13] Reports have demonstrated relatively consistent identification of malignant processes.[114, 260, 265, 264] However, lack of specificity for localization of the growth and inconsistencies in the performance of the technique itself relegate the procedure at this time to that of a research tool.

PATHOLOGY

By far the commonest malignant lesion in the colon and rectum is adenocarcinoma. The tumor arises from the glandular epithelium. It can invade microscopic blood vessels and metastasize to distant organs, most commonly the liver. It can spread by way of the lymphatics to regional lymph nodes and ultimately pass into the systemic circulation. It can extend locally into adjacent organs.

Histologically, the cancer may appear well differentiated (Fig. 10-11), moderately differentiated (Fig. 10-12), or poorly differentiated (Fig. 10-13). The tumor may produce so much mucin that the nucleus is pushed to one side of the cell, creating a signet ring appearance (Fig. 10-14).

Macroscopically, the tumor can display a number of forms (Figs. 10-15 to 10-22). Generally, the more poorly differentiated tumors are more invasive at the time of diagnosis; the more invasive the tumor, the poorer the prognosis.

(Text continues on p. 282)

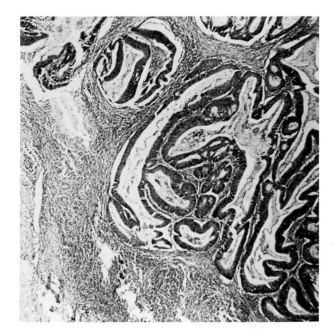

FIG. 10-11. Well-differentiated adenocarcinoma. The neoplastic glands display somewhat oriented epithelium and resemble crypts in their overall architecture. (Original magnification × 250. Courtesy of Rudolf Garret, M.D.)

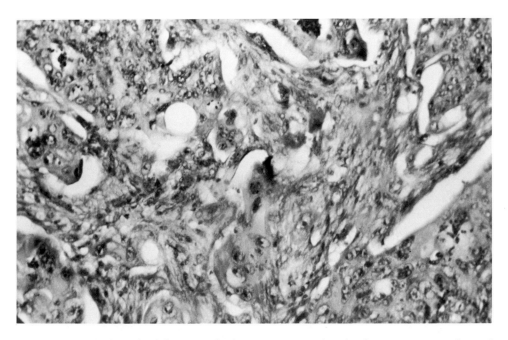

FIG. 10-12. Moderately differentiated adenocarcinoma. The glands are more irregular and exhibit less orientation of the epithelium. (Original magnification × 250. Courtesy of Rudolf Garret, M.D.)

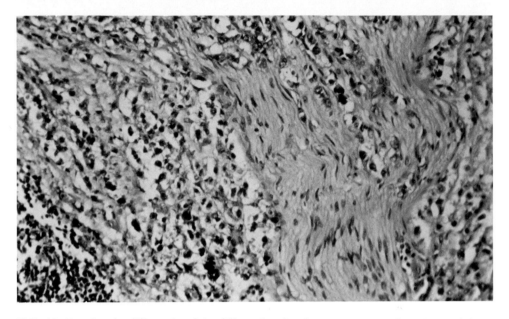

FIG. 10-13. Poorly differentiated (undifferentiated) adenocarcinoma. There is no definite formation of glands. (Original magnification × 250. Courtesy of Rudolf Garret, M.D.)

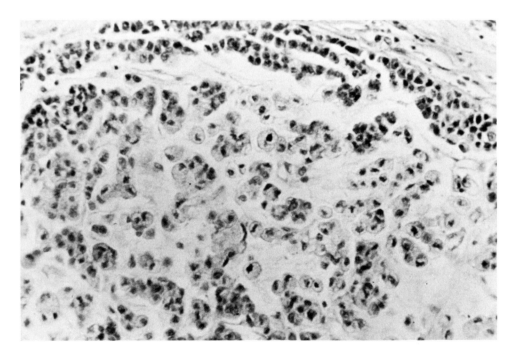

FIG. 10-14. Signet ring carcinoma. In this highly malignant variant, mucin displaces the nucleus to one side. This is occasionally seen in right-sided lesions and when carcinoma arises in ulcerative colitis. (Original magnification × 600. Corman ML, Veidenheimer MC, Swinton NW: Diseases of the Anus, Rectum and Colon. Part I: Neoplasms. New York, Medcom, 1972)

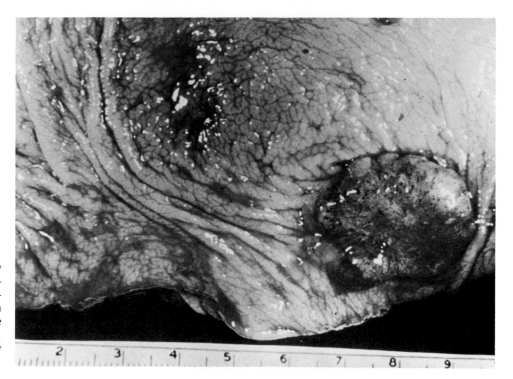

FIG. 10-15. Relatively small polypoid carcinoma. (Corman ML, Veidenheimer MC, Swinton NW: Diseases of the Anus, Rectum and Colon. Part I: Neoplasms. New York, Medcom, 1972)

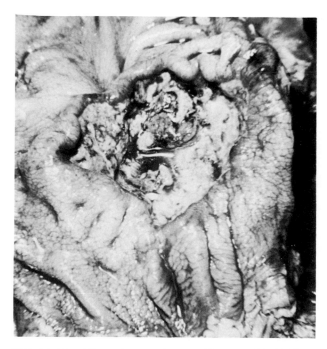

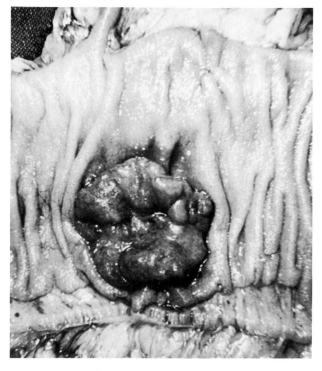

FIG. 10-16. Ulcerating carcinoma. (Corman ML, Veidenheimer MC, Swinton NW: Diseases of the Anus, Rectum and Colon. Part I: Neoplasms. New York, Medcom, 1972)

FIG. 10-17. Polypoid carcinoma with ulceration. (Corman ML, Veidenheimer MC, Swinton NW: Diseases of the Anus, Rectum and Colon. Part I: Neoplasms. New York, Medcom, 1972)

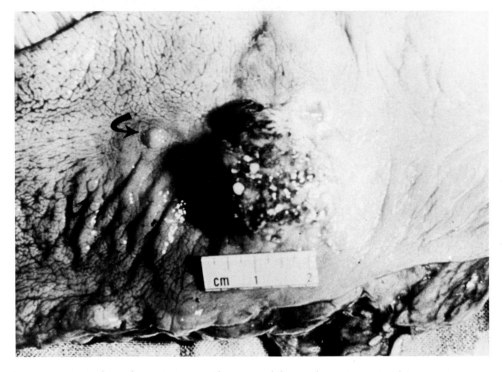

FIG. 10-18. Polypoid carcinoma with mucosal hyperplasia *(arrow)*. This association is commonly seen. (Corman ML, Veidenheimer MC, Swinton NW: Diseases of the Anus, Rectum and Colon. Part I: Neoplasms. New York, Medcom, 1972)

Carcinomas of the colon and rectum are relatively slow-growing tumors. Symptoms usually appear early in the development of the disease, and metastases occur relatively late. Tumor growth and spread are subject to considerable variation, owing partly to histologic grading (based on cellular arrangement and differentiation), increased ameboid action of some cancer cells, such enzymes as hyaluronidase, decreased adhesiveness of the tumor cells, size of the lesion at the primary site, and the length of time the lesion has been present.[109, 258] Additional variables include location of the tumor, indeterminate host factors, manipulation at surgery, and the age and sex of the person.[10, 44, 70, 138, 236]

The first opportunity to measure the growth of colonic cancer at its site of origin was reported in 1961 by Spratt and Ackerman.[252] In this study, nine air contrast enemas were performed over a period of 7.5 years.[251] Radiographic measurements of the tumor were taken, and by appropriate plotting on a graph the growth curve was shown to conform to an exponential increase in volume. The tumor was calculated to have a doubling time of 636.5 days. When desquamation from the surface was taken into account it was postulated that a net increase of only 1 cell per 1000 cells a

day was adequate to account for the observed rate of growth. Further observation of radiographic studies on other patients confirmed these findings.

Doubling time of pulmonary metastases from colon and rectal carcinomas has been calculated radiographically and found to be 109 days.[250] Metastatic tumors increase their cellular complement six times faster than primary cancers.[251] It is theorized that the absence of desquamation in the metastatic site accounts for this observed difference.

The metastatic behavior of neoplasms varies. According to Spratt, examination of the cancer–host interface is helpful in determining the behavioral pattern of the tumor. A tumor that is less likely to metastasize exhibits a well-circumscribed, intact margin; the tumor that is more likely to metastasize to lymph nodes has a loose or infiltrating margin with little inflammatory reaction.

The importance of tumor invasion and its prognostic implications was postulated by Dukes in 1930 and subsequently revised by him in 1932.[64, 65] This has come to be known as Dukes' classification; it was originally directed toward rectal cancer (Table 10-1). After performing numerous meticulous dissections of resected

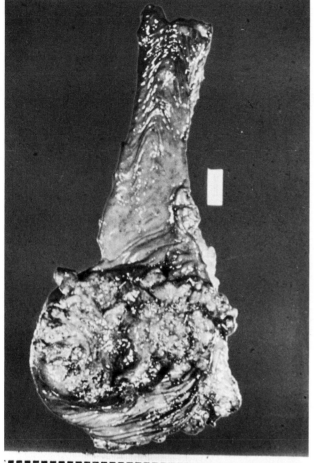

FIG. 10-19. Large polypoid carcinoma. Despite its size, the prognosis is better with this tumor than with a smaller invasive lesion. (Corman ML, Veidenheimer MC, Swinton NW: Diseases of the Anus, Rectum and Colon. Part I: Neoplasms. New York, Medcom, 1972)

Table 10-1. Dukes' Classification of Rectal Cancer (1932)

Stage	Classification
A	Carcinoma limited to wall of rectum
B	Carcinoma spread by direct continuity to extrarectal tissues; no lymph node metastases
C	Metastases present in regional lymph nodes

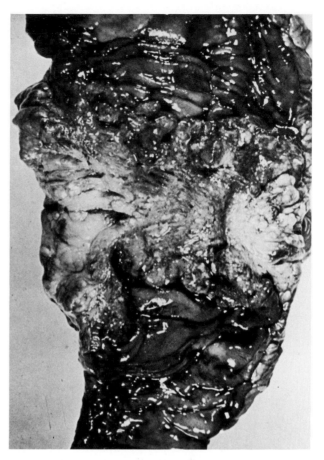

FIG. 10-20. Scirrhous or infiltrating carcinoma is associated with a poor prognosis. (Corman ML, Veidenheimer MC, Swinton NW: Diseases of the Anus, Rectum and Colon. Part I: Neoplasms. New York, Medcom, 1972)

specimens to identify metastases to lymph nodes, Dukes further modified his classification in 1944.[66] Those tumors with lymph node involvement but with a negative node at the ligation of the inferior mesenteric artery he called C_1. Lesions classified C_2 had metastases to the node at the level of the ligature (Table 10-2).

Table 10-2. Dukes' Classification of Rectal Cancer (1944)

Stage	Classification
A	Carcinoma confined to wall of rectum
B	Carcinoma spread by direct continuity to perirectal tissue; no lymph node metastasis
C_1	Metastasis present in nodes but not to ligature
C_2	Metastasis present in nodes to level of ligature

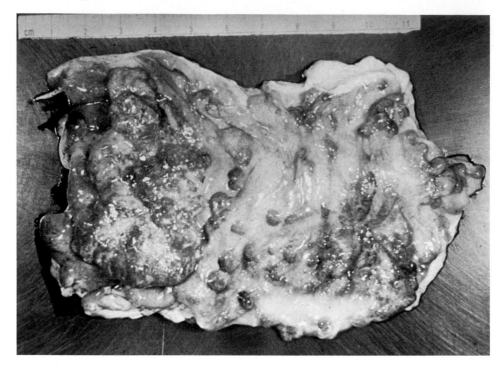

FIG. 10-21. Colloid carcinoma. Prognosis is poor with this variant of carcinoma. Note the gelatinous appearance. (Corman ML, Veidenheimer MC, Swinton NW: Diseases of the Anus, Rectum and Colon. Part I: Neoplasms. New York, Medcom, 1972)

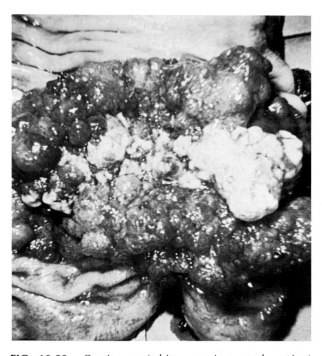

FIG. 10-22. Carcinoma *(white area in central portion)* arising in villous adenoma. (Corman ML, Veidenheimer MC, Swinton NW: Diseases of the Anus, Rectum and Colon. Part I: Neoplasms. New York, Medcom, 1972)

Others have introduced their own classifications, expanding and subdividing Dukes' classification and broadening it to include colon cancer and disseminated metastases.[9, 115, 154, 269, 291] The addition of the D category has been fairly well accepted as representative of tumor beyond the reach of potential surgical curability (Table 10-3). Figure 10-23 illustrates the more popular staging systems. I agree with Goligher that the various classifications proposed can only create confusion and mislead the reader when interpreting the surgical results from one institution to another.[99] I believe that the clinicopathologic classification of Dukes fulfills the criteria for reasonable prognostication.

The importance of lymph node involvement by tumor has been well established.[85, 90, 105, 112] By special

Table 10-3. Clinicopathologic Classification of Colorectal Cancer (Modified Dukes')

Stage	Classification
A	Carcinoma confined to wall of bowel
B	Carcinoma spread by direct continuity to perirectal or pericolonic tissue; no lymph node metastasis
C	Metastasis present in regional lymph node
D	Omental implant; peritoneal seeding; metastasis beyond the confines of surgical resection

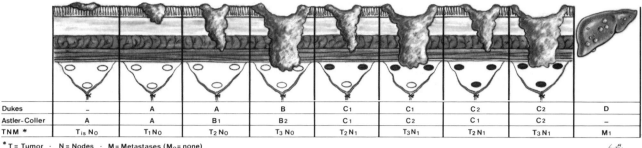

Dukes	–	A	A	B	C₁	C₁	C₂	C₂	D
Astler-Coller	A	A	B₁	B₂	C₁	C₂	C₁	C₂	–
TNM *	T$_{is}$N$_0$	T$_1$N$_0$	T$_2$N$_0$	T$_3$N$_0$	T$_2$N$_1$	T$_3$N$_1$	T$_2$N$_1$	T$_3$N$_1$	M$_1$

*T = Tumor · N = Nodes · M = Metastases (M$_0$= none)

FIG. 10-23.   Comparison of staging classifications for colorectal carcinoma.

clearing techniques a greater number of lymph nodes have been identified, thereby improving our ability to suggest prognosis.[112, 214] I have not routinely employed this approach but believe that if all laboratories vigorously pursued lymph node identification, greater consistency in reporting the results of treatment would be achieved.

Recently Tsakraklides and colleagues evaluated the histologic morphology of lymph nodes in an attempt to improve prognostic ability.[268] They found a higher rate of survival (which was not statistically significant) in patients whose nodes showed germinal center predominance compared with those whose nodes showed lymphocyte predominance, the "unstimulated pattern."

Compared with lymph node involvement the importance of blood vessel invasion (Fig. 10-24) has been emphasized to a much lesser extent.[25, 45, 75] However, the prognostic implication of blood vessel invasion is real[52] and has stimulated different approaches to the

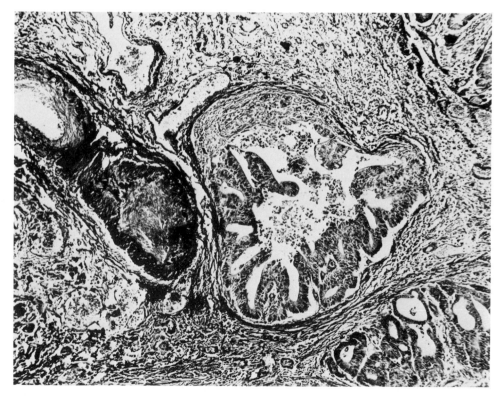

FIG. 10-24.   Blood vessel invasion by colonic adenocarcinoma. Note the extensive growth of tumor inside the vein that has thin, black elastica in its wall and fibrous thickening of the intima in the artery to the left. (Original magnification × 80. Corman ML, Swinton NW Sr, O'Keefe DD et al: Colorectal carcinoma at the Lahey Clinic, 1962–1966. Am J Surg 1973; 125:424–428)

technique of surgical removal of the lesion.[16, 75, 234, 269] The pathologist should seek to identify and report invasion of blood vessels with the same concern used to identify involvement of lymph nodes.

Colitis Proximal to a Partially Obstructing Carcinoma of the Colon

A nonspecific type of ulcerative colitis proximal to a partially obstructing carcinoma is an uncommon condition. It is a clinical and pathologic entity that must be distinguished from idiopathic ulcerative colitis from which a carcinoma may subsequently develop.[74, 232, 265, 280, 287] The colitis is invariably located proximal to the tumor with the bowel distal to the tumor normal. In almost all reported cases a short segment of normal mucosa separates the colitis from the tumor. The pathologic description of the colitis varies from involvement of the entire bowel wall with hemorrhagic necrosis to superficial mucosal ulcerations only.

The colitis is frequently unsuspected and discovered only at the time of surgery for the colonic tumor. Although often apparent from the macroscopic appearance of the proximal intestine and mesentery, the extent of the inflammatory process may not be fully appreciated until the bowel is opened. The extent of resection will be dictated not only by the requirement of an adequate cancer operation but also by the length of the inflamed bowel.

ANATOMIC DISTRIBUTION

A number of reports seem to show a change in the distribution of colorectal carcinoma.[1, 33, 107, 192] It had previously been thought that 75% of colorectal cancers were within the range of the proctosigmoidoscope. More recent data suggest that the figure should be closer to 60%.

Whether the trend in more proximal location of tumors will continue is impossible to say. Figure 10-25 illustrates the distribution of tumors based on our most recent 10-year report.[49] In the beginning and at the end of the decade we noted no change in the location of cancers. Rectal and sigmoid lesions together encompassed 67% in the previous 5-year study and 69% in the most recent report. Ascending colonic lesions were present in 18% of the patients in each group.

Cady and associates reviewed almost 6000 resected specimens of the large bowel that had been removed over a 40-year period (1928–1967).[33] During this time the incidence of cancer of the right colon increased from 7% to 22%, and the incidence of rectosigmoid, sigmoid, and rectal carcinomas fell from 80% to 62%. These changes represent statistically significant differences. A trend to smaller tumors was also evident, with less frequent lymph node involvement of the distal lesions, possibly reflecting an improvement in early detection.

SURGICAL TREATMENT

Historical Perspective

Resection of the bowel with intestinal anastomosis is a relatively recent operation. In 1818, Zang declared that "every intestinal suture is a mighty procedure in a highly vulnerable organ, and therefore a dangerous, yes, a very dangerous undertaking."[80] Exteriorization was the method of treatment for intestinal disease and injury, a technique which had remained essentially unchanged for over two millenia.

Reybard of Lyons (1833) was the first to perform a successful resection of the sigmoid colon; for this he was criticized by the Paris Academy of Medicine.[4] Colostomy was advocated as a palliative procedure as early as 1839. Before this time an occasional obstructing carcinoma of the colon was relieved by the spontaneous formation of a fecal fistula, if it were relieved at all. Before 1889 the mortality rate for colonic resection was 60%, but this figure had been reduced to 37% by 1900.[191] Because of the high mortality for intra-abdominal resection and anastomosis, the staged extraperitoneal operation was devised.[20, 211, 274]

The initial attempts to coapt ends of intestine involved insertion of various objects into the lumens of the cut ends of the bowel, with or without the addition of sutures. These procedures included the use of a reed pipe, goose trachea, cardboard smeared with sweet oil, a cylinder of fish glue, a wax ring, and a silver ring, to name a few.[80, 157] Perhaps the most famous internal stent was the Murphy "button" (Fig. 10-26).[194] Introduced in 1892, it quickly became the primary method of anastomosing bowel.

Travers (1812) is felt to have been the pioneer in the use of sutures to effect intestinal anastomoses.[267] Lembert (1826) is eponymously associated with a type of intestinal suturing that produces serosa-to-serosa apposition.[159] In 1887, Halsted reported an experimental study which demonstrated that the submucosa was the primary layer responsible for a safe and secure anastomosis.[125] This was confirmed in a subsequent report.[126] Later Connell described his continuous inverting suture.[211]

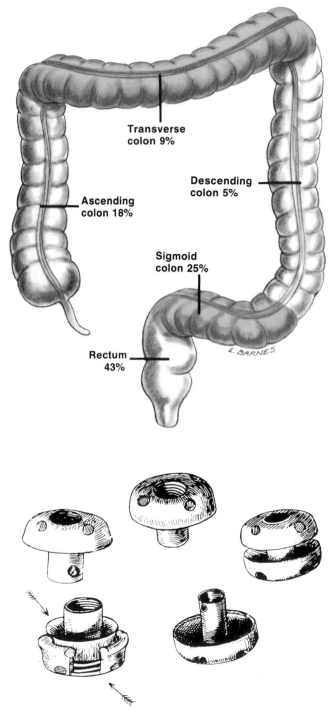

FIG. 10-25. Distribution of colon and rectal cancer.

Numerous articles have been written that address the means to avoid fecal contamination with bowel resection (closed anastomosis with noncrushing clamps, the use of rubber-shod clamps) and to avoid inverting too much tissue (*e.g.*, the Gambee suture[82]). To further complicate the issue, Getzen and associates advocated that eversion produced a more secure anastomosis than inversion.[84] Although this contention was initially supported by some studies,[36, 127, 134, 165] other reports refuted this observation[103, 230]; currently the eversion technique is in disfavor.

In the 20th century, resection of the colon with primary anastomosis did not become generally used until the antibiotic era. In fact, in many centers, resection of the sigmoid colon was not attempted without a diversionary colostomy until the 1950s.

Preoperative Preparation

For elective colonic resection patients are admitted to the hospital 2 days before surgery. The need for prolonged hospitalization to prepare the bowel is no longer

FIG. 10-26. Murphy button with and without spring cup attachment. (Murphy JB: Cholecysto-intestinal, gastro-intestinal and entero-intestinal anastomosis, and approximation without sutures. Med Rec NY 1892; 42:665–676)

necessary. Preparation consists of appropriate dietary restriction, mechanical cleansing, and antibiotics.

On the day of admission the patient is given a full liquid diet, and on the day before surgery, a clear liquid diet. The mechanical preparation begins at 4 P.M. the day before surgery. A vigorous cathartic is administered at this time so that its effect will have ended by early morning. The choice of laxative is often a matter of the surgeon's personal experience or prejudice, because when adjusted for dosage most laxatives have the same effect. Patients may prefer the taste of one to another or think that one causes less cramping than another. Castor oil (2 oz), magnesium citrate (10 oz), and X-Prep liquid (2.5 oz) are relatively equivalent in obtaining the desired results. Others prefer "whole-gut" irrigation (see Chap. 1).[131] More important than the cathartic, however, is colonic irrigation. I advise a tap-water enema until the returns are clear in the morning prior to surgery.

Nonabsorbable antibiotics are also administered. The regimen advocated by Nichols and co-workers has been successful.[200] This consists of neomycin (1 g) and erythromycin base (1 g) at 2 P.M., 3 P.M., and 10 P.M. the day before surgery. The use of a broad-spectrum systemic antibiotic immediately preoperatively, intraoperatively, and for one or two doses postoperatively may be advisable. However, Condon and associates, in a cooperative Veterans Administration study, demonstrated no discernible benefit from adding parenteral antibiotic prophylaxis in elective colon surgery if mechanical cleansing and neomycin and erythromycin are employed.[46] In the poorly prepared bowel, in the presence of obstruction, perforation, abscess, or fecal contamination, with a prolonged operative time, and with considerable blood loss, I believe that antibiotics should be continued beyond the first postoperative day. Any patient with valvular heart disease or a prosthetic heart valve also requires systemic antibiotic prophylaxis.

An integral part of the preoperative evaluation of the patient who is to undergo bowel surgery is preoperative *intravenous pyelography.* I have been impressed by the unexpected findings identified through the routine use of intravenous pyelography (see Tables 1-1 and 1-2). In our experience ureteral duplication was seen in 2.2% of patients, in addition to a number of other congenital anomalies and serendipitous findings.[216] Also, the course of the ureters and the presence of ureteral obstruction can be ascertained, and the postvoiding residual can be estimated. This latter information is important in patients who are to have extensive pelvic dissection. If one routinely employs preoperative intravenous pyelography, the likelihood of ureterovesical injury will be reduced.

The placement of *ureteral catheters* has been advised prior to colon resection. However, I limit their use to those patients who are to have reoperative pelvic surgery; otherwise, I do not use the catheters routinely. They may aid in identifying the ureters (by palpation), but care must be taken not to rely too much on them. The caution that the ureters should be sought and carefully dissected away from the area of the surgical extirpation should be heeded, regardless of the ease or difficulty of the dissection, or the presence or absence of ureteral catheters.

An indwelling *urinary catheter* is placed for all bowel operations. It may be removed the day after surgery if there has been no pelvic dissection. For an abdominoperineal resection or low pelvic operation, the urinary catheter should remain in place a minimum of 7 days.

Overnight *intravenous hydration* prior to surgery is advisable in any patient who might be prone to adverse cardiac or renal consequences of excessive fluid loss. Oral hydration during catharsis is also helpful.

Hyperalimentation has been advocated before operation for the nutritionally depleted patient in order to prepare for the assault on the patient's metabolic processes. Many patients with colorectal cancer have lost weight, are anemic and hypoalbuminemic, or have a variety of fluid and electrolyte problems. With the exception of weight loss, however, laboratory abnormalities can usually be corrected in 2 or 3 days of appropriate therapy. Delaying surgical intervention for a week or more to administer hyperalimentation is an expensive, time-consuming extravagance that has an associated morbidity. I am impressed by the salutary effects of surgery following the expeditious removal of disease. The patient can usually start a regular diet by the sixth postoperative day.

The routine use of a *nasogastric tube* is discouraged for colon resections. It does not protect the anastomosis and merely causes patient discomfort. Obviously, on a therapeutic basis (intestinal obstruction, postoperative vomiting), gastric drainage is usually required.

Other areas in the preoperative evaluation that might delay elective surgery or necessitate additional treatment include a history of corticosteroid therapy, hypoprothrombinemia, and the presence of cardiac, pulmonary, or renal disease.

Operative Technique

General Principles

As with all operations for carcinoma, the objective in surgical treatment of carcinoma of the colon is removal of the growth with an adequate margin, including the associated vascular pedicle and lymph-bearing structures. All colon surgery should be performed through a midline incision; this permits ready access to both sides of the abdomen and allows rapid entry into the peritoneal cavity. Furthermore, it leaves both sides of the abdomen free should a colostomy or ileostomy be required. The wounds heal strongly and are easily closed in a single layer.

A self-retaining (Balfour) retractor is inserted for retraction of the abdominal wall; I no longer use a wound protector. The abdominal contents are examined carefully for the presence of metastatic disease and for any other incidental lesion.

The tumor itself is examined last. It is important to determine whether the tumor is freely movable or fixed, whether sepsis or perforation is present, whether the mesentery is invaded by tumor, whether seeding of the peritoneal cavity has occurred, and, of course, whether metastatic disease is present. It is often difficult to determine by inspection whether lymph nodes contain tumor or are uninvolved. Large, firm nodes may prove to be inflammatory when examined under the microscope.

Resection for colon cancer consists of wide excision of the tumor-bearing area with attention to the blood supply to that segment (Fig. 10-27), removal of the associated lymph-bearing area, and performing an anastomosis without tension.

For *wound closure*, I prefer a single layer of interrupted long-term absorbable sutures (Dexon or Vicryl), placed through all layers except the skin. In a controlled trial of three different suture materials for abdominal wound closure (a nonabsorbable monofilament suture, a nonabsorbable multifilament suture, and a long-term absorbable suture) no statistically significant difference was seen in the incidence of wound infection, wound dehiscence, and incisional hernia.[50]

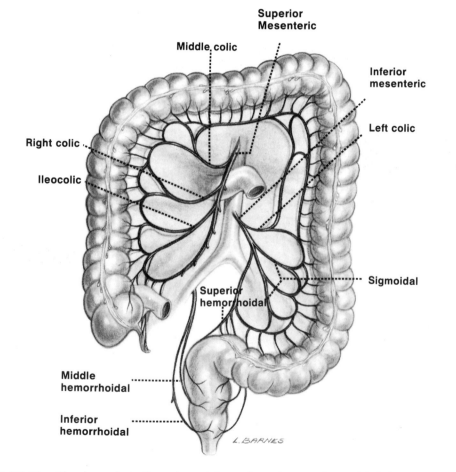

FIG. 10-27.   Blood supply to the colon originates from the superior and inferior mesenteric arteries.

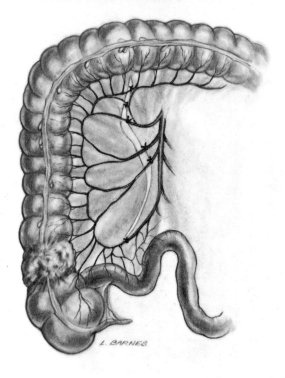

L. BARNES

FIG. 10-28. Right hemicolectomy. Early ligation of the vascular supply to the right colon is illustrated.

It was felt that closure of the abdominal wall with long-term absorbable suture is the preferred method. Needless to say, other surgeons involved in other trials concluded that different materials and methods are preferred.[101, 178, 227]

The operations that are generally employed for cancer above the rectum include right colectomy, transverse colectomy, left colectomy, sigmoid colectomy, high anterior resection, subtotal colectomy, and total colectomy. Other more limited resections are occasionally undertaken for palliation, but these usually should be condemned because of the problems of inadequate blood supply, insufficient mesenteric removal, and tension on the anastomosis.

Right Hemicolectomy

Lesions of the cecum, ascending colon, and hepatic flexure usually are treated by right hemicolectomy since the blood supply to this area comes from the ileocolic and right colic arteries. Because the most difficult aspect of the dissection is usually at the hepatic flexure, the incision should be relatively higher in the

epigastrium rather than low in the hypogastrium. The dissection is expedited if the surgeon stands on the patient's left side. Resectability of the tumor is evaluated with a minimum of manipulation. The small bowel is packed into the left half of the abdominal cavity, and the root of the mesentery and the base of the transverse mesocolon are exposed. Many surgeons ligate the right colic and right branch of the middle colic arteries and veins as the initial maneuver (Fig. 10-28). This procedure is not difficult unless the patient is obese, in which case preliminary ligation of the blood vessels may not be safe. The small incision in the root of the mesentery required for this preliminary main trunk ligation is now extended to the point on the transverse colon and ileum where division of the bowel is to take place. The vessels in the mesentery and mesocolon are ligated; the entire blood supply to the tumor is divided before any handling of the bowel itself.

Although I am not an advocate of the no-touch technique (see later), it certainly makes sense not to manipulate the bowel or handle the tumor unnecessarily. However, I believe that one may still adhere to this principle and yet expedite the operation by initially mobilizing the colon. The terminal ileum and right colon are elevated from the retroperitoneal structures by dividing the peritoneum along the lateral gutter (Fig. 10-29). Included in the resected specimen is any lateral and posterior peritoneum involved by serosal tumor. Care must be taken to avoid injury to the ureter, spermatic or ovarian vessels, and inferior vena cava.

The next structure of concern is the second portion of the duodenum. This must be displaced carefully as the colon is freed from its retroperitoneal attachments. The developmental adhesions from the gall bladder and liver to the hepatic flexure are incised. When the head of the pancreas is in view (Fig. 10-30), the duodenum is sufficiently clear from the dissection so that clamping of the blood supply can be accomplished with safety. This can be performed by passing the hand around the vessels in the avascular plane (Fig. 10-31).

It is often advisable to enter the lesser sac, dividing the gastrocolic omentum as far to the left as possible. This maneuver expedites entrance into the sac and permits the posterior wall of the stomach to be dropped away. The remainder of the gastrocolic omentum is then divided until the hepatic flexure is no longer tethered. The omentum is incised longitudinally to the point where the anastomosis will be performed. With all the blood supply divided to the segment, the bowel is resected, leaving the ends open that are to be anastomosed (Fig. 10-32).

Occasionally, discrepancy exists in the size of the lumen between the ileum and the transverse colon, the latter being considerably larger. Under such circum-

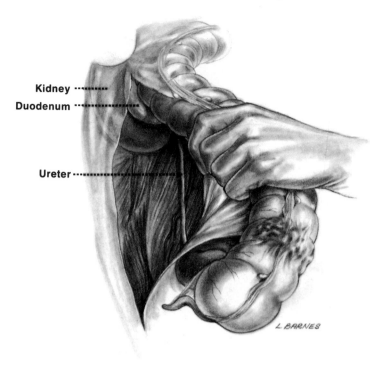

Kidney ....
Duodenum ....

Ureter ....

FIG. 10-29. Right hemicolectomy. The dissection proceeds along the right paracolic gutter, and the retroperitoneal structures are identified and preserved.

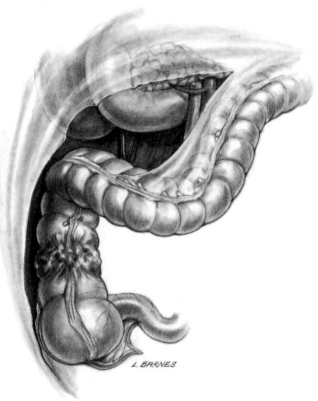

FIG. 10-30. Right hemicolectomy. The hepatic flexure is mobilized, exposing the duodenum and the head of the pancreas.

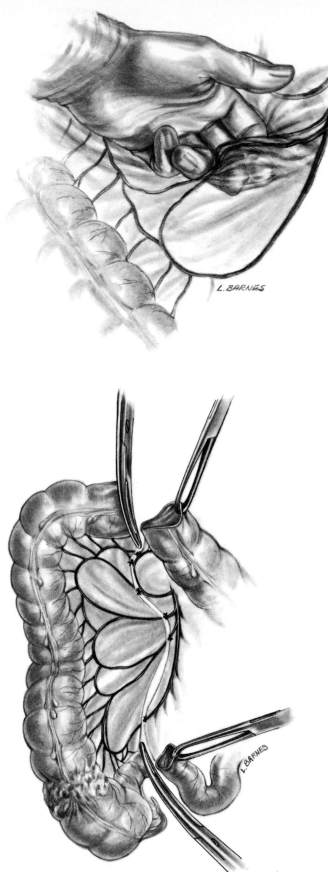

FIG. 10-31. Right hemicolectomy: technique of identification and manual isolation of major blood supply to right colon.

FIG. 10-32. Right hemicolectomy. After ligation of the vascular supply and mobilization of the bowel, crushing clamps are applied to the ileum and transverse colon, and the bowel is divided with a scalpel, leaving the ends open for anastomosis.

stances it is usually advisable to make a Cheatle cut into the antimesenteric portion of the ileum to avoid this discrepancy (Fig. 10-33, *A*). I do not advocate a side-to-end anastomosis for lesions of the right colon.

All colonic anastomoses should be performed by the interrupted inverting technique (Fig. 10-33). Small bites of the mucosa are taken with a relatively deeper passage through the seromuscular layer. Although the submucosal layer is the most important, there is very little consequence of incorporating a small amount of mucosa. The use of a second row of seromuscular sutures is not advised; it adds nothing to the security of the anastomosis, and only inverts more tissue, thereby narrowing the lumen. Anastomosis is effected with a single layer of interrupted 3-0 Dexon or Vicryl sutures. Prolene and wire are tedious to tie, and the braided sutures create more tissue reaction and can serve as a nidus for sepsis. Catgut is acceptable, but objectively has no advantage over one of the long-term absorbable sutures. Some differences of opinion exist over choice of suture material and technique (whether a single or double layer is preferable); few surgeons disagree, however, that an interrupted, inverting approach is the proper one for all colonic anastomoses.

After a satisfactory anastomosis has been secured, the mesenteric defect is closed with either an interrupted or continuous technique. This prevents herniation of small bowel through the defect in the mesentery. It is also useful to wrap omentum around all colonic anastomoses to protect further against leakage.

Surgery for Carcinoma of the Transverse Colon

Carcinoma of the transverse colon often presents a challenge in the choice of operative procedure. The blood supply to this area is derived from the middle colic artery as well as the right and left colic vessels. Anastomosis in the region of the splenic flexure poses some risk for compromise of the blood supply to the bowel, because with the middle colic artery divided the blood supply must come from the inferior mesenteric artery. In the region of the hepatic flexure, however, blood supply is not usually a problem because of the ileocolic and right colic vessels.

In addition to the concerns about blood supply with anastomoses in the transverse colon, another problem is the lymph-bearing area. A carcinoma in this area can spread to regional lymphatics through the middle colic, right colic, and left colic branches. Because of this it has been advocated that subtotal colectomy be performed.

My own philosophy for removing carcinomas of the transverse colon depends on the location of the tumor. For proximal lesions, right hemicolectomy is advised;

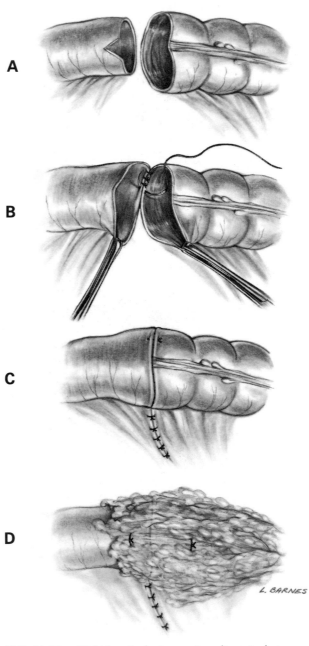

A

B

C

D

L. BARNES

FIG. 10-33.   Right hemicolectomy. Any disparity between the luminal ends can be corrected by dividing the smaller segment of bowel along its antimesenteric border (**A**). The anastomosis is accomplished using a single layer of interrupted sutures (**B**). Note the single mattress suture used to effect final closure. The rent in the mesentery is closed (**C**). Omentum is placed around the anastomosis (**D**).

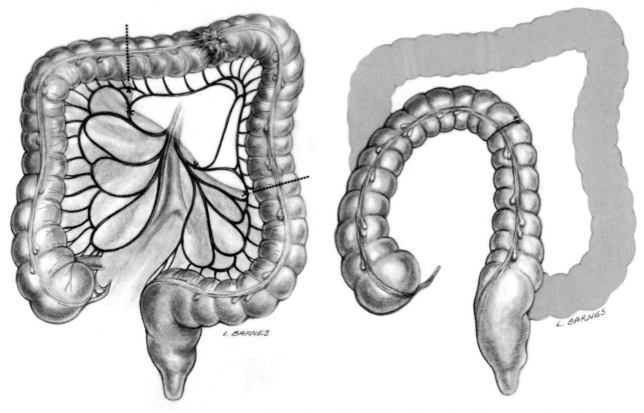

FIG. 10-34. Left partial colectomy. Tumors of the left portion of the transverse colon require resection of the descending colon to obtain a safe anastomosis while removing lymphatic drainage areas.

FIG. 10-35. Left partial colectomy. Anastomosis between the midtransverse colon and the upper sigmoid is usually possible without difficulty, except in the very obese patient.

for distal lesions, left partial colectomy (Fig. 10-34), with anastomosis of the transverse colon to the upper sigmoid (Fig. 10-35); and for lesions of the midtransverse colon, limited transverse colectomy. However, if tension or technical difficulty prevents a safe anastomosis between the proximal and distal transverse colon (Fig. 10-36), subtotal or total colectomy and ileosigmoid or ileorectal anastomosis are suggested. The danger of too much tension on a transverse colon anastomosis is illustrated in Figure 10-37.

Tumors of the splenic flexure usually are not amenable to wide excision unless the spleen and tail of the pancreas are removed. Retroperitoneal extension of tumor can also involve the left kidney and suprarenal areas.

Mobilization of the splenic flexure is facilitated by, first, division of the gastrocolic omentum to within a few centimeters of the flexure, and, second, by incision

of the lateral peritoneal attachments along the descending colon (Fig. 10-38). As the splenic flexure is approached, the spleen is seen and the lienocolic ligament divided (Fig. 10-39). Only one clamp should be used in order to avoid tearing the splenic capsule. The splenic flexure is delivered into the wound, and any back-bleeding can be clamped at this point without concern about injury to the spleen (Fig. 10-40). The technique of anastomosis does not differ from that already described.

When the tumor invades upward and perhaps even into the spleen, it is necessary to perform a splenectomy. Removal of the spleen in conjunction with a colonic anastomosis is associated with a high morbidity (Fig. 10-41). Drains should not be used except in the presence of sepsis or obvious contamination. Under such circumstances a sump suction drain is employed for 5 to 7 days.

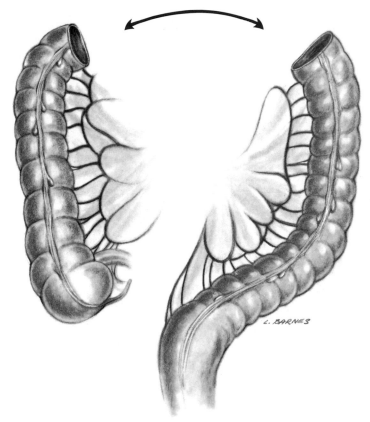

FIG. 10-36. Transverse colon resection. Anastomosis may not be feasible because of tension.

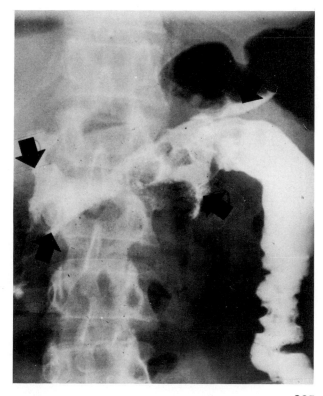

FIG. 10-37. Anastomotic leak *(arrows)* demonstrated on postoperative barium enema study, 2 weeks after transverse colectomy for carcinoma. At the second operation the ends of the bowel were found to have separated completely.

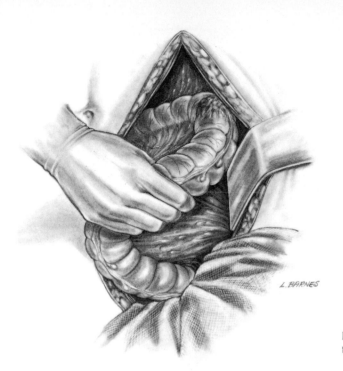

FIG. 10-38. Mobilization of the splenic flexure is facilitated by freeing the descending colon.

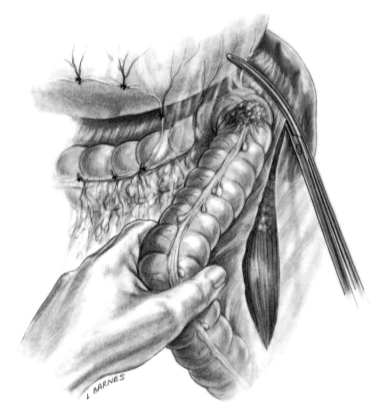

FIG. 10-39. The lienocolic ligament is divided. Back-bleeding can be dealt with as the splenic flexure is brought into the wound.

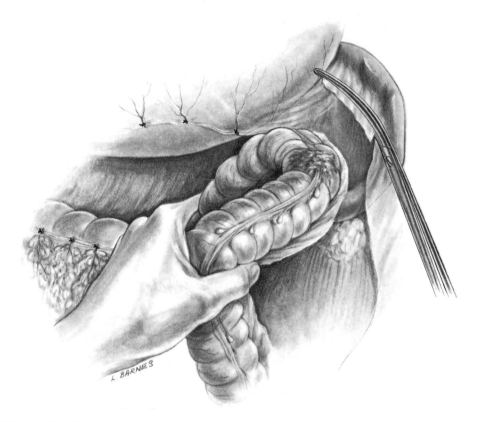

FIG. 10-40.   With traction on the transverse colon and descending colon, the splenic flexure is delivered from its retroperitoneal attachment.

Left Partial Colectomy

Left partial colectomy is the operation of choice for tumors involving the distal transverse colon, splenic flexure, and descending colon. The left branch of the middle colic artery should be intact proximally; the left colic artery is ligated, care being taken to preserve the inferior mesenteric artery (Fig. 10-42). The anastomosis is effected between the midtransverse colon and the upper sigmoid. In most instances sufficient redundancy of the sigmoid colon is present to permit an anastomosis without tension. Occasionally, with an obese patient or with someone who has undergone resection previously, such an anastomosis is not possible. Under these circumstances total or subtotal colectomy is recommended.

Sigmoid Colectomy and High Anterior Resection (Anastomosis into the Upper Rectum)

Removal of the sigmoid colon for carcinoma is the standard operation for tumors in this location. With respect to blood supply, the operation preserves the left colic artery, dividing only the sigmoidal branches of the inferior mesenteric artery (IMA). Some surgeons stress the importance of high ligation of the IMA (on the aorta). However, if a node at this level harbors cancer, the chance for cure is very remote indeed. Viability of the distal bowel should present no problem because of the usually excellent blood supply from the middle hemorrhoidal arteries and the lower sigmoidal vessels. The proximal blood supply is usually adequate by way of the left colic artery. It is my belief that left hemicolectomy is rarely justified for a sigmoid lesion. The additional dissection necessary, the possibility of injury to the spleen, and the technical difficulty associated with a transverse colorectal anastomosis all militate against this approach.

In mobilization of the sigmoid colon a great concern is to avoid trauma to the left ureter. Most injuries to this structure take place at the level of the iliac vessels. The left ureter is bluntly dissected laterally, displacing it from the area of resection (Fig. 10-43). The surgeon's left hand is passed beneath the inferior mesenteric ves-

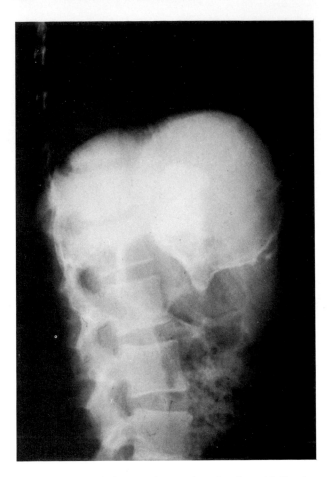

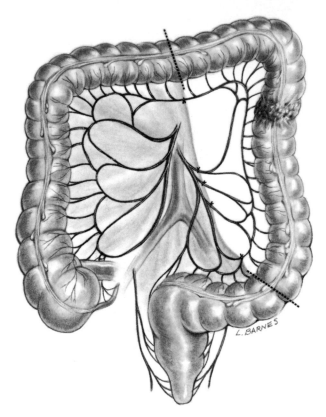

FIG. 10-42. Left partial colectomy: areas of resection for descending colon lesion preserving sigmoid and rectal vessels.

FIG. 10-41. Subphrenic abscess that developed following colectomy and splenectomy.

sels, and the peritoneum is incised on the right side (Fig. 10-44). The left hand is then withdrawn and passed beneath the vessels and through the defect between the left colic artery and the sigmoidal vessels (Fig. 10-45). The inferior mesenteric vessels are cross-clamped, divided, and ligated, and the arcade vessels to the upper sigmoid are divided. Rather than perform an anastomosis between the upper sigmoid and lower sigmoid (because of a potential problem with distal blood supply) I prefer a high anterior resection, anastomosing the bowel to the upper rectum at or just below the peritoneal reflection. For distal sigmoid lesions it may be necessary to mobilize the rectum slightly and preserve a portion of proximal sigmoid to effect a safe anastomosis without tension. Conversely, for proximal sigmoid lesions I prefer to preserve the

distal sigmoid and perform an anastomosis between the lower descending colon and the distal sigmoid colon rather than mobilize the splenic flexure to obtain desired length.

The technique that many surgeons use for dividing the mesorectum is unnecessarily nitpicking. A right-angle clamp is placed into the mesorectum; by exerting vigorous proximal traction the mesentery is divided (Fig. 10-46). This maneuver effectively strips the bowel in preparation for the anastomosis.

Left Hemicolectomy

Left hemicolectomy should rarely be performed for left colon lesions. I do not believe that the potential advantage of radical removal of the lymphatics justifies the risks of splenic injury, prolonged operative time, and tension on the anastomosis.

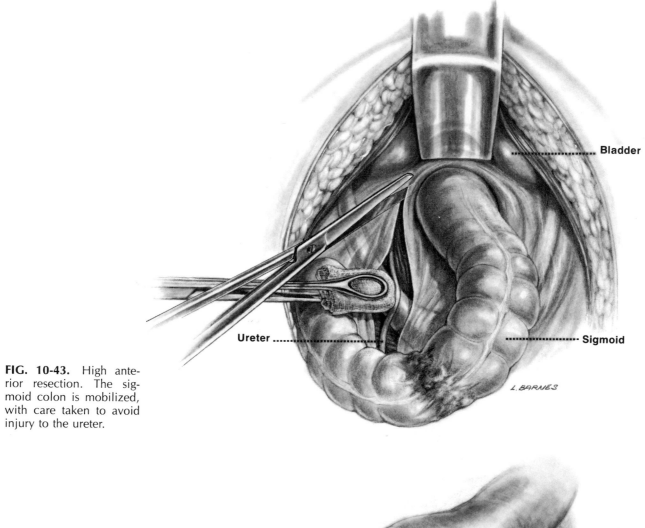

Bladder

Ureter

Sigmoid

L. BARNES

FIG. 10-43. High anterior resection. The sigmoid colon is mobilized, with care taken to avoid injury to the ureter.

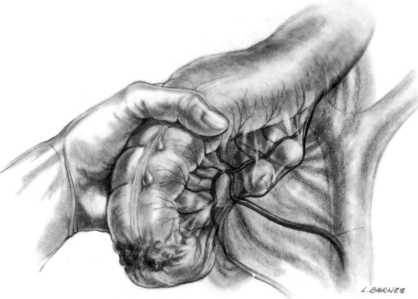

L. BARNES

FIG. 10-44. High anterior resection. The left hand is passed behind the bowel and beneath the vessels.

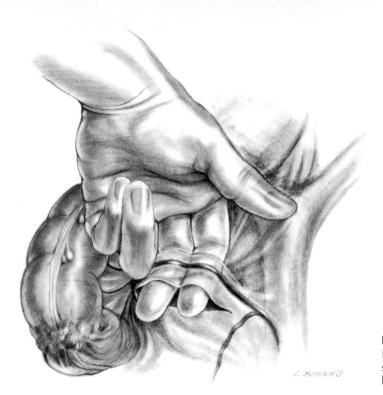

FIG. 10-45. High anterior resection. The left hand is repositioned to pass around the mesenteric vessels. The vascular pedicle is clamped as it is held by the left hand.

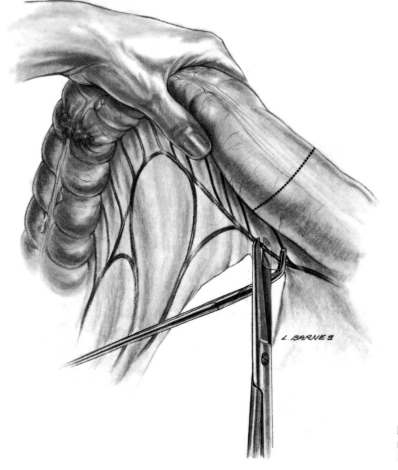

FIG. 10-46. High anterior resection. The mesentery is clamped with vigorous cephalad traction as the mesocolon is divided.

Subtotal or Total Colectomy

Removal of all or most of the colon and anastomosing the bowel to the upper rectum or sigmoid colon is a more extensive operation but permits a technically simple anastomosis. It also has the theoretical advantage of maximal removal of lymph-bearing tissue. The procedure is indicated when tumors are found synchronously on the left and on the right side of the colon (Fig. 10-47), when multiple tumors (benign or malignant or both) are present, when resection has been performed previously for colonic cancer, when the distal colon is obstructed (see Treatment of Obstruction), or when technical factors preclude a limited bowel resection.[24, 91, 110, 147]

Usually an end-to-end anastomosis can be performed easily between the ileum and the rectum or sigmoid colon, but occasionally, because of discrepancy between the lumens of the bowel or the angulation of the mesentery when the ileum is turned down onto the rectum, a side-to-end anastomosis may be advisable (Fig. 10-48).

No-Touch Technique

In 1954 Cole and associates and others prompted Turnbull and associates to ligate the vascular pedicle before mobilizing the colon and to develop the method known as the no-touch technique.[45, 75, 269] In Turnbull's operation the cancer-bearing segment is mobilized last.

Although the theoretical value of early ligation of the vascular pedicle seems reasonable, it is difficult to understand how the excellent cure rates reported by the Cleveland Clinic group are achieved solely by this maneuver. Many patients already harbor inapparent tumor above the ligature; they obviously would not be cured by this technique. One possible explanation for Turnbull's results is that a somewhat different classification is used for staging cancers of the colon. In my opinion, the value of the no-touch technique has been greatly overstated.

Stapling Colonic Anastomoses

De Petz was not the first person to describe a stapling device, but he is generally felt to have produced the initial practical instrument, employing it for gastrectomy.[58] The Russians, however, were responsible for the development of a number of stapling devices. The impetus arose from the problems associated with performing vascular anastomoses during World War II.[80] They and others performed anastomoses that were sometimes everting and sometimes inverting.[5, 219, 220]

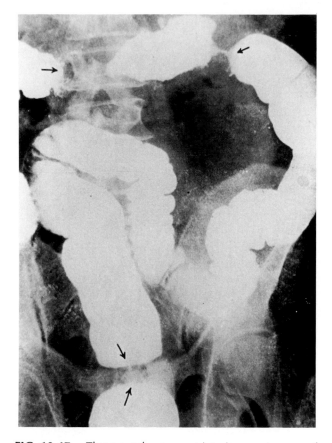

FIG. 10-47. Three synchronous, stricturing carcinomas of the colon: mid-transverse, at the splenic flexure, and at the rectum. (Corman ML, Veidenheimer MC, Swinton NW: Diseases of the Anus, Rectum and Colon. Part I: Neoplasms. New York, Medcom, 1972)

Ultimately, the Russian SPTU gun was described; it produced an inverting end-to-end anastomosis by means of a circular row of staples placed within the lumen of the bowel. The United States Surgical Corporation was the initial developer of stapling instruments in this country, and other American companies produced further modifications. Reports of their successful application are myriad.[100, 102, 133, 221, 223]

There are three types of stapling devices available to perform intestinal anastomoses: the TA series, which applies two rows of staggered staples (Fig. 10-49); the gastrointestinal anastomosis stapler (GIA; Fig. 10-50), which applies four rows of staggered staples and divides the tissue by means of a contained knife; and the end-to-end anastomosis stapler (EEA and ILS; see Figs.

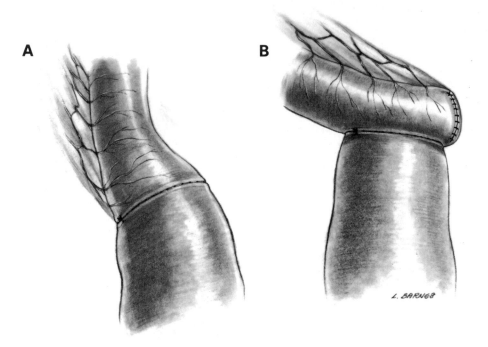

FIG. 10-48.   Ileorectal anastomosis can usually be accomplished end to end, with or without a Cheatle cut of the ileum **(A)** or as a side-to-end anastomosis **(B).**

11-66 and 11-67), which secures two rows of staples from within the lumen of the bowel to produce an inverting anastomosis in a circular fashion.

Stapling of the bowel requires greater attention to stripping the mesentery and fat from the ends of the intestine. This should be carried out for a distance of approximately 5 mm.[223] Anastomosis of the bowel can be accomplished by a number of methods. Figure 10-51 demonstrates the application of the TA stapler by a triangulation technique. The staple lines should cross each other. This produces an everting anastomosis that, despite criticism when applied to conventional suture technique, does not seem to be a problem with the stapling device. An alternate approach is to invert the posterior row, everting the two anterior limbs (Fig. 10-52).

Another alternative is to use the GIA stapler; this creates a side-to-side anastomosis, but the tissue is di-

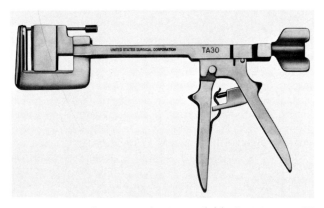

FIG. 10-49.   The TA stapler is available in 30 mm, 55 mm, and 90 mm. (Courtesy of the United States Surgical Corporation)

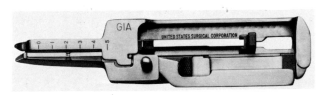

FIG. 10-50.   GIA stapler, reusable or disposable. (Courtesy of the United States Surgical Corporation)

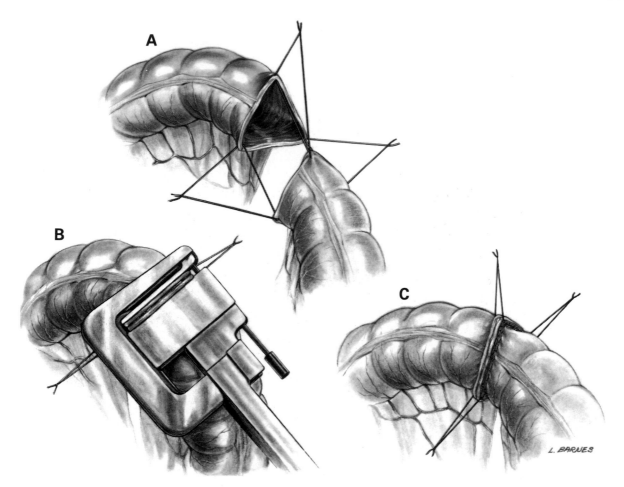

FIG. 10-51. Everting anastomosis using three stay sutures **(A)**, the TA stapler **(B)**, and triangulation **(C)**. (After Reiling RB: Staplers in gastrointestinal surgery. Surg Clin North Am 1980; 60:381–397)

vided, producing a functional end-to-end. Figure 10-53 illustrates the closed technique with closure of the enterotomies (Fig. 10-54). Alternatively, the open technique can be employed (Figs. 10-55 and 10-56).

The circular stapling device can be used to effect colonic anastomoses. Figure 10-57 demonstrates this procedure. Other methods of application are illustrated in Chapter 11.

Irrespective of the technique employed to anastomose bowel, the rates of complications (fecal fistula, hemorrhage, stricture) are approximately the same.[39,153,224,276,278] However, Dunn and co-workers, in a study on dogs, felt that the one-layer anastomosis was superior.[69] Reiling and associates, in a controlled

trial, reported that operating time, nasogastric intubation, and total length of hospitalization were about the same for both techniques.[224] This implies that the variables responsible for complications have less to do with the method of anastomosis than with other factors—tension on the anastomosis, blood supply, presence of sepsis, and nutritional state of the patient.

Comment

Stapling instruments have replaced conventional suture techniques for many surgeons today. In fact, in some teaching centers surgical residents have only minimal exposure to the conventional approach. It is prob-

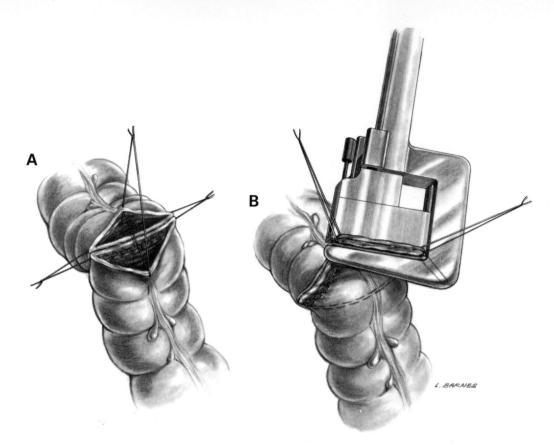

FIG. 10-52. Inversion of the posterior (mesenteric) wall **(A)** and eversion of the anterior walls **(B)**, using triangulation and the TA stapler. (After Reiling RB: Staplers in gastrointestinal surgery. Surg Clin North Am 1980; 60:381–397)

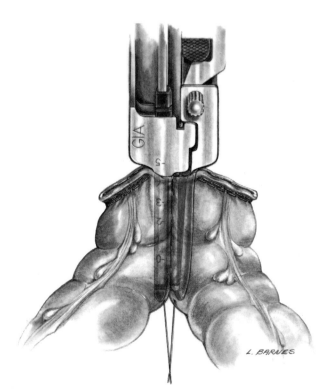

FIG. 10-53. Functional end-to-end anastomosis by the closed technique after creation of two enterotomies for insertion of the separate limbs of the GIA stapler. (After Reiling RB: Staplers in gastrointestinal surgery. Surg Clin North Am 1980; 60:381–397)

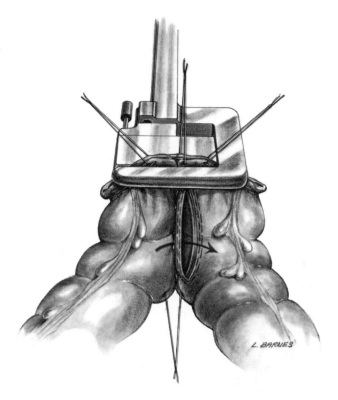

FIG. 10-54. Closure of the enterotomies using the TA stapler. (After Reiling RB: Staplers in gastrointestinal surgery. Surg Clin North Am 1980; 60:381–397)

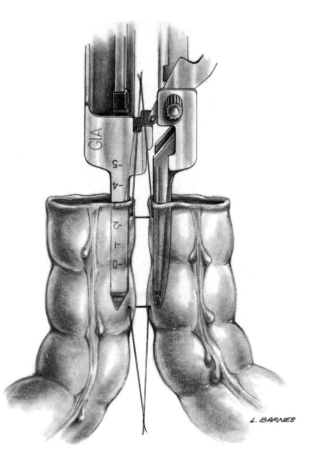

FIG. 10-55. Functional end-to-end anastomosis by the open technique with the GIA stapler. (After Reiling RB: Staplers in gastrointestinal surgery. Surg Clin North Am 1980; 60:381–397)

ably true that as experience is gained an anastomosis may be constructed somewhat more quickly with a stapling instrument. It is difficult to believe, however, that operative times can, as has been stated, be reduced by 25% and even 50%. The fact is that the performance of the anastomosis itself represents only a small part of the time invested in the whole operation. Opening and exploring the abdomen, dissecting out the bowel, resecting the specimen, and closing the abdomen represent efforts that may require considerable expenditure of time. Intestinal stapling does nothing to expedite these. I believe that the stapling device offers no great advantage over the conventional suture technique. Perhaps it is familiarity or simply intransigence that causes me to persist in using standard suture technique for the performance of intestinal anastomoses, but I must confess that I enjoy sewing.

Treatment of Obstruction

Obstructing carcinoma of the proximal colon (Fig. 10-58) usually can be treated by resection and primary anastomosis without a diversionary procedure. Technically, the resection can be relatively easily performed and an anastomosis effected between the ileum and the distal bowel.

When the ileocecal valve is intact, the distal ileum is usually of normal calber without muscular hypertrophy. Even when the small bowel is dilated an anastomosis should be performed. Whenever carcinoma of the right and transverse colon presents with obstruction, the resection proximal to the lesion should always include the colon to the ileum. The obstructed large bowel should never be used for an anastomosis unless a proximal diversion is employed. If the surgeon believes that diversion of a proximal colonic obstruction is necessary as the first stage, or if a protective stoma after ileocolonic anastomosis is indicated, loop ileostomy is the diversionary procedure of choice (see Figs. 16-55 to 16-57).

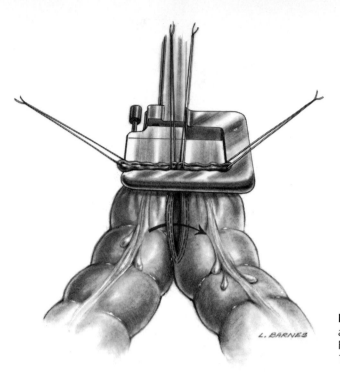

FIG. 10-56. Closure of the bowel ends with the TA stapler after open functional end-to-end anastomosis. (After Reiling RB: Staplers in gastrointestinal surgery. Surg Clin North Am 1980; 60:381–397)

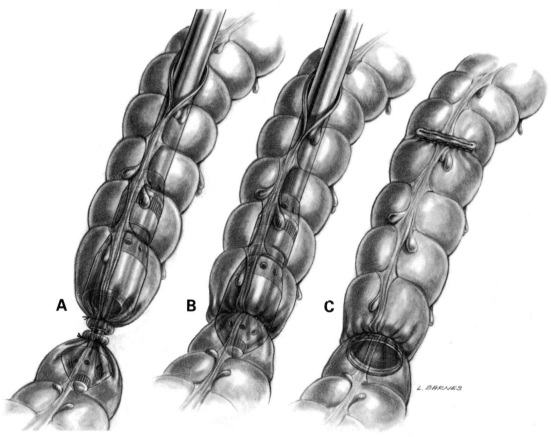

A   **B**   **C**

FIG. 10-57. Steps of EEA stapler use in colonic anastomosis through a proximal colotomy **(A, B).** Note stapled closure of the colotomy **(C)** converting the longitudinal incision to a transverse closure. (After Reiling RB: Staplers in gastrointestinal surgery. Surg Clin North Am 1980; 60:381–397)

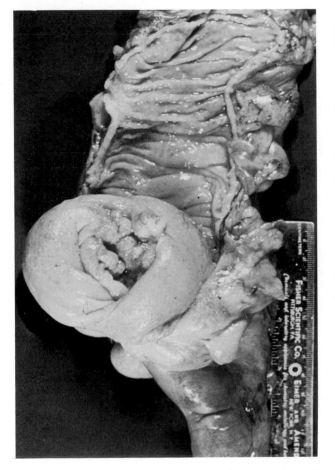

FIG. 10-58. Ileocecal intussusception from cecal carcinoma producing intestinal obstruction. (Courtesy of Rudolf Garret, M.D.)

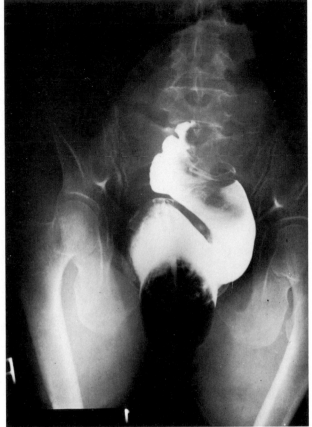

FIG. 10-59. Partial colonic obstruction secondary to carcinoma of the sigmoid with intussusception. Note the characteristic "coiled-spring" appearance of the intussusceptum.

When carcinoma precipitates a left-sided obstruction, the surgeon faces a more difficult decision. Should primary resection be undertaken? Should an anastomosis be performed? Should a diversion be created? It is difficult to answer these questions dogmatically because nuances in the presentation or in the findings might lead the surgeon to take a different course of action.

One of the important considerations is to note whether the obstruction is complete or partial (Figs. 10-59 and 10-60). If the patient continues to have bowel movements, pass flatus, or have gas distal to the site of obstruction demonstrable on plain film of the abdomen, the obstruction is not complete. Conversely, if the patient has not passed flatus or defecated for many hours or even days, and no gas is visible distally,

the obstruction is undoubtedly complete. At exploratory laparotomy the degree of dilatation of the proximal bowel can be assessed and the choice of operation determined.

If the dilatation is minimal or moderate and the resection can be accomplished without tedious dissection (as with a sigmoid lesion), resection might be advisable. It would be ideal to remove the tumor in the first instance and obtain a pathology report. An anastomosis may then be considered. If this is done, however, a proximal colostomy should be performed. Not to do this in a situation in which the bowel is unprepared and the colon is dilated invites disaster. Conversely, the surgeon may elect to defer anastomosis in favor of, for example, a sigmoid colostomy and mucus fistula, a safe, acceptable alternative. It should be

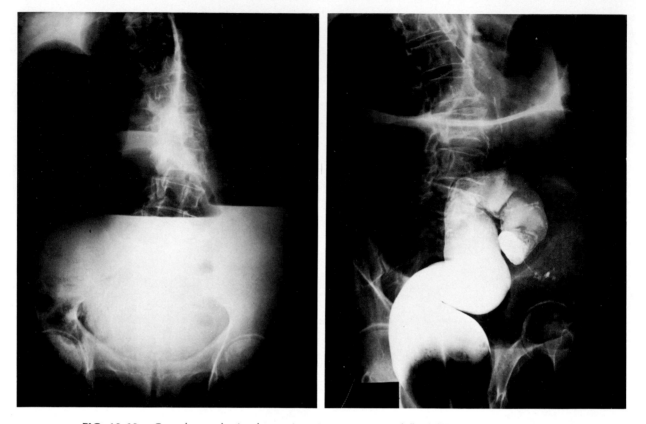

FIG. 10-60. Complete colonic obstruction. **A.** Huge gas and fluid-filled loops of colon are characteristic of mechanical obstruction. **B.** Barium enema demonstrates sigmoid obstruction.

remembered, however, that a dilated stoma (especially a sigmoid colostomy) tends to retract. An extra length should be delivered to avoid this complication. When left-sided obstruction produces sufficient dilatation to contraindicate resection, or when considerable dissection may be required for removal (as with lesions of the splenic flexure, upper descending colon, or distal transverse colon), loop transverse colostomy should be performed. Ten days to two weeks later, elective resection is undertaken. The diversionary stoma may or may not be disconnected at the same time as the resected specimen since the rate of wound infection for the combined procedures is high. I do not advise closing the colostomy synchronously with a distal anastomosis. Two colonic anastomoses are dangerous; the colostomy should be closed not sooner than six weeks later.

Another way of dealing with an obstructed colon and of avoiding a temporary colostomy is to perform subtotal or total colectomy and ileosigmoid or ileorectal anastomosis.[24,91] This obviously requires more dissec-

tion, but in selective circumstances this may be used. More commonly, however, this procedure should be directed to the treatment of perforation, in which case it is much more important to remove the bowel.

Bypass Procedure

Enteroenterostomy is a reasonably safe alternative for patients with obstructing or unresectable tumors when future obstruction is a possibility (Fig. 10-61). To effect a safe bypass the enterostomy should be at least 20 cm from the lesion proximally and distally, and the anastomosis should be clear of areas of tumor implantation if this is possible. A colocolostomy is the preferred approach whenever it can be accomplished, to save as much useful bowel as possible and to avoid diarrhea (Fig. 10-61, *B*). For right-sided lesions, an ileocolostomy is usually very effective (Fig. 10-61, *A*), but if the entire colon is in jeopardy for recurrence,

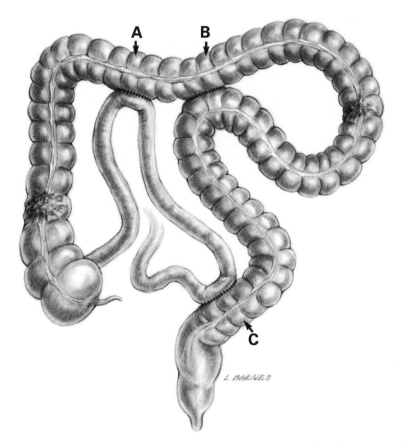

FIG. 10-61. Bypass procedures. **A.** Ileotransverse colostomy. **B.** Colocolostomy. **C.** Ileosigmoidostomy.

ileorectal or ileosigmoid bypass is indicated (Fig. 10-61, *C*).

Colostomy or ileostomy obviously bypasses the lesion, but I prefer to avoid a stoma if the rectum is spared. When a stoma is employed for obstruction it should either be a loop or be divided with the distal end exteriorized. If the distal end is closed, subsequent obstruction may lead to perforation of the oversewn bowel. Loop ileostomy is an alternative to transverse colostomy and may be easier to manage. I do not use cecostomy except for colonic ileus (Olgilvie's syndrome; see Chap. 17); it is tedious to manage and diverts inadequately.

Treatment of Perforation

Carcinoma of the colon with perforation is another challenging surgical problem. More often than not, the pathologic diagnosis is not clearly established. The patient may present with pneumoperitoneum, a rigid abdomen, and generalized peritonitis. Surgery often is required without benefit of gastrointestinal investigation or even a meaningful patient history. Even though extravasation is demonstrated on a limited Gastrografin enema, the differential diagnosis (especially for a sigmoid lesion) always includes diverticulitis. Colonoscopy often fails to reach the site of the disease because of inadequate bowel preparation, the general condition of the patient, and the inflammatory reaction in the area.[57] Failure to demonstrate a carcinoma by means of colonoscopy at or near the site of a known perforation does not exclude the diagnosis.

The establishment of a diagnosis can usually be confirmed with certainty only by exploratory laparotomy and resection of the involved segment of bowel. It should be emphasized repeatedly to all surgical trainees that limited exploration and blind diversionary procedures for suspected colonic perforation are to be condemned. Passing the hand into the pelvis to attempt diagnosis in the presence of inflammatory reaction, adhesions, pus, or feces is a gesture in futility. A transverse colostomy for a perforated cecal carcinoma is a totally preventable tragedy. For all patients suspected of having a perforation of the bowel, the lesion should clearly be demonstrable before embarking on operative treatment.

The operative approach for perforation is somewhat more direct than for obstruction. The goal should be to remove the diseased segment; if a colostomy and drainage procedure is performed for a sigmoid lesion the cause may not clearly be defined for many weeks. If carcinoma is diagnosed and not removed, resection should be undertaken in 10 to 14 days. If diverticular disease is the cause, resection theoretically may be deferred for many months (see Chap. 14). Another reason for resecting the lesion initially is to remove the septic process. Even with drainage and proximal diversion the contamination will continue, because a foot or more of stool-filled bowel may be found between the stoma and the perforation. Finally, desquamated cells from the tumor itself may continue to seed the abdomen and further worsen the already grim prognosis. Surgical procedures for removal of perforated areas include resection of the disease-bearing segment, anastomosis if convenient, always a protective colostomy or ileostomy, and drainage of the area of contamination.

With a right-sided perforation the surgeon may elect to perform an end ileostomy and mucus fistula of the colon, ileocolic anastomosis with protective loop ileostomy, or end ileostomy with closure of the colonic stump. With more distal lesions the surgeon can use an anastomosis with protective loop colostomy or loop ileostomy, end stoma with mucus fistula, or end stoma with closure of the distal stump.

Subtotal or total colectomy with ileosigmoid or ileorectal anastomosis is another alternative for the treatment of perforation. It fulfills the criterion of removing the disease, and it permits an easier anastomosis for left-sided perforations. But dissection in the upper part of the abdomen in the presence of a hypogastric perforation incurs the risk of spreading the septic process under the diaphragms and under the liver. Even with a technically safe anastomosis, loop ileostomy should be considered when contamination has occurred. Although possibly applicable in a number of situations, in one circumstance subtotal colectomy is the procedure of choice: when obstructing carcinoma of the left colon produces perforation of the right colon. Under these circumstances this operation is preferred despite the extensive dissection required.

When a primary resection is performed, blunt dissection should be employed as often as possible. Unless invasion by the tumor has caused fixation of the bowel, it should be mobilized by this method. Sharp dissection invites injury to the ureter and other retroperitoneal structures. If difficulties are encountered, the area should be drained with proximal diversion of the fecal stream. Although this is not the optimal course of action, it can be an acceptable alternative. In addition, because of poor prognosis of perforating carcinomas of the colon and the high risk of local recurrence, silver clips should be applied to serve as markers for subsequent radiotherapy. I believe that adjuvant postoperative radiotherapy should be employed for the perforating tumor (see later).

Finally, vigorous irrigation of the peritoneal cavity should be performed with many liters of saline.[11,150,183,187] Continuous postoperative lavage is also useful for up to 72 hours. I do not employ antibiotics or povidone-iodine in the solution.

Managing Liver Metastases

What to do with metastatic liver disease at the time of resection is a problem that often confronts the surgeon. Recent studies have demonstrated some success in resection for liver metastasis. Fortner and associates estimated that 15% to 25% of patients with metastatic disease are candidates for this procedure.[77] The Mayo Clinic group analyzed 60 patients with hepatic metastases from colorectal cancer.[3,281] Two thirds were solitary lesions. The results were "unexpectedly favorable." Forty-two percent of patients with apparent solitary lesions survived 5 years; there were no survivors among patients with multiple metastases. Others also report improved survival rates.[78,166,217] Foster and Berman, however, reported an 18% 5-year survival in 88 patients who underwent resection.[79]

In my own experience it is the rare patient indeed who is found to harbor an isolated liver lesion at the time of resection. The following protocol for treatment is recommended when a hepatic metastatic tumor is identified:

If a small focus of disease is present on the margin of the liver and no other lesion can be palpated, it should be removed. For any other lesion resection is not carried out; the location and size are determined. A CT scan (Fig. 10-62) is obtained during the postoperative convalescence. If multiple or bilobar disease is present, no operative intervention takes place. If solitary or unilobar disease is seen on the first scan, the study is repeated in 4 weeks. If only localized disease persists, the patient is admitted to the hospital for selective hepatic angiography. If there is still no evidence

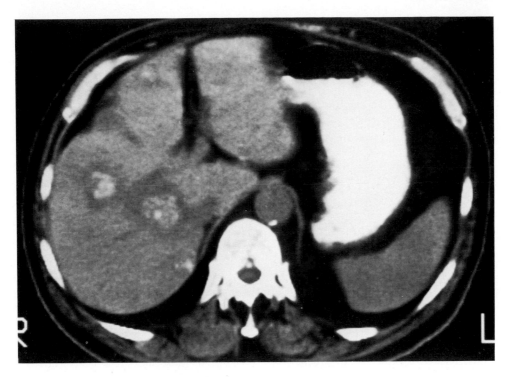

FIG. 10-62.   CT scan demonstrating multiple defects in the liver parenchyma consistent with metastases.

of extension, exploratory laparotomy and resection are recommended.

Excision in Continuity

Resection of adjacent small or large intestine, bladder wall, uterus, tubes and ovaries, stomach, spleen, tail of pancreas, duodenum, kidney, and portions of the abdominal wall may be performed for cure or to offer better palliation. Because of the differences in the biologic nature of neoplasms, occasionally a tumor will invade locally and not metastasize until late in the course of the disease. If the locally invasive tumor is not removed, the patient may experience many months or years of pain, intestinal obstruction, and visible protrusion of the tumor.

When other organs are involved in conjunction with the primary lesion, every effort should be made to remove the disease if technically possible. However, I do not advocate major abdominal wall resection, alloplasty, hemicorporectomy, or total pelvic exenteration to increase curability. The morbidity and mortality rates associated with these operations are so high that they preclude potential benefit.

Postoperative Care

For colon resection, patients are given no oral alimentation until flatus is passed, at which time a progressive diet is initiated. Initially, clear liquids are begun, followed by full liquids, and then a regular diet. On average, fluids are commenced on the third or fourth postoperative day, with discharge of the patient on the seventh or eighth day following surgery.

Complications

Complications of colon and rectal surgery are discussed in Chapter 11.

Results of Treatment

We reported 1008 patients who underwent definitive treatment for carcinoma of the colon and rectum.[49] Of these, 15 patients (1.5%) did not undergo operation. Thirty-nine operative deaths occurred, a mortality rate of 3.9%. Operative mortality in patients operated upon for cure was 1.8%. These data are summarized below.

Results of Operation for Colorectal Carcinoma (1962–1971)

Number of patients:	1008
Men:	548
Women:	460
Mean Age:	63 years
Men:	63
Women:	62
Not operated:	15
Operated:	993
Not resected:	51
Resectability:	95%
Operative mortality:	39 (3.9%)

(Corman ML, Veidenheimer MC, Coller JA: Colorectal carcinoma: A decade of experience at the Lahey Clinic. Dis Colon Rectum 1979; 22:477–479)

Considerable difficulty is encountered in analyzing the results of survival after resection for colorectal carcinoma from various institutions. Many reports are now using actuarial methods, correcting the data for the age of the patient, thereby giving more accurate survival statistics. For example, only a few patients over age 90 whose disease is cured survive 5 years. If a patient in this age group dies of carcinoma of the colon 4 years after resection, this is considered a cure. Another method commonly employed to analyze results of surgical treatment groups patients who have had surgery into two categories: those who have had resection and in whom the surgeon believes disease is potentially curable, and those whose disease is considered incurable and in whom the operations are palliative. A third method of analysis is to determine the crude survival rate, which is calculated on the basis of the number of patients alive 5 years after treatment. Obviously, this may not be a true estimate of the number of deaths from cancer, since the patient may have died from another cause during the 5-year period. Determinate survivors are those patients who die within 5 years with no evidence of recurrent disease. Some institutions employ this means for reporting data, with the obvious implication that the survival figures will be better if patients are considered cured if they die free of disease before 5 years have elapsed.

A need exists for uniformity in reporting the results of treatment for colorectal cancer and for the use of similar classifications of staging. The prognostic implication of Dukes' classification has been well estab-

Table 10-4.   Survival Rate by Dukes' Classification (1962–1971)

Dukes' Classification	Uncorrected No.	Uncorrected Percent	Corrected* (Percent)
A	225	81	95
B	332	62	90
C	204	35	55
D	247	0	1
	1008		

* United States National Center for Health Statistics: Table of Expectation of Life and Mortality Rates from Vital Statistics for the United States (1974), Vol 2, Section 5, Life Tables. Washington, DC, US Government Printing Office, 1976 (Corman ML, Veidenheimer MC, Coller JA: Colorectal carcinoma: A decade of experience at the Lahey Clinic. Dis Colon Rectum 1979; 22:477–479)

lished. When the lesion is confined to the bowel wall the chance of cure is great. In our experience the uncorrected survival rate for a patient with a Dukes' A lesion is 81%.[49] For Dukes' B lesions the uncorrected rate is 62%, and for Dukes' C lesions, 35%. Actuarially corrected rates are 95%, 90%, and 55%, respectively (Table 10-4). Table 10-5 compares our results with those of others.

Survival rates generally correlate with increasing lymph node involvement. Table 10-6 illustrates the survival rate versus the number of positive lymph nodes. If more than three nodes were positive the overall survival rate was 18 percent. These results lend further support to the contention that ultraradical resection for colorectal carcinoma is not justifiable. The number of positive nodes in the specimen would appear to be as important as the level of nodes involved.

In addition to lymph node involvement we have been particularly interested in the presence or absence of blood vessel invasion. Table 10-7 shows the uncorrected survival rate in patients with Dukes' C lesions with and without blood vessel invasion. The survival rate with blood vessel invasion is 31%, compared with 43% without blood vessel invasion. These differences are not statistically significant, but they do suggest that the combination of blood vessel invasion with lymph node involvement is associated with a poorer prognosis for survival than lymph node involvement alone. The importance of blood vessel invasion is evident in Table 10-8. With Dukes' B lesions, 5-year survival was 70% in patients without blood vessel invasion but only 55% in those with such invasion. This difference is statistically significant ($P < 0.05$). The mean age of patients with and without blood vessel invasion, alive or dead, was identical.

Table 10-5.   5-Year Survival

	Source	Study Years	Number of Patients	Uncorrected 5-Year Survival (Percent)
Dukes' Classification A	Gilbertsen[86]	1940–1959	359	67
	Dukes and Bussey[67]	1928–1952	308	81
	Corman and co-workers[49]	1962–1971	225	81
Dukes' Classification B	Dukes and Bussey[67]	1928–1952	692	64
	Corman and co-workers[49]	1962–1971	332	62
	Gilbertsen[86]	1940–1959	174	51
Dukes' Classification C	Dukes and Bussey[67]	1928–1952	1037	32
	Grinnell[111]	1936–1945	221	36
	Corman and co-workers[49]	1962–1971	204	35
	Gilbertsen[86]	1940–1950	173	33
	Botsford and co-workers[21]	1960–1965	146	44

Table 10-6.   Survival vs Number of Lymph Nodes Involved (1962–1971)

Number of Positive Lymph Nodes	Total	Deaths	5-Year Survival Number	5-Year Survival Percent
1	71	39	32	45
2	47	33	14	30
3	30	15	15	50
4	20	16	4	20
5	11	9	2	18
6	8	6	2	25
7	7	6	1	14
8 or more	9	8	1	11
Totals	203	132	71	35

(Corman ML, Veidenheimer MC, Coller JA: Colorectal carcinoma: A decade of experience at the Lahey Clinic. Dis Colon Rectum 1979; 22:477–479)

Table 10-7.   Uncorrected Survival Rate, Dukes' C Colorectal Carcinoma (1962–1966)

Blood Vessel Invasion	5-Year Survival	Deaths	Living Total	Living Percent
Present	19	43	62	31
Absent	24	32	56	43

(Corman ML, Veidenheimer MC, Coller JA: Colorectal carcinoma: A decade of experience at the Lahey Clinic. Dis Colon Rectum 1979; 22:477–479)

Table 10-8. Uncorrected Survival Rate, Dukes' B Colorectal Carcinoma (1962–1966)

Blood Vessel Invasion	Living	Deaths	Total	Living (Percent)
Present	32	26	58	55
Absent	82	35	117	70
Total	114	61	175	65

(Corman ML, Swinton NW Sr, O'Keefe DD et al: Colorectal carcinoma at the Lahey Clinic, 1962–1966. Am J Surg 1973; 125:424–428)

Mzabi and colleagues undertook a retrospective study to determine the factors associated with mortality and survival after resection for colonic cancer.[195] As might be expected, patients who presented for operation with no symptoms had a statistically significant better rate of survival than those patients who presented with symptoms. Furthermore, the authors demonstrated that rectal bleeding as a symptom was a better prognostic sign than the other presenting symptoms of colonic cancer.

Obstructing and Perforating Carcinoma

Patients who present with obstruction or perforation have a poorer prognosis than other patients with colorectal carcinoma. The operative morbidity and the operative mortality are much higher. As previously mentioned, perforated carcinoma should be treated by primary resection whenever possible; primary resection also should be carried out for proximal obstructing lesions. Gennaro and Tyson reported an overall operative mortality of 14% for obstructing carcinoma.[83] The uncorrected survival rate at 5 years was approximately 9%, and 18% of patients who underwent curative resection survived 5 years.

Glenn and McSherry reported an operative mortality of 13% in patients with obstruction, and a 5-year survival rate of approximately 20%.[92] Their experience with perforated carcinoma revealed an equally grim prognosis. The operative mortality was 15%, and the 5-year survival rate, 28%.[92]

Carcinoma in Young Patients

Colorectal carcinoma is associated with a poor prognosis when it develops in young patients. Although the incidence is much lower in the younger age group, it is particularly imperative for the physician to investigate anyone who presents with symptoms suggestive of a bowel tumor (rectal bleeding or change in bowel habits). Because of the symptoms at presentation and the difficulty in interpreting their significance, delay in diagnosis and treatment undoubtedly is the major factor responsible for the poor survival rates.

Even for the same stage of lesion, however, younger persons do poorly when compared with older patients. Recalde and associates reported a 13% 5-year survival rate in 40 patients 35 years of age or younger.[222] Furthermore, they noted that no 5-year survivors were found among patients who had lymph node metastases, visceral metastases, or tumors larger than 5 cm in diameter. Sanfelippo and Beahrs reported on 118 patients under 40 years of age who underwent resection for colorectal carcinoma.[237] Their overall 5-year survival rate was 39%. Patients with Dukes' C lesions had a 5-year survival rate of 21%.

Carcinoma of the colon is extremely uncommon in children. In contrast to adults, the most frequent symptom is abdominal pain, often with vomiting. Pemberton reported on a cure of a 9-year-old child and noted that no other report is found in the literature of a survivor in whom the disease developed at such an early age.[212] He noted that in children the colon is affected more frequently by cancer than any other part of the digestive system.

Palliative Resection

Because carcinoma of the colon is a relatively slow-growing tumor, I strongly advocate that a palliative resection be performed whenever possible. Even with extensive metastatic disease, patients may live a relatively long time and be free of the often miserable sequelae associated with an untreated primary lesion. Of our patients, 8.5% had hepatic metastases at the time of laparotomy for treatment of the primary tumor.

Cady and co-workers reported that during the years 1941 to 1960, patients with liver metastases diagnosed at operation survived a mean of 13 months.[32] Factors that adversely influenced survival included weight loss, intestinal symptoms, ascites, peritoneal seeding, extension of the primary cancer to other viscera, histologic involvement of lymph nodes or blood vessels, and extent of surgical treatment.[32] Takaki and associates noted a mean survival time of approximately 12 months in 59 patients who underwent palliative resection.[259] Goslin and colleagues reported a similar median survival.[104] Patients whose tumors were poorly differentiated or with weight loss greater than 10% at presentation survived a median of only 6 months.

Exceptions to performing palliative resection include the presence of ascites, massive peritoneal seeding, jaundice, or severe debilitation. Obviously, the decision to carry out such a procedure is a matter of surgical judgment.

Follow-Up Evaluation

How to follow up patients who have undergone resection for carcinoma of the colon is a subject worthy of some discussion. Methods of evaluation include physical examination, proctosigmoidoscopy, colonoscopy, barium enema examination, chest radiography, carcinoembryonic antigen, liver function studies, liver scan, computerized tomography, and exploratory laparotomy at an interval after operation.

In addition to the types of examinations and procedures that are available to evaluate the cancer patient postoperatively, the frequency with which such examinations and tests should be undertaken is also the subject of debate. One school of thought postulates that the patient should be discharged after recovery from surgery and only report if symptoms develop, so pessimistic is the belief of many physicians and surgeons that earlier diagnosis and treatment of recurrent disease result in a sufficient survival rate to justify the cost and effort.

My experience is that very few patients are salvaged in whom a recurrence of cancer develops. However, in a number of patients cure can still be achieved, or at least life-style can be improved, if recurrent tumor is recognized early. In one area, at least, there appears to be little disagreement: that there is increased risk of the development of a second cancer. If for no other reason than this, the patient should never be discharged from follow-up study but should be evaluated periodically for the development of a second primary tumor in the bowel. Heald and Lockhart-Mummery showed that the chance of cure was much improved in those patients who attended follow-up clinic at the time of the occurrence of a second growth.[132]

Physical Examination

Physical examination is most unrewarding in my opinion for identifying an early recurrence. By the time palpation of the abdomen reveals a tumor in the liver or a recurrent lesion in the peritoneal cavity, the cancer is always unresectable. Therefore, palpation of the abdomen and supraclavicular nodes and pelvic examination serve primarily to reassure the patient and the physician. The only value of such examinations is to follow the response to supplementary treatment when a lesion has been identified.

Proctosigmoidoscopy

On an annual basis, proctosigmoidoscopy is of value, particularly if the anastomosis can be seen with the instrument. Recurrence at the suture line, which most often results from inward growth of the tumor from the pelvis and not from residual tumor in the bowel wall, may be identified and may permit re-resection for possible cure. If the lesion is not within range of the sigmoidoscope the only purpose of the examination is to identify a metachronous lesion.

Colonoscopy

Colonoscopy should be employed to evaluate the entire residual colon following resection if the procedure was not performed or if it was unsuccessful in visualizing the bowel preoperatively. Many studies have demonstrated the high incidence of benign and malignant lesions harbored in the residual colon, presumably missed at the time of resection.[81, 155, 198, 271] Reilly and associates performed perioperative colonoscopy on 92 patients.[225] Synchronous cancers were found in almost 8%. Approximately 3½ years following treatment of the index cancer, an additional 8% demonstrated a metachronous malignancy.

The procedure is also of value in identifying recurrent disease at the anastomosis. Colonoscopy is advisable every 3 years once the bowel has been demonstrated to be completely neoplasm-free.[208]

Barium Enema Examination

The barium enema examination is of limited benefit in the follow-up evaluation of the patient with colorectal cancer. It is unlikely that recurrent disease at the suture line will be identified more readily by this technique than by colonoscopy. However, an extrinsic lesion might be perceived more easily with a barium enema study than by means of colonoscopy. In follow-up evaluation colonoscopy appears to be the preferred tool.

Chest Radiography

Chest radiography should be performed annually to identify patients with pulmonary metastasis; some of these patients may be operated on for cure (see Treatment of Metastases: Resection for Isolated Metastases).

Carcinoembryonic Antigen

Although the studies of Gold and Freedman demonstrated that elevated titers of carcinoembryonic antigen (CEA) preceded clinical signs of disease by 2 weeks to 10 months, Moertel and co-workers opined that the CEA test is grossly insensitive in the diagnosis of recurrent colorectal carcinoma.[94, 95, 190] They performed testing on 36 patients with histologically demonstrable recurrent or residual malignant disease after resection but with no clinical evidence of distant metastases. Only nine patients (25%) had abnormal CEA levels despite the fact that most patients had symptoms of recurrence for several months. Sugarbaker and colleagues studied the serial monthly CEA determinations of 33 patients after resection for large bowel cancer.[256] Confirmed recurrent malignant disease subsequently developed in 12 of these patients. A rising titer was the first evidence of recurrence in only 4 of these 12, and all 4 had distant metastases.

Despite objections about the lack of specificity of CEA and its questionable ability to diagnose early recurrent disease, most researchers generally agree that increasing levels are found with more advanced disease, that a failure of elevated levels of carcinoembryonic antigen to return to normal after resection is associated with a poor prognosis, and that elevated levels usually appear before any clinical evidence of recurrence.[8, 164, 167, 175–177, 201, 249, 290]

I believe that the carcinoembryonic antigen determination is useful in the follow-up evaluation of patients who have undergone resection for colon and rectal cancer. However, I have not been convinced that the determination has diagnosed recurrence early enough to permit surgical excision for possible cure except in the rare case.

One other possible application of the carcinoembryonic antigen determination has been reported by Patt and co-workers.[210] Using selective angiographic techniques a carcinoembryonic antigen concentration gradient can be determined by sampling from appropriate vessels. Identification of the site of recurrence might be possible with this method. More work must be done, however, before its true value can be assessed.

Liver Function Studies

Liver function studies are useful to follow up the patient for the development of recurrent disease. In my experience the alkaline phosphatase determination has been about as effective in diagnosing liver metastases as has the carcinoembryonic antigen.

Liver Scan

Liver scan is commonly used preoperatively by some surgeons to identify liver metastases. I do not believe this is a useful exercise, however. The presence of metastases does not contraindicate surgery, and I do not advocate synchronous liver resection with bowel resection (see Surgical Treatment, Operative Technique: Managing Liver Metastases). Postoperatively, however, with known liver metastases, the liver scan is useful to confirm the location and presence of the lesion or lesions. In the absence of a positive carcinoembryonic antigen determination or elevated level of alkaline phosphatase, this study has no place in postoperative screening.

Computed Tomography

Computed tomography (CT) offers a simple, noninvasive method for the evaluation of metastatic colon tumor by visualization of the liver, pelvis, retroperitoneum, and adrenal glands (see Fig. 10-62). Some have suggested that it be employed as a baseline study following surgery and then used at intervals to detect local recurrence.[71] It has proved valuable in the evaluation of patients for supplemental therapy. CT-guided aspiration technique is also useful for obtaining cytologic confirmation of malignancy. Computed tomography is a rapidly advancing modality and will probably develop into the procedure of choice for evaluation of the extent of disease.

Second-Look Operation

When recurrence of tumor is discovered, surgical resection offers the best possible chance for cure in those patients who have localized disease. Wangensteen first proposed the second-look procedure in the management of colorectal cancer in 1949 in an attempt to increase the cure rate for patients with nodal disease at the time of resection.[275] These patients were subjected to an exploratory laparotomy 6 months to 1 year after operation. Obviously, this meant that a number of patients were explored who had no evidence of recurrent disease; only 15% of Wangensteen's patients actually had recurrence at the time of exploratory laparotomy. For this reason the second-look concept was abandoned until the development of carcinoembryonic antigen.

Minton and associates reoperated 36 patients on the basis of progressive elevation of the carcinoembryonic antigen determination and found recurrent tumor in 30 of them.[188] The last 11 patients were able to have the tumor removed. They attributed their later improved results to a decrease in the time delay between identification of an appreciable rise in carcinoembryonic antigen and reoperation. They recommend serial carcinoembryonic antigen determination every 2 months. Whether these patients have been cured is another matter. Most studies do not yet report 5-year follow-up evaluations after reresection. Steele and associates reported on 75 patients with Dukes' B and C lesions followed for a median of 24 months.[255] Of 15 patients found to have a tumor at a second-look operation (based on successive increased elevations of the carcinoembryonic antigen value), 4 were resected. Tong and colleagues performed a laparotomy on 64 patients with known recurrent disease.[266] Seventeen percent underwent attempted curative resection; "prolonged" survival was achieved in three.

Whether the morbidity, mortality, and cost of the second-look procedure is justified remains an unanswered question.

TREATMENT OF METASTASES

Pulmonary Metastases

Solitary lung metastases have been resected for cure more often than metastases to all other sites combined.[229] Cahan and co-workers reported that in a patient with a history of colorectal carcinoma, a solitary lung lesion will be metastatic from that primary one half of the time.[34] It still should be remembered that primary lung cancer is the commonest visceral cancer in men and that isolated pulmonary metastases should not contraindicate radical surgical removal of the bowel tumor. Conversely, a solitary lung lesion that is metastatic from a colon primary carcinoma has a better chance of cure if resected than does a primary bronchogenic carcinoma. Bronchoscopy, mediastinoscopy, and sputum cytology are useful in identifying the histologic nature of the neoplasm. Lung tomograms are required to rule out the presence of additional nodules. In the experience of McCormack and Attiyeh, the 5-year survival rate was 22%, and this was significantly increased when the primary colonic cancer was a Dukes' A or B lesion.[182]

I believe in a vigorous approach to the treatment of solitary pulmonary metastases. Wedge resection, preserving as much lung tissue as possible, is usually performed, although resection of the lobe is sometimes necessary to remove the lesion completely.

Ovarian Metastases

The ovary may be the only site of macroscopic spread of disease; it is a site of metastases in 3% to 5% of patients. Bilateral oophorectomy has been recommended on a prophylactic basis in all women over 40 years of age who have colorectal cancer because of the risk of harboring a metastatic focus, but the major benefit probably is to prevent the subsequent development of ovarian carcinoma (see Chap. 11).

Liver Metastases

See Surgical Treatment, Operative Technique: Managing Liver Metastases.

Osseous Metastases

Osseous metastases from colonic and rectal cancer are relatively uncommon. In the experience of the Memorial Sloan-Kettering Cancer Center, 6.9% of patients with disseminated colorectal carcinoma had osseous metastases.[16, 17] Most of these patients had metastatic spread to bone in association with widespread metastases elsewhere. A few patients had only skeletal metastases. Treatment is palliative and essentially limited to radiotherapy for bone pain. This is usually quite effective.

Cerebral Metastases

Metastatic carcinoma to the brain is uncommon and is usually associated with metastatic disease elsewhere, especially in the lung. Rarely will a metastatic focus be present in the brain with no other evidence of metastases. Under these circumstances an aggressive approach by craniotomy is indicated to remove the metastatic lesion. One can expect good palliation of neurologic signs and symptoms. Nakajima and associates reported on a patient who had removal of a metastatic lesion of the brain; at postmortem examination 2 years later, no evidence was found of intracranial metastases.[196] I have had a similar experience.

CHEMOTHERAPY

Colorectal cancer has proved extremely resistant to chemotherapeutic agents. Practically every available agent has had extensive trials, but only a few drugs are still being used. The antimetabolites, 5-fluorouracil (5-FU) and 5-fluorodeoxyuridine (5-FUDR), are the most commonly employed and have had the best results. Second most commonly used are the nitrosoureas and then mitomycin C. Other drugs have been administered, but none has been particularly successful.

Recently an *in vitro* test for determining sensitivity of cancer cells to a chemotherapeutic agent, the tumor stem cell assay (clonogenic chemosensitivity test), has been developed.[233, 242] Although the assay may predict responsiveness to a given drug, the fact is that there is no truly effective chemical for the treatment of this cancer.

The standard treatment with 5-FU consists of a 5-day loading course by intravenous injection and then maintenance therapy, either with a 5-day treatment once a month or by weekly injection. A Hickman catheter is frequently inserted to provide vascular access in patients who undergo intravenous therapy.[288] Oral administration has been found to be unreliable because of variable absorption. Pumps and reservoirs have been surgically implanted for infusion.[15, 130] Hepatic artery infusion is sometimes recommended; it produces higher regression rates and slightly longer remissions than other techniques.[31] However, these advantages are at the cost of increased morbidity, time in the hospital, and technical difficulties, which make this route less than desirable. Usually hepatic artery infusion is applied to those patients who have failed to show improvement with conventional systemic techniques.

Patients who respond to 5-FU (20%) have an improved quality of life compared with nonresponders and untreated controls. However, when all patients treated by 5-FU are considered and compared with untreated controls, no evidence of increased survival is found. Patients with slowly growing tumors and younger patients have a higher response rate.

The combination of chemotherapy and multiple drugs has also been rather disappointing. Many combinations of drugs have been evaluated, but most studies have shown that the length of remission produced is no better than with single agents. Another disadvantage is that combination chemotherapy may produce more side-effects.

Chemotherapeutic agents, especially 5-FU, have been used in combination with other modalities of treatment, such as surgery, radiation, and immunotherapy. The value of chemoimmunotherapy has been evaluated, and in preliminary studies from the M.D. Anderson Hospital and the Southwest Oncology Group, 5-FU plus bacille Calmette Guérin (BCG) has been shown to produce a longer disease-free period with increased survival in some patients.[14, 117] These studies have not yet been confirmed by randomized controlled trials from other institutions.

When 5-FU is combined with radiation therapy, a modest improvement takes place in length of remission and survival compared with results of radiation therapy alone in patients with local, inoperable, or recurrent disease.

The agents 5-FU and 5-FUDR have been evaluated extensively in adjuvant trials after surgery in patients with Dukes' B and C lesions. Statistically significant data indicating more prolonged survival with these regimens have yet to be published.

Immunotherapy

Immunotherapy with bacille Calmette Guérin (BCG) is most effective when the tumor mass is reduced to a minimum, when it is administered directly into or close to the tumor, when the patient is able to respond to BCG, and when a large enough dose is given. Routes of administration include directly into the tumor, intradermally (by skin scarification), intracavitarily, and orally.[137, 173]

Although the number of colorectal patients reported on in whom BCG immunotherapy has been used is still small, this regimen has produced increased survival, most striking in patients with liver metastases. Mavligit and co-workers reported on 83 patients with Dukes' C colorectal carcinoma who received postoperative BCG alone or in combination with orally administered 5-FU.[179] The BCG had been administered by the scarification method at weekly intervals. Patients had been followed for as long as 30 months with an appreciable prolongation of both disease-free interval and overall survival. The conclusion of this group is that adjuvant immunotherapy without chemotherapy improves the prognosis of patients with surgically treated Dukes' C colorectal carcinoma. Further studies and control trials need to be done before the true value of this approach to supplementary treatment is understood.

RADIOTHERAPY

Radiotherapy has been applied primarily in the treatment of rectal cancer (see Chap. 11). However, Gunderson and associates reported a unique method of administering radiation treatment.[116] For treatment of inoperable, residual, or recurrent colorectal cancer, doses in excess of 60 Gy (6000 rads) were given using an intraoperative technique at the time of laparotomy. This required transporting the patient to a different area of the hospital for radiation therapy, anesthetized, with the abdomen open. The authors postulate that if this technique proves feasible it might be possible to ablate tumor by radiation therapy, a result that could not be expected with lower dose radiation levels. I have had no experience with this technique but await the results of long-term follow-up.

Radiotherapy is used by conventional external means when macroscopic tumor is left behind or when fixity of the lesion might be attributable to tumor. The area is marked with silver clips. Usually 45 Gy (4500 rads) is administered over a period of 5 weeks. I believe that this reduces the chance for local recurrence.

COMMENT

In reviewing the experience with colorectal carcinoma for the past 40 years it seems apparent that no significant improvement in operative mortality and cure rate has taken place. It appears, then, that surgery has accomplished all it possibly can for this condition. Any further improvement in survival rates will depend on bringing patients to operation earlier and on the effectiveness of other modalities of therapy.

REFERENCES

1. Abrams JS: Elective resection for colorectal cancer in Vermont: 1971–1975. Am J Surg 1980; 139:78–83
2. Abrams JS, Anton JR, Dreyfuss DC: The absence of a relationship between cholecystectomy and the subsequent occurrence of cancer of the proximal colon. Dis Colon Rectum 1983; 26:141–144
3. Adson MA, Van Heerden JA: Major hepatic resections for metastatic colorectal cancer. Ann Surg 1980; 191:576–683
4. d'Allaines F, Morgan CN, Lloyd-Davis OV: Discussion on conservative resection in carcinoma. Proc R Soc Med 1950; 43:697–710
5. Androsov PI: Experience in the application of instrumental suture in surgery of the stomach and rectum. Acta Chir Scand 1970; 136:57–63
6. Aries V, Crowther JS, Drasar BS et al: Bacteria and the aetiology of cancer of the large bowel. Gut 1969; 10:334–335
7. Armstrong B, Doll R: Environmental factors and cancer incidence and mortality in different countries, with special reference to dietary practices. Int J Cancer 1975; 15:617–631
8. Arnaud JP, Koehl C, Adloff M: Carcinoembryonic antigen (CEA) in diagnosis and prognosis of colorectal carcinoma. Dis Colon Rectum 1980; 23:141–144
9. Astler VB, Coller FA: Prognostic significance of direct extension of carcinoma of colon and rectum. Ann Surg 1954; 139:846–852
10. Ault GW: Carcinoma of rectum: Factors responsible for recurrent or residual disease. Am Surg 1953; 19:1035–1044
11. Aune S, Norman E: Diffuse peritonitis treated with continuous peritoneal lavage. Acta Chir Scand 1970; 136:401–404
12. Axtell LM, Cutler SJ, Myers MH (eds): End Results in Cancer. Report No. 4. Publication No (NIH) 73-272, p 217. Bethesda, US Department of Health, Education, and Welfare, 1972
13. Ayeni AO, Thomson DMP, MacFarlane JK: A comparison of tube leukocyte adherence inhibition assay and standard physical methods for diagnosing colorectal cancer. Cancer 1981; 48:1855–1862
14. Baker LH, Matter R, Talley R et al: 5-FU vs 5-FU and Me CCNU in gastrointestinal cancers: A phase III study of the South West Oncology Group (abstr). Proc Am Assoc Cancer Res 1975; 16:229
15. Balch CM, Urist MM, McGregor ML: Continuous regional chemotherapy for metastatic colorectal cancer using a totally implantable infusion pump: A feasibility study in 50 patients. Am J Surg 1983; 145:285–290
16. Barringer PL, Dockerty MB, Waugh JM et al: Carcinoma of the large intestine: A new approach to the study of venous spread. Surg Gynecol Obstet 1954; 98:62–72
17. Besbeas S, Stearns MW Jr: Osseous metastases from carcinomas of the colon and rectum. Dis Colon Rectum 1978; 21:266–268
18. Bjelke E: Epidemiologic Studies of Cancer of the Stomach, Colon, and Rectum: With Special Emphasis on the Role of Diet. Abstracts and Literature Review. Oslo, Universitets Forlaget, 1974
19. Bjelke E: Epidemiologic studies of cancer of the stomach, colon, and rectum; with special emphasis on the role of diet. Scand J Gastroenterol (Suppl) 1974; 9:1–235
20. Bloch OT: Om extra-abdominal behandlung af cancer intestinalis (rectum derfra undtaget) med en frem stilling af de for denne sygdom foretagne operationer og deres resultater. Nord Med Ark 1892; 24:1–10
21. Botsford TW, Aliapoulios MR, Fogelson FS: Results of treatment of colorectal cancer at the Peter Bent Brigham Hospital from 1960 to 1965. Am J Surg 1971; 121:398–402
22. Boyd JT, Langman M, Doll R: The epidemiology of gastrointestinal cancer with special reference to causation. Gut 1964; 5:196–200
23. Brendel TH, Kirsh IE: Lack of association between inguinal hernia and carcinoma of the colon. N Engl J Med 1971; 284:369–370
24. Brief DK, Brener BJ, Goldenkranz R: An argument for increased use of subtotal colectomy in the management of carcinoma of the colon. Am Surg 1983; 49:66–72

25. Brown CE, Warren S: Visceral metastasis from rectal carcinoma. Surg Gynecol Obstet 1938; 66:611–620

26. Burbank F: Patterns in cancer mortality in the United States: 1950–1967. Natl Cancer Inst Monogr 1971; 33:1–594

27. Burkitt DP: Relationship as a clue to causation. Lancet 1970; 2:1237–1240

28. Burkitt DP: Epidemiology of cancer of the colon and rectum. Cancer 1971; 28:3–13

29. Burkitt DP: Some neglected leads to cancer causation. J Natl Cancer Inst 1971; 47:913–919

30. Burkitt DP, Walker AR, Painter NS: Effect of dietary fibre on stools and the transit-times, and its role in the causation of disease. Lancet 1972; 2:1408–1412

31. Cady B, Oberfield RA: Regional infusion chemotherapy of hepatic metastases from carcinoma of the colon. Am J Surg 1974; 127:220–227

32. Cady B, Monson DO, Swinton NW Sr: Survival of patients after colonic resection for carcinoma with simultaneous liver metastases. Surg Gynecol Obstet 1970; 131:697–700

33. Cady B, Persson AV, Monson DO et al: Changing patterns of colorectal carcinoma. Cancer 1974; 33:422–426

34. Cahan WG, Castro El B, Hajdu SI: The significance of a solitary lung shadow in patients with colon carcinoma. Cancer 1974; 33:414–421

35. Camp TF Jr, Connolly JM: Colorectal polypoid lesions. Arch Surg 1966; 93:625–630

36. Canalis F, Ravitch MM: Study of healing of inverting and everting intestinal anastomoses. Surg Gynecol Obstet 1968; 126:109–114

37. Cancer of the colon and rectum. CA 1980; 30:208–215

38. Cederlöf R, Friberg L, Hrubec Z et al: The Relationship of Smoking and Some Social Covariables to Mortality and Cancer Morbidity: A Ten Year Follow up in a Probability Sample of 55,000 Swedish Subjects Age 18 to 69. Stockholm, Karolinska Mediko-Kirurgiska Institutet, 1975

39. Chassin JL, Rifkind KM, Sussman B et al: The stapled gastrointestinal tract anastomosis: Incidence of postoperative complications compared with the sutured anastomosis. Ann Surg 1978; 188:689–696

40. Chen W-F, Patchefsky AS, Goldsmith HS: Colonic protection from dimethylhydrazine by a high fiber diet. Surg Gynecol Obstet 1978; 147:503–506

41. Clark TW, Schor SS, Elsom KE et al: The periodic health examination: Evaluation of routine tests and procedures. Ann Intern Med 1961; 54:1209–1222

42. Clemmesen J: Statistical studies in the aetiology of malignant neoplasms. Acta Pathol Microbiol Scand 1974; (Suppl) 247:1–266

43. Clemmesen J, Nielsen A: Social distribution of cancer in Copenhagen, 1943 to 1947. Br J Cancer 1951; 5:159–171

44. Cohn I Jr: Implantation in cancer of the colon. Surg Gynecol Obstet 1967; 124:501–508

45. Cole WH, Packard D, Southwick HW: Carcinoma of the colon with special reference to prevention of recurrence. JAMA 1954; 155:1549–1554

46. Condon RE, Bartlett JG, Greenlee H et al: Efficacy of oral and systemic antibiotic prophylaxis in colorectal operations. Arch Surg 1983; 118:496–502

47. Cook PJ, Doll R, Fellingham SA: A mathematical model for the age distribution of cancer in man. Int J Cancer 1969; 4:93–112

48. Corman ML, Coller JA, Veidenheimer MC: Proctosigmoidoscopy—age criteria for examination in the asymptomatic patient. CA 1975; 24:286–290

49. Corman ML, Veidenheimer MC, Coller JA: Colorectal carcinoma: A decade of experience at the Lahey Clinic. Dis Colon Rectum 1979; 22:477–479

50. Corman ML, Veidenheimer MC, Coller JA: Controlled clinical trial of three suture materials for abdominal closure after bowel resections. Am J Surg 1981; 141:510–513

51. Corman ML, Veidenheimer MC, Swinton NW: Diseases of the Anus, Rectum and Colon. Part I: Neoplasms. New York, Medcom, 1972

52. Corman ML, Swinton NW Sr, O'Keefe DD et al: Colorectal carcinoma at the Lahey Clinic, 1962–1966. Am J Surg 1973; 125:424–428

53. Correa P, Llanos G: Morbidity and mortality from cancer in Cali, Colombia. J Natl Cancer Inst 1966; 36:717–745

54. Creagan ET, Fraumeni JF Jr: Cancer mortality among American Indians. J Natl Cancer Inst 1972; 49:959–967

55. Cutler SJ, Young JL Jr (eds): The third national cancer survey: Incidence data. Cancer morbidity. Natl Cancer Inst Monogr 1975; 41:1–454

56. Davis WC, Jackson FC: Inguinal hernia and colon carcinoma. CA 1968; 18:143–145

57. Dean ACB, Newell JP: Colonoscopy in the differential diagnosis of carcinoma from diverticulitis of the sigmoid colon. Br J Surg 1973; 60:633–635

58. de Petz A: Aseptic technic of stomach resections. Ann Surg 1927; 86:388–392

59. Doll R: The geographical distribution of cancer. Br J Cancer 1969; 23:1–8

60. Doll R, Hill AB: Mortality in relation to smoking:

Ten years' observations of British doctors. Br Med J 1964; 1:1399–1410

61. Doll R, Muir C, Waterhouse J (eds): Cancer Incidence in Five Continents. Technical Reports International Union Against Cancer. New York, Springer-Verlag, 1970

62. Drexler J: Asymptomatic polyps of the colon and rectum. 3. Proximal and distal polyp relationships. Arch Intern Med 1971; 127:466–469

63. Drexler J: Proctosigmoidoscopy: When and why? N Engl J Med 1972; 286:668–669

64. Dukes CE: The spread of cancer of the rectum. Br J Surg 1930; 17:643–648

65. Dukes CE: The classification of cancer of the rectum. J Pathol Bacteriol 1932; 35:323–332

66. Dukes CE: The surgical pathology of rectal cancer. (President's address.) Proc R Soc Med 1944; 37:131–144

67. Dukes CE, Bussey HJ: The spread of rectal cancer and its effect on prognosis. Br J Cancer 1958; 12:309–320

68. Dunham LJ, Bailar JC 3rd: World maps of cancer mortality rates and frequency ratios. J Natl Cancer Inst 1968; 41:155–203

69. Dunn DH, Robbins P, Decanini C, Goldberg S, Delaney JP: A comparison of stapled and hand-sewn anastomoses. Dis Colon Rectum 1978; 21:636–639

70. Dwight RW, Higgins GA, Keehn RJ: Factors influencing survival after resection in cancer of the colon and rectum. Am J Surg 1969; 117:512–522

71. Ellert J, Kreel L: The value of CT in malignant colonic tumors. CT 1980; 4:225–240

72. Enstrom JE: Cancer mortality among Mormons. Cancer 1975; 36:825–841

73. Eraklis AJ, Folkman MJ: Adenocarcinoma at the site of ureterosigmoidostomies for exstrophy of the bladder. J Pediatr Surg 1978; 13:730–734

74. Feldman PS: Ulcerative disease of the colon proximal to partially obstructive lesions: Report of two cases and review of the literature. Dis Colon Rectum 1975; 18:601–612

75. Fisher ER, Turnbull RB Jr: The cytologic demonstration and significance of tumor cells in the mesenteric venous blood in patients with colorectal carcinoma. Surg Gynecol Obstet 1955; 100:102–108

76. Fleiszer D, MacFarlane J, Murray D et al: Protective effect of dietary fibre against chemically induced bowel tumours in rats. Lancet 1978; 2:552–553

77. Fortner JG, Kim DK, Barrett MK et al: Eight years' experience with surgical management of 321 patients with liver tumors. In Fox BW (ed): Advances in Medical Oncology Research and Education, Vol 5, Basis for Cancer Therapy I, pp 257–261. Oxford, Pergamon Press, 1979

78. Foster JH: Survival after liver resection for secondary tumors. Am J Surg 1978; 135:389–394

79. Foster JH, Berman M: Solid Liver Tumors. Philadelphia, WB Saunders, 1977

80. Fraser I: An historical perspective on mechanical aids in intestinal anastomosis. Surg Gynecol Obstet 1982; 155:566–574

81. Gabrielsson N, Granqvist S, Ohlsén H: Recurrent carcinoma of the colon in the anastomosis diagnosed by roentgen examination and colonoscopy. Endoscopy 1976; 8:47–52

82. Gambee LP: Single-layer open intestinal anastomosis applicable to small as well as large intestine. West J Surg 1951; 59:1–5

83. Gennaro AR, Tyson RR: Obstructive colonic cancer. Dis Colon Rectum 1978; 21:346–351

84. Getzen LC, Roe RD, Holloway CI: Comparative study of intestinal anastomotic healing in inverted and everted closures. Surg Gynecol Obstet 1966; 123:1219–1227

85. Gilbertsen VA: Improving the prognosis for patients with intestinal cancer. Surg Gynecol Obstet 1967; 124:1253–1259

86. Gilbertsen VA: The earlier diagnosis of adenocarcinoma of the large intestine: A report of 1,884 cases, including 5-year follow-up survival data, results of surgery for the disease, and effect on survival prognosis of treatment earlier in the development of the disease. Cancer 1971; 27:143–149

87. Gilbertsen VA: Proctosigmoidoscopy and polypectomy in reducing the incidence of rectal cancer. Cancer 1974; (Suppl) 34:936–939

88. Gilbertsen VA: The detection of colorectal cancers. Presented at the International Symposium on Colorectal Cancer, New York, March, 1979

89. Gilbertsen VA, Williams SE, Schuman L et al: Colonoscopy in the detection of carcinoma of the intestine. Surg Gynecol Obstet 1979; 149:877–878

90. Gilchrist RK, David VC: A consideration of pathological factors influencing 5 year survival in radical resection of the large bowel and rectum for carcinoma. Ann Surg 1947; 126:421–438

91. Glass RL, Smith LE, Cochran RC: Subtotal colectomy for obstructing carcinoma of the left colon. Am J Surg 1983; 145:335–336

92. Glenn F, McSherry CK: Obstruction and perforation in colorectal cancer. Ann Surg 1971; 173:983–992

93. Go VLW: Carcinoembryonic antigen: Clinical application. Cancer 1976; 37:562–566

94. Gold P, Freedman SO: Demonstration of tumor-specific antigens in human colonic carcinomata by immunological tolerance and absorption techniques. J Exp Med 1965; 121:439–462

95. Gold P, Freedman SO: Specific carcinoembryonic antigens of the human digestive system. J Exp Med 1965; 122:467–481

96. Goldenberg DM, DeLand FH, Kim E et al: Use of radiolabeled antibodies to carcinoembryonic antigen for the detection and localization of diverse cancers by external photoscanning. N Engl J Med 1978; 298:1384–1388

97. Goldenberg DM, Kim EE, Bennett SJ et al: Carcinoembryonic antigen radioimmunodetection in the evaluation of colorectal cancer and in the detection of occult neoplasms. Gastroenterology 1983; 84:524–532

98. Goldenberg DM, Kim EE, DeLand FH et al: Radioimmunodetection of cancer with radioactive antibodies to carcinoembryonic antigen. Cancer Res 1980; 40:2984–2992

99. Goligher JC: The Dukes' A, B and C categorization of the extent of spread of carcinomas of the rectum. Surg Gynecol Obstet 1976; 143:793–794

100. Goligher JC: Use of circular stapling gun with peranal insertion of anorectal purse-string suture for construction of very low colorectal or colo-anal anastomoses. Br J Surg 1979; 66:501–504

101. Goligher JC, Irvin TT, Johnston ID et al: A controlled clinical trial of three methods of closure of laparotomy wound. Br J Surg 1975; 62:823–829

102. Goligher JC, Lee PWR, Macfie J et al: Experience with the Russian model 249 suture gun for anastomosis of the rectum. Surg Gynecol Obstet 1979; 148:517–524

103. Goligher JC, Morris C, McAdam WAF, de Dombal FT, Johnston D: A controlled trial of inverting versus everting intestinal suture in clinical large-bowel surgery. Br J Surg 1970; 57:817–822

104. Goslin R, Steele G, Zamcheck N et al: Factors influencing survival in patients with hepatic metastases from adenocarcinoma of the colon or rectum. Dis Colon Rectum 1982; 25:749–754

105. Gray JH: The relation of lymphatic vessels to the spread of cancer. Br J Surg 1939; 26:462–495

106. Greegor DH: Occult blood testing for detection of asymptomatic colon cancer. Cancer 1971; 28:131–134

107. Greene FL: Distribution of colorectal neoplasms. Am Surg 1983; 49:62–65

108. Greenwald P, Korns RF, Nasca PC et al: Cancer in United States Jews. Cancer Res 1975; 35:3507–3512

109. Grinnell RS: The spread of carcinoma of the colon and rectum. Cancer 1950; 3:641–652

110. Grinnell RS: The rationale of subtotal and total colectomy in the treatment of cancer and multiple polyps of the colon. Surg Gynecol Obstet 1958; 106:288–292

111. Grinnell RS: Results of ligation of inferior mesenteric artery at the aorta in resections of carcinoma of the descending and sigmoid colon and rectum. Surg Gynecol Obstet 1965; 120:1031–1046

112. Grinnell RS: Lymphatic block with atypical and retrograde lymphatic metastasis and spread in carcinoma of the colon and rectum. Ann Surg 1966; 163:272–280

113. Gross L: Incidence of appendectomies and tonsillectomies in cancer patients. Cancer 1966; 19:849–852

114. Grosser N, Thomson DMP: Cell-mediated antitumor immunity in breast cancer patients evaluated by antigen-induced leukocyte adherence inhibition in test tubes. Cancer Res 1975; 35:2571–2579

115. Gunderson LL, Sosin H: Areas of failure found at reoperation (second or symptomatic look) following "curative surgery" for adenocarcinoma of the rectum: Clinicopathologic correlation and implications for adjuvant therapy. Cancer 1974; 34:1278–1292

116. Gunderson LL, Cohen AM, Welch CE: Residual, inoperable or recurrent colorectal cancer: Interaction of surgery and radiotherapy. Am J Surg 1980; 139:518–525

117. Gutherman JU, Mavligit GM, Blumenshein G et al: Immunotherapy of human solid tumors with bacillus Calmette-Guérin: Prolongation of disease-free interval and survival in malignant melanoma, breast and colorectal cancer. Ann NY Acad Sci 1976; 277:135–159

118. Haenszel W: Cancer mortality among the foreign-born in the United States. J Natl Cancer Inst 1961; 26:37–132

119. Haenszel W: Cancer mortality among U.S. Jews. Isr J Med Sci 1971; 7:1437–1450

120. Haenszel W, Correa P: Cancer of the colon and rectum and adenomatous polyps: A review of epidemiological findings. Cancer 1971; 28:14–24

121. Haenszel W, Dawson EA: A note on the mortality from cancer of the colon and rectum in the United States. Cancer 1965; 18:265–272

122. Haenszel W, Kurihara M: Studies of Japanese migrants. I. Mortality from cancer and other diseases among Japanese in the United States. J Natl Cancer Inst 1968; 40:43–68

123. Haenszel W, Berg JW, Segi M et al: Large-bowel

cancer in Hawaiian Japanese. J Natl Cancer Inst 1973; 51:1765–1779

124. Haenszel W, Correa P, Cuello C: Social class in differences among patients with large-bowel cancer in Cali, Colombia. J Natl Cancer Inst 1975; 54:1031–1035

125. Halsted WS: Circular suture of the intestine—an experimental study. Am J Med Sci 1887; 94:436–461

126. Halsted WS: Intestinal anastomosis. Bull Johns Hopkins Hosp 1891; 2:1–4

127. Hamilton JE: Reappraisal of open intestinal anastomoses. Ann Surg 1967; 165:917–923

128. Hammond EC: Smoking in relation to the death rates of one million men and women. Natl Cancer Inst Monogr 1966; 19:127–204

129. Haney MJ, McGarity WC: Ureterosigmoidostomy and neoplasms of the colon: Report of a case and review of the literature. Arch Surg 1971; 103:69–72

130. Hardy TG, Hartmann RF, Samson RB et al: Percutaneous intrahepatic chemotherapy via indwelling portal vein catheter and subcutaneous injection reservoir. Dis Colon Rectum 1982; 25:292–296

131. Hares MM, Alexander-Williams J: The effect of bowel preparation on colonic surgery. World J Surg 1982; 6:175–181

132. Heald RJ, Lockhart-Mummery HE: The lesion of the second cancer of the large bowel. Br J Surg 1972; 59:16–19

133. Heald RJ, Leicester RJ: The low stapled anastomosis. Br J Surg 1981; 68:333–337

134. Healey JE Jr, McBride CM, Gallagher HS: Bowel anastomosis by inverting and everting techniques. J Surg Res 1967; 7:299–304

135. Herberman RB: Immunologic approaches to the diagnosis of cancer. Cancer 1976; 37:549–561

136. Herbst CA Jr, Sessions JT, Lapis JL: Fiberoptic colonoscopic examination in surgical patients with colorectal cancer. South Med J 1980; 73:548–550

137. Hersh EM, Gutterman JU, Mavligit GM et al: BCG vaccine and its derivatives: Potential, practical considerations, and precautions in human cancer immunotherapy. JAMA 1976; 235:246–250

138. Herter FP, Slanetz CE Jr: Preoperative intestinal preparation in relation to the subsequent development of cancer at the suture line. Surg Gynecol Obstet 1968; 127:49–56

139. Hertz RE, Deddish MR, Day E: Value of periodic examinations in detecting cancer of the rectum and colon. Postgrad Med 1960; 27:290–294

140. Higginson J: Etiological factors in gastrointestinal

cancer in man. J Natl Cancer Inst 1966; 37:527–545

141. Higginson J: Etiology of gastrointestinal cancer in man. Natl Cancer Inst Monogr 1967; 25:191–198

142. Higginson J, Oettle AG: Cancer incidence in the Bantu and "Cape Colored" races of South Africa: Report of a cancer survey for the Transvaal (1953–1955). J Natl Cancer Inst 1960; 24:589–671

143. Hill MJ, Drasar BS, Aries V et al: Bacteria and aetiology of cancer of large bowel. Lancet 1971; 1:95–100

144. Howell MA: Factor analysis of international cancer mortality data and per capita food consumption. Br J Cancer 1974; 29:328–336

145. Howell MA: Diet as an etiological factor in the development of cancer of the colon and rectum. J Chronic Dis 1975; 28:67–80

146. Howie JGR, Timperley WR: Cancer and appendectomy. Cancer 1966; 19:1138–1142

147. Hughes ESR, Cuthbertson AM: Subtotal colectomy for obstructing carcinoma of the upper left colon. Dis Colon Rectum 1965; 8:411–412

148. Hyams L, Wynder EL: Appendectomy and cancer risk: An epidemiological evaluation. J Chronic Dis 1968; 21:391–415

149. Irvin TT, Greaney MG: Duration of symptoms and prognosis of carcinoma of the colon and rectum. Surg Gynecol Obstet 1977; 144:883–886

150. Jennings WC, Wood CD, Guernsey JM: Continuous postoperative lavage in the treatment of peritoneal sepsis. Dis Colon Rectum 1982; 25:641–643

151. Jenson CB, Shahon DB, Wangensteen OH: Evaluation of annual examinations in the detection of cancer: Special reference to cancer of the gastrointestinal tract, prostate, breast, and female generative tract. JAMA 1960; 174:1783–1788

152. Kahn HA: The Dorn study of smoking and mortality among U.S. veterans: Report on eight and one-half years of observation. Natl Cancer Inst Monogr 1966; 19:1–125

153. Khoury GA, Waxman BP: Large bowel anastomoses. I. The healing process and sutured anastomoses. A review. Br J Surg 1983; 70:61–63

154. Kirklin JW, Dockerty MB, Waugh JM: Role of peritoneal reflection in prognosis of carcinoma of rectum and sigmoid colon. Surg Gynecol Obstet 1949; 88:326–331

155. Kronborg O, Hage F, Deichgraeber E: The remaining colon after radical surgery for colorectal cancer: The first three years of a prospective study. Dis Colon Rectum 1983; 26:172–176

156. Labow SB, Hoexter B, Walrath DC: Colonic ad-

enocarcinomas in patients with ureterosigmoid-ostomies. Dis Colon Rectum 1979; 22:157–158

157. Lanfrank: Science of Chirurgerie. Fleischhaker R (trans): London, Early English Text Society, Kegan Paul, Trench, Trubner and Co, 1894

158. Leadbetter GW Jr, Zickerman P, Pierce E: Uterosigmoidoscopy and carcinoma of the colon. J Urol 1979; 121:732–735

159. Lembert A: Memoire sur l'enterorrhaphie avec la description d'un procede nouveau pour pratiquer cette operation chirurgicale. Rep Gen Anat Physio Path 1826; 2:100–107

160. Lemon FR, Walden RT: Death from respiratory system disease among Seventh-Day Adventist men. JAMA 1966; 198:117–126

161. Lemon FR, Walden RT, Woods RW: Cancer of the lung and mouth in Seventh-Day Adventists: Preliminary report on a population study. Cancer 1964; 17:486–497

162. Levin ML, Haenszel W, Carroll BE et al: Cancer incidence in urban and rural areas of New York State. J Natl Cancer Inst 1960; 24:1243–1257

163. Lightdale CJ, Sternberg SS, Posner G et al: Carcinoma complicating Crohn's disease: Report of seven cases and review of the literature. Am J Med 1975; 59:262–268

164. Livingstone AS, Hampson LG, Shuster J et al: Carcinoembryonic antigen in the diagnosis and management of colorectal carcinoma: Current status. Arch Surg 1974; 109:259–264

165. Loeb MJ: Comparative strength of inverted, everted and end-on-intestinal anastomoses. Surg Gynecol Obstet 1967; 125:301–304

166. Logan SE, Meier SJ, Ramming KP: Hepatic resection of metastatic colorectal carcinoma. Arch Surg 1982; 117:25–28

167. Lo Gerfo P, Herter FP: Carcinoembryonic antigen and prognosis in patients with colon cancer. Ann Surg 1975; 181:81–84

168. Lovett E: Family studies in cancer of the colon and rectum. Br J Surg 1976; 63:13–18

169. Lynch HT, Guirgis H, Swartz M et al: Genetics and colon cancer. Arch Surg 1973; 106:669–675

170. Lynch PM, Lynch HT, Harris RE: Hereditary proximal colonic cancer. Dis Colon Rectum 1977; 20:662–668

171. Lyon JL, Klauber MR, Gardner JW et al: Cancer incidence in Mormons and non-Mormons in Utah, 1966–1970. N Engl J Med 1976; 294:129–133

172. MacDougall IPM: The cancer risk in ulcerative colitis. Lancet 1964; 2:655–658

173. MacGregor AB, Falk RE: Immunotherapy of malignant disease (part 2). J R Coll Surg Edinb 1976; 21:43–49

174. MacGregor AMC: Mucus-secreting adenomatous polyp at the site of ureterosigmoidostomy: A case report and review of the literature. Br J Surg 1968; 55:591–594

175. Mach J-P, Jaeger P, Bertholoet M-M et al: Detection of recurrence of large bowel carcinoma by radioimmunoassay of circulating carcinoembryonic antigen (CEA). Lancet 1974; 2:535–540

176. Martin EW Jr, James KK, Hurtubise PE et al: The use of CEA as an early indicator for gastrointestinal tumor recurrence and second-look procedures. Cancer 1977; 39:440–446

177. Martin EW Jr, Kibbey WE, DiVecchia L et al: Carcinoembryonic antigen: Clinical and historical aspects. Cancer 1976; 37:62–81

178. Martyak SN, Curtis LW: Abdominal incision and closure, a systems approach. Am J Surg 1976; 131:476–480

179. Mavligit GM, Burgess MA, Seibert GB et al: Prolongation of postoperative disease-free interval and survival in human colorectal cancer by B.C.G. or B.C.G. plus 5-fluorouracil. Lancet 1976; 1:171–185

180. Maxwell JW Jr, Davis WC, Jackson FC: Colon carcinoma and inguinal hernia. Surg Clin North Am 1965; 45:1165–1171

181. Mayo WJ: The cancer problem. Lancet 1915; 35:339–343

182. McCormack PM, Attiyeh FF: Resected pulmonary metastases from colorectal cancer. Dis Colon Rectum 1979; 22:553–556

183. McKenna JP, Currie DJ, MacDonald JA: The use of continuous postoperative peritoneal lavage in the management of diffuse peritonitis. Surg Gynecol Obstet 1970; 130:254–258

184. McVay JR Jr: The appendix in relation to neoplastic disease. Cancer 1964; 17:929–937

185. Michener WM, Gage RP, Sauer WG et al: The prognosis of chronic ulcerative colitis in children. N Engl J Med 1961; 265:1075–1079

186. Milham S Jr: Occupational mortality in Washington state, 1950–1971, Vols 2 and 3. Cincinnati, US Dept of Health, Education, and Welfare, Public Health Service, Center for Disease Control, National Institute for Occupational Safety and Health, Division of Surveillance, Hazard, Evaluation, and Field Studies, 1976

187. Minervini A, Bentley S, Young D: Prophylactic saline peritoneal lavage in elective colorectal operations. Dis Colon Rectum 1980; 23:392–394

188. Minton JP, James KK, Hurtubise PE et al: The use of serial carcinoembryonic antigen determinations to predict recurrence of carcinoma of the colon and the time for a second-look operation. Surg Gynecol Obstet 1978; 147:208–210

189. Moertel CG, Hill JR, Dockerty MB: The routine proctoscopic examination: A second look. Mayo Clin Proc 1966; 41:368–374

190. Moertel CG, Schutt AJ, Go VLW: Carcinoembryonic antigen test for recurrent colorectal carcinoma. JAMA 1978; 239:1065–1066

191. Morgan CN: The management of carcinoma of the colon. Ann R Coll Surg Engl 1952; 10:305–323

192. Morgenstern L, Lee SE: Spatial distribution of colonic carcinoma. Arch Surg 1978; 113:1142–1143

193. Morowitz DA, Block GE, Kirshner JB: Adenocarcinoma of the ileum complicating chronic regional enteritis. Gastroenterology 1968; 55:397–402

194. Murphy JB: Cholecysto-intestinal, gastro-intestinal and entero-intestinal anastomosis, and approximation without sutures. Med Rec NY 1892; 42:665–676

195. Mzabi R, Himal HS, Demers R et al: A multiparametric computer analysis of carcinoma of the colon. Surg Gynecol Obstet 1976; 143:959–964

196. Nakajima N, Ramadan H, Lapi N et al: Rectal carcinoma with solitary cerebral metastasis: Report of a case and review of the literature. Dis Colon Rectum 1979; 22:252–255

197. National Board of Health and Welfare: Cancer Incidence in Sweden, 1959–1965. Stockholm, Swedish Cancer Registry, 1971

198. Nava HR, Pagana TJ: Postoperative surveillance of colorectal carcinoma. Cancer 1982; 49:1043–1047

199. Newill VA: Distribution of cancer mortality among ethnic subgroups of the white population of New York City, 1953–1958. J Natl Cancer Inst 1961; 26:405–417

200. Nichols RL, Broido P, Condon RE et al: Effect of preoperative neomycin-erythromycin intestinal preparation on the incidence of infectious complications following colon surgery. Ann Surg 1973; 178:453–459

201. Nicholson JR, Aust JC: Rising carcinoembryonic antigen titers in colorectal carcinoma: An indication for the second-look procedure. Dis Colon Rectum 1978; 21:163–164

202. Nigro ND: A strategy for prevention of cancer of the large bowel. Dis Colon Rectum 1982; 25:755–758

203. Nigro ND, Bull AW, Klopfer BA et al: Effect of dietary fiber on azoxymethane-induced intestinal carcinogenesis in the rat. J Natl Cancer Inst 1979; 62:1097–1102

204. Nitschke J, Richter H, Herguth D et al: Acute appendicitis and postoperative fecal fistula:

Symptoms of an unrecognized carcinoma of the colon. Dis Colon Rectum 1976; 19:605–610

205. Nivatvongs S, Gilbertsen VA, Goldberg SM et al: Distribution of large-bowel cancers detected by occult blood test in asymptomatic patients. Dis Colon Rectum 1982; 25:420–421

206. Occupational Morality: Decennial Supplement England and Wales. Population Censuses & Surveys Office, 1970–1972, London, HM Stationery Office, 1978

207. Ostrow JD, Mulvaney CA, Hansell JR et al: Sensitivity and reproducibility of chemical tests for fecal occult blood with an emphasis on false-positive reactions. Am J Dig Dis 1973; 18:930–940

208. Overholt BF: Colonoscopy and colon cancer: Current clinical practice. CA 1982; 32:180–186

209. Painter NS, Burkitt DP: Diverticular disease of the colon: a deficiency disease of Western civilization. Br Med J 1971; 2:450–454

210. Patt YZ, Màvligit G, Chuang VP et al: Arteriovenous carcinoembryonic antigen gradient: Determination by selective angiography for localization of metastatic colorectal cancer. Arch Surg 1980; 115:1122–1124

211. Paul FT: Colectomy. Br Med J 1895; 1:1136–1139

212. Pemberton M: Carcinoma of the large intestine with survival in a child of nine and in his father: A study of carcinoma of the colon with particular reference to children. Br J Surg 1970; 57:841–846

213. Phillips RL: Role of life-style and dietary habits in risk of cancer among Seventh-Day Adventists. Cancer Res 1975; (Suppl II:Part 2) 35:3513–3522

214. Pickren JW: Nodal clearance and detection. JAMA 1975; 231:969–971

215. Portes C, Majarakis JD: Proctosigmoidoscopy—incidence of polyps in 50,000 examinations. JAMA 1957; 163:411–413

216. Prager E, Swinton NW, Corman ML et al: Intravenous pyelography in colorectal surgery. Dis Colon Rectum 1973; 16:479–481

217. Rajpal S, Dasmahapatra KS, Ledesma EJ et al: Extensive resections of isolated metastasis from carcinoma of the colon and rectum. Surg Gynecol Obstet 1982; 155:813–816

218. Raskin HF, Pleticka S: The cytologic diagnosis of cancer of the colon. Acta Cytol (Baltimore) 1964; 8:131–140

219. Ravitch MM, Lane R, Cornell WP et al: Closure of duodenal, gastric and intestinal stumps with wire staples: Experimental and clinical studies. Ann Surg 1966; 163:573–579

220. Ravitch MM, Steichen FM: Technics of staple suturing in the gastrointestinal tract. Ann Surg 1972; 175:815–837

221. Ravitch MM, Steichen FM: A stapling instrument for end-to-end inverting anastomoses in the gastrointestinal tract. Ann Surg 1979; 189:791–797

222. Recalde M, Holyoke ED, Elias EG: Carcinoma of the colon, rectum, and anal canal in young patients. Surg Gynecol Obstet 1974; 139:909–913

223. Reiling RB: Staplers in gastrointestinal surgery. Surg Clin North Am 1980; 60:381–397

224. Reiling RB, Reiling WA Jr, Bernie WA et al: Prospective controlled study of gastrointestinal stapled anastomoses. Am J Surg 1980; 139:147–152

225. Reilly JC, Rusin LC, Theuerkauf FJ Jr: Colonoscopy: Its role in cancer of the colon and rectum. Dis Colon Rectum 1982; 25:532–538

226. Reynoso G, Chu TM, Holyoke D et al: Carcinoembryonic antigen in patients with different cancers. JAMA 1972; 220:361–365

227. Richards PC, Balch CM, Aldrete JS: Abdominal wound closure: A prospective study of 571 patients comparing continuous vs. interrupted suture techniques. Ann Surg 1983; 197:238–243

228. Rosato FE, Shelley WB, Fitts WT Jr et al: Nonmetastatic cutaneous manifestations of cancer of the colon. Am J Surg 1969; 117:277–281

229. Rubin P, Green J: Solitary Metastases. Springfield, Charles C Thomas, 1968

230. Rusca JA, Bornside GH, Cohn I: Everting versus inverting gastrointestinal anastomoses: Bacterial leakage and anastomotic disruption. Ann Surg 1969; 169:727–735

231. Saeed W, Kim S, Burch BH et al: Development of carcinoma in regional enteritis. Arch Surg 1974; 108:376–379

232. Saegesser F, Sandblom P: Ischemic lesions of the distended colon. Am J Surg 1975; 129:309–315

233. Salmon SE, Hamburger AW, Soehnlen B et al: Quantitation of differential sensitivity of human tumor stem cells to anticancer drugs. N Engl J Med 1978; 298:1321–1327

234. Salsbury AJ, McKinna JA, Griffiths JD et al: Circulating cancer cells during excision of carcinomas of the rectum and colon with high ligation of the inferior mesenteric vein. Surg Gynecol Obstet 1965; 120:1266–1270

235. Sandler RS, Sandler DP: Radiation-induced cancers of the colon and rectum: Assessing the risk. Gastroenterology 1983; 84:51–57

236. Sanfelippo PM, Beahrs OH: Factors in the prognosis of adenocarcinoma of the colon and rectum. Arch Surg 1972; 104:401–406

237. Sanfelippo PM, Beahrs OH: Carcinoma of the colon in patients under forty years of age. Surg Gynecol Obstet 1974; 138:169–170

238. Schwartz D, Flamant R, Lellouch J et al: Results of a French survey on the role of tobacco, particularly inhalation, in different cancer sites. J Natl Cancer Inst 1961; 26:1085–1108

239. Scudamore HH: Cancer of the colon and rectum—general aspects, diagnosis, treatment, and prognosis: A review. Dis Colon Rectum 1969; 12:105–114

240. Segi M: Cancer Mortality for Selected Sites in 24 Countries: 1950–1957. Sendai, Japan, Department of Public Health, Tohoku University School of Medicine, 1960

241. Seidman H: Cancer death rates by site and sex for religious and socioeconomic groups in New York City. Environ Res 1970; 3:234–250

242. Selby P, Buick RN, Tannock I: A critical appraisal of the human tumor stem-cell assay. N Engl J Med 1983; 308:129–134

243. Shahon DB, Wangensteen OH: Early diagnosis of cancer of the gastrointestinal tract. Postgrad Med 1960; 27:306–311

244. Shapiro A, Berlatsky Y, Lijovetsky G et al: Carcinoma of colon after ureteric anastomosis. Urology 1979; 13:617–620

245. Sheil F O'M, Clark CG, Goligher JC: Adenocarcinoma associated with Crohn's disease. Br J Surg 1968; 55:53–58

246. Silverberg E: Cancer statistics, 1983. CA 1983; 33:16–17

247. Smith RL: Recorded and expected mortality among the Japanese of the United States and Hawaii, with special reference to cancer. J Natl Cancer Inst 1956; 17:459–473

248. Smith RL: Recorded and expected mortality among the Indians of the United States with special reference to cancer. J Natl Cancer Inst 1957; 18:385–396

249. Sorokin JJ, Sugarbaker PH, Zamcheck N et al: Serial carcinoembryonic antigen assays: Use in detection of cancer recurrence. JAMA 1974; 228:49–53

250. Spratt JS Jr: The rates and patterns of growth of neoplasms of the large intestine and rectum. Surg Clin North Am 1965; 45:1103–1115

251. Spratt JS Jr: Gross rates of growth of colonic neoplasms and other variables affecting medical decisions and prognosis. In Burdette WJ (ed): Carcinoma of the Colon and Antecedent Epithelium, pp 66–77. Springfield, Charles C Thomas, 1970

252. Spratt JS Jr, Ackerman LV: The growth of a

colonic adenocarcinoma. Am Surg 1961; 27: 23–28

253. Staszewski J, McCall MG, Stenhouse NS: Cancer mortality in 1962–66 among Polish migrants to Australia. Br J Cancer 1971; 25:599–610

254. Statistical Review of England and Wales. Supplement on Cancer, 1968–1970. London, HM Stationery Office, 1975

255. Steele G Jr, Zamcheck N, Wilson R et al: Results of CEA-initiated second-look surgery for recurrent colorectal cancer. Am J Surg 1980; 139:544–548

256. Sugarbaker PH, Zamcheck N, Moore FD: Assessment of serial carcinoembryonic antigen (CEA) assays in postoperative detection of recurrent colorectal cancer. Cancer 1976; 38:2310–2315

257. Swinton NW Sr, Scherer WP: The value of proctosigmoidoscopic examinations. CA 1968; 18:88–91

258. Swinton NW Sr, Nahra KS, Khazei AM et al: The evolution of colorectal cancer. Dis Colon Rectum 1968; 11:413–419

259. Takaki HS, Ujiki GT, Shields TS: Palliative resections in the treatment of primary colorectal cancer. Am J Surg 1977; 133:548–550

260. Tataryn DN, MacFarlane JK, Murray D et al: Tube leukocyte adherence inhibition (LAI) assay in gastrointestinal (GIT) cancer. Cancer 1979; 43:898–912

261. Teppo L, Hakamd M, Hakulinen T et al: Cancer in Finland, 1953–1970: Incidence, Mortality, Prevalence. Copenhagen, Munksgaard, 1975

262. Terezis NL, Davis WC, Jackson FC: Carcinoma of the colon associated with inguinal hernia. N Engl J Med 1963; 268:774–776

263. Thomson DMP, Krupey J, Freedman SO et al: The radioimmunoassay of circulating carcinoembryonic antigen of the human digestive system. Proc Natl Acad Sci USA 1969; 64:161–167

264. Thomson DMP, Tataryn DN, Lopez M et al: Human tumor-specific immunity assayed by a computerized tube leukocyte adherence inhibition. Cancer Res 1979; 39:638–643

265. Tietjen GW, Markowitz AM: Colitis proximal to obstructing colonic carcinoma. Arch Surg 1975; 110:1133–1138

266. Tong D, Russell AH, Dawson LE et al: Second laparotomy for proximal colon cancer: Sites of recurrence and implications for adjuvant therapy. Am J Surg 1983; 145:382–386

267. Travers B: An inquiry into the process of nature in repairing injuries of the intestine. London, Longmans, Green and Co, Ltd 1812

268. Tsakraklides V, Wanebo HJ, Sternberg SS et al: Prognostic evaluation of regional lymph node morphology in colorectal cancer. Am J Surg 1975; 129:174–180

269. Turnbull RB Jr, Kyle K, Watson FR et al: Cancer of the colon: The influence of the *no-touch isolation* technic on survival rates. Ann Surg 1967; 166:420–427

270. Turunen MJ, Kivilaakso EO: Increased risk of colorectal cancer after cholecystectomy. Ann Surg 1981; 194:639–641

271. Unger SW, Wanebo HJ: Colonoscopy: An essential monitoring technique after resection of colorectal cancer. Am J Surg 1983; 145:71–76

272. Urdaneta LF, Duffell D, Creevy CD et al: Late development of primary carcinoma of the colon following ureterosigmoidostomy: Report of three cases and literature review. Ann Surg 1966; 164:503–513

273. Vernick LJ, Kuller LH, Lohsoonthorn P et al: Relationship between cholecystectomy and ascending colon cancer. Cancer 1980; 45:392–395

274. von Mikulicz J: Chirurgische erjahrun uber das darmcarcinom. Arch f Klin Chir Berl 1903; 69:28–47

275. Wangensteen OH: Cancer of the colon and rectum: With special reference to (1) earlier recognition of alimentary tract malignancy; (2) secondary delayed re-entry of the abdomen in patients exhibiting lymph node involvement; (3) subtotal primary excision of the colon; (4) operation in obstruction. Wis Med J 1949; 48:591–597

276. Wassner JD, Yohai E, Heimlich HJ: Complications associated with the use of gastrointestinal stapling devices. Surgery 1977; 82:395–399

277. Waterhouse J, Muir C, Correa P et al (eds): Cancer Incidence in Five Continents. Vol III, International Union Against Cancer. New York, Springer-Verlag, 1976

278. Waxman BP: Large bowel anastomoses. II. The circular staplers. Br J Surg 1983; 70:64–67

279. Whitaker RH, Pugh RC, Dowe D: Colonic tumours following uretero-sigmoidostomy. Br J Urol 1971; 43:562–575

280. Whitehouse GH, Watt J: Ischemic colitis associated with carcinoma of the colon. Gastrointest Radiol 1977; 2:31–35

281. Wilson SM, Adson MA: Surgical treatment of hepatic metastases from colorectal cancers. Arch Surg 1976; 111:330–334

282. Winawer SJ: The role of CEA in the diagnosis of colonic cancer and other lesions. Natl Large Bowel Cancer Proj Newsl 1975; 3:7

283. Winawer SJ: Screening for colorectal cancer. Pre-

sented at the International Symposium on Colorectal Cancer, New York, March, 1979

284. Winawer SJ: Colon Cancer. In Hunt RH, Waye JD (eds): Colonoscopy: Techniques, Clinical Practice and Colour Atlas, pp 327–342. London, Chapman & Hall, 1981

285. Winawer SJ, Leidner SD, Hajdu SI et al: Colonoscopic biopsy and cytology in the diagnosis of colon cancer. Cancer 1978; 42:2849–2853

286. Winawer SJ, Leidner SD, Miller DG et al: Results of a screening program for the detection of early colon cancer and polyps using fecal occult blood testing (abstr). Gastroenterology 1977; 72:A–127

287. Wolloch Y, Zer M, Lurie M et al: Ischemic colitis proximal to obstructing carcinoma of the colon. Am J Proctol 1979; 30:17–22

288. Wool NL, Straus AK, Roseman DL: Hickman catheter placement simplified. Am J Surg 1983; 145:283–284

289. Young JL Jr, Devesa SS, Cutler SJ: Incidence of cancer in United States blacks. Cancer Res 1975; 35:3523–3536

290. Zamcheck N, Moore TL, Dhar P et al: Immunologic diagnosis and prognosis of human digestive-tract cancer: Carcinoembryonic antigens. N Engl J Med 1972; 286:83–86

291. Zinkin LD: A critical review of the classifications and staging of colorectal cancer. Dis Colon Rectum 1983; 26:37–43

292. Zinkin LD, Brandwein C: Adenocarcinoma in Crohn's colitis. Dis Colon Rectum 1980; 23:115–117

CHAPTER 11

Carcinoma of the Rectum

329

The treatment of cancer of the rectum has been and continues to be among the most debated of surgical discussions. There are a number of procedures available that can, under particular circumstances, be the optimal approach for a given patient (see the list below).

Choices of Operation for Cancer of the Rectum

Abdominoperineal resection
Low anterior resection
Colostomy or ileostomy
Hartmann resection
Abdomino-anal pull-through
Abdominosacral (coccygeal) resection
Transsacral resection (Kraske)
Transanal excision (local excision)
Transsphincteric excision (Mason)
Electrocoagulation
Cryosurgical destruction
Radiation*

* Obviously this is not an operation, but it can be the sole modality of treatment in some instances.

This chapter addresses several surgical decisions (when to employ a procedure, when not to implement it, and how to proceed) and the results.

SIGNS AND SYMPTOMS

The signs and symptoms of cancer of the rectum have been discussed in the previous chapter. Bleeding is the most common complaint (35% to 40%), followed by diarrhea, change in bowel habits, and abdominal pain. Rectal pain as a presenting symptom is quite uncommon. There is, however, a potential area of confusion in the diagnosis: one must be wary of the rectal mass that is due to invasion by carcinoma of the prostate. It can produce obstructive symptoms, may ulcerate, or may even appear circumferential. In a review by Fry and associates of 13 patients, 6 had rectal bleeding, and all had constipation.[59] In 10 cases the lesion was annular.

Biopsy may show adenocarcinoma, but if poorly differentiated, special staining may be required to establish the tumor to be of prostatic origin. Because of the frequency of both conditions, the two tumors may occur synchronously (Fig. 11-1). If a pyelogram is performed, a consistent finding is the presence of ureteral dilatation.[59]

The significance of an incorrect diagnosis cannot be overestimated since the treatment for the two conditions is obviously so different.

HISTORICAL NOTES

Colostomy as a diverting procedure has its origins in antiquity. Praxagoras (c. 400 B.C.) was alleged to have employed some form of decompression maneuver for ileus. Littré is usually credited with performing the first colostomy (1710),[127] but the procedure did not achieve a significant role until Amussat (1839), a French sur-

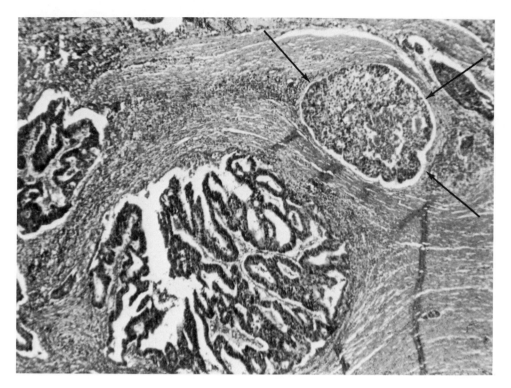

FIG. 11-1. Prostatic carcinoma *(arrows)* invading the rectal wall with an associated primary rectal cancer. This is known as a "collision tumor." (Original magnification × 250. Courtesy of Rudolf Garret, M.D.)

geon, urged that colostomy be employed routinely for rectal cancer.[184]

The treatment of carcinoma of the rectum by some form of excisional or amputative procedure dates back over 250 years, but it was not until 1826 that Lisfranc successfully excised the rectum for this condition.[126] His was a perineal approach and, as such, was of necessity used only for low-lying rectal lesions. The results of the perineal operation were poor; there was frequent incontinence, a high recurrence rate, and a high mortality rate. In 1884, Czerny was unable to remove a rectal cancer and combined the extirpation with an abdominal operation, thus becoming the first person to perform an abdominoperineal resection.[43]

In 1885, Kraske removed the coccyx and part of the sacrum (a maneuver which had been done many times as an extension of the perineal proctectomy), but he preserved the anus and sphincters to effect an anastomosis.[110] The operation became extremely popular but ultimately fell into disrepute because of the complications of sepsis, anastomotic leak, and recurrent disease.

In 1908, Miles described his modification of Czerny's operation, placing emphasis on meticulous dissection and removing the zone of upward spread of the cancer (Fig. 11-2).[158] He concluded as follows:

. . . (1) that an abdominal anus is a necessity; (2) that the whole of the pelvic colon, with the exception of the part from which the colostomy is made, must be removed because its blood-supply is contained in the zone of upward spread; (3) that the whole of the pelvic mesocolon below the point where it crosses the common iliac artery, together with a strip of peritoneum at least an inch wide on either side of it, must be cleared away; (4) that the group of lymph nodes situated over the bifurcation of the common iliac artery are in all instances to be removed; and lastly (5) that the perineal portion of the operation should be carried out as widely as possible so that the lateral and downward zones of spread may be effectively extirpated.

Although initially presenting 12 patients, with an operative mortality of 42%, Miles felt that with improved technique and further experience the operation could be performed relatively safely. He was quite prescient: the "Miles" resection has become the standard operation for the treatment of cancers of the low rectum.

The first documented attempt at abdominal resection with restoration of continuity is generally attrib-

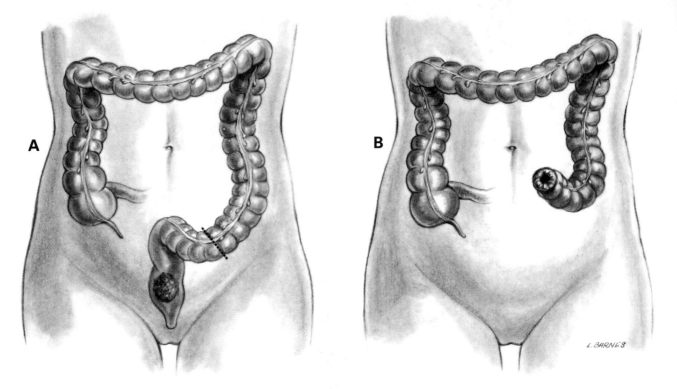

FIG. 11-2. A. Extent of removal in classical abdominoperineal resection **B.** The sigmoid colostomy is created in the left iliac fossa.

uted to Reybard of Lyon.[185] He performed a partial sigmoid resection, the patient surviving approximately 10 months. In 1892, Maunsell described a technique using an anastomotic method employed by Hochenegg in what has come to be called the "pull-through" procedure.[92, 152] The fear of sepsis and anastomotic leak inspired Murphy to create his ingenious "button" in 1892 (see Fig. 10-26).[169] The staged procedures of Bloch and von Mikulicz obviated some of the difficulties, but were not appropriate for the treatment of rectal cancer.[20, 157] The familiar operation of resection and primary anastomosis evolved over the first half of the 20th century and is still changing (*e.g.*, everting versus inverting technique, interrupted versus continuous suture, and stapled versus hand-sewn anastomoses).

FACTORS INDICATING THE CHOICE OF OPERATION

To save or not to save the sphincter is a perennial question. Is there a level below which an anastomosis should not be attempted? When is an abdominoperineal resection inappropriate or an anterior resection

the operation of choice? Unfortunately, there is no consistent answer to these questions. Some would advise with the simple adage, "If you can feel the lesion you should not perform a sphincter-saving operation"—*the rule of the index finger.* But this is much too simplistic an approach and may prejudice the surgeon to embark upon the wrong operation.

Too often, surgeons, in a zealous effort to avoid a colostomy and reestablish intestinal continuity, compromise on the margins of resection. The consequences are often tragic: recurrent disease, anastomotic obstruction, unremitting pelvic pain, and the requirement for subsequent surgery, including a colostomy. Obviously, an abdominoperineal resection is no panacea, but it is an operation that can be relatively safely accomplished and is at least as effective as any other modality of treatment for curing carcinoma of the rectum.

The alternatives to abdominoperineal resection are numerous and are discussed individually. However, if another resective procedure is contemplated, it should rarely be other than an *anterior resection*. If one embarks upon what may be called an *esoteric sphincter-saving operation* (*e.g.*, abdomino-anal pull-through, abdominosacral resection, electrocoagulation, transanal excision, transcoccygeal excision), one must be able to justify it as the optimal treatment of the patient under the circumstances.

Factors that are helpful in determining the choice of operation are summarized in the list below.

Determining Factors in the Choice of Operation for Cancer of the Rectum

Level
Macroscopic appearance (ulcerated, polypoid, *etc.*)
Extent of circumferential involvement
Fixity
Degree of differentiation
Presacral adenopathy
Body habitus
Sex
Age
Metastatic disease
Other systemic disease
Other conditions that might preclude colostomy (e.g., blindness, severe arthritis, mental incapacity)

Level of the Lesion

The distance of the lower edge of the tumor from the anal verge is probably the single most important variable that aids the surgeon in the choice of operation. Using the rigid proctosigmoidoscope, the distance between the anal verge and the lower edge of the tumor should be carefully measured and the result recorded (Fig. 11-3). When measuring, care must be taken to spread the buttocks so that the instrument can be seen emerging from the anus, not from the buttock fat.

The preconceived notion that a tumor which is 7 cm from the anal verge requires abdominoperineal resection, but the one at 8 cm can be treated by anterior resection is erroneous. Other factors may prove the opposite to be true in both cases (*e.g.,* the tumor may be intussuscepting from a higher level).

Macroscopic Appearance

Generally, the distal margin of resection should be approximately 4 cm below the tumor, but for infiltrative carcinomas one may not be "safe" from the risk of anastomotic recurrence with a margin less than 7 cm. Conversely, a small, exophytic lesion may be adequately removed with a 1-cm cuff of normal distal bowel. Ascertaining the appearance of the lesion, whether ulcerated, scirrhus (infiltrative), or polypoid, is very helpful in aiding the surgeon in the choice of operation.

Extent of Circumferential Involvement

Usually, more highly aggressive tumors tend to involve a greater circumference of the bowel wall when they present. Therefore, a greater margin of resection is required when the tumor encompasses the whole of the bowel circumference. An anterior resection may be a poor choice in this situation, even though resection and anastomosis can be technically effected.

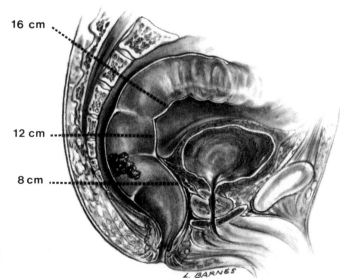

FIG. 11-3. Schematic illustration of rectal cancer. Tumors of the upper third (12 cm–16 cm) are amenable to anterior resection. Tumors of the lower third (to 8 cm) usually require an abdominoperineal resection. It is the middle third tumor that most often represents the management problem.

Fixity

Fixity of the tumor in the pelvis implies a poor prognosis. There is a great likelihood of residual tumor following resection, and anastomotic recurrence is a frequent sequela. An abdominoperineal resection, although no guarantee of obviating the problem of recurrent disease, would probably offer better palliation, because the need for subsequent reoperation would be less likely. The presence of a fixed tumor might also encourage the surgeon to consider preoperative radiotherapy (see later).

Degree of Differentiation

A biopsy is, of course, mandatory, and is done routinely, usually at the time of initial discovery of the lesion. All too often, however, the surgeon pays scant attention to the details of the report, except for noting whether the tumor is indeed malignant. However, it is important to be aware of the histologic appearance of a malignant tumor. Is it a poorly differentiated, a moderately well-differentiated, or a well-differentiated tumor (see Figs. 10-11 to 10-13)? The more anaplastic, the more aggressive is the lesion; and the more aggressive, the greater the resection margin required. The chance of local recurrence is much higher with a poorly differentiated cancer than with one that is well differentiated. If the pathologist fails to supply this information he should be asked to review the slides and to amend the report.

Presacral Adenopathy

By careful palpation of the rectum, feeling for masses outside the wall, the surgeon can occasionally identify a hard lesion, a lymph node with metastasis. Such a finding can aid the surgeon by suggesting (although by no means proving) that the tumor has spread beyond the bowel wall and that recurrence is, therefore, more likely. A sphincter-saving operation is liable to result in recurrence. This is another situation in which preoperative radiotherapy may be of benefit.

The previous factors concerned the tumor itself. The following variables that may influence the choice of operation are related to the patient.

Body Habitus

A rectal resection carried out on an asthenic patient usually permits a technically lower anastomosis than an operation for the same level of lesion in an obese patient. In preoperative evaluation and counseling of the patient, the factor of body habitus may lead the surgeon to present an optimistic or pessimistic view of the likelihood of reestablishing intestinal continuity.

Sex

An anastomotic procedure for resection is more likely to be favored in women than in men. The broad pelvis, furthermore, usually permits a wider resection, whereas a narrow pelvis tends to impede adequate dissection and limit the use of conventional anastomotic techniques. This is particularly true in the performance of a low anterior resection.

Age

A resection involving an anastomosis is a higher-risk procedure than an abdominoperineal resection; morbidity is greater, and operative mortality is higher. Furthermore, the possibility of a second operation (*e.g.*, closure of a colostomy) increases the risk still further. Although it is not an absolute contraindication in elderly patients, they are less suitable for staged operations.

Metastatic Disease

Anastomotic procedures are often mistakenly embarked upon in the presence of metastatic disease in order to avoid colostomy during the terminal phase of the patient's illness. All too often, however, even if the procedure is initially successful, the patient returns to have a colostomy because of complications related to pelvic recurrence. Operative mortality, furthermore, is much higher for palliative resections, including abdominoperineal resection. A colostomy or a Hartmann resection may be adequate,[85] or a local procedure (especially electrocoagulation) may be the best choice if symptoms can be controlled by this means.

Systemic Disease

Any patient, regardless of age, is at an increased risk for surgery if systemic disease (*e.g.,* cardiovascular, pulmonary, renal) is present. Such patients are more safely treated by a procedure that does not involve an anastomosis. The surgeon must balance the risks against the advantages of avoiding a colostomy.

Other Conditions

Avoiding a colostomy in a patient who cannot cope with an appliance or a stoma is an unusual, albeit legitimate, reason for choosing an alternative procedure. The quality of life may be poor, indeed, if a patient must be relegated to a nursing home or terminal care facility because he cannot cope at home managing a stoma. This can happen if the patient is blind, has severe impairment in the use of hands (*e.g.,* arthritis), or cannot be taught. Obviously, alternatives exist to support the patient, such as care by a family member, a visiting nurse, or a home helper. Of course, there may be no alternative except a stoma to cure the disease or to effectively palliate the condition.

In the choice of operation, the surgeon must consider all of the above factors and make a recommendation based upon what is the appropriate procedure for the given person. A tumor in one patient may require quite a different treatment than the same lesion in the same location in another.

Each operation for carcinoma of the rectum is discussed on its own merits.

ABDOMINOPERINEAL RESECTION

The description in 1908 by W. Ernest Miles of the abdominoperineal approach to tumors of the rectum was a landmark in the history of large bowel surgery.[159] This operation involved an abdominal dissection and mobilization of the rectum; the rectum was then buried beneath the reconstituted pelvic floor. It was then excised through the perineal route, classically in the left lateral position. Since the original publication, only minor modifications in the surgical technique have been introduced.[153, 183]

Others (*e.g.,* Lahey) felt that if the operation were divided into two stages, it might be better tolerated by the patient.[116] The first stage consisted of making a median incision, dividing the sigmoid colon, and creating a left iliac colostomy with a mucous fistula of the distal segment delivered through the lower part of the abdominal incision. Care was taken to preserve the superior hemorrhoidal artery to the distal bowel. In the second stage the proctectomy was carried out.

Although the two-stage procedure was successful in reducing morbidity and mortality prior to blood transfusion and in the pre-antibiotic era, it was gradually abandoned because of the progressive improvement in the results of the one-stage approach.

J. P. Lockhart-Mummery of St. Mark's Hospital introduced an extended perineal excision with preliminary colostomy and reported an improved mortality rate.[135] This method, however, did not remove the in-

ferior mesenteric lymph nodes, nor was the technique applicable for higher rectal growths. But it was used for over 80% of the excisions of the rectum at that institution from 1928 to 1932, the Miles operation being used for the remainder.

In 1939, Lloyd-Davies reaffirmed the value of the synchronous combined (two-team) abdominoperineal resection which had been originally suggested by Mayo.[128, 154] By 1963, at the St. Mark's Hospital, the Lloyd-Davies technique was by far the most commonly employed approach, and the operative mortality had been reduced to under 3%.[163] This is my preferred approach for low-lying carcinomas of the rectum.

The technique involves two teams operating synchronously once the resectability of the tumor has been ascertained by the abdominal surgeon. This permits easier access to the pelvis and allows an attack on the area from two directions. It is particularly helpful when one is confronted with a bulky or fixed tumor, or in a patient with a narrow pelvis. In spite of the fact that Miles stated that his operation took only from an hour and a quarter to an hour and a half and that his patients suffered ''no more shock than after an ordinary perineal excision,'' blood loss *can* be reduced and operative time decreased by using a two-team method.[158]

Indications

When tumors are less than 8 cm from the anal verge, the usual and customary treatment is abdominoperineal resection. Higher lesions may permit restoration of intestinal continuity, usually by low anterior resection. As a palliative procedure (even in the presence of metastatic disease), if the patient's life expectancy may be several months or more, greater patient comfort can often be achieved than with a diversionary procedure alone. This is particularly true when the tumor invades the sphincter mechanism to produce tenesmus, or extends to the perineum, or bleeds. It is the most consistently successful operation for carcinoma and is the procedure against which alternative sphincter-saving operations must be compared.

Preoperative Preparation

The routine screening studies are discussed in Chapter 10. Evaluation of the proximal bowel by means of air-contrast barium enema examination (to look for synchronous lesions) should be undertaken routinely except when the rectal tumor appears virtually obstructing. An intravenous pyelogram should also be required. The bowel preparation consists of laxatives, enemas, and nonabsorbable antibiotics (see Chap. 10).

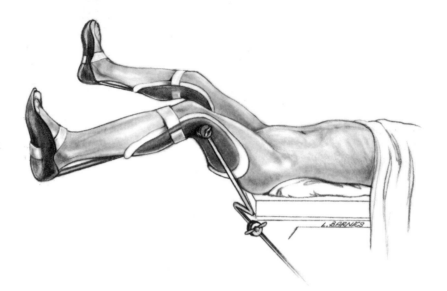

FIG. 11-4. Perineolithotomy (Lloyd-Davies) position: the thighs are abducted and extended, and the knees are flexed.

Anesthesia

A general, endotracheal anesthetic is preferred for this procedure, but a spinal anesthetic can also be used. Continuous cardiac monitoring, as with all major surgery, is advisable. A size-16 Foley catheter with a 5-ml bag is inserted into the bladder in the operating room. A Silastic catheter is preferred because there is less tissue reactivity and it is less likely to cause a urethral stricture. No nasogastric tube is advised.

Technique

The patient is placed in the perineolithotomy position with the legs in stirrups (Fig. 11-4). The leg supports should be similar to those described by Lloyd-Davies[128] and not those that are usually employed for gynecologic procedures, although obstetric or urologic stirrups may be substituted (Fig. 11-5). Support of the thighs and feet is required. The knees can be flexed, but the hips should be relatively extended and the thighs abducted in order to allow access to the abdomen and to the perineum. Too much hip flexion can interfere with the abdominal operator's maneuverability. Furthermore, if a second assistant is required for the pelvic dissection, he may be unable to be used near the sur-

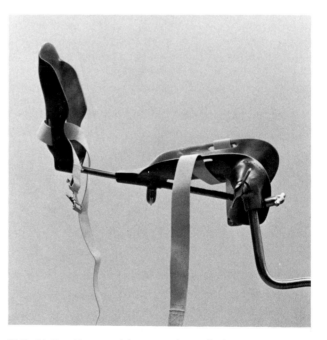

FIG. 11-5. Knee and foot crutch to eliminate pressure on the popliteal area. (Courtesy of American Sterilizer Co.)

geon. A moderate degree of Trendelenburg (head-down) tilt aids in the dissection.

The Mayo stand should be placed over the patient's head as low as the anesthesiologist will permit. No ether screen is employed; sterility on the cephalad aspect of the operative field is obtained using IV poles.

A pursestring suture is placed around the anus using a nonabsorbable retention suture (Fig. 11-6). The abdomen and perineum are then cleansed with an antiseptic solution. Draping can be expedited by using a ''thyroid'' or split sheet in a reverse fashion in order to limit the amount of bulky covering over the perineum. Mayo-stand covers over the legs also simplify the draping.

The location of the incision is important, not only for the obvious reason of access to the abdomen, but also to avoid interference with the subsequent placement of the stoma. A midline hypogastric incision is advised, extending through the umbilicus if necessary. The colostomy ideally should be placed over the rectus muscle and brought through the split thickness of the muscle. Paracolostomy herniation is less likely to occur if the stoma is brought through the rectus muscle than in a pararectus location. It should never be brought out through the incision. Therefore, a left paramedian incision is relatively contraindicated. Furthermore, the stoma should be situated beneath the belt line at a distance from bony promontories and umbilicus (Fig. 11-7; see also Chap. 16).

The technique of abdominoperineal resection requires identification and control of the inferior mesenteric vessels, the middle hemorrhoidal arteries (which pass adjacent to the lateral ligaments of the rectum), and the inferior hemorrhoidal vessels (Fig. 11-8).

After the insertion of a self-retaining (Balfour) retractor, the abdomen is explored for evidence of metastatic disease, the presence of a synchronous colon lesion, or other pathology. The small intestine is packed into the upper abdomen using three moist pads: one over the cecum, one along the descending colon, and the third from side to side across the abdomen. Rarely should it be necessary to exteriorize the bowel. By keeping the viscera warm and moist and within the abdomen there is less likelihood of postoperative ileus, and a nasogastric tube can be avoided.

Mobilization of the sigmoid colon and rectosigmoid commences along the left colic gutter, lysing the developmental adhesions in order to obtain sufficient mobility to deliver the bowel to the abdominal wall at the level of the proposed colostomy.

The peritoneum on the left lateral aspect is incised, and the left ureter is identified and retracted laterally (see Fig. 10-43). Injury to the ureter most commonly

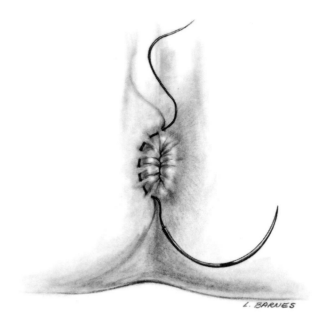

FIG. 11-6. Abdominoperineal resection: a pursestring suture is secured, closing the anus.

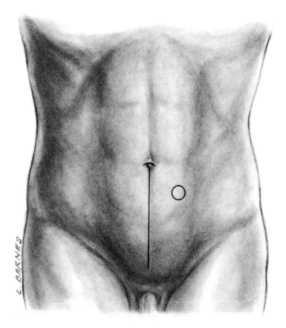

FIG. 11-7. The proper position of the sigmoid colostomy site for abdominoperineal resection is away from bony promontories, the umbilicus, scars, and skin folds, and within the rectus muscle.

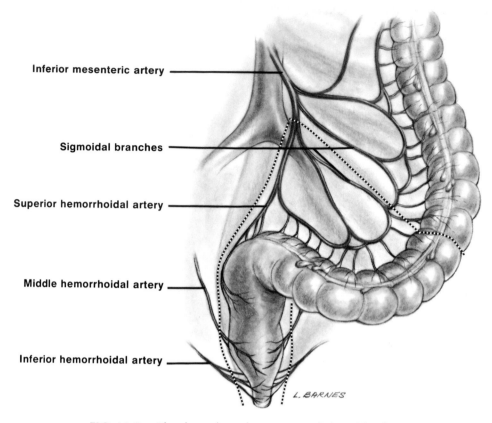

Inferior mesenteric artery

Sigmoidal branches

Superior hemorrhoidal artery

Middle hemorrhoidal artery

Inferior hemorrhoidal artery

L. BARNES

FIG. 11-8. Blood supply to the rectum and sigmoid colon.

occurs during this point in the operation, at the level of the iliac artery; it must always be visualized and protected. Incision of the peritoneum is continued anteriorly to the base of the bladder.

The left hand is then passed beneath the inferior mesenteric vessels, and the peritoneal incision is performed in a similar fashion on the right side (see Fig. 10-44). The mesenteric vascular pedicle is ligated between clamps; one should always check to be certain that the left ureter has not been incorporated (see Fig. 10-45). The importance of the right ureter is not meant to be deemphasized, but it should not be involved in this aspect of the dissection unless there is a congenital anomaly or a history of previous surgery that caused medial deviation of this structure. Injury to the right ureter is usually caused at the time of pelvic floor reconstruction by mobilization and suture of the peritoneum on that side.

Ligation of the inferior mesenteric artery at its origin is unnecessary because in my experience nodal involvement at that level is found only in patients with incurable cancer. Ligation distal to the first branch of

the inferior mesenteric artery ensures a viable blood supply to the bowel from which the stoma will be created. Pelvic peritoneal incisions are then joined across the base of the bladder (or at the vaginal apex in women).

Attention is then turned to the retrorectal space; this space should be entered by sharp dissection (Fig. 11-9). Often, surgeons commence blunt dissection at the level of the sacral promontory. When doing this, the plane may be improperly entered, and the presacral vessels can be torn. Gentle anterior traction is placed on the rectosigmoid and the scissors inserted anterior to the sacral promontory. The presacral space is relatively avascular and usually readily entered. The loose areolar tissue is identified and incised.

Once the presacral space has been demonstrated, the right hand is inserted into this region, and the presacral dissection is carried out by means of blunt finger dissection and gentle anterior displacement of the rectum (Fig. 11-10). It is often helpful to drape a sponge over the fingers to facilitate this maneuver. The rectum is freed from the anterior sacral fascia to the

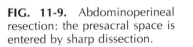

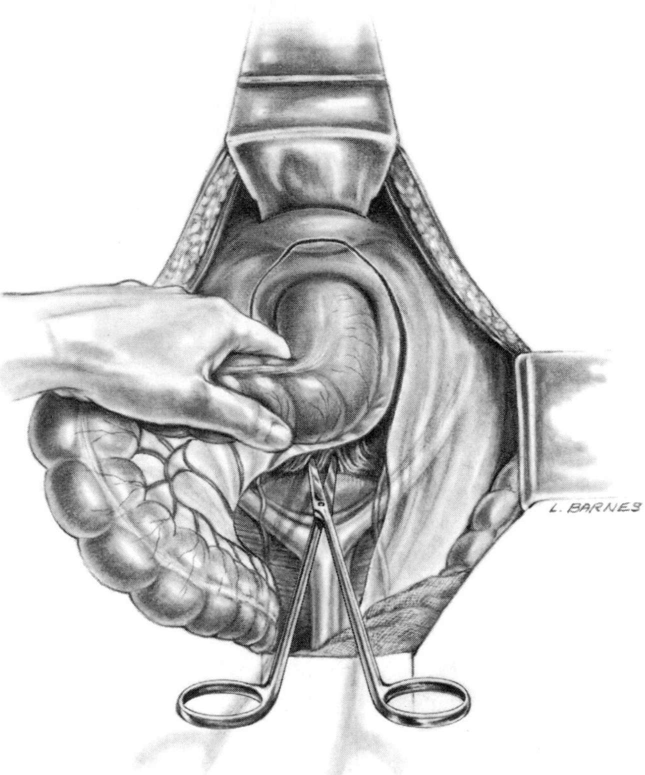

FIG. 11-9. Abdominoperineal resection: the presacral space is entered by sharp dissection.

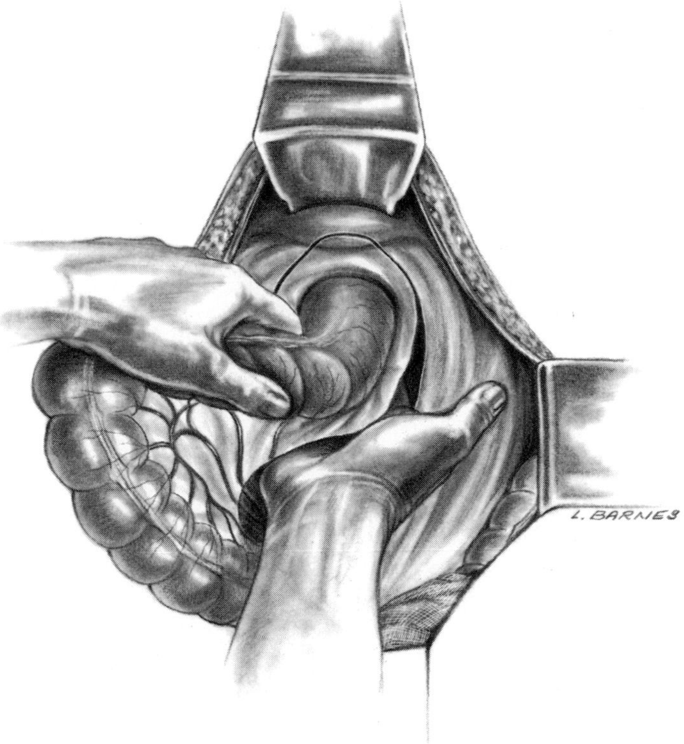

FIG. 11-10. Abdominoperineal resection: the rectum is mobilized from the lower pelvic adhesions by blunt dissection; this produces a characteristic "sucking" sound.

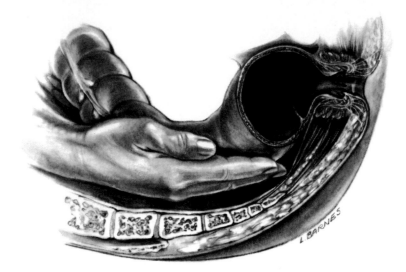

FIG. 11-11.   Abdominoperineal resection: the lateral view illustrates that, ideally, the sacral fascia is not breached when the rectum is bluntly dissected.

level of the tip of the coccyx distally. The dissection is performed in a plane anterior to the fascia, and thus damage to the presacral veins is avoided (Fig. 11-11). When bleeding vessels are encountered, attempt at ligation may be unsuccessful, especially if bleeding exudes directly from bone. Rather than attempting to electrocoagulate and continuing to lose blood, direct pressure for a few minutes with a large pad is suggested. If posterior mobilization of the rectum is impeded by tumor extension, the abdominal operator should wait for the perineal surgeon to develop a plane rather than proceeding blindly. If a synchronous combined procedure is not being performed, or if no plane can be developed from either direction, the surgeon must dissect wherever he presumes the plane to have been, fully realizing that the possibility for cure may be compromised. If one is performing a synchronous approach, it is at this point in the operation that the abdominal operator meets the perineal surgeon (in the posterior midline), when the rectococcygeus ligament has been divided.

Attention is then turned to the anterior part of the dissection. The posterior wall of the bladder and seminal vesicles (or uterus and posterior vaginal wall in women) are demonstrated using a St. Mark's pattern retractor (7 inch with turned-back lip), and by a combination of sharp and blunt dissection (Fig. 11-12). Denonvillier's fascia must be incised in order to separate the rectum completely from the prostate and the seminal vesicles. By means of retraction of the bladder and prostatic area and countertraction of the rectum, the dissection is carried distally until the apex of the

prostate and the urethra with its contained catheter can be palpated. In women, the posterior vaginal wall is swept away to the point where the posterior vaginal wall is to be excised (Fig. 11-13). Dissection is facilitated by placing the left hand and compressing the anterior rectal wall as distally as possible.

Attention is then turned to the lateral ligaments and to the middle hemorrhoidal arteries. Using a long scissors the space is entered distal to the lateral ligaments, and the scissors are spread in the anterior–posterior plane. The index finger of the left hand is then passed behind the ligament and adjacent vessls on the right side. There is often a firm fascial band that needs to be traversed bluntly. The ligament is then straddled by the index and long fingers of the left hand and retracted medially (Fig. 11-14). A single crushing clamp is used, and the lateral ligament and the middle hemorrhoidal vessel transected medial to the clamp. Back-bleeding from the artery rarely occurs but can easily and safely be controlled by rotating the rectum and directly visualizing the bleeding point. With the lateral ligament divided, the rectum is readily mobilized.

The left lateral ligament is divided similarly, but the maneuver is slightly more difficult to perform. The left index and long finger again straddle the structures, but the rectum is pushed away toward the right side, and the clamp is applied behind the hand (Fig. 11-15). Upon completion of this step in the procedure, the rectum is completely isolated anteriorly, laterally, and posteriorly. A few fibrous strands may require division, but no important vascular structures need to be controlled in order to complete the pelvic dissection.

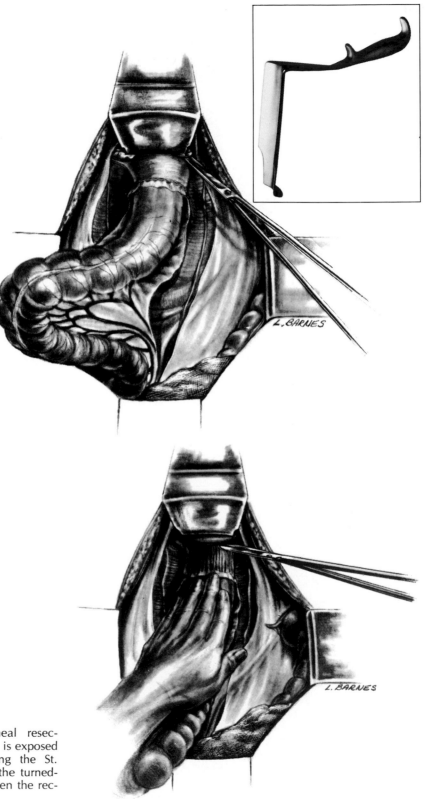

FIG. 11-12. Abdominoperineal resection: the anterior peritoneal dissection in the male reveals the seminal vesicles and prostate. The mobilization is facilitated by use of the St. Mark's pattern retractor *(inset)*.

FIG. 11-13. Abdominoperineal resection: the posterior vaginal wall is exposed below the retractor. By using the St. Mark's pattern retractor with the turned-back lip, the dissection between the rectum and vagina is facilitated.

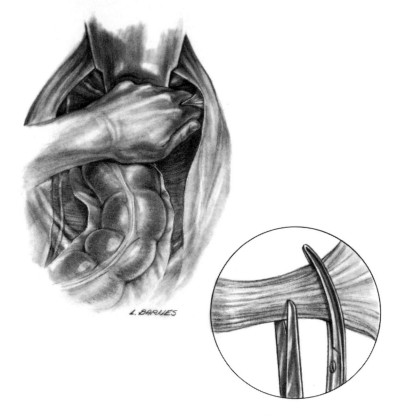

FIG. 11-14. Abdominoperineal resection: the right lateral ligament is isolated between the index and long fingers of the left hand. The ligament and middle hemorrhoidal artery are clamped laterally and divided on the rectal side *(inset).*

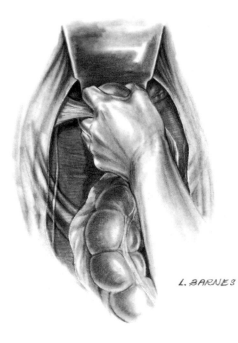

FIG. 11-15. Abdominoperineal resection: the left lateral ligament is isolated with the left hand, and the rectum is "pushed" toward the right side. A single clamp is then placed laterally.

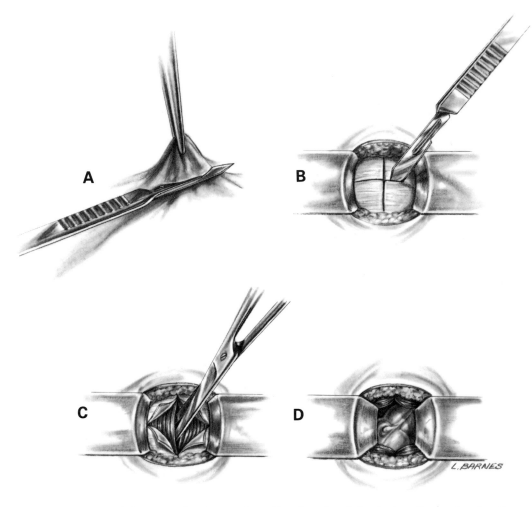

FIG. 11-16. Abdominoperineal resection: Creating the abdominal wall opening for the colostomy. **A.** A disk of skin is excised. **B.** A cruciate incision is made in the anterior rectus fascia. **C.** The rectus muscle is split longitudinally. **D.** The completed abdominal wall opening.

The sigmoid colon is then held up to the abdominal wound and a point (usually at the apex) is selected for creation of the colostomy. If the abdominal wall is very thick, a slightly more distal point is selected. If the sigmoid colon is redundant, a more cephalad site is chosen. The arcade vessel is then divided.

The site of the colostomy is now prepared by grasping the skin with a Kocher clamp and excising a circular segment of skin, the diameter of which should approximate the diameter of the sigmoid colon to be used for the colostomy (Fig. 11-16, *A*). The subcutaneous, fatty tissue is bluntly retracted and the anterior sheath of the rectus muscle is incised in a cruciate fashion (Fig. 11-16 *B, C*). The rectus muscle fibers are then split in a longitudinal direction, and the peritoneal cavity is entered with scissors (Fig. 11-16, *D*). The colostomy aperture in the peritoneum, muscle, and skin must permit two fingers.

The surgeon should now inspect the abdominal wall for possible injury to the inferior epigastric vessels. Frequently, an attempt is made to control bleeding from the colostomy site by clamping through the skin opening. Since the vascular structures lie just above the peritoneum, this is often a futile exercise. By placing a sponge through the future stomal opening and out the abdominal incision, exposure of the epigastric artery and vein is facilitated (Fig. 11-17). Hemostasis can be readily established.

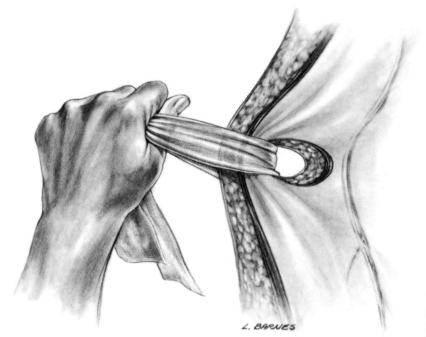

L. BARNES

FIG. 11-17. Abdominoperineal resection: exposure of the epigastric vessels by sponge retraction.

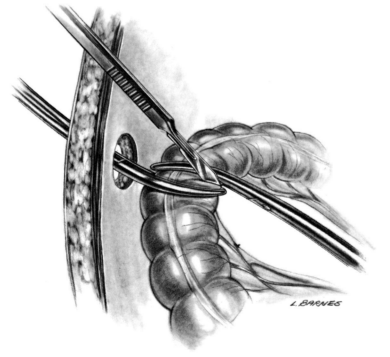

L. BARNES

FIG. 11-18. Abdominoperineal resection: a clamp is passed through the abdominal wall opening to grasp the bowel at the site for the creation of the colostomy. This maneuver eliminates one step and reduces the risk of fecal spillage when both clamps are placed within the abdomen.

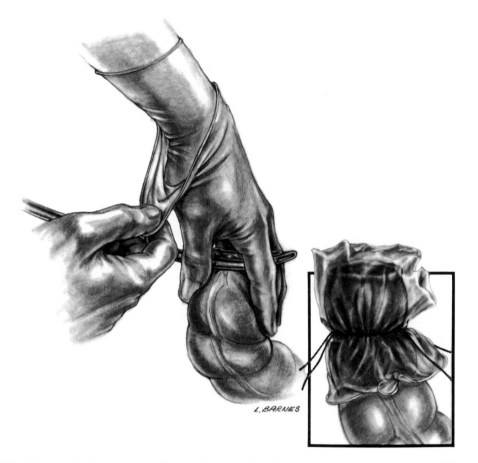

FIG. 11-19. Abdominoperineal resection: the distal colonic stump is encompassed by a rubber glove. It is then everted and secured with heavy ligatures *(inset).*

A crushing clamp is passed through the colostomy wound into the abdominal cavity to grasp the prepared colon at the site of the proposed colostomy (Fig. 11-18). The distal rectosigmoid is also clamped, and the bowel is divided between these two clamps. The proximal bowel is withdrawn through the abdominal wall to lie without tension on the anterior abdominal surface.

The divided distal bowel is sealed from contamination by grasping it in a doubly-gloved hand and tying the removed outer glove over the stump of the rectosigmoid as the clamp is removed (Fig. 11-19). Doubled No. 2 silk or catgut is used. The rectum is then delivered through the perineal opening (in a synchronous combined operation) or buried in the pelvic cavity (as in the classical Miles approach).

Kocher clamps are then placed on the cut edge of the peritoneum, and by finger dissection the lateral peritoneum is mobilized to a degree that will permit closure with a continuous absorbable suture (Fig. 11-20). Closure of the lateral paracolostomy opening (gutter) is not recommended. Too often, a narrow opening results when a suture cuts through or breaks. A large opening is preferred to a narrow one.

Following abdominal wound closure the redundant bowel is excised and the colostomy primarily "matured" by using approximately eight sutures of 4-0 chromic catgut through the full thickness of the bowel and the skin (Fig. 11-21).

Concomitant Hysterectomy

Although hysterectomy concomitant with abdominoperineal resection should not be routinely employed, occasionally the tumor breaches the seromuscular wall

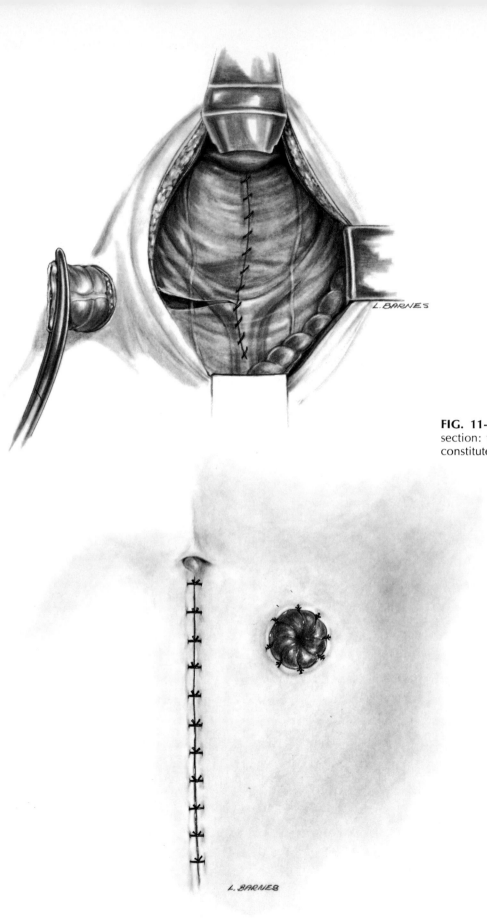

FIG. 11-20. Abdominoperineal resection: the floor of the pelvis is reconstituted.

FIG. 11-21. Abdominoperineal resection: the wound is closed and the colostomy "matured."

with invasion of the cervix, lower uterine segment, or body of the uterus. Under such circumstances an in-continuity hysterectomy must be performed in order to adequately extirpate the tumor.

The incision of the peritoneum in the floor of the pelvis must of necessity be wider than that for abdominoperineal resection (Fig. 11-22). Both ureters are in greater danger of injury when this operation is performed. They should, therefore, be clearly identified throughout their lengths. Anteriorly, the peritoneal flap is dissected off the uterus, and the bladder is bluntly pushed away from the cervix and vaginal wall. The infundibulopelvic and round ligaments are cross-clamped, divided, and ligated (Fig. 11-23). The broad ligament is dissected away from the pelvic wall, exposing the uterine artery. By retraction of the uterus to the contralateral side, the uterine artery is cross-clamped, divided, and ligated. Division of the cardinal ligament poses the greatest threat to the ureter. If the tumor approaches this area, the cardinal ligament must be clamped close to the pelvic wall, and the ureter must be clearly visualized (Fig. 11-24). I prefer to use a curved Kocher clamp placed on only one side, a maneuver analogous to the technique employed for division of the lateral ligaments.

When the dissection has been completed on both sides, the anterior vaginal wall is incised and the posterior vaginal wall removed with the proctectomy.

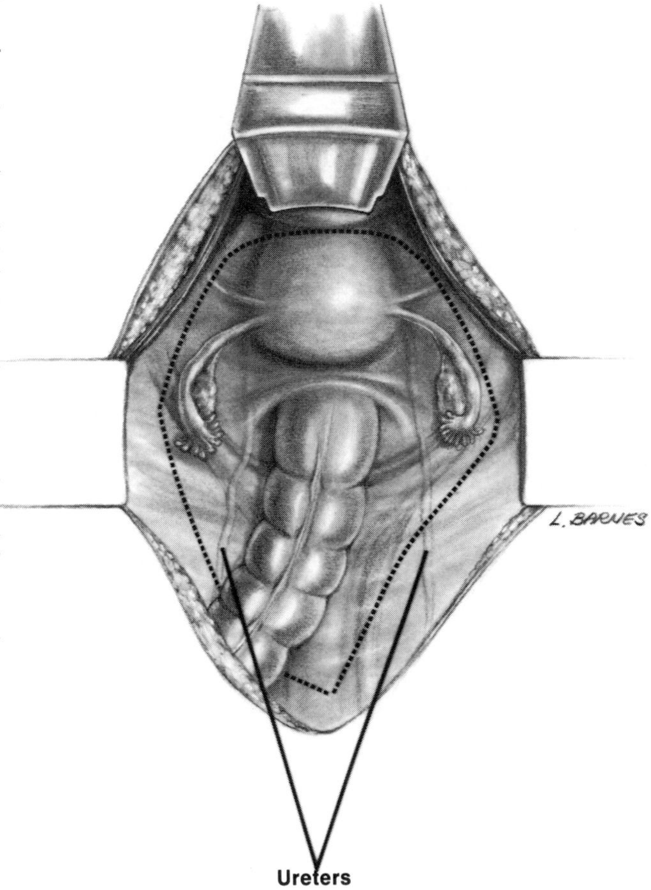

Incidental Appendectomy

Incidental appendectomy is not recommended with proctectomy or with any bowel resection. It is difficult enough to evaluate postoperative lower abdominal signs and symptoms, fever, and leukocytosis, without adding unnecessary variables.

Prophylactic Oophorectomy

Metastatic disease apparent at the time of surgery obviously is an indication for *therapeutic* oophorectomy, but the value of *prophylactic* oophorectomy has been the subject of considerable debate.[3, 17, 18, 108, 139] Metastatic colorectal carcinoma to the ovary, even when resectable for cure, is associated with only a 5% 5-year survival. Even with microscopic involvement, prognosis is poor (20% to 30%). With the low incidence of microscopic metastatic involvement, it is difficult to justify prophylactic oophorectomy in the premenopausal age group, but removal of the ovaries in the postmenopausal patient appears a reasonable course. In

FIG. 11-22. In hysterectomy concomitant with abdominoperineal resection, the peritoneal incision *(dotted line)* must be quite wide to incorporate the uterus and rectum for removal in continuity.

reality, however, the prevention of primary ovarian cancer is probably the main benefit.[41] Parenthetically, oophorectomy is as appropriate for cecal carcinoma as it is for a rectal or sigmoid lesion.

Sacrectomy and Exenteration

Sugarbaker has advocated *en bloc* excision of rectal cancer with sacrectomy for lesions that are fixed posteriorly.[221] In reporting his experience with six patients, four survived more than 3 years. Others have demonstrated that pelvic exenteration (abdominoperineal resection and cystectomy) in selected patients may produce a 30% 5-year survival.[107]

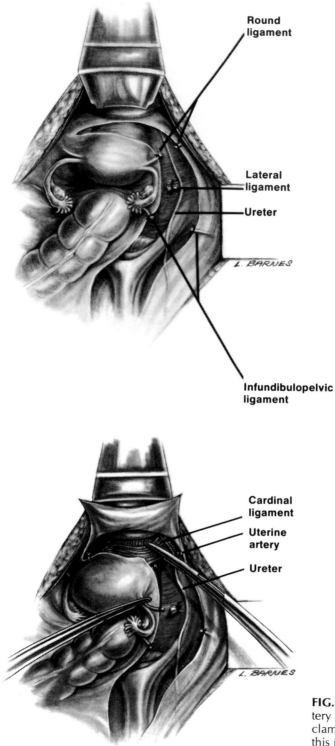

FIG. 11-23.   Concomitant hysterectomy: the uterus and rectum are mobilized on the right side by division of the round, infundibulopelvic, and lateral ligaments.

FIG. 11-24.   Concomitant hysterectomy: the uterine artery has been divided, and the cardinal ligament is clamped. The ureter is extremely vulnerable to injury at this point.

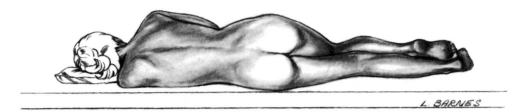

FIG. 11-25. Perineal dissection is carried out with the patient in the left lateral position in the classical Miles' operation. The surgeon can be seated.

Although there probably is an occasional patient who may be a candidate for one of the more aggressive extirpations, I have not as yet found such an individual. Perhaps my pessimism concerning the likelihood of success with this type of surgery is responsible for my lack of experience in this area.

Perineal Dissection

In the synchronous-combined excision, the perineal dissection is commenced as soon as the abdominal operator determines that the lesion is resectable. If two teams are not available, the perineal portion of the operation is done after the entire abdominal operation has been completed and the pelvic peritoneum has been closed above the stump of the rectosigmoid. Under no circumstances should the perineal operation be undertaken initially. If the perineal proctectomy is performed with the patient in the left lateral position (the classic Miles approach) it is usually more comfortable if the surgeon is seated. The light is directed from the foot, and the first assistant stands on a platform on the opposite side (Fig. 11-25). The following illustrations, however, demonstrate the procedure in the perineolithotomy position, although the principles are the same.

An elliptical incision is made outside of the sphincter muscle, including a generous margin of perianal skin (Fig. 11-26). The edges of the perianal skin are grasped on each side with serial Kocher clamps. The dissection is carried out at least initially with electrocautery, and the assistant clamps any bleeding vessel with a curved hemostat. By touching the tip of the electrocautery to the hemostat one can continue dissecting without the need for frequent scraping of debris off the coagulating tip. Usually two vascular bundles are identified lying anteriorly and posteriorly on either side in the ischiorectal fat. These are the inferior hemorrhoidal vessels (Fig. 11-27).

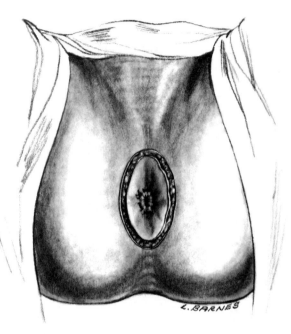

FIG. 11-26. Perineal dissection: an elliptical incision is made outside the anus.

Once the ischiorectal fossa has been entered a self-retaining (Lace) retractor facilitates the exposure. The anterior dissection is deepened by incising the deep transverse perineal muscle (Fig. 11-28).

The presacral space is now entered by dividing the rectococcygeus, commencing at the level of the tip of the coccyx (Fig. 11-29, A). The coccyx is not removed unless the tumor proves to be so large that it cannot be delivered through the perineal opening. To remove the coccyx, a scalpel is inserted into the joint by flexing the bone with the thumb (Fig. 11-29, B). It is then separated and removed by using a knife or heavy scissors. Care should be taken to dissect sufficiently anterior to the sacrum; all too often the perineal procedure

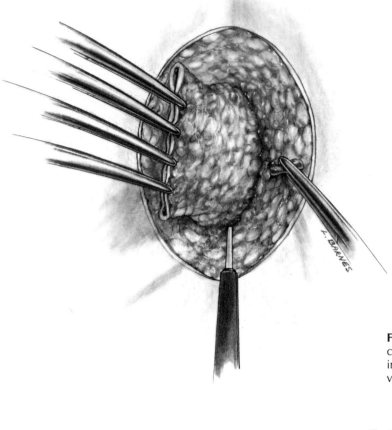

FIG. 11-27. Perineal dissection: serial Kocher clamps are applied to the perianal skin and the incision is deepened. The inferior hemorrhoidal vessels are clamped and divided.

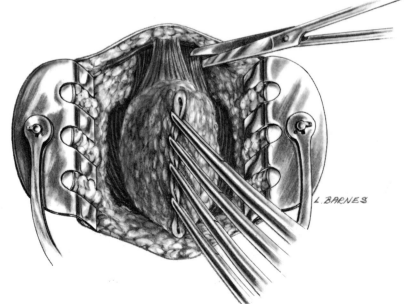

FIG. 11-28. Perineal dissection: the rectum is freed anteriorly by dividing the transverse perineal muscle.

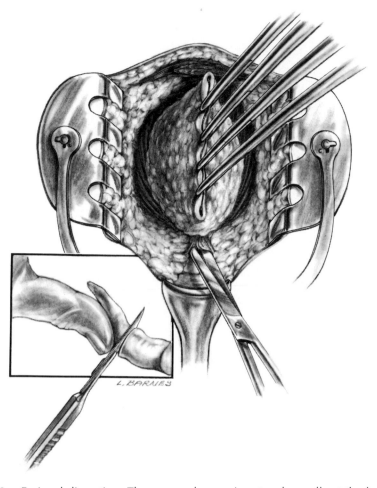

L. BARNES

FIG. 11-29. Perineal dissection. The presacral space is entered, usually at the level of the tip of the coccyx. If necessary, the coccyx can be disarticulated (inset).

is carried out too close to the sacrum, stripping the presacral fascia and causing considerable bleeding. Conversely, one must be careful not to dissect too far anteriorly because of the risk of entering the rectum. This is particularly likely to occur if the tumor is relatively fixed posteriorly. With the synchronous combined operation, the abdominal operator can direct the perineal surgeon into the proper plane. The rectum and anus should now be free in the midline posteriorly.

After the presacral space is entered, a finger is swept across the superior aspect of the levator muscles on the left and right sides of the pelvis. The levatores are then divided along their pelvic wall attachments with scissors or electrocautery. This is a relatively avascular dissection (Fig. 11-30).

Sometimes one or both lateral ligaments are divided

from below. The perineal operator must take care to avoid injury to the ureter by this maneuver. The distal ureter is cut more frequently by the perineal operator during combined abdominoperineal resection than by the abdominal surgeon.

The proximal rectum may now be delivered from the pelvic defect. By vigorous anterior traction the remaining attachments of the rectourethralis muscle and fascia in the region of the urethra are sharply divided. There is no plane in which this can be undertaken bluntly (Fig. 11-31). By feeling the indwelling catheter the surgeon's palpating finger should be able to determine the location of the urethra and avoid it.

If the perineal surgeon moves along expeditiously, or if the abdominal surgeon is delayed mobilizing the rectum, the anterior perineal dissection should be con-

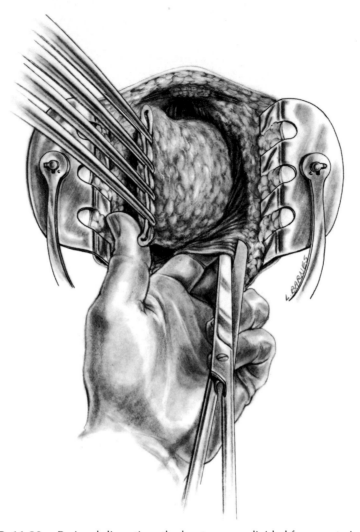

FIG. 11-30.   Perineal dissection: the levatores are divided from posterior to anterior on each side.

tinued. By posterior retraction on the rectum the muscles are further divided with scissors (Fig. 11-32). In men, it is dangerous to use electrocautery because of the risk of injuring the urethra. There may be a tendency for some surgeons to dissect too far anteriorly in men, thereby risking injury to the urethra and prostate as well as producing hemorrhage. Dissecting too far posteriorly risks entering the rectum or performing an inadequate cancer operation. If one can draw an imaginary line to the promontory of the sacrum and dissect in that direction, dividing the transverse perineal and rectourethralis muscles anteriorly, the posterior aspect

of the prostate gland will be clearly identified. With the division of the fascia of Denonvilliers, the peritoneal cavity is entered.

Posteriorly, the proximal dissection may be in some instances carried to the level of the sacral promontory if necessary, and the lateral ligaments can be clamped and divided by the perineal operator. Again, care must be taken to avoid injury to the ureter. It has been said that a skilled surgeon operating in the perineum can do everything but perform a high ligation of the inferior mesenteric artery.

After the bowel has been removed, the perineal

wound is copiously irrigated with saline and the skin closed. No attempt is made to reapproximate the levatores. A suction drain (*e.g.*, Jackson-Pratt) is placed into the pelvic cavity and brought out through the wound (Fig. 11-33, *A*). An alternative closure involves the same procedure, but the drain is brought out through a stab wound in the buttock (Fig. 11-33, *B*). In either case the wound is closed primarily.

Occasionally, diffuse bleeding from pelvic veins may persist. This may be due to difficulty encountered because of tumor extension, prior pelvic surgery, or dissection in the improper plane. Under these circum-

stances, packing the pelvis with gauze, Kling, or Kerlex, will usually control the source of the bleeding.

Perineal Dissection in Women

Unless the tumor is quite small and exophytic, or localized only to the posterior wall of the rectum, a posterior vaginectomy should always be performed coincident with an abdominoperineal resection. For very distal lesions, excision of the lower third or the lower half of the posterior vaginal wall may be all that is required, but for more extensive or more proximal

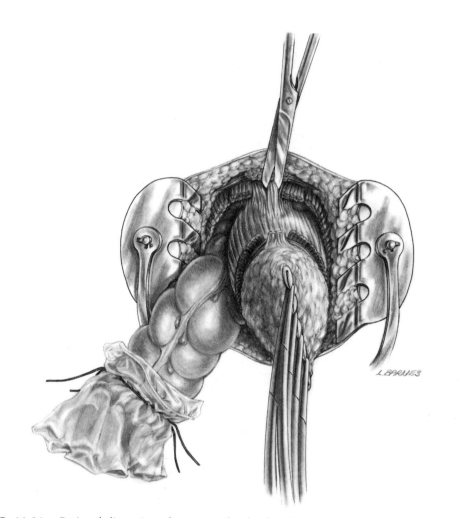

FIG. 11-31.   Perineal dissection: the proximal colon has been delivered through the pelvic defect. The rectourethralis muscle and the visceral fascia are the only structures remaining to be divided.

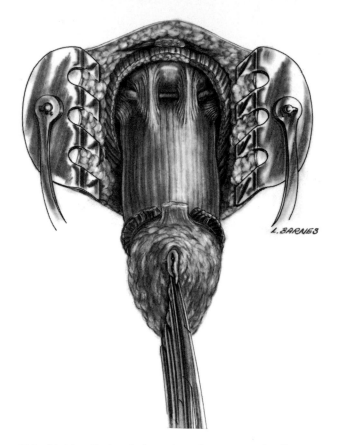

FIG. 11-32. Perineal dissection: the rectourethralis muscle has been divided, exposing the prostate. With the division of the fascia of Denonvilliers the peritoneal cavity can be entered anteriorly.

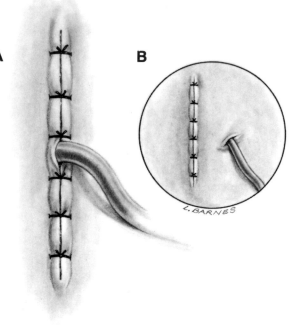

FIG. 11-33. Perineal dissection: the wound is closed primarily and the pelvis drained, either through the incision (**A**) or through a stab wound (**B**).

tumors, the vagina should be excised to the posterior cul-de-sac (Fig. 11-34). A transverse incision is made at the cephalad limit of the dissection connecting the two lateral incisions.

Following posterior vaginectomy the perineal closure is carried out until the forchette has been reconstructed. A drain is brought out through the defect in the posterior vaginal wall (Fig. 11-35).

Postoperative Care

An indwelling catheter should be left in place for one full week, longer if the patient has had a history of difficulty voiding or has prostatic hypertrophy. In fact, in those patients whose prostatic enlargement has seriously interfered with urinary function preoperatively,

transurethral resection of the prostate may ultimately be necessary. I prefer to defer such a procedure for some weeks, even if it is necessary for the patient to be discharged with an indwelling catheter. Generally, women have fewer problems with micturition following abdominoperineal resection than men.

A nasogastric tube is not routinely employed. With reasonably expeditious surgery and no intraoperative complications or extenuating circumstances, the great majority of patients tolerate the lack of the tube quite well. Occasionally a patient complains of nausea, but antiemetic medication usually suffices. If vomiting ensues, a nasogastric tube should be placed until the colostomy functions or gastric output is minimal.

Nothing is permitted by mouth until flatus is passed through the colostomy. This usually takes from 48 to 96 hours. A progressive oral intake is instituted beginning with clear liquids, advancing through full liquids, and then to a selected diet. This encompasses 2 to 3 days.

Early ambulation is advised following abdominoperineal resection. Patients may be asked to sit or stand the evening of surgery and encouraged to walk on the first postoperative day. Fear of evisceration through the perineal wound is not justified.

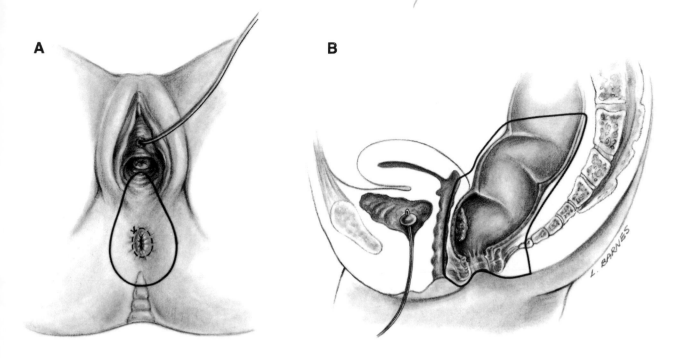

FIG. 11-34. Perineal dissection in women. Outline of the incision for excising the posterior vaginal wall **(A).** Lateral view showing the extent of removal **(B).**

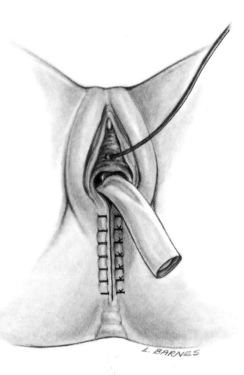

FIG. 11-35. Perineal dissection in women: the skin wound is completely closed and the perineal body reconstructed. The drain is placed in the pelvis and brought out through the defect in the posterior vaginal wall.

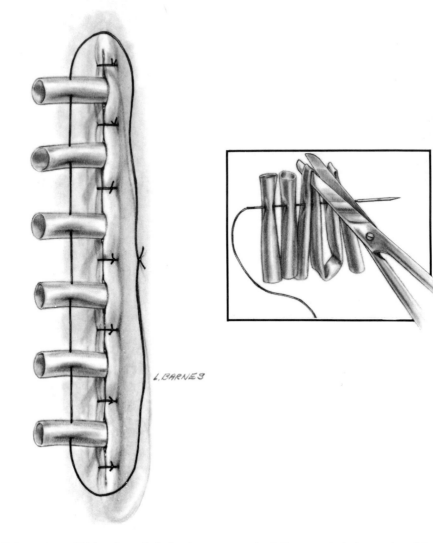

FIG. 11-36. ''Picket-fence'' drains (one-quarter-inch Penrose drains) are placed in the subcutaneous tissue for most colon operations. They are removed in approximately 3 days.

Any abdominal, subcutaneous drains are removed by the third postoperative day (Fig. 11-36). At this time the perineal drain is removed, and the wound is vigorously irrigated with saline, three times daily. If the wound appears foul, one-half strength Dakin's solution or povidone-iodine (Betadine) is used. Sitz baths are also useful for comfort and are advised immediately following the irrigation. Sitz baths alone, however, are inadequate for cleansing the perineal cavity. Hematoma, pus, and debris are effectively removed only by irrigation.

If the perineal wound required packing, the pack is removed at 72 hours. This is done at the bedside and usually requires a parenteral narcotic. Rarely is it necessary to return the patient to the operating room for an anesthetic in order to have the pack removed.

During the hospital stay the colostomy is managed with a disposable transparent bag that is changed daily (see Chap. 16). By the sixth day the patient is involved in stomal care, appliance changes, and irrigation techniques. Spontaneous evacuation versus irrigation is always a subject of debate, but I believe that the patient should have the choice. Accordingly, the patient is instructed in both management techniques if he or she is willing to learn (see Chap. 16).

Complications

Intraoperative Complications

Injury to small bowel usually is easily dealt with by standard reparative techniques, as long as the problem is recognized at the time of surgery. Likewise, *slippage of ligatures on vessels* or *injury to vessels* can be readily addressed by conventional hemostatic maneuvers.

By far the greatest fear that confronts the surgeon performing an abdominoperineal resection is that of *injury to the ureter.* However, the operator can take some solace in the fact that in most cases recognition of the injury at that time will usually lead to a good functional result through the application of proper principles of repair. The degree of difficulty in effecting delayed repair is much greater, and the results of such maneuvers are not as successful if the injury is not initially recognized.

Ureteral Injury

In spite of advances in the surgical treatment of patients, ureteral injuries still occur frequently during the performance of pelvic operations, especially hysterectomy and abdominoperineal resection. Injury to the ureter occurs usually at one of three places during the procedure of removal of the rectum.

First, during the ligation of the inferior mesenteric vessels, the left ureter can be incorporated in the ligature or divided when the vessels themselves are divided. Care must be taken to displace the left ureter laterally, away from the vascular pedicle. Also, when dividing the inferior mesenteric vessels, one should always look a second time to be certain that the left ureter is out of harm's way.

The second area of injury occurs deep in the pelvis and is usually coincident with the division of the lateral ligaments. The ureter is particularly exposed to danger if a synchronous hysterectomy is carried out. The risk of injury can obviously be reduced by retracting both ureters laterally and visualizing them throughout their lengths. However, this is often cumbersome and unnecessary if the growth is not adherent to the pelvic wall or if there has not been prior surgery that might have caused displacement. A preoperative intravenous pyelogram is most useful in identifying the anatomy and course of the structures. A practical means for avoiding ureteral injury during the course of division of the lateral ligaments is to employ only one clamp. Less exposure is required, so there is less likelihood of incorporating the ureter in the laterally placed hemostat. Back-bleeding is rarely present but can be easily controlled by separate applications of a clamp, with the rectum freed and the vascular area rotated anteriorly (see earlier, under Technique).

The use of indwelling ureteral catheters does not necessarily protect the ureter from injury. However, when repeat pelvic surgery is necessary or when a difficult dissection is expected, indwelling ureteral catheters may aid the surgeon in identifying the structures.

Injury to the lower ureter is more likely to occur during synchronous-combined abdominoperineal resection than in the single-team approach.[79] This is because a more extensive perineal operation is performed by the perineal surgeon. If the lateral ligaments are divided from below or blind scissors dissection is employed, the ureter can be unknowingly injured. Great care must be taken by the perineal surgeon when dividing the ligaments or when dissecting in the supralevator area.

The third area of vulnerability occurs during the mobilization of the peritoneum and the closure of the pelvic peritoneal floor. Both ureters may be divided as the peritoneum is elevated, or they may be incorporated in the suture during the closure. It is imperative that the ureters be clearly visualized during mobilization of the peritoneum and that they be displaced laterally.

Only 20% to 30% of ureteral injuries are recognized at the time of operation.[242] If one is concerned about the possibility of ureteral injury during a difficult pelvic dissection, identification of the injury site may be revealed by injecting 12.5 g of mannitol intravenously followed by the intravenous administration of 5 ml of indigo carmine dye. The presence of a blue stain in the operative field is diagnostic of injury. If the distal ureter cannot be identified, a cystotomy should be made and a ureteral catheter placed through the ureteral orifice until it presents in the operative field. If ligation without penetration is suspected, a proximal linear ureterotomy permits antegrade insertion of a ureteral catheter to test patency.[243]

As suggested, most ureteral injuries go unrecognized, and indeed may forever be unrecognized if a single ureter has been ligated. Flank pain, fever, leukocytosis, and tenderness are the most often presenting signs and symptoms of ureteral ligation during the early postoperative period. Urinary fistula can be suspected if there is copious serous or serosanguineous perineal wound drainage in the early postoperative period. A blue stain appearing on the perineal or abdominal wound dressing after intravenous administration of indigo carmine confirms the diagnosis.

Late urinary fistula can occur because of necrosis to the ureter from devascularization injury or from urinary fistula from the membranous urethra or from the base of the bladder.

Treatment. With crush injury from a hemostat or with partial ligation, removing the ligature and performing a *limited repair* or *tube decompression* requires careful patient selection in order to avoid postoperative complications. Occasionally, if the patient's poor general condition precludes prolonging the operation by the performance of a definitive reconstruction, a temporary feeding-tube proximal diversion can be employed.[242] Proximal *ureteral ligation* with the expectation of renal death in the poor-risk patient who has a limited life expectancy is generally to be condemned because of the complications of sepsis and fistula formation.[242]

Injury to the Lower Ureter. *Uretero-neocystotomy* is the procedure of choice for injuries of the pelvic ureter. Injuries within 5 cm of the bladder and often at greater distances are suitable for this approach. The technique has been described by Politano and Leadbetter and by others.[124, 125, 180] The procedure achieves an antireflux-ing ureteral anastomosis. The following operations have been advocated by Libertino and Zinman.[124, 125]

A midline cystotomy is made and 3 ml of saline are injected through a 23-gauge needle, raising a small bleb of mucosa (Fig. 11-37). An ellipse of mucosa is excised, and a 3 cm submucosal tunnel is created with a right angle clamp (Fig. 11-38). The clamp is then rotated to point through the bladder wall, and the detrusor muscle is pierced. The distal ureter is pulled through the tunnel with the aid of traction sutures, and spatulated for approximately 1 cm.[125] A No. 6 or No. 8 French catheter is inserted to make certain that the ureter pursues a direct course. The ureter is then sutured to the bladder with interrupted 5-0 chromic catgut sutures. Deep bites of detrusor must be included in the two distal sutures at the 5- and 7-o'clock positions to help restore normal ureterovesical function.[124] A No. 5 feeding tube is used as a ureteral stent and is brought out alongside a suprapubic cystotomy catheter. It is removed at 7 days.

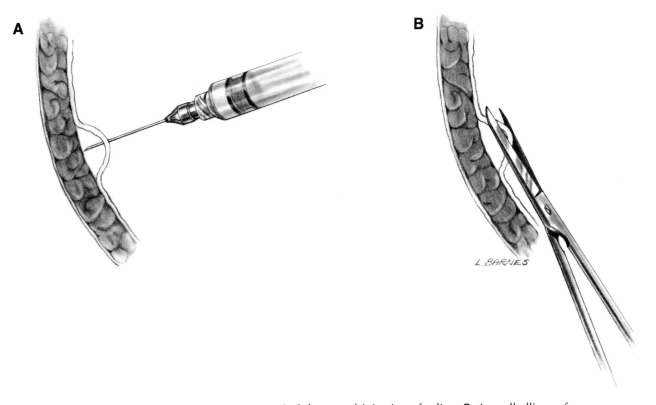

FIG. 11-37. Ureteroneocystotomy. **A.** Submucosal injection of saline. **B.** A small ellipse of bladder mucosa is excised to allow creation of a submucosal tunnel. (After Libertino JA, Zinman L: Technique for uretero-neocystotomy in renal transplantation and reflux. Surg Clin North Am 1973; 53:459–463)

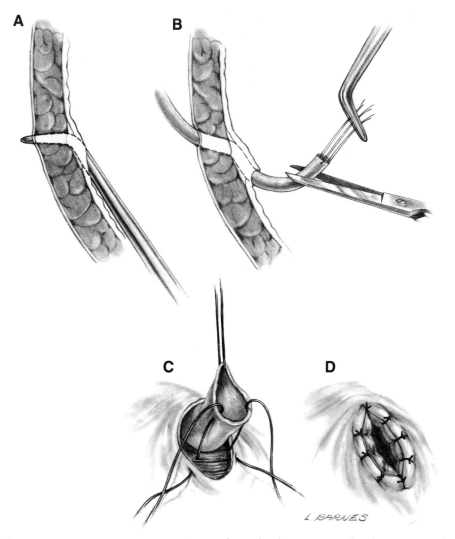

FIG. 11-38. Ureteroneocystotomy. **A.** A right-angle clamp pierces the detrusor muscle. **B.** The ureter is pulled through the submucosal tunnel; the distal ureter is cut at 45° angle, creating a new ureteral meatus. **C.** The ureter is anchored to the bladder detrusor muscle. **D.** Completion of the anastomosis to the bladder mucosa. (After Libertino JA, Zinman L: Technique for uretero-neocystotomy in renal transplantation and reflux. Surg Clin North Am 1973; 53:459–463)

Ureteral reimplantation into the bladder is the best method of restoring continuity following ureteral injury; every effort should be made to accomplish this. If the ureter cannot be brought down without tension, a Boari bladder flap tube technique can be employed, or preferably a so-called psoas bladder hitch maneuver can be used.[19, 226] These techniques are best accomplished by a urologist who is familiar with the special-

ized approaches to ureterovesical surgery. It is always wise to take advantage of the availability of urologic consultation when injury to the urinary tract has occurred.

Transureteroureterostomy is another technique that may be employed for the injured ureter. Hodges and co-workers reported a large, successful experience with this technique,[93] but because of the possibility of injury

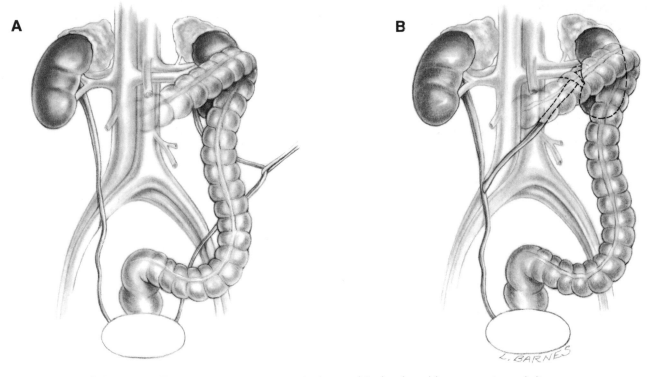

FIG. 11-39. Transureteroureterostomy. **A.** A tunnel is developed by retroperitoneal dissection after exposure of the upper ureter lateral to the colon. **B.** The ureter is brought across the retroperitoneal space and anastomosed. (After Libertino JA, Zinman L: Technique for ureteroneocystotomy in renal transplantation and reflux. Surg Clin North Am 1973; 53:459–463)

to the recipient ureter it should be used only sparingly and then limited to injuries of the *upper pelvic ureter* when reimplantation cannot be accomplished.[125] The technique is described in Fig. 11-39. The injured ureter should be resected at a point of certain viability, with care being taken to preserve the adventitia and blood supply, and the recipient ureter should not be mobilized from its bed.

Injury to the Mid and Upper Ureter. Injuries to the proximal ureter are the most difficult and least satisfactory to treat. Fortunately, this is a rare complication of bowel surgery. Because of the distance, reimplantation into the bladder is not possible, and the blood supply is less adequate. Direct repair by end-to-end *ureteroureterostomy* is the treatment of choice. With loss of ureteral length from excision or necrosis, up to 8-cm defects can be traversed by this method using a renal lowering technique.[125] If direct repair is not possible, one can consider the highly specialized techniques of *ileal interposition* and *autotransplantation. Ne-*

phrectomy may be used if the surgeon is satisfied that contralateral kidney function is adequate and calculous disease or other conditions that might affect the kidney are not present.

Whenever a direct repair of a ureteral injury is performed, proximal diversion is required. Zinman and associates recommend a No. 6 to a No. 8 French Silastic catheter with a 2-cm diverting ureterostomy approximately 5 cm above the anastomosis (Fig. 11-40, *A*).[242] The cut edges of the ureter are debrided and spatulated, and the kidney, ureter, or both are adequately mobilized.[125] The ureter is spatulated on opposing sides of each end to prevent stricture (Fig. 11-40, *B*). Anastomosis is effected with interrupted 5-0 chromic catgut sutures placed full thickness, with the knots on the outside, inverting the mucosa (Fig. 11-40, *C*). Noncrushing vascular forceps can be used to grasp the tissue, and the presence of a catheter within the lumen facilitates the procedure. A continuous suture should never be employed. The ureter can be wrapped in omentum if the anastomosis is felt to be precarious. A

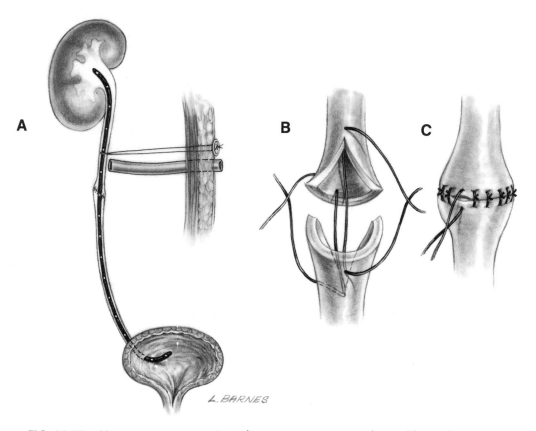

L. BARNES

FIG. 11-40. Ureteroureterostomy. **A.** Midureteroureterostomy is diverted by a Silastic stent secured by a ligature with linear ureterotomy above anastomosis. The suture is tied loosely to button on skin to prevent spontaneous passage of the stent by ureteral peristalsis. **B.** The ureters are spatulated on opposing sides of each end to achieve oblique anastomosis. **C.** The edges are approximated with interrupted fine catgut sutures placed through the full thickness of the ureteral wall, inverting the mucosa. (After Libertino JA, Zinman L: Technique for ureteroneocystotomy in renal transplantation and reflux. Surg Clin North Am 1973; 53:459–463)

soft rubber drain (Penrose) is placed at the site of the diverting ureterotomy and brought out through a stab wound. The stent is removed on the 10th postoperative day, followed by the drain 48 hours later (if no urine drainage is present).

Prior to discharge, an intravenous pyelogram should be performed for all patients who undergo ureteral repair, to determine the adequacy of the reconstruction.

Bladder Injury

Bladder injury that is recognized at the time of surgery can usually be repaired by means of a layered closure of 2-0 chromic catgut. When injury to the bladder neck or trigone has occurred, great care must be taken to avoid incorporating the distal ureters in the suture. A cystotomy with insertion of small catheters in a retrograde fashion through the ureteral orifices is useful in preventing this complication. Drainage of the area is advised. Suprapubic cystotomy is prudent when the injury is to the bladder neck or trigone.

Urethral Injury

Injury to the urethra occurs most often as a result of too vigorous electrocoagulation of the prostatic area. Also, tumor extension anteriorly may invade the prostate, and in an attempt to perform a curative resection the prostatic urethra can be entered. External trauma can create a delayed urethral stricture, which may require catheterization or subsequent reconstruction. If injury to this area is recognized at the time of proctectomy, direct repair or urethroplasty may be indicated. A urologist should be consulted if the surgeon is not experienced with reparative approaches.

Urethral stricture may require dilatation, internal urethrotomy, or reconstructive urethroplasty.[241] Here again, one should seek the advice of someone who has expertise in the management of such a complication.

Postoperative Complications

Perineal Hemorrhage

Bleeding from the perineal wound in the recovery room has a characteristic scenario. It usually begins with the surgeon noting "moderate pelvic oozing" in the operating room. After some effort at clamping vessels in the sacral area, under the raised peritoneal flap, in the prostatic bed, the lateral ligaments, levators, and subcutaneous tissue, it is decided to close and drain or to pack the area. The bleeding is often noticed by the circulating nurse while the patient is still in the operating room; frequently, however, the surgeon directs that the patient be removed to the recovery area in the expectation that the bleeding will cease.

Returning the patient to the operating room is certainly a defeat for the surgeon and a risk to the patient. Fortunately, perineal hemorrhage can usually be controlled by opening the wound and finding the bleeding vessel. Occasionally, however, laparotomy must be undertaken again.

This complication is usually preventable. Perineal wound hemostasis should be adequate before the patient is permitted to leave the operating room. If the bleeding is so diffuse that a specific vessel cannot be identified, packing with or without a supplementary hemostatic agent may be necessary.

Necrotic Colostomy

I have mentioned that I do not advocate a high ligation of the inferior mesenteric artery because it does not increase the likelihood of cure. Furthermore, by preserving the first branch of the artery, blood supply to the descending colon and residual sigmoid colon is less likely to be impaired. In spite of this precaution, division of the inferior mesenteric artery or one of its major branches may result in necrosis or frank gangrene of the bowel.[101, 200] This occurs when the colon receives much or all of its vascular supply from the inferior mesenteric artery. Goligher demonstrated that approximately 25% of patients who underwent high ligation of the inferior mesenteric artery during rectal excision developed gangrene or sloughing.[72] Some have suggested the use of Doppler ultrasound to determine the adequacy of the blood supply to the intes-

tine at the time of surgery,[32–34, 239] but such a relatively esoteric study is unnecessary, for bowel ischemia can usually be assessed adequately by clinical inspection.

In spite of careful attention to the viability of the intestine, the colostomy at the time of abdominal wound closure may appear ischemic. This is usually noted when the surgeon has difficulty creating the stoma, either because of the patient's obesity or because of tension on the bowel itself. By making certain that there is sufficient bowel available to create the stoma without such tension, and by preparing a large enough opening in the abdominal wall, this difficulty can be avoided. All too often, however, the surgeon does not place sufficient importance on the creation of the stoma; to the patient it is the most important part of the operation.

If the bowel looks ischemic, it probably is ischemic. If the mucosa looks blue, it probably is blue. The optimal time to redo the stoma is at the time of the laparotomy, not 2 or 3 days later, when it has retracted into the peritoneal cavity or has become gangrenous. The treatment of stomal problems is addressed in Chapter 16.

Intestinal Obstruction

Small bowel obstruction is not uncommon following abdominoperineal resection. Some element of ileus is normally present for a few days following surgery, but if flatus fails to pass by the sixth or seventh postoperative day, one must entertain the possibility that obstruction is present. Goligher and co-workers reported an incidence of obstruction of approximately 3% in 1302 patients who underwent abdominoperineal resection.[77]

Obstruction is most commonly caused by adhesions between loops of bowel, a complication that can occur after laparotomy for any purpose, but there are two specific situations that are directly related to abdominoperineal resection: herniation below the pelvic floor and herniation through the lateral colostomy space. The former usually occurs when the suture breaks or pulls out of the peritoneum, leaving a hole through which a loop of small intestine descends and becomes entrapped. Repair requires liberation of the bowel and closure of the defect. Rarely, the loop of bowel descends to the perineal skin or actually through the wound. Gangrene can occur, but this is also quite unusual. Small bowel resection under such circumstances would obviously be required.

Harshaw and colleagues advocate leaving the peritoneum open and closing the skin primarily, thereby avoiding this complication[84]; however, it is preferable to close the pelvic floor if for no other reason than to keep the small bowel out of the pelvis should postoperative radiotherapy be deemed advisable (see Post-operative Radiotherapy).

Herniation of the small bowel through the defect in the lateral gutter can produce small bowel obstruction. Although some recommend a pursestring, interrupted, or continuous suture to close the space, and others prefer an extraperitoneal approach, I like to leave the defect widely patent, on the theory that entrapment is less likely to take place if the opening is large enough. In my experience those patients who subsequently developed obstruction had undergone closure of the lateral space. At surgery, the suture was found to have either broken or pulled out.

If surgery is required, the bowel is reduced and the opening enlarged. If the gutter *had* been left widely open and herniation with obstruction did occur, it is probably wiser to close the defect.

Urinary Retention

Urinary tract infection and urinary retention are the most common complications following abdominoperineal resection. Marks and Ritchie reported an incidence of 34%.[147] Urinary retention may be due to injury to the sympathetic or parasympathetic nerves to the bladder, the result of postoperative distension, local trauma, prostatic hypertrophy, or prolapse of the bladder into the pelvis. By evaluating preoperatively the urologic situation in a systematic way, Leadbetter and Leadbetter felt that they could selectively perform prostatectomy at the time of the abdominoperineal resection and decrease the incidence of postoperative urinary retention.[120]

From a limited experience with this approach, I feel that such a combined operation should be condemned. There is an associated high incidence of urinary tract infection, pelvic sepsis, and urinary–perineal fistula (Fig. 11-41).

The most important preventive maneuver that one may employ is to retain a Foley catheter in place for a minimum of 1 week. The effects of direct trauma to the bladder necessitate a period of recovery. The catheter is removed at 6:00 A.M. and the voiding pattern carefully observed. If the patient is unable to void or urinates frequently in small amounts, a residual urine determination should be made. If it is greater than 300 ml, the catheter should be reinserted and left for a minimum of 5 days. During this interval it is reasonable to place the patient on Urecholine, 25 to 50 mg, four times daily. This is suggested in an effort to improve detrusor tone. If after removal of the catheter the patient is unable to void, urodynamic studies are suggested.

A cystometrogram usually will demonstrate a flaccid type of bladder. The urethral pressure profile will prob-

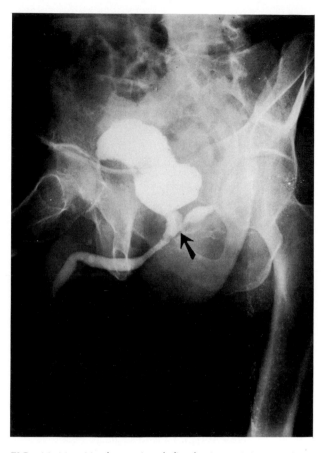

FIG. 11-41. Urethroperineal fistula *(arrow)* is a serious consequence of an ill-advised concomitant proctectomy and prostatectomy.

ably be normal. What is important is to determine the external sphincter electromyogram (EMG). Very often after an abdominoperineal resection the internal pudendal nerve is compromised, and the patient loses the innervation of the external sphincter. Continence, therefore, is maintained by the internal sphincter or bladder neck mechanism only. The cystometrogram, urethral pressure profile, and external sphincter EMG should be correlated with the anatomic findings of cystourethroscopy. If the patient has an obstructed prostate and a normal sphincter EMG, then it is reasonable to carry out a transurethral resection. It is safer, however, to defer prostatectomy for 6 weeks in a patient who has recently undergone abdominoperineal resection, in order to minimize the risk of a urinary–perineal fistula. If the external sphincter EMG shows a flaccid external sphincter, one would be loath to carry out a transurethral resection of the prostate or any form of

Table 11-1. Predisposing Factors for the Development of Wound Infections After Colonic Surgery

	Percent Infections	Statistical Significance
Preoperative irradiation	22.2	p < 0.04
Serum albumin < 2.9 g/dl	20.1	p < 0.02
Preoperative stoma	19.1	p < 0.001
Blood loss > 2 units	17.4	p < 0.03
Crohn's disease	14.3	p < 0.002
Bowel preparation		
Other than mechanical preparation plus nonabsorbable antibiotic	14.1	p < 0.001
Antibiotic other than erythromycin base and neomycin	7.7	p < 0.001
Operative time > 2 hours	11.7	p < 0.06

(After DeGennaro V, Corman ML, Coller JA, Veidenheimer MC: Wound infections after colectomy. Dis Colon Rectum 1978; 21:567–572)

prostatectomy for fear of making the patient incontinent. Under these circumstances it is advisable to leave the catheter in place for a period of 6 weeks to 2 months, or to instruct the patient in the use of intermittent catheterization. Hopefully, this respite will allow the bladder residual urine to be of small enough volume not to overdistend the bladder and decompensate the detrusor musculature. Intermittent catheterization is preferable to patient incontinence.

Current urological practice discourages clamping and unclamping the catheter in an attempt to restore detrusor tone. What is important is to make certain that the bladder is empty, and the detrusor tone will return ultimately.

In women the procedure should be essentially the same as that described above. If the woman has difficulty voiding after further catheter drainage and treatment with Urecholine, she should be taught the technique of intermittent self-catheterization until the bladder tone returns and normal voiding occurs.

Perineal Wound Sepsis

Perineal sepsis is not uncommon following abdominoperineal resection. It may be caused by contamination at the time of proctectomy from injury to the rectal wall, fecal spillage, the presence of a perforated carcinoma, or the presence of perineal disease (*e.g.*, fistula or abscess). It may be the result also of an infected hematoma. Furthermore, there is an association between a prolonged operative time and the subsequent development of sepsis.

Characteristically, the patient develops a low-grade fever on the fourth or fifth postoperative day, which progresses to a higher spiking fever elevation. In the absence of another obvious source for pyrexia, the perineal wound should be carefully explored with a gloved finger. Loculations should be broken and, if necessary, the wound reopened. Irrigating with one-half strength Dakin's solution (using a rubber catheter) is important to remove clot and debris. A sitz bath, even with the wound widely open, is inadequate for treating or preventing perineal sepsis. There is a means for obviating the difficulty, and that is to leave the perineal wound widely open to heal by second intention. The disadvantage of delayed healing (not infrequently for 4 or more months) makes this approach inadvisable. Conversely, primary closure without drainage is contraindicated because of the high likelihood of sepsis.

A satisfactory compromise is to close the skin and to bring a drain through the wound or through a separate incision. A suction catheter (*e.g.*, Shirley, Jackson-Pratt) drains more effectively and probably reduces the likelihood of pelvic sepsis.

Abdominal Wound Infection

Although wound infection alone is rarely fatal, it adds considerably to morbidity and prolongs the patient's hospital stay. The incidence of wound infection following abdominoperineal resection is the same as that for any colon resection. We reported an incidence of 8.6%, a rate comparable to others for colonic operations.[14, 37, 38, 47, 196, 215, 236]

The necessary ingredients for wound infection are contamination with pathogenic organisms and a susceptible host. Because of the nature of colonic and rectal surgery, some contamination is present in all patients, but a number of factors are known to predispose to this complication (Table 11-1).

Many methods have been devised to decrease the incidence of wound infection in contaminated incisions; numerous bowel preparations and antibiotics have been used.[30, 31] The lowest incidence of wound infection in our experience occurred among patients who were administered the combination of oral erythromycin and neomycin, as popularized by Nichols and associates.[172] Recent evidence suggests that perioperative broad-spectrum antibiotics may also be of benefit in reducing the incidence of wound infections.[25, 89, 102, 170, 193, 222, 233] By using these approaches, my wound infection rate for colon surgery irrespective of the presence of pus or gross contamination is less than 2%. Although still a subject of controversy, the use of drainage of the subcutaneous tissue (see Fig. 11-36) is recommended because of the impressive amount of serosanguinous drainage apparent on the dressing in the first 48 hours when this technique is employed. With adequate hemostasis, debridement of devitalized tissue, copious saline irrigation, careful tissue handling, and reduction of the operative time, wound infection should be an infrequent complication.

Impotence and Infertility

Impotence following proctectomy for carcinoma of the rectum is the rule rather than the exception.[234] The resection requires extensive pelvic dissection, which may result in injury to the parasympathetic nerves (nervi erigentes). Also, the patient's preoperative sexual function may have been less than adequate, and even minimal trauma may be sufficient to precipitate impotence. This may be an important explanation for why young patients who undergo proctectomy for inflammatory bowel disease rarely have such difficulties when compared with older cancer patients.

In men, infertility can result even if tumescence is not impaired, because of injury to the sympathetic nerves and because of retrograde ejaculation. Women seem less likely to experience problems with orgasm, although most studies include a high number of widowed or elderly women who have no sexual partners.

Should the risk of impotence or infertility be discussed prior to surgery? In this litigious era the doctrine of informed consent would seem to indicate that it *should* be mentioned. However, when an older or elderly man is already burdened with the knowledge that he has cancer, it seems appropriate that the subject of impotence should be addressed more casually. However, in a relatively young man undergoing abdominoperineal resection, it is important to discuss the possibility. Such a patient has occasionally elected to "bank" his sperm prior to undergoing this operation, or he may elect alternative therapy (*e.g.*, electrocoagulation).

Organic impotence has been rather unsuccessfully treated with drugs, but in order that the patient may satisfy a sexual partner and gain an element of self-satisfaction, penile prosthetic implants have been used.[11, 55, 61, 136, 179, 180] The procedure should not be performed, however, for at least 1 year after abdominoperineal resection, because of the possibility of return of this function.

Perineal Hernia

Perineal hernia is a rare, late compliation of abdominoperineal resection (Fig. 11-42). Only a handful of cases have been reported in the literature.[23, 81] It is more common in women. It may produce few symptoms, may ulcerate, or may be associated with an

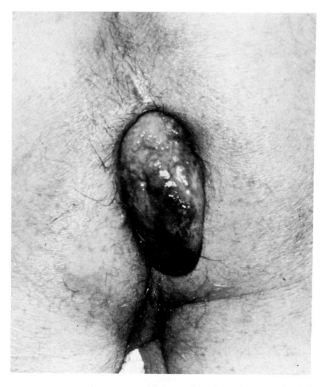

FIG. 11-42. This perineal hernia developed 6 months following abdominoperineal resection. Treatment of such hernias requires laparotomy and reconstruction of the pelvic floor.

evisceration. Treatment is best directed to a synchronous abdominal and perineal approach. delivering the bowel out of the pelvis and reconstituting the pelvic floor.[194] The redundant skin should be excised and the pelvis drained.

Stomal Problems

Colostomy retraction, stenosis, prolapse, and hernia, as well as peristomal dermatitis and appliance management problems, are discussed in Chapter 16.

Results

The operative mortality rate following abdominoperineal resection has remained unchanged for the past 40 years. My colleagues and I reported in-hospital mortality to be between 1% and 2% during this period.[187] Others relate a mortality of 2% to 6.5% (Table 11-2).

Most institutions report a high complication rate[56, 204]; we have reported an incidence of complications of

Table 11-2. Operative Mortality Following Abdominoperineal Resection

Author, year	Percent
Lockhart-Mummery and co-workers, 1976[134]	2.1
Localio and co-workers, 1978[131]	2.3
Deddish and Stearns, 1961[46]	2.0
Bordos and co-workers, 1974[21]	2.9
Williams and co-workers, 1966[237]	4.3
Palumbo and Sharpe, 1968[172]	4.4
Glenn and McSherry, 1966[68]	4.7
Walz and co-workers, 1977[228]	3.2
MacLennan and co-workers, 1976[140]	3.2
Stearns, 1974[209]	3.5
Strauss and co-workers, 1978[220]	3.5
Slanetz and co-workers, 1972[204]	5.4
Enker and co-workers, 1979[54]	6.4
Zollinger and Sheppard, 1971[243]	6.5

(Rosen L, Veidenheimer MC, Coller JA, Corman ML: Mortality, morbidity, and patterns of recurrence after abdominoperineal resection for cancer of the rectum. Dis Colon Rectum 1982; 25:202–208)

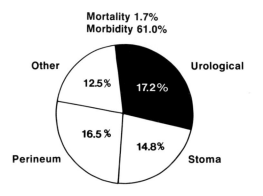

FIG. 11-43. Morbidity and mortality following abdominoperineal resection in 230 patients. (Rosen L, Veidenheimer MC, Coller JA, Corman ML: Mortality, morbidity, and patterns of recurrence after abdominoperineal resection for cancer of the rectum. Dis Colon Rectum 1982; 25:202–208)

61% (Fig. 11-43).[187] Urologic problems are the most frequently seen (Table 11-3). Lapides reported a 15% incidence of poor micturition following the procedure.[119] In fact, Gerstenberg and associates recommend the routine application of urinary flow measurements and cystometry in all postoperative patients who undergo abdominoperineal resection in order to detect potential problems at an early stage.[62]

The uncorrected 5-year survival in our experience between 1963 and 1976 is shown in Table 11-4 ac-

Table 11-3. Complications Following Abdominoperineal Resection

Complication	Number of Patients	Percent*
Urologic		
Benign prostatic hypertrophy requiring TURP	13	8.1
Urinary tract infection	13	5.6
Neurogenic bladder	8	3.5
Orchitis	2	1.2
Urethral stricture	1	0.4
Fistula		
Vesicovaginal	1	
Vesicoperineal	1	0.4
Ureteroperineal	1	0.4
Perineal		
Abscess	26	11.3
Hemorrhage	10	4.3
Hernia	2	0.9
Stomal operation		
Stenosis, retraction, or prolapse	25	10.9
Hernia	7	3.0
Abscess	2	0.9
Miscellaneous		
Abdominal wound infection	6	2.6
Wound evisceration	7	3.0
Small bowel obstruction	10	4.3
Myocardial infarction	1	2.6
Atrial fibrillation	1	2.6
Hepatitis	1	2.6
Pulmonary embolism	1	2.6
Iliac vein injury	1	2.6
Pelvic abscess	1	2.6

* Percentages are calculated according to the number of men (160) and the number of women (70) in the series, when applicable.
(Rosen L, Veidenheimer MC, Coller JA, Corman ML: Mortality, morbidity, and patterns of recurrence after abdominoperineal resection for cancer of the rectum. Dis Colon Rectum 1982; 25:202–208)

Table 11-4. Survival Following Abdominoperineal Resection

Dukes' Classification	Number of Patients	Uncorrected 5-year Survival (Percentage)
A	45	86
B	75	65
C	60	33
D	20	0
Total	200	54

(Rosen L, Veidenheimer MC, Coller JA, Corman ML: Mortality, morbidity, and patterns of recurrence after abdominoperineal resection for cancer of the rectum. Dis Colon Rectum 1982; 25:202–208)

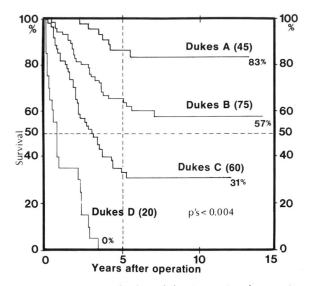

FIG. 11-44. Survival after abdominoperineal resection. (Rosen L, Veidenheimer MC, Coller JA, Corman ML: Mortality, morbidity, and patterns of recurrence after abdominoperineal resection for cancer of the rectum. Dis Colon Rectum 1982; 25:202–208)

cording to Dukes' classification (see Fig. 10-23). The mean age of patients was 62 years. The uncorrected 5-year survival approaches 90% in patients with Dukes' A lesions. This falls to 65% for Dukes' B and 33% for Dukes' C lesions. This was essentially the same as the uncorrected survival rate for colon resections during

Table 11-5. Abdominoperineal Resection: Five-Year Survival Rate

Author, year	Dukes' Lesion		
	A	B	C
Dukes, 1940[51]	93	65	23
Gilbertsen, 1960[63]	80	50	23
Slanetz and co-workers, 1972[205]	81	52	33
MacLennan and co-workers, 1976[140]	91	59	25
Strauss and co-workers, 1978[221]	82	40	15
Walz and co-workers, 1977[229]	78	45	22

(Rosen L, Veidenheimer MC, Coller JA, Corman ML: Mortality, morbidity, and patterns of recurrence after abdominoperineal resection for cancer of the rectum. Dis Colon Rectum 1982; 25:202–208)

the same period. The uncorrected survival rate for all patients who underwent abdominoperineal resection was 54%. The 10-year survival rate is illustrated in Fig. 11-44. There is no significant falloff in survival after 5 years. This implies that it is the rare patient who dies of recurrent cancer of the rectum after this period of time. The survival rate from other institutions is shown in Table 11-5.

We analyzed retrospectively the patterns of recurrence in 180 of our patients who underwent an abdominoperineal resection for cure.[187] Seventy-eight (43%) developed recurrent cancer (Fig. 11-45). In 18 of these patients the initial recurrence was local, whereas in 60 the initial manifestation of the recurrence was in a distant location. No patient who had a

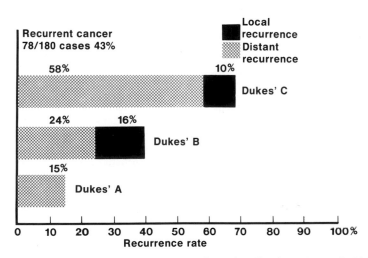

FIG. 11-45. Rate of recurrence according to Dukes' classification. (Rosen L, Veidenheimer MC, Coller JA, Corman ML: Mortality, morbidity, and patterns of recurrence after abdominoperineal resection for cancer of the rectum. Dis Colon Rectum 1982; 25:202–208)

Table 11-6.   Survival According to Initial Site of Recurrence

Site	Dukes' Stage	Number of Patients	Median Time From Operation to Recurrence (Months)	Median Time From Recurrence to Death (Months)	Overall Median Survival (Months)
Local (23%)	A	0			
	B	12	21.5	17	38.5
	C	6	6	10.5	16.5
Distant (77%)	A	7	20	18	44
	B	18	12	11.5	22.5
	C	35	12	9	24

(Rosen L, Veidenheimer MC, Coller JA, Corman ML: Mortality, morbidity, and patterns of recurrence after abdominoperineal resection for cancer of the rectum. Dis Colon Rectum 1982; 25:202–208)

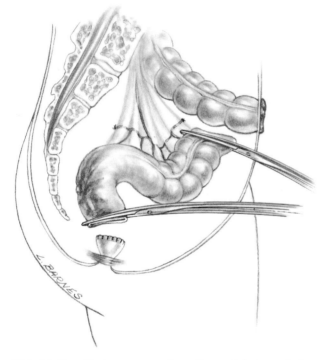

FIG. 11-46. Hartmann resection: the rectal stump is inverted by conventional suture technique or closed with a TA stapler distal to the tumor. A sigmoid colostomy is created.

Dukes' A lesion initially developed a local recurrence (Table 11-6). Penetration through the bowel wall with residual tumor in the pelvis is the most important factor contributing to pelvic and perineal recurrent disease.

Local recurrence appears much earlier in patients with Dukes' C lesions than in patients who initially had a Dukes' B tumor. However, once recurrence develops there is no statistically significant difference in median survival time between the two groups of patients. Furthermore, there is no statistically significant difference in survival time irrespective of whether the initial recurrence was local or distant.

Palliative Resection

Palliative abdominoperineal resection has been advocated by a number of authors.[8, 21, 133] Others have suggested that alternative forms of therapy should be considered because of the high morbidity and mortality rates.[142, 182] Careful patient selection is required. Individuals who have extensive liver metastases, lung metastases, or disseminated disease to the bone or the brain are poor candidates. Patients with ascites or multiple peritoneal implants are also high operative mortality risks. But because the mean survival time in patients with Dukes' D lesions approximates 1 year, there is a group of patients who should be considered for a palliative resection, including those with perineal pain, tenesmus, or hemorrhage. If the tumor can be extirpated, a better quality of life can be anticipated.

Occasionally, a patient with metastatic disease can be adequately treated by the so-called *Hartmann resection* (Fig. 11-46).[85] ReMine and Dozios reported on 107 procedures, approximately half of which were considered palliative; they were able to perform a subsequent colorectal anastomosis on only 10% of their patients.[184]

The procedure has the advantage of removing the tumor mass. However, when the operation is undertaken for cure, the colostomy is usually permanent. It is more convenient to manage, though, than a transverse colon stoma. Although several techniques have been devised to simplify the process,[35, 143, 181] a major procedure is required to reestablish intestinal continuity. It is for this reason that I do not recommend the Hartmann resection in cancer patients who are potentially curable.

Treatment of Local Recurrence

The treatment of metastatic disease following resection of colorectal carcinoma is presented in Chapter 10. The discussion that follows is limited to the specific problems of recurrence encountered following abdominoperineal resection.

Unfortunately, there is no satisfactory treatment for perineal or pelvic recurrence (Fig. 11-47). There is, however, the rare instance when perineal (suture line) recurrence develops secondary to implantation or to inadequate skin excision. The patient may still be curable by reexcision of the perineal wound. However, with recurrent pelvic malignancy, rarely can resection be successfully effected. Stearns, in a report on the experience at the Memorial Sloan-Kettering Cancer Center in New York, stated, "Pelvic recurrence, in our experience, has not been curable by surgical excision or by any other modality of treatment."[210]

With perineal recurrence, patients complain of a painful lump. Biopsy usually confirms the diagnosis. With pelvic recurrence, patients may be asymptomatic, have deep-seated pelvic pain that can radiate to the lower back and buttocks or a sciatic distribution. If the tumor involves the bladder, prostate, or urethra, urinary symptoms (including hematuria) may develop. Urethral obstruction can supervene, but the most troubling, indeed disabling, complaint is the pain.

Diagnosis can be made without studies and without positive biopsy evidence of recurrence, so characteristic is the syndrome. Knowledge of a previously "unfavorable" pathology report is helpful. A mass may be felt in the perineum or in the vagina. Recently, computerized tomography (CT) has been used successfully to delineate both the presence of a tumor mass and the extent of pelvic spread.[96] It has also been suggested as potentially valuable in the follow-up of patients for the development of recurrence before symptoms appear. CT has been demonstrated to be a useful tool for establishing the histologic diagnosis of recurrent carcinoma in the pelvis by means of percutaneous biopsy with computed tomography guidance.[122, 240] But as stated, the implementation of therapy does not need to await the results of esoteric diagnostic endeavors. Carcinoembryonic antigen (CEA) elevations are certainly suggestive of recurrent disease, but all too often are unreliable. Patients with local recurrence tend to have normal values as compared with those patients who have liver or other organ involvement.

Surgical extirpation for pelvic recurrence has been used primarily for palliation,[229, 230] but radiation has also been shown to be an effective treatment modality for these patients. Wang and Schulz reported a palliative benefit lasting from several months up to 10 years.[231] This might imply an increased survival rate, but our patients survived a median of only 15 months

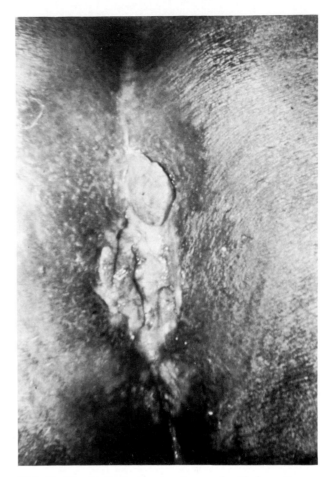

FIG. 11-47. Unhealed perineal wound with fungating recurrent rectal carcinoma following proctectomy. (Courtesy of Daniel Rosenthal, M.D.)

following radiotherapy for local recurrence, the same as the median survival rate reported by Moosa and coworkers with no radiotherapy.[162, 187]

Postoperative radiotherapy can be administered up to 6000 rads (depending on whether the patient received preoperative treatment; see later). Radiation therapy can be effective in the treatment of pain in approximately three quarters of patients. It may also decrease the size of a mass, and for an ulcerating lesion, the amount of perineal or vaginal drainage. The Memorial Sloan-Kettering group prefers short treatments of 2000 rads when symptoms develop rather than a large-dose course.[210, 214] I concur, and believe further that complications of treatment (skin irritation, micturition problems) are less frequent with this protocol.

Other treatment modalities include radium implantation and chemotherapy. Although some have suggested the possibility of improved response to radiotherapy in combination with chemotherapy, I have witnessed no such benefit.

For the pain that cannot be effectively treated by radiotherapy and which is no longer responsive to narcotic analgesics, neurosurgical consultation is advised. Intrathecal alcohol or chordotomy may be appropriate alternatives in the intractable situation.

LOW ANTERIOR RESECTION

The first resection of the sigmoid colon was performed in 1833 by Reybard of Lyons,[185] but for the next 100 years practically all operative approaches to the treatment of carcinoma either involved extirpation of the rectum or another sphincter-saving procedure, such as the various modifications of the pull-through operation. Murphy introduced his button in 1882 to perform a rapid and safe anastomosis,[169] but it was not until the 1940s, and even the 1950s in some centers, before conventional anastomotic techniques were felt safe enough to be employed for most cases of carcinoma of the rectum when intestinal continuity might be reestablished. Generally, it was the work of Dixon and of Wangensteen that contributed so much to the ultimate success of this operation.[49, 232]

Indications

The most important factor that determines the likelihood of performing an anastomosis is the level of the lesion. Although favorable factors such as good differentiation, small size, and polypoid configuration may safely reduce the distal margin of resection to 1 or 2 cm, it is the rare patient who should be considered for a low anterior resection when the tumor is below 8 cm from the anal verge. When compared with other resective sphincter-saving operations, the low anterior resection is the one that is preferred. To embark upon an esoteric approach, one must believe rather strongly that an abdominoperineal resection is inappropriate and a low anterior resection is technically impossible to accomplish.

Technique

There is often confusion about what constitutes a low anterior resection. This operation requires complete mobilization of the rectum from the hollow of the sacrum and division of the lateral ligaments and the middle hemorrhoidal arteries. Anastomosis is effected in the rectum distal to the visceral peritoneum. Unless these criteria are met, the procedure is *not* by definition a low anterior resection.

The patient may be positioned in the perineolith-

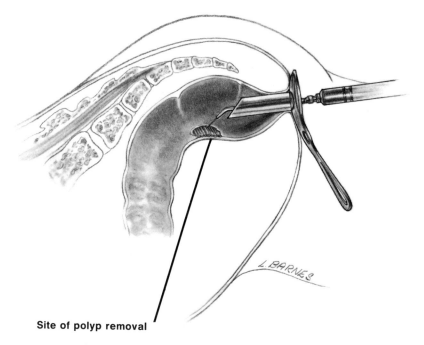

Site of polyp removal

FIG. 11-48.   Technique of India ink injection of a previously removed tumor area.

otomy (Lloyd-Davies) position or supine on the operating table. When the surgeon feels confident that an anterior abdominal approach will permit anastomosis by conventional means, the supine position is preferred. However, if there is some doubt whether an anastomosis can be effected readily from above, the perineolithotomy position should be utilized. By using this approach, alternative anastomotic techniques can be employed if necessary (see Other Anastomotic Techniques). Furthermore, an abdominoperineal resection can be synchronously performed should an anastomotic procedure be considered unwise or technically impossible to accomplish. I do not believe in the value of irrigating the rectum prior to resection; this is not in itself an indication for using this position.

An exploratory laparotomy is performed and a determination made of the possibility and advisability of performing a resection; this decision is based on the presence or absence of metastatic disease and the fixity of the tumor in the pelvis. It may not be possible, though, to determine resectability until the rectum has been fully mobilized.

On occasion, the surgeon may elect to perform a resection on a patient who had previously undergone polypectomy and who was found to have invasive carcinoma. At laparotomy it is sometimes impossible to identify the site of the lesion; this may necessitate a "blind" resection. To avoid this sequela, the area from which the tumor had been previously excised is infiltrated with India ink (Fig. 11-48). This produces a

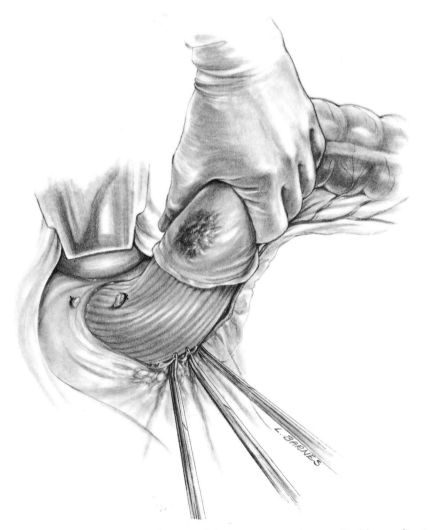

FIG. 11-49. Anterior resection: division of the mesorectum is expedited by application of right-angle clamps and vigorous cephalad tension as the mesentery is cut.

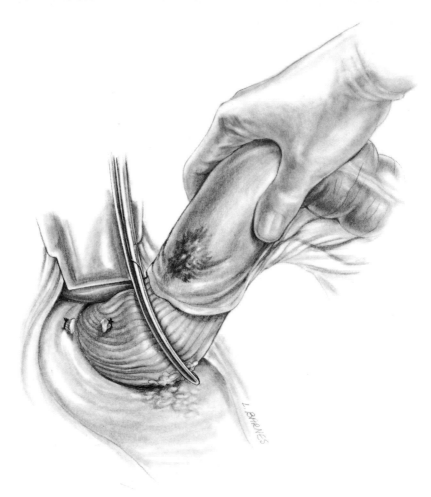

FIG. 11-50.   Anterior resection: an angled or curved clamp is applied at an adequate distance below the tumor.

black pigment in the lymphatics and permits ready identification of the tumor area from within the pelvis.

The initial steps of the procedure are identical to that described for abdominoperineal resection; the splenic flexure is *not* routinely mobilized.

Having been satisfied that an anastomosis can be performed, the next step is to divide the mesorectum; the more distal the anastomosis, the less mesorectum there is to divide. Right angle clamps are placed posteriorly and the mesentery divided above the clamps. Tension on the proximal bowel permits separation of the posterior rectal wall (Fig. 11-49). With a very low anastomosis there is usually little or no mesentery to divide.

A crushing clamp is applied, usually 5 cm below the distal margin of the tumor; an angled or curved clamp

placed in the anteroposterior plane is preferred (Fig. 11-50). Only one is used.

Anchoring sutures are placed and the bowel is divided distal to the clamp. Long Allis clamps may be used to visualize the cut edge of the rectum (Fig. 11-51). With the proximal bowel divided and the specimen removed, an open end-to-end anastomosis is performed. Interrupted 3-0 long-term absorbable sutures are recommended, but the type of suture material is of less importance than is the technique employed. Simple, interrupted sutures are placed as a single layer, taking deeper bites in the muscularis and minimal mucosa (the rectum has no serosa at this level). With a low anatomosis it is easier to place all of the sutures into the posterior row initially, before tying (Fig. 11-52). It is usually more convenient to place the initial

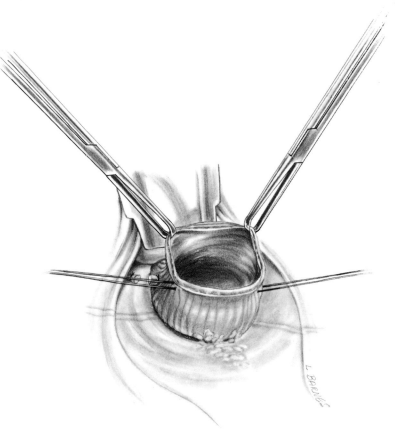

FIG. 11-51. Anterior resection: the open distal rectum is prepared for anastomosis. Allis clamps and guide sutures are helpful.

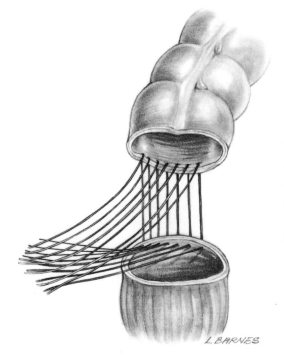
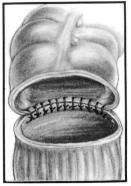

FIG. 11-52. Anterior resection: sutures are initially placed in the posterior row but not secured. The inset demonstrates the posterior row completed.

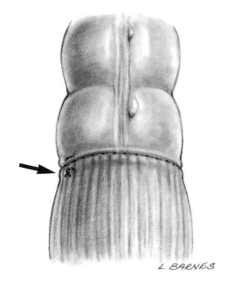

FIG. 11-53. Anterior resection: anastomosis completed. Note the final inverting mattress suture *(arrow)*.

suture through the sigmoid on the ventral aspect of the mesenteric side and then through the right anterolateral part of the rectum. The knots are then secured and the anterior row completed. The last suture is usually a horizontal mattress suture, in order to invert the mucosa (Fig. 11-53). A single layer is considered adequate, although the surgeon may prefer to pull the anterior peritoneum over the anastomosis with Lembert sutures. The floor of the pelvis is not reconstituted, however. Vigorous irrigation of the pelvis with saline is advised.

A useful step in the procedure is to place or secure omentum around the anastomosis.[69, 70, 118, 156] This can be accomplished by freeing it from the transverse colon with care to avoid injury to the blood supply (Fig. 11-54). The appropriately tailored omentum is then brought down the lateral gutter into the pelvis, and an anchoring suture is placed below and posterior to the anastomosis to secure it (Fig. 11-55). No drains are advised.

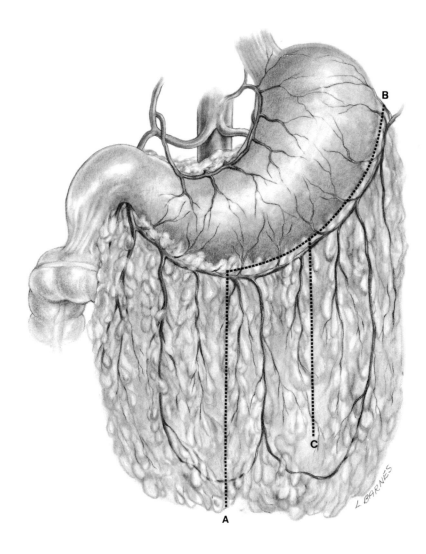

FIG. 11-54. Tailoring of the omentum: adequate length can usually be achieved if the apron is divided along lines *a* and *b*. If more is required, another incision *(c)* will usually suffice.

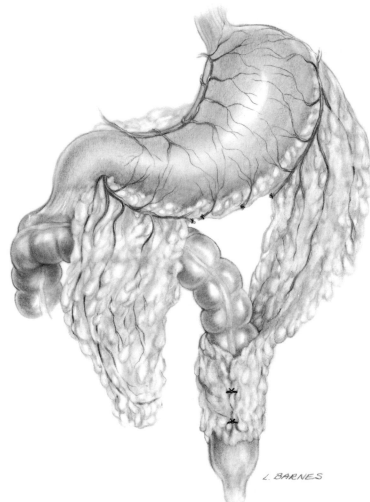

L. BARNES

FIG. 11-55. Tailoring of the omentum: the omentum is brought down the lateral gutter posterior to the anastomosis. It is then wrapped anteiorly and fixed to the rectum and pelvic floor.

Concomitant Colostomy

The decision whether to perform a protective colostomy at the time of low anterior resection is often not a matter of objective analysis but one of emotion. "The operation was technically difficult to perform, there was considerable blood loss, the tumor was stuck in the pelvis, the patient had multiple medical problems, metastases were present, metastases weren't present, the anastomosis looked tenuous, there was some tension on the suture line, I didn't feel good about it, I'll be able to sleep better tonight"—all are reasons expressed for protecting the anastomosis with a transverse colostomy. With proper technique, however, proximal diversion should rarely be necessary.

Probably the commonest reason for subsequent anastomotic complications is tension on the suture line. This may compromise healing, not only because of distraction of the anatomosis itself, but because of vas-

cular insufficiency (Fig. 11-56). Although mobilizing the splenic flexure is rarely necessary in the performance of a low anterior resection, every effort must be made to free the proximal bowel so that there is no tension on the anastomosis; placing the omentum helps to minimize the risk of leak.

If the above precautions are taken, a transverse colostomy is usually unnecessary. Pelvic sepsis, blood loss, other systemic disease, and poor nutritional status, however, are relative indications for protecting the anastomosis. But if the patient is felt to have a limited survival, a Hartmann resection is preferred. By leaving a sigmoid colostomy rather than a more difficult-to-manage transverse colostomy (a stoma which under such circumstances all too often is permanent), better palliation is achieved.

Finally, the creation of a transverse colostomy as well as the closure are not without complications. Overall morbidity rates in our experience were 21%

375

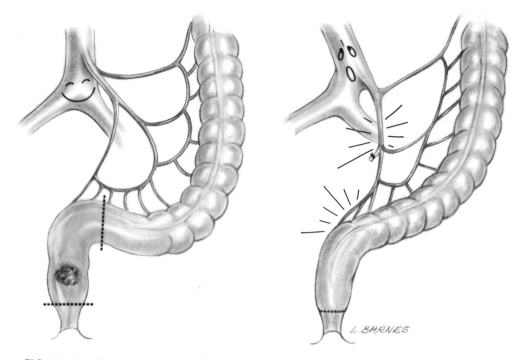

FIG. 11-56. Cartoonist's view of the etiology of anastomotic leaks: tension on the suture line with vascular compromise (as suggested by John A. Coller, M.D.).

Table 11-7. Interval Between Colostomy and Closure and Its Relation to Complications

Interval (Months)	Number of Patients	Number with Complications	Percent with Complications
0– 3	41	21	51.2
4– 6	35	12	34.2
7–12	26	9	34.6
> 12	16	3	18.8
	118	45	

(Mirelman D, Corman ML, Veidenheimer MC, Coller JA: Colostomies—indications and contraindications: Lahey clinic experience, 1973–1974. Dis Colon Rectum 1978; 21:172–176)

for colostomy construction and 49% for colostomy closure.[161] Closure of the colostomy without resection produces the lowest incidence of complications when compared with other types of closure. If a colostomy is created the interval between creation and closure should be at least 6 weeks. The longer the subsequent closure is deferred, the safer the procedure will be (Table 11-7).

The techniques for creating and closing a transverse colostomy are discussed in Chapter 16.

Postoperative Care

There are no specific postoperative care areas unique to low anterior resection. A nasogastric tube is not advised on a prophylactic basis. An indwelling urinary catheter, however, is required for approximately 1 week. The amount of manipulation necessary to extirpate the rectum and effect a low anastomosis is equivalent to that for an abdominoperineal resection. A progressive diet is instituted after the patient has passed flatus. The patient is discharged after the diet has been established and bowel and bladder function is relatively normal. This usually takes between 7 and 10 days.

Complications

Intraoperative Complications

With the exception of the complications resulting from the creation of a stoma and the perineal wound, the intraoperative problems encountered with a low anterior resection are identical to those of abdominoperineal resection.

Postoperative Complications

Anastomotic Bleeding

Hemorrhage from the anastomosis is seen in approximately 1% of patients.[145] This may be due to inadequate hemostasis at the suture line itself or to rupture of a hematoma in the pelvis through the posterior wall of the anastomosis. The former situation usually presents within the first 48 hours, whereas the latter may not become apparent for 10 days to 2 weeks. The problem may be managed expectantly, although one must be concerned about an anastomotic dehiscence. The presence of fever, leukocytosis, and peritoneal signs might cause the surgeon to consider abdominal drainage and proximal diversion.

Obstruction at the Anastomosis

Obstruction at the anastomosis without evidence of sepsis is not commonly seen, but when colonic ileus is associated with an "intact" ileocecal valve, perforation can result (Fig. 11-57). Usually conservative treatment (nasogastric tube) will suffice, and rarely is it necessary to perform a laparotomy. Digital rectal examination may be helpful, but the use of a rectal tube is relatively contraindicated because of the danger of perforating the anastomosis. If unrelieved, this may be one of the few indications for cecostomy (see Chap. 16).

Anastomotic Leak

Anastomotic sepsis and fecal fistula are among the more serious concerns in the postoperative period and are the primary causes of operative mortality (Fig. 11-58). A number of factors have been associated with these complications, and include disease (inflammation) of the bowel itself, inadequate blood supply, tension on the suture line, inaccurate suture placement,

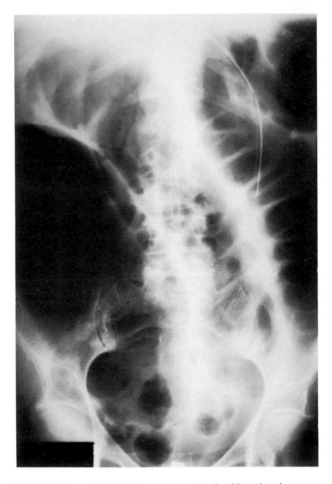

FIG. 11-57. Colonic ileus: a massively dilated colon (especially the cecum) in a patient who underwent a low anterior resection. With an "intact" ileocecal valve there is danger of perforation.

trauma, and failure to obtain a watertight seal.[44, 86, 196] Our results in a study of 152 patients indicate that diseases that affect local blood flow and response to infection (anemia, atherosclerotic disease, and diabetes) are important risk factors (Table 11-8).[145]

The complication rate of anastomotic leak following anterior resection has been variously reported from 15% to 77%.[24, 44, 52, 76, 86, 97, 145, 165, 196, 199] More recently, however, reports would seem to indicate a trend to lower rates (less than 10%).[88, 95] For anastomoses below the peritoneal reflection, protection is afforded if the peritoneal cavity is left open and omental wrapping is employed. The presence of drains is associated with an increased incidence of anastomotic complications, although it is possible that only less secure

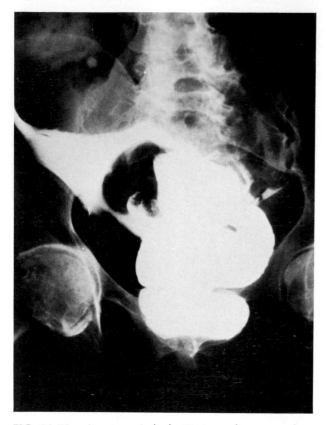

FIG. 11-58. Anastomotic leak: Gastrografin enema demonstrates extravasation into the pelvis 1 week following anterior resection.

Table 11-8. Significance of Related Factors in Anastomotic Complications (Obstruction, Sepsis, and Fistula)—152 Patients

Factor*	Significance
Atherosclerotic disease	$p < 0.001$
Anemia	$p < 0.001$
Anastomosis below the peritoneal reflection	$p < 0.001$
Obstruction and perforation	$p < 0.001$
Anastomosis below the closed peritoneum	$p < 0.005$
Use of drains, anastomosis below the peritoneal reflection	$p < 0.01$
Diabetes	$p < 0.019$
Increased age	$p < 0.02$
Use of drains, entire series	$p < 0.05$

* The following factors were not significant for anastomotic complications: operative transfusions, $p < 0.1$; abnormal serum albumin levels, $p < 0.2$; cancer in the margin of resection, $p < 0.3$; other organ involvement, $p < 0.3$; all other abnormal liver function tests, $p < 0.5$; other colonic disease (diverticulitis, diverticulosis) in specimen, $p < 0.5$; extent of disease (Dukes), $p < 0.5$; operative blood loss, $p < 0.5$; anesthesia time, $p < 0.5$; sex, $p < 0.5$; abnormal prothrombin time, $p < 0.6$. Sample size for history of previous radiation therapy, for use of steroids, and for other debilitating diseases was too small for accurate calculations.
(Manson PN, Corman ML, Coller JA, Veidenheimer MC: Anterior resection for adenocarcinoma: Lahey Clinic experience from 1963 through 1969. Am J Surg 1976; 131:434–441)

anastomoses are drained. There is certainly support for the concept that drains adversely affect anastomotic healing.[71, 146]

Obstructed or perforated tumors are frequently associated with a high incidence of anastomotic breakdown. Therefore, the implementation of proximal colostomy or delayed anastomosis in these patients would be appropriate. The routine use of proximal colostomy with low anterior resection, however, has been shown to reduce mortality but not the morbidity of anastomotic septic and fistula complications.[76, 196] Proximal colostomy not only prolongs the recovery period but also has its own morbidity and mortality in the construction and subsequent closure. Therefore, as previously stated, colostomy should be limited to those patients who have an increased risk for development of anastomotic complications. The determination of all factors preoperatively will facilitate operative decision making by indicating which patients are at high risk for the development of these septic and fistula complications.

Pelvic Abscess

Pelvic abscess should be a rare complication if the pelvic floor has not been reconstituted. Treatment may be unnecessary if the abscess spontaneously drains through the anastomosis or through the vagina. If surgical drainage is required it is usually accomplished from below (see Figs. 4-11 and 4-12). If signs of peritonitis are present, laparotomy is required for drainage, and a concomitant colostomy should also be performed.

Fecal Fistula

Abdominal fecal fistula in the absence of sepsis, and with the patient having bowel movements, can usually be treated expectantly. Without distal obstruction or persistent tumor, the fistula will usually close within a matter of a few weeks. If drainage is considerable, a colostomy appliance may be used (see Chap. 16).

Late Complications

Stricture

Benign stricture following anterior resection is usually secondary to anastomotic breakdown and subsequent fibrosis (Fig. 11-59). If there is an anastomotic dehiscence of 50% or more of the circumference, healing will usually result in stricture formation.

Medical treatment consists of the use of stool softeners, enemas, or suppositories. Dilatation of the stricture can be performed manually if it is within reach of the finger. For higher strictures (*viz.* 8–12 cm) a double-ended Hegar's dilator (17–18 mm) may be used (Fig. 11-60).

If a symptomatic stricture persists, transanal lysis in the posterior midline may ameliorate the condition, although continued dilatation is usually required for a number of weeks. If all such treatments are of no avail, re-resection may be indicated. It must be kept in mind, however, that a possible etiology of the stricture is malignant recurrent disease. The use of CT scan may be helpful, but biopsy is mandatory.

Incontinence and Irregular Bowel Function

Low anterior resection, irrespective of anastomotic technique, may be transiently associated with control problems and other bowel management difficulties. Inflammatory reaction, narrowing at the anastomosis, sensory impairment, and bowel denervation all may play a role. As long as the anal canal and sphincter muscles have been preserved, the symptoms usually resolve in a matter of a few weeks. "Slowing" medications should rarely be used because of the risk of precipitating a fecal impaction. Most patients are able to regulate themselves by paying slightly more attention to their diet than had been their custom. Eventually, all such restrictions become unnecessary in most instances.

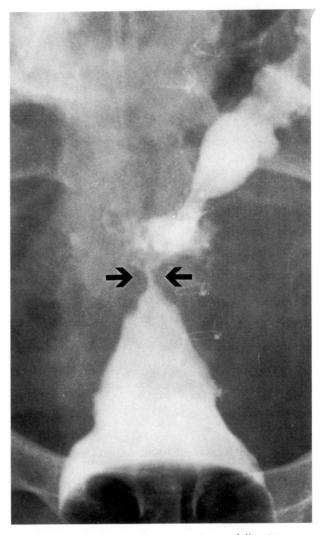

FIG. 11-59. Rectal anastomotic stricture following anterior resection. Multiple biopsies failed to reveal tumor.

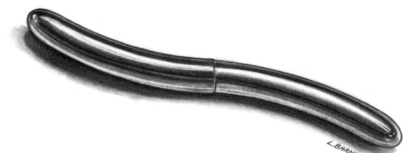

FIG. 11-60. The double-ended Hegar's dilator is a useful tool in the treatment of strictures in the mid and upper rectum.

Results

We reported our experience with high and low anterior resection in 152 patients.[145] The mean age for both men and women was 62 years. There were two in-hospital deaths, a mortality rate of 1.3%. The most common complication involved the urinary tract (14%). The wound infection rate was 6%, and pelvic abscess requiring drainage was seen in 1.3%.

Survival data according to Dukes' classification is shown in Table 11-9. There was no statistically significant difference in survival rates between abdomino-perineal resection and anterior resection in patients with Dukes' A and Dukes' B lesions. However, patients with Dukes' C lesions who underwent abdominoperineal resection had a significantly poorer survival rate than patients who had a lesion proximal enough to permit an anterior resection.

The most difficult problem following anterior resection is recurrent disease and its management (Fig. 11-61). It is possible to identify preoperatively the patient at high risk for recurrence and not elect to perform a sphincter-saving operation on that individual. For example, in our experience there was a dramatic decrease in the frequency of recurrence when the lesion was more than 13 cm from the anal verge.[144] Furthermore, most subsequent recurrences involved tumors that initially penetrated the rectal wall and extended into the surrounding tissue. Eighty-eight percent of recurrent malignant lesions in "curative" cases followed resections for this type of tumor.[144] Table 11-10 lists those variables that are statistically significant in their association with increased risk of anastomotic recurrence. Table 11-11 shows the incidence of recurrence versus the histology. Table 11-12 compares the recurrence rate

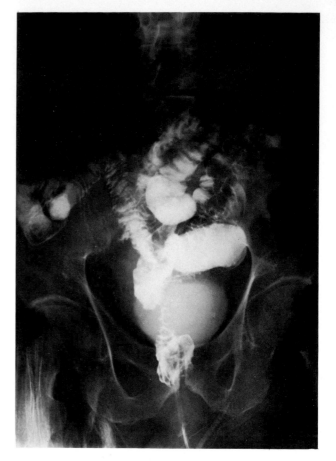

FIG. 11-61. Rectal stenosis due to anastomotic recurrence. Note also reflux of barium into the small intestine due to ileal fistula at the site of colorectal anastomosis. (Cystogram has been performed also.)

Table 11-9. Five-Year Survival for Anterior Resection According to Dukes' Classification

Dukes' Stage	Number of Patients	Percent of Series	Number of 5-Year Survivors	Uncorrected 5-Year Survival (%)	Actuarially Corrected 5-Year Survival (%)
A	49	32.2	37	75.5	86.1
B	45	29.6	31	68.8	78.8
C	39	25.7	20	51.3	57.0
D	19	12.5	0	0.0	0.0
A,B,C	133	87.5	88	66.2	71.7
All stages	152	100.0	88	57.9	72.8

(Manson PN, Corman ML, Coller JA, Veidenheimer MC: Anterior resection for adenocarcinoma: Lahey Clinic experience from 1963 through 1969. Am J Surg 1976; 131:434–441)

with Dukes' classification, and Table 11-13, the recurrence rate versus the distal margin of resection.

In summary, the incidence of anastomotic recurrence

Increases with more distal lesions.
Increases with resection margins less than 6 cm.
Is higher with ulcerating tumors.
Is low with exophytic lesions.
Is prohibitively high with poorly differentiated growths.
Is low with well-differentiated tumors.
Is low when the tumor does not penetrate the bowel.
Is high with Dukes' B and C lesions and in the presence of metastatic disease.

Therefore, in selecting patients for sphincter-saving procedures, the preoperative assessment is most important. If the tumor is low-lying (less than 8 cm from the anal verge) or is poorly differentiated (if it appears fixed, infiltrative or ulcerating), then a sphincter-saving operation may be relatively contraindicated.

Recurrence has been attributed to unresected tumor

Table 11-10. Anastomotic Recurrence After Anterior Resection: Related Factors

Factor	Significance
Penetration of coats of bowel by cancer	$p < 0.003$
Increased dedifferentiation	$p < 0.005$
Ulcerating cancer	$p < 0.005$
Tumor below peritoneal reflection	$p < 0.01$
Distal margin of resection	$p < 0.01$
Distal margin of resection less than 6 cm	$p < 0.05$

The following factors were not significant for anastomotic recurrence: Lymph node involvement, $p < 0.07$; size of lesion, $p < 0.3$; proximal margin of resection, $p < 0.3$; previous colonic cancer, $p < 0.5$; polyps in specimen, $p < 0.5$; extent of disease (Dukes), $p < 0.5$; other organ involvement, $p < 0.5$; blood vessel invasion, $p < 0.5$; age, $p < 0.5$; sex, $p < 0.6$.

(Manson PN, Corman ML, Coller JA, Veidenheimer MC: Anterior resection for adenocarcinoma: Lahey Clinic experience from 1963 through 1969. Am J Surg 1976; 131:434–441)

Table 11-11. Anterior Resection for Carcinoma: Anastomotic Recurrence Versus Histology

Type	Number of Patients	Number of Recurrences	Percent of Recurrences
Well differentiated	107	5	4.7
Moderately differentiated	33	6	18.2
Poorly differentiated	5	4	80.0
Villous	7	3 (2 benign)	42.9
Total	152	18	11.8

(Manson PN, Corman ML, Coller JA, Veidenheimer MC: Anastomotic recurrence after anterior resection for carcinoma: Lahey clinic experience. Dis Colon Rectum 1976; 19:219–224)

Table 11-12. Anterior Resection for Carcinoma: 5-Year Survival (Uncorrected)

Dukes' Stage	Number of Patients	Number Survived	Percent Survived
A	49	38	77.6
B	45	30	66.6
C	39	19	48.7
D	19	1	5.3
All stages	152	88	57.9

(Manson PN, Corman ML, Coller JA, Veidenheimer MC: Anastomotic recurrence after anterior resection for carcinoma: Lahey clinic experience. Dis Colon Rectum 1976; 19:219–224)

Table 11-13. Anterior Resection for Carcinoma: Anastomotic Recurrence Versus Distal Margin of Resection

Distal Margin (cm)	Number of Patients	Number of Recurrences	Percent of Recurrences
0	2	0	0.0
1	10	1	10.0
2	17	3	17.6
3	23	2	8.7
4	24	3	12.5
5	31	6	19.4
6	16	2	12.5
7	14	1	7.1
> 7	15	0	0.0

(Manson PN, Corman ML, Coller JA, Veidenheimer MC: Anastomotic recurrence after anterior resection for carcinoma: Lahey clinic experience. Dis Colon Rectum 1976; 19:219–224)

(in the pelvis or the bowel wall itself),[46, 64, 65, 66, 129, 137, 154, 159, 204, 207] to a zone of potentially malignant mucosa,[137] to a new primary tumor,[74, 137, 138] to spillage of viable malignant cells,[26–29, 74, 137, 155, 205, 227] and to implantation by suture material.[57]

Although tumor at the margin of resection or in adjacent lymph nodes, or a second primary lesion are other sources of recurrent disease, they are in all probability quite uncommon causes of recurrence. It is my belief that the overwhelming majority of suture-line recurrences are due to residual tumor left behind in the pelvis that subsequently grows into the lumen through the anastomosis.

Measures to control recurrence from implantation have been reported to reduce recurrence rates,[74, 90, 115,] [164, 189, 205, 225] but in these nonrandomized studies one wonders if the alleged improved results are due to patient selection and attention to other concerns, such as a wide resection.

The only effective prevention is to select out those patients who are at increased risk for the subsequent development of recurrence, and either to perform an abdominoperineal resection or to consider the possibility of entering the patient into a controlled study of adjuvant radiotherapy or chemotherapy.

Treatment of Recurrence

When anastomotic recurrence develops, it usually presents within 2 years following resection. The patient

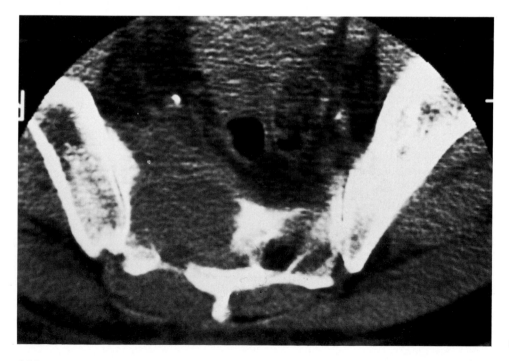

FIG. 11-62. Recurrent rectal cancer: CT scan shows bony erosion.

usually has no new symptoms, but the suspicious area is identified either by palpation (digital examination) or by proctosigmoidoscopy as part of the follow-up of a cancer patient. Occasionally the patient may report bleeding, change in the caliber of the stool, or pelvic, abdominal, or sacral pain. Biopsy usually will confirm the suspicion, but barium enema examination and CT scan also may be helpful (Fig. 11-62). Most patients who present with recurrent cancer in the pelvis do not have disseminated disease. The CEA is often not elevated.

The only hope for cure is re-resection; this usually involves an abdominoperineal resection (Fig. 11-63). It is imperative when resective surgery is contemplated to study the urinary tract; ureteral obstruction is common (Fig. 11-64).[91] In fact, nonvisualization of a kidney secondary to long-standing obstruction is not rare. It is helpful to insert ureteral catheters prior to laparotomy. Although no guarantee that ureteral injury will be avoided, their presence may permit easier palpation

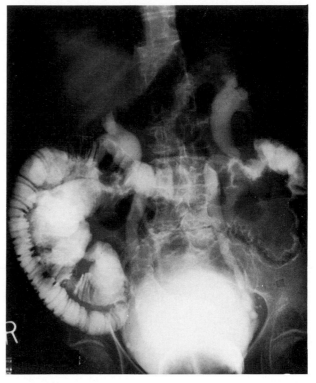

FIG. 11-64. Recurrent rectal cancer with ureteral obstruction.

of the structures when visualization may be difficult; they can be removed at the end of the operation.

The perineolithotomy position is advised for a two-team approach. Once resectability has been ascertained, synchronous dissection can be initiated.

Studies of abdominoperineal resection following anastomotic recurrence have limited numbers of patients and are difficult to interpret.[198] Overall cure rates are certainly less than 50% in those considered resectable for cure. It is my feeling that cure is rarely achieved except in those patients in whom a second primary lesion developed, or when the pathologist reports that the recurrence is confined to, but does not breach, the bowel wall.

OTHER ANASTOMOTIC TECHNIQUES

Side-to-End Anastomosis

Baker advocated side-to-end anastomosis of the colon to the rectum in order to deal with the disparity between the two lumens.[9] Others have also found this to be a useful technique.[105]

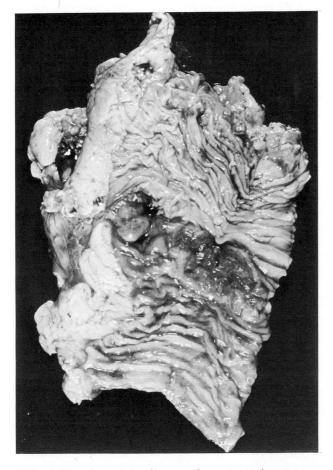

FIG. 11-63. A portion of resected specimen showing suture line recurrence of tumor.

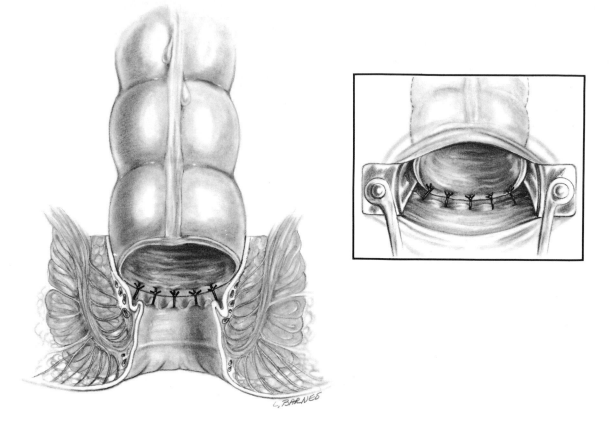

FIG. 11-65. Coloanal anastomosis: a Parks retractor facilitates the insertion of sutures *(inset)*.

I do not believe that this approach serves a useful purpose. Anastomosis can be more readily accomplished in an end-to-end fashion, with the addition of a Cheatle cut if necessary to deal with the lumenal discrepancies (see Fig. 10-48).

Transanal Anastomosis

An alternative technique for reestablishing intestinal continuity is the transanal or coloanal anastomosis, described initially by Parks in 1972.[176] A round-bodied modification of a Turner-Warwick urethroplasty needle may be used, or a long-term absorbable suture on a five-eighths circle needle. Using a Parks self-retaining, three-bladed anal retractor or paired Gelpé retractors placed at right angles to each other, a transanal anastomosis can be effected (Fig. 11-65). This is the technique employed for reestablishing continuity after colectomy, mucosal proctectomy, and ileal pouch for inflammatory bowel disease (see Chap. 15). The sutures incorporate the full thickness of the colon with the anal canal and the underlying internal sphincter.

Parks reported 76 patients who underwent rectal excision for carcinoma with restoration of bowel continuity by coloanal anastomosis.[177] Ten developed pelvic sepsis, two with anastomotic breakdown. Sixty-nine of 70 patients reviewed had a good functional result. Although not all patients were followed for 5 years, Parks felt that the preliminary survival data was comparable to that for patients treated by abdominoperineal resection. Rudd reported an 80% incidence of perfect continence in his series.[191]

Comment

Although this technique is at least as tedious as the various pull-through procedures (see later), it may be usefully applied in the rare situation in which intestinal continuity cannot be reestablished by a more conventional means. It must be remembered, however, that the purpose of the operation is to cure the patient. If an anastomotic technique compromises the margins of resection, then preserving the patient's ability to defecate through the anus is indeed a pyrrhic victory. As of this writing I have found no indication for this technique in the treatment of malignant disease.

Magnetic Ring Anastomosis

A modification of the Murphy button has been described by Jansen and co-workers by which an anastomotic apparatus consisting of two magnetic rings embedded in polyester progressively compresses and necroses the intervening bowel by increasing magnetic force while healing takes place.[99] After 7 to 12 days, the magnets cut through and are eliminated through the stool.

I have had no experience with this technique, but can see no great advantage over the conventional anastomotic procedures.

Stapled Anastomosis

The application of stapling anastomoses is discussed in Chapter 10, but the creation of a low rectal anastomosis is not possible with the conventional instruments and maneuvers described in that chapter.

In 1978 the United States Surgical Corporation introduced a circular stapling device (similar to the Russian stapler, PKS) which is uniquely advantageous in effecting low colorectal anastomoses. The end-to-end anastomosis (EEA) stapler (Fig. 11-66) and the intraluminal stapler (ILS; Fig. 11-67), both reusable and disposable, create an inverted, circular anastomosis

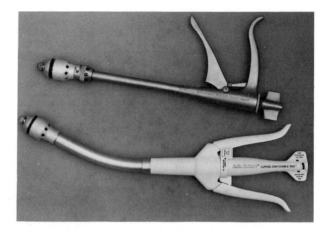

FIG. 11-66. End-to-end anastomotic (EEA) staplers, reusable and disposable. (Courtesy of United States Surgical Corp.)

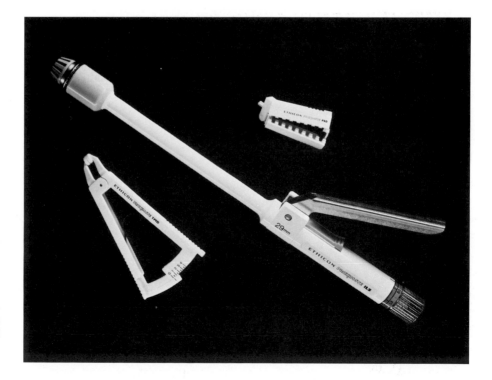

FIG. 11-67. Intraluminal stapler (proximate ILS) with tissue measuring device (TMD) and pursestring device (PSD). (Courtesy of Ethicon, Inc.)

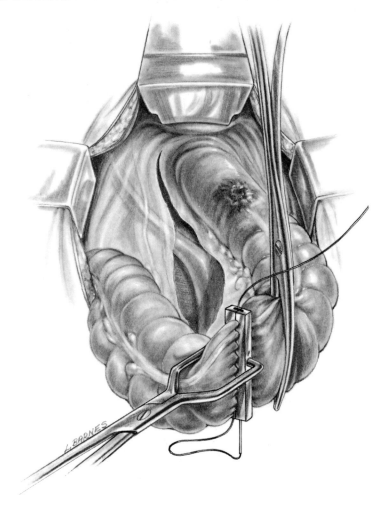

FIG. 11-68.   Circular stapled anastomosis: application of pursestring instrument.

with two staggered rows of staples, and remove a "donut" of bowel from each end to create an adequate lumen. Cartridges are available in several diameters: 31 mm, 28 mm, and 25 mm.

Technique

The patient is placed in the perineolithotomy position in order to facilitate access to the anus and to the abdomen. After the bowel has been mobilized above and below the tumor and the blood supply has been divided, the proximal site for the anastomosis is prepared. In contrast to conventional suturing technique, the bowel must be meticulously debrided of all fat for

1.5 cm to 2 cm. A crushing clamp is placed distally and a pursestring suture proximally. If the pursestring instrument is used, a straight Keith needle of 2-0 Prolene is passed through both channels (Fig. 11-68). A monofilament nonabsorbable suture is required in order to prevent dragging when the pursestring is secured. The bowel is then divided between the clamps.

In like manner, the distal bowel below the tumor is freed and the mesentery debrided. Ideally, the pursestring clamp is placed below the tumor (Fig. 11-69). Unfortunately, the applicator often cannot be usefully employed for anastomoses low in the pelvis. This is the single most important reason for my relative lack of enthusiasm for the circular stapling device. The pursestring must be applied in this situation manually.

A crushing clamp is placed on the bowel distal to the tumor. It is helpful to apply a noncrushing intestinal clamp or vascular clamp on the distal rectal stump to use as a handle, or to place several guide sutures to elevate the rectum. The bowel is then divided, and the specimen is removed. A monofilament, nonabsorbable, pursestring suture is then inserted in an "over-and-over" fashion (Fig. 11-70), although the more tedious "weaving" suture may be used (Fig. 11-71, *A*). Moseson and associates facilitate the application of the suture by elevation of the rectal cuff with traction on a Foley catheter.[167]

An alternative technique involves inverting the rectal stump with the aid of guide sutures and passing it to the perineal operator. If the rectum is of sufficient length it is sometimes possible to apply the pursestring device outside the anal verge (Fig. 11-71, *B*). Realistically, though, if there is so much rectum remaining to permit this maneuver, it should be possible to apply

the instrument through the abdomen. But there is the occasional situation in which this can be a useful modification. After the suture has been placed, the rectum is returned to the pelvis.

Attention is then turned to the cartridge. With experience, the surgeon should be able to select the appropriate size; the largest (31 mm) should be used whenever possible. The sigmoid colon usually has the smaller lumen, but with the aid of a sizer–dilator, the lumenal discrepancy may be somewhat obviated. When bowel spasm presents a problem, the intravenous administration of 2 mg of glucagon has been recommended, as has the use of a Foley catheter balloon.[83, 160]

The perineal surgeon dilates the anus, and the well-lubricated instrument is inserted into the rectum. The abdominal surgeon should guide the instrument anteriorly, because there is a tendency for the perineal operator to direct the instrument into the sacrum. The

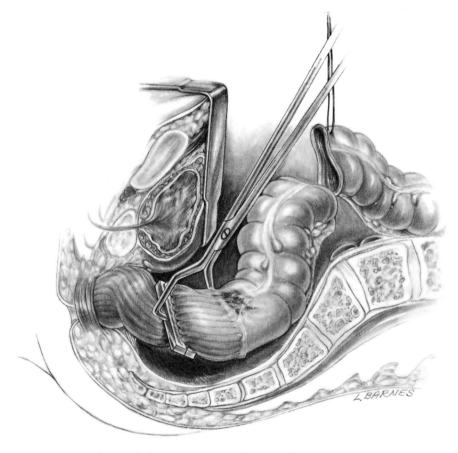

FIG. 11-69. Circular stapled anastomosis: application of pursestring instrument distal to the tumor. The proximal suture is in place. Clamps are omitted for ease of illustration.

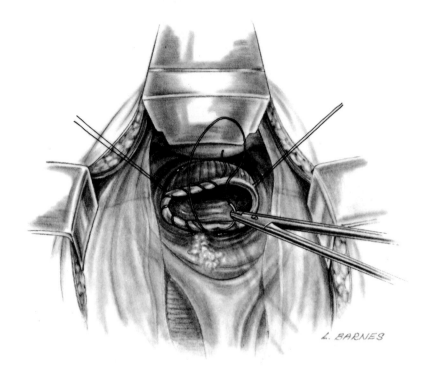

FIG. 11-70. Circular stapled anastomosis: a hand-sewn pursestring suture is placed in the rectal stump.

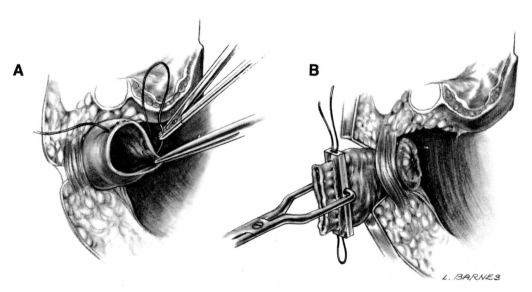

FIG. 11-71. Circular stapled anastomosis. **A.** Hand-sewn pursestring suture placed using "weaving" technique. **B.** Pursestring applicator employed on inverted rectal stump.

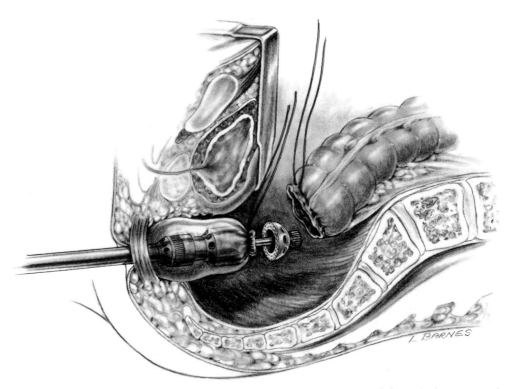

FIG. 11-72.   Circular stapled anastomosis: the instrument is inserted through the anus and the distal pursestring secured.

wing nut is turned counterclockwise, and the anvil is advanced from the cartridge into the pelvis. The pursestring suture is then tied over the shaft (Fig. 11-72).

Then, using Babcock forceps, the proximal bowel is eased over the anvil and the proximal pursestring suture secured. Both sutures are then cut (Fig. 11-73). The perineal surgeon then tightens the wing nut, and the bowel ends are approximated. The abdominal surgeon makes certain that no tissue comes between the anvil and the cartridge. The safety catch is released, and the handle grip is tightened to fire the staples and cut the redundant bowel (Fig. 11-74). The safety catch is reapplied and the anvil advanced. Using a gentle rotational movement, the instrument is withdrawn with careful guidance by the abdominal operator.

Finally, the excised ''donuts,'' which are the cut edges of both ends of the anastomosis (with the pursestring sutures), are examined for the presence of intact rings (Fig. 11-75). If the rings are not intact, the anastomosis will have to be redone or reinforced with sutures.

The anastomosis should be inspected by placing sa-

line in the pelvis and looking for bubbles when air is insufflated into the rectum. Proctosigmoidoscopic visualization of the adequacy of the lumen may also be helpful. If the technique has been properly performed, no reinforcing sutures are necessary.

The indications for proximal colostomy should be the same as those following hand-sewn anastomosis. Stenosis is a particularly troublesome problem if a diversionary procedure is performed when the stapling technique is used.[78]

Complications

The three most common complications following stapled end-to-end anastomosis are hemorrhage, stricture, and breakdown.

Hemorrhage was thought to be a problem with a single row of staples associated with the Russian instrument. But with the American double row of interlocking staples, bleeding is a rare complication.[87]

Stricture at the anastomosis has been reported, but is probably secondary to breakdown and fibrosis rather

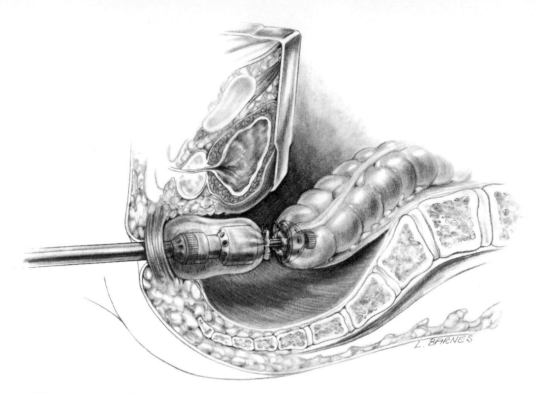

FIG. 11-73. Circular stapled anastomosis: proximal and distal pursestring sutures are secured.

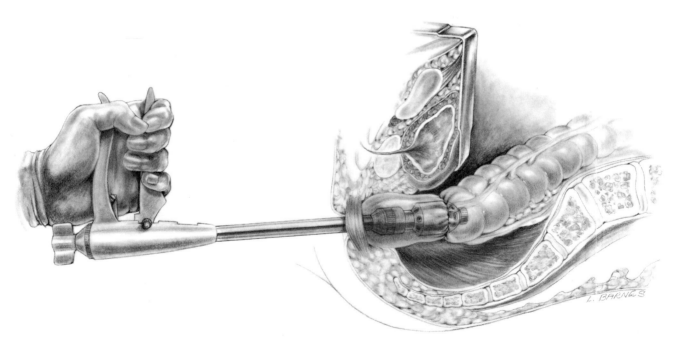

FIG. 11-74. Circular stapled anastomosis: the instrument is fired after the ends of the bowel have been approximated.

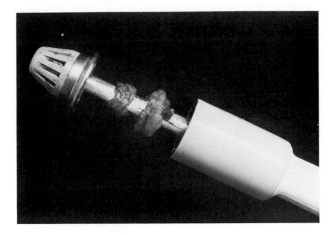

FIG. 11-75. Circular stapled anastomosis: intact donuts indicate complete anastomosis. (Courtesy of Ethicon, Inc.)

than to an intrinsic problem associated with the instrumentation or the staples. Treatment is the same as that for stricture following conventional sutured anastomosis.

The incidence of *anastomotic breakdown* following stapled anastomoses has been reported by Heald and Leicester.[87] They noted 13 clinical leaks in 100 stapled anastomoses. They attributed their high breakdown rate primarily to the low level of the anastomosis (all occurred below 7 cm). They caution that blood supply is more adequate if the left colon is fully mobilized and used for the anastomosis rather than the sigmoid colon (conserving the inferior mesenteric artery).

The Mayo Clinic group reported a controlled randomized trial.[10] Sixty percent of the hand-sewn anastomoses were considered difficult, whereas only 36% of the stapled anastomoses fell into this category. The time for anastomosis was significantly different for hand-sewn (19 minutes) and stapled (11 minutes): p = 0.01. The authors felt that approximately 12% of their patients had their rectums preserved by stapling.

Marti and associates reported three clinical and seven radiologic leaks in 79 patients anastomosed with the EEA stapler, and others noted 11 complications in 19 low anterior resections performed with this technique.[148, 195] Lack of experience is the suggested reason for the poor results. Eleven anastomotic leaks in 100 patients were reported by Detry and Kestens[48]; Kennedy and associates experienced a 20% incidence of stapler-related complications in 265 patients; there was a 3% incidence of clinical anastomotic leaks.[103] Other complications include rectovaginal fistula, serosal tears, incomplete donuts, instrument failure, and difficulty extracting.[123]

Comment

Although the end-to-end circular stapling instruments permit reestablishment of intestinal continuity in the rare situation in which conventional technique cannot be applied, they are no panacea. The same principles of cancer removal must prevail. Margins needed for resection are the same. Tension on the suture line and the blood-supply concerns are identical. Even in the most experienced hands they save very little operating time when compared with the duration of the entire procedure. Stapling should be considered merely another tool in our surgical armamentarium; each clinical situation must be evaluated individually. The circular stapling device is not appropriate for every patient with cancer of the rectum.

Abdomino-Anal Pull-Through Procedures

Another alternative means for reestablishing intestinal continuity following rectal resection is the pull-through procedure. There are several methods of accomplishing anal anastomosis by this technique.

The procedure was initially described by Maunsell in 1892 and supported by Weir in 1901.[152, 235] It was developed as an alternative to the transsacral excision of Kraske (see Sacral Resection) and the Murphy anastomotic button.[111, 169]

Pull-through procedures in general are applied for anastomoses below 7 cm, but are relatively infrequently employed today because of other techniques (*viz.* circular stapling) and other treatment modalities (*e.g.,* electrocoagulation). The surgeon must be wary of using the pull-through procedure for malignant disease lest in his ardor to effect an anastomosis he compromises on the margin of resection.

Eversion Techniques

The patient is placed in the perineolithotomy position if consideration is to be given to performing a pull-through procedure. The operation proceeds as if for a low anterior resection. However, when a pull-through operation is undertaken, greater length of proximal colon needs to be liberated. In most cases the splenic flexure requires mobilization. The bowel is divided as low as is possible and the specimen resected.

The safest anastomosis and the one that offers the best functional result is accomplished with the Weir procedure; the rectal stump is everted, the proximal bowel "pulled-through," and the anastomosis performed by the perineal operator with interrupted 3-0

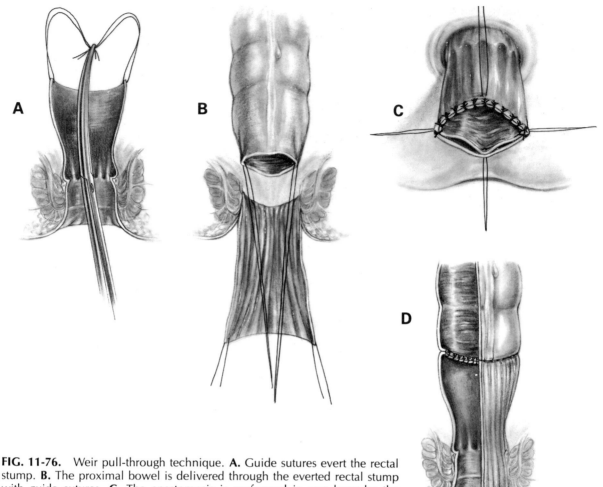

FIG. 11-76. Weir pull-through technique. **A.** Guide sutures evert the rectal stump. **B.** The proximal bowel is delivered through the everted rectal stump with guide sutures. **C.** The anastomosis is performed in one layer by the perineal surgeon. **D.** The bowel returns to the pelvis.

long-term absorbable sutures (Fig. 11-76). The anastomotic area returns to the pelvis spontaneously. The pelvic peritoneal floor is left open; no drains are usually employed, but a proximal colostomy is advised.

A modification of the Weir technique has been described by Turnbull and Cuthbertson and by Cutait and Figliolini.[40, 224] The rectal stump is everted, but the bowel is pulled through and left to project on the perineum for 7 or 8 cm. The cut edge of the rectum is sutured to the seromuscular surface of the intussuscepting colon, not penetrating the lumen (Fig. 11-77). A catheter is secured into the protruding bowel. After 10 days to 2 weeks, the redundant colon is amputated and the anastomosis resutured; the rectum retracts into the pelvis.

Comment

The advantage of the Weir (Maunsell) procedure is that it is tidier, since the anastomosis is performed primarily. The staged operation creates an uncomfortable, often frightening, foul-smelling, necrotic perineal protrusion, but it can accomplish an anastomosis safely, without the need for a diversionary procedure; hence, it has this advantage. The fact of the matter is, however, that both procedures are rarely useful alternatives to low anterior resection with or without the stapling instrument. In order to evert the rectum sufficiently to deliver it to the perineum, a minimum of 6 cm of residual rectum is required. The tethering of the levatores tends to draw the bowel back into the pelvic cavity. Most patients are able to have continuity reestablished by more conventional means (if reestablishment is considered advisable) with so much rectum remaining. With less rectum available eversion is virtually impossible.

A much lower anastomosis can be effected using the Babcock, Bacon, or Black techniques.[4, 5, 7, 16]

Delayed Union–Amputation Techniques

Babcock described his technique for one-stage abdominoperineal proctosigmoidectomy with perineal anus in 1932.[4] After a generous posterior sphincterotomy has been performed, the bowel is amputated at the top of the anal canal and pulled through. This allegedly reduces the risk of necrosis of the exteriorized colon. Healing takes place between the cut edge of the anorectum and the serosa of the colon. Amputation of the stump is performed 2 weeks later.

In the Black modification no sphincterotomy is undertaken.[16]

Bacon first described his alternative in 1945.[7] He removed the anal canal by way of the perineal route, dividing the bowel at or above the levators. This permits a wider surface area to come in contact with the pulled-through bowel, a theoretical advantage in that healing may be more effective. As with the other procedures, the redundant bowel is amputated approximately 2 weeks later.

Comment

The delayed union, amputative techniques permit a lower anastomosis than can be achieved through eversion. Hence, they can effect an anastomosis in situations when an anterior abdominal approach with any suture technique is impossible. However, the anastomosis may be less secure, and subsequent continence may not be as satisfactory as with the former methods. With the temporary, perineal "colostomy," a proximal diversion, however, should be unnecessary.

One problem in my experience has been that of the wet anus (see Fig. 7-2). The mucosal ectropion associated with nonanastomotic pull-through procedures can be a source of considerable discharge and discomfort.

One must be skeptical of the frequent application of an esoteric operation when most other surgeons use another, more standard approach. Although I hesitate to accuse surgeons who favor esoteric operations of provincialism or of unwarranted enthusiasm, I have difficulty in placing great credence on the value of their reports.

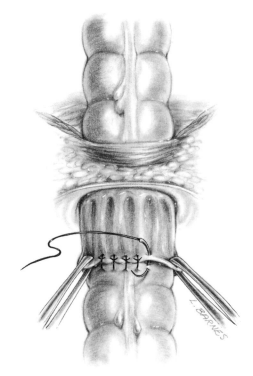

FIG. 11-77. Pull-through by eversion and seromuscular suture (first stage).

Rather than abstract the results of the moderately extensive literature on the subject, I have appended a list of references.[6, 12, 13, 15, 75, 106, 112, 113, 208, 224] All studies are uncontrolled or, at best, relate only to historical controls. Morbidity is generally higher than with abdominoperineal resection, as is the length of hospitalization. Mortality rates are also higher with the pull-through procedures. Cure rates and problems with pelvic recurrence are comparable, however, Continence generally is good.[117]

In my opinion the operation should be performed rarely for malignant disease and essentially relegated to the individual who refuses colostomy and in whom no other resective or local procedure is possible.

Sacral Resection

Sacral excision had been performed by Kocher in 1875.[109] However, it has been associated with the name of Kraske ever since he described the technique in detail to the Fourteenth Congress of the German Association of Surgeons in 1884.[110]

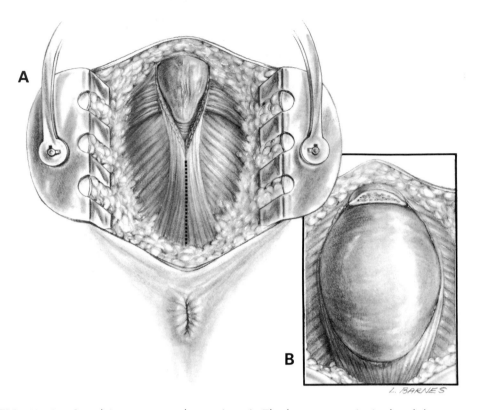

L. BARNES

FIG. 11-78. Sacral (transcoccygeal resection. **A.** The levatores are incised and the coccyx exposed. **B.** The posterior rectal wall is visualized and the coccyx removed. Further exposure can be achieved by removing the lower sacral segments.

Technique

Routine bowel preparation is carried out as if for an anterior resection. The operation is performed with the patient in the prone position and with the buttocks taped. Some surgeons prefer the lateral position, but the prone jackknife is easier. An incision is made in the midline from just above the anal verge to the lower sacrum and carried through the subcutaneous tissue to expose the levator ani muscle and coccyx (Fig. 11-78). The levator ani muscle is then divided, exposing the posterior wall of the rectum. The coccyx is then freed from its muscular attachments, disarticulated, and re-moved. If it is apparent that sufficient exposure has been achieved, then no part of the sacrum is removed. However, if further exposure is necessary, the lower portion (two sacral segments) are excised using a Gigli saw. It is imperative when dividing the sacrum that the third sacral nerve on one side be preserved in order to avoid problems with incontinence.

The rectum is then completely mobilized. Care must be taken to avoid injuring the anterior rectum where it is adherent to the vagina or to the prostate. A Penrose drain is placed around the rectum for traction and the dissection is completed. The peritoneum may be opened anterior to the rectum. The bowel is then drawn downward as far as is possible and the superior hemorrhoidal vessels divided. The bowel is divided at the desired level and an anastomosis is effected with interrupted 3-0 long-term absorbable sutures as a sin-gle layer. Classically, the bowel was brought out by establishing a sacral anus at the posterior end of the wound, amputating the entire distal rectum. This, in essence, was a sacral colostomy.

A Jackson-Pratt drain is placed through a stab wound of the buttock into the presacral space. It is usually left in place for 48 to 72 hours or until drainage ceases.

Postoperatively, the treatment is essentially the same as that for a low anterior resection. When flatus is passed a progressive diet is instituted. During the time of convalescence the patient is instructed on perineal strengthening exercises. A degree of incontinence occurs for several days to a few weeks, but in all cases virtually normal control will be restored eventually.

Comment

The Kraske operation usually permits resection of 8 to 10 cm of rectum without difficulty. Sacral excision rapidly became the most popular modality of treatment for carcinoma of the rectum toward the end of the 19th century, but the problems of anastomotic breakdown, fecal fistula, wound sepsis, and tumor recurrence have caused the procedure to fall into disrepute. Certainly, by modern standards, the surgery must be regarded as inadequate for the treatment of cancer in that it does nothing to remove the ''zone of upward spread.''

While some surgeons are still recommending this operation for malignant disease (particularly if the cancer is small), I believe that the operation is contraindicated for this condition. It does, however, have application in carefully selected cases of benign disease: villous adenoma, benign rectal stricture, rectovaginal fistula, and rectoprostatic fistula.

Abdominosacral Resection

Kraske was the first to suggest a combined abdominosacral resection to overcome the disadvantage of failure to remove the lymphatics of the rectum and rectosigmoid. More recently, Donaldson and co-workers and Localio and Stahl have revived the interest in this approach for the treatment of rectal cancer.[50, 132]

Technique

In the modification described by Localio and Stahl, access to the abdomen and the sacrum is achieved simultaneously by placing the patient in the right lateral position (Fig. 11-79).[132] Two teams can then operate independently on the abdomen and the sacrum. I have found this approach cumbersome and much prefer the patient placed in the perineolithotomy position and the abdominal phase completed as if for a low anterior resection. The lateral stalks are divided, and the surgeon then decides on the advisability of reestablishing continuity and the choice of operation to accomplish this. If the sacral approach is elected the abdomen is closed. It is important to fully mobilize the entire left colon and splenic flexure so that the bowel can be easily delivered and so there is no tension on the subsequent anastomosis. The bowel is *not* divided during the abdominal phase of the procedure. A transverse loop colostomy is routinely performed.

The patient is then placed in the prone jackknife position, and the Kraske approach is used (see Fig. 11-78). With the rectum already fully mobilized, the bowel containing the tumor can be delivered through the incision and resected (Fig. 11-80). Anastomosis is accomplished with an interrupted single-layer technique. The muscles are repaired with zero long-term absorbable sutures, and a Jackson-Pratt drain is placed into the hollow of the sacrum and brought out through a stab wound in the buttock.

Results

Localio and colleagues have probably the largest experience with this operation.[130, 131] Most recently they reported the results on 427 patients for carcinoma of

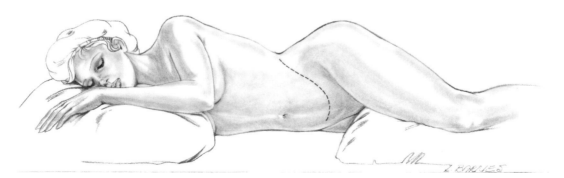

FIG. 11-79. Abdominosacral resection: position of the patient for synchronous resection and anastomosis (not recommended).

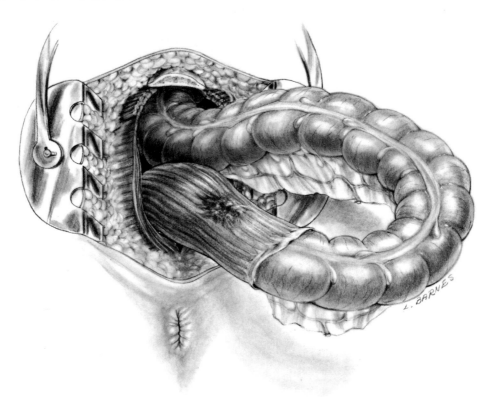

FIG. 11-80. Abdominosacral resection: the colon is delivered through the sacral defect and resected. Anastomosis is readily performed through the sacral wound.

the rectum. Preoperative assessment was made to determine the type of operation that the patient would require: abdominoperineal resection, anterior resection, or abdominosacral resection. One hundred abdominosacral resections were performed. Although recurrence rates and mortality rates were comparable for the three procedures, the morbidity of abdominosacral resection was much higher. Twelve percent of the patients developed either a fecal fistula or peritonitis. Because of these complications the authors advise that a colostomy should always be performed.

Comment

Although I have had only a limited experience with this operation, and that primarily for benign conditions, I am not enthusiastic about its value in the treatment of rectal cancer. It is true that the procedure effectively removes the cancer-bearing segment and lymphatics and that a low anastomosis can satisfactorily be achieved, but a candidate for its application is infrequent indeed. The fact that the patient must contend with a sacral wound as well as an abdominal incision causes me to look for other alternative means

of preserving the anal sphincter when such an approach is desirable.

Transsphincteric Excision

Mason reported his experience of removing cancer of the rectum by means of a transsphincteric, local excision.[149]

With the patient in the prone jackknife position, the levator ani and external sphincter muscles are completely divided in the posterior midline. The bowel is opened, offering excellent exposure of the mid and lower rectum (Fig. 11-81). Although tumors on the anterior wall are the easiest to demonstrate, those on the posterior or lateral walls can be brought into view by fully mobilizing the rectum.

In an experience on 14 patients, Mason reported a recurrence rate of 13%.[150]

Allgöwer and co-workers reported 36 patients with rectal cancers treated by a sphincter-splitting approach.[1, 2] There were no operative deaths but there were 9 recurrences. The authors recommend frozen

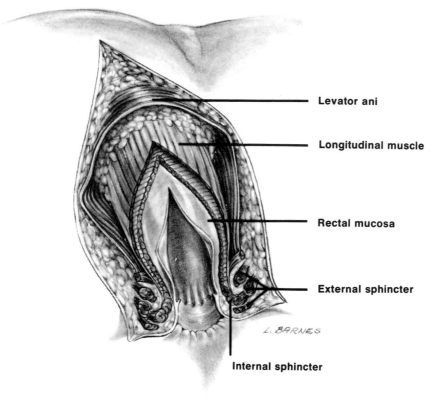

Levator ani

Longitudinal muscle

Rectal mucosa

External sphincter

L. BARNES

Internal sphincter

FIG. 11-81. Transsphincteric excision: the rectum is opened like a book in the posterior midline.

section examination of the surgical margins and depth of penetration by the tumor.

Although I have had no experience with this technique, the obvious criticism of failure to remove the associated lymphatics would relegate this procedure to one of palliation in the poor-risk patient. I have no reservations, however, about dividing the sphincter muscles, because good results can be expected with direct repair.

Mason reported an alternative means of effecting an anastomosis following an abdomino-anal pull-through.[151] By dividing the sphincter muscles as was previously described, an anastomosis can be performed quite readily at the anal verge.

As with other esoteric sphincter-saving approaches, it is not difficult for me to temper my enthusiasm.

TRANSANAL (LOCAL) EXCISION

Transanal excision with a cold knife through an operating proctoscope or by dilating the anus and using retractors, has been advocated by surgeons for the occasional, small, exophytic, movable, well-differentiated lesion.[42, 45, 166] Hager and associates reported 95 patients treated by local excision.[82] The 5-year survival rate for tumors confined to the mucosa and submucosa was 90%, and 78% when the cancer invaded the muscularis propria. Despite reasonably favorable results by this approach with the restricted indications mentioned, I believe that electrocoagulation should be the modality used for local treatment, because it is less likely to seed viable tumor cells.

ELECTROCOAGULATION

Destruction of tumors by electric current has been reported virtually since electricity was harnessed. In 1913, Strauss advocated electrocoagulation for palliation in poor-risk patients with carcinoma of the rectum and in those patients with extensive lesions.[216–219] His indications were gradually broadened to include almost all stages of carcinoma of the rectum. Subsequent reports advocating electrosurgical destruction have dotted the literature, but their authors emphasized that the primary value of the procedure was in those patients who had incurable carcinoma or in those who refuse colostomy.[98, 104, 188] Despite Strauss' results, which were reported to be at least as satisfactory as those for surgically resected carcinomas, the use of this technique failed to have any significant impact on surgical thinking until Madden and Kandalaft reported their series in 1967.[141] They believed electrocoagulation to be the preferred treatment for carcinoma of the rectum. Subsequently, they updated their study in 1971, and Crile and Turnbull reported a series with favorable results in 1972.[36, 142] Others have been encouraged with the selective application of this technique.[114, 192, 238] Because of these reports, many surgeons have begun to use this treatment not only for palliation, but also for the potentially surgically curable lesion.

The decision to avoid abdominoperineal resection, a surgical procedure that has been reasonably successful in the primary treatment of carcinoma of the rectum for more than 70 years, requires careful consideration. It would be helpful if there were a prospective, randomized, controlled clinical study comparing abdominoperineal resection with electrocoagulation. However, it is unlikely that we shall ever see one.

The classic way to perform a randomized, prospective trial of two operative techniques is to "draw a card" after the operation has begun, and thus decide which procedure to employ. Imagine the surgeon's moral dilemma if he were confronted with an 85-year-old patient with a 1-cm carcinoma of the rectum and were "directed" to perform an abdominoperineal resection. On the other hand, performing an electrocoagulation on a 35-year-old patient who has a large, ulcerating carcinoma might indeed be unconscionable.

But even in the absence of a controlled study, enough evidence has accumulated to warrant adoption of a policy of advising electrocoagulation for selected patients with carcinoma of the rectum.

Indications

Electrocoagulation may be considered when the tumor encompasses less than 50% of the circumference of the bowel wall, when the lesion is exophytic and well-differentiated (or of a low grade malignancy), when the patient with known metastases can have symptoms effectively palliated, when debilitating disease is present, or when the patient refuses or cannot manage a colostomy. Relative contraindications to the procedure include a circumferential lesion, a poorly differentiated

or highly anaplastic tumor, deeply ulcerating growth, an anterior lesion in a woman, or a tumor that extends above the peritoneal reflexion. Certainly, if the growth is high enough to be removed by anterior resection, this is the treatment of choice.

Prior to operation the surgeon must explain to the patient the alternative forms of therapy available and the pros and cons of each procedure. If electrocoagulation is contemplated, the importance of close follow-up examination and the possibility of readmission to the hospital must be stressed. This places a considerable emotional burden on both the patient and the surgeon, and this must clearly be recognized at the outset. It is much easier for a surgeon to perform an abdominoperineal excision knowing that he has little more to offer the patient from the surgical point of view if the tumor recurs. When tumor recurs it is extremely difficult to judge when electrocoagulation should be abandoned and when abdominoperineal excision should be undertaken, for even after unsuccessful electrocoagulation the patient may be cured by radical surgery many months after the initial therapy.

Technique

All patients are treated in the hospital, *not* as outpatients. Regional or general anesthesia is required.

The technique has been described by Madden and Kandalaft.[141] The patient is placed in the prone position if the tumor is primarily anterior, and in the lithotomy position if the tumor is essentially posterior. Following sphincter stretch a plastic operating anoscope of appropriate diameter and length is inserted (Fig. 11-82). These instruments were initially advocated by Schultz and Muldoon and by Muldoon and Capehart for use in excision of polyps of the colon and rectum.[168, 197] However, I have found them ideal for exposing the tumor preparatory to electrocoagulation. Salvati and Rubin suggest the use of local infiltration with bupivacaine and epinephrine to improve anal relaxation and to limit the depth of anesthesia required.[192]

The goal of electrocoagulation is to destroy by coagulating current the entire tumor and a margin of normal tissue both deep to and around it (Fig. 11-83). A standard electrocautery unit is used with the needle tip adapter, and only coagulating current is employed. The tip is plunged into the tumor while the current is applied, and the process is repeated until the entire area has been treated. Necrotic tissue is removed by scraping with the aid of an electrified wire-loop or endometrial curette. When normal tissue is encountered (muscular wall or perirectal adipose tissue) the procedure is terminated (Fig. 11-84). The operative

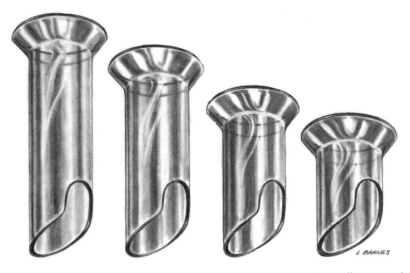

FIG. 11-82. Plastic retractors of varied lengths and diameters permit excellent visualization for electrocoagulation.

time varies according to the size of the lesion and the degree of penetration; it may be as long as 2 hours. By no means should it be considered a minor undertaking. Multiple sessions are frequently required, each necessitating hospitalization and an anesthetic.

After the tumor has been ablated the patient is confined in the hospital for 10 days, at which time further biopsies are taken, and a repeat coagulation is performed if necessary. The patient is seen at monthly intervals for the first 6 months and readmitted to the hospital for biopsy and electrocoagulation if a recurrent tumor is suspected. After 6 months without evidence of tumor, the intervals between office visits are gradually lengthened to a minimum of 4 times a year (Fig. 11-85).

Complications

The commonest postoperative complication is *pyrexia*. An oral temperature of 103° F (39.4° C) on the evening after surgery is almost the rule rather than the exception. It is because of this problem that broad-spectrum antibiotic treatment is recommended preoperatively and postoperatively for 48 to 72 hours. Pelvic peritonitis may occur without rectal perforation, but abdominal exploration, drainage, or colostomy are rarely indicated.

Hemorrhage at the time of surgery may necessitate multiple blood transfusions. All patients should have blood available when electrocoagulation is performed.

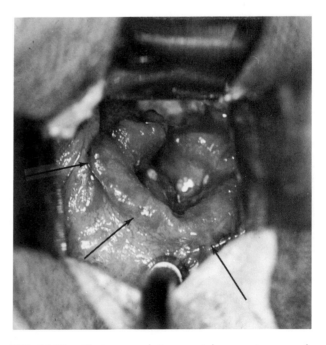

FIG. 11-83. Electrocoagulation: rectal cancer is exposed. (Courtesy of John L. Madden, M.D.)

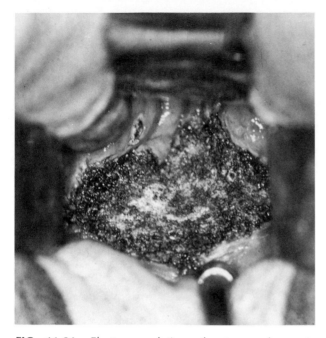

FIG. 11-84. Electrocoagulation: the tumor shown in Fig. 11-83 has been completely electrocoagulated. (Courtesy of John L. Madden, M.D.)

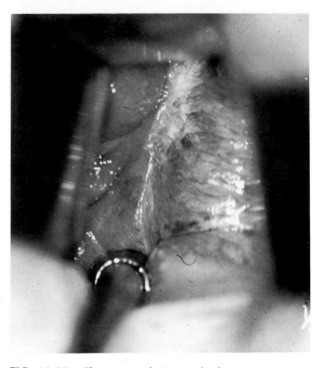

FIG. 11-85. Electrocoagulation: only the scar remains 2 months following treatment. (Courtesy of John L. Madden, M.D.)

Late hemorrhage can occur up to several weeks after the procedure, probably secondary to sloughing of the eschar. This often requires readmission to the hospital and transfusion, and has been reported to occur in as many as 22% of patients who undergo electrocoagulation.[142] Five of 48 patients (10%) had severe enough hemorrhage to require transfusion in our experience.[94]

Rectal stricture may result from electrocoagulation if more than 50% of the bowel wall is involved by tumor. Repeat therapy increases the likelihood of the development of this complication and impedes the ability of the surgeon to visualize the area for possible recurrence. Benign stricture may be treated by lysis and the frequent insertion by the patient of a Hegar's dilator (see Fig. 11-60). Strictures occurred in 8% of our patients.[94]

In women, *rectovaginal fistula* may result from vigorous burning of an anterior lesion. Electrocoagulation should be performed only for small, exophytic lesions when they occur in this location.

Results

In our experience of electrocoagulation in the treatment of carcinoma of the rectum, 39 patients were operated upon for cure.[94] Twenty-one were men, and 18 were women. The median age was 70 years (range, 48 to 89 years), as compared with a median age of 62 years for the group of patients who underwent abdominoperineal resection. Ten patients were 80 years or older. The approximate size of the lesion was 2 cm or less in 14 patients, 3 cm in 13 patients, 4 cm in 8 patients, and 6 or more cm in 4 patients. Twenty-four patients had exophytic tumors, and 15 patients had ulcerative lesions. Only three of the exophytic tumors were more than 3 cm, whereas nine of the ulcerating tumors were more than 3 cm. Thirty-seven patients had well-differentiated or moderately well-differentiated tumors. The remaining two patients had poorly differentiated lesions. Ten patients required only a single session for treatment. Nine patients underwent two sessions, four patients underwent four sessions, and four patients underwent six or more sessions. There were two operative deaths related to cardiac problems, which should remind the surgeon that this is not a benign procedure.

In 27 of the 39 patients (69%), no evidence of disease was apparent at the end of the follow-up period. Twenty patients were alive, and seven had died of causes unrelated to the rectal cancer. Of the 24 patients with exophytic tumors, 22 (92%) had no evidence of the disease. However, only 5 of the 15 patients with ulcerative tumors (33%) had no evidence of disease (Table 11-14). Forty percent of patients who initially had ulcerative lesions could not have their local disease controlled by electrocoagulation; 27% required abdominoperineal resection.

Palliation. I remain unconvinced that electrocoagulation is an effective modality of therapy for the incurable patient. In seven such patients whom we treated, four required a colostomy.[94] The median number of operative sessions was three, hardly a promising experience. The report of Salvati and Rubin was better.[192] Colostomy was avoided in all but 3 of the 19 patients so treated for palliation.

Comment

In order for electrocoagulation to be successfully employed, careful preoperative assessment must be made. Tumors should be mobile, exophytic, and well-differentiated or moderately well-differentiated. The chance of lymph node metastases is considerably reduced if this protocol is followed.[36, 67, 80] The greatest dilemma is what to do if the tumor recurs. When should one abandon this modality of treatment? The answer, in my experience, lies in the quality of the doctor–patient relationship. The patient who accepts electrocoagulation in the first instance will often help to guide the surgeon in making future operative decisions.

CRYOSURGERY

Gage reported on the use of cryotherapy for palliation of symptoms in seven patients with inoperable rectal cancer and in one with perineal recurrence of cancer after abdominoperineal resection.[60] Bleeding was controlled, obstruction was relieved, and colostomy was not required. These benefits were felt to be related to the reduction of tumor bulk. Gage concluded that cryotherapy can compete successfully with irradiation and electrocoagulation in the management of selected cases of inoperable rectal cancer.

Fritsch treated 219 patients with this technique but only for palliation.[58] Six months to seven years following treatment, local tumor was eradicated in 30% and reduced in size sufficiently to relieve symptoms in 52 patients. Fourteen percent experienced hemorrhage, and 26% developed stenoses; other major complications (including peritonitis) were seen in 8%. Disad-

Table 11-14. Results of Electrocoagulation on Morphologic Appearance of the Lesion

Results	Exophytic	Ulcerative
Median age	68	73
Size (cm)		
Less than 3	21	6
More than 3	3	9
Median treatments		4
No evidence of disease	92%	33%
Disease not controlled	4%	40%
Subsequent abdominoperineal resection	4%	27%

(Hughes EP, Veidenheimer MC, Corman ML, Coller JA: Electrocoagulation of rectal cancer. Dis Colon Rectum 1982; 25:215–218)

vantages included frequent discharge of necrotic tissue and malodorous secretions, plus the extensive, costly equipment.

I have had no experience with this technique. Cautious consideration may be given to the application of the modality in patients who harbor symptomatic rectal cancers too proximal to electrocoagulate and in whom metastatic disease is present.

ENDOCAVITARY IRRADIATION

Although radiation therapy has been employed in the palliative treatment of incurable or recurrent rectal cancer for over 25 years, it was not until Papillon reported his initial experience in 1973 that this modality of treatment was applied as an alternative to surgery for a potentially curable lesion.[173]

Technique

The procedure requires a special device that can be inserted through a large-diameter proctoscope. The contact unit, manufactured by Phillips (Fig. 11-86), develops a high radiation output (1000 to 2000 rad/min) with low-voltage (50 kv) x-rays. The effective area is approximately 3 cm in diameter, with absorption of the x-rays essentially limited to a depth of 2 cm. Papillon recommends 3000 to 4000 rads at each treatment, administered within 3 minutes.[174] Treatments are repeated from 1 to 3 weeks later for a total dose of between 8000 and 15000 rads over a period of 4 to 10 weeks. Most patients can be treated outside a hospital setting. No anesthesia is usually required.

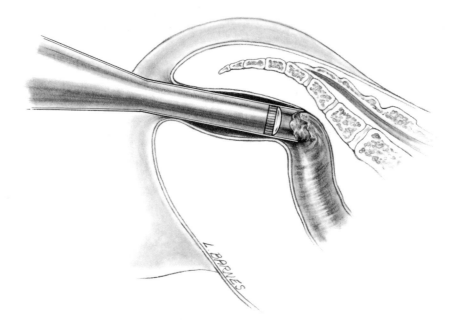

FIG. 11-86.   Endocavitary irradiation: the unit is introduced by means of a rectoscope.

Patient Selection

According to Papillon, a number of criteria must be met if a patient is to be considered for this form of treatment[174]:

> Accessibility of the entire lesion
> Small size
> Noninfiltrating
> Histologically well differentiated
> Palpable
> Movable

Results

Papillon reported initially on 106 patients, 70% of whom were alive and free of disease after 5 years.[174, 175] Local recurrence developed in 14 patients (13%). Sixteen patients (15%) died of malignant disease. Sischy and Remington reported 23 of 25 patients to have responded to treatment and to be free of disease, but the follow-up period was considerably shorter.[201]

Complications

Very few complications are attributable to the treatment. Jelden reported short periods of mild proctitis and occasional bleeding.[100] Rectovaginal fistula has also been seen. Deaths directly related to the therapy have not been reported.[202]

Comment

As with electrocoagulation, it is difficult to assess the results of endocavitary radiation by comparison with standard resective treatment. Only those patients who have the most favorable prognoses are selected. A patient who undergoes abdominoperineal resection for a Dukes' A lesion has a chance of cure that approaches 90%, so that claiming a cure rate close to this figure does not represent a great breakthrough in the treatment of cancer of the rectum. Furthermore, as with electrocoagulation, one wonders if some patients are being deprived of the only possibility for cure if they harbor lymph node metastases. Even with careful patient selection, the application of local treatments requires preoperative counseling and close follow-up care.

RADIOTHERAPY

The use of radiotherapy in the management of rectal cancer has received considerable press in recent years as treatment adjunctive to surgery, either preoperatively or postoperatively. Theoretically, if used preoperatively, the tumor might be reduced in size enough to enable the surgeon to extirpate it completely, or at least to decrease the depth of invasion. In the postoperative patient who is known to have a less favorable lesion (Dukes' B or C), radiotherapy might decrease the likelihood of pelvic recurrence.

Preoperative Radiotherapy

The recent impetus for the application of preoperative radiotherapy has come from the Memorial Hospital in New York.[121, 206, 211–213] Although the initial reports indicated improved survival, in a prospective study the overall survival rate was not improved, but the incidence of failure due to local recurrence was reduced.[213] Stearns and colleagues used external radiation through opposing anterior and posterior portals, 250 rads daily, to 2000 rads. The resection was carried out from 2 days to 6 weeks following treatment.

The frequently quoted Veterans Administration (VA) study of 700 men randomly allocated either to surgery or to preoperative radiotherapy plus surgery revealed a statistically significant decreased incidence of positive nodes in the irradiated group and a lower incidence of recurrent disease in those who died.[53, 190] Roswit and associates used 2000 rads over 2 weeks, with a booster dose of 500 rads when the tumor was less than 9 cm from the anal verge.

Increasing preoperative dosage levels to 4000 or 5000 rads has been suggested, but thus far there have been no controlled studies to substantiate the statement that preoperative radiation for rectal cancer increases the chance for cure. Cummings and associates treated 123 patients with 4000 rads of external beam radiation as primary treatment.[39] The overall 5-year survival rate was 21%.

Comment

I believe that unless one is to participate in a well-controlled, randomized clinical trial, preoperative radiotherapy should be limited to those patients in whom the surgeon believes a chance for cure by resection is unlikely: for example, when the tumor is fixed or deeply ulcerating, or when firm lymph nodes are palpated in the presacral space. If radiotherapy is to be considered under these circumstances, it should be carried to approximately 4500 rads over 5 or 6 weeks, with resection performed (with or without anastomosis) 2 or 3 weeks later.

Postoperative Radiotherapy

Patients with Dukes' B and C tumors have a high incidence of local recurrence following resection.

Romsdahl and Withers delivered a total of 5500 rads following abdominoperineal resection to patients who were found to have such lesions.[186] The local recurrence rate was 8%, as compared with a 27% rate in historical controls.

Comment

Unfortunately, there are no reports of controlled clinical studies of postoperative radiotherapy for rectal cancer. In the absence of such a study, my attitude is to advise this modality of supplementary therapy for patients who are at a high risk for recurrence: those with poorly differentiated tumors and those with Dukes' B or C lesions.

The treatment should be begun not sooner than 1 month following surgery in order to avoid problems with wound healing. The dosage range should be from 5000 to 6500 rads.

Radiotherapy is not without significant complications: urinary tract infection, diarrhea, small bowel injury, and skin and wound breakdown. Therefore, before embarking on such treatment one must consider other factors, such as the age of the patient and the quality of life anticipated.

PALLIATIVE IRRADIATION

Radiotherapy can be uniquely beneficial in the treatment of patients with recurrent disease who have pelvic pain. So obvious is the symptom complex (deep-seated pelvic, perineal or sacral pain, or tenderness) that pathologic evidence should not be required to initiate treatment.

CHEMOTHERAPY

The role of chemotherapy in colorectal cancer is discussed in Chapter 10.

COMBINED CHEMOTHERAPY AND RADIOTHERAPY

Preliminary reports have been somewhat encouraging on the use of combined modalities of treatment with chemotherapy and radiotherapy.[22, 203] We all wait with interest the results of long-term, randomly controlled prospective studies in this area. As stated in the previous chapter, further improvements in survival rates will depend upon bringing the patient to surgery sooner and upon applying additional modalities of therapy.

REFERENCES

1. Allgöwer M: Sphincter-splitting approach to the rectum. Am J Surg 1983; 145:5–7
2. Allgöwer M, Dürig M, von Hochstetter A, Huber A: The parasacral sphincter-splitting approach to the rectum. World J Surg 1982; 6:539–548
3. Antoniades K, Spector HB, Hecksher RH Jr: Prophylactic oophorectomy in conjunction with large-bowel resection for cancer: Report of two cases. Dis Colon Rectum 1977; 20:506–510
4. Babcock WW: Experiences with resection of the colon and the elimination of colostomy. Am J Surg 1939; 4:186–203
5. Babcock WW: Radical single-stage extirpation for cancer of the large bowel, with retained functional anus. Surg Gynecol Obstet 1947; 85:1–7
6. Bacon HE: Abdominoperineal proctosigmoidectomy with sphincter preservation: Five-year and ten-year survival after "pull-through" operation for cancer of rectum. JAMA 1956; 160:628–634
7. Bacon HE: Evaluation of sphincter muscle preservation and re-establishment of continuity in the operative treatment of rectal and sigmoidal cancer. Surg Gynecol Obstet 1945; 81:113–127
8. Bacon HE, Martin PV: The rationale of palliative resection for primary cancer of the colon and rectum complicated by liver and lung metastasis. Dis Colon Rectum 1964; 7:211–217
9. Baker JW: Low end to side rectosigmoidal anastomosis: Description of technique. Arch Surg 1950; 67:143–157
10. Beart RW Jr, Wolff BG: The use of staplers for anterior anastomoses. World J Surg 1982; 6:525–530
11. Beheri GE: Surgical treatment of impotence. Plast Reconstr Surg 1966; 38:92–97
12. Bennett RC: The place of pull-through operations in treatment of carcinoma of the rectum. Dis Colon Rectum 1976; 19:420–424
13. Bennett RC, Hughes ES, Cuthbertson AM: Long-term review of function following pull-through operations of the rectum. Br J Surg 1972; 59:723–725
14. Bernard HR, Cole WR: The prophylaxis of surgical infection: The effect of prophylactic antimicrobial drugs on the incidence of infection following potentially contaminated operations. Surgery 1964; 56:151–157
15. Black BM, Botham RJ: Combined abdominoendorectal resection: A critical reappraisal based on 91 cases. Surg Clin North Am 1957; 37:989–997
16. Black BM, Kelly AH: Recurrent carcinoma of the rectum and rectosigmoid: Results of treatment after continence preserving procedures. Arch Surg 1955; 71:538–542
17. Blamey SL, McDermott FT, Pihl E, Hughes ESR: Resected ovarian recurrence from colorectal adenocarcinoma. Dis Colon Rectum 1981; 24:272–275
18. Blamey S, McDermott F, Pihl E et al: Ovarian involvement in adenocarcinoma of the colon and rectum. Surg Gynecol Obstet 1981; 153:42–44
19. Bischoff PF: Boari-plasty and vesicorenal reflux. In Whitehead ED (Ed): Current Operative Urology, pp 708-723. New York, Harper and Row, 1975
20. Bloch O: Extraabdominal resektion af hele colon descendens og et stykke af colon transversum for cancer. Hosp Tid Kjobenh 1894; 4(2):1053
21. Bordos DC, Baker RR, Cameron JL: An evaluation of palliative abdominoperineal resection for carcinoma of the rectum. Surg Gynecol Obstet 1974; 139:731–733
22. Buroker T, Nigro N, Correa J et al: Combination preoperative radiation and chemotherapy in adenocarcinoma of the rectum: A preliminary report. Dis Colon Rectum 1976; 19:660–663
23. Cawkwell I: Perineal hernia complicating abdominoperineal resection of the rectum. Br J Surg 1963; 50:431–433
24. Clark CG, Harris J, Elmasri S et al: Polyglycolic-acid sutures and catgut in colonic anastomosis. A controlled clinical trial. Lancet 1972; 2:1006–1007
25. Clarke JS, Condon RE, Bartlett JG et al: Preoperative oral antibiotics reduce septic complications of colon operations: Results of prospective, randomized, double-blind clinical study. Ann Surg 1977; 185:251–259
26. Cohn I: Implantation in cancer of the colon. Surg Gynecol Obstet 1967; 124:501–508
27. Cohn I: Cause and prevention of recurrence following surgery for colon cancer. Cancer 1971; 28:183–189
28. Cole WH: Recurrence in carcinoma of colon and proximal rectum following resection for carcinoma. Arch Surg 1952; 65:264–270
29. Cole WH, Packard D, Southwick W: Carcinoma of the colon with special reference to prevention of recurrence. JAMA 1954; 155:1549–1553
30. Condon RE: Antibiotic preparation of the colon or rectum for elective resection. Infect Surg 1982; 1:15–60
31. Condon RE, Bartlett JG, Greenlee H et al: Efficacy of oral and systemic antibiotic prophylaxis in colorectal operations. Arch Surg 1983; 118:496–502
32. Cooperman M, Martin EW Jr, Evans WE, Carey LC: Assessment of anastomotic blood supply in operations upon the colon by Doppler ultrasound. Surg Gynecol Obstet 1979; 149:15–16

33. Cooperman M, Martin EW Jr, Keith LM, Carey LC: Use of Doppler ultrasound in intestinal surgery. Am J Surg 1979; 138:856–859

34. Cooperman M, Pace WG, Martin EW Jr et al: Determination of viability of ischemic intestine by Doppler ultrasound. Surgery 1978; 83:705–710

35. Criado FJ, Wilson TH Jr: Technique for reestablishing continuity after the Hartmann operation. Am Surg 1981; 47:366–367

36. Crile G Jr, Turnbull RB Jr: The role of electrocoagulation in the treatment of carcinoma of the rectum. Surg Gynecol Obstet 1972; 135:391–396

37. Cruse PJ: Incidence of wound infection on the surgical services. Surg Clin North Amer 1975; 55:1269–1275

38. Cruse PJ, Foord R: A five-year prospective study of 23,649 surgical wounds. Arch Surg 1973; 107:206–210

39. Cummings BJ, Rider WD, Harwood AR et al: Radical external beam radiation therapy for adenocarcinoma of the rectum. Dis Colon Rectum 1983; 26:30–36

40. Cutait DE, Figliolini FJ: A new method of colorectal anastomosis in abdominoperineal resection. Dis Colon Rectum 1961; 4:335–342

41. Cutait R, Enker WE: Prophylactic oophorectomy in surgery for large-bowel cancer. Dis Colon Rectum 1983; 26:6–11

42. Cuthbertson AM, Kaye AH: Local excision of carcinomas of the rectum, anus and anal canal. Aust NZ J Surg 1978; 48:412–415

43. Czerny V: Casuistische Mittheilugen aus der Chirurg, p 11. Klin zu Heidelberg. Munch med Wchnschr, 1894

44. Debas HT, Thomson FB: A critical review of colectomy with anastomosis. Surg Gynecol Obstet 1972; 135:747–752

45. Deddish MR: Local Excision. Surg Clin North Am 1974; 54:877–880

46. Deddish MR, Stearns MW Jr: Anterior resection for carcinoma of the rectum and rectosigmoid area. Ann Surg 1961; 154:961–966

47. DeGennaro V, Corman ML, Coller JA, Veidenheimer MC: Wound infections after colectomy. Dis Colon Rectum 1978; 21:567–572

48. Detry RJ, Kestens PJ: Colorectal anastomoses with the EEA stapler. World J Surg 1981; 5:739–742

49. Dixon CF: Anterior Resection for malignant lesions of the upper part of the rectum and lower part of the sigmoid. Ann Surg 1948; 128:425–442

50. Donaldson GA, Rodkey GV, Behringer GE: Resection of the rectum with anal preservation. Surg Gynecol Obstet 1966; 123:571–580

51. Dukes CE: Cancer of the rectum: An analysis of 1000 cases. J Pathol Bacteriol 1940; 50:527–539

52. Dunphy JE: The cut gut. Presidential address. Amer J Surg 1970; 119:1–8

53. Dwight RW, Higgins GA, Roswit B et al: Preoperative radiation and surgery for cancer of the sigmoid colon and rectum. Am J Surg 1972; 123:93–103

54. Enker WE, Laffer UT, Block GE: Enhanced survival of patients with colon and rectal cancer is based upon wide anatomic resection. Ann Surg 1979; 190:350–360

55. Fein RL, Needell MH, Winton L: An orderly approach to the impotent male and the dorsal approach for insertion of the Jonas penile prosthesis. Cont Surg 1983; 23:93–99

56. Fitzgibbons RJ Jr, Harkrider WW, Cohn I Jr: Review of abdominoperineal resections for cancer. Am J Surg 1977; 134:624–629

57. Franklin R, McSwain B: Carcinoma of the colon, rectum, and anus. Ann Surg 1970; 171:811–818

58. Fritsch A, Seidl W, Walzel C et al: Palliative and adjunctive measures in rectal cancer. World J Surg 1982; 6:569–577

59. Fry DE, Amin M, Harbrecht PJ: Rectal obstruction secondary to carcinoma of the prostate. Ann Surg 1979; 189:488–492

60. Gage AA: Cryotherapy for inoperable rectal cancer. Dis Colon Rectum 1968; 11:36–44

61. Gee WF, McRoberts JW, Ansell JS: Penile prosthetic implant for the treatment of organic impotence. Am J Surg 1973; 126:698–700

62. Gerstenberg TC, Nielsen ML, Clausen S et al: Bladder function after abdominoperineal resection of the rectum for anorectal cancer: Urodynamic investigations before and after operation in a consecutive series. Ann Surg 1980; 191:81–86

63. Gilbertsen VA: Adenocarcinoma of the rectum: Incidence and locations of recurrent tumor following present-day operations performed for cure. Ann Surg 1960; 151:340–348

64. Gilbertsen VA: The results of surgical treatment of cancer of the rectum. Surg Gynecol Obstet 1962; 114:313–319

65. Gilchrist RK, David VC: Consideration of pathological factors influencing five year survival in radical resection of large bowel and rectum for carcinoma. Ann Surg 1947; 126:421–438

66. Gilchrist RK, David VC: Prognosis in carcinoma of bowel. Surg Gynecol Obstet 1948; 86:359–371

67. Gingold BS, Mitty WF Jr, Tadros M: Importance of patient selection in local treatment of carcinoma of the rectum. Am J Surg 1983; 145:293–295

68. Glen F, McSherry CK: Carcinoma of the distal

large bowel: 32-year review of 1,026 cases. Ann Surg 1966; 163:838–849

69. Goldsmith HS: Protection of low rectal anastomosis with intact omentum. Surg Gynecol Obstet 1977; 144:584–586

70. Goldsmith HS: Use of the omentum in the presacral space. Dis Colon Rectum 1978; 21:405–407

71. Goldstein M, Duff JH: Reconsideration of colostomy in elective left colon resection. Surg Gynecol Obstet 1972; 134:593–594

72. Goligher JC: The adequacy of the marginal blood-supply to the left colon after high ligation of the inferior mesenteric artery during excision of the rectum. Br J Surg 1954; 41:351–353

73. Goligher JC: Further reflections on preservation of the anal sphincters in the radical treatment of rectal cancer. Proc R Soc Med 1962; 55:341–346

74. Goligher JC, Dukes CE, Bussey HJR: Local recurrences after sphincter-saving excisions of carcinoma of rectum and rectosigmoid. Br J Surg 1951; 39:199–211

75. Goligher JC, Duthie HL, DeDombal FT et al: Abdomino-anal pull-through excision for tumors of the mid-third of the rectum: A comparison with low anterior resection. Br J Surg 1965; 52:323–334

76. Goligher JC, Graham NG, DeDombal FT: Anastomotic dehiscence after anterior resection of rectum and sigmoid. Br J Surg 1970; 57:109–118

77. Goligher JC, Lloyd-Davies OV, Robertson CT: Small-gut obstructions following combined excision of rectum, with special reference to strangulation around the colostomy. Br J Surg 1951; 38:467–473

78. Graffner H, Fredlund P, Olsson S-A et al: Protective colostomy in low anterior resection of the rectum using the EEA stapling instrument—a randomized study. Dis Colon Rectum 1983; 26:87–90

79. Graham JW, Goligher JC: The management of accidental injuries and deliberate resections of the ureter during excision of the rectum. Br J Surg 1954; 42:151–160

80. Greaney MG, Irvin TT: Criteria for the selection of rectal cancers for local treatment: A clinicopathologic study of low rectal tumors. Dis Colon Rectum 1977; 20:463–466

81. Gregory JS, Muldoon JP: Perineal herniation—a late complication of abdominoperineal resection of the rectum: Report of a case. Dis Colon Rectum 1969; 12:33–35

82. Hager Th, Gall FP, Hermanek P: Local excision of cancer of the rectum. Dis Colon Rectum 1983; 26:149–151

83. Harford FJ: Use of glucagon in conjunction with

the end-to-end anastomosis (EEA) stapling device for low anterior anastomoses. Dis Colon Rectum 1979; 22:452–454

84. Harshaw DH, Gardner B, Vives A, Sundaram KN: The effect of technical factors upon complications from abdominal perineal resections. Surg Gynecol Obstet 1974; 139:756–758

85. Hartmann H: Nouveau procede d'ablation des cancers de la partie terminale du colon pelvien, pp 411–414. Trentième Congres de Chirurgie, Strasbourg, France, 1921

86. Hawley PR: Infection—the cause of anastomotic breakdown: An experimental study. Proc R Soc Med 1970; 63:752

87. Heald RJ, Leicester RJ: The low stapled anastomosis. Dis Colon Rectum 1981; 24:437–444

88. Heberer G, Denecke H, Pratschke E, Teichmann R: Anterior and low anterior resection. World J Surg 1982; 6:517–524

89. Herter FP, Colacchio TA: The influence of antibiotics on infection and anastomotic recurrence after colon resection for cancer. World J Surg 1982; 6:188–194

90. Herter FP, Slanetz CA Jr: Preoperative intestinal preparation in relation to the subsequent development of cancer at the suture line. Surg Gynecol Obstet 1968; 127:49–56

91. Hickey RC, Romsdahl MM, Johnson DE et al: Recurrent cancer and metastases. World J Surg 1982; 6:585–595

92. Hochenegg J: Die Sakrale Methode der Exstirpation von Mastdarmkrebsen nach Prof. Kraske. Wien Klin Wschr 1888; 1:254

93. Hodges CV, Moore RJ, Lehman TH et al: Clinical experiences with transureteroureterostomy. J Urol 1963; 90:552–562

94. Hughes EP, Veidenheimer MC, Corman ML, Coller JA: Electrocoagulation of rectal cancer. Dis Colon Rectum 1982; 25:215–218

95. Hunt TK: Anastomotic failure. In Simmons RL (ed): Topics in Intraabdominal Surgical Infection, p 101. Appleton-Century-Crofts, Norwalk, 1982

96. Husband JE, Hodson NJ, Parsons CA: The use of computed tomography in recurrent rectal tumors. Radiology 1980; 134:677–682

97. Irvin TT, Goligher JC: Aetiology of disruption of intestinal anastomoses. Br J Surg 1973; 60:461–464

98. Jackman RJ: Conservative management of selected patients with carcinoma of the rectum. Dis Colon Rectum 1961; 4:429–434

99. Jansen A, Brummelkamp WH, Davies GAG et al: Clinical applications of magnetic rings in colorectal anastomosis. Surg Gynecol Obstet 1981; 153:537–545

100. Jelden GL: Presentation to American Society of Therapeutic Radiologists, Miami Beach (as reported in Medical News). JAMA 1981; 246:2419

101. Karmody AM, Jordan FR, Zaman SN: Left colon gangrene after acute inferior mesenteric artery occlusion. Arch Surg 1976; 111:972–975

102. Keighley MRB, Crapp AR, Burdon DW et al: Prophylaxis against anaerobic sepsis in bowel surgery. Br J Surg 1976; 63:538–541

103. Kennedy HL, Rothenberger DA, Goldberg SM et al: Colocolostomy and coloproctostomy utilizing the circular intraluminal stapling devices. Dis Colon Rectum 1983; 26:145–148

104. Kergin FG: Diathermy fulgurization in treatment of certain cases of rectal carcinoma. Can Med Assoc J 1953; 69:14–17

105. Khubchandani IT, Trimpi HD, Sheets JA: Low end-to-side rectoenteric anastomosis with single-layer wire. Dis Colon Rectum 1975; 18:308–310

106. Kirwan WO, Turnbull RB Jr, Fazio VW, Weakley FL: Pullthrough operation with delayed anastomosis for rectal cancer. Br J Surg 1978; 65:695–698

107. Kiselow M, Butcher HR Jr, Bricker EM: Results of the radical surgical treatment of advanced pelvic cancer: A fifteen-year study. Ann Surg 1967; 166:428–436

108. Knoepp LF, Ray JE, Overby I: Ovarian metastases from colorectal carcinoma. Dis Colon Rectum 1973; 16:305–311

109. Kocher T: Quoted in Rankin FW, Bargen JA, Buie LA (eds): The Colon, Rectum and Anus. Philadelphia, WB Saunders, 1932

110. Kraske P: Ueber die Entstehung sek undarer Krebsqeschwüre durch Impfung. Zentralbl Chir 1884; 11:801

111. Kraske P: Zur exstirpation hochsitzendes Mastdarmkrebses. Verhandl Deutsch gesellsch Chir 1885; 14:464

112. Kratzer GL: The pull-through operaton. Dis Colon Rectum 1967; 10:112–117

113. Kratzer GL: Modification of the pull-through operation Dis Colon Rectum 1972; 15:288–291

114. Kratzer GL, Onsanit T: Fulguration of selected cancers of the rectum. Dis Colon Rectum 1972; 15:431–435

115. Labow SB, Salvati EP, Rubin RJ: Suture-line recurrences in carcinoma of the colon and rectum. Dis Colon Rectum 1975; 18:123–125

116. Lahey FH: Two-stage abdominoperineal removal of cancer of the rectum. Surg Gynecol Obstet 1930; 51:622–669

117. Lane RHS, Parks AG: Function of the anal sphincters following colo-anal anastomosis. Br J Surg 1977; 64:596–599

118. Lanter B, Mason RA: Use of omental pedicle graft to protect low anterior colonic anastomosis. Dis Colon Rectum 1979; 22:448–451

119. Lapides J: Urologic complications of abdominoperineal surgery. Cont Surg 1974; 5:81–87

120. Leadbetter GW, Leadbetter WF: A new approach to the problem of urinary retention following abdominoperineal resection for carcinoma of the rectum. Surg Gynecol Obstet 1958; 107:333–338

121. Leaming RH, Stearns MW, Deddish MR: Preoperative irradiation in rectal carcinoma. Radiology 1961; 77:257–263

122. Leer JWH, Scholten RE, Heslinga-T, Binswanger RO: Role of computed tomography in the diagnosis and radiotherapy planning of recurrent rectal carcinoma. Diagn Imaging 1980; 49:208–213

123. Leff EI, Hoexter B, Labow SB et al: The EEA stapler in low colorectal anastomoses: Initial experience. Dis Colon Rectum 1982; 25:704–707

124. Libertino JA, Rote, AR, Zinman L: Ureteral reconstruction in renal transplantation. Urology 1978; 12:641–644

125. Libertino JA, Zinman L: Technique for ureteroneocystotomy in renal transplantation and reflux. Surg Clin North Am 1973; 53:459–463

126. Lisfranc J: Mémoire sur l'excision de la partie inférieure du rectum devenue carcinomateuse. Rev Méd Franç 1826; 2:380

127. Littré A: Mémoire de l'academie des sciences. 1710; 10:36

128. Lloyd-Davies OV: Lithotomy-Trendelenburg position for resection of rectum and lower pelvic colon. Lancet 1939; 2:74–76

129. Localio SA: Curative surgery of midrectal cancer with preservation of the sphincters. Surg Ann 1974; 6:213–245

130. Localio SA, Baron B: Abdomino-transsacral resection and anastomosis for mid-rectal cancer. Ann Surg 1973; 178:540–546

131. Localio SA, Eng K, Gouge TH, Ranson JHC: Abdominosacral resection for carcinoma of the mid-rectum: Ten years experience. Ann Surg 1978; 188:475–480

132. Localio SA, Stahl WH: Simultaneous abdominotranssacral resection and anastomosis for mid-rectal cancer. Am J Surg 1969; 117:282–289

133. Lockhart-Mummery HE: Surgery in patients with advanced carcinoma of the colon and rectum. Dis Colon Rectum 1959; 2:36–39

134. Lockhart-Mummery HE, Ritchie JK, Hawley PR: The results of surgical treatment for carcinoma of the rectum at St. Mark's Hospital from 1948 to 1972. Br J Surg 1976; 63:673–677

135. Lockhart-Mummery JP: Two hundred cases of cancer of the rectum treated by perineal excision. Br J Surg 1926; 14:110–124

136. Loeffler RA, Sayegh ES: Perforated acrylic implants in the management of organic impotence. J Urol 1960; 84:559–561

137. Lofgren EP, Waugh JM, Dockerty MB: Local recurrence of carcinoma after anterior resection of the rectum and the sigmoid: Relationship with the length of normal mucosa excised distal to the lesion. Arch Surg 1957; 74:825–838

138. Long JW, Mayo CW, Dockerty MB et al: Recurrent versus new and independent carcinomas of the colon and rectum. Mayo Clin Proc 1950; 25:169–178

139. MacKeigan JM, Ferguson JA: Prophylactic oophorectomy and colorectal cancer in premenopausal patients. Dis Colon Rectum 1979; 22:401–405

140. MacLennan G, Stogryn RD, Voitk AJ: Abdominoperineal resection: Treatment of choice for carcinoma of the rectum. Cancer 1976; 38:953–956

141. Madden JL, Kandalaft S: Electrocoagulation: A primary and preferred method of treatment for cancer of the rectum. Ann Surg 1967; 166:413–419

142. Madden JL, Kandalaft S: Clinical evaluation of electrocoagulation in the treatment of cancer of the rectum. Am J Surg 1971; 122:347–352

143. Madura JA, Fiore AC: Reanastomosis of a Hartmann rectal pouch: A simplified procedure. Am J Surg 1983; 145:279–280

144. Manson PN, Corman ML, Coller JA, Veidenheimer MC: Anastomotic recurrence after anterior resection for carcinoma: Lahey clinic experience. Dis Colon Rectum 1976; 19:219–224

145. Manson PN, Corman ML, Coller JA, Veidenheimer MC: Anterior resection for adenocarcinoma: Lahey clinic experience from 1963 through 1969. Am J Surg 1976: 131:434–441

146. Manz CW, LaTendresse C, Sako Y: The detrimental effects of drains on colonic anastomosis: An experimental study. Dis Colon Rectum 1970; 13:17–25

147. Marks CG, Ritchie JK: The complications of synchronous combined excision for adenocarcinoma of the rectum at St. Mark's Hospital. Br J Surg 1975; 62:901–905

148. Marti MC, Fiala JM, Rohner A: EEA stapler in large bowel surgery. World J Surg 1981; 5:735–737

149. Mason AY: Surgical access to the rectum—a transsphincteric exposure. Proc R Soc Med 1970; 63:91–94

150. Mason AY: The place of local resection in the treatment of rectal carcinoma. Proc R Soc Med 1970; 63:1259–1261

151. Mason AY: Trans-sphincteric exposure for low rectal anastomosis. Proc R Soc Med 1972; 65:974

152. Maunsell HW: A new method of excising the two upper portions of the rectum and the lower segment of the sigmoid flexure of the colon. Lancet 1892; 2:473–476

153. Mayo CH: Cancer of the large bowel. Med Sent 1904; 12:37

154. Mayo CW, Schlicke CP: Carcinoma of the colon and rectum: A study of metastasis and recurrences. Surg Gynecol Obstet 1942; 74:83–91

155. McGrew EA, Laws JF, Cole WH: Free malignant cells in relation to recurrence of carcinoma of colon. JAMA 1954; 154:1251–1254

156. McLachlin AD: Anastomotic leakage below the peritoneal reflection, a study in the dog. Dis Colon Rectum 1978; 21:400

157. Mikulicz JV: Chirurgische Erfahrung über das Darmcarcinom. Arch F Klin Chir 1903; 69:28

158. Miles WE: A method of performing abdominoperineal excision for carcinoma of the rectum and the terminal portion of the pelvic colon. Lancet 1908; 2:1812–1813

159. Miles WE: Cancer of the rectum. Trans Med Soc Lond 1923; 46:127

160. Minichan DP Jr: Enlarging the bowel lumen for the EEA stapler. Dis Colon Rectum 1982; 25:61

161. Mirelman D, Corman ML, Veidenheimer MC, Coller JA: Colostomies—indications and contraindications: Lahey clinic experience, 1973–1974. Dis Colon Rectum 1978; 21:172–176

162. Moosa AR, Ree PC, Marks JE et al: Factors influencing local recurrence after abdominoperineal resection for cancer of the rectum and rectosignoid. Br J Surg 1975; 62:727–730

163. Morgan CN: Carcinoma of the rectum. Ann R Col Surg Engl 1965; 36:73–97

164. Morgan CN, Lloyd-Davies OV: Discussion on conservative resection in carcinoma of the rectum. Proc R Soc Med 1950; 43:701

165. Morgenstern L, Yamakawa T, Ben-Shashkan M et al: Anastomotic leakage after low colonic anastomosis: Clinical and experimental aspects. Am J Surg 1972; 123:104–109

166. Morson BC, Bussey HJ, Samoorian S: Policy of local excision for early cancer of the colorectum. Gut 1977; 18:1045–1050

167. Moseson MD, Salvati EP, Rubin RJ, Eisenstat TE: Technique for placement of distal pursestring. Dis Colon Rectum 1982; 25:59–60

168. Muldoon JP, Capehart RJ: Two scope technique for the transrectal removal of lesions high in the rectum and sigmoid colon. Surg Gynecol Obstet 1973; 137:1019–1022

169. Murphy JB: Cholecysto-intestinal, gastro-intestinal, entero-intestinal anastomosis, and approximation without sutures. Med Record 1892; 42:665–676

170. Nichols RL: Postoperative wound infection. N Eng J Med 1982; 307:1701–1702

171. Nichols RL, Broido P, Condon RE et al: Effect of preoperative neomycin-erythromycin intestinal preparation on the incidence of infectious complications following colon surgery. Ann Surg 1973; 178:453–459

172. Palumbo LT, Sharpe WS: Anterior versus abdominoperineal resection: Resection for rectal and rectosigmoid carcinoma. Am J Surg 1968; 115:657–660

173. Papillon J: Endocavitary irradiation of early rectal cancers for cure: A series of 123 cases. Proc R Soc Med 1973; 66:1179–1181

174. Papillon J: Endocavitary irradiation in the curative treatment of early cancers. Dis Colon Rectum 1974; 17:172–180

175. Papillon J: Intracavitary irradiation of early rectal cancer for cure: A series of 186 cases. Cancer 1975; 36:696–701

176. Parks AG: Transanal technique in low rectal anastomosis. Proc R Soc Med 1972; 65:975–976

177. Parks AG: Per-anal anastomosis. World J Surg 1982; 6:531–538

178. Pearman RO: Treatment of organic impotence by implantation of a penile prosthesis. J Urol 1967; 97:716–719

179. Pearman RO: Insertion of a Silastic penile prosthesis for the treatment of organic sexual impotence. J Urol 1972; 107:802–806

180. Politano VA, Leadbetter WF: An operative technique for the correction of vesicoureteral reflux. J Urol 1958; 79:932–941

181. Ramirez OM, Hernandez-Pombo J, Marupudi SR: New technique for anastomosis of the intestine after the Hartmann's procedure with the end-to-end anastomosis stapler. Surg Gynecol Obstet 1983; 156:367–368

182. Ramsey WH: Treatment of inoperable cancer of the rectum by fulguration. Dis Colon Rectum 1963; 6:114–117

183. Rankin FW, Graham AS: Cancer of the Colon and Rectum, p 248. Springfield, Charles C Thomas, 1939

184. ReMine SG, Dozois RR: Hartmann's procedure: Its use with complicated carcinomas of sigmoid colon and rectum. Arch Surg 1981; 116:630–633

185. Reybard JF: Mémoire sur une tumeur cancéreuse affectant l'iliaque du colon: Ablation de la tumeur et de l'intestin. Bull Acad Roy de Méd 1833; 296

186. Romsdahl M, Withers H: Radiotherapy combined with curative surgery: Its use as therapy for carcinoma of the sigmoid colon and rectum. Arch Surg 1978; 113:446–453

187. Rosen L, Veidenheimer MC, Coller JA, Corman ML: Mortality, morbidity, and patterns of recurrence after abdominoperineal resection for cancer of the rectum. Dis Colon Rectum 1982; 25:202–208

188. Rosenthal II, Turell R: Surgical diathermy (electrothermia) of cancer of the rectum. JAMA 1958; 167:1602–1605

189. Rosi PA, Cahill WJ, Carey J: A ten year study of hemicolectomy in the treatment of carcinoma of the left half of the colon. Surg Gynecol Obstet 1962; 114:15–24

190. Roswit B, Higgins G, Keehn R: Preoperative irradiation for carcinoma of the rectum and rectosigmoid colon: Report of a National Veterans Administration randomized study. Cancer 1975; 35:1597–1602

191. Rudd WWH: The transanal anastomosis: A sphincter-saving operation with improved continence. Dis Colon Rectum 1979; 22:102–105

192. Salvati EP, Rubin RJ: Electrocoagulation as primary therapy for rectal carcinoma. Am J Surg 1976; 132:583–586

193. Sandusky WR: Use of prophylactic antibiotics in surgical patients. Surg Clin North Am 1980; 60:83–92

194. Sarr MG, Stewart JR, Cameron JC: Combined abdominoperineal approach to repair of postoperative hernia. Dis Colon Rectum 1982; 25:597–599

195. Schaeffer CJ, Giordano JM: Complications associated with EEA stapler in performance of low anterior resections. Am Surg 1981; 47:426–428

196. Schrock TR, Deveney CW, Dunphy JE: Factors contributing to leakage of colonic anastomoses. Ann Surg 1973; 177:513–518

197. Schultz PE, Muldoon JP: A transrectal approach to the high-lying lesion in the rectosigmoid. Dis Colon Rectum 1969; 12:417–420

198. Segall MM, Nivatvongs S, Balcos E et al: Abdominoperineal resection for recurrent cancer following anterior resection. Dis Colon Rectum 1981; 24:80–84

199. Sehapayak S, McNatt M, Carter HG et al: Continuous sump-suction drainage of the pelvis after low anterior resection: A reappraisal. Dis Colon Rectum 1973; 16:485–489

200. Shaw RS, Green TH: Massive mesenteric infarction following inferior mesenteric-artery ligation in resection of the colon for carcinoma. N Engl J Med 1953; 248:890–891

201. Sischy B, Remington JH: Treatment of carcinoma of the rectum by intracavitary irradiation. Surg Gynecol Obstet 1975; 141:562–564

202. Sischy B, Remington JH, Sobel SH: Treatment of rectal carcinomas by means of endocavity irradiation. Cancer 1978; 42:1073–1076

203. Sischy B, Remington JH, Sobel SH, Savlov ED: Treatment of carcinoma of the rectum and squamous carcinoma of the anus by combination chemotherapy, radiotherapy and operation. Surg Gynecol Obstet 1980; 151:369–371

204. Slanetz CA Jr, Herter FP, Grinnell RS: Anterior resection versus abdominoperineal resection for cancer of the rectum and rectosigmoid: An analysis of 524 cases. Am J Surg 1972; 123:110–117

205. Southwick HW, Harridge WH, Cole WH: Recurrence at the suture line following resection for carcinoma of the colon. Incidence following preventive measures. Am J Surg 1962; 103:86–89

206. Stearns MW Jr: Preoperative radiation in carcinoma of the rectum. Proc Natl Cancer Conf 1964; 5:489–493

207. Stearns MW Jr: Surgical management of colorectal cancer. Proc Natl Cancer Conf 1973; 7:481–485

208. Stearns MW Jr: The choice among anterior resection, the pull-through, and abdominoperineal resection of the rectum. Cancer 1974; 34:969–971

209. Stearns MW Jr: Carcinoma of the rectum: Results of abdominoperineal resection (symposium). Dis Colon Rectum 1974; 17:586–587

210. Stearns MW Jr: Diagnosis and management of recurrent pelvic malignancy following combined abdominoperineal resection. Dis Colon Rectum 1980; 23:359–361

211. Stearns MW Jr, Bert JW, Deddish MR: Preoperative irradiation of cancer of the rectum. Dis Colon Rectum 1961; 4:403–408

212. Stearns MW Jr, Deddish MR, Quan SHQ: Preoperative roentgen therapy for cancer of the rectum. Surg Gynecol Obstet 1959; 109:225–229

213. Stearns MW Jr, Deddish MR, Quan SHQ, Leaming R: Preoperative roentgen therapy for cancer of the rectum and rectosigmoid. Surg Gynecol Obstet 1974; 138:584–586

214. Stearns MW Jr, Whiteley HW Jr, Leaming RH, Deddish MR: Palliative radiation therapy in patients with localized cancer of the colon and rectum. Dis Colon Rectum 1970; 13:112–115

215. Stone HH, Hooper CA, Kolb LD et al: Antibiotic prophylaxis in gastric, biliary and colonic surgery. Ann Surg 1976; 184:443–452

216. Strauss AA: Immunologic Resistance to Carcinoma Produced by Electrocoagulation; Based on Fifty-seven Years of Experimental and Clinical Results, p 6. Springfield, Charles C Thomas, 1969

217. Strauss AA, Appel M, Saphir O et al: Immunologic resistance to carcinoma produced by electrocoagulation. Surg Gynecol Obstet 1965; 121:989–996

218. Strauss AA, Strauss SF, Crawford RA et al: Surgical diathermy of carcinoma of rectum: Its clinical end results. JAMA 1935; 104:1480–1484

219. Strauss AA, Strauss SF, Strauss HA: New method and end results in treatment of carcinoma of stomach and rectum by surgical diathermy (electrical coagulation). South Surg 1936; 5:348–359

220. Strauss RJ, Friedman M, Platt N, Wise L: Surgical treatment of rectal carcinoma: Results of anterior resection vs abdominoperineal resection at a community hospital. Dis Colon Rectum 1978; 21:269–276

221. Sugarbaker PH: Partial sacrectomy for *en bloc* excision of rectal cancer with posterior fixation. Dis Colon Rectum 1982; 25:708–711

222. Törnquist A, Ekelund G, Forsgren A et al: Single dose doxycycline prophylaxis and preoperative bacteriological culture in elective colorectal surgery. Br J Surg 1981; 68:565–568

223. Turnbull RB Jr: Cancer of the colon: The five- and ten-year survival rates following resection utilizing the isolation technique. Ann R Coll Surg Engl 1970; 46:243–250

224. Turnbull RB Jr, Cuthbertson A: Abdominorectal pull-through resection for cancer and for Hirschsprung's disease: Delayed posterior colorectal anastomosis. Cleve Clin Q 1961; 28:109–115

225. Turnbull RB Jr, Kyle K, Watson FR et al: Cancer of the colon: The influence of the no-touch isolation technic on survival rates. Ann Surg 1967; 166:420–427

226. Turner-Warwick R, Worth PH: The psoas bladder-hitch procedure for the replacement of the lower third of the ureter. Br J Urol 1969; 41:701

227. Vink M: Local recurrence of cancer in large bowel: Role of implantation metastases and bowel disinfection. Br J Surg 1954; 41:431–433

228. Walz BJ, Lindstrom ER, Butcher HR Jr, Baglan RJ: Natural history of patients after abdominal perineal resection: Implications for radiation therapy. Cancer 1977; 39:2437–2442

229. Wanebo HJ: Resection of pelvic recurrence of rectal cancer. Cont Surg 1982; 21:21–33

230. Wanebo HJ, Marcove RC: Abdominal sacral resection of locally recurrent rectal cancer. Ann Surg 1981; 194:458–471

231. Wang CC, Schulz MO: The role of radiation therapy in the management of carcinoma of the sigmoid, rectosigmoid, and rectum. Radiology 1962; 79:1–5

232. Wangensteen OH: Primary resection (closed anastomosis) of rectal ampulla for malignancy with preservation of sphincteric function together with further account on primary resection of colon and rectosigmoid and note on excision of hepatic metastases. Surg Gynecol Obstet 1945; 81:1–24

233. Washington JA, Dearing WH, Judd ES et al: Effect of preoperative antibiotic regimen on development of infection after intestinal surgery: Prospective, randomized, double-blind study. Ann Surg 1974; 180:567–572

234. Weinstein M, Roberts M: Sexual potency following surgery for rectal carcinoma. Ann Surg 1977; 185:295–300

235. Weir RF: An improved method of treating high-seated cancers of the rectum. JAMA 1901; 37:801–803

236. Welch CE, Hedberg SE: Complications in surgery of the colon and rectum. In Artz CP, Hardy JD (eds): Management of Surgical Complications, 3rd ed, p 600. Philadelphia, WB Saunders, 1975

237. Williams RD, Yurko AA, Kerr G, Zollinger RM: Comparison of anterior and abdominoperineal resections for low pelvic colon and rectal carcinoma. Am J Surg 1966; 111:114–119

238. Wilson E: Local treatment of cancer of the rectum. Dis Colon Rectum 1973; 16:194–196

239. Wright CB, Hobson RW: Prediction of intestinal viability using Doppler ultrasound technics. Am J Surg 1975; 129:642–645

240. Zelas P, Haaga JR, Fazio VW: The diagnosis by percutaneous biopsy with computed tomography of a recurrence of carcinoma of the rectum in the pelvis. Surg Gynecol Obstet 1980; 151:525–527

241. Zinman LM, Libertino JA: Surgical management of urethral strictures. Surg Clin North Am 1973; 53:465–472

242. Zinman LM, Libertino JA, Roth RA: Management of operative ureteral injury. Urology 1978; 12:290–303

243. Zollinger RM, Sheppard MH: Carcinoma of the rectum and the rectosigmoid: A review of 729 cases. Arch Surg 1971; 102:335–338

CHAPTER 12

Malignant Tumors of the Anal Canal

Carcinoma of the anal canal and perianal skin are uncommon clinical entities that account for 2% or fewer of all colorectal carcinomas. At the Memorial Sloan Kettering Cancer Center, between 1929 and 1974 approximately 400 uncommon neoplasms were found in this area, an incidence of 4%, as compared with almost 10,000 adenocarcinomas of the rectum.[40]

Anal canal cancer is almost three times more common than carcinoma of the anal margin.[32] Anal canal cancer is more frequently seen in women (3:2), and carcinoma of the anal margin is more common in men (4:1). Morson and Pang note, however, the same median age (57 years).[32]

ANATOMY AND HISTOLOGY

The anal canal is defined as the distal segment of the intestinal tract that lies between the termination of the rectal mucosa above and the beginning of the perianal skin below (Fig. 12-1). It is divided into a proximal transitional zone encompassing the columns and sinuses of Morgagni and a distal zone lined by squamous epithelium (Fig. 12-2). The transitional zone derives from the embryonic cloaca and separates the rectal mucosa from the squamous epithelium of the distal anal canal. The anal ducts arise from this area (Fig. 12-3) and are lined by stratified columnar epithelium.

This chapter was written in collaboration with Roger C. Haggitt, M.D.

The transitional zone contains epithelium resembling that found in the urethra, but much variability exists in the region; patches of squamous epithelium are frequently present, especially over the crests of the columns of Morgagni. The junction between the transitional zone and squamous mucosa lies at the inferior limit of the columns of Morgagni and has been referred to as the dentate or pectinate line; however, some authors place the dentate line at the proximal limit of the anal canal, at the junction between the rectal mucosa and transitional zone.[24, 27] The more distal zone of the anal canal is lined by stratified squamous epithelium and can be differentiated histologically from perianal skin by the absence of the epidermal appendages found in the skin. Thus, a finger examining the anal canal first passes the perianal skin, the squamous epithelium of the distal anal canal, the transitional zone, and finally reaches the rectal mucosa. Separating tumors that arise in the anal canal from those of perianal skin is important because their biologic behavior, and consequently their treatment, is distinctly different.

CARCINOMA OF THE PERIANAL SKIN

Neoplasms of the anal margin and perianal skin include squamous cell carcinoma, Bowen's disease, Paget's disease, and basal cell carcinoma. They are discussed in Chapter 8. It is self-evident that any suspicious lesion around the anus should be biopsied. If it is confirmed

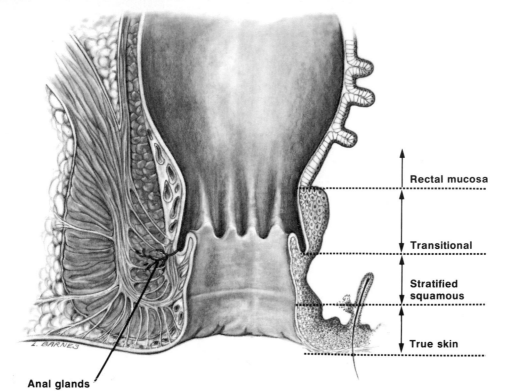

FIG. 12-1. Anatomy of the anus.

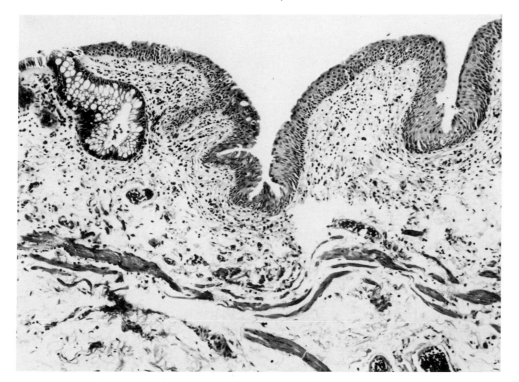

FIG. 12-2. Normal anal canal at the junction between the glands of the rectal mucosa and the transitional zone *(left)*. The epithelium of the transitional zone *(center and right)* resembles the transitional epithelium of the lower genitourinary tract. (Original magnification × 100)

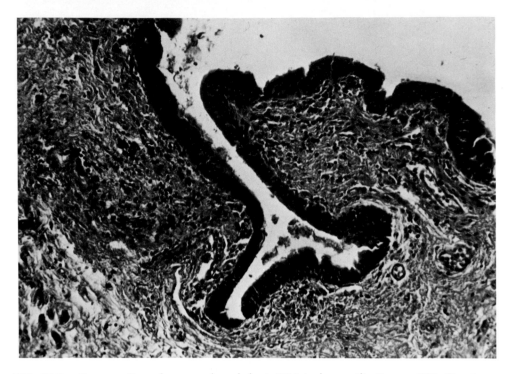

FIG. 12-3. Cross section of a normal anal duct. (Original magnification × 250. Courtesy of Rudolf Garret, M.D.)

to be a malignant neoplasm, the treatment of choice is wide local excision, since these lesions tend not to metastasize. The defect created by excision can be left to granulate, covered by a split-thickness skin graft, or in some instances, may be closed by rotating a flap of adjacent skin, such as is described in Chapter 6.

CLASSIFICATION OF ANAL CANAL TUMORS

Three histologic types of tumors are identified in the anal canal: epidermoid (squamous cell) and mucoepidermoid carcinoma, transitional–cloacogenic carcinoma, and malignant melanoma. Some physicians regard transitional–cloacogenic carcinoma simply as a manifestation of epidermoid carcinoma,[36, 38] whereas others believe it is a distinctly separate entity that arises from the transitional zone of the anal canal and therefore has different morphologic and clinical features.[20, 27] Transitional–cloacogenic carcinomas are generally recognizable morphologically as a distinct group of tumors. However, they overlap to some extent with standard epidermoid carcinomas, and, therefore, form one part of a spectrum that ranges from pure transitional–cloacogenic tumors through lesions with mixtures of squamous elements to those with purely squamous differentiation. With the exception of melanoma, the clinical behavior of carcinoma of the anal canal appears to be relatively independent of the morphologic subtype when compared stage for stage and grade for grade.

Epidermoid (squamous cell) carcinoma accounted for the majority of the tumors in our series (almost two thirds), transitional–cloacogenic carcinomas composed approximately one fourth, and melanomas made up the remainder (14%).[14]

Epidermoid (Squamous Cell) Carcinoma of the Anus

Incidence

Epidermoid carcinoma of the anus is a rare condition. It can be multifocal in the anal canal as well as the perianal skin, perineum, and vulvar areas. Most physicians report a limited experience. Failes and Morgan reported 59 patients over a 20-year period[19]; Sawyers and co-workers reported 42 patients over a period of 35 years (2.4% of cancers of the colon, rectum, and anus), and Cattell and Williams reported a 1.7% incidence of epidermoid carcinoma in 600 rectal and anal neoplasms.[10, 44] Grinnell reported a 1.8% incidence of epidermoid carcinoma in colorectal cancers.[23] Golden and Horsley reported on 26 patients, an incidence of 1.8% of all colorectal cancers.[22] Beahrs and Wilson at the Mayo Clinic reported on 113 patients with epidermoid carcinoma, an incidence of approximately 1% of all colorectal carcinomas seen during the 20-year review.[4] Stearns and Quan reported an experience of 234 epidermoid carcinomas, which represented approximately 3.9% of all malignant tumors detected in the terminal 18 cm of the alimentary tract.[49]

Age and Sex

Epidermoid carcinoma can occur at almost any age but usually is seen in the sixth and seventh decades. As mentioned, most studies have shown a preponderance of carcinoma of the anal canal in women; however, in our experience, the sex incidence was approximately the same (15 women and 14 men).[14] The mean age of the 29 patients was 59 years, with a range of 39 to 84 years.

Pathology

Epidermoid carcinoma originates from the stratified squamous epithelium of the distal anal mucosa and therefore morphologically resembles similar carcinomas arising from the buccal mucosa, esophagus, cervix uteri, and so forth. The tumor is composed of squamous epithelial cells that resemble normal anal mucosa to a varying extent, depending on their degree of differentiation (Fig. 12-4). The more differentiated tumors have readily apparent keratin formation, either as pearls or as individual cell keratinization. The lesions can be graded on the basis of the degree of keratinization and the nuclear morphology, and this grade correlates with the behavior of the tumor: that is, well-differentiated tumors tend to be less deeply invasive and are less likely to metastasize.

A careful search using mucin stains may disclose a focus of mucin-producing cells in as high as 10% to 15% of patients.[33] Such tumors have been classified separately as mucoepidermoid carcinomas, but little evidence exists that differences in the behavior of this subgroup warrant its separation.

Signs and Symptoms

Symptoms of anal canal carcinoma include rectal bleeding, pruritus, mucous discharge, tenesmus, the sensation of a lump in the anus, and a change in bowel habits (Fig. 12-5). Occasionally, a patient may present with a mass in the groin, a manifestation of a metastasis, before the primary tumor causes significant symptoms.

Examination and Biopsy

Rectal examination reveals an ulcerating, hard, tender, bleeding mass in the anal canal or lower rectum. The lesion can fungate through the anal canal and appear

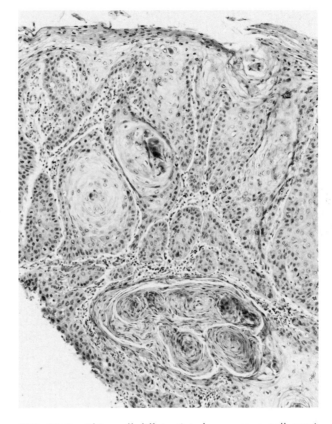

FIG. 12-4. This well-differentiated squamous cell carcinoma resembles normal squamous epithelium and is producing keratin pearls *(bottom)*. Less well-differentiated lesions lose their resemblance to squamous epithelium, lack keratin pearls, and behave more aggressively. (Original magnification × 100)

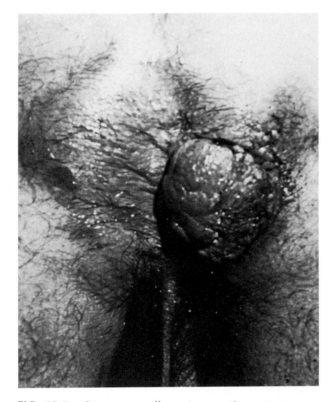

FIG. 12-5. Squamous cell carcinoma: the patient complained of a lump. (Corman ML, Veidenheimer MC, Swinton NW: Diseases of the Anus, Rectum and Colon. Part I: Neoplasms. New York, Medcom, 1972)

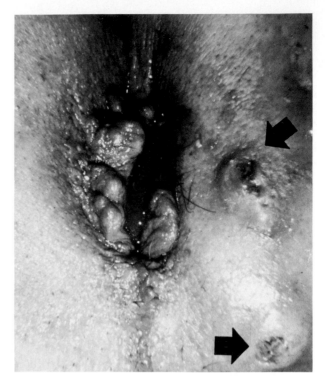

FIG. 12-6. Two fistulous openings *(arrows)* from anal canal carcinoma. Biopsy of the tracts confirmed the presence of tumor. (Corman ML, Veidenheimer MC, Swinton NW: Diseases of the Anus, Rectum and Colon. Part I: Neoplasms. New York, Medcom, 1972)

on the perianal skin or present through a chronic draining anal fistula (Fig. 12-6). Proctosigmoidoscopic examination usually shows that the tumor is confined to the anal canal. Late in the course of the disease the tumor may extend upward high enough to involve the rectum. A carcinoma in the anal canal may rarely represent carcinoma of the rectum that has spread downward (Fig. 12-7). Biopsy of the lesion will establish its histologic nature.

Carcinoma in a Hemorrhoidectomy Specimen

The problem of what to do when the pathologist reports a focus of carcinoma in a hemorroidectomy specimen is one of the quandaries that occasionally confronts the surgeon (Fig. 12-8). Some have criticized the technique of rubber ring ligation for hemorrhoids, be-

cause it fails to obtain a specimen that might harbor an occult neoplasm. However, I sometimes think that the knowledge of a focus of carcinoma in the excised tissue is something I would prefer not to have. The histology should at least be reviewed and the depth of invasion ascertained if possible. Rarely is it helpful to examine the patient again until the wounds are healed. The following protocol is recommended:

1. Reexamine the patient under anesthesia in 4 to 6 weeks when his wounds are healed, and perform multiple biopsies, mapping the source in the anus from which the biopsies are taken.
2. If results of the biopsies are negative, follow the patient's status at 3-month intervals for 1 year, and biopsy any suspicious areas.
3. If no recurrence develops by 1 year, the patient is considered cured. If a persistent tumor or recurrence is identified, the patient should undergo standard surgical treatment.

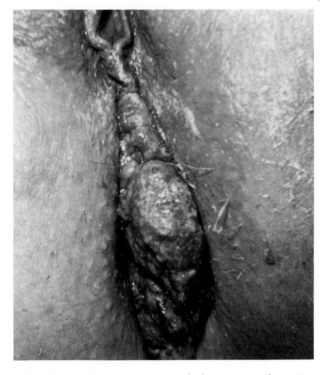

FIG. 12-7. Adenocarcinoma of the rectum fungating through the anal canal. (Corman ML, Veidenheimer MC, Swinton NW: Diseases of the Anus, Rectum and Colon. Part I: Neoplasms. New York, Medcom, 1972)

Treatment

Conventional Surgical Treatment

The two surgical approaches to carcinoma of the anal canal are local excision and abdominoperineal resection. The choice of therapy depends on the stage of the tumor as determined by depth of invasion. For carcinoma confined to the mucosa (carcinoma in situ; Fig. 12-9), and submucosa, wide local excision with or without anoplasty will usually be curative. For tumors invading the muscularis propria (the internal sphincter), local excision, including the internal sphincter, usually achieves cure. However, for tumors that invade more deeply than the internal sphincter, abdominoperineal resection has been the treatment of choice. These differences in therapy based on the stage of the tumor require precise preoperative evaluation, including careful digital examination to assess the depth of invasion.

The technique of abdominoperineal resection is described in Chapter 11. An important principle to remember is that when the anal margin is involved by tumor, a wider excision of perianal skin is required than is customary for adenocarcinoma of the rectum (Fig. 12-10).

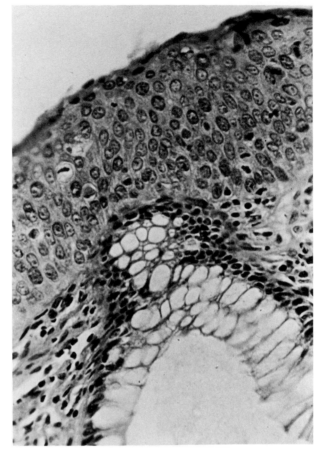

FIG. 12-8. Squamous cell carcinoma in situ, discovered in a hemorrhoidectomy specimen. Note the atypical squamous cells occupying the full thickness of the epithelium. Normally, surface mucosa consists of columnar cells, as in the gland seen here. (Original magnification × 250. Corman ML, Veidenheimer MC, Swinton NW: Diseases of the Anus, Rectum and Colon. Part I: Neoplasms. New York, Medcom, 1972)

Results. Singh and associates reported 65 patients from Roswell Park Memorial Institute, two thirds of whom had epidermoid carcinoma of the anal canal.[47] The remainder harbored cloacogenic cancers. The overall survival rate depended on the depth of invasion, but was approximately 50% in both groups. Wide local

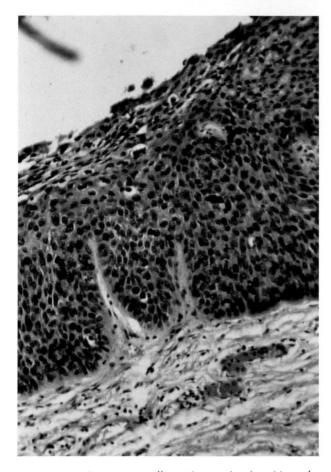

FIG. 12-9. Squamous cell carcinoma in situ. Note the complete destruction of the architecture of the squamous epithelium with absence of maturation and preserved basement membrane. (Original magnification × 250. Courtesy of Rudolf Garret, M.D.)

excision for tumors that invaded through the submucosa was accompanied by a recurrence rate of 100%. Of all surgical approaches, abdominoperineal resection with posterior exenteration had the lowest recurrence rate.

Welch and Malt noted a 30% recurrence rate in the perineums of 37 patients who underwent abdominoperineal resection.[54] Carcinoma was present in 20% of the resection margins. The authors, therefore, appropriately caution the surgeon to perform posterior vaginectomy in women as well as wide excision of the perianal skin. Madden and colleagues reported a 21% survival rate in 29 patients after 5 years.[30]

In our experience, all patients who had disease confined to the mucosa or submucosa were cured by local excision or abdominoperineal resection. Likewise, all patients who had abdominoperineal resection were cured (without supplemental therapy) if the disease was confined to muscle.[14]

With lymph node involvement or invasion into the perirectal or perianal fat, the prognosis is much less optimistic. With the exception of malignant melanoma, it is uniformly agreed that the depth of invasion and the presence or absence of lymph node involvement are the major criteria for determining length of survival. The prognosis after resection for transitional–cloacogenic carcinoma is essentially the same as that for epidermoid carcinoma for the same depth of invasion. In analysis of survival with regard to cell differentiation, no relationship is apparent except that the more poorly differentiated lesions tend to present at a more advanced stage. With lymph node involvement, we have observed a 29% 5-year survival rate.[14]

Radical Groin Dissection

Radical groin dissection has been advocated in the past as a valuable adjunctive procedure in the primary treatment of carcinoma of the anal canal because of the possibility of spread to inguinal nodes. More recent reports are highly critical of this approach.[4, 14, 49, 54] Because of its high morbidity, and because it is an unnecessary operation in the vast majority of patients, radical groin dissection as a therapeutic modality should be employed only when adenopathy is subsequently discovered.[43] Even though the cure rate is still very low, some authors feel that this procedure reduces the risk of groin complications from tumor growth.[43] However, I prefer to implement chemotherapy and radiotherapy in these patients, in light of the responsiveness of this tumor to such an approach (see Radiotherapy and Newer Approaches).

Pelvic Lymphadenectomy

Pelvic lymphadenectomy in conjunction with abdominoperineal resection may be performed relatively easily in some patients. The value of obtaining nodes to determine prognosis and the advisability of additional therapy justifies this approach, but it should not be performed if the dissection is difficult.

Radiotherapy

The place of radiotherapy in the treatment of carcinoma of the anal canal is not well established. However, squamous cell carcinoma is a radiosensitive tumor, and this modality may even be used as the definitive treatment. Cummings and associates, in a retrospective review of 51 patients who were treated

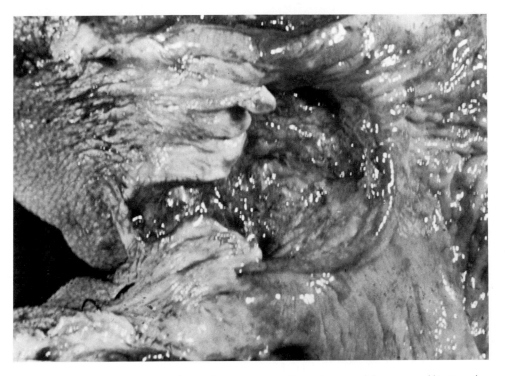

FIG. 12-10. Proctectomy specimen of squamous cell carcinoma of the anus infiltrating the pectinate line. (Courtesy of Rudolf Garret, M.D.)

with radiation therapy, with surgery reserved for those with residual carcinoma, noted a survival rate of 59%.[18] Over one half of the patients' tumors were controlled by radiation alone. Twenty-three of 30 long-term survivors did not require a colostomy.

Preoperative radiotherapy (in the range of 4500 to 5500 rads) should be considered in patients with suspected invasion into the perirectal or perianal soft tissue. *Postoperatively,* if invasion was proved at operation, a dose of 6000 rads may be appropriate. Radiotherapy in this dose range is also advised for patients who are found to have lymph node involvement by pathologic confirmation.

Summary

The following protocol is recommended for *conventional* management of carcinoma of the anal canal based on the depth of invasion:

1. Local excision is the procedure of choice for patients with invasion into the submucosa only. Close follow-up evaluation should be pursued and biopsies of suspicious areas should be taken. Abdominoperineal resection is unnecessarily radical.

2. Abdominoperineal resection is the treatment of choice for patients with tumors that invade muscle. Radiotherapy is not advised.

3. Patients with suspected invasion into the perirectal or perianal soft tissue should undergo preoperative radiotherapy in the range of 4500 to 5000 rads or, postoperatively, if invasion is discovered at surgery, to a dose of 6000 rads. Radiotherapy in this dose range is also advised for patients who are found to have lymph node involvement in the resected specimen.

4. If suspicious nodes are present in the groin or develop subsequently, radical groin dissection is suggested in addition to the preceding radiotherapy regimen.

Newer Approaches

Interstitial Curie Therapy. In 1973 Papillon reported on 98 epidermoid carcinomas treated by interstitial Curie therapy over a 20-year period.[37] This was usually accomplished under general anesthesia, using radium needles inserted either through the skin or anal mucosa. The dose was less than 4000 rads in 2 or 3 days. A second implant was usually performed for residual tumor 2 months after the first implant. External irradiation may be given coincident with implantation. Sixty-four patients were followed up for more than five years, 44 of whom were alive and free of disease (68%). Papillon cautions that treatment must be planned carefully to avoid radionecrosis. Although he is selective in his choice of patients for this procedure, including only those with the most favorable prognosis, the results are impressive and are worthy of further study.

Combined Therapy. In 1974, Nigro and associates reported dramatic results in the treatment of epidermoid carcinoma of the anus by means of radiation therapy and chemotherapy before operation.[35] Subsequent reports from Nigro's unit at Wayne State University School of Medicine reveal continued enthusiasm.[7, 8, 34] Their experience is worth describing in some detail.

Nineteen patients with squamous cell cancer involving the dentate line had been treated. All lesions were ulcerated and moderately to poorly differentiated. There was no evidence of disseminated disease or inguinal adenopathy. All but four tumors were 5 cm or smaller. Following radiation and chemotherapy, there was no evidence of gross tumor in 15 patients. In the other four patients, at least a 50% decrease in size was noted. Of 12 patients who underwent abdominoperineal resection, seven had no gross or microscopic evidence of tumor. Seven patients (the most recently treated) underwent only wide excision of the scar, since there was no macroscopic evidence of tumor. No microscopic tumor was found, and abdominoperineal resection was *not* performed. Their experience has convinced the authors that abdominoperineal resection can be avoided if the tumor disappears and biopsy is negative.[34]

Others have also reported a very favorable experience.[17, 42, 48] Quan and co-workers demonstrated greatly reduced tumor sizes in 9 of 10 patients so treated.[42] Sischy and co-workers reported 15 patients who received chemotherapy and radiotherapy with a complete response, thereby avoiding an abdominoperineal resection.[48] Cummings and associates achieved tumor control in all six patients by the protocol, and Wanebo and associates had a favorable experience even in patients with recurrent and locally advanced disease.[17, 52]

The protocol consists of preoperative radiation (3000 rads) to the rectum and nodal areas in 15 treatments over a 3-week period. The day radiotherapy is commenced, the patient is given 5-fluorouracil in 5% glucose, 100 mg/m², daily for 4 days as a continuous 24-hour infusion. In addition, the patient is given mitomycin-C, 15 mg/m², as a single bolus on day one. Biopsy or local excision is performed 6 weeks after completion of therapy. With this regimen thrombocytopenia and leukopenia were of mild degree.

Comment. Although the number of patients submitted to this procedure is small, preliminary results are so impressive that serious consideration should be given to applying this approach to all patients having epidermoid carcinoma of the anal region. Thus far no reports have appeared on the effects of such combined treatment for patients with transitional–cloacogenic carcinoma.

Transitional–Cloacogenic Carcinoma

In 1955 Grinvalsky and Helwig published a study of the anatomy of the anal canal in which they detailed the features of the transitional or "cloacogenic" zone and suggested that tumors arising in this zone differed from the usual epidermoid carcinomas originating in the squamous epithelium of the distal anal canal.[24] They proposed the term *transitional–cloacogenic* for tumors arising in this zone. Subsequent studies confirmed that tumors arising in the anal canal had a morphology different from the usual squamous carcinomas.[27, 36] Cooper and co-workers reported four cases in anal-receptive homosexual men.[12]

Transitional–cloacogenic carcinomas may resemble carcinomas of urothelium to a certain extent, or they may have patterns similar to those of basal cell carcinoma of skin—hence the term *basaloid* for this subgroup. Those tumors resembling urothelial carcinomas are composed of islands or nests of cells that have indistinct borders and oval nuclei (Fig. 12-11). A focus of keratinization is often present, and, as stated before, mixtures of varying amounts of squamous elements produce a spectrum of lesions ranging from purely transitional through mixed varieties to purely squamous lesions. Occasional tumors have a distinct resemblance to basal cell carcinomas of the skin because the cells at the periphery of cell nests are arranged in an orderly, palisaded fashion (Fig. 12-12). This subgroup has been designated basaloid, but it must not be confused with basal cell carcinoma of skin, because the former is a malignant tumor that frequently metastasizes. Some examples of transitional–cloacogenic carcinoma occur that appear to arise in the lower part of the rectum above the transitional zone; others may not involve the mucosa. The probable explanation for these phenomena is that such tumors may arise from the transitional epithelium lining anal ducts and thus may

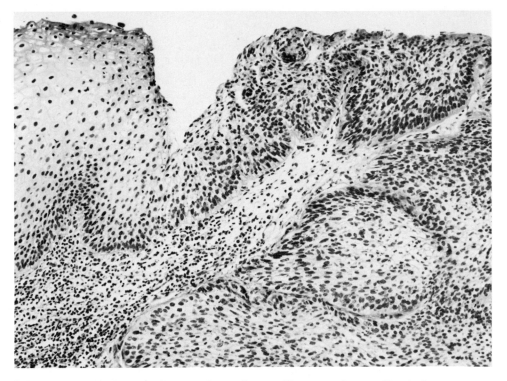

FIG. 12-11. Transitional–cloacogenic carcinoma: The tumor has an "in situ" component *(upper right)* resembling a transitional cell carcinoma of the urinary bladder, hence its name. (Original magnification × 125)

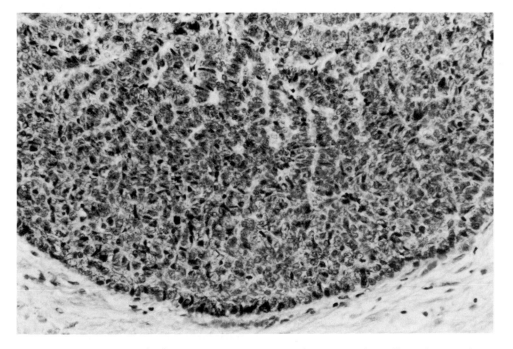

FIG. 12-12. Transitional–cloacogenic carcinoma: In this tumor, the cells at the periphery tend to arrange themselves in a palisade, thus resembling basal cell carcinoma of the skin. This variant of transitional–cloacogenic carcinoma is sometimes called basaloid carcinoma. (Original magnification × 80)

take their origin deep to the mucosa or in proximal ramifications of the ducts beneath rectal mucosa.

As stated before, transitional–cloacogenic tumors form a morphologically recognizable subgroup of anal canal carcinomas, but on the basis of grade and stage of the lesions, their behavior appears to be comparable to epidermoid carcinomas of similar grade and stage.

Treatment

Treatment is abdominoperineal resection for invasive lesions (Fig. 12-13). However, there is some thought that the Nigro protocol should be applied to this tumor also. Results following resection are the same for the

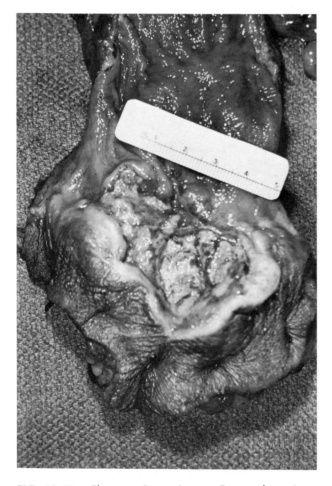

FIG. 12-13. Cloacogenic carcinoma: Resected specimen of ulcerated tumor impinging on the pectinate line. (Courtesy of Rudolf Garret, M.D.)

same stage of lesion as epidermoid carcinoma, the 5-year survival rate being approximately 50%.[16, 26, 45]

Malignant Melanoma

Although the anal canal represents the commonest site for the development of malignant melanoma in the alimentary tract, it is an extremely rare condition. The tumor is presumed to arise from melanocytes present in the squamous mucosa of the lower anal canal. Less than 300 cases have been reported. Cooper and associates analyzed 255 cases and added 12 of their own.[13] One of the largest series is from Memorial Hospital and was reported by Quan and co-workers.[41] Twenty-one cases were seen over a period of 25 years. Mason and Helwig reviewed 17 cases seen at the Armed Forces Institute of Pathology and concluded that all the evidence militates against any melanoma arising from the rectal mucosa.[31] Other authors, however, have claimed that melanoma may be primary in the lower rectum as well as in the anal canal.[1]

Symptoms

Many patients note a feeling of a lump or "hemorrhoid." Rectal bleeding, change in bowel habits, and discomfort are also commonly reported. A mass in the groin may be a presenting complaint.

Physical Findings

Findings on physical examination vary from a small hemorrhoid-like, pigmented lesion to a deeply ulcerating or fungating mass. Pigment may readily be apparent, but Quan and associates reported an incidence of 29% histologically amelanotic lesions, an incidence similar to that reported by Cooper and associates.[13, 41]

Histology

The cells composing the lesion usually assume either a polygonal or a spindle shape (Fig. 12-14) and are often arranged in nests to produce an alveolar pattern. If the mucosa overlying the lesion is not ulcerated, evidence of a junctional component, such as nests of melanoma cells within the squamous epithelium, may be found. This finding confirms the squamous mucosa of the anal canal as the primary site of origin. Identification of melanin within the tumor cells permits diagnosis of the lesion as a melanoma rather than a poorly differentiated carcinoma. Melanin pigmentation was readily apparent in 11 of the 17 tumors reported by Mason and Helwig and was demonstrable by special staining techniques in four additional lesions.[31] Electron mi-

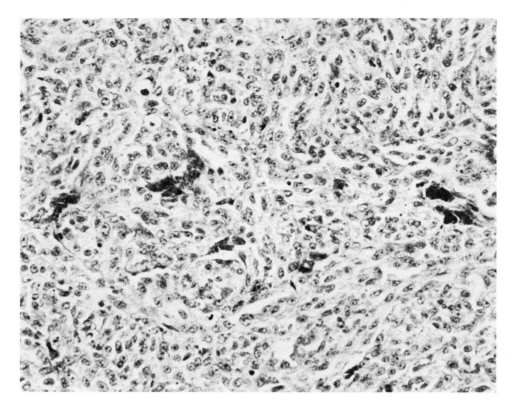

FIG. 12-14. Melanoma of the anus: This very poorly differentiated tumor is recognizable as a melanoma only because of the black pigment being produced. (Original magnification × 250)

croscopy can be of value in identifying apparently amelanotic melanomas by demonstrating melanosomes within the tumor cells.

Treatment and Results

Abdominoperineal resection is the treatment of choice, but the prognosis is so grim that a case might even be made for no treatment at all or a local procedure only. Quan and associates reported one survivor (5%).[41] Most series report few cures.[3, 5, 11, 14, 46, 53] Cooper and associates noted no statistical difference in determinate survivals of patients treated for cure by local excision versus abdominoperineal resection.[13]

Supplementary treatment with radiotherpy has been of no benefit, nor have the various chemotherapeutic agents helped. Immunotherapy for malignant melanoma in other sites has been employed, usually with BCG vaccine, but reports of its value with malignant melanoma of the anal canal have been anecdotal and discouraging.

Miscellaneous Conditions

Verrucous Squamous Carcinoma

A very rare tumor, verrucous squamous carcinoma has come to be known as the tumor of Buschke and Loewenstein because of their description of it in 1925.[9] The lesion is frequently confused with benign anal conditions, especially condylomas. It may appear as a pale, pink, cauliflower-like mass on the perianal skin or in the anal canal (Fig. 12-15).

Histologically, the tumor is so well differentiated that it closely resembles benign proliferative lesions of squamous epithelium, and it may not be recognizable as a carcinoma until invasion of underlying structures can be identified. For this reason, superficial biopsies of verrucous squamous cell carcinomas are not infrequently undiagnosable as carcinoma. Diagnostic biopsies should be taken from the base of the lesion to demonstrate invasion.

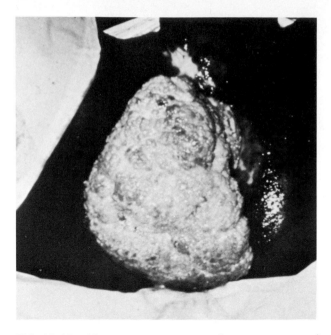

FIG. 12-15. Verrucous squamous carcinoma, or tumor of Buschke-Loewenstein. (Corman ML, Veidenheimer MC, Swinton NW: Diseases of the Anus, Rectum and Colon. Part I: Neoplasms. New York, Medcom, 1972)

Treatment consists of wide local excision or abdominoperineal resection for invasive tumors.[21, 29, 50] Radiation therapy has not proved valuable.

Epidermoid (Squamous Cell) Carcinoma of the Colon

Epidermoid carcinoma of the colon is extremely rare, less than 40 cases having been reported in the English literature.[51] Burgess and co-workers reviewed 15 cases in 1979 and added one of their own.[6] Balfour believed that this entity was either a metastatic lesion or degeneration of a poorly differentiated adenocarcinoma.[2] Vezeridis and colleagues offered a number of possible explanations for its pathogenicity, including mucosal injury, chronic irritation, embryonal nests, metaplasia of an adenocarcinoma, and differentiation in an adenoma.[51] In the absence of metastases, the lesion should be treated in the same manner as adenocarcinoma in that location would be treated.

Pseudosarcomatous Carcinoma

Pseudosarcoma has been described in the esophagus, larynx, oral cavity, and other areas, but Kuwano and associates reported the first and only case of such a tumor in the anal canal.[28] The patient presented with a pedunculated 4-cm mass in the anal canal. Microscopic examination of the locally excised specimen revealed epithelial elements in sarcoma-like areas. No recurrence was noted after a 25-month follow-up.

Carcinoma of the Anal Glands and Ducts

Colloid or mucinous adenocarcinoma of anal glandular or ductal origin is a rare entity.[25, 55, 56] Parks stated, however, that although the condition is extremely uncommon it may not be as infrequent as the literature suggests.[39] This, he postulates, is explained by the fact that the site of origin is destroyed early by the malignant growth. Since this is a highly malignant variant, abdominoperineal resection is recommended.

Basal Cell Carcinoma, Bowen's Disease, Paget's Disease

See Chapter 8.

REFERENCES

1. Alexander RM, Cone LA: Malignant melanoma of the rectal ampulla: Report of a case and review of the literature. Dis Colon Rectum 1977; 20:53–55
2. Balfour TW: Does squamous carcinoma of the colon exist? Br J Surg 1972; 59:410–412
3. Baskies AM, Sugarbaker EV, Chretien PB et al: Anorectal melanoma: The role of posterior pelvic exenteration. Dis Colon Rectum 1982; 25:772–777
4. Beahrs OH, Wilson SM: Carcinoma of the anus. Ann Surg 1976; 184:422–428
5. Braastad FW, Dockerty MB, Dixon CF: Melanoepithelioma of anus and rectum: Report of cases and review of literature. Surgery 1949; 25:82–90
6. Burgess PA, Lupton EW, Talbot IC: Squamous-cell carcinoma of the proximal colon: Report of a case and review of the literature. Dis Colon Rectum 1979; 22:241–244
7. Buroker TR, Nigro N, Bradley G et al: Combined therapy for cancer of the anal canal: A follow-up report. Dis Colon Rectum 1977; 20:677–678
8. Buroker T, Nigro N, Correa J et al: Combination preoperative radiation and chemotherapy in adenocarcinoma of the rectum: Preliminary report. Dis Colon Rectum 1976; 19:660–663
9. Buschke A, Loewenstein L: Condylomata acuminata simulating cancer on penis. Klin Wochenschr 1925; 4:1726–1728

10. Cattell RB, Williams AC: Epidermoid carcinoma of the anus and rectum. Arch Surg 1943; 46:336–349

11. Chiu YS, Unni KK, Beart RW Jr: Malignant melanoma of the anorectum. Dis Colon Rectum 1980; 23:122–124

12. Cooper HS, Patchefsky AS, Marks G: Cloacogenic carcinoma of the anorectum in homosexual men: An observation of four cases. Dis Colon Rectum 1979; 22:557–558

13. Cooper PH, Mills SE, Allen MS Jr: Malignant melanoma of the anus; report of 12 patients and analysis of 255 additional cases. Dis Colon Rectum 1982; 25:693–703

14. Corman ML, Haggitt RC: Carcinoma of the anal canal. Surg Gynecol Obstet 1977; 145:674–676

15. Corman ML, Veidenheimer MC, Swinton NW: Diseases of the Anus, Rectum and Colon. Part I: Neoplasms. New York, Medcom, 1972

16. Cullen PK Jr, Pontius EE, Sanders RJ: Cloacogenic anorectal carcinoma. Dis Colon Rectum 1966; 9:1–12

17. Cummings BJ, Harwood AR, Keane TJ et al: Combined treatment of squamous cell carcinoma of the anal canal: Radical radiation therapy with 5-fluorouracil and mitomycin-C, a preliminary report. Dis Colon Rectum 1980; 23:389–391

18. Cummings BJ, Thomas GM, Keane TJ et al: Primary radiation therapy in the treatment of anal canal carcinoma. Dis Colon Rectum 1982; 25:778–782

19. Failes D, Morgan BP: Squamous-cell carcinoma of the anus. Dis Colon Rectum 1973; 16:397–401

20. Gillespie JJ, MacKay B: Histogenesis of cloacogenic carcinoma: Fine structure of anal transitional epithelium and cloacogenic carcinoma. Hum Pathol 1978; 9:579–587

21. Gingrass PJ, Bubrick MP, Hitchcock CR et al: Anorectal verrucose squamous carcinoma: Report of two cases. Dis Colon Rectum 1978; 21:120–122

22. Golden GT, Horsley JS 3d: Surgical management of epidermoid carcinoma of the anus. Am J Surg 1976; 131:275–280

23. Grinnell RS: An analysis of 49 cases of squamous cell carcinoma of the anus. Surg Gynecol Obstet 1954; 98:29–39

24. Grinvalsky HT, Helwig EB: Carcinoma of the anorectal junction: Histological considerations. Cancer 1956; 9:480–488

25. Hagihara P, Vazquez MT, Parker JC, Griffen WO Jr: Carcinoma of anal duct origin: Report of a case. Dis Colon Rectum 1976; 19:694–701

26. Kheir S, Hickey RC, Martin RG: Cloacogenic carcinoma of the anal canal. Arch Surg 1972; 104:407–415

27. Klotz RG Jr, Pamukcoglu T, Souilliard DH: Transitional cloacogenic carcinoma of the anal canal: Clinicopathologic study of three hundred seventy three cases. Cancer 1967; 20:1727–1845

28. Kuwano H, Iwashita A, Enjoji M: Pseudosarcomatous carcinoma of the anal canal. Dis Colon Rectum 1983; 26:123–128

29. Lock MR, Katz DR, Samoorian S et al: Giant condyloma of the rectum: Report of a case. Dis Colon Rectum 1977; 20:154–157

30. Madden MV, Elliot MS, Botha JBC, Louw JH: The management of anal carcinoma. Br J Surg 1981; 68:287–289

31. Mason JK, Helwig EB: Ano-rectal melanoma. Cancer 1966; 19:39–50

32. Morson BC, Pang LSC: Pathology of anal cancer. Proc R Soc Med 1968; 61:623–624

33. Morson BC, Volkstadt H: Muco-epidermoid tumours of the anal canal. J Clin Pathol 1963; 16:200–205

34. Nigro ND, Vaitkevicius VK, Buroker T et al: Combined therapy for cancer of anal canal. Dis Colon Rectum 1981; 24:73–75

35. Nigro ND, Vaitkevicius VK, Considine B Jr: Combined therapy for cancer of the anal canal: A preliminary report. Dis Colon Rectum 1974; 17:354–356

36. Pang LS, Morson BC: Basaloid carcinoma of the anal canal. J Clin Pathol 1967; 20:128–135

37. Papillon J: Radiation therapy in the management of epidermoid carcinoma of the anal region. Dis Colon Rectum 1974:17:181–187

38. Paradis P, Douglass HO Jr, Holyoke ED: The clinical implications of a staging system for carcinoma of the anus. Surg Gynecol Obstet 1975; 141:411–416

39. Parks TG: Mucus-secreting adenocarcinoma of anal gland origin. Br J Surg 1970; 57:434–436

40. Quan SHQ: Anal and para-anal tumors. Surg Clin North Am 1978; 58:591–603

41. Quan SHQ, White JE, Deddish MR: Malignant melanoma of the anorectum. Dis Colon Rectum 1959; 2:275–283

42. Quan SHQ, Magill GB, Leaming RH et al: Multidisciplinary preoperative approach to the management of epidermoid carcinoma of the anus and anorectum. Dis Colon Rectum 1978; 21:89–91

43. Sawyers JL: Current management of carcinoma of the anus and perianus. Am Surg 1977; 43:424–429

44. Sawyers JL, Herrington JL Jr, Main FB: Surgical considerations in the treatment of epidermoid carcinoma of the anus. Ann Surg 1963; 157:817–824

45. Shindo K, Bacon HE: Transitional-cell cloacogenic carcinoma of the perianal region, anal canal, and

rectum: Report of seven cases. Dis Colon Rectum 1971; 14:222–225

46. Sinclair DM, Hannah G, McLaughlin IS et al: Malignant melanoma of the anal canal. Br J Surg 1970; 57:808–811

47. Singh R, Nime F, Mittleman A: Malignant epithelial tumors of the anal canal. Cancer 1981; 48:411–415

48. Sischy B, Remington JH, Hinson EJ et al: Definitive treatment of anal-canal carcinoma by means of radiation therapy and chemotherapy. Dis Colon Rectum 1982; 25:685–688

49. Stearns MW Jr, Quan SH: Epidermoid carcinoma of the anorectum. Surg Gynecol Obstet 1970; 131:953–957

50. Sturm JT, Christenson CE, Uecker JH et al: Squamous-cell carcinoma of the anus arising in a giant condyloma acuminatum: Report of a case. Dis Colon Rectum 1975; 18:147–151

51. Vezeridis MP, Herrera LO, Lopez GE et al: Squamous cell carcinoma of the colon and rectum. Dis Colon Rectum 1983; 26:188–191

52. Wanebo HJ, Futrell W, Constable W: Multimodality approach to surgical management of locally advanced epidermoid carcinoma of the anorectum Cancer 1981; 47:2817–2826

53. Wanebo HJ, Woodruff JM, Farr GH, Quan SH: Anorectal melanoma. Cancer 1981; 47:1891–1900

54. Welch JP, Malt RA: Appraisal of the treatment of carcinoma of the anus and anal canal. Surg Gynecol Obstet 1977; 145:837–841

55. Wellman KF: Adenocarcinoma of anal duct origin. Can J Surg 1962; 5:311–318

56. Winkleman J, Grosfeld J, Bigelow B: Colloid carcinoma of anal-gland origin: Report of a case and review of the literature. Am J Clin Path 1964; 42:395–401

CHAPTER 13

Less Common Tumors and Tumor-Like Lesions of the Colon, Rectum, and Anus

429

Although adenoma and adenocarcinoma constitute the most commonly seen neoplasms of the colon, rectum, and anus, many other tumors and tumor-like conditions in this anatomic region have been described. Of these, some represent extraordinarily rare lesions and may thus be the source of difficult decisions in the therapeutic approach to the patient. Others are important because they represent benign conditions that may be mistaken for a malignant process. Many lesions present a similar clinical picture despite their diverse pathologic nature. Understanding the biology of each is vital to sound therapeutic intervention; the importance of adequate pathologic examination cannot be overstressed.

The classification scheme on p. 431 organizes diseases essentially by their tissue of origin.

TUMORS OF EPITHELIAL ORIGIN

Carcinoid Tumor

Carcinoid tumors have been described for more than 100 years, but the term *carcinoid* was not introduced until 1907.[180] It was believed that the tumor was similar to carcinoma because metastasis could occur, but the clinical course tended to be relatively more benign. Carcinoids arise from the Kultchitsky or basogranular enterochromaffin cells located in the crypts of Lieberkühn (Fig. 13-1). In the past few decades various investigators have suggested that the histochemical, chemical, and clinical characteristics vary depending on the site of origin.[31, 186, 266] The current classification relates to the anatomic site of the tumor and the reactivity to silver incorporation by cytoplasmic granules.[33] A positive argentaffin reaction involves the reduction of ionic to metallic silver by strong endogenous reducing substances.[247] Argentaffinity usually implies that the argyrophil reaction will be positive, but the mechanism for the latter reaction is unknown.[247] Two distinctive types of neurosecretory granules have been observed by electron microscopy.[274] A relatively small granule appears to be associated with argyrophil carcinoids and a larger one with argentaffin (Fig. 13-2).

Midgut carcinoids (mid-duodenum to mid-transverse colon) are usually both argyrophil and argentaffin positive, are frequently multicentric in origin, and often are associated with the carcinoid syndrome. Hindgut carcinoids have been reported to be rarely argyrophil or argentaffin positive, are usually unicentric, and are not associated with the carcinoid syndrome.[186] Saegesser and Gross, however, reported the carcinoid syndrome in a patient with carcinoid of the rectum, and Taxy and co-workers noted in 23 patients that most rectal carcinoids are argyrophil if the more sensitive Grimelius method is employed.[215, 247] In this same group of patients only three were argentaffin positive. The authors concluded that the Grimelius argyrophil stain is the most accurate, light-microscopic means for confirming the diagnosis of a rectal carcinoid.

Determination of urine 5-hydroxyindoleacetic acid (5-HIAA) excretion is not helpful in defining metastatic disease in rectal tumors, since hindgut lesions are generally argentaffin negative and do not produce a detectable increase in tryptophan metabolites.[31]

Classification of Unusual Tumors and Tumor-Like Conditions

Tumors of epithelial origin
  Carcinoid tumor
  Bowen's disease
  Perianal Paget's disease
  Basal cell carcinoma
  Cloacogenic carcinoma
  Malignant melanoma
  Squamous cell carcinoma
Tumors of lymphoid origin
  Lymphoid hyperplasia (benign lymphoma, lymphoid
    polyp)
  Malignant lymphoma
  Plasmacytoma
Mesenchymal tumors
  Fibrous tissue origin
    Fibroma
    Inflammatory fibroid polyp
    Fibrosarcoma
    Malignant fibrous histiocytoma
  Smooth muscle origin
    Leiomyoma
    Leiomyosarcoma
  Adipose tissue origin
    Lipoma
Tumors of neural origin
  Neurofibroma
  Neurilemmoma (schwannoma)
  Ganglioneuroma
  Granular cell tumor
Vascular lesions
  Hemangioma
  Lymphangioma
  Hemangiopericytoma
Heterotopias and hamartomas
  Endometriosis
  Hamartoma
  Dermoid cyst
  Colitis cystica profunda (enterogenous cysts)
Exogenous, extrinsic, and miscellaneous tumors
  Metastatic tumor
  Barium granuloma
  Oleoma
  Malacoplakia
  Sacrococcygeal chordoma
  Pneumatosis cystoides intestinalis

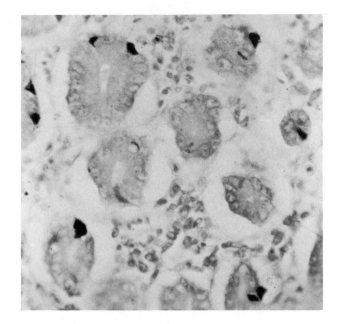

FIG. 13-1. Normal bowel showing dark-staining argyrophilic granules (in Kulchitsky cells) from which carcinoid tumors arise. (Original magnification × 600. Courtesy of Rudolf Garret, M.D.)

Gastrointestinal carcinoid tumors arise most commonly in the appendix and are found in 0.26% of appendectomy specimens.[43] The next most common location is the small intestine, followed by the rectum and stomach. Colonic involvement is infrequent, comprising 2.5% of gastrointestinal carcinoids.[43] Orloff collected 3000 cases of gastrointestinal carcinoids from the literature and reported 38 patients with rectal tumors.[186] Morson reported only 21 cases of rectal carcinoids seen at St. Mark's Hospital in 25 years.[172] The condition occurs most commonly in patients in their sixth and seventh decades; the mean age in Orloff's series was 55.[186]

Carcinoid tumors are frequently asymptomatic. Moertel and co-workers advised that the presence of an abdominal mass on the right side and a long history of weight loss and diarrhea should raise suspicion of a carcinoid in the small intestine.[169] Colonic carcinoids usually grow to a large size before they become symptomatic. Even then they are less likely to cause obstruction or rectal bleeding than adenocarcinoma of the colon. Thirty-two percent of Orloff's patients were asymptomatic, and an additional 21% had symptoms that were due to another condition. When the lesion produces symptoms, they are indistinguishable from those caused by adenocarcinoma (bleeding, change in bowel habits, abdominal pain, *etc*).

In the rectum, a carcinoid tumor usually presents as a small, circumscribed, yellowish, submucosal nodule, 1 cm or less in diameter. It is often found incidentally, either in the course of pathologic examination of an excised rectum for another condition, or in the course of clinical examination for other complaints (Figs. 13-3 and 13-4).

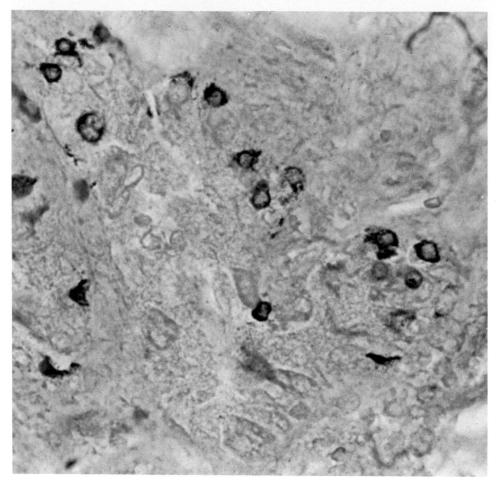

FIG. 13-2. Carcinoid tumor showing argyrophilic granules in the cytoplasm, Fontana stain. (Original magnification × 600. Courtesy of Rudolf Garret, M.D.)

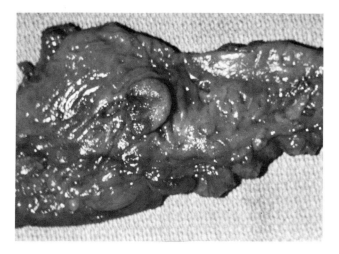

FIG. 13-3. Carcinoid tumor: an ulcerated nodule protruding from the rectum in a resected specimen. (Courtesy of Rudolf Garret, M.D.)

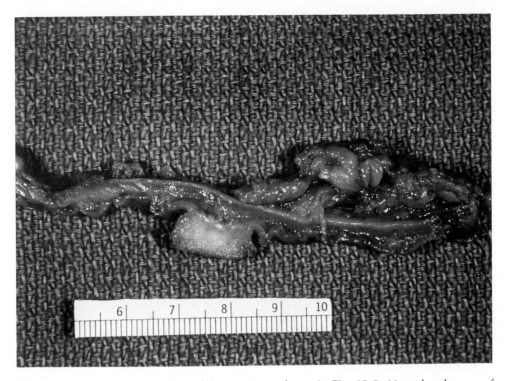

FIG. 13-4. Longitudinal section of the specimen shown in Fig. 13-3. Note the absence of infiltration of muscularis. (Courtesy of Rudolf Garret, M.D.)

Radiologic evaluation of colonic carcinoids reflects the appearance of the presenting lesion (Fig. 13-5). For larger tumors, it is virtually impossible to distinguish the histologic nature from that of an adenocarcinoma.

Microscopically, it is very difficult to differentiate between benign and malignant carcinoid. The usual criteria of malignancy, such as mitotic activity or pyknotic nuclei, are often lacking. The incidence varies from 8% to 40%, with the evidence of malignancy based on the presence of local extension or metastasis.[264] The tumor is composed of uniform, small, round or polygonal cells with prominent, round nuclei and eosinophilic cytoplasmic granules (Fig. 13-6 through 13-8).

Patients with carcinoid tumors seem to have an increased incidence of gastrointestinal adenocarcinoma.[25, 38, 199] Thorough evaluation of the gastrointestinal tract is advised in all patients found to harbor a carcinoid. Nelson has demonstrated a possible association with myelofibrosis, and postulates that evaluation of the bowel in a patient with hematologic disease may be a useful exercise.[175]

Treatment for colonic carcinoid is resection. These tumors are relatively slow growing, and metastatic disease is not a contraindication to resection of the primary lesion. Metastatic disease occurs more frequently with carcinoids of the colon than with carcinoids of the small bowel. Perhaps this can be explained by the fact that carcinoid tumors may attain a considerable size before they become symptomatic.

In the rectum, the size of the carcinoid is the distinguishing feature that determines treatment. Most tumors smaller than 2 cm in diameter require only local, transanal excision. However, tumors that are demonstrably invasive or 2 or more cm in diameter should probably be treated by a cancer type of resection. Orloff applied this therapeutic principle, and all 23 of his patients with lesions smaller than 2 cm survived 5 years.[186] The survival rate of the 15 patients with lesions measuring 2 cm or more in diameter was 40%.

According to Berardi, the average length of survival after resection of colonic carcinoids is 26 months.[27] Welch and Donaldson stated that the 5-year survival rate for patients with colonic carcinoids is similar to that for patients with carcinoma of the colon and rectum.[265] When a distinction is made between cecal and other colonic sites, the former is found to be associated with a 71% incidence of metastasis, while the latter has a 33% incidence.[219]

(Text continues on p. 436)

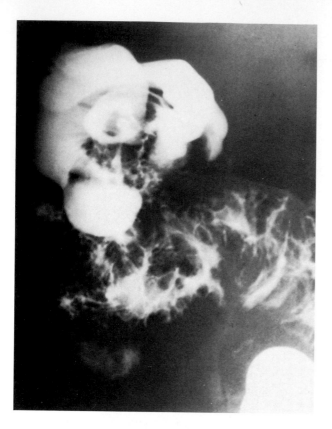

FIG. 13-5. Carcinoid of the colon: hepatic flexure spot film on barium enema reveals distension with thickened folds. This appearance is caused by intense fibrosis and desmoplastic response produced by the carcinoid tumor.

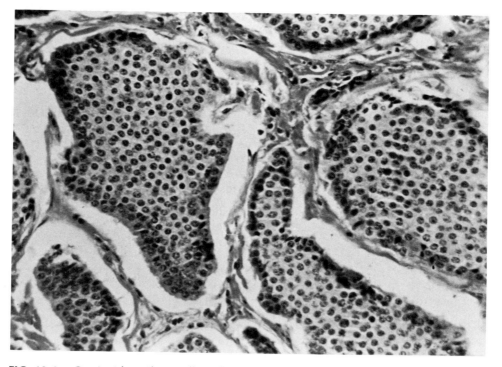

FIG. 13-6. Carcinoid: uniform cells with minimal variation of cell nuclei in clusters within the lymphatic spaces. (Original magnification × 280. Corman ML, Veidenheimer MC, Swinton NW: Diseases of the Anus, Rectum and Colon. Part I: Neoplasms. New York, Medcom, 1972)

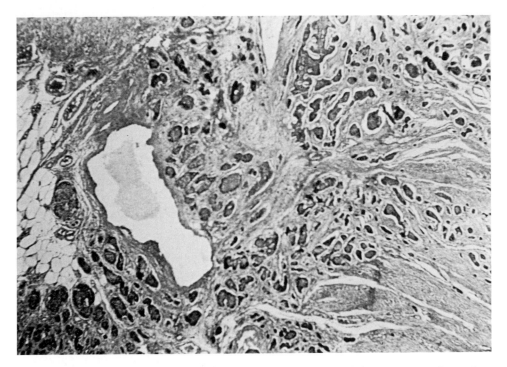

FIG. 13-7. Malignant carcinoid infiltrating the whole wall of the rectum and invading adipose tissue. Note the cluster of tumor cells in tissue spaces and lymphatics. (Original magnification × 80. Courtesy of Rudolf Garret, M.D.)

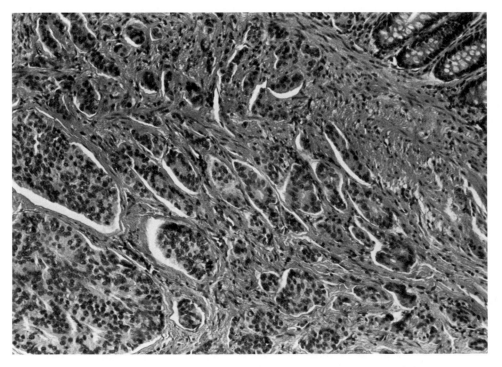

FIG. 13-8. Malignant carcinoid: uniform cells in tissue spaces, some forming abortive glandular structures. (Original magnification × 280. Courtesy of Rudolf Garret, M.D.)

Moertel and associates recommended appendectomy as adequate treatment for appendiceal carcinoids of less than 2 cm in diameter, even if lymphatic invasion is noted on subsequent histologic examination.[168] They found no recurrence in a group of more than 100 patients who had microscopic evidence of lymphatic invasion and who were so treated.

Anderson and Bergdahl reported results of treatment of carcinoid of the appendix in 25 children under the age of 15 years.[10] All underwent appendectomy, but one patient was subjected to right hemicolectomy because of tumor in the margin of the resected appendix. Despite serosal extension in nine children and lymph node metastases in one, no signs of recurrence were seen with a mean follow-up period of 12 years.

Radiotherapy and chemotherapy have not proved to be effective in the treatment of carcinoid of the colon and rectum. Adequate surgical excision remains the treatment of choice.

Bowen's Disease, Perianal Paget's Disease, and Basal Cell Carcinoma

See Chapter 8.

Cloacogenic Carcinoma and Malignant Melanoma

See Chapter 12.

Squamous Cell Carcinoma

Primary squamous cell carcinoma of the colon and rectum is an extremely rare tumor; approximately 50 cases have been reported (8 by Comer and associates and 6 by Vezeridis and associates).[49,256] The incidence of this tumor is believed to be approximately 1 per 3000 malignant tumors of the bowel.[49,256]

A number of theories have been postulated about the etiology and pathogenicity of squamous cell carcinoma. These include metaplasia of glandular epithelium, embryonal rests, squamous metaplasia of existing adenoma or adenocarcinoma, damaged epithelium from toxic substance, and basal cell anaplasia.[49, 150, 256] Specific predisposing factors that have been associated with the condition are ulcerative colitis, radiotherapy, and schistosomiasis.[49,150]

Symptoms are the same as that for adenocarcinoma, especially bleeding and change in bowel habits. Evaluation of the patient should proceed in the manner outlined in the chapters on cancer of the colon and rectum. Total colonoscopy is suggested because of the not uncommon association of synchronous benign and malignant tumors.

Histologic examination may demonstrate squamous metaplasia of the colon mucosa with the squamous cell carcinoma.

Treatment is surgical extirpation, but consideration should be given to the implementation of the multimodality approach described in the previous chapter, especially if abdominoperineal resection appears to be the operative alternative.

TUMORS OF LYMPHOID ORIGIN

Lymphoid Hyperplasia (Benign Lymphoma, Lymphoid Polyp)

Lymphoid hyperplasia is a benign, focal or diffuse condition that occurs typically where clusters of lymphoid follicles are present (terminal ileum, rectum).[53, 54, 65, 115] Although the etiology is not known, the possibility of an inflammatory reaction, as well as hereditary predisposition, are suggested. Lymphoid hyperplasia is characterized radiographically by small, uniform, localized or generalized polypoid lesions. A fleck of barium may be seen in the center of the polyp on contrast study, representing umbilication at the apex of the lymphoid nodule. A central dimple in the nodule is considered good evidence for benign lymphoid hyperplasia.[129]

The macroscopic and microscopic appearance of the lesion may resemble malignant lymphoma or Hodgkin's disease. In fact, the condition has been regarded by some as a form of malignant lymphoma and has even been designated as pseudolymphoma.[245] However, the lesion lacks the infiltrating and destructive characteristics of malignant lymphoma and does not become disseminated. In the benign lymphoid polyp a follicular pattern with a clearly defined germinal center is seen (Fig. 13-9), whereas malignant lymphoma shows a poorly defined and irregular pattern with no germinal centers.[198] The condition also can resemble leukemic infiltration of the bowel, but in leukemia the lesion tends to have a segmental distribution (Fig. 13-10). In addition, evidence of the disease is usually apparent in the peripheral blood smear.

One of the earliest reports of benign lymphoid hyperplasia was by Cohnheim, who, in 1865, introduced the term *gastrointestinal pseudoleukemia*.[46] He pointed out hyperplasia of the lymphoid follicles of the gastrointestinal tract with polyp formation but without the blood picture of lymphatic leukemia.

In 1940, Ewing stated that "the gastro-intestinal tract is the seat of a remarkable form of primary lymphoid hyperplasia which lacks the destructive character

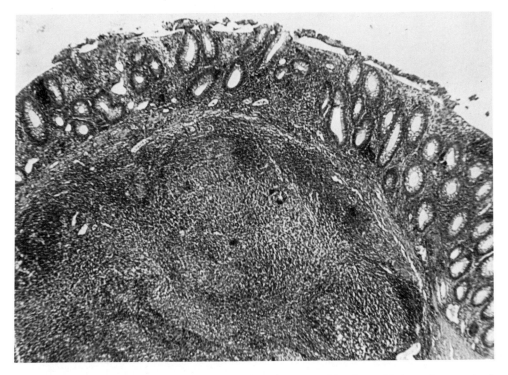

FIG. 13-9. Lymphoid polyp of the rectum: lymphocytic infiltration with irregular germinal centers in the submucosa. (Original magnification × 250. Courtesy of Rudolf Garret, M.D.)

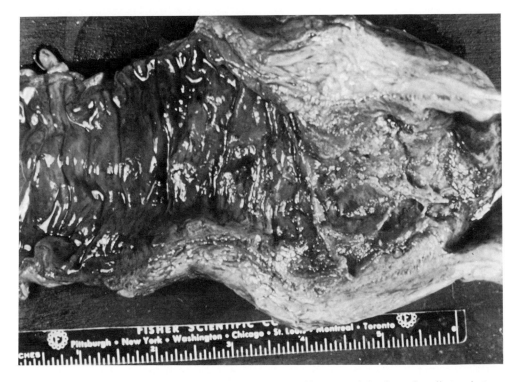

FIG. 13-10. Autopsy specimen showing leukemic infiltration of the bowel wall simulating scirrhous carcinoma. (Courtesy of Rudolf Garret, M.D.)

of lymphosarcoma and fails to give lymphocytosis in the blood."[73] He pointed out that lesions of the gastrointestinal tract may be limited or diffuse and sometimes are associated with widespread lymphoid hyperplasia but never with leukemia. Symmers confirmed these findings in 1948.[245] Since that time, isolated cases have been reported sporadically, all of which confirm the benign nature of the disease.[37, 48, 55, 125]

In 1961, Cornes and co-workers reviewed 100 cases.[54] The tumors were described as usually single and most frequent in the lower third of the rectum. They may be seen in a patient at any age but most commonly are found during the third and fourth decades.[37, 54, 198] They are usually small, firm, and sessile but occasionally may be large and may become pedunculated. When removed and sectioned, the tumors are found to be composed of well-differentiated lymphoid tissue with follicles separated by white fibrous bands and covered by rather thin mucous membrane.

Gruenwald has suggested that the lesions are congenital malformations or hamartomas.[103] This is supported by the occasional familial occurrence of the lesions. Granet has reported solitary benign lymphomas in identical twins.[98] Keeling and Beatty have reported the lesions in three siblings, ages 6, 7, and 9 years.[132] Others have reported an association with familial polyposis.[102, 255]

Collins and associates have reported a case in which the clinical presentation was identical to that of neurofibromatosis with neurovisceral involvement.[48] However, no similarity exists between the bowel lesions of lymphoid hyperplasia and neurofibromatosis.

Although it may produce no symptom if located in the rectum, a lymphoid polyp may cause considerable pain when it occurs in the anal canal. Colonic lesions may cause bleeding, abdominal pain, change in bowel habits, and symptoms related to intussusception.

Local excision is indicated and adequate for isolated or scattered lesions.[54, 111, 123] Removal is important to differentiate the condition from other neoplasms. In 100 patients so treated by Cornes and associates only 5 had recurrences, even though a number of polyps were incompletely removed.[54]

Patients with lymphoid polyposis have been treated by colectomy with and without ileorectal anastomosis.[48, 55] In other instances less extensive bowel resections have been performed in patients with lymphoid hyperplasia who were misdiagnosed preoperatively.[84, 241] It is crucial that an awareness of this entity exists and that it is differentiated from multiple polyposis.

Since radiotherapy and cytotoxic agents are often beneficial in the treatment of malignant lymphomas of the gastrointestinal tract, similar treatment has been proposed for benign lymphoid polyposis.[53] Symmers stated that radiation is the accepted method of treating

lymphoid polyposis.[245] Cosens claimed that the lesions may respond well to roentgen therapy, although no response occurred in his own case.[55] In my opinion, in the absence of symptoms, management should be expectant; spontaneous regression may occur without treatment.

Malignant Lymphoma

Malignant lymphoma, as a primary lesion or as part of a generalized malignant process, may involve the gastrointestinal tract. As a primary tumor, lymphoma comprises between 1% and 4% of all gastrointestinal malignancies,[163] but only 0.5% of colonic and 0.1% of rectal cancers.[224] Gastric involvement is more common than that of small or large intestinal lymphoma and carries a better prognosis.[50] Colonic lymphoma preferentially involves the cecum and the rectum; however, concurrent tumors elsewhere in the large bowel, the small bowel, and the stomach have been reported.

In most series the incidence is greater in men than in women by a ratio of 2 to 1.[167, 272] Most patients are over 50 years of age at diagnosis, but the condition can occur at any age. Many patients complain of abdominal pain that is usually crampy and localized to the area of the tumor. Other prominent symptoms include weight loss, change in bowel habits, weakness, nausea, vomiting, anorexia, bleeding, and fever. Discrete intra-abdominal masses are generally not appreciated until late in the course of the disease.

The symptoms produced by *rectal involvement* are variable and largely depend on whether the growth has become ulcerated. In early stages, with an intact mucosa, symptoms consist of a bearing-down sensation or a feeling of fullness in the rectum, with some rectal irritability and low backache. When ulceration of the underlying mucosa has developed, bleeding and mucous discharge may be noticed; later, pain and soreness are described if the growth begins to encroach on the anal canal. Obstructive symptoms are not likely to occur because the primary growth often remains fairly localized to one quadrant and does not usually extend in an annular fashion, as is seen with carcinoma.

Macroscopic examination of the tumor reveals a polypoid or ulcerated mass resembling carcinoma or a diffuse process extending over a large segment of colon, sometimes with numerous polypoid intraluminal excrescences. The bowel wall is thickened and rubbery in consistency, and its cut surface demonstrates a greatly thickened mucosa, often with prominent convoluted folds resembling the surface of brain and reaching a thickness of 1 or 2 cm (Fig. 13-11). The submucosa is markedly thickened as a result of infiltration by closely packed tumor cells. Deep ulceration and

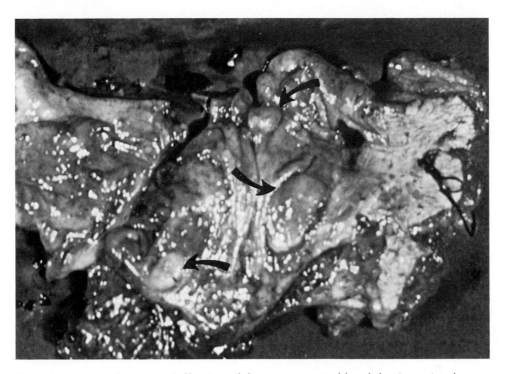

FIG. 13-11. Lymphomatous infiltration of the rectum treated by abdominoperineal resection. Multiple lesions are noted *(arrows)*. (Courtesy of Rudolf Garret, M.D.)

perforation are uncommon, in contrast to disease in the small bowel; however, superficial ulceration and necrosis may be seen. Rectal biopsy with microscopic examination readily distinguishes lymphoma from other malignancies.[117]

Regional lymph nodes are involved in approximately half of the patients at the time of laparotomy. The presence of enlarged nodes may, however, represent reactive lymphoid hyperplasia and must be examined histologically to document the presence of tumor. Associated leukemia has been described, thereby mandating total and differential white blood cell counts as part of a workup. Since involvement beyond a single segment of bowel and its regional nodes excludes the diagnosis of primary lymphoma, a careful search for diseased nodes elsewhere is necessary.

It is thought that malignant lymphoma starts in the submucosal lymphoid tissue, which in places extends into the mucosa. It is not known whether it begins multicentrically or arises from a single area and later spreads by direct extension or through lymphatic channels. At presentation, a large segment of colon may be involved in a uniform and continuous fashion. Submucosal infiltration often extends beyond the area of obvious involvement, and additional lesions may be found apart from that region. Marked involvement is commonest in the ileocecal or the rectosigmoid area, where tumors sometimes become confluent and form a large conglomerate mass. This may cause intussusception and intestinal obstruction. In the ileocecal region the process usually extends into the appendix and into the ileum for a variable distance. When the rectum is the site of the tumor, inguinal nodes may be enlarged and palpable. Extensive serosal or retroperitoneal involvement is not characteristic of diffuse lymphoma.

Malignant lymphoma is classified on the basis of its cellular morphology and immunologic surface markers. Included are the following histologic types: lymphocytic lymphoma, lymphosarcoma, reticulum cell sarcoma, giant follicular lymphoma, and Hodgkin's disease. Hodgkin's disease of the colon or rectum is the rarest.

Tumors are also classified on the basis of extent of involvement:

Class I.   Confined to bowel wall
Class II. Regional node involvement within drainage area of bowel primary
Class III. Para-aortic node involvement; direct extension to adjacent viscera

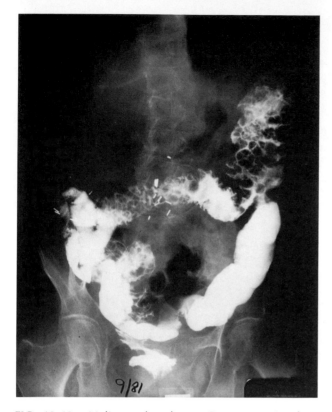

FIG. 13-12. Malignant lymphoma. Post-evacuation barium enema demonstrates multiple polypoid filling defects of varying size with areas of ulceration.

tric dilatation of the lumen, and a polypoid filling defect of the terminal ileum and ileocecal valve (Fig. 13-12).[106]

The presence of a nonulcerated, submucous tumor in the rectal wall requires differentiation from benign lesions, such as lipoma, myoma, and nodular lymphoid hyperplasia, and also from an inflammatory condition, such as a submucosal or intermuscular abscess. Thus, biopsy and histologic examination are crucial to the evaluation of such lesions (Figs. 13-13 and 13-14).

Malignant lymphoma of the colon has been reported in association with a variety of other entities, especially those of altered immune status.[61, 74, 124, 134, 142, 176, 183, 192, 240, 259] Waldenström pointed out considerable overlap between macroglobulinemia, lymphoma, and lymphocytic leukemia.[259] This was exemplified by a case reported by Levy and co-workers in which cecal lymphoma developed in an 81-year-old patient while the patient was receiving immunosuppressive therapy for

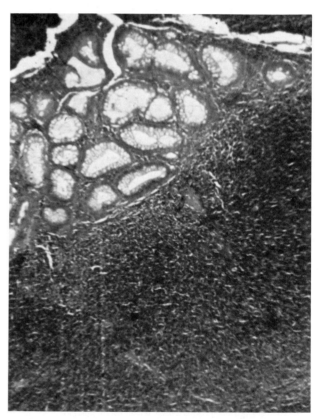

FIG. 13-13. Lymphoma of the sigmoid colon. Note the heavy infiltrate of lymphocytic tumor cells involving the mucosa and submucosa. (Original magnification × 80. Courtesy of Rudolf Garret, M.D.)

As pointed out by Wychulis and associates and by others, the prognosis of primary extranodal lymphoma in the colon or rectum is not clearly related to cell type but is primarily affected by stage.[144, 216, 272]

Clinical and radiographic diagnosis of colonic and rectal lymphoma may be obscured by the variety of appearances it may assume. Usher reported 10 cases of rectal lymphoma at the Mayo Clinic and observed that in all cases the lesion was visualized on proctoscopic examination.[254] In no instance could a definite diagnosis of lymphoma be made on the appearance of the lesion. Usually, it was described as a polypoid tumor, diffuse proctitis, a submucous nodule, or carcinoma.

From the radiologic point of view, diffuse lymphoma of the colon must be differentiated from familial polyposis, ulcerative colitis with pseudopolyposis, granulomatous colitis, nodular lymphoid hyperplasia, and schistosomiasis. Although radiologic differentiation from carcinoma may be impossible, Halls points out that certain presentations strongly suggest lymphoma: presence of a bulky extracolonic component, concen-

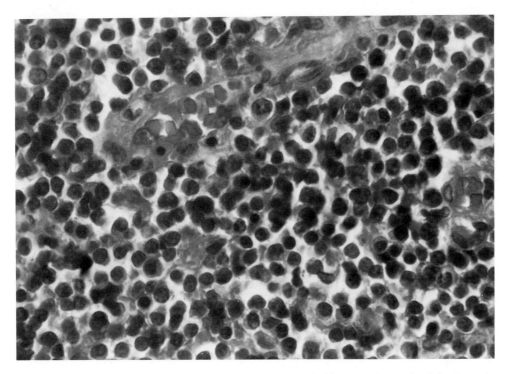

FIG. 13-14. Lymphoma of the cecum. Note the lymphoblasts in the wall of the bowel. (Original magnification × 600. Courtesy of Rudolf Garret, M.D.)

macroglobulinemia.[142] An association with chronic ulcerative colitis, Crohn's disease, and celiac disease has also been observed.[144]

The treatment of malignant lymphoma primary to the colon and rectum is resection followed by radiotherapy. In those tumors considered unresectable, radiation therapy is of definite benefit. A combined program with chemotherapy is recommended for systemic disease.

Contreary and colleagues reported a 50% 5-year survival in those patients operated upon for cure.[50] When the tumor was confined to the bowel or involved only local nodes, the survival rates in both situations were also 50%. When regional nodes were involved, 5-year survival fell to 12%. Although this was not a controlled study, the difference in survival rates between those patients operated upon for cure with supplementary radiotherapy and without it was 83% versus 16%. Moertel reported an overall 5-year survival rate of 55%.[167]

Plasmacytoma

Primary plasmacytoma is a localized plasma cell tumor that is most commonly found in the nasopharynx, although it has been described in many parts of the body. The condition involves the colon extremely rarely, less than 10 cases having been reported as a primary disease. Plasma cell neoplasms are classified in five categories: multiple myeloma, solitary myeloma, extramedullary plasmacytoma (with multiple myeloma), plasma cell leukemia, and primary plasmacytoma.[226]

Disseminated multiple myeloma is often diagnosed in patients who have a localized plasmacytoma if these patients are followed up for a long enough period. A number of reported tumors have involved the bowel secondarily and as apparent primary tumors in the gastrointestinal tract.[97, 108, 114] Primary and secondary colorectal plasmacytoma is commoner in men than in women by a ratio of 3 to 2.

Presenting symptoms include abdominal pain, bleeding, anorexia, nausea, vomiting, and weight loss. The tumor can be single or multiple and consist of diffuse cellular infiltrates or of polypoid or nodular protrusions. Microscopic examination demonstrates the characteristic population of plasma cells (Fig. 13-15); the use of immunoperoxidase studies has also been advised.[93]

Treatment ideally consists of total excision when possible. If, for example, a gastrointestinal lesion was

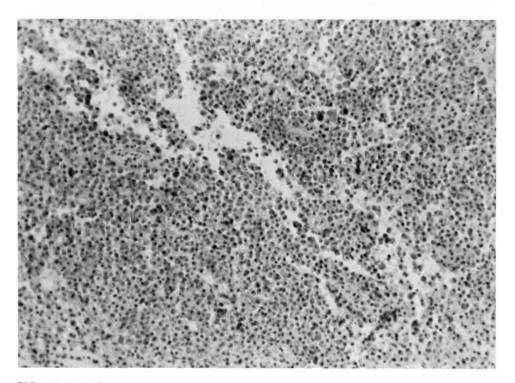

FIG. 13-15. Plasmacytoma, a tumor consisting of many plasma cells, some of which demonstrate hyperchromatic nuclei. (Original magnification × 280. Courtesy of Rudolf Garret, M.D.)

excised for purposes of diagnosis and the entire lesion was removed, probably no additional treatment would be indicated. Of the cases reviewed by Sidani and associates none metastasized to any organ other than lymph nodes.[226] Plasmacytomas that are not readily resectable might be responsive to radiotherapy. The use of chemotherapy is restricted to disseminated disease.

MESENCHYMAL TUMORS

Fibroma

Fibroma of the colon is a very rare tumor belonging to the uncommon spindle cell group of benign tumors of the colon that also includes leiomyomas.[233] Its incidence is only one tenth that of leiomyoma.[35]

Although many authors use the terms *fibroma, leiomyoma,* and *fibromyoma* interchangeably, Rose emphasized that differential histologic tissue staining techniques distinguish the true fibroma from other spindle cell tumors.[211] According to Aird, the tumor may originate in any layer of the bowel wall but arises most frequently in the submucosa.[4] Fibromas have been reported in the appendicular stump and near the mesentery.[78, 251] Reports of fibroma of the colon are few.[16, 75, 185, 211] Abdominal pain and distension may be noted. Resection is the treatment of choice.

Fibroma of the anorectal region is very rare. It may arise from an hypertrophied papilla or by fibrous infiltration of a large prolapsing internal hemorrhoid, generally as a result of repeated attacks of thrombosis and strangulation without sloughing. It is encapsulated, firm, slightly movable, ovoid, of small to moderate size, and has little tendency to ulcerate. It is usually situated in the wall. In time, the covering of columnar epithelium becomes converted into squamous epithelium. A smooth, pale fibrous polyp results. The tumor may remain in the wall of the rectum or become polypoid and extend into the lumen. In general, it is single and of slow growth. However, fibrous polyps may be multiple, so a careful proctoscopy is essential.

Symptoms include tenesmus and a sense of heaviness in the rectum. If ulceration has occurred (an exception), bleeding may be noted. The diagnosis is seldom made without microscopic examination. Transanal excision is the appropriate treatment.

Inflammatory Fibroid Polyp

Inflammatory fibroid polyp is a rare, focal lesion, occurring in the submucosa of the gastrointestinal tract, least commonly in the colon.[130, 145, 196] Only a handful of cases have been reported.[162, 187, 257] Another term for the condition is *eosinophilic granuloma*. Although the etiology is uncertain, the observation of the proliferation of submucosal mesenchymal fibrous tissue as well as variable eosinophilic infiltration suggest the effect of an inflammatory stimulus (Fig. 13-16).[145]

Rectal bleeding, tenesmus, and change in bowel habits are the commonest symptoms. Intussusception has been reported.[145] Since malignant degeneration has

not been noted, endoscopic removal is suggested. However, lesions may be sessile and submucosal and have a tendency to bleed readily. If colonoscopic resection is unsuccessful or inadvisable, colectomy or colotomy and polypectomy should be performed.

Fibrosarcoma

Of the sarcomas involving the gastrointestinal tract, fibrosarcoma is one of the rarest. Stoller and Weinstein reported 21 cases of fibrosarcoma of the rectum in the literature from 1927 until 1954 and added 2 cases of their own.[236] The mean age of the patients in this series was 51 years. All tumors were situated in the rectum within 10 cm of the pectinate line. Only two cases of fibrosarcoma of the colon have been reported.[24, 121] Espinosa and Quan reported the only case of *anal* fibrosarcoma.[71] The lesion apparently arose at the site of a previous fistulectomy incision.

The commonest presenting symptom of fibrosarcoma of the rectum is difficulty with defecation. Pain is the second commonest symptom, and bleeding,

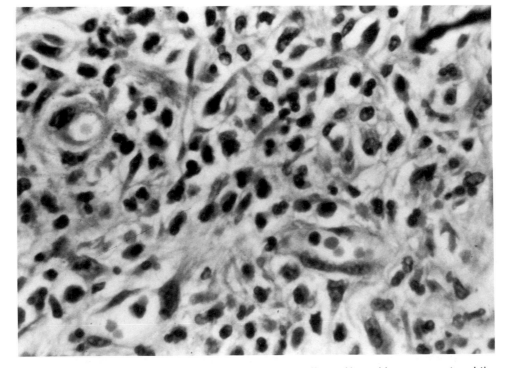

FIG. 13-16.   Inflammatory fibroid polyp. The bowel wall is infiltrated by many eosinophils. Note some fibroblasts and small blood vessels lined by prominent endothelial cells. (Original magnification × 280. Courtesy of Rudolf Garret, M.D.)

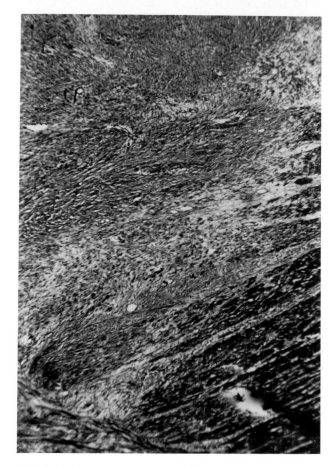

FIG. 13-17. Fibrosarcoma: a well-differentiated tumor infiltrating the wall of the bowel. (Trichrome stain; original magnification × 80. Courtesy of Rudolf Garret, M.D.)

third.[236] Proctosigmoidoscopic examination may reveal the tumor to be consistent with an adenocarcinoma, and only histologic determination can establish the definitive diagnosis.

Microscopically, the tumor is characterized by strands of fibrous tissue that infiltrate the adjacent structures of the bowel wall but tend to spare the mucosa until late in the disease (Figs. 13-17 and 13-18).[236] The presence of mitoses is helpful in establishing the diagnosis if it is fibrosarcoma.

Treatment is essentially the same as that for adenocarcinoma: radical resection of the involved rectum either with or without a sphincter-saving approach. Radiotherapy or chemotherapy has not been helpful in the management of this rare condition.

Malignant Fibrous Histiocytoma

Malignant fibrous histiocytoma is an extremely rare fibrosarcoma variant in which histiocytic-like cells are present.[223, 260] The term was originally proposed by O'Brien and Stout to describe tumors composed of both fibroblasts and histiocytes (Fig. 13-19).[181] The lesion is usually found in the lower extremity.

It is difficult to present a meaningful evaluation of the signs, symptoms, diagnosis, therapy, and prognosis with such an uncommon lesion. Tumors tend to be large, present with obstructive symptoms, and are thought to be adenocarcinomas clinically. Treatment is radical resection; prognosis is presumably poor.

Leiomyoma

Smooth muscle tumors of the alimentary tract are rare, and benign smooth muscle tumors of the colon are exceedingly uncommon. Stout conducted a 50-year study in which he found 30 leiomyomas in 200 benign neoplasms.[237] In a 15-year study, Ferguson and Houston reported two leiomyomas in 67 benign tumors.[77] Skardalakis and colleagues reviewed 59 cases of leiomyomas, and MacKenzie and co-workers collected reports of 19 cases from the literature and added 8 cases of their own.[152, 228]

Lookanoff and Tsapralis observed that the sigmoid and transverse colon seemed to be the commonest sites and that very few leiomymas were found in the cecum.[148] The tumor may be an incidental finding in an asymptomatic patient, or the patient may present with pain or a lump. Perforation, intestinal obstruction (secondary to the tumor itself or to intussusception), and hemorrhage have been reported.[173]

Smooth muscle tumors are found in patients of all ages with a gradual increase in frequency and malignant degeneration up to sixth decade.[133] The tumor is classified according to its appearance and direction of growth. The intracolonic type may be pedunculated or sessile. The extracolonic type grows away from the lumen of the bowel and lies in the abdominal cavity attached to the wall. The dumbbell type grows into the lumen and into the abdominal cavity simultaneously. This type of tumor accounts for 4% of all smooth tumors of the gastrointestinal tract. These usually reach a much larger size than those with unilateral spread. The constrictive type encircles a variable length of bowel.

Macroscopically, the tumor appears well encapsulated. On cross section, leiomyomas have a fleshy ap-

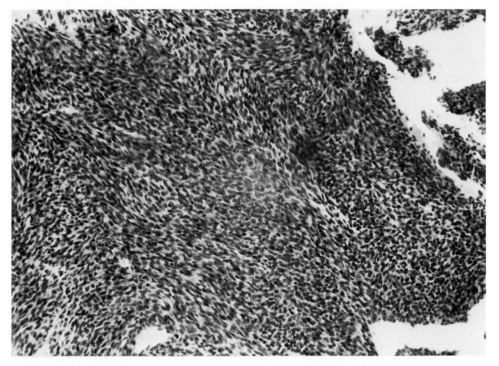

FIG. 13-18. Fibrosarcoma: cellular tumor consisting of bundles of undifferentiated fibroblasts. (Original magnification × 280. Courtesy of Rudolf Garret, M.D.)

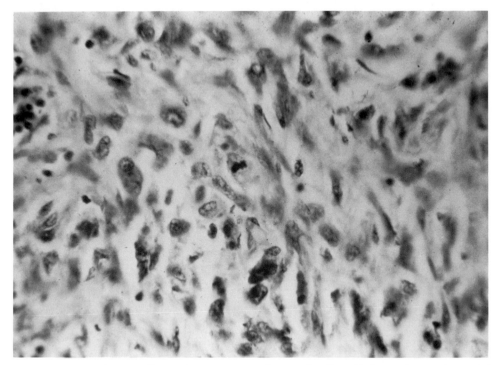

FIG. 13-19. Malignant fibrous histiocytoma: elongated cells with hyperchromatic nuclei and some mitotic figures. Some cells demonstrate large amounts of cytoplasm suggesting histiocytic origin. (Original magnification × 600. Courtesy of Rudolf Garret, M.D.)

445

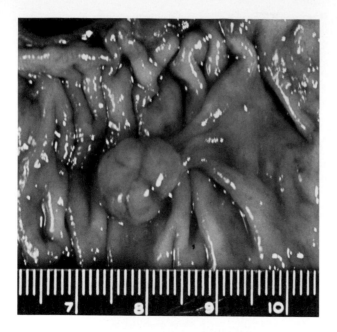

FIG. 13-20. Pedunculated leiomyoma.

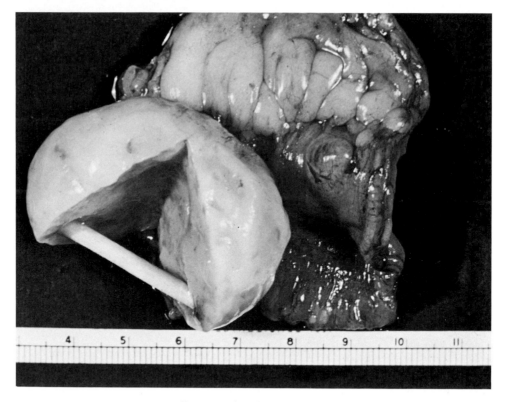

FIG. 13-21. Leiomyoma: a well-encapsulated mass in the bowel wall. (Courtesy of Rudolf Garret, M.D.)

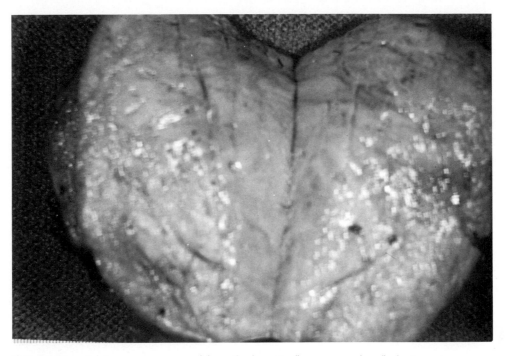

FIG. 13-22.   A leiomyoma removed from the hepatic flexure reveals a fleshy tumor on cross section. (Courtesy of Rudolf Garret, M.D.)

pearance; since the tumor is under pressure it tends to protrude (Figs. 13-20, 13-21, and 13-22).

Most investigators believe that the mitotic rate is the single most important criterion for diagnosis of malignancy (Fig. 13-23).[28, 34, 72, 238] Other indicators are a variation in nuclear size and shape, hyperchromasia,[28] frequent bizarre cells, and difficulty in identification of longitudinal myofibrils.[34, 72] If the mitotic rate is high, if the growth is rapid, if an ulcer is present, or if the lesion is more than 2.5 cm in diameter, malignant degeneration should be suspected. Smooth muscle tumors are usually locally invasive, but metastasis from a primary tumor in the gastrointestinal tract has been described.[34]

Radiologic features vary, depending on whether the tumor is intramural, submucosal, subserosal, or dumbbell shaped.[20] Surgery results in cure unless the tumor is extraperitoneal or rectal. Complete excision should be attempted regardless of the radiologic appearance or of probable inoperability.

Swerdlow and co-workers reported a case of an elderly patient with a benign leiomyoma of the cecum that had ulcerated and perforated the bowel wall.[243] The patient presented with an acute abdomen. Since it is generally not possible to distinguish benign from malignant lesions preoperatively, a standard cancer op-

eration should be performed under such circumstances.

Only a handful of cases of *rectal leiomyomas* have been reported.[11, 178, 220] Smaller myomas usually cause no symptoms, can be found on routine rectal examination, and are usually removed with a diathermy snare or by transanal excision. Large tumors may cause interference with defecation, a sense of fullness in the rectum, and a frequent desire to defecate. Because of these distressing symptoms and the possibility of obstruction and malignant degeneration, removal of the growth is indicated. When the tumor is extrarectal, it is best to excise it from outside rather than through the rectum. These tumors tend to arise from the internal anal sphincter.

Large tumors may be treated by local excision, but if any clinical suspicion of malignancy exists, such as ulceration, hemorrhage, or extrarectal fixation, radical surgical treatment by excision of the rectum is indicated. Biopsies are difficult to interpret in such cases.

Leiomyosarcoma

Leiomyosarcoma of the *large bowel* is a very rare lesion; the total number of published cases is probably fewer than 50.[14, 18, 20, 39, 45, 201, 209, 222, 234] No age predilection

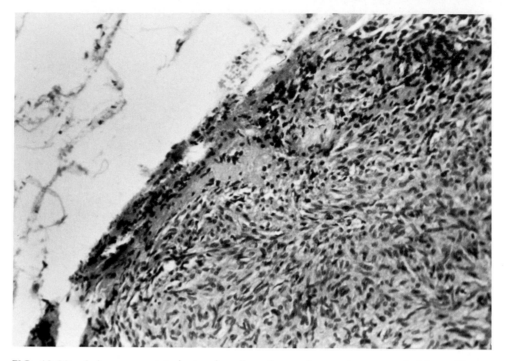

FIG. 13-23. Leiomyoma: interlacing bundles of smooth muscle surrounded by a fibrous capsule. No mitoses are evident. (Original magnification × 260. Courtesy of Rudolf Garret, M.D.)

for this disease is apparent. It affects the sexes equally and is more than twice as common in the rectum as it is in the rest of the colon.

Leiomyosarcoma arises from the smooth muscle of the bowel wall (Fig. 13-24). A very insidious disease, it can remain asymptomatic for a long period. Weight loss is almost never recorded, but pain is a common symptom. Tarry stools and the sequelae of anemia are the most frequent presentations (Fig. 13-25). A palpable tumor is almost always present when the lesion occurs in the rectum, and, in some instances, obstruction is also seen.

Diagnosis of this lesion preoperatively is extremely difficult because it resembles carcinoma of the colon in its radiographic appearance. The tumor may project into the lumen of the bowel, grow outward, or present as a dumbbell-type tumor.[210] An interesting radiologic finding may be demonstrated when tracks of barium extend into subserosal tumors.[39] Sonographic features may include a thick echogenic rim with central cavitation.[131] Colonoscopy and biopsy are useful in establishing the diagnosis.

Most of the reported cases have been managed by resection of the tumor-bearing portion of the colon.

Leiomyosarcoma is usually a tumor of low-grade malignancy. Patients who have been treated by resection have lived many years despite residual tumor or metastases.[95] The lungs and regional lymph nodes are rarely involved, but the tumor does have a tendency to metastasize to the liver.

An attempt to stage the disease for the sake of better management has been reported by Astarjian and co-workers, as follows[14]:

Stage I. Tumor confined to the intestinal wall; no invasion, no ulceration
  A. Submucosal tumors
  B. Subserosal tumors
Stage II. Tumor extending beyond the wall of the colon
  A. Intraluminal ulceration
  B. Infiltration into adjacent extracolonic tissues
Stage III. Tumor with distant metastases

Based on this staging and on the slow-growing nature of colonic leiomyosarcoma, these investigators

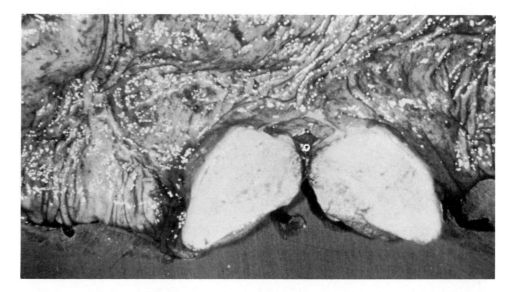

FIG. 13-24.   Leiomyosarcoma. This tumor of the bowel wall looks well encapsulated, but histologic examination revealed frequent mitotic figures. (Corman ML, Veidenheimer MC, Swinton NW: Diseases of the Anus, Rectum and Colon. Part I: Neoplasms. New York, Medcom, 1972)

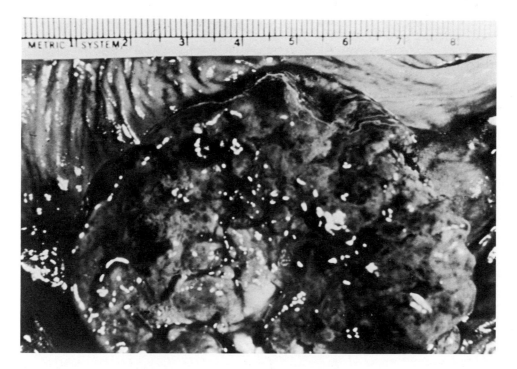

FIG. 13-25.   Leiomyosarcoma: ulcerating lesion producing hematochezia. The absence of infiltrating margins indicate that it is less likely to be adenocarcinoma. (Corman ML, Veidenheimer MC, Swinton NW: Diseases of the Anus, Rectum and Colon. Part I: Neoplasms. New York, Medcom, 1972)

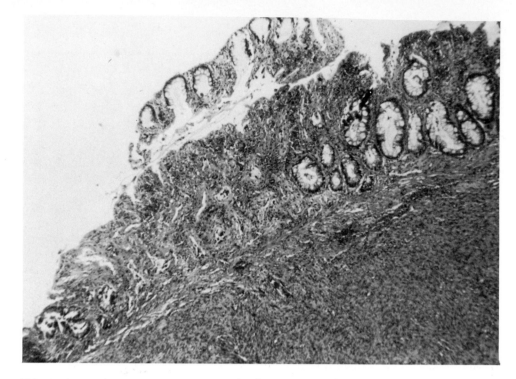

FIG. 13-26. Leiomyosarcoma: a mass of cells consisting of smooth muscle fibers adjacent to the muscularis mucosae of the rectum. (Original magnification × 80. Courtesy of Rudolf Garret, M.D.)

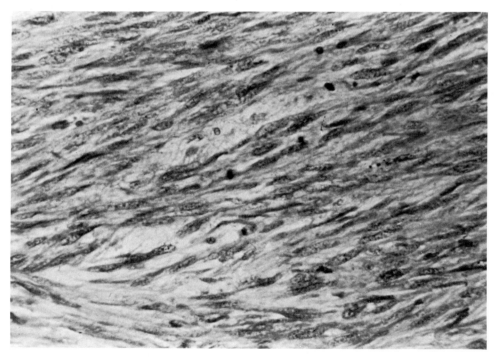

FIG. 13-27. Leiomyosarcoma: smooth muscle fibers showing at least six mitotic figures. (Original magnification × 600. Corman ML, Veidenheimer MC, Swinton NW: Diseases of the Anus, Rectum and Colon. Part I: Neoplasms. New York, Medcom, 1972)

suggest prognosis for patients with this tumor as follows:

Stage I-A and B: Excellent
Stage II-A: Excellent
Stage II-B: Fair
Stage III: Poor

The accuracy of prognosis based upon the degree of differentiation has been described by the Mayo Clinic group.[5] Grade 1 tumors have a greater abundance of cells than leiomyomas; mitotic activity is minimal with no pleiomorphism or anaplasia. With Grade 2 tumors, mitoses are noted in one of five high-power fields. In Grade 3 leiomyosarcoma, a mitosis is seen in every high-power field. Grade 4 lesions demonstrate marked cellularity, pleomorphism, and three or more mitoses per high-power field.

More than 100 cases of *rectal leiomyosarcoma* have been recorded in the literature.[11, 15, 29, 69, 82, 171, 200, 218, 231, 232, 242, 250, 275] The tumor arises in the smooth muscle of the rectal wall. Most of these tumors are seen in the lower third of the rectum and more commonly in men than in women. The tumor may present as a nodular or protuberant swelling with some central ulceration that appears to arise in the deeper layers of the bowel wall. Most of these tumors are large and consist microscopically of interlacing bands of smooth muscle fibers that are well differentiated and histologically of a low-grade malignancy (Figs. 13-26 and 13-27). Extensive direct spread into the perirectal tissue is a characteristic feature. This may make surgical removal so difficult that local recurrence even after excision of the rectum is not uncommon.

Smooth muscle sarcomas of the rectum do not usually metastasize to regional lymph nodes unless they are poorly differentiated; an exception was described by Thorlakson and Ross in a case with lymphatic spread to one hemorrhoidal lymph node and with venous involvement.[250]

Morson pointed out that although the majority of leiomyosarcomas are of a low-grade malignancy, the ultimate prognosis is very poor.[171] This is essentially because of late diagnosis and extensive local spread by the time of surgery. Rectal disease has an overall survival rate of 20%.[69] Apart from local recurrence, metastasis to the liver and lungs is the commonest cause of death. Many of these patients give a rather long history of symptoms before coming to treatment.[5] Their general clinical course confirms the histologic observation that these smooth muscle tumors are mostly well differentiated and of a low-grade malignancy. Local excision is liable to be followed by recurrence, even though this may be delayed for some years.[60, 76] A standard cancer resection is the recommended treatment for all operable lesions. Although the tumor is not radiosensitive, chemotherapy with vincristine, cyclophosphamide, actinomycin D, and adriamycin has been advocated because of the poor prognosis.[12]

Lipoma

Excluding hyperplastic polyps, lipoma is the second most common benign tumor of the colon (after adenomatous polyp) and the commonest intramural tumor; however, it is still a relatively rare entity. Weinberg and Feldman reviewed over 60,000 autopsy reports and found only 135 lipomas of the colon (0.2%).[263] Haller and Roberts found only 11 lipomas in over 3400 autopsies (0.3%).[105]

Colonic lipomas are well-differentiated, benign fatty tumors arising from deposits of adipose connective tissue in the bowel wall (Fig. 13-28); malignant change has not been reported. Approximately 90% are submucosal and 10% subserosal. The submucosal lipoma is covered by mucosa and occasionally by muscularis mucosae, and grows toward the intestinal lumen (Figs. 13-29 and 13-30). The mucosa covering the tumor

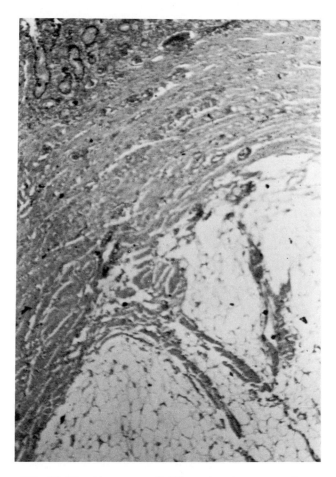

FIG. 13-28. Lipoma: well-differentiated mature adipose tissue in the wall of the bowel. (Original magnification × 260. Courtesy of Rudolf Garret, M.D.)

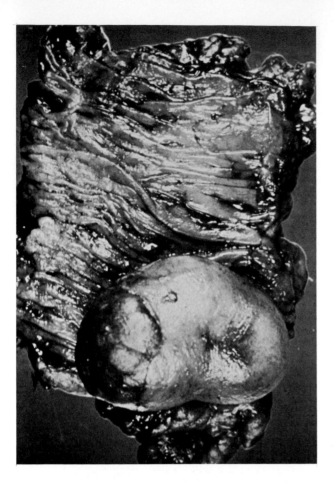

FIG. 13-29. Submucosal lipoma in the region of the ileocecal valve. (Corman ML, Veidenheimer MC, Swinton NW: Diseases of the Anus, Rectum and Colon. Part I: Neoplasms. New York, Medcom, 1972)

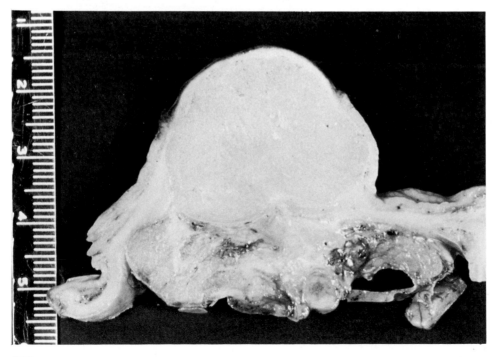

FIG. 13-30. Lipoma: a formalin-fixed specimen of a well-circumscribed mass in the wall of the large bowel. (Courtesy of Rudolf Garret, M.D.)

cending colon, and sigmoid colon. Pemberton and McCormack found 50 tumors in the right colon, 15 in the transverse colon, and 37 in the left colon and rectum.[191] Castro and Stearns reported 45 tumors, 31 of which were in the right colon (69%).[40] Eleven of their patients (26%) had two or more lipomas, and four had three or more. All multiple lipomas were found in the right half of the colon. Swain and co-workers reported a child with lipomatous polyposis throughout the entire colon, and Ling and associates resected the colon of a 60-year-old woman with 107 lipomas.[146, 239]

Radiographically, colonic lipomatosis must be differentiated from numerous benign and malignant conditions (Figs. 13-32 through 13-34). These include familial polyposis,[158] juvenile polyposis,[227] Gardner's

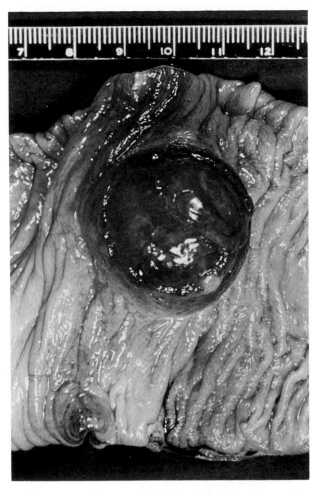

FIG. 13-31. Submucosal lipoma of the transverse colon. Rectal bleeding is explained by the hemorrhagic appearance of the lesion. (Courtesy of Rudolf Garret, M.D.)

may become atrophic, congested, ulcerated, or even necrotic, or it may retain its normal yellowish appearance. The subserosal type usually originates from the appendices epiploicae and grows toward the peritoneal cavity.

Most colonic lipomas are asymptomatic and are found at autopsy or incidentally during operation for some other problem. Symptoms may include constipation, diarrhea, abdominal pain, and rectal bleeding (Fig. 13-31). Colonic lipomas usually occur in patients between the ages of 50 and 70 years with about an equal sex distribution. The average age is similar to that of patients with colonic carcinoma. However, patients with colonic lipoma do not appear ill nor do they experience anorexia, weight loss, or anemia.

The commonest sites for lipoma are the cecum, as-

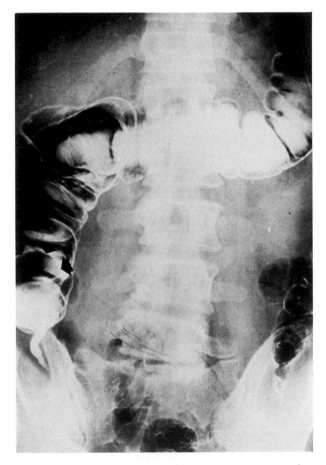

FIG. 13-32. Lipoma: barium enema demonstrates a characteristic filling defect in the proximal ascending colon (*arrows*). The smooth, spherical outline is practically pathognomonic of this disease. (Corman ML, Veidenheimer MC, Swinton NW: Diseases of the Anus, Rectum and Colon. Part I: Neoplasms. New York, Medcom, 1972)

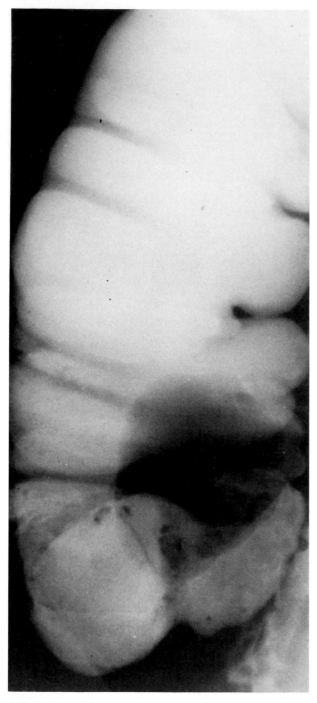

FIG. 13-33.   A lipoma of the ileocecal valve that produced abdominal pain and vomiting.

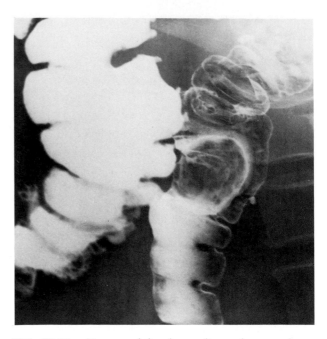

FIG. 13-34.   Lipoma of the descending colon: a submucosal polypoid mass without mucosal irregularity or destruction. The patient complained of left upper abdominal pain.

syndrome,[276] Cronkhite-Canada syndrome,[56] Peutz-Jegher's syndrome,[94] nodular lymphoid hyperplasia,[83] inflammatory bowel disease with pseudopolyposis, lymphosarcoma,[270] ganglioneurofibromatosis,[36] malacoplakia,[214] pneumatosis coli, and colitis cystica profunda.[262] A water enema with low kilovoltage technique may take advantage of the different absorption coefficients of fat and water; fat-containing lesions will appear relatively radiolucent.[157]

Mucosal lipomas can also be diagnosed by the colonoscope.[59] Occasionally, they may be removed by means of this instrument.[22, 261] This approach is usually limited to symptomatic patients and those in whom the lesion is somewhat pedunculated (Figs. 13-35 and 13-36).

Colonic lipomas do not require treatment except when they ulcerate. Once the diagnosis has been established and carcinoma has been ruled out, the patient need only be reassured. However, in the symptomatic patient, a limited resection or colotomy and lipomectomy is usually advised.

Lipoma of the rectum is extremely rare. When it can be reached digitally, it usually is felt as a soft, smooth, lobulated mass. If it is seen with the aid of a proctoscope, the yellow color of the fat of which it is composed is usually apparent through the mucosa. The

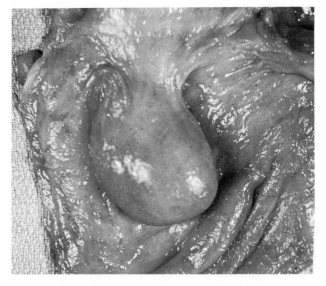

FIG. 13-35. Pedunculated lipoma treated by bowel resection. (Courtesy of Rudolf Garret, M.D.)

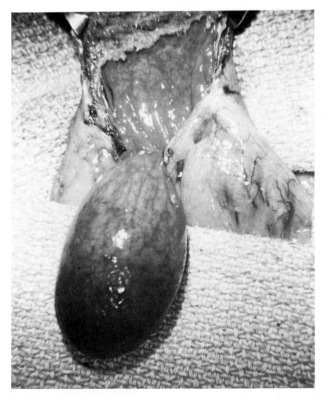

FIG. 13-36. Pedunculated lipoma at laparotomy, treated by colotomy and lipomectomy. Attempt at colonoscopic removal was unsuccessful.

most frequent site in the rectal area is the perianal region, in which case the tumor develops from the subcutaneous tissue.

Lipomas in the perianal region and buttocks usually cause no symptoms unless they become quite large, and the overlying skin becomes irritated. Situated in the rectum and the sigmoid, they may produce symptoms because of their size or when traumatized. Tenesmus may be produced when the growth is in the lower rectum and involves the internal sphincter.

Ligation of the base and removal may be performed when the tumor is pedunculated. Incision and enucleation may be employed if the lipoma is confined to the rectal wall.

TUMORS OF NEURAL ORIGIN

Neurofibroma, Neurilemoma (Schwannoma), and Ganglioneuromatosis

Von Recklinghausen first described multiple neurofibromatosis in 1882.[258] Subcutaneous neurofibromas were noted; the condition has since been known as von Recklinghausen's disease. Visceral involvement in disseminated neurofibromatosis is considered rare, yet reports appeared as early as 1930.[64] The possibility of this disease should be considered if gastrointestinal bleeding or intestinal obstruction occurs in a patient known to have generalized neurofibromatosis.[23, 101, 141, 155, 197] However, it may be seen in the alimentary tract and nowhere else.

The lesions in the intestinal tract arise in the submucosa or muscularis (Figs. 13-37 and 13-38).[90] As the neurofibroma enlarges, the overlying mucosa becomes ulcerated and bleeds. Intussusception can produce intestinal obstruction. Sarcomatous degeneration is a recognized complication.[141]

Local excision is preferred unless a large cluster is noted in one segment; under these circumstances resection may be advisable.

Donnelly and colleagues reported a 9-year-old boy who underwent total colectomy because of multiple colonic polyps that caused severe rectal bleeding.[63] Of the two kinds of polyps found, one was largely composed of groups of ganglion cells and nerve fibers in trunks and networks, and the other resembled retention polyps. Ganglion cells, nerve fiber networks, or both were also found in the nonpolypoid colonic mucosa and in the mucosa of the stalks of the retention polyps. These authors selected the term *ganglioneuromatosis* for its descriptive value, and suggested that this

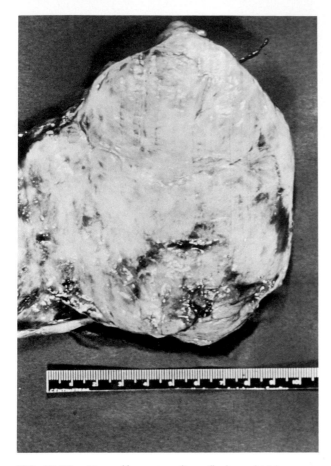

FIG. 13-37. Neurofibroma: a firm, fleshy, whitish tumor attached to wall of the bowel. (Courtesy of Rudolf Garret, M.D.)

lesion is probably akin to neurofibromatosis and should be distinguished from ganglioneuroma, although its precise relationship to the former is not definitely established. Normann and Otnes reported a case of diffuse intestinal ganglioneuromatosis in which severe diarrhea was the predominant symptom.[179]

Ganglioneuromas are neuroectodermal tumors that are rarely found in the colon (Fig. 13-39). They are composed of nerve fibers, Schwann sheath elements, and ganglion cells (Fig. 13-40 and 13-41.).[30] When solitary, they may resemble a carcinoma radiologically. Treatment is local excision or resection.

Neurogenic tumors have been reported to be the cause of masses in the presacral space. Kovalcik and co-workers removed a 13-cm *neurilemoma* by means of a combined abdominotranssacral approach.[139]

Granular Cell Tumor

Granular cell tumor is an uncommon tumor of uncertain histogenesis. It was first described in 1926 by Abrikossoff, who named the tumor because of its resemblance to primitive myoblasts and its proximity to striated muscle.[2] He believed that neoplastic cells were formed from damaged adult muscle cells in the process of regeneration. Willis regarded the process as nonneoplastic and regenerative in nature.[268] However, Klinge suggested that the tumor could arise from heterotopic rests of myoblasts, a theory that was later accepted by Abrikossoff and Murray.[3, 137, 174]

Fisher and Wechsler, using electron microscopy and histochemical studies, concluded that the tumor had a definite neural pattern most closely resembling a damaged Schwann cell.[80] They believed that it was not similar to muscular tissue and noted that the tumor had a more histiocytic than neoplastic nature (Fig. 13-42). I have elected to place this tumor in the classification under neural origin for these reasons.

Usually the tumor involves the tongue (33%), skin and subcutaneous soft tissues (10%), and skeletal muscle (5%). About 50% of the tumors occur in the oral cavity and nasopharynx.[47] However, it has also been reported in most other organ systems. Involvement of the gastrointestinal tract is rare. Yanai-Inbar and associates, in their review of the literature, found 17 cases involving the large intestine, mainly in the proximal portion of the colon.[273] Only two tumors were identified in the rectum. Anal and perianal lesions have also been reported.[151, 205, 212, 269]

In the colon, granular cell tumors appear as yellowish-white submucosal nodules, usually less than 2 cm in diameter. Most are found incidentally, but abdominal pain and bleeding can occur. Malignant degeneration may result, but this is unusual, and the possibility of such an association is still controversial.

Treatment classically has been local excision if possible, or resection. Recent success with colonoscopic removal may prove to be the optimal therapy for most lesions.[153]

VASCULAR LESIONS

Hemangioma

Vascular malformations of the gastrointestinal tract have been reported since 1839 with Phillips' initial description of a lesion in the rectum.[194] These tumors

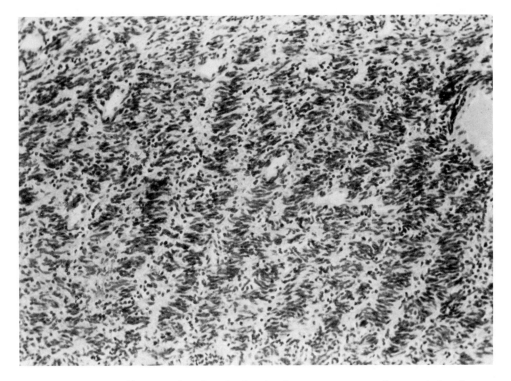

FIG. 13-38. Neurofibroma, showing the herring-bone appearance characteristic of nerve tissue tumor. (Original magnification × 260. Courtesy of Rudolf Garret, M.D.)

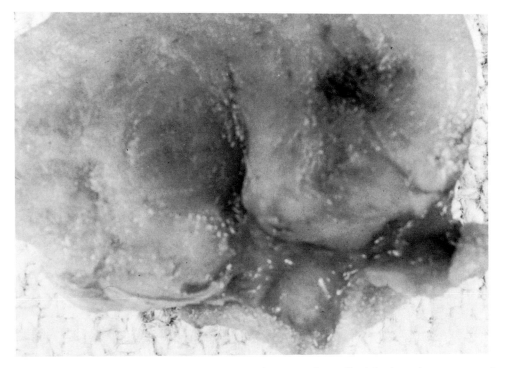

FIG. 13-39. Neurilemoma: a well-demarcated mass in the wall of the bowel. (Courtesy of Rudolf Garret, M.D.)

457

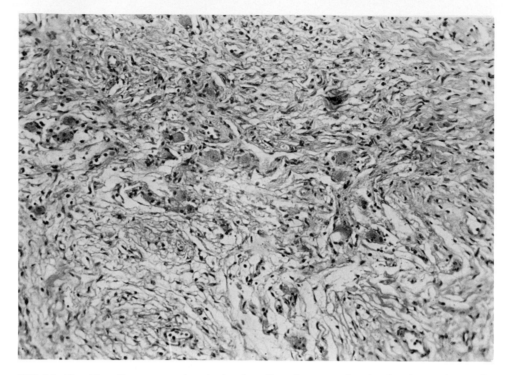

FIG. 13-40. Ganglioneuroma: interlacing bundles of nerve cells mixed with ganglion cells. (Original magnification × 260. Courtesy of Rudolf Garret, M.D.)

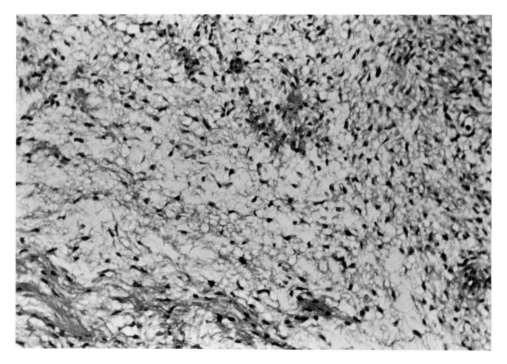

FIG. 13-41. Neurilemoma: edematous cells (Antoni A pattern) characteristic of schwannoma. (Original magnification × 260. Courtesy of Rudolf Garret, M.D.)

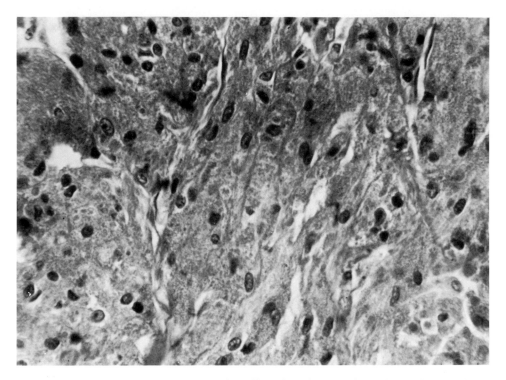

FIG. 13-42. Granular cell tumor: granular cells with uniform nuclei and granular cytoplasm. (Original magnification × 280. Courtesy of Rudolf Garret, M.D.)

are found in virtually every organ of the body; the skin is a particularly common location. However, hemangioma is one of the rarest tumors found in the colon. Gentry and associates reviewed the world literature through 1945 and found reports of 293 benign vascular tumors of the gastrointestinal tract.[89] Only 31 of these tumors were hemangiomas of the colon. Rissier reviewed 18 cases in 1960.[206] Thirteen additional reports of this lesion appeared in the literature between 1957 and 1971.[66, 79, 96, 136, 164, 170, 184, 188, 204, 213, 225, 235, 253] The Armed Forces Institute of Pathology included venous angiomas in its list of benign vascular malformations as well as arteriovenous angiomas (racemose aneurysms), plexiform angiomas, and several other variants of hemangiomas.[140]

The pathogenesis of these tumors is not well defined. However, they are generally agreed to be congenital, with their origin in embryonic sequestrations of mesodermal tissue. Enlargement occurs by projection of budding endothelial cells. Whether these growths are neoplastic or congenital is a matter of controversy.

The capillary hemangioma consists of small, thin-walled, closely packed vessels with a well-differentiated, hyperplastic endothelial lining. These tumors are distributed equally throughout the gastrointestinal tract. They comprise 6% of benign vascular tumors, arise from the submucosal vascular plexus, and are often encapsulated. Mucosal ulceration occurs in one half of these lesions.

The cavernous hemangioma is composed of large, thin-walled vessels that are much larger than those of the capillary hemangioma. The supporting stroma contains scant connective tissue and may contain smooth muscle fibers (Fig. 13-43). These lesions may be of the ''multiple phlebectasia'' type, characterized by a multitude of discrete tumors less than 1 cm in diameter. Although they represent one third of all the benign vascular tumors of the gastrointestinal tract, they are frequently overlooked. The simple polypoid type of cavernous hemangioma constitutes 10% of benign vascular intestinal malformations and is usually of sufficient size to produce such symptoms as obstruction and hemorrhage. The diffuse, expansive type varies widely in shape and size, and often involves 20 to 30 cm of intestine, occasionally in multiple locations. Diffuse cavernous hemangiomas, which produce severe symptoms at a relatively early age, account for 20% of intestinal angiomas.

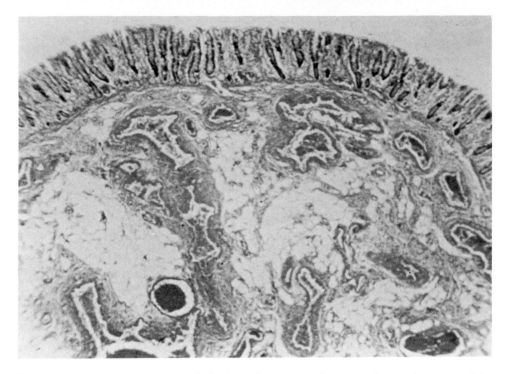

FIG. 13-43. Hemangioma: irregularly shaped arteries and veins in the areolar tissue of the submucosa. (Corman ML, Veidenheimer MC, Swinton NW: Diseases of the Anus, Rectum and Colon. Part I: Neoplasms. New York, Medcom, 1972)

Venous angiomas are often confused with cavernous hemangiomas. Both are composed of large, thin-walled vessels with large lumens. However, the walls of venous angiomas contain varying amounts of smooth muscle and usually resemble veins. Many of these tumors are extensive, especially those found in the extremities. Thrombosis is common in venous as well as in cavernous hemangiomas, and calcification frequently occurs in these thrombi and in the surrounding interstitial tissue.

Enlarged hemangiomas may produce symptoms of obstruction or hemorrhage. The obstructive symptoms may be caused by the tumor, volvulus, or intussusception. Intussusception has most frequently been reported from eastern Europe.

The commonest complication of hemangioma of the colon is bleeding; the incidence in colorectal hemangioma is 60% to 90%. Early onset and frequency of hemorrhage often lead to diagnosis in adolescence or early adulthood. Characteristically, colonic hemangiomas bleed episodically, slowly, and persistently; the symptoms are melena and the results of anemia: fatigue and weakness. Cavernous hemangiomas tend to bleed massively much more frequently than capillary hemangiomas. Melena begins in childhood, is recurrent throughout adolescence, and results in intermittent symptomatic anemia. Bleeding tends to become more severe with each recurrent episode. Although early onset of bleeding with recurrence usually leads to definitive diagnosis and treatment during adolescence, hemangiomas of the colon may be difficult to diagnose before laparotomy. A positive family history may be helpful.

Physical examination is often unremarkable, but the presence of hemangiomas of the skin or mucous membrane should raise a suspicion that a similar lesion might be present in the colon.

Barium enema examination may reveal a filling defect, and phleboliths may be noted within the filling defect (Fig. 13-44). Hollingsworth first documented the association of narrowing of the sigmoid colon on barium enema examination with an area of surrounding phleboliths.[122] The occurrence of phleboliths is probably related to thrombosis within the tumor and is seen particularly with cavernous hemangioma of the colon.[19, 122, 184] Selective angiography may also reveal a

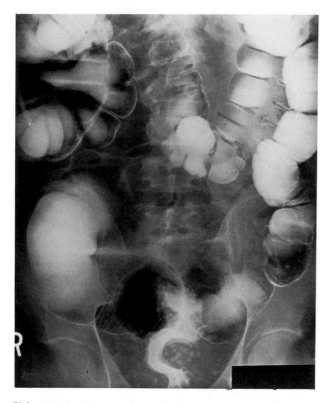

FIG. 13-44. Hemangioma: barium enema reveals extrinsic compression of the left wall of the rectum and irregularity of the rectosigmoid wall. The surrounding soft tissue mass contains multiple calcifications.

vascular malformation, particularly in the late vascular phase (see Figs. 14-31 and 14-32), although the differential diagnosis of angioma and A–V malformation is confusing.

Resection of a bleeding colonic hemangioma is optimal treatment. If the benign nature of the tumor can be determined at laparotomy and confirmed by adequate frozen section examination, local excision of the hemangioma is sufficient. If malignancy cannot be excluded, resection of the involved segment should be undertaken

Malignant vascular tumors include hemangioendothelioma, angiosarcoma, Kaposi's sarcoma, and benign metastasizing hemangioma, and represent approximately 13% of all vascular lesions of the colon and rectum.

Only 75 cases of *hemangioma of the rectum* had been reported in the world literature before 1978.[128] Treatments that have been proposed include sclerosing agents,[67] ligation of the feeding vessels,[85] local exci-

sion,[112] abdominoperineal resection,[113] and, most recently, coloanal anastomosis.[127]

Since radiation has been reported as a successful treatment for hemangiomas of the neck and face, Chaimoff and Lurie applied this technique in a woman who presented with a low-lying perirectal hemangioma.[41, 120, 221] Nearly 2 years after treatment, consisting of five successive sessions of 300 rads each (for a total of 1500 rads), the patient was asymptomatic.

Skovgaard and Sorensen reported an instance of hemangioma of the sigmoid colon in an 8-year-old boy whose tumor was diagnosed by colonoscopy.[229] These investigators believe that since hemangioma can be diagnosed radiographically only if it is large, and can easily be overlooked at exploratory laparotomy, colonoscopy should be used in evaluating all children with lower intestinal hemorrhage of unknown cause. Endoscopic diagnosis usually is not difficult; the tumor will appear deep red or purple. Hasegawa and colleagues performed colonoscopic polypectomy for a polypoid lesion, but their article was followed by an editorial comment cautioning the reader to be wary of the possibility of inducing uncontrolled hemorrhage.[109]

Lymphangioma

Lymphangioma of the gastrointestinal tract is a very rare lesion, and the colon is the least frequent site involved. Fleming and Carlson reported on nine lymphatic cysts of the abdomen diagnosed at the Mayo Clinic between 1959 and 1968.[81] Of these, three arose submucosally in the gastrointestinal tract, and one originated in the colon. Only eight lymphangiomas of the colon have been reported, one in the ascending colon, one in the hepatic flexure, four in the transverse colon, and two in the descending colon.[9, 13, 91, 100, 118, 138, 182]

The lesion originates in the lymphatic plexus within the submucosa into which the lacteals of the villi empty. In 1958, Willis noted the frequent association of lymphangioma with smooth muscle and believed that these cysts, like angiomas, are hamartomas rather than true tumors.[268]

Another theory considers lymphangiomas secondary to obstructed mesenteric lymph nodes, with subsequent stasis and dilation caused by a rise in pressure in the nodes, a mechanism similar to the production of postoperative lymphocysts.[62] If this theory were valid, one would expect an increased incidence of such lymphangiomatous cysts after laparotomy and abdominal node dissection; this finding has not been reported.

Lymphangiomas of the colon may be submucosal or pedunculated. The small number of documented submucosal lymphangiomas of the gastrointestinal tract does not permit satisfactory analysis of the radiologic characteristics.

The first report of lymphangioma of the rectum in an English-language journal was that of Chisholm and Hillkowitz in 1932.[44] In 1973 we reported the case of a woman with rectal bleeding.[51] A hemorrhoidectomy had been performed for this complaint. Proctosigmoidoscopy revealed numerous extramucosal cystic masses scattered from the anorectal ring to approximately 9 cm from the anal verge, and appearing to contain clear fluid.

After a gastrointestinal investigation produced negative findings, the cystic masses were excised through the operating proctoscope. Pathologically, a noncapsulated, poorly circumscribed mass of cavernous, thinwalled vascular channels occupied the submucosa.

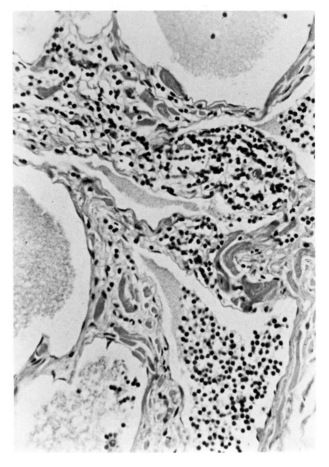

FIG. 13-46. Lymphangioma: endothelial-lined spaces, some of which contain lymphocytes. (Original magnification × 300. Corman ML, Veidenheimer MC, Swinton NW: Diseases of the Anus, Rectum and Colon. Part I: Neoplasms. New York, Medcom, 1972)

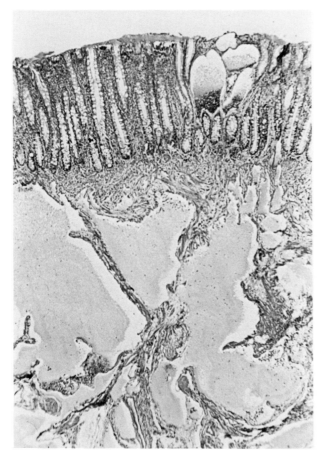

FIG. 13-45. Lymphangioma: endothelial-lined, irregular spaces in the submucosa of the bowel. (Original magnification × 80. Corman ML, Veidenheimer MC, Swinton NW: Diseases of the Anus, Rectum and Colon. Part I: Neoplasms. New York, Medcom, 1972)

These channels were irregular in size and shape. They had walls or septa formed of fibrous tissue and were lined by a single layer of flattened endothelium. Although the mucosal surface was intact throughout, focal discontinuities in the muscularis mucosa permitted some of the dilated lymphatic vessels to extend into the lamina propria. Homogeneous pink material, presumably lymph, filled most of the vessels (Fig. 13-45). A few contained erythrocytes. Accumulations of lymphocytes were present both within the lymphatic channels and in the thin septa between them. The diagnosis of lymphangioma was made because of the presence of lymphocytes within the vessel and septa, the scarcity of elastic tissue, and the predominance of lymphatic elements (Fig. 13-46).

The presence of blood vessels within many lesions designated as lymphangioma is well recognized and has been taken as evidence that these lesions actually represent vascular malformations or hamartomas rather than true neoplasms. Differentiation from hemangioma may be impossible in those lesions that lack abundant intraluminal and interstitial lymphocytes as evidence of their lymphatic origin.

Apart from lymphangioma, the histologic differential diagnosis includes lesions that may produce cystic spaces in the submucosal region of the bowel. The epithelial lining of colitis cystica profunda usually permits its easy recognition. However, the giant-cell lining that remains behind after dissolution of the oils in an oil granuloma (oleoma) may be more difficult to recognize. Gas cysts of recent origin may lack a lining. When they are chronic they are lined by giant cells similar to those of the oil granuloma.

None of the reported lymphangiomas of the colon and rectum has infiltrated the muscularis propria. However, such infiltration did occur in a lymphangioma of the small bowel reported by Wood.[271]

Excision biopsy with careful visualization under suitable anesthesia is the recommended procedure for rectal lesions. Colonoscopy is a valuable adjunct in the diagnosis of more proximal lesions. Colonoscopic polypectomy for pedunculated lymphangiomas appears to be satisfactory treatment, but a limited resection should be considered for all sessile or infiltrative tumors.

Hemangiopericytoma

Hemangiopericytoma is an extremely rare tumor that arises from pericytes and is usually found in the soft tissue of the trunk and extremities. A review of English-language publications revealed only two cases involving the colon. The small intestine is the commonest gastrointestinal site.[17, 87] Abdominal pain, intestinal obstruction, intussusception, and rectal bleeding are associated with intestinal tumors. Malignant degeneration is usually based on the clinical course (recurrence or metastases) rather than the histologic picture. Microscopically, the tumor is characterized by multiple endothelial-lined capillaries or capillary buds (Fig. 13-47). Resection is the treatment of choice.[87]

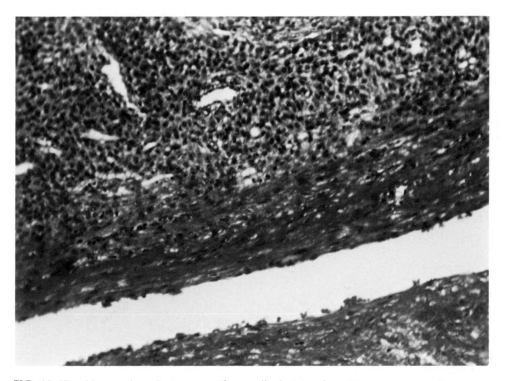

FIG. 13-47. Hemangiopericytoma: uniform cells deriving from Zimmermann pericytes surrounding the vascular spaces. (Original magnification × 260. Courtesy of Rudolf Garret, M.D.)

HETEROTOPIAS AND HAMARTOMAS

Endometriosis

Endometriosis is a disorder resulting from the presence of actively growing and functioning endometrial tissue, both glandular and stromal, in sites outside the uterus. The pathogenesis of this common disorder is not clearly understood. In 1897, Pfannenstiel reported the case of a patient with aberrant endometrium that involved the rectovaginal septum.[193] In 1909, Meyer reported the first case of bowel endometriosis; the patient ultimately required resection.[165] In 1922, Blair-Bell, in reporting a series of cases of aberrant endometrium, first used the terms *endometriosis* and *endometrioma*, the former for the disease, the latter for the individual cystic lesion.[32]

Many theories have been proposed to explain this disease. Sampson believed that fragments of endometrium regurgitated with the menstrual blood through the oviducts in a retrograde fashion and implanted onto peritoneal surfaces and pelvic and abdominal structures.[217] These eroded into the subserosal tissues with viable cells growing and functioning and in turn possibly leading to further implantation. This is the theory of tubal reflux and implantation.

Another theory proposed is that of coelomic epithelial metaplasia; it assumes that dormant, immature cellular elements of müllerian origin are known to persist into adult life, particularly throughout the central region of the pelvis. After menarche, repeated cyclic ovar-

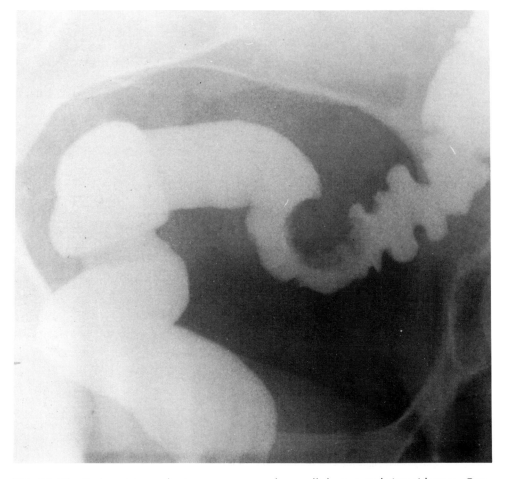

FIG. 13-48.   Endometrioma: barium enema reveals a well-demarcated sigmoid mass. Confusion with carcinoma should not occur because the lesion demonstrated here has an intact overlying mucosa.

ian stimulation of these elements with their totipotential capacities for differentiation could result in the metaplastic formation of functioning endometrial tissue in ectopic sites.

Other theories have been suggested, including lymphatic dissemination of endometrial cells and deportation of normal endometrium by way of venous channels. These do not seem to offer a satisfactory explanation for the pathology.

Endometriosis is seen almost exclusively in women; in 75% it occurs between the ages of 20 and 40 years, and in 25%, up to the age of menopause. Isolated case reports of endometriosis in men with prostatic cancer who are receiving estrogen therapy have appeared.[195]

The classic history is one of acquired or secondary dysmenorrhea. The pain is related to, but does not necessarily occur simultaneously with, each menstrual period. Pelvic discomfort associated with endometriosis is more likely to begin a day or two before the onset of menstrual flow, although its intensity may increase during the early days of menstruation. It tends to be a deep-seated ache or bearing-down pain in the lower part of the abdomen, posterior pelvis, vagina, or back, and often radiates into the rectal and perineal areas with tenesmus and symptoms of an irritable bowel. When, as is often the case, endometrioma of one or both ovaries is present, dull unilateral or bilateral lower abdominal pain, often with radiation to the thighs, may be noted.

The discomfort tends to abate after 2 or 3 days, subsiding completely toward the end of or just after the menstrual period. The patient will then be comfortable once more until a day or two before the onset of the next menstrual flow. However, as the disease progresses, pain tends to increase in severity and may last most of each cycle.

Not all patients with endometriosis have pain, however. Despite extensive disease palpable on pelvic examination or found at laparotomy, 15% to 20% of patients report no discomfort whatever. They may have other manifestations of the pathologic process, notably infertility or the presence of a mass. Other symptoms include dyspareunia, cyclic bowel disturbances with painful defecation, rectal bleeding, and intestinal obstruction. Although rectal bleeding is not a common presenting symptom of endometriosis, when associated with menses, colon endometriosis should be considered. Leakage or rupture of an enlarging ovarian endometrioma may produce generalized peritonitis and an acute abdominal problem. Spillage of the contents of a "chocolate" endometrial cyst produces an intense local irritation and inflammatory response that results in chemical peritonitis.

A characteristic, almost diagnostic, physical finding is the hard, fixed, fibrotic nodule in the uterosacral ligaments, cul-de-sac, or posterior surface of the lower uterine wall or cervix. This nodularity is almost universally present in patients with endometriosis and is pathognomonic of the disease. In endometriosis of the rectovaginal septum, bidigital rectovaginal examination helps to define the nature of the pathologic condition.

If the history is characteristic but the physical findings minimal and equivocal, laparoscopy or culdoscopy may prove valuable in establishing a definite diagnosis. When a trial of medical therapy is being considered, pelvic endoscopy using the laparoscope or culdoscope is important in establishing a precise diagnosis before treatment.

Endometriosis is frequently first discovered at the time laparotomy is performed for some other reason or with another diagnosis in mind. Other diagnostic tests include barium enema (Figs. 13-48 and 13-49), intravenous pyelography to determine location and degree of obstruction (if involvement of the ureters or periureteral tissue is suspected), and cystoscopy (during the menstrual period) to reveal the characteristic bluish-black, submucosal, cystic lesions if endometriosis of the bladder is suspected.

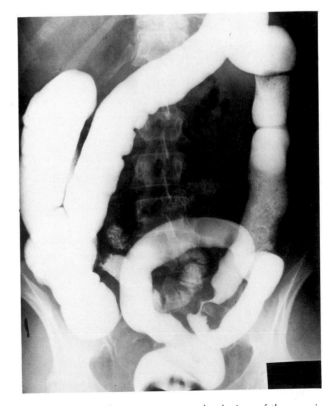

FIG. 13-49. Endometrioma: annular lesion of the proximal sigmoid. Since there is no mucosal abnormality, the lesion is either intramural or extrinsic.

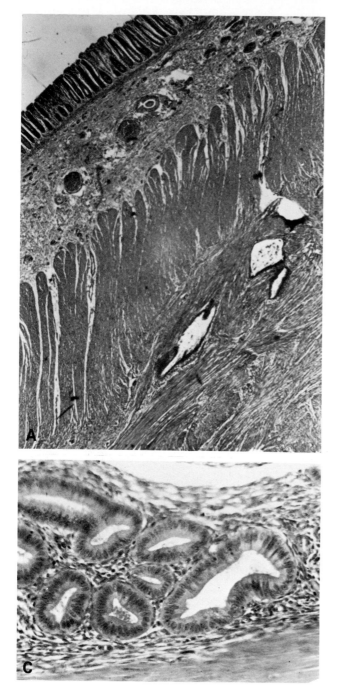

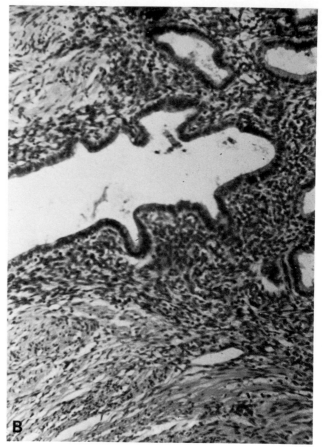

FIG. 13-50. Endometrial glands and stroma within the wall of the bowel. **A.** Original magnification × 80. **B.** Original magnification × 260. **C.** Original magnification × 400.

The three diagnostic histologic features of endometriosis are endometrial glands, endometrial stroma (Fig 13-50), and evidence of fresh hemorrhage (red cells and hemosiderin pigment) or old hemorrhage (hemosiderin-laden macrophages).

Because of its microscopic resemblance to normal endometrium and its known response to ovarian hormonal stimulation, the functioning epithelium of an endometrioma sometimes closely duplicates phases of the normal intrauterine endometrium, showing proliferative changes in the preovulatory or progestational phase. However, more often, the ectopic endometrial tissues are out of phase with the normal endometrium and are found in the proliferative stage even during the secretory phase of the normal menstrual cycle. This may be due to the difference in blood supply and the effects of increasing tissue fibrosis surrounding the endometriosis.

In the ovary the process is almost always bilateral. The tendency is for the formation of cystic structures varying from tiny bluish or dark brown blisters to large "chocolate" cysts. Usually present are considerable fibrosis and puckering of the ovarian surface in the region of the cyst, and adherence to neighboring structures.

Kistner observed that endometrial implants disappear after administration of large doses of progestins and estrogen.[135] Riva and associates likewise reported the beneficial effects of these compounds as observed by culdoscopy but cautioned about the rapidity of recurrence in some instances.[207] Gunning and Moyer, after using medroxyprogesterone acetate (Depo-Provera), demonstrated by culdoscopy and laparoscopy the shrinkage of endometrial tissue and confirmed microscopically that the endometriosis had disappeared.[104] The action of these therapies has not been completely elucidated. Endometriosis disappears, but follow-up studies have shown considerable variation in the rate of reappearance. The use of progestin alone or in combination with estrogen has become the standard method of hormonal treatment of endometriosis.

The most recent addition to the medical management of endometriosis is danazol (Danocrine).[99] In doses of 200 to 800 mg per day, studies showed that the pituitary inhibiting action resulted in suppression of ovulation, abolition of the midcycle increase of luteinizing hormone, and amenorrhea. The recommended dosage schedule for danazol in the treatment of endometriosis is 200 mg four times a day for at least 6 months. A maintenance dose of 200 to 400 mg daily may control pain after the initial treatment. Menstruation ceases with the commencement of therapy and returns promptly after the treatment has been discontinued. The pain of endometriosis is usually relieved in at least 80% of patients.

When endometriosis involves the small or large bowel it may be excised by careful dissection. Resection and anastomosis of the bowel is advisable for obstructing lesions (Fig. 13-51). However, caution is suggested against extensive dissection beneath the peritoneal reflection, in the posterior cul-de-sac, or in the rectovaginal septum. Fistula complicating low anterior resection for endometriosis is not an uncommon occurrence.

If pelvic endometriosis is so extensive that complete resection or fulguration is impossible or inadvisable, and if childbearing has been completed, bilateral oophorectomy is curative, since recurrence or progression

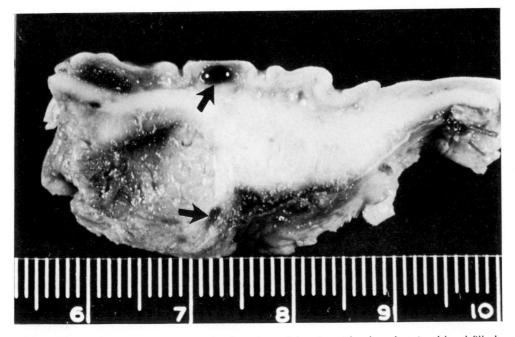

FIG. 13-51. Endometriosis: longitudinal section of the sigmoid colon showing blood-filled cysts *(arrows)*.

depends on cyclic ovarian hormone production. Natural menopause, if imminent, may also be relied on to cure the process. The most difficult therapeutic decisions arise when young women with extensive disease would like to retain reproductive potential. Reasonable efforts should be made to eradicate the disease surgically in these women. Postoperatively, patients should be advised to commence childbearing as soon as possible. Since pregnancy eliminates menstruation for a period of 9 months, some therapeutic benefit may be expected. When childbearing is completed, definitive surgical therapy is less emotionally traumatic. If childbearing is not a practical alternative, the patient should be given hormone therapy designed to prevent menstruation. Oral contraceptive pills given in a cyclic manner to allow intermittent withdrawal bleeding are not beneficial therapeutically. Birth control pills given daily and in sufficient potency to prevent breakthrough bleeding will result in softening, resorption, and necrobiosis of the endometrial glands. Medroxyprogesterone acetate, 100 to 150 mg, given by intramuscular injection every 2 to 3 months, will suppress menstruation. Its main disadvantages are occasional troublesome breakthrough bleeding requiring the addition of estrogen for control and, in a small percentage of women, permanent anovulation and resultant sterility. Medroxyprogesterone acetate is not generally recommended in patients who are interested in further childbearing; danazol is the treatment of choice.

In the experience of most physicians, hormone therapy does not always cure the process, but it gives the patient time to consider alternatives and to complete childbearing before progression of the disease or before increased symptoms and complications require the only successful therapy: bilateral oophorectomy with hysterectomy. After surgical castration for relief of endometriosis, estrogen replacement therapy to prevent menopausal symptoms should be instituted. Medroxyprogesterone acetate used for the first 6 to 9 months after surgery alleviates menopausal symptoms and promotes further necrobiosis of any residual endometriosis.

Perineal endometrioma is a special situation in which implantation of viable endometrial cells occurs in episiotomy incisions. A tender nodule producing cyclic symptoms at the site of an episiotomy is highly suggestive of the diagnosis.[107] Local excision is the treatment of choice, although suppressive therapy may be employed.

Hamartoma

Albrecht introduced the term *hamartoma* to describe tumor-like malformations that result from inborn errors of tissue development; they are characterized by abnormal mixtures of mature tissue indigenous to that area.[6] Hamartomas may be derived from any of the germinal layers, and any type of tissue may predominate.

According to Willis, the term *hamartoma* should be applied only to lesions for which evidence of a developmental anomaly is definite.[269] This includes either actual malformation with tissue excess present at birth or an inborn tissue anomaly that manifests itself by excessive growth continuing until puberty. The nomenclature depends on the tissue type that predominates: with vascular predominance, it is *angiomatous;* with fatty tissue, it is *lipomatous;* and with lymphoid tissue, it is *lymphomatous.*

Eichel and Hallberg have differentiated hamartomas from teratomas and dermoids.[68] The term *teratoma* describes a spontaneous, autonomous new growth derived from pluripotential tissues. It is foreign to the region in which it occurs and is composed of elements of all three germinal layers. A dermoid tumor has the same histogenesis but differs in that it is usually cystic. Unlike a teratoma, it originates from only two germinal layers, the ectoderm and the mesoderm. Clinically, it is difficult to differentiate between teratomas, dermoids (especially when small), and hamartomas.

Suspicion of hamartoma may be aroused by a small but definite funnel-shaped dimple in the posterior midline at the anal margin or the midanal level. This anal dimple associated with a higher lesion has been reported only once, although it must have been encountered many times.[249]

Complete surgical removal is the only effective treatment for retrorectal cystic hamartoma. The surgical approach may be either through the anal canal or posteriorly, transcoccygeally. However, in those instances in which a large cyst lies at a very high level, an abdominal approach is indicated.

Dermoid Cyst

Dermoid cysts are tumors of epithelial origin believed to be caused by faulty inclusion of ectoderm when the embryo coalesces. They generally do not appear until adult life and are commoner in women than in men.[126,177,244]

Galletly published a report in 1924 in which he stated "simple presacral cysts, lined by squamous or columnar epithelium, probably originate from cells of the neurenteric canal."[86] He included in his study 17 cases reported by Skutsch, all alleged to be dermoids.[230] Thomason reported on one patient with a deep suppurating sinus extending from an anal dimple into the presacral region, who required three operations.[249] Microscopic section showed a cyst lined with columnar epithelium and mucous glands in its wall. Robertson and Wride reported on a patient who had a tumor with a draining sinus at the base of the spine with a foul-smelling discharge.[208] The sinus had a convoluted pattern, was anterior to the sacrum and coccyx, and was lined with columnar epithelium of a mucous type. Gius and Stout reported on two patients, one of whom had three operations for multilocular lesions; the other underwent operation for an asymptomatic cystic tumor situated anterior to the coccyx.[92]

Patients may be asymptomatic but have an extra-rectal mass as an incidental finding on rectal examination. A cyst may become infected and mimic an anorectal abscess or fistula. Intraluminal cysts may produce varied rectal symptoms including hair protruding from the anus. A plain abdominal radiograph may be helpful.

Jackman and co-workers recognized the possibility that recurrent fistula may be associated with an infected dermoid cyst.[126] They believed that the cyst may arise from remnants of the neurenteric canal.

Two cases of malignant change in retrorectal cystic lesions have been reported. One patient had a sacro-coccygeal adenocarcinoma in a cyst lined by columnar epithelium and probably originating from remnants of postanal gut.[21] The second patient had an adenocarcinoma in a presacral enterogenous cyst.[57]

Resection of the mass can frequently be performed by means of a posterior approach, disarticulating the coccyx. An abdominal or abdominosacral approach may be required for more extensive or more proximal lesions. Prognosis is excellent; recurrence after surgery, however, is possible if the lesion is incompletely removed.

Dermoid cysts can occur in the rectum, but this is even more unusual than the postanal or presacral locations. Aldridge and colleagues identified only 12 cases.[7] The case they reported contained respiratory epithelium; the patient presented with rectal bleeding and prolapse of the mass. Transanal excision is the recommended approach.

Colitis Cystica Profunda (Enterogenous Cysts)

Colitis cystica profunda is a non-neoplastic condition characterized by the presence of mucous cysts deep to the muscularis mucosa and usually confined to the sigmoid colon and rectum. The commonest symptoms are rectal bleeding, passage of mucus, and diarrhea. It must be differentiated from mucus-producing adenocarcinoma.

Wayte and Helwig divided colitis cystica profunda into two groups: localized, in which the cysts are con-

fined to a distinct area of the rectum, and diffuse, in which the cysts are located in extensive areas.[262] The histogenesis of this benign condition remains in dispute. Based on differences in the evaluation of clinical and pathologic findings, the following descriptive terms have been used:

Colitis cystica profunda[70, 262]
Solitary ulcer of the rectum (see Chap. 17)[110, 127, 154]
Syndrome of the descending perineum (see Chap. 7)[189]
Enterogenous cysts of the rectum[246]
Hamartomatous inverted polyp of the rectum[8]

Colitis cystica profunda of the localized type may

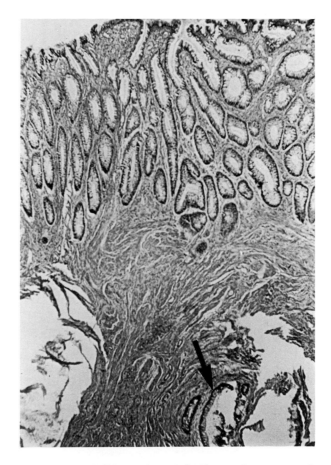

FIG. 13-52. Colitis cystica profunda: cystic structures in the wall of the bowel, one of which is lined by columnar epithelium *(arrow)*. The other cyst has lost epithelium. (Original magnification × 80. Corman ML, Veidenheimer MC, Swinton NW: Diseases of the Anus, Rectum and Colon. Part I: Neoplasms. New York, Medcom, 1972)

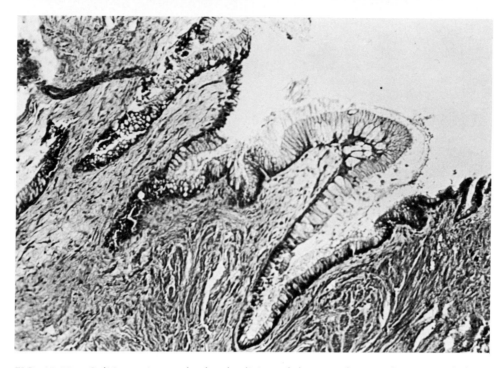

FIG. 13-53. Colitis cystica profunda: the lining of the cyst shows columnar epithelium. (Original magnification × 260. Corman ML, Veidenheimer MC, Swinton NW: Diseases of the Anus, Rectum and Colon. Part I: Neoplasms. New York, Medcom, 1972)

protrude slightly into the lumen of the bowel as a polypoid mass and can thus mimic carcinoma of the rectum.

The etiology of the condition is unknown. However, a number of patients have a history of prior rectal trauma, especially removal of a large polyp. Madigan and Morson described the correlation between anorectal dysfunction and this disease.[154] Epstein and associates theorized that the most probable primary factor was a weakness or defect in muscularis mucosa resulting in mucosal herniation.[70]

Differentiation by biopsy may be difficult.[8] In Madigan and Morson's series, 31 of 51 patients had lesions with histologic appearance suggestive of solitary ulcer or colitis cystica profunda (Figs. 13-52 and 13-53).[154]

Transanal excision of the lesion is the proper therapy if technically it can be performed. A transsacral approach may also be possible. Martin and associates reviewed the Mayo Clinic experience of 66 patients with this condition.[159] Less than three quarters were asymptomatic after local excision. Not uncommonly, the lesion is unresectable, except by radical abdominoperineal resection. Such treatment is contraindicated, however, for this benign condition. Reassurance and periodic proctosigmoidoscopy are suggested.

EXOGENOUS, EXTRINSIC, AND MISCELLANEOUS TUMORS

Metastatic Tumor

Metastatic tumor to the colon and rectum can produce obstructive symptoms, abdominal pain, bleeding, and change in bowel habits. Although usually producing extrinsic compression of the bowel on barium enema examination, ulceration may mimic primary carcinoma of the colon (Fig. 13-54). Tumors of adjacent organs that may invade the colon and rectum include prostate, uterus (Figs. 13-55 and 13-56), ovary (Fig. 13-57), kidney, stomach, duodenum, and pancreas. Metastatic disease can occur from breast, malignant melanoma, hypernephroma, and pulmonary origins.

Barium Granuloma

A submucosal rectal nodule that can be confused with a neoplastic condition, especially a carcinoid, may be due to a barium granuloma. Such lesions appear in the

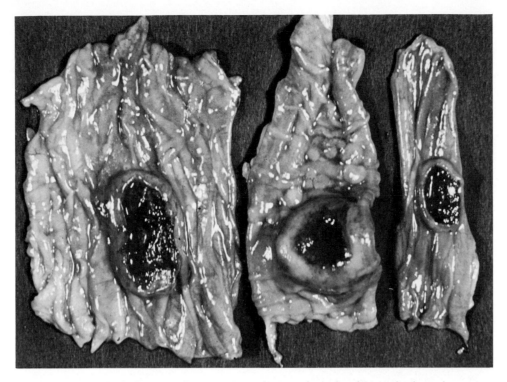

FIG. 13-54. Multiple lesions of metastatic melanoma from the skin to the bowel mucosa; normal mucosa surrounds the deep ulcer in the center. (Courtesy of Rudolf Garret, M.D.)

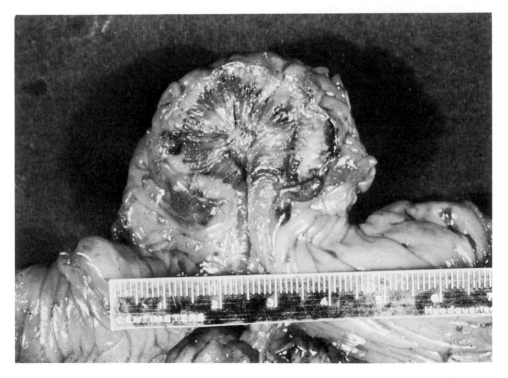

FIG. 13-55. Tumor on the serosa of the sigmoid from extension of uterine cervical cancer. (Courtesy of Rudolf Garret, M.D.)

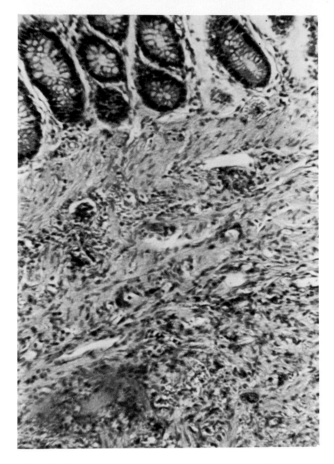

FIG. 13-56. Metastatic adenocarcinoma from the uterine cervix. Note the normal overlying colonic epithelium. The wall is infiltrated by tumor cells forming small glandular structures. (Original magnification × 260. Courtesy of Rudolf Garret, M.D.)

lower rectum, usually as submucosal white or yellowish plaques, and are usually asymptomatic. A break in the continuity of the rectal mucosa is the probable initiating factor. Transanal excision is mandatory for differential diagnosis.

Rand studied the effects of injection of barium in the rectal wall of dogs.[203] He produced a granulomatous ulcer that healed spontaneously despite retained barium in the tissues. Histologically, presence of barium in the tissue produces a typical foreign body granulomatous reaction.

Care in the introduction of the enema catheter and caution with the use of the balloon tip are clearly indicated for prevention of barium granuloma. A num-

ber of cases of rupture of the bowel with barium peritonitis have been reported when barium enema examination has followed rectal biopsy.[116] Margulis and Burhenne stated that a double-contrast examination of the colon should not be performed for at least 2 weeks after rectal biopsy.[156] I believe that if a polyp excision is contemplated on a patient who is to have a barium enema examination, the patient should initially complete the contrast study and then return for the other procedure.

Oleoma (Eleoma)

Oleoma, also known as oleogranuloma or paraffinoma, is a rare entity that occurs in the gastrointestinal tract or skin as a result of an injection of mineral oil (paraffin), enema oil, or vegetable oil. Although the lesion produced is not a true neoplasm, it is considered in this chapter because it may easily be confused with a benign growth. The differential diagnosis must be confirmed by biopsy to rule out other neoplastic and inflammatory conditions.

The clinical manifestations may develop very rapidly or may not present for many years after oil enters the tissue. The injection site usually appears as one or more irregular, firm nodules. In the gastrointestinal tract oleomas are usually found proximal to the dentate line in the lower portion of the rectum. The lesion may be defined as an intramural pseudotumor that develops as a foreign body reaction secondary to injection of any oily substance, usually mineral oil, for the treatment of hemorrhoids or oil enemas for constipation. The lesion is occasionally cystic and may be termed an oleocyst.

An oleoma is usually localized to the submucosa. However, considerable inflammation of the mucosa and even the perianal skin may be present. Histologically, oleomas are typified by large mononuclear phagocytes, epithelioid cells, eosinophilic leukocytes, and multinucleated giant cells of the foreign body type surrounding large, clear spaces that give the tissue a swiss-cheese appearance under low-power magnification. Histologic staining with oil red O verifies the presence of the lipid.

Mazier and associates reported four cases of oleoma.[160] All patients recovered after simple excision.

Malacoplakia

In 1902 Michaelis and Gutmann described malacoplakia as a rare chronic inflammatory disorder most

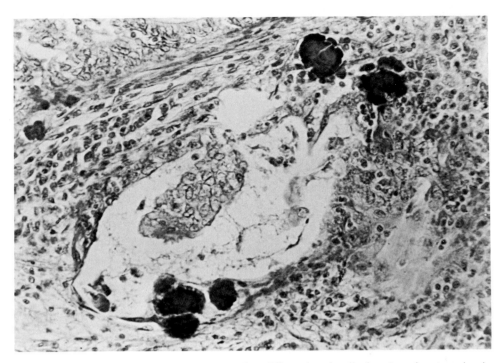

FIG. 13-57. Metastatic tumor consisting of undifferentiated cells forming abortive glands with psammoma bodies. The tumor was metastatic from an ovary. (Corman ML, Veidenheimer MC, Swinton NW: Diseases of the Anus, Rectum and Colon. Part I: Neoplasms. New York, Medcom, 1972)

commonly affecting the urinary bladder and other portions of the genitourinary tract.[166] In 1965, Terner and Lattes reported the first case of colonic involvement.[248] This was followed in the literature by several such cases.[202]

Clinical presentation is varied, but rectal bleeding, diarrhea, and obstructive symptoms are most commonly described. The lesion may be observed as an incidental finding. There is a preponderance of women among patients with the genitourinary lesion, but this is not the case among patients with colonic involvement.

The macroscopic lesion appears as a mucosal thickening or plaque and may assume a polypoid configuration. Histologically, one observes a proliferation of eosinophilic, coarsely granular histiocytes that often contain laminated calcific concretions, the so-called Michaelis-Gutmann bodies that are virtually pathognomonic of this entity (Fig. 13-58). The histiocytic proliferation is accompanied by a chronic inflammatory infiltrate and sometimes by fibrosis (Fig. 13-59).

Although the pathogenesis is not fully understood,

ultrastructural evidence suggests that altered heat response to certain species of gram-negative bacteria may be involved.[143] Abdou and co-workers have demonstrated a reversible lysosomal defect that might impair lysosomal bacterial killing in this disorder.[1] Sound ultrastructural evidence implies that the Michaelis-Gutmann body is a morphologic by-product of impaired lysosomal function.[149]

McClure reviewed the world literature in 1981 of malacoplakia of the gastrointestinal tract.[161] There were 34 recorded cases with 86 sites involved, most commonly in the rectum and colon.

Although the lesions are for the most part self-limited or responsive to antibiotic therapy, occasionally surgical intervention becomes necessary because of bleeding, the development of nonhealing fistulas, or localized anatomic complications. Biopsy and histologic examination are necessary to differentiate this lesion from carcinoma, which it may resemble clinically. It is of interest that malacoplakia has been associated, as an incidential finding, with colonic carcinoma.[161, 202]

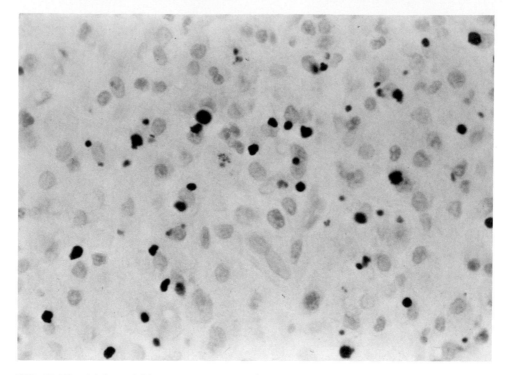

FIG. 13-58. Malacoplakia: von Kossa stain showing Michaelis-Gutmann bodies. (Original magnification × 600. Courtesy of Rudolf Garret, M.D.)

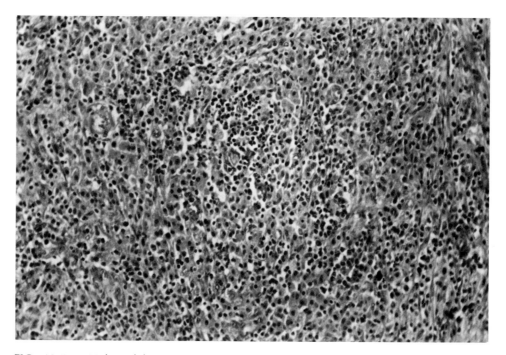

FIG. 13-59. Malacoplakia: many macrophages and lymphocytes are evident. (Original magnification × 260. Courtesy of Rudolf Garret, M.D.).

474

Sacrococcygeal Chordoma

Sacrococcygeal chordoma, a rare tumor of the fetal notochord, is characterized by a slow but inexorable progressive growth that usually spans a period of years. It invades by direct extension. Irrespective of the method of treatment chosen, the prognosis is poor. This tumor, thought by many to remain a local disease, has been reported to demonstrate distant metastases in up to 43% of patients.[88, 119]

Symptoms are produced as the tumor proliferates, often reaching considerable size before the diagnosis is made. Surrounding soft tissue and viscera are at first simply displaced. Adjacent bone is gradually eroded (Fig. 13-60).

The commonest initial symptom is pain; it is so gradual in onset and of such indefinite character that patients with this complaint often experience a delay in diagnosis of months to years. Constipation is the second commonest presenting symptom. The most significant physical finding is a firm, smooth, presacral mass with overlying intact rectal mucosa. There may be a history of prior treatment for a neurologic, orthopedic, or urologic disorder.

Bone destruction, a soft tissue mass, and anterior displacement of the rectum are the characteristic radiographic signs. These tumors often involve far more soft tissue than the osseous deformity would imply, and at operation, bone destruction is likely to be more extensive than was evident from the radiographic studies.[131]

The usual sites of distribution of chordoma are sacrococcygeal, 50%; spheno-occipital, 35%; and vertebral, 15%; there are rare examples of extranotochordal origin.[106]

Radiographic examination, including CT scan (Fig. 13-61), is the only investigative procedure of value in making the diagnosis of chordoma. Needle biopsy is to be condemned because of the possibility of implanting viable tumor cells (Figs. 13-62 and 13-63).

Cure of sacrococcygeal chordoma depends on complete extirpation of the tumor. I favor en bloc removal of the coccyx and the lower sacral segments with the lesion (Figs. 13-64, 13-65 and 13-66). The limiting factor in the extent of resection performed is mainly the second sacral segment, since removal of this will lead to permanent neurologic damage, and fecal and urinary incontinence. It is helpful to have neurosurgical consultation available in the operating room. The patient must understand the risk of nerve injury in spite of all precautions. In addition to neurologic impairment, resections more extensive than the lower three sacral segments may also result in instability and collapse of the pelvis and descent of the lumbar spine.[26, 190]

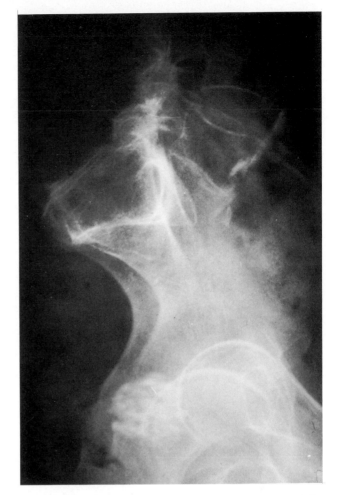

FIG. 13-60. Sacrococcygeal chordoma: invasion of the sacrum produces complete destruction, as seen on lateral projection.

Some surgeons favor a more radical approach, including abdominosacral resection or even posterior exenteration and sacrectomy.[147] Because of the high likelihood of recurrence,[42, 58, 119] my attitude is rather fatalistic; if the tumor cannot be excised by the posterior route alone, I do not believe the disease can be controlled by any means. I do not advocate radiation, because the tumor is not radiosensitive. If recurrence develops, surgical debulking may palliate pain symptoms; with radiated skin, healing may be considerably delayed or the wound may not heal at all. For unremitting pain, uncontrolled by medication, chordotomy may be necessary.

(Text continues on p. 479)

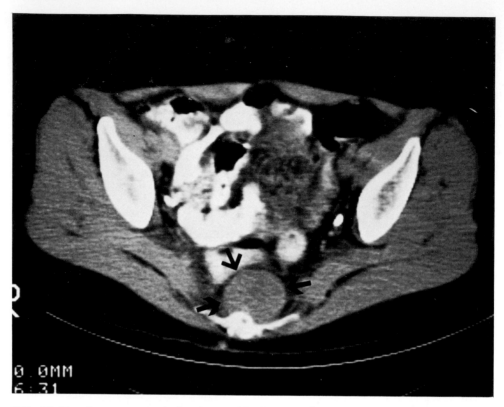

FIG. 13-61. Sacrococcygeal chordoma: this CT scan demonstrates a well-circumscribed mass invading the sacrum.

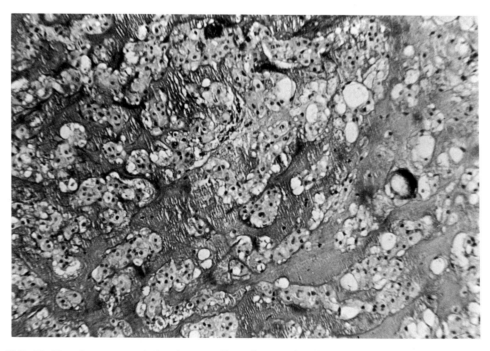

FIG. 13-62. Sacroccygeal chordoma: cells with vacuolated cytoplasm resembling chondrocytes. (Original magnification × 280. Courtesy of Rudolf Garret, M.D.)

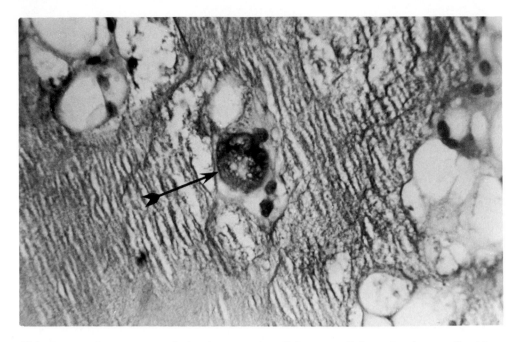

FIG. 13-63. Sacrococcygeal chordoma: a physaliphorous cell *(arrow)*, a large cell with a lobulated, large nucleus, is evident in the chordoma. (Original magnification × 600. Courtesy of Rudolf Garret, M.D.)

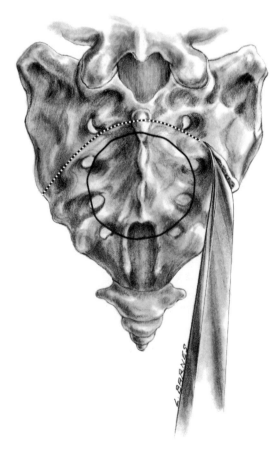

FIG. 13-64. Technique of removing the sacrum with an osteotome.

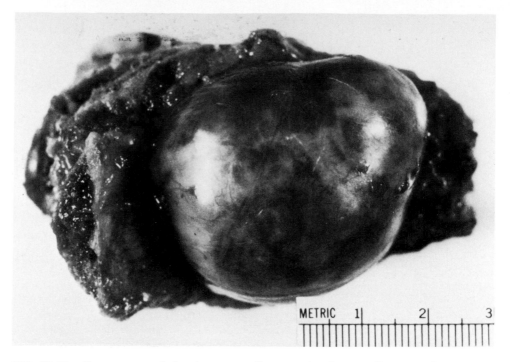

FIG. 13-65. Sacrococcygeal chordoma: a well-encapsulated mass adherent to the sacrum.

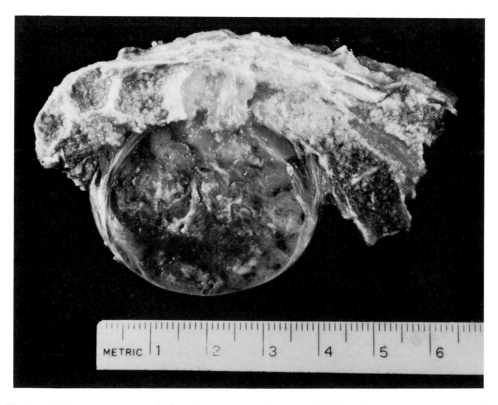

FIG. 13-66. Sacrococcygeal chordoma: cut section reveals the gelatinous appearance of the tumor.

478

Pneumatosis Cystoides Intestinalis

Pneumatosis cystoides intestinalis is discussed in Chapter 17.

REFERENCES

1. Abdou NI, Napombejara C, Sagawa A et al: Malakoplakia: Evidence for monocyte lysosomal abnormality correctable by cholinergic antagonist in vitro and in vivo. N Engl J Med 1977; 297:1413–1419

2. Abrikossoff AI: Über Myome, ausgehend von der quergestreiften willkürlichen Muskalatur. Virchows Arch [Path Anat] 1926; 260:215–233

3. Abrikossoff AI: Weitere Untersuchungen über Myoblastenmyome. Virchows Arch [Path Anat] 1931; 280:723–740

4. Aird I: A companion in Surgical Studies, 2nd ed, p 844. E & S Livingstone, Edinburgh, 1957

5. Akwari OE, Dozois RR, Weiland LH, Beahrs OH: Leiomyosarcoma of the small and large bowel. Cancer 1978; 42:1375–1384

6. Albrecht E: Ueler Hamartome. Verh Dtsch Ges Pathol 1904; 7:153–157

7. Aldridge MC, Boylston AW, Sim AJW: Dermoid cyst of the rectum. Dis Colon Rectum 1983; 26:333–334

8. Allen MS Jr: Hamartomatous inverted polyps of the rectum. Cancer 1966; 19:257–265

9. Alvich JP, Lepow HI: Cystic lymphangioma of hepatic flexure of colon: Report of a case. Ann Surg 1960; 152:880–884

10. Anderson Å, Bergdahl L: Carcinoid tumors of the appendix in children: A report of 25 cases. Acta Chir Scand 1977; 143:173–175

11. Anderson PA, Dockerty MB, Buie LA: Myomatous tumors of the rectum (leiomyomas and myosarcomas). Surgery 1950; 28:642–650

12. Angerpointner Th A, Weitz H, Haas RJ, Hecker W Ch: Intestinal leiomyosarcoma in childhood—case report and review of the literture. J Pediatr Surg 1981; 16:491–495

13. Arnett NL, Friedman PS: Lymphangioma of the colon; roentgen aspects: A case report. Radiology 1956; 67:881–885

14. Astarjian NK, Tseng CH, Keating JA et al: Leiomyosarcoma of the colon: Report of a case. Dis Colon Rectum 1977; 20:139–143

15. Asuncion CM: Leiomyosarcoma of the rectum: Report of two cases. Dis Colon Rectum 1969; 12:281–287

16. Atlay RD, Cuschieri A: Torsion of a colonic fibroma complicating pregnancy. Aust NZ J Obstet Gynecol 1969; 9:262–263

17. Ault GW, Smith RS, Castro CF: Hemangiopericytoma of the sigmoid colon: Case report. Surgery 1951; 30:523–527

18. Bacon HE: Cancer of the Colon, Rectum and Anal Canal, p 956. Philadelphia, JB Lippincott Co, 1964

19. Bailey JJ, Barrick CW, Jenkinson EL: Hemangioma of the colon. JAMA 1956; 160:658–659

20. Baker HL Jr, Good CA: Smooth-muscle tumors of the alimentary tract: Their roentgen manifestations. AJR 1955; 74:246–255

21. Ballantyne EN: Sacrococcygeal tumors: Adenocarcinoma of a cystic congenital embryonal remnant. Arch Pathol 1932; 14:1–9

22. Bar-Meir S, Halla A, Baratz M: Endoscopic removal of colonic lipoma. Endoscopy 1981; 13:135–136

23. Barton AD, Inglis K: Neurofibromatosis with both cutaneous and visceral lesions. J Coll Surg Australasia 1931; 3:397–402

24. Bassler A, Peter AG: Fibrosarcoma, an unusual complication of ulcerative colitis, report of a case. Arch Surg 1949; 59:227–231

25. Bates HR Jr: Carcinoid tumors of the rectum. Dis Colon Rectum 1962; 5:270–280

26. Beaugie JM, Mann CV, Butler EC: Sacrococcygeal chordoma. Br J Surg 1969; 56:586–588

27. Berardi RS: Carcinoid tumors of the colon (exclusive of the rectum): Review of the literature. Dis Colon Rectum 1972; 15:383–391

28. Berg J, McNeer G: Leiomyosarcoma of the stomach: A clinical and pathological study. Cancer 1960; 13:25–33

29. Bhargava KS, Lahiri B, Gupta RC et al: Leiomyosarcoma of the rectum. J Indian Med Assoc 1964; 42:228–230

30. Bibro MC, Houlihan RK, Sheahan DG: Colonic ganglioneuroma. Arch Surg 1980; 115:75–77

31. Black WC III: Enterochromaffin cell types and corresponding carcinoid tumors. Lab Invest 1968; 19:473–486

32. Blair-Bell W: Endometrioma and endometriomyoma of ovary. J Obstet Gynecol Br Emp 1922; 29:443–446

33. Bluth I: Gastrointestinal carcinoid tumors: Roentgen features. Radiology 1960; 74:573–580

34. Botting AJ, Soule EH, Brown AL Jr: Smooth muscle tumors in children. Cancer 1965; 18:711–720

35. Braasch JW, Denbo HE: Tumors of the small intestine. Surg Clin North Am 1964; 44:791–809

36. Brodey PA, Hoover HC: Polypoid ganglioneurofibromatosis of the colon. Br J Radiol 1974; 47:494–495

37. Byrne WJ, Jiminez JF, Euler AR, Golladay ES: Lymphoid polyps (focal lymphoid hyperplasia) of the colon in children. Pediatrics 1982; 69:598–600

38. Caldarola VT, Jackman RJ, Moertel CG, Dockerty MB: Carcinoid tumor of the rectum. Am J Surg 1964; 107:844–849

39. Calem SH, Keller RJ: Leiomyosarcoma of the sigmoid colon. Mt Sinai J Med (NY) 1973; 40:818–824

40. Castro EB, Stearns MW: Lipoma of the large intestine: A review of 45 cases. Dis Colon Rectum 1972; 15:441–444

41. Chaimoff C, Lurie H: Hemangioma of the rectum: Clinical appearance and treatment. Dis Colon Rectum 1978; 21:295–296

42. Chambers PW, Schwinn CP: Chordoma: A clinicopathologic study of metastasis. Am J Clin Pathol 1979, 72:765–776

43. Cheek RC, Wilson H: Carcinoid tumors. Curr Probl Surg 1970; pp 4–31

44. Chisholm AJ, Hillkowitz P: Lymphangioma of the rectum. Am J Surg 1932; 17:281–282

45. Cho KC, Smith TR: Multiple leiomyosarcoma of the transverse colon: Report of a case and discussion. Dis Colon Rectum 1980; 23:118–121

46. Cohnheim J: Ein Fall von Pseudoleukämie. Virchows Arch [Path Anat] 1865; 33:451–454

47. Colberg JE: Granular cell myoblastoma. Int Abstr Surg, Surg Gynecol Obstet 1962; 115:205–213

48. Collins JO, Falk M, Guibone R: Benign lymphoid polyposis of the colon: A case report. Pediatrics 1966; 38:897–899

49. Comer TP, Beahrs OH, Dockerty MB: Primary squamous cell carcinoma and adenoacanthoma of the colon. Cancer 1971; 28:1111–1117

50. Contreary K, Nance FC, Becker WF: Primary lymphoma of the gastrointestinal tract. Ann Surg 1980; 191:593–598

51. Corman ML, Haggitt RC: Lymphangioma of the rectum: Report of a case. Dis Colon Rectum 1973; 16:524–529

52. Corman ML, Veidenheimer MC, Swinton NW: Diseases of the Anus, Rectum and Colon. Part I: Neoplasms. New York, Medcom, 1972

53. Cornes JS: Multiple lymphomatous polyposis of the gastrointestinal tract. Cancer 1961; 14:249–257

54. Cornes JS, Wallace MH, Morson BC: Benign lymphomas of the rectum and anal canal: A study of 100 cases. J Pathol Bacteriol 1961; 82:371–382

55. Cosens CG: Gastro-intestinal pseudoleukemia: A case report. Ann Surg 1958; 148:129–133

56. Cronkhite LW Jr, Canada WJ: Generalized gastrointestinal polyposis: Unusual syndrome of polyposis, pigmentation, alopecia and onychotropia. N Engl J Med 1955; 252:1011–1015

57. Crowley LV, Page HG: Adenocarcinoma arising in presacral enterogenous cyst. Arch Pathol 1960; 69:64–66

58. Dahlin DC, MacCarty CS: Chordoma: A study of fifty-nine cases. Cancer 1952; 5:1170–1178

59. DeBeer RA, Shinya H: Colonic lipomas. An endoscopic analysis. Gastrointest Endosc 1975; 22:90–91

60. Diamante M, Bacon HE: Leiomyosarcoma of the rectum: Report of a case. Dis Colon Rectum 1967; 10:347–351

61. Doak PB, Montgomerie JZ, North JD et al: Reticulum cell sarcoma after renal homotransplantation and azathioprine and prednisone therapy. Br Med J 1968; 4:746–748

62. Dodd GD, Rutledge R, Wallace S: Postoperative pelvic lymphocysts. AJR 1970; 108:312–323

63. Donnelly WH, Sieber WK, Yunis EJ: Polypoid ganglioneurofibromatosis of the large bowel. Arch Pathol 1969; 87:537–541

64. Dudley GS: Visceral neurofibroma. Surg Clin North Am 1930; 10:539–540

65. Dukes C, Bussey HJR: The number of lymphoid follicles of the human large intestine. J Pathol Bacteriol 1926; 29:111–116

66. Dzioba H, Kabza R: Naczyniaki jelita grubego. Pol Tyg Lek 1965; 20:147–148

67. Edgerton MT: The treatment of hemangiomas: With special reference to the role of steroid therapy. Ann Surg 1976; 183:517–532

68. Eichel BS, Hallberg OE: Hamartoma of the middle ear and eustachian tube: Report of a case. Laryngoscope 1966; 76:1810–1815

69. Eitan N, Auslander L, Cohen Y: Leiomyosarcoma of the rectum: Report of three cases. Dis Colon Rectum 1978; 21:444–446

70. Epstein SE, Ascari WQ, Ablow RC et al: Colitis cystica profunda. Am J Clin Pathol 1966; 45:186–201

71. Espinosa MH, Quan SHQ: Anal fibrosarcoma: Report of a case and review of literature. Dis Colon Rectum 1975; 18:522–527

72. Evans N: Malignant myomas and related tumors of the uterus. (Report of seventy-two cases occurring in a series of 4000 operations for uterine fibromyomas.) Collected Papers of the Mayo Clinic 1919; 11:349–375

73. Ewing J: Neoplastic Diseases: A Treatise on

Tumors, 4th ed. Philadelphia, WB Saunders, 1940

74. Fahey JL: Cancer in the immunosuppressed patient. Ann Intern Med 1971; 75:310–312

75. Fayemi AO, Toker C: Gastrointestinal fibroma: A clinicopathological study. Am J Gastroenterol 1974; 62:250–254

76. Feldtman RW, Oram-Smith JC, Teears RJ, Kircher T: Leiomyosarcoma of the rectum: The military experience. Dis Colon Rectum 1981; 24:402–403

77. Ferguson EF Jr, Houston CH: Benign and malignant tumors of the colon and rectum. South Med J 1972; 65:1213–1220

78. Ferrarese R: Fibroma semplice del mesentere in sede ileo-cecale. Arch Ostet Ginecol 1968; 73:94–103

79. Figliolini FJ, Cutait DE, de Oliveira MR et al: Rectosigmoidal hemangioma: Report of two cases. Dis Colon Rectum 1961; 4:349–355

80. Fisher ER, Wechsler H: Granular cell myoblastoma—a misnomer: Electron microscopic and histochemical evidence concerning its Schwann cell derivation and nature (granular cell schwannoma). Cancer 1962; 15:936–954

81. Fleming MP, Carlson HC: Submucosal lymphatic cysts of the gastrointestinal tract: A rare cause of submucosal mass lesion. AJR 1970; 110:842–845

82. Fontaine R, Suhler A, Babin S et al: A propos de deux nouveaux cas de leiomyosarcome du rectum: Revue de la littérature. Ann Chir 1965; 19:1353–1357

83. Franken EA Jr: Lymphoid hyperplasia of the colon. Radiology 1970; 94:329–334

84. Freeman FJ: Lymphoid hyperplasia and gastrointestinal bleeding in children. Guthrie Clin Bull 1964; 33:175–179

85. Gabriel WB: The Principles and Practice of Rectal Surgery, 5th ed, p 481. Springfield, Charles C Thomas, 1963

86. Galletly A: Presacral tumors of congenital origin. Proc R Soc Med (Sect: Gynaecol Obstet) 1924; 17:105–122

87. Genter B, Mir R, Strauss R et al: Hemangiopericytoma of the colon: Report of a case and review of literature. Dis Colon Rectum 1982; 25:149–156

88. Gentil F, Coley BL: Sacrococcygeal chordoma. Ann Surg 1948; 127:432–455

89. Gentry RW, Dockerty MB, Clagett OT: Collective review: Vascular malformations and vascular tumors of the gastrointestinal tract. Int Abstr Surg, Surg Gynecol Obstet 1949; 88:281–323

90. Ghrist TD: Gastrointestinal involvement in neurofibromatosis. Arch Int Med 1963; 112:357–362

91. Girdwood TG, Philip LD: Lymphatic cysts of the colon. Gut 1971; 12:933–935

92. Gius JA, Stout AP: Perianal cysts of vestigial origin. Arch Surg 1938; 37:268–287

93. Gleason TH, Hammar SP: Plasmacytoma of the colon: Case report with lambda light chain demonstrated by immunoperoxidase studies. Cancer 1982; 50:130–133

94. Godard JE, Dodds WF, Phillips JC et al: Peutz-Jeghers syndrome: Clinical and roentgenographic features. AJR 1971; 113:316–324

95. Golden T, Stout AP: Smooth muscle tumors of the gastrointestinal tract and retroperitoneal tissues. Surg Gynecol Obstet 1941; 73:784–810

96. Goldlust D, Chalut J, Rault JJ et al: L'hémangiomatose recto-sigmoidienne. J Radiol Electrol Med Nucl 1971: 52:108–111

97. Goldstein WB, Poker N: Multiple myeloma involving the gastrointestinal tract. Gastroenterology 1966; 51:87–93

98. Granet E: Simple lymphoma of the sphincteric rectum in identical twins. JAMA 1949; 141:990–991

99. Greenblatt RB, Dmowski WP, Mahesh VB et al: Clinical studies with an antigonadotropin—Danazol. Fertil Steril 1971; 22:102–112

100. Greene EI, Kirshen MM, Greene JM: Lymphangioma of the transverse colon. Am J Surg 1962; 103:723–726

101. Grill J, Kuzma JF: Recklinghausen's disease with unusual symptoms from intestinal neurofibroma. Arch Pathol 1942; 34:902–910

102. Gruenberg J, Mackman S: Multiple lymphoid polyps in familial polyposis. Ann Surg 1972; 175:552–554

103. Gruenwald P: Abnormal accumulation of lymph follicles in the digestive tract. Am J Med Sci 1942; 203:823–829

104. Gunning JE, Moyer D: The effect of medroxyprogesterone acetate on endometriosis in the human female. Fertil Steril 1967; 18:759–774

105. Haller JD, Roberts TW: Lipomas of the colon: A clinicopathologic study of 20 cases. Surgery 1964; 55:773–781

106. Halls JM: Lymphomas of the large intestine. In Greenbaum EI: Radiographic Atlas of Colon Disease, pp 303-309. Chicago, Year Book Medical Publishers, 1980

107. Hambrick E, Abcarian H, Smith D: Perineal endometrioma in episiotomy incisions: Clinical features and management. Dis Colon Rectum 1979; 22:550–552

108. Hampton JM, Gandy JR: Plasmacytoma of the gastrointestinal tract. Ann Surg 1957; 145:415–422

109. Hasegawa K, Lee W-Y, Noguchi T et al: Colonscopic removal of hemangiomas. Dis Colon Rectum 1981; 24:85–89

110. Haskell B, Rovner H: Solitary ulcer of the rectum. Dis Colon Rectum 1965; 8:333–336

111. Hayes HT, Burr HB: Benign lymphomas of the rectum. Am J Surg 1952; 84:545–550

112. Head HD, Baker JQ, Muir RW: Hemangioma of the colon. Am J Surg 1973; 126:691–694

113. Hellstrom J, Hultborn KA, Engstedt L: Diffuse cavernous hemangioma of the rectum. Acta Chir Scand 1955; 109:277–283

114. Hellwig CA: Extramedullary plasma cell tumors as observed in various locations. Arch Pathol 1943; 36:95–111

115. Helwig EB, Hansen J: Lymphoid polyps (benign lymphoma) and malignant lymphoma of the rectum and anus. Surg Gynecol Obstet 1951; 92:233–243

116. Hemley SD, Kanick V: Perforation of the rectum: A complication of barium enema following rectal biopsy: Report of 2 cases. Am J Dig Dis 1963; 19:882–884

117. Heule BV, Taylor CR, Terry R, Lukes RJ: Presentation of malignant lymphoma in the rectum. Cancer 1982; 49:2602–2607

118. Higgason JM: Lymphatic cyst of the transverse colon: Report of a case. AJR 1958; 79:850–853

119. Higinbotham NL, Phillips H, Farr W et al: Chordoma: Thirty-five year study at Memorial Hospital. Cancer 1967; 20:1841–1850

120. Hoehn JG, Farrow GM, Devine KD et al: Invasive hemangioma of the head and neck. Am J Surg 1970; 120:495–500

121. Hoehn JL, Hamilton GH, Beltaos E: Fibrosarcoma of the colon. J Surg Oncol 1980; 13:223–225

122. Hollingsworth G: Haemangiomatous lesions of the colon. Br J Radiol 1951; 24:220–222

123. Holtz F, Schmidt LA III: Lymphoid polyps (benign lymphoma) of the rectum and anus. Surg Gynecol Obstet 1958; 106:639–642

124. Immunology and cancer. (Annotation). Lancet 1968; 1:1298–1299

125. Jackman RJ, Beahrs OH: Tumors of the Large Bowel. Philadelphia, WB Saunders 1968

126. Jackman RJ, Clark PL III, Smith ND: Retrorectal tumors. JAMA 1951; 145:956–962

127. Jalan KN, Brunt PW, Maclean N et al: Benign solitary ulcer of the rectum—a report of 5 cases. Scand J Gastroenterol 1970; 5:143–147

128. Jeffery PJ, Hawley PR, Parks AG: Colo-anal sleeve anastomosis in the treatment of diffuse cavernous haemangioma involving the rectum. Br J Surg 1976; 63:678–682

129. Johnson RC, Bleshman MH, DeFord JW: Benign lymphoid hyperplasia manifesting as a cecal mass. Dis Colon Rectum 1978; 21:510–513

130. Johnstone JM, Morson BC: Inflammatory fibroid polyp of the gastrointestinal tract. Histopathology 1978; 2:349–361

131. Kaftouri JK, Aharon M, Kleinhaus U: Sonographic features of gastrointestinal leiomyosarcoma. J Clin Ultrasound 1981; 9:11–15

132. Keeling WM, Beatty GL: Lymphoid polyps of the rectum: Report of 3 cases in siblings. Arch Surg 1956; 73:753–756

133. Khanna KK, Chandra RK, Veliath AJ et al: Leiomyoma of the cecum. Am J Dis Child 1968; 116:675–677

134. Kim HH, Williams TJ: Endometrioid carcinoma of the uterus and ovaries associated with immunosuppressive therapy and anticoagulation: Report of a case. Mayo Clin Proc 1972; 47:39–41

135. Kistner RW: The use of newer progestins in the treatment of endometriosis. Am J Obstet Gynecol 1958; 75:264–278

136. Kitoraga NF: Hemangioma of the large intestine causing profuse hemorrhage. Vestn Khir 1962; 88:125–126

137. Klinge F: Ueber die sogenannten ureifen, nicht guergestreiften Myoblastenmyome. Verh Dtsch Ges Pathol 1928; 23:376–382

138. Koenig RR, Claudon DB, Byrne RW: Lymphatic cyst of the transverse colon: Report of a case radiographically simulating neoplastic polyp. Arch Pathol 1955; 60:431–434

139. Kovalcik PJ, Simstein NL, Cross GH: Benign neurilemmoma manifesting as a presacral (retrorectal) mass: Report of a case. Dis Colon Rectum 1978; 21:199–202

140. Landing BH, Farber S: Tumors of the cardiovascular system. In Atlas of Tumor Pathology, section 3, fascicle 7, p 45. Washington, DC, Armed Forces Institute of Pathology, 1956

141. Levy D, Khatib R: Intestinal neurofibromatosis with malignant degeneration: Report of a case. Dis Colon Rectum 1960; 3:140–144

142. Levy M, Stone AM, Platt N: Reticulum cell sarcoma of the cecum and macroglobulinemia: A case report. J Surg Oncol 1976; 8:149–153

143. Lewin KJ, Harell GS, Lee AS et al: Malacoplakia. An electron-microscopic study: Demonstration of bacilliform organisms in malacoplakic macrophages. Gastroenterology 1974; 66:28–45

144. Lewin KJ, Ranchod M, Dorfman RF: Lymphomas of the gastrointestinal tract: A study of 117 cases

presenting with gastrointestinal disease. Cancer 1978; 42:693–707

145. Lifschitz O, Lew S, Witz M, et al: Inflammatory fibroid polyp of sigmoid colon. Dis Colon Rectum 1979; 22:575–577

146. Ling CS, Leagus C, Stahlgren LH: Intestinal lipomatosis. Surgery 1959; 46:1054–1059

147. Localio SA, Francis KC, Rossaro PG: Abdominosacral resection of sacrococcygeal chordoma. Ann Surg 1967; 166:394–402

148. Lookanoff VA, Tsapralis PC: Smooth-muscle tumors of the colon: Report of a case involving the cecum and ascending colon. JAMA 1966; 198:206–207

149. Lou TY, Teplitz C: Malacoplakia; pathogenesis and ultrastructural morphogenesis: A problem of altered macrophage (phagolysosomal) response. Hum Pathol 1974; 5:191–207

150. Lyttle JA: Primary squamous carcinoma of the proximal large bowel: Report of a case and review of the literature. Dis Colon Rectum 1983; 26:279–282

151. Ma WH: Myoblastoma: Report of a case with review of 287 cases collected from literature. Chin Med J 1952; 70:35–45

152. MacKenzie DA, McDonald JR, Waugh JM: Leiomyoma and leiomyosarcoma of the colon. Ann Surg 1954; 139:67–75

153. Madiedo G, Komorowski RA, Dhar GH: Granular cell tumor (myoblastoma) of the large intestine removed by colonoscopy. Gastrointest Endosc 1980; 26:108–109

154. Madigan MR, Morson BC: Solitary ulcer of the rectum. Gut 1969; 10:871–881

155. Manley KA, Skyring AP: Some heritable causes of gastrointestinal disease: Special reference to hemorrhage. Arch Intern Med 1961; 107:182–203

156. Margulis AR, Burhenne HJ (eds): Alimentary Tract Roentgenology, Vol 2, p 730. St Louis, CV Mosby, 1967

157. Margulis AR, Jovanovich A: The roentgen diagnosis of submucous lipomas of the colon. AJR 1960; 84:1114–1120

158. Marshak RH, Moseley JE, Wolf BS: The roentgen findings in familial polyposis with special emphasis on differential diagnosis. Radiology 1963; 80:374–382

159. Martin JK Jr, Culp CE, Weiland LH: Colitis cystica profunda. Dis Colon Rectum 1980; 23:488–491

160. Mazier WP, Sun KM, Robertson WG: Oil-induced granuloma (eleoma) of the rectum: Report of four cases. Dis Colon Rectum 1978; 21:292–294

161. McClure J: Malakoplakia of the gastrointestinal tract. Postgrad Med J 1981; 57:95–103

162. McGee HJ Jr: Inflammatory fibroid polyps of the ileum and cecum. Arch Pathol 1960; 70:203–207

163. McSwain B, Beal JM: Lymphosarcoma of the gastrointestinal tract: Report of 20 cases. Ann Surg 1944; 119:108–123

164. Mendoza CC: Arteriovenous angioma of the colon. South Med J 1962; 55:40–41

165. Meyer R: Ueber entzündliche heterotope Epithel vucherungen im weiblichen Genitalgebiete und uber eine bis in die Wurzel des Mesocolon ausgedehnte benigne Wucherung des Darmepithels. Virchows Arch [Pathol Anat] 1909; 195:487

166. Michaelis L, Gutmann C: Ueber Einschlusse in Blasentumoren. Klin Med (Mosk) 1902; 47:208–215

167. Moertel CG: Large Bowel. In Holland JF, Frei E III (eds): Cancer Medicine, pp 1597-1627. Philadelphia, Lea and Febiger, 1973

168. Moertel CG, Dockerty MB, Judd ES: Carcinoid tumors of the vermiform appendix. Cancer 1968; 21:270–278

169. Moertel CG, Sauer WG, Dockerty MB et al: Life history of the carcinoid tumor of the small intestine. Cancer 1961; 14:901–912

170. Morl FK, Dortenmann J: Hämangiome des Dickdarms. Med Welt 1968; 45:2483–2485

171. Morson BC: In Dukes CE (ed): Cancer of the Rectum, Vol 3, p 92. Edinburgh, E & S Livingstone, 1960

172. Morson BC: Pathology of carcinoid tumours. In Jones FA (ed): Modern Trends in Gastro-enterology, pp 107–117. London, Butterworth and Co, 1958

173. Murphy B: Leiomyoma of intestine. J Ir Med Assoc 1973: 66:153

174. Murray MR: Cultural characteristics of 3 granular-cell myoblastomas. Cancer 1951; 4:857–865

175. Nelson RL: The association of carcinoid tumors of the rectum with myelofibrosis: Report of two cases. Dis Colon Rectum 1981; 24:548–549

176. Neoplasms: A complication of organ transplants? JAMA 1968; 206: 246–247

177. Nigam R: A case of dermoid arising from the rectal wall. Br J Surg 1947; 35:218–219

178. Norbury L: Specimen of post-rectal fibro-leiomyoma. Proc R Soc Med 1934; 27:930–931

179. Normann T, Otnes B: Intestinal ganglioneuromatosis, diarrhoea and medullary thyroid carcinoma. Scand J Gastroenterol 1969; 4:553–559

180. Oberndorfer-München S: Ueber die "kleinen Dünndarmcarcinome." Verh Dtsch Ges Pathol 1907; 11:113–116

181. O'Brien JE, Stout AP: Malignant fibrous xanthomas. Cancer 1964; 17:1445–1455

182. Ochsner SF, Ray JE, Clark WH Jr: Lymphangioma of the colon: A case report. Radiology 1959; 72:423–425

183. Okano H, Azar HA, Osserman EF: Plasmacytic reticulum cell sarcoma: Case report with electron microscopic studies. Am J Clin Pathol 1966; 46:546–555

184. Olnick HM, Woodhall JP Jr, Clay CB Jr: Hemangioma of the colon. J Med Assoc Georgia 1957; 46:383–384

185. Orda R, Bawnik JB, Wiznitzer T et al: Fibroma of the cecum: Report of a case. Dis Colon Rectum 1976; 19:626–628

186. Orloff MJ: Carcinoid tumors of the rectum. Cancer 1971; 28:175–180

187. Pardo MV, Rodriquez TI: Eosinophilic granuloma of the colon. Arch Hosp Univ Habana 1952; 4:248

188. Paris J, Goudemand M, Leduc M et al: Angiome isole du colon droit avec hemorragies digestives repetées pendant 15 ans. Lille Med 1967; 12:592–594

189. Parks AG, Porter NH, Hardcastle J: The syndrome of the descending perineum. Proc R Soc Med 1966; 59:477–482

190. Pearlman AW, Friedman M: Radical radiation therapy of chordoma. AJR 1970; 108:332–341

191. Pemberton J, McCormack CJ: Submucous lipomas of colon and rectum. Am J Surg 1937: 37:205–218

192. Penn I, Starzl TE: Immunosuppression and cancer. Transplant Proc 1973; 5:943–947

193. Pfannenstiel J: Über die Adenomyome des Genitalstrangs. Verh Dtsch Ges Gynaek 1897; 7:195–200

194. Phillips B: Lectures on the Principles and Practices of Surgery. London Med Gaz 1839; 1:608–617

195. Pinkert TC, Catlow CE, Straus R: Endometriosis of the urinary bladder in a man with prostatic carcinoma. Cancer 1979; 43:1562–1567

196. Pitchumoni CS, Dearani AC, Burke AV, Floch MH: Eosinophilic granuloma of the gastrointestinal tract. JAMA 1970; 211:1180–1182

197. Poate H, Inglis K: Ganglioneuromatosis of the alimentary tract. Br J Surg 1928; 16:221–225

198. Price AB: Benign lymphoid polyps and inflammatory polyps. In Morson BC: The Pathogenesis of Colorectal Cancer, pp 33-42. Philadelphia, WB Saunders, 1978

199. Quan SH, Bader G, Berg JW: Carcinoid tumors of the rectum. Dis Colon Rectum 1964; 7:197–206

200. Quan SH, Berg JW: Leiomyoma and Leiomyosarcoma of the rectum. Dis Colon Rectum 1962; 5:415–425

201. Rao BK, Kapur MM, Roy S: Leiomyosarcoma of the colon: A case report and review of literature. Dis Colon Rectum 1980; 23:184–190

202. Ranchod M, Kahn LB: Malacoplakia of the gastrointestinal tract. Arch Pathol 1972; 94:90–97

203. Rand AA: Barium granuloma of the rectum. Dis Colon Rectum 1966; 9:20–32

204. Reiss H, Ryć K: Roxlegly naczyniak jelita grubego i odbytnicy o mieszenej budowie. Pol Przegl Chir 1971; 43:115–118

205. Rickert RR, Larkey IG, Kantor EB: Granular-cell tumors (myoblastomas) of the anal region. Dis Colon Rectum 1978; 21:413–417

206. Rissier HL Jr: Hemangiomatosis of the intestine: Discussion, review of the literature and report of two new cases. Gastroenterologia 1960; 93:357–385

207. Riva HL, Kawasaki DM, Messinger AJ: Further experience with norethynodrel in treatment of endometriosis. Obstet Gynecol 1962; 19:111–117

208. Robertson FN, Wride GE: Case of persistent cyst of post-anal gut origin in an adult. Can Med Assoc J 1934; 31:535–537

209. Roo T de: Leiomyosarcoma of the colon, a rare tumour: Three case reports and review. Radiol Clin Biol 1974; 43:187–195

210. Roo T de, Vaas F: Leiomyosarcoma of the transverse and descending colon: Two case reports and review. Am J Gastroenterol 1969; 52:150–156

211. Rose TF: True fibroma of the caecum. Med J Aust 1972: 1:532–533

212. Rosenberg I: Perianal granular cell myoblastoma: Report of a case. J Int Coll Surg 1960; 33:346–349

213. Ruiz-Moreno F: Hemangiomatosis of the colon: Report of a case. Dis Colon Rectum 1962; 5:453–456

214. Rywlin AM, Ravel R, Hurwitz A: Malakoplakia of the colon. Am J Dig Dis 1969; 14:491–499

215. Saegesser F, Gross M: Carcinoid syndrome and carcinoid tumors of the rectum. Am J Proctol 1969; 20:27–32

216. Saltzstein SL: Extranodal malignant lymphomas and pseudolymphomas. Pathol Annu 1969; 4:159–184

217. Sampson JA: Intestinal adenomas of endometrial type. Arch Surg 1922; 5:217–280

218. Sanders RJ: Leiomyosarcoma of the rectum: Report of six cases. Ann Surg 1961; (Suppl) 154:150–154

219. Sanders RJ, Axtell HK: Carcinoids of the gas-

trointestinal tract. Surg Gynecol Obstet 1964; 119:369–380

220. Sanger BJ, Leckie BD: Plain muscle tumours of the rectum. Br J Surg 1959; 47:196–198

221. Schlernitzauer DA, Font RL: Sebaceous gland carcinoma of the eyelid following radiation therapy for cavernous hemangioma of the face. Arch Ophthalmol 1976; 94:1523–1525

222. Schumann F: Leiomyosarcoma of the colon: Report of a case and review of treatment and prognosis. Dis Colon Rectum 1972; 15:211–216

223. Sewell R, Levine BA, Harrison GK et al: Primary malignant fibrous histiocytoma of the intestine: Intussusception of a rare neoplasm. Dis Colon Rectum 1980; 23:198–201

224. Sherlock P, Winawer SJ, Goldstein MJ et al: Malignant lymphoma of the gastrointestinal tract. In Glass GB (ed): Progress in Gastroenterology, vol 2, pp 367-391. New York, Grune & Stratton, 1970

225. Shklovskii GS, Kadyrov FA: Gemangioma tolst oi kishki s invaginatsiei. Vestn Khir 1964; 93:114

226. Sidani MS, Campos MM, Joseph JI: Primary plasmacytomas of the colon. Dis Colon Rectum 1983; 26:182–187

227. Silverberg SG: "Juvenile" retention polyps of the colon and rectum. Am J Dig Dis 1970; 15:617–625

228. Skardalakis JE, Gray SW, Shepard D et al: Smooth Muscle Tumors of the Alimentary Tract: Leiomyomas and Leiomyosarcomas—A Review of 2525 Cases, p 155. Springfield, Charles C Thomas, 1962

229. Skovgaard S, Sorensen FH: Bleeding hemangioma of the colon diagnosed by coloscopy. J Pediatr Surg 1976; 11:83–84

230. Skutsch: Zeit f Geburschülfe und Gunäkol, XI, p 353. Stuttgart, 1899 (quoted by Galletly A, Ref 86)

231. Smith G: Leiomyosarcoma of the rectum. Br J Surg 1963; 50:633–635

232. Somervell JL, Mayer PF: Leiomyosarcoma of the rectum. Br J Surg 1971; 58:144–146

233. Starr GF, Dockerty MB: Leiomyomas and leiomyosarcomas of the small intestine. Cancer 1955; 8:101–111

234. Stavorovsky M, Jaffa AJ, Papo J, Baratz M: Leiomyosarcoma of the colon and rectum. Dis Colon Rectum 1980; 23:249–254

235. Stening SG, Heptinstall DP: Diffuse cavernous haemangioma of the rectum and sigmoid colon. Br J Surg 1970; 57:186–189

236. Stoller R, Weinstein JJ: Fibrosarcoma of the rectum: A review of the literature and the presen-

tation of 2 additional cases. Surgery 1956; 39:565–573

237. Stout AP: Tumors of the colon and rectum (excluding carcinoma and adenoma). Surg Clin North Am 1955; 35:1283–1288

238. Stout AP, Hill WT: Leiomyosarcoma of the superficial soft tissues. Cancer 1958; 11:844–854

239. Swain VA, Young WF, Pringle EM: Hypertrophy of the appendices epiploicae and lipomatous polyposis of the colon. Gut 1969; 10:587–589

240. Swanson MA, Schwartz RS: Immunosuppressive therapy: The relation between clinical response and immunologic competence. N Engl J Med 1967; 277:163–170

241. Swartley RN, Stayman JW Jr: Lymphoid hyperplasia of the intestinal tract requiring surgical intervention. Ann Surg 1962; 155:238–240

242. Swartzlander FC: A clinico-pathological review of submucosal rectal nodules. University of Minnesota, 1955

243. Swerdlow DB, Pecora C, Gradone F: Leiomyoma of the cecum presenting as an acute surgical abdomen: Report of a case. Dis Colon Rectum 1975; 18:438–440

244. Swinton NW, Lehman G: Presacral tumors. Surg Clin North Am 1958; 38:849–857

245. Symmers D: Lymphoid disease: Hodgkin's granuloma, giant follicular lymphadenopathy, lymphoid leukemia, lymphosarcoma and gastrointestinal pseudoleukemia. Arch Pathol 1948; 45:73–131

246. Talerman A: Enterogenous cysts of the rectum (colitis cystica profunda). Br J Surg 1971; 58:643–647

247. Taxy JB, Mendelsohn G, Gupta PK: Carcinoid tumors of the rectum: Silver reactions, fluorescence, and serotonin content of the cytoplasmic granules. Am J Clin Path 1980; 74:791–795

248. Terner JY, Lattes R: Malakoplakia of colon and retroperitoneum: Report of a case with a histochemical study of the Michaelis-Gutmann inclusion bodies. Am J Clin Pathol 1965; 44:20–31

249. Thomason TH: Cysts and sinuses of the sacrococcygeal region. Ann Surg 1934; 99:585–592

250. Thorlakson RH, Ross HM: Leiomyosarcoma of the rectum. Ann Surg 1961; 154:979–984

251. Toti A, Tedeschi M: Fibroma cecale insorto su monocone appendicolare invaginato. Minerva Chir 1952; 7:420–422

252. Turell R: Diseases of the Colon and Anorectum, 2nd ed. Philadelphia, WB Saunders, 1969

253. Upson JF, Bunnell I, Kokkinopoulis E: Hemangioma of the cecum—diagnosis by angiography. JAMA 1971; 217:1104–1105

254. Usher FC: Lymphosarcoma of the intestines. University of Minnesota, 1940

255. Venkitachalam PS, Hirsch E, Elguezabal A, Littman L: Multiple lymphoid polyposis and familial polyposis of the colon: A genetic relationship. Dis Colon Rectum 1978; 21:336–341

256. Vezeridis MP, Herrera LO, Lopez GE et al: Squamous-cell carcinoma of the colon and rectum. Dis Colon Rectum 1983; 26:188–191

257. Vitolo RE, Rachlin SA: Inflammatory fibroid polyp of large intestine: Report of a case. J Int Coll Surg 1955; 23:700–709

258. Von Recklinghausen FH; Ueber die multiplen Fibrome der Haut und ihre Beziehung zu den multiplen Neuromen. Berlin, Festrschrift for Vichow, A Hirschwald, 1882

259. Waldenström JG: Studies on conditions associated with disturbed gamma globulin formation (gammopathies). Harvey Lect 1960–1961; 56:211–231

260. Waxman M, Faegenburg D, Waxman JS, Janelli DE: Malignant fibrous histiocytoma of the colon associated with diverticulitis. Dis Colon Rectum 1983; 26:339–343

261. Waye JD, Frankel A: Removal of pedunculated lipoma by colonoscopy. Am J Gastroenterol 1974; 61:221–222

262. Wayte DM, Helwig EB: Colitis cystica profunda. Am J Clin Pathol 1967; 48:159–169

263. Weinberg T, Feldman M: Lipomas of the gastrointestinal tract. Am J Clin Pathol 1955; 25:272–281

264. Welch CE, Hedberg SE: Polypoid Lesions of the Gastrointestinal Tract, 2nd ed, pp 121-143. Philadelphia, WB Saunders, 1975

265. Welch JP, Donaldson GA: Recent experience in the management of cancer of the colon and rectum. Am J Surg 1974; 127:258–266

266. Williams ED, Sandler M: The classification of carcinoid tumours. Lancet 1963; 1:238–239

267. Williams GT, Blackshaw AJ, Morson BC: Squamous carcinoma of the colorectum and its genesis. J Pathol 1979; 129:139–147

268. Willis RA: The Borderland of Embryology and Pathology, pp 348–350. London, Butterworth & Co, 1960

269. Willis RA: Pathology of Tumors, 3rd ed. London, Butterworth & Co, 1960

270. Wolf BS, Marshak RH: Roentgen features of diffuse lymphosarcoma of the colon. Radiology 1960; 75:733–740

271. Wood DA: Tumors of the intestines. In Atlas of Tumor Pathology, section 6, fascicle 22, p 52. Washington, DC, Armed Forces Institute of Pathology, 1967

272. Wychulis AR, Beahrs OH, Woolner LB: Malignant lymphoma of the colon: A study of 69 cases. Arch Surg 1966; 93:215–225

273. Yanai-Inbar I, Odes HS, Krugliak P et al: Granular cell myoblastoma of the sigmoid colon. Dig Dis Sci 1981; 26:852–854

274. Yoshida A, Yano M, Fujinaga Y et al: Argentaffin carcinoid tumor of the rectum. Cancer 1981; 48:2103–2106

275. Yoshikawa O: A case of leiomyosarcoma of the rectum. Arch Jap Chir 1969; 38:342–345

276. Ziter FMH Jr: Roentgenographic findings in Gardner's syndrome. JAMA 1965; 192:1000–1002

CHAPTER 14

Diverticular Disease

Diverticular disease (diverticulitis and diverticulosis) were rare conditions prior to the end of the 19th century. Although the manifestations were described accurately by such renowned 19th century surgeons and pathologists as Cruveilhier, Rokitansky, Cripps, and Virchow, the condition was regarded as a surgical curiosity.[93] The disease has become progressively more pervasive in the 20th century and virtually epidemic in Western countries. Today, the risk of developing diverticular disease by the age of 60 in the United States approximates 50%. However, probably not more than 10% of those with colonic diverticula develop symptoms, and of these only a small proportion ever require surgery.[95]

PATHOGENESIS

Diverticula occur most commonly on the antimesenteric surface of the bowel, usually the sigmoid, between the teniae at the point where the blood vessels penetrate the bowel wall (Fig. 14-1). The circular muscle is weakened by the tunnels that are formed by the blood vessels.[92] It is presumed that the diverticula become manifest as a result of a high intracolonic pressure impacting on these areas of weakness.

Study of physiology of the normal colon by means of pressure tracings reveals that the principal wave form represents a slow change of pressure, waxing and waning over about 30 seconds.[25] Complete quiescence may normally be present for several hours. Usually, the waves are not transmitted to adjacent areas of the colon, but occasionally the transport of material over considerble distance does occur.[25] Radiologically, this is seen as a loss of haustration succeeded by movement of the contents over a number of centimeters.

Motor studies in patients with diverticular disease reveal an exaggerated response to pharmacologic stimuli, increased intraluminal pressures, and faster frequency waves and rapid contractions (more than 5 per minute).[25]

Increased pressure is brought about through progressive colonic narrowing and segmentation. When contraction occurs in a segment that is relatively narrowed, considerble intraluminal pressure develops, causing the colon to hypertrophy. The pressure is related to the narrowness or spasticity of the involved segment. According to the law of Laplace, the tension in the wall of a hollow cylinder is proportional to its radius multiplied by the pressure within the cylinder. This implies that the intraluminal pressure is greater when the lumen is narrowed, and explains the increased likelihood that diverticula will develop in this particular area.[25] The thickened colonic muscle becomes uneven, with resultant herniation through the

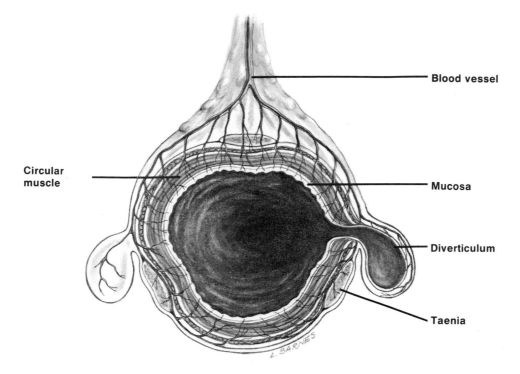

FIG. 14-1. Cross section of colon showing areas of weakness through which the diverticula become manifest.

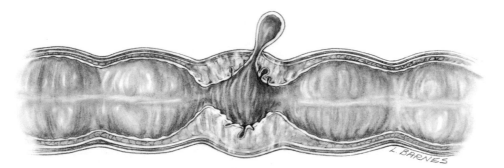

FIG. 14-2. Mechanism of segmental contraction with elevated, localized intracolonic pressure and resultant diverticulum.

weakened parts of its wall (Fig. 14-2).[92] Since the sigmoid has to propel the most formed fecal material, it is the most frequent site for the occurrence of diverticular disease (Figs. 14-3 and 14-4).[92] Microscopically, the diverticula are of the pulsion type, consisting only of mucous membrane and peritoneum. The muscle shows thickening but no evidence of cellular hypertrophy or hyperplasia.[83] Antimesenteric diverticula have only a very thin layer of investing longitudinal muscle, mucous membrane, and muscularis mucosae separating the fecal contents of the bowel from the peritoneal cavity (Fig. 14-5).[83]

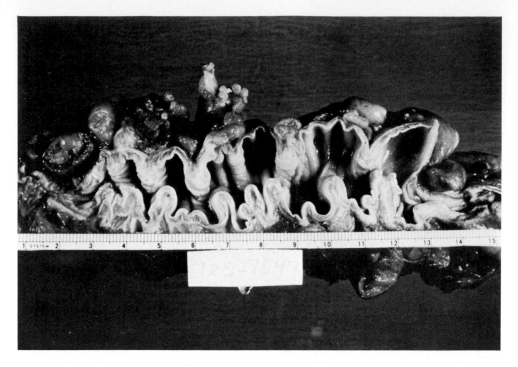

FIG. 14-3. Resected portion of the sigmoid colon demonstrating multiple "little bladders" or "rooms" resulting from hypertrophy and segmentation.

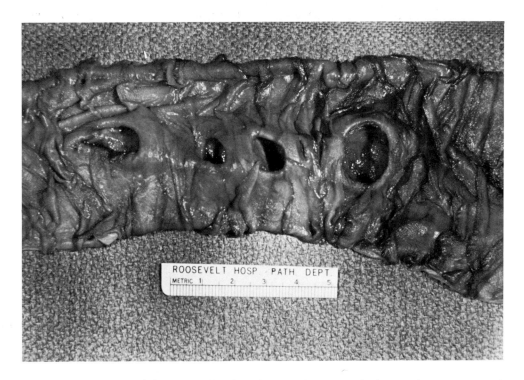

FIG. 14-4. Portion of the sigmoid colon showing large-mouth diverticula. (Courtesy of Rudolf Garret, M.D.)

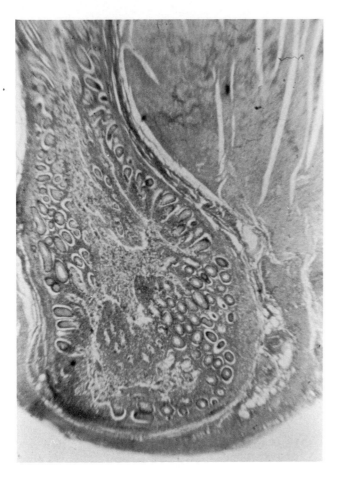

FIG. 14-5. Diverticulum demonstrating only mucous membrane, muscularis mucosae, and peritoneum separating the lumen from the peritoneal cavity. (Original magnification × 80).

ETIOLOGY AND EPIDEMIOLOGY

Painter and Burkitt are the two individuals most responsible for our current concepts of the etiology and epidemiology of diverticular disease.[20, 21, 90-93] Since the condition was extremely rare in the 19th century and became relatively commonly observed in Western countries only after 1920, the authors believed that a change in the dietary habits in those Western countries was the incriminating factor. During the years 1870 and 1880, the grist mills for grinding wheat into whole meal flour were replaced by the much more efficient roller mills. This new process succeeded in crushing the grain so effectively that a very pure white flour was produced. At about the same time, with the advent of effective refrigeration and canning, consumption of refined sugar, fat, and protein increased. The result was a critical decrease in the amount of fiber available in the diet. Painter stated that the greatest change in our diet in the past 100 years has been a reduction in the amount of cereal fiber consumption to as little as one tenth that previously eaten.[92] Because of this very sudden change, within a matter of approximately 40 years diverticular disease has become pervasive.

Theoretically, a high-fiber diet produces a large, bulky stool that requires less "effort" by the bowel to propel the contents. Muscular hypertrophy does not occur, and segmentation is much less likely to develop. Transit time is considerbly reduced. The result of this phenomenon is the probable explanation for the infrequent development of colon and rectal carcinoma in people who have a high-fiber diet (see Chap. 10)

Burkitt and associates compared the transit times and stool weights of various ethnic groups.[21] They were particularly interested in the low incidence of colorectal disease in rural African natives. Ugandan villagers passed over 400 g of stool within 35 hours, whereas the shore-based United Kingdom naval personnel produced 100 g of constipated stool with a transit time of approximately 5 days.[91] Gear and co-workers reported the results of barium enema examination in vegetarians and nonvegetarians.[39] The mean intake of dietary fiber was twice as great in the former group. Vegetarians were found to have a 12% incidence of diverticular disease, compared with a 33% incidence among nonvegetarians.

With economic development, affluence, and Westernization of diet, an increased incidence of diverticular disease has been noted among native Africans.[116] Other studies have demonstrated an increased frequency of diverticular disease in immigrants to Western countries from less developed nations. The addition of fiber has been shown to be effective in the treatment of symptomatic patients with uncomplicated diverticular disease.[19, 29, 56, 91, 92]

Fiber

Fiber is that portion of the dietary intake that is not absorbed; this is usually in the form of cellulose. One of the highest fiber items is the outer covering of any cereal grain, the bran. Certain vegetables and fruits are also relatively high in fiber. Milk and milk products, chicken, fish, meat, eggs, fats, and beverages have no fiber. The highest fiber content in vegetables is in the legumes. Enthusiasm for their consumption, however, is somewhat muted; daily beans can be rather tedious, and the troublesome consequence of flatulence is a distinct disadvantage also. Many people believe that by eating a salad each day they should be achieving adequate fiber intake; however, a whole head of lettuce is not quite the equivalent of one serving (one-third cup) of a bran cereal in nonabsorbed fiber. But in spite of the availability of high-fiber foods, most people find them either unpalatable or intolerably repetitious.

An alternate approach would be to employ one of a number of proprietary preparations, the so-called bulk laxatives. These are made from the outer covering of the psyllium grain. Over-the-counter preparations containing psyllium include Hydrocil, Konsyl, Konsyl-D, and Metamucil. A daily whole-grain cereal or bran bread may become rather monotonous, but most people have a glass of juice in the morning. By adding one of the psyllium preparations to juice or a glass of water, once or twice daily, an effective fiber supplement to the diet can be achieved.

SIGNS AND SYMPTOMS

The vast majority of people who harbor diverticular disease do not have symptoms specifically related to the condition. This means that surgical extirpation of the affected bowel will not ameliorate the patient's condition. The patient's complaint probably has a physiologic basis: the so-called *irritable bowel syndrome.* Other names, including functional gastrointestinal disorder, psychophysiologic gastrointestinal disturbance, splenic flexure syndrome, and spastic colon, have all been used. Patients with irritable bowel symptoms constitute the majority of those seen by gastroenterologists. It is also the commonest single diagnosis reported by major referral clinics. In England, one fifth of a sample from the general population had experienced abdominal pain more than six times in one year.[67] Approximately one fourth of a similar sample in the United States reported abdominal pain more than six times in that year.[67] The term *irritable bowel syndrome* suggests that these patients have an abnormality in the intestine, but the symptoms can develop without any anatomic abnormality, and certainly in the absence of diverticulosis. It is important to recognize the distinction between the two often-concurrent conditions and findings, and to initiate the appropriate medical therapy for the illness. The problem is to distinguish between those patients who harbor diverticula and whose symptoms are related to the presence of this anatomic abnormality, and those patients whose symptoms are unrelated (Figs. 14-6 and 14-7).

Patients with *diverticulitis* complain primarily of abdominal pain. The pain is usually located in the left

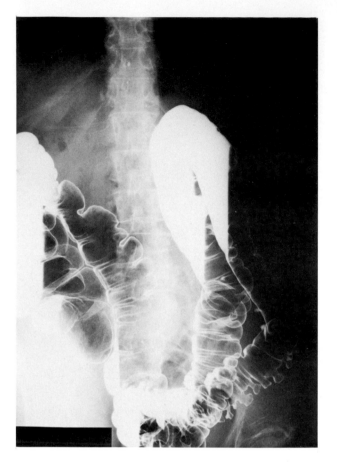

FIG. 14-6. Air-contrast barium enema demonstrates extensive sigmoid diverticulosis without colonic narrowing. The patient's abdominal complaint is unlikely to be relieved by resection.

lower quadrant and tends to be constant rather than colicky in nature. The pain may radiate to the back, left flank, groin, and leg. The duration and severity of symptoms are quite variable, depending on whether the patient has a localized or diffuse process. Nausea and vomiting are not commonly seen, unless there is some element of intestinal obstruction. Change in bowel habits is frequently observed; there may be absence of bowel movements or the patient may experience diarrhea.

Urinary symptoms (dysuria, urgency, frequency, nocturia) are frequently observed in patients with acute diverticular disease because of impingement of the inflammatory mass on the wall of the bladder.

Rectal bleeding has been thought to be part of the symptom complex of diverticulosis when there is no

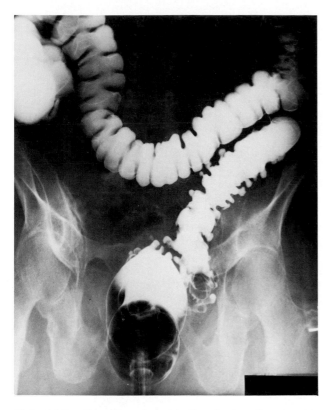

FIG. 14-7. Extensive sigmoid diverticular disease with slight spasm but no stigmata of acute inflammation. In the absence of objective symptoms and signs of diverticulitis, surgery is not advised.

acute abdominal inflammation, but there is some confusion on this issue. Massive lower gastrointestinal bleeding in the presence of diverticular disease may be due to a vascular malformation rather than diverticulosis. However, there is evidence to suggest that some patients *do* bleed from diverticular disease (see Complications: Hemorrhage).

Fever is also commonly observed in patients with acute diverticulitis. This is usually of low grade, but if peritonitis develops or if there is an abscess present, pyrexia can be considerably elevated.

The duration and the nature of symptoms have an important bearing on the outcome of the disease. Parks noted that half of the patients with diverticular disease of the colon were in good health until less than 1 month prior to hospitalization, and three quarters had symptoms for less than 1 year.[94] Patients with some of the most serious complications were essentially asymptomatic until just prior to admission.

Physical examination will reveal tenderness, voluntary guarding, and, in the presence of peritonitis, absent bowel sounds, a board-like abdomen, and all the signs and symptoms of an acute abdominal catastrophe. Tenderness and a mass in the pelvis from a sigmoid phlegmon may be noted on rectal examination. Proctosigmoidoscopic examination is usually quite limited because of tenderness and because of the presence of the mass. Negotiation of the rectosigmoid is usually impossible with a rigid instrument.

There is some controversy about whether endoscopy should be performed in the presence of acute inflammation. There is a risk of disturbing a walled-off perforation with the use of the instrument or by insufflation of air. Although proctosigmoidoscopic examination can be carried out with minimal air use, considerable caution must be employed with air insufflation when using the fiberoptic instrument. There is far more likelihood of injuring an acutely inflamed bowel with flexible sigmoidoscopy or colonoscopy, but direct visualization may be very helpful if one is to distinguish between diverticulitis and other pathologic conditions (*e.g.*, ischemic colitis, carcinoma, inflammatory bowel disease).

MEDICAL MANAGEMENT

Patients who present with tenderness and a suggestion of a sausage-like mass in the left lower quadrant can, in the absence of systemic signs and symptoms, be initially treated as outpatients. A low-residue diet is suggested during the acute phase of the illness. One prefers to place the bowel at relative rest until such time as the inflammatory process has resolved. A broad-spectrum oral antibiotic is advised (a cephalosporin, tetracycline, or ampicillin); this should be continued for 10 days. If the patient's symptoms continue to improve, elective evaluation is undertaken when the acute process has resolved. If the patient's symptoms fail to improve, inpatient therapy is recommended.

For a person who has more severe abdominal signs and symptoms, who has a pyrexia, or who appears systemically ill, hospitalization is indicated. Medical management includes the usual supportive measures. Oral intake is permitted unless the patient's symptoms suggest the need for imminent operation; clear liquids in his circumstance would be reasonable. It is not usually necessary to employ a nasogastric tube unless intestinal obstruction or vomiting is apparent. In the inpatient setting, systemic antibiotics are warranted. These are given intravenously and should include an agent to which anaerobic organisms are susceptible. As the patient's symptoms improve, a progressive diet is instituted, supplemented by a stool softener. Although the observed hypermotility of the sigmoid colon in many symptomatic patients with diverticular disease provides a rationale for the common use of anticholinergic drugs, their efficacy has never been clearly documented.[5] I have not found them particularly useful; hence, I do not employ them in the medical management of the resolving acute inflammatory condition. With aggressive medical management, the patient's symptoms should considerably improve within 24 to 48 hours. As long as consistent improvement is observed, investigation can be deferred until the process has resolved. However, if the patient's symptoms persist unchanged for a period of 2 days, I prefer to perform radiologic investigation to try to confirm the diagnosis.

DIFFERENTIAL DIAGNOSIS

The most valuable and most commonly employed study to evaluate patients with diverticular disease is the barium enema examination. In the acute situation, the study should be performed with extreme caution. Should a perforation be present or should one be created by the instillation of the barium, barium peritonitis may result, an often fatal complication (see Chap. 1). If there is some concern on the part of the surgeon or radiologist, a gentle, water-soluble (Gastrografin) enema should be used.

Carcinoma

The most important aspect of the differential diagnosis, and the reason for performing a barium enema in the first place, is to rule out the presence of a cancer as the cause of the patient's symptoms. If a carcinoma is present, surgical intervention will become necessary within a relatively short period of time, irrespective of the fact that the patient's symptoms may not have completely resolved. On the other hand, if one is satisfied that the patient's findings are due to diverticulitis, surgery may be delayed as long as the clinical condition improves.

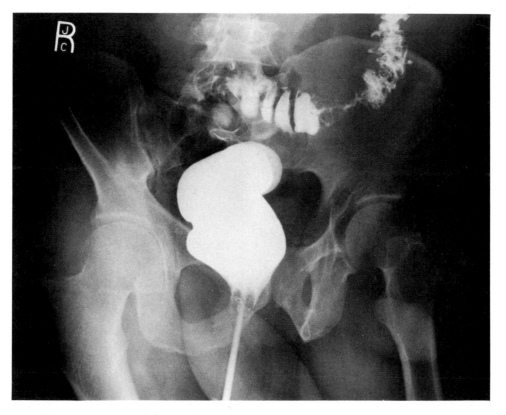

FIG. 14-8. Sigmoid diverticulitis: proximal sigmoid stricture with intact mucosa.

Unfortunately, differentiation between sigmoid diverticulitis and carcinoma is not always readily established.

The *sine qua non* for distinguishing the two conditions is the presence of intact colonic mucosa (Figs. 14-8 through 14-10). In my opinion, this is the most valuable radiologic finding in permitting differentiation. It is extremely important to fill the bowel lumen on both sides of the stricture. An attempt at filling the colon may be impossible because of significant sigmoid narrowing. Whereas the x-ray shown in Figure 14-11 probably reveals a normal mucosa in spite of inadequate proximal filling, the obstruction shown in Figure 14-12 would preclude an accurate diagnosis.

The length of the narrowed segment has also been felt to be an important differential diagnostic radiologic finding. In patients with carcinoma, the stricture is usually quite short, whereas with diverticulitis, strictures usually are longer (Fig. 14-13).

The presence of a mass in the wall of the bowel with the mucosa intact is a third diagnostic point consistent with diverticulitis. An intramural or mesenteric abscess is the commonest complication of diverticular disease (Figs. 14-14 and 14-15).

The presence of associated diverticula within or around the segment of narrowing has also been thought to be reasonable circumstantial evidence for benign disease. However, because carcinoma of the colon and diverticular disease are frequently seen in association, too much emphasis should not be placed on this finding. Figure 14-16 illustrates a diverticulum within a segment of narrowing that proved to be a carcinoma. Pseudodiverticula can be present due to the deformity of the invasive cancer. Overhanging margins are highly suspicious of cancer, as well as destruction of the mucosa itself. But none of the observations described is an infallible aid for establishing the diagnosis. Figure 14-17 reveals overhanging edges and an element of mucosal destruction; following resection, pathologic evaluation revealed this to be sigmoid diverticulitis.

As mentioned, flexible fiberoptic sigmoidoscopy and colonoscopy may be usefully employed to differentiate between diverticulitis and carcinoma. The problem,

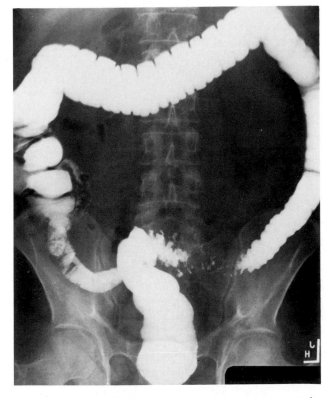

FIG. 14-9. Sigmoid diverticulitis: a mass containing multiple diverticula with preservation of mucosa.

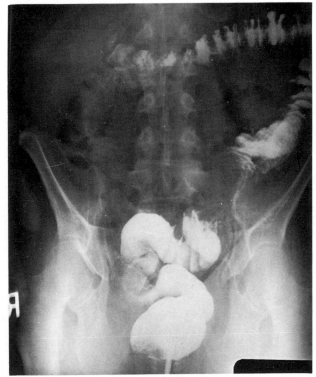

FIG. 14-10. Sigmoid diverticulitis: a large mass with suspicious ''overhanging'' margins but with normal mucosa.

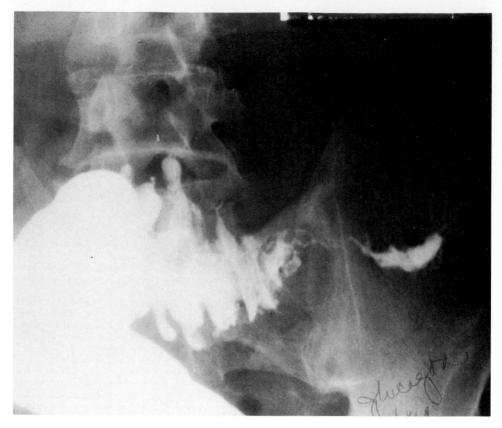

FIG. 14-11. Sigmoid diverticulitis: presumed mucosal preservation in an inadequately studied colon.

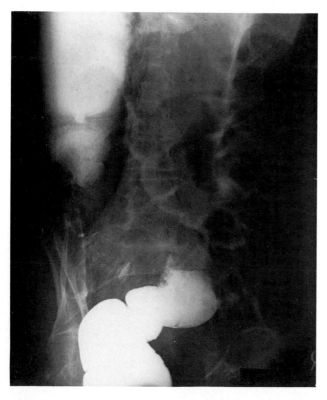

FIG. 14-12. Sigmoid colon obstruction: differential diagnosis between carcinoma and diverticulitis is impossible. The lesion eventually proved to be diverticulitis.

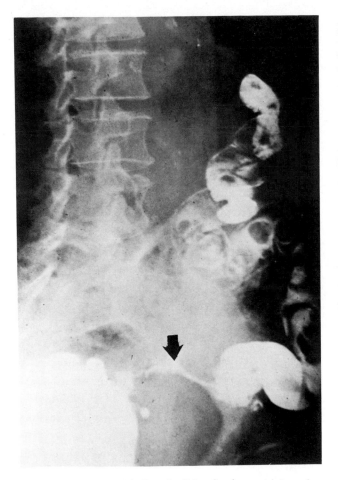

FIG. 14-13. Sigmoid diverticulitis: the long stricture *(arrow)* is more consistent with inflammatory change than neoplasm.

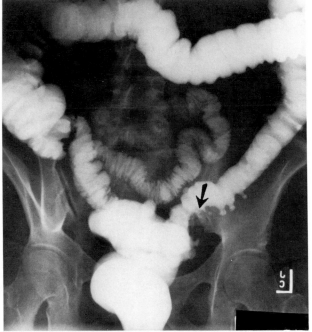

FIG. 14-14. Sigmoid diverticulitis: intramural abscess *(arrow)* of the proximal sigmoid with intact mucosa.

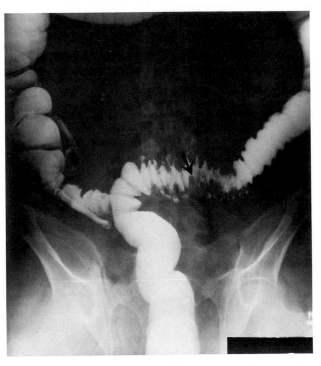

FIG. 14-15. Sigmoid diverticulitis: an irregular mass in the wall of the bowel *(arrow)* with extensive associated diverticulosis and with mucosal preservation.

however, is to satisfactorily negotiate the sigmoid colon without causing injury. Even in the noninflamed bowel, the sigmoid colon may be quite narrow because of thickening of the muscularis. The surgeon can feel assured only if the entire mucosa has been visualized and appears intact, and the openings of the diverticula are identified (Fig. 14-18). Erythema and edema of the bowel wall are usually seen, and occasionally pus may be observed to exude from one of the orifices.

A number of studies have been recently published advocating colonoscopy as an effective tool in the differentiation of carcinoma and diverticulitis.[28, 34, 75, 124] As mentioned, the risk of injury from the instrument itself is only one problem; less obvious is the hidden hazard of air pressure in causing overt perforation through a thin-walled diverticulum or walled-off abscess.[124] For these reasons only the most courageous

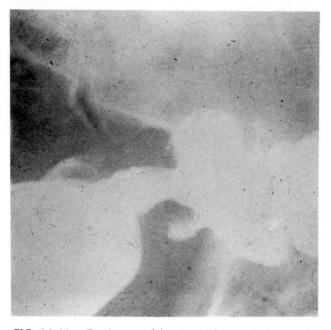

FIG. 14-16. Carcinoma of the sigmoid. Pseudodiverticula or even true diverticula may be frequently associated with cancer of the sigmoid colon.

endoscopist would embark upon this procedure in the acutely ill patient. Examination under such circumstances is probably contraindicated, but as the patient's symptoms improve, endoscopic evaluation should be considered if the differential diagnosis is still in question.

Dean and Newell reported 36 patients in whom barium enema examination had suggested the possibility of carcinoma in a segment of diverticular disease.[28] All of the patients were examined at least 6 weeks following an acute exacerbation of the condition. The authors found that the procedure was particularly difficult to perform, having failed to visualize the diseased segment in approximately half of the cases. However, they were able through colonoscopy to establish the diagnosis of carcinoma in four patients and exclude it in five. Max and Knutson performed colonoscopic evaluation on 26 patients in whom radiologic examination disclosed an area of spasm or diverticulitis that raised a suspicion of carcinoma.[75] In 19 patients the questionable area was completely visualized; in every patient successfully examined the diagnosis was proved correct in 100%.

In patients who fail to respond despite vigorous medical management and who are found on the basis of radiologic studies or ultrasonography to have a localized abscess, consideration may be given to percutaneous drainage of the septic process. Greco and

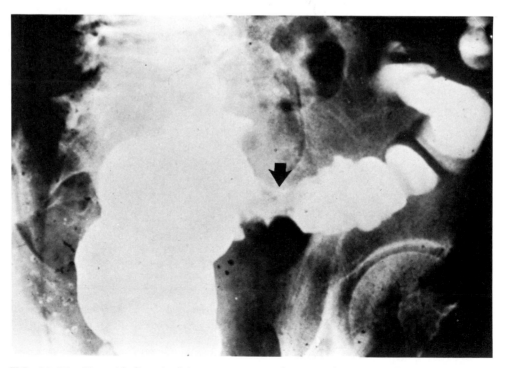

FIG. 14-17. Sigmoid diverticulitis: apparent ''napkin-ring'' lesion, overhanging margins, and mucosal irregularity. The lesion proved to be benign.

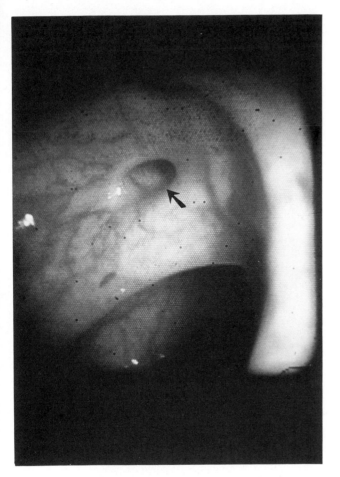

FIG. 14-18. Diverticular opening in sigmoid colon seen through a flexible instrument.

co-workers performed percutaneous drainage of a peridiverticular abscess by means of sonography-guided catheter placement.[44] This was subsequently followed by successful primary colonic resection.

Other Diseases

As mentioned, the most important differential diagnosis, and the one that presents the most difficulty, is that of carcinoma. Other diseases may present with signs, symptoms, and findings that may mimic diverticulitis; these include Crohn's disease, ulcerative colitis, acute appendicitis, ischemic colitis, pelvic inflammatory disease, and urinary tract disorders (infection, nephrolithiasis).

It is sometimes quite difficult to differentiate *Crohn's disease* from diverticulitis. Symptoms which may lead the surgeon to suspect underlying Crohn's disease are diarrhea and rectal bleeding. Presence of anal disease (fissure, fistula) is also more suggestive of Crohn's disease. Sigmoidoscopic examination reveals a normal rectum in diverticulitis, whereas in Crohn's disease the rectum may or may not be spared. Even at the time of laparotomy it may be impossible to distinguish between the two conditions. Usually, however, the pathologist has little difficulty in making the distinction. In true diverticulitis the mucous membrane, although edematous, is otherwise normal. Evidence of granularity or ulceration is indicative of inflammatory bowel disease. The presence of granulomas does not necessarily distinguish Crohn's disease, because foreign body giant cells as a reaction to pericolonic abscess can be seen in diverticulitis.[83]

In our experience during the period 1957 through 1978 in patients who required colonic resection for "diverticulitis" a second time, all 25 patients eventually proved to have combined diverticulitis and Crohn's disease.[15] In many instances the diagnosis of Crohn's colitis was suspected but unproved until a subsequent resection provided histopathologic proof of combined diverticulitis and Crohn's disease. Symptoms and signs of recurrent illness were similar to those present when the patient was initially seen, that is, prior to the first operation. In these patients there was often a history of smoldering illness, in contrast to the more episodic nature of the symptoms in patients with diverticulitis. The age of the patient was not particularly helpful in distinguishing the two conditions, because in the older age groups Crohn's disease tends to involve the large bowel.

The distinction between the two diseases is extremely important, since medical and surgical treatment differs. In retrospect, the development of extracolonic manifestations (*e.g.*, pyoderma, arthritis), unusual technical difficulty in performing the resection, and failure of decompression to result in resolution of the colonic inflammatory process should lead the surgeon to suspect that he is dealing with Crohn's disease.

The distinction between acute diverticulitis and a complication of *ulcerative colitis* should not be difficult. Proctosigmoidoscopic examination always reveals disease in the rectum in patients with ulcerative colitis (see Chap. 15). However, the rectum is spared with diverticulitis. Although the two conditions can certainly coexist, it is difficult to imagine how one might be able to distinguish acute diverticulitis superimposed upon acute ulcerative colitis. The importance of performing a sigmoidoscopic examination prior to embarking upon surgery for acute diverticulitis cannot be overestimated. The presence of inflammatory changes in the rectum or a high index of suspicion of inflammatory bowel disease would dictate an alternative operative approach.

Ischemic colitis may pose a problem in differential diagnosis. This is particularly true if the ischemic changes include the rectosigmoid. However, patients who have disease limited to this location usually present with frequent bowel movements and rectal bleeding. Abdominal pain is suggestive of a more fulminant manifestation and a more extensive one. The presence of thumb printing on the barium enema film and the involvement of the process particularly in the region of the splenic flexure suggest ischemia (see Fig. 17-7).

COMPLICATIONS

Free Perforation

Free perforation with generalized peritonitis is an uncommon complication of diverticulitis. When it occurs it can have catastrophic consequence. Patients are critically ill and demonstrate the usual signs and symptoms of septicemia. The history may be one of rather sudden onset of abdominal pain, usually in the lower abdomen, progressing to generalized pain. Marked abdominal distention may be noted, due to pneumoperitoneum (Fig. 14-19). Abdominal rigidity is usually observed. An upright film of the abdomen or a lateral decubitus x-ray film will reveal the presence of free gas (Fig. 14-20). It has been sometimes suggested that the amount of gas present on the roentgenogram will lead the surgeon to suspect either a colonic or a gastroduodenal perforation: the more gas present, the greater the likelihood of it being a colonic perforation. This may be a helpful distinguishing feature in determining the area where the incision will be made.

Phlegmon or Abscess

The most common complication of sigmoid diverticulitis is a walled-off perforation or abscess. An acute inflammatory reaction usually involves the sigmoid colon and its mesentery. Signs and symptoms are usually confined to the left lower quadrant of the abdomen. Varying degrees of peritoneal irritation may be manifested. Radiologic evaluation may reveal the changes

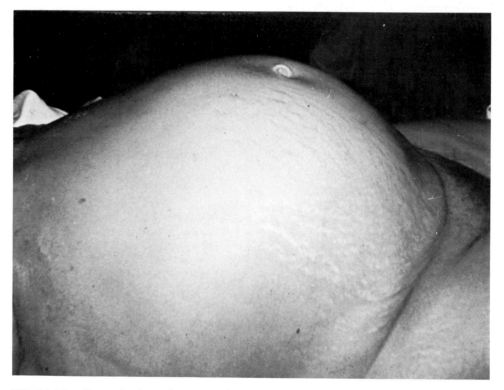

FIG. 14-19. Free colonic perforation with pneumoperitoneum producing profound abdominal distension.

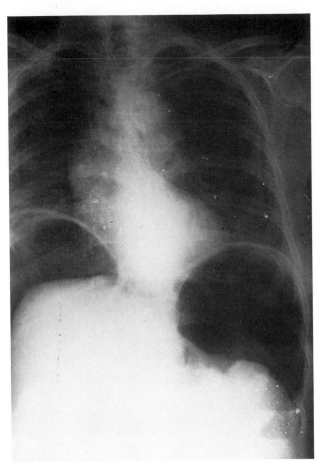

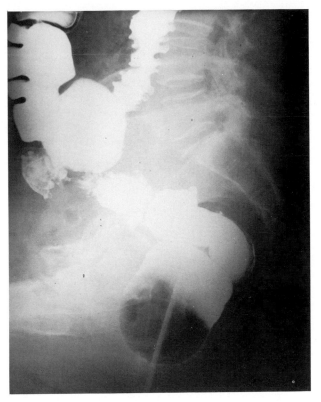

FIG. 14-21. Diverticulitis with abscess seen on barium enema in lateral projection.

FIG. 14-20. Upright abdominal roentgenogram reveals free gas under both hemidiaphragms. Perforation of the colon secondary to diverticulitis was found.

already described, but in addition there may be tracking of the barium into other areas. The barium may fill an abscess cavity adjacent to the perforation (Fig. 14-21) track down into the pelvis to present as an ischiorectal abscess (Fig. 14-22), lead to a pelvic abscess with consequent rectal narrowing and deviation (Fig. 14-23 and 14-24), perforate into the abdominal wall (Fig. 14-25), or track into quite distant areas (Fig. 14-26). Whereas surgical intervention in a case of free perforation is mandatory, and a decision easily reached, this is not necessarily true of the patient with an acute phlegmonous diverticulitis or localized abscess. The aforementioned medical measures are usually instituted, but in patients who have a continued nidus for sepsis (an undrained abscess), persistent pain, fever, white blood count elevation, or failure to achieve successful oral alimentation, the surgeon should suspect this complication.

Fistula

The commonest cause of *colovesical fistula* is diverticulitis. In the experience of Colcock and Stahmann, this manifestation accounted for half of all fistulas secondary to diverticulitis.[24] The second most common fistula was colocutaneous, followed by colovaginal, coloenteric, and other unusual manifestations (coloureteric, colouterine, *etc.*). In our experience, of the 55 patients found to have colovesical fistulas, 30 fistulas were due to diverticulitis (55%).[62] Other causes included malignant tumors from several organs, inflammatory bowel disease, and radiation therapy. Sixty-nine percent presented symptoms related to the urinary tract. Pneumaturia was the most frequent complaint, followed by frequency of urination, dysuria, fecaluria, and hematuria. Complaints unrelated to the urinary tract included lower abdominal pain and fever; less than a quarter of patients experienced these symptoms, however. Passage of urine through the rectum is exceedingly rare and probably the result of bladder outflow obstruction.

(Text continues on p. 504)

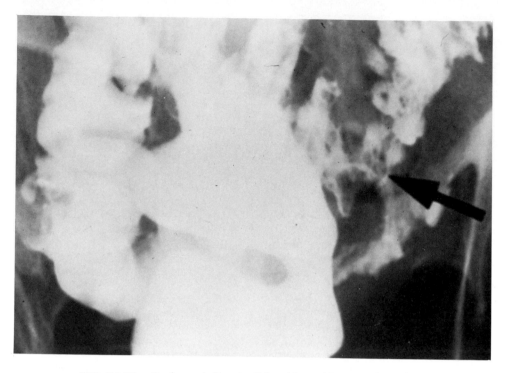

FIG. 14-22.   Perforated diverticulitis with tracking into the pelvis.

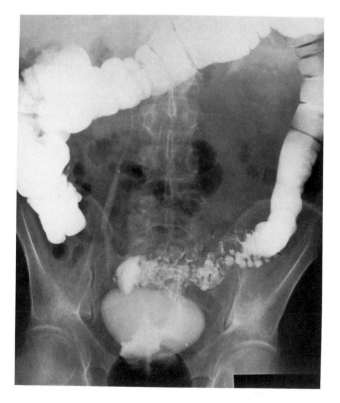

FIG. 14-23.   Perforated diverticulitis with a pelvic mass and rectal deviation.

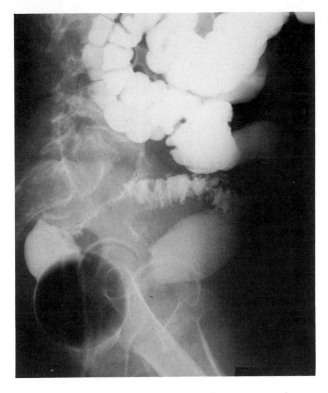

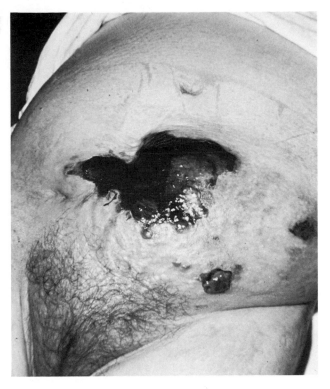

FIG. 14-24. Pararectal and pelvic abscess secondary to diverticulitis producing rectal narrowing.

FIG. 14-25. Gangrene of the abdominal wall from perforation of the sigmoid underlying the area.

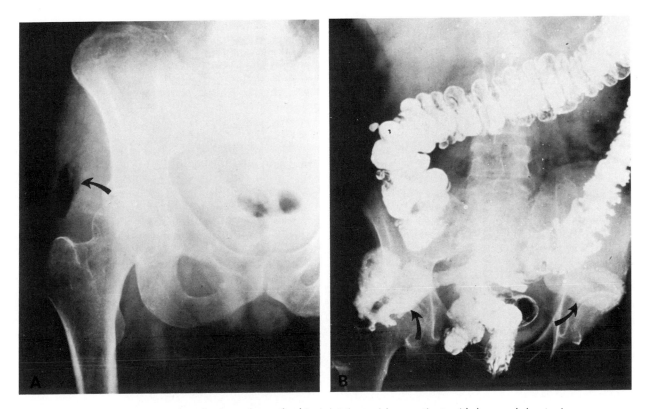

FIG. 14-26. **A.** Gas shadow above the hip joint *(arrow)* in a patient with lower abdominal pain. **B.** Subsequent barium enema reveals extravasation in both acetabula *(arrows)*.

503

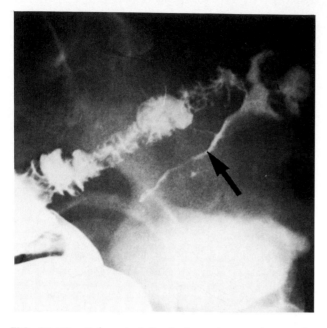

FIG. 14-27. Colovesical fistula *(arrow)* secondary to diverticulitis.

Colovaginal fistula may be a late consequence of acute diverticulitis, after the abdominal signs and symptoms subside. Discharge of feces, blood, pus, mucus, or gas are the usual complaints. Pelvic examination usually reveals an opening or granular area at the apex of the vagina, most commonly on the left side. Barium enema may identify the communication (see Fig. 4-37), or alternative diagnostic means may be employed (see Chap. 4).

The procedures employed to evaluate patients suspected of colovesical fistula include urinalysis, urine culture, barium enema, cystoscopy, cystography, intravenous pyelography, and endoscopy. Occasionally, other techniques, such as methylene blue dye administered rectally during cystoscopy, are employed. The study with the greatest frequency of identifying the site of the fistula is the barium enema examination (Fig. 14-27). Although sigmoidoscopy is useful in evaluating the presence or absence of inflammatory bowel disease, in our experience it failed to disclose a single fistula. Flexible fiberoptic endoscopy was not available in our study, so its applicability to the evaluation of this complication could not be assessed.

The surgical management of acute diverticular disease is discussed later, but the unique features of colovesical or colovaginal fistula necessitate discussion of the operative approach at this point. Frequently an operation must be undertaken on the basis of clinical suspicion without definitive endoscopic or radiologic evidence of a fistula.

Characteristically, at laparotomy the sigmoid colon is seen to be tethered in the pelvis, fixed to the bladder wall, or, in a woman whose uterus is surgically absent, adherent to the apex of the vagina. Usually the fistula can be divided by blunt dissection, pinching the area between the colon and the bladder or vagina. Occasionally, when a long-standing fistula causes extensive fibrosis, sharp dissection and division of the communication is required. It is not necessary to close a vaginal opening; a drain may be placed through the vagina into the pelvis if the surgeon prefers, but this is not mandatory. However, it is usually advisable to close the bladder opening with interrupted absorbable sutures, in two layers if possible. Excision of the bladder, formally closing the organ in an area where there is no fibrosis, is an unnecessarily meddlesome technique. The bowel is resected and a primary anastomsis is performed to the upper rectum. No protecting colostomy is advised.

Hool and colleagues reviewed over 2300 patients with diverticular disease, 80 of whom required operative treatment.[53] Four coloenteric fistulas were noted, an incidence of 5%. Pheils and co-workers noted that 25% of 80 patients for whom elective resection was performed had a fistula, a very high incidence.[97] Ten percent of the 144 patients who underwent resection for diverticular disease (elective and emergency) in the series of Orebaugh and associates had a colonic fistula.[88]

In our review of surgery for diverticular disease, 51 patients were operated upon for colonic fistula.[50] There were 3 deaths (6%; Table 14-1).

Hemorrhage

Massive lower gastrointestinal bleeding has been generally attributed to diverticular disease, usually without any evidence of diverticulitis.[40, 86, 125] However, recent evidence would seem to suggest that unexplained massive lower intestinal bleeding, even in the presence of known diverticulosis, is most likely due to an arteriovenous malformation (angiodysplasia) rather than diverticular disease[4, 10, 11] With the advent of angiography, and the ability to indentify preoperatively the site of bleeding, arteriovenous malformations have not uncommonly been observed in areas where diverticulosis is present.

Baer demonstrated 20 of 22 patients to have had a pathologically proved ruptured vasa recta within a diverticulum as the source of lower gastrointestinal hemorrhage.[9] Theoretically, the vasa recta is in intimate contact with the dome of the diverticulum and can

Table 14-1.   Surgery for Diverticular Disease: Morbidity and Mortality

Presentation	Number of Patients	Number of Complications*	Number of Deaths	Percent Mortality
Phlegmon	99	56	7	7
Fistula	51	44	3	6
Abscess	33	31	2	6
Obstruction	9	6	1	10
Perforation	7	9	1	14
Total	155	146	14	9

*Some patients had more than one complication.
(Helbraun MA, Corman ML, Coller JA, Veidenheimer MC: Diverticular disease. Reported at the annual meeting of the American Society of Colon and Rectal Surgeons, 1979)

rupture either at the apex of the diverticulum or at the neck on the antimesenteric border as the vessel proceeds into the submucosa of the colon. The problem, however, is that most lower gastrointestinal hemorrhage comes from the right side of the colon, where there are few or no diverticula. Since vascular ectasia is most commonly seen in the right colon, and this is the commonest site for lower gastrointestinal hemorrhage, one must presume that vascular malformation is the most frequent cause of lower intestinal hemorrhage. The bleeding associated with ectasia is usually less severe, tends to be intermittent, and is probably due to venous encroachment of the mucosa as compared with the ruptured vasa rectum of a bleeding diverticulum.

Symptoms

Patients usually present with no antecedent history, and they frequently have no abdominal pain. Blood from the rectum may be bright red or maroon, and may contain clots. If the bleeding is severe enough, hypotension may ensue, with the requirement for resuscitative measures. Usually, however, the patient's condition is relatively stable, permitting time for evaluation.

Physical examination is usually unrewarding. Often the bleeding ceases spontaneously; the administration of an enema prior to endoscopic examination or a barium enema study has frequently been therapeutic.[1] But proceeding directly to barium enema examination is not advised; a contrast study will preclude the possibility of performing an adequate angiographic study for perhaps several days. Although barium enema may succeed in identifying an intraluminal lesion, the presence of diverticula does not indicate that they are the source of the bleeding. One would be hard pressed to identify which diverticulum was the site of the hemorrhage in Figure 14-28, if bleeding were coming from

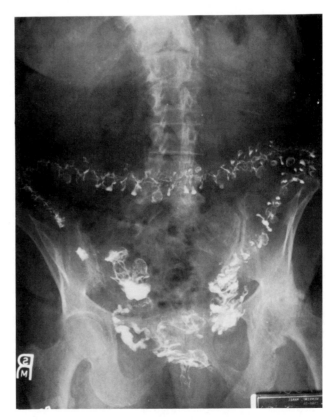

FIG. 14-28.   Post-evacuation barium enema in a patient with massive intestinal hemorrhage shows extensive diverticulosis. Identification of the source of bleeding is impossible.

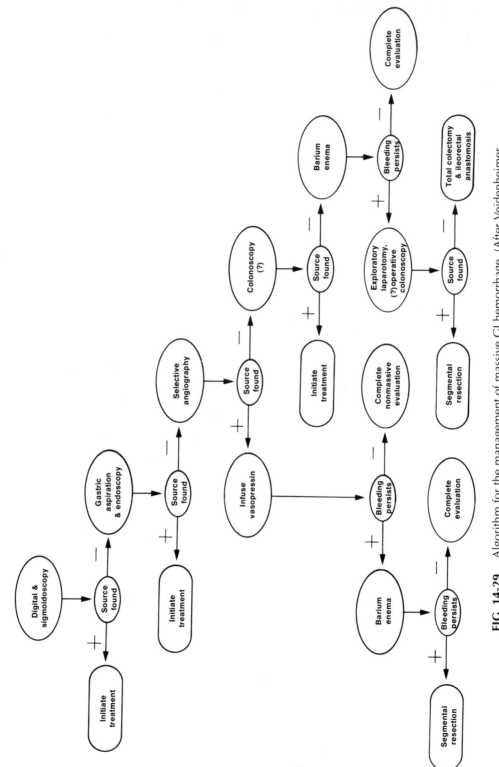

FIG. 14-29. Algorithm for the management of massive GI hemorrhage. (After Veidenheimer MC, Corman ML, Coller JA: Colonic hemorrhage. Surg Clin North Amer 1978; 58:581-590).

one of them in the first place. An organized approach to the evaluation of the patient with massive hemorrhage of presumed colonic origin is suggested. An algorithm is presented in Figure 14-29 that provides an overview for carrying out the proper sequence of studies in the hemorrhaging patient.

Having identified the source of bleeding by means of rectal examination, sigmoidoscopy, or upper gastrointestinal endoscopy, appropriate therapy can be instituted. Unfortunately, in patients who massively bleed from the colon, these studies are usually not diagnostic. The next investigative procedure that should be performed is selective angiography. Unless the technique is not available at a hospital, the patient should not be taken to the operating room without this radiologic investigation. Direct selective catheterization of the celiac, superior mesenteric, and inferior mesenteric artery is accomplished by way of the groin using a modified Seldinger technique.[110] In suspected lower gastrointestinal bleeding, the superior mesenteric artery is injected first because of the higher incidence of colonic bleeding from the right side.[41] If the source of bleeding is not found, the inferior mesenteric artery is then studied. Finally, if no source is identified, a celiac injection should be made, because, rarely, upper gastrointestinal bleeding may appear to come from the colon. Radiographic abnormalities include extravasation (Fig. 14-30), arteriovenous malformation (Fig. 14-31), and an early filling vein (Fig. 14-32).

If the bleeding point is identified, it may be possible to control the hemorrhage by means of either an embolization technique or the infusion of Pituitrin (vasopressin). The use of vasopressin to control gastrointestinal hemorrhage has several disadvantages, however. First, the drug has the side-effects, which include decreased cardiac output, hypertension, and arrhythmias.[41] The mechanism of effectiveness of the drug is due to vasoconstriction with decreased flow to the area. Since many of these patients are elderly and perhaps have an unstable cardiovascular condition, it is important to carefully monitor the intake and output; vasopressin has a profound antidiuretic effect. In addition, there are problems related to prolonged catheter use: embolism, hemorrhage around the puncture site, hematoma, and limitation of activity. An arterial pump is needed in order to administer the drug. The position of the catheter has to be checked daily by means of a portable x-ray. Many papers have been published that deal with the efficacy of vasopressin in the treatment of gastrointestinal hemorrhage.[12, 30, 99]

The use of embolization has been reported to be an acceptable alternative to infusing a vasoconstrictor.[42, 74, 81, 107, 112] Diagnostic angiography is followed by selective embolization with Gelfoam strips or autologous

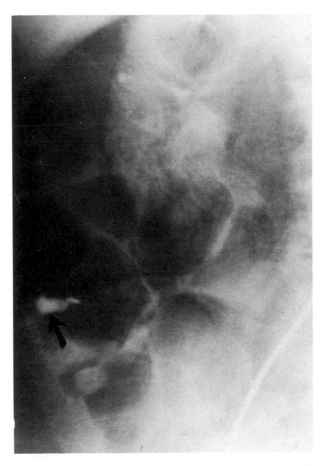

FIG. 14-30. SMA injection: contrast collects in the right colon *(arrow)*. A bleeding diverticulum was found at resection. (Courtesy of Brian A. Schnier, M.D.)

clotted blood through the same catheter. Since Gelfoam particles have a low coefficient of friction and therefore are readily injectable through comparatively small catheters, injection can take place satisfactorily even through relatively small bleeding arterial branches.[74] Not every patient is suitable for such therapy, nor is the technique readily available in all medical centers. However, for those patients deemed appropriate, if a satisfactory response is achieved, operative intervention may be avoided or at least delayed so that it might be performed at an elective time.

Although the value of *colonoscopy* is undeniable in the investigation of a patient with undiagnosed rectal bleeding,[59, 114] its use during an episode of massive colonic hemorrhage is considerably limited. The instrument may, in fact, induce hemorrhage that may have

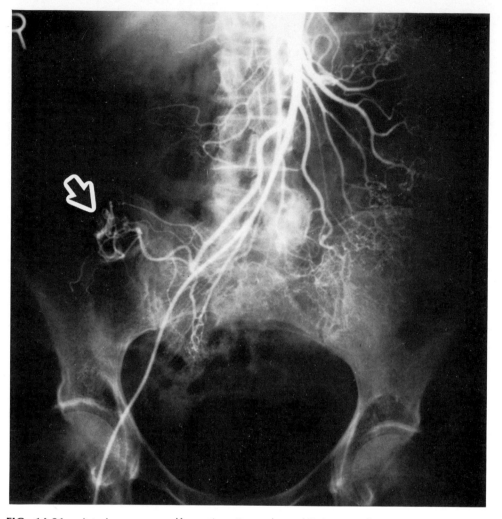

FIG. 14-31. Arteriovenous malformation "vascular tuft" *(arrow)* demonstrated by SMA injection. (Courtesy of Brian A. Schnier, M.D.)

ceased previously. The procedure is technically complex and should be performed only by the most experienced operators. Instruments with large-bore suction channels, additional aspirating–irrigating equipment, and fluoroscopic control are mandatory.[118]

Examination within 24 to 36 hours after cessation of active massive hemorrhage enables the endoscopist to perform the examination without a complete bowel preparation.[118] Forde reported the results of colonoscopy performed on 25 patients during or soon after an episode of active rectal bleeding, when the barium enema or mesenteric angiography was either not fea-

sible or when the results were negative.[35] He advises frequent changing of the patient's position; by this technique, the instrument can be passed while the liquid blood is in a rather dependent portion of the bowel. He found five patients to be bleeding from diverticular disease, three from unsuspected carcinomas, and two each from polyps, ischemic colitis, and arteriovenous malformations. Results of five examinations were negative. There was one perforation that was recognized immediately. Although Forde's results were impressive, he cautions that the technique is not terribly valuable when bleeding is active, but it is most usefully per-

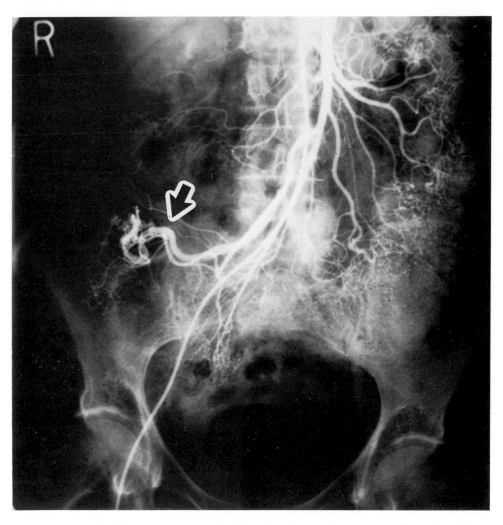

FIG. 14-32. Early filling vein *(arrow)* draining from the arteriovenous malformation shown in Fig. 14-31. (Courtesy of Brian A. Schnier, M.D.)

formed soon after the onset or cessation of hemorrhage. He also emphasizes the requirement for more experience and skill than is usually necessary for routine colonoscopy.

Surgical Treatment

As implied from the foregoing, if the bleeding point is identified by means of angiography, endoscopy, or barium enema examination, the appropriate therapy can be instituted: medical management or resection, depending on the nature of the lesion and the patient's clinical course. What is the proper treatment if the patient continues to bleed, and if the source has not been identified? In the past, patients were submitted to exploratory laparotomy in the hope that a lesion could be identified at the operating table. Multiple colotomies were undertaken to identify the proximal limit of the bleeding and to perform operative coloscopy. In the high-risk patient, a prolonged operative procedure exposes the patient to increased mortality as well as further morbidity due to infection from contamination. Alternatively, blind left colectomy had been advocated for a time (Figs. 14-33 and 14-34), and more recently,

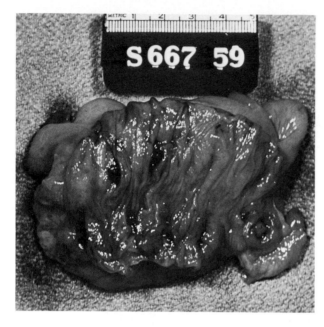

FIG. 14-33. "Blind" sigmoid colectomy reveals clot in several diverticula.

right colectomy. Another alternative involves a combination of laparotomy and colonoscopy using a two-team approach. The abdominal surgeon assists the colonoscopist in the passage of the instrument in order to make one final attempt to identify a discrete bleeding point.[118] If one is seen, it may be dealt with through the instrument, or it may be effectively treated by a less-than-total abdominal colectomy. But if a bleeding point is not identified at the time of surgery and the bleeding appears to be of lower intestinal origin, total abdominal colectomy is advised. However, it is important to search vigorously for the cause of the bleeding in accordance with the algorithm described in Figure 14-29. With the diagnostic studies available today, the surgeon should rarely have to resort to blind resection.

SURGICAL TREATMENT OF ACUTE DIVERTICULITIS

If the patient fails to respond to medical measures or if the patient's condition is deteriorating, urgent surgical intervention should be performed. Obviously, in the patient with generalized peritonitis and pneumoperitoneum, emergency operation is indicated.

There are basically six operations available for the treatment of acute sigmoid diverticulitis (Fig. 14-35):

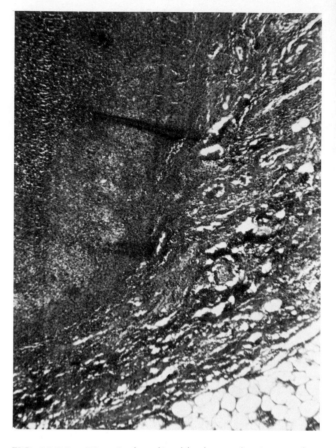

FIG. 14-34. Diverticulum lined by hemorrhagic granulation tissue in a patient who had massive lower GI hemorrhage. (Original magnification × 260. Courtesy of Rudolf Garret, M.D.)

1. Transverse colostomy and drainage of the perforation
2. Exteriorization of the involved segment
3. Resection, sigmoid or descending colon colostomy, and mucous fistula
4. Resection, end colostomy, and closure of rectal stump (Hartmann)
5. Resection, primary anastomosis, and protecting transverse colostomy
6. Resection and primary anastomosis (no stoma)

Transverse Colostomy and Drainage

Staged operation has been advocated for the treatment of acute diverticulitis for many years. This consists of a diversionary colostomy and drainage, elective resection, and, finally, closure of the colostomy. This procedure had been advocated by Mayo in 1907, by Rankin and Brown, and Smithwick.[77, 101, 111] Until recently, intestinal diversion was felt to be the safest surgical procedure for carrying the patient through the critical phase of his illness. A transverse loop colostomy is performed, and drainage of the infected area is established (Fig. 14-35, *A*). (The technique is described in Chap. 16). Although the operation has been successful in the acute management of these patients, morbidity and mortality for the three stages are quite high. The patient must contend for some time with a difficult stoma. In addition, the nidus of sepsis may persist for many weeks or even months. In essence, the entire left colon is available to drain through the perforation if the opening is still present free in the peritoneal cavity. Furthermore, inadequate external drainage may not have been established in the first instance. Placing a drain on top of an inflamed sigmoid colon does not permit adequate drainage. If an abscess is present it will obviously remain untreated. When the surgeon decides to embark on a staged procedure, it is imperative that the inflammatory mass be mobilized sufficiently in order to break up any loculations and to effect adequate drainage.

If the patient succeeds in recovering from this initial operation, he still must look forward to at least two more procedures. The diseased bowel must ultimately be resected and an anastomosis performed. Closure of the colostomy is the final step in the three-stage approach. Each one of these procedures has its attendant morbidity and mortality.

The question remains of when to intervene and resect the colon after the fecal stream has been diverted. My own preference is to wait approximately 6 weeks. I have not uncommonly found the dissection quite easy at this stage and do not believe that further delay simplifies the subsequent operation. In fact, I have been in the position of struggling to perform a resection 6 months or even 1 year following the initial acute episode. I do not advocate this operation for the treatment of acute diverticular disease, especially perforation. However, this *is* a reasonable alternative for a surgeon to use if he does not feel comfortable with colon resection even under elective circumstances; this is certainly not the time to embark upon emergency colectomy. Another reason for performing initial drainage and diversion is when the colon cannot be mobilized safely. However, when the surgeon finds himself in this predicament, he should consider the possibility that there is an underlying carcinoma or that the patient has Crohn's disease.

One must differentiate between perforated diverticulitis with fecal peritonitis and that of a walled-off perforation or phlegmon in deciding whether to divert or to resect. In the former situation, colostomy and drainage is inappropriate, whereas with the latter, one may be reasonably content.

In 1980, Thompson stated in Maingot's textbook of abdominal operations that any perforation should be sutured and covered with adjacent appendix epiploica and a transverse colostomy performed.[115] Alexander-Williams reviewed four series and noted a mean mortality rate of 45% following perforated diverticular disease treated by drainage and colostomy.[3] His own experience from the Birmingham General Hospital during the period 1969 through 1973 (a total of 333 patients) revealed 68 deaths, a mortality rate of 22%. It was his opinion that this mortality rate was excessively high, implying that simply drainage and transverse colostomy is an inadequate operation for perforated diverticular disease, especially in the presence of generalized peritonitis or gross fecal contamination. Griffen cautions that although each patient should be individualized, the standard three-stage technique of right transverse colostomy, followed by resection of the involved colon, and finally closure of the transverse colostomy should be used rarely, if at all.[46]

When presenting the results of the three-stage resection, it is inaccurate for an author to state that his patients survived the initial insult, and then compare his mortality statistics with other operations that initially involved resection. The total morbidity and mortality of the three stages must be considered if one is to fairly compare the various techniques. Unfortunately, many studies fail to do this. The fact of the matter is that all too often staged operations with an initial colostomy are not carried through to the final procedure. Patients may be lost to follow-up, become too ill to undergo a secondary or tertiary procedure, refuse further surgery because they are well, be too great a risk for another operative procedure, or have expired in the interim. The surgeon should consider in his selection of the operation what is the likelihood of eventually reestablishing intestinal continuity in that individual.

Greif and associates reviewed over 1300 cases of acute perforated sigmoid diverticulitis from the literature, using 19 references from 1965 through 1979.[45] Criteria for selection of the cases included the presence of an abscess with localized or diffuse peritonitis. The surgery was performed during the acute illness, and the operative mortality was clearly stated. Among patients who had perforated diverticulitis with abscess and localized peritonitis (510 patients), those who were initially resected were found to have a 2% operative mortality, whereas those who underwent a proximal diverting colostomy (306 patients) had a 12% operative mortality; these differences were statistically significant. Over 800 patients with perforated diverticulitis

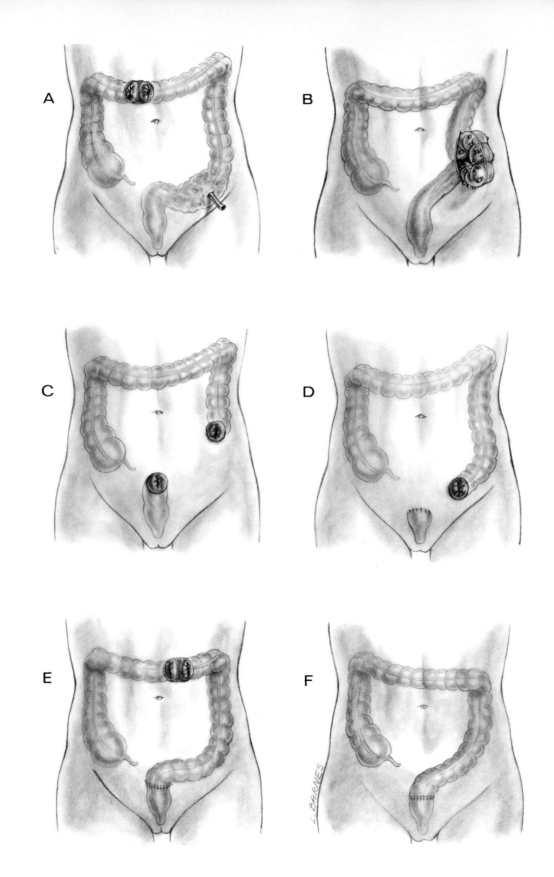

and generalized peritonitis underwent emergency surgery. The combined operative mortality was 12% for patients undergoing resection initially, against 29% who underwent colostomy and drainage.

Classen and co-workers reported a retrospective review of a 10-year experience with the three-stage operation.[23] Only patients with fecal or generalized peritonitis, or pelvic peritonitis with abscess were included in the study. Over 200 patients were considered. The operative mortality after the first stage was 8.5%, at the second stage, 0.7%, and at the third stage, 4%; therefore, the overall mortality rate was 11%.

Wara and associates ascertained the outcome of staged operations for complicated sigmoid diverticulitis for the 10-year period ending in 1979.[120] Of the 83 patients in the study, only 58% subsequently underwent a resection of the diseased segment, and fewer (46%) eventually had their intestinal continuity restored. Eleven of 25 patients died from generalized peritonitis when managed by proximal colostomy and drainage only (one third of those with purulent peritonitis and over 80% of those with fecal peritonitis).

Exteriorization and Resection with Colostomy and Mucous Fistula

Colonic exteriorization has been advocated for cancer since the end of the 19th century (Fig. 14-35, *B*). Eponymous operations have been associated with Bloch, Paul, and von Mikulicz.[17, 80, 96] Traditionally, resection was subsequently undertaken, and anastomosis was effected often with some form of spur-crushing clamp (Fig. 14-36). This operation succeeds in removing the nidus of sepsis from the peritoneal cavity, the single most important aim of surgery for complicated sigmoid diverticulitis. Today, however, it is not necessary to delay resection after the peritoneal cavity has been "sealed." The bowel is removed at the same time (see Fig. 14-35, *C*).

A sigmoid colostomy is an eminently satisfactory stoma to manage. The stool is formed and can be handled with a conventional colostomy appliance; the patient may elect to irrigate and employ only a small dressing (see Chap. 16). If the colostomy for one reason or another must be permanent, the patient should not

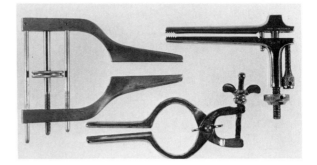

FIG. 14-36. Von Mikulicz's clamps. (Courtesy of Thomas J. Anglem, M.D.)

be significantly inconvenienced, at least not to the extent that he or she would be had the colostomy been located in the transverse colon. Transverse colostomies have all the disadvantages of colostomy and ileostomy, including a relatively liquid and malodorous effluent. After a period of time, most loop transverse colostomies will prolapse; even dividing the stoma is no guarantee of the subsequent development of this complication.

Another advantage of exteriorization–resection is the fact that the procedure requires only two stages to effect restoration of intestinal continuity; the second operation is relatively simple because the distal bowel can be easily identified.

The difficulty with recommending colostomy and mucous fistula following resection is that the disease rarely occurs at a sufficiently proximal location in the bowel to enable the distal colon to be delivered to the level of the skin. Far more commonly, the inflammatory reaction is confined to the sigmoid colon, usually almost to the level of the peritoneal reflection. Under these circumstances it is impossible to bring the distal bowel out to the abdominal wall. Thus, although the concept of resection with colostomy and mucous fistula is a good one, its application is quite limited.

Over the years there have been a number of advocates of this procedure[113, 121, 122]; its relatively limited application, however, implies that one must seek other alternatives for the treatment of acute sigmoid diverticulitis if one is to succeed in decreasing morbidity and mortality.

FIG. 14-35. Choice of operations for acute sigmoid diverticulitis. **A.** Loop transverse colostomy and drainage. **B.** Exteriorization. **C.** Resection, colostomy, and mucous fistula. **D.** Resection, colostomy, and rectal closure (Hartmann). **E.** Resection, anastomosis, and colostomy. **F.** Resection and anastomosis (no stoma).

Resection with Sigmoid Colostomy and Closure of Rectal Stump (Hartmann)

It is now generally agreed that if one is able to remove the source of the infection at the initial operation, this would be the most satisfactory operative approach. In 1923 Henri Hartmann published a two-paragraph observation that succeeded in achieving for him eponymous immortality.[48] His operation can perhaps best be described by the author himself in my somewhat liberal translation:

> It is the rule that, in order to remove cancers of the distal pelvic colon, it is necessary to perform a very serious operation when removing the rectum by means of abdominal perineal resection. In two patients who underwent colostomy for intestinal obstruction, at the second operation I limited resection to the intermediate portion of the colon between the artificial anus and the rectum including the corresponding area of innervation. Following this I closed the upper end of the rectum and reperitonealized it, without reconstructing the perineal floor.

> Following the operation both cases were as uneventful as that for an operation for a cold appendix. The conservation of a small cul-de-sac of the rectum above the sphincter did not present a particular problem, and follow-up 9 and 10 months later revealed the patients to be quite well.

Although the operation is infrequently performed for cancer, it has become in the United States the most commonly employed resective surgical procedure for the treatment of acute diverticulitis (see Fig. 14-35, *D*).

The operation involves a resection of the inflammatory bowel, end-sigmoid colostomy, and closure of the rectal stump. The procedure effectively removes the source of sepsis from the peritoneal cavity, creates a most satisfactory stoma, and obviates the risk for anastomosis under septic conditions. It does, however, have one major disadvantage: the second stage of the operation performed 6 or more weeks later requires a major abdominal procedure.

The colostomy must be excised and the proximal bowel liberated. Often this necessitates mobilizing the splenic flexure, a procedure that poses some risk for splenic injury. The so-called Hartmann pouch may be difficult to identify and may be considerably retracted. Even if satisfactory mobilization of the proximal and distal bowel can be achieved, there is still the risk of a

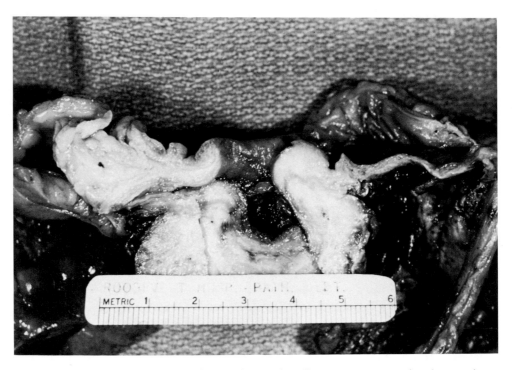

FIG. 14-37. Acute and chronic diverticulitis with inflammatory mass. The diverticulum simulates ulcerating carcinoma. (Courtesy of Rudolf Garret, M.D.)

complication related to the anastomosis itself. Since the operation is of some magnitude, many high-risk patients are deprived of the opportunity of having intestinal continuity reestablished. All too often, therefore, the Hartmann operation results in a permanent stoma.

The technique of removing the colon during the acute phase is worthy of some discussion. Many times when entering the peritoneal cavity the surgeon is confronted with what appears to be a large, fixed, unresectable mass (Fig. 14-37). However, one should not be overwhelmed by first appearances. The acute inflammatory reaction can often be dealt with by careful blunt dissection without fear of injuring vital retroperitoneal structures such as a ureter. Mobilization at a later time may be impossible without using sharp dissection. Under such circumstances the ureter is much more likely to be injured. If one begins the dissection by gently passing the left hand lateral to the inflammatory mass and easing the bowel away from the parietal peritoneum, one may be pleasantly surprised at how readily the mass seems to come free. An occasional fibrous band may be snipped with the scissors, but virtually the entire dissection is carried out bluntly with the tips of the fingers, either pushing to identify the plane of dissection or pinching adherent areas. When the bowel is delivered into the abdominal cavity, the surgeon can usually identify 1 or 2 cm of distal rectosigmoid that seem to be spared of inflammatory reaction (Fig. 14-38). This is an important point, because it is this sparing of the rectosigmoid that permits a relatively safe anastomosis, should one elect to perform it at that time. However, if the surgeon prefers the Hartmann operation, the bowel is resected, a colostomy is created, and the rectal stump is closed. Stump closure can be effected by conventional suture technique or by stapling with a TA stapler.

Bell suggests as an alternative to closing the rectal stump that every effort be made to create a mucous fistula.[13] In order to permit sufficient length to enable the surgeon to effect this, he suggests that less sigmoid colon be resected, even if it means leaving some element of residual disease or inflammation. At the second stage the remainder of the sigmoid can be resected and anastomosis created in the normal rectum. I have had no experience with this technique, but in the situations in which I have found myself, the large phlegmon would not permit preservation of sufficient bowel to create a mucous fistula. If one were to do this, in most cases this would necessitate leaving behind a potential source for sepsis.

A number of procedures have been devised to simplify subsequent reanastomosis of the Hartmann rectal pouch. Madure and Fiore advise the use of the TA-55 stapling device as well as permanently marking the two "corner" areas with 2-0 polypropylene (Prolene) su-

tures, leaving the ends trimmed to a length of 1 or 2 inches.[71] They found that the procedure effectively identified the pouch in all 30 patients in whom the technique was used. Alternative methods to identify the rectal stump include the use of a Foley catheter inserted into the rectum or a firm rectal tube.[27]

Another technique is the use of the circular stapling instrument. Ramirez and associates recommended initially inserting a rigid sigmoidoscope into the rectum with the distal end of the instrument pointed against the apex of the pouch.[100] The illuminated scope tip serves as the identification point for creating a small stab wound in the rectal wall. A No. 18 French urethral catheter with beveled tip is passed through the stab wound and out the rectum. The catheter is then attached to the pin end of the circular stapling device (Fig. 14-39, *A*). The instrument is then introduced into the rectum until the pin is passed through the opening that was created in the rectal pouch. No distal pursestring is required. After removing the catheter, the proximal bowel segment is drawn over the anvil, and the previously applied proximal pursestring suture is

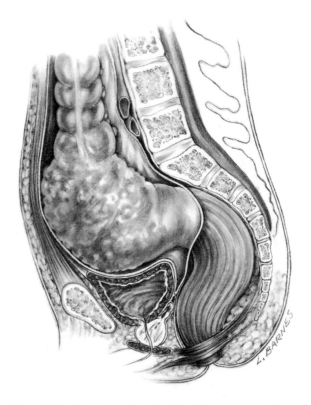

FIG. 14-38. Sigmoid diverticulitis. The mass usually terminates distally in relatively normal, uninflamed bowel, just above the peritoneal reflection.

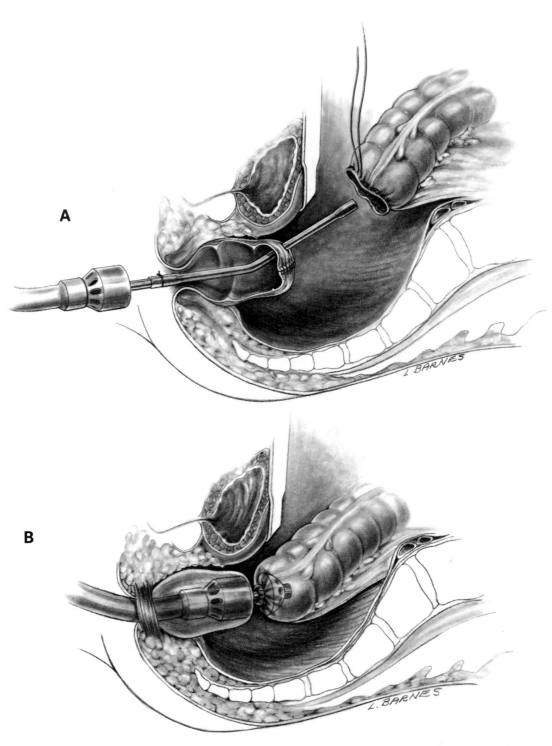

FIG. 14-39.   Circular staple technique for Hartmann pouch anastomosis. **A.** The stapler is introduced and guided by catheter (the head has been removed). **B.** The proximal bowel is brought down to effect anastomosis.

tied. The parts of the instrument are then reconnected and the stapling gun is fired, creating an end-to-end anastomosis without rectal mobilization (Fig. 14-39, B).

In analyzing the results of the Hartmann resection for acute and perforated diverticular disease, again it is inadequate to talk merely in terms of the first stage. In calculating the overall morbidity and mortality, one must consider the subsequent procedure or procedures. Unfortunately, much of the literature (which is voluminous) fails to deal with the entire spectrum of surgery required to effect complete resolution of the disease process, including reestablishment of intestinal continuity.

Nunes and colleagues performed a Hartmann resection on 25 patients for complications of acute diverticulitis.[87] Five failed to undergo a second-stage procedure (20%). There were two deaths after the first operation, a mortality rate of 8%. No deaths were reported after the second stage; however, three anastomotic leaks developed (15%), necessitating transverse colostomy. Approximately two thirds of the patients had essentially an uneventful postoperative course after the second operation. Labow and associates reported a complication rate of 67% in 15 patients treated by the Hartmann procedure, but there were no deaths.[63] Laimon reported only one death in 36 patients.[64]

Howe and co-workers compared their experience with the three-stage procedure and the Hartmann resection in patients with colon perforation secondary to diverticular disease.[54] An overall morbidity of 71% was noted after the three-stage operation, and 37% after the Hartmann. Wound infection comprised the major morbidity. The operative mortality in the former was 5%, versus approximately 6% in the latter. Only four additional surgical procedures were required in the Hartmann group, whereas 34 operations were additionally required in the three-stage group. Others also have reported favorable results with Hartmann's operation for perforated diverticulitis.[31, 68, 106]

Resection With Anastomosis With or Without Transverse Colostomy

The primary disadvantages of the previously mentioned Hartmann operation are the difficulty and the risk of subsequently reestablishing intestinal continuity. An alternative approach would be to effect an anastomosis at the initial operation and protect it with a transverse colostomy (see Fig. 14-35, E). The second stage procedure is, therefore, greatly simplified, although it, too, is not without morbidity (see Chap. 16). The resection and anastomosis can be performed in accordance with the principles outlined, recognizing that there is vir-

tually always a rim of relatively uninvolved rectum that will permit a safe anastomosis (see Fig. 14-38).

Another advantage of performing colorectal anastomosis at the first stage is that adequate mobility can usually be achieved without liberating the splenic flexure. Since further bowel usually must be sacrificed at the second stage of the Hartmann resection, splenic flexure mobilization is not uncommonly required.

The protecting colostomy is placed in the transverse colon on the *left* side (see Fig. 14-35, E). In truth, there is no advantage to a right transverse colostomy. The stool is theoretically more liquid on the right side, and the location predisposes to efferent limb prolapse. A left transverse colostomy is performed as far to the left as possible, so that the splenic flexure tethers the efferent limb, making prolapse virtually impossible. The colostomy should, however, be delivered through the split rectus muscle (see Chap. 16).

Should the colostomy be divided? In my opinion the answer is *no*. A properly constructed loop-ostomy stoma should not retract and is, therefore, completely diverting. Stool does not appear from the proximal limb, look around, and disappear into the distal opening. However, my major criticism of a divided colostomy is that it requires a formal resection and anastomosis, compared with simple closure of the anterior wall with the loop-ostomy.

The timing of the closure of the colostomy is always a subject for discussion among surgeons. A colostomy should not be undertaken whimsically (see Chap. 11). There is a considerable morbidity associated with its creation as well as its closure. Furthermore, it is not a convenient stoma to manage. But, having embarked upon this approach, the colostomy should remain at least 6 weeks. The morbidity of closure prior to this time is excessively high, probably because of the amount of inflammatory reaction.

Prior to closure, the anastomosis should be examined by means of the rigid proctosigmoidoscope or flexible fiberoptic instrument. The presence of pus suggests the possibility of a dehiscence. Barium enema is also suggested to ascertain whether the anastomosis is intact. Not uncommonly, a short track may be present, usually extending posteriorly (Fig. 14-40). Rarely should this pose a problem, and colostomy closure usually can be safely performed. The exception to this is when a communication exists to the abdominal wall (Fig. 14-41). In this situation a fecal fistula may be a consequence of closure. Reresection of the anastomosis may be required if healing does not take place within 3 or 4 months. However, no generalization can be made on this issue; some will close spontaneously, others will heal following development of a fecal fistula, and still others will never become manifest, never become symptomatic.

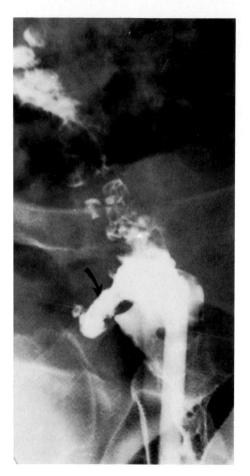

FIG. 14-40.   Barium enema demonstrates posterior dehiscence 8 weeks following low anterior resection *(arrow)*.

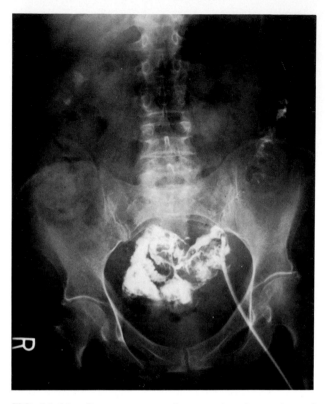

FIG. 14-41.   Status post anterior resection for perforated diverticulitis: a fistulogram through the abdominal wall reveals communication with the colon as well as the small bowel.

The treatment of perforated lesions of the sigmoid colon by primary resection with anastomosis and no colostomy (see Fig. 14-35, *F*) was initially advocated by Madden and Tan in 1961.[70] Although stating that "treatment. . .is admittedly contrary to the generally accepted surgical principles," the authors felt that their results suggested that this would be the preferred treatment. By 1966, however, Madden, although still adhering to the concept of resection at the first stage, felt that colostomy *should* be employed, particularly in cases of diffuse peritonitis and of gross contamination, and in situations in which the rectum was mobilized.[69]

Evaluation of reported series is difficult. Some investigators use the term "primary resection" interchangeably with "primary anastomosis (no colostomy)," "primary anastomosis (with colostomy)," and "Hartmann resection." Many authors equate primary resection with staged resection, and the reader never is told whether a protecting colostomy was employed.

Farkouh and associates performed primary resection and anastomosis without colostomy on 15 patients with perforation and peritonitis.[33] The operation was restricted to those whose bowel demonstrated no obstruction, was empty of feces, and was minimally edematous. Further criteria included normal distal bowel above the peritoneal reflection, no fecal contamination, and good general health of the patient. There was one death and one anastomotic leak. In reviewing a total of nine series with 73 patients so treated, these authors noted an operative mortality of 8.2%. Auguste and Wise suggest that colostomy is not necessary if a pericolic abscess is confined to the mesentery or if the abscess is localized to the pelvis.[8] With generalized peritonitis or fecal contamination, a colostomy in their opinion is mandated. Others have advised that patients who are receiving steroids should have a protective colostomy created.[108]

Comment

My preferred operative approach to the mangement of acute diverticular disease is to remove the inflammation at the first operation. Ideally, an anastomosis should be effected at the initial procedure. The Hartmann resection is used if technical factors preclude satisfactory anastomosis or if the patient's condition is tenuous.

A protecting colostomy is usually not used if the bowel is relatively well prepared (a not uncommon situation when the patient has been hospitalized for a number of days prior to operation). Also, if the perforation is into the mesentery or if the abscess is relatively small and localized to the pelvis, a colostomy is not a requisite. However, with peritonitis, poorly prepared bowel, obstruction, or fecal contamination, a protecting loop, left-transverse colostomy is indicated.

Drainage is recommended if there is an abscess present. Continued irrigation with large volumes of Ringer's lactate solution is advised for fecal peritonitis for 48 hours following the procedure. Since anaerobes are usually the predominant organism (*Bacteroides* is almost always present), along with coliforms and enterococci, systemic antibiotic therapy with metronidazole, clindamycin, or one of the newer cephalosporins is suggested. The addition of ampicillin and an aminoglycoside is recommended in the patient with massive contamination or generalized peritonitis.

ELECTIVE RESECTION

The decision of when to intervene surgically in a patient with uncomplicated sigmoid diverticular disease is a matter of considerable controversy, and is often a source of debate and conflict between internists and surgeons. It has been mentioned that diverticulosis in the absence of one of the described complications is unlikely to be the source of the patient's symptoms (bloating, cramps, abdominal pain, constipation, *etc.*). The antecedent history of a complication of diverticulitis somewhat simplifies the operative recommendation, but many patients who might benefit from resection do not have such a prior history. Radiologic evaluation that reveals narrowing, deformity, or even partial obstruction may help one decide in favor of the procedure, but one can never be certain that symptoms will resolve following resection unless acute disease is found at laparotomy. If colonoscopy reveals edema, stricture, or pus, resection would be indicated. Conversely, if colonoscopic evaluation is unremarkable, resection of the sigmoid colon is less likely to resolve the patient's complaints. Rennie and associates demonstrated a low complication rate in 88 patients who underwent elective resection for uncomplicated diverticular disease, but persistent symptoms were evident in 86%.[104]

It has been previously stated that surgery for complicated diverticulitis is associated with a high morbidity and mortality. If a patient recovers from an acute attack, the question must be addressed of whether the patient should undergo an elective resection. In our retrospective review, 133 patients underwent resection for diverticular disease as a planned, elective operation; there were no deaths, and only 10 complications were noted.[50] During the same period, 155 patients underwent an operation for complicated diverticular disease; the overall operative mortality was 9% (see Table 14-1). The complication rate was also extremely high.

Based on these observations, an "aggressive" attitude to elective surgical intervention in patients who have experienced a complication of diverticulitis is recommended. Elective resection is advised under the following circumstances:

- One or more attacks of left lower quadrant pain associated with fever, leukocytosis, and radiologic evidence of diverticulitis, especially if
    The patient is less than 55 years of age [22, 89]
    There is radiologic evidence of leak
    There are urinary tract symptoms (suggests possible impending fistula)
    There is evidence of obstruction
- Radiologic and endoscopic changes that cannot exclude cancer

Resection should be performed with the anastomosis placed into the rectum. Splenic flexure mobilization is not usually necessary, and attempt at removal of all diverticula is meddlesome and not helpful. Wolff and co-workers presented the Mayo Clinic experience with 505 elective resections for sigmoid diverticular disease between 1971 and 1976.[126] In reviewing the barium enema studies of 61 of these patients from 5 to 9 years postresection, only 9 (14.7%) showed progression of diverticula, and this was felt to be minimal in all cases. However, 7 patients (11.4%) developed signs and symptoms of recurrent diverticulitis. Although the authors felt there was no benefit in resecting all of the diverticula-bearing colon, the results are somewhat disturbing. Since the authors describe the operation as a "sigmoid resection," the explanation for their less-than-optimal results might be that the anastomosis was not placed into the rectum and that a zone of increased pressure was permitted to remain distal to the anastomosis. It should be remembered also that even in the elective situation there may be an unexpected abscess, phlegmon, fistula, or sealed perforation. The fact is that diverticular disease is associated with a higher operative complication rate than is resection for cancer.[18, 32]

MYOTOMY

Reilly, in 1964, recommended the performance of sigmoid myotomy in the treatment of diverticular disease.[102] In a more recent report he stated that the primary indication for the procedure is long-standing uncomplicated diverticular disease that has not responded to standard medical measures.[103] These patients composed 75% of his 104 reported cases. The remainder represent those patients who exhibited complications of sigmoid diverticulitis and who underwent elective myotomy following resolution of the acute process, sometimes following colostomy and drainage.

The procedure involves division of the antimesenteric tenia and underlying circular muscle from the rectosigmoid junction for "whatever distance is necessary," sometimes 60 cm. The mucosa is permitted to pout. If the lumen of the bowel is entered, Reilly recommends closure of the mucosa with catgut.

It is difficult to interpret the author's experience. In the uncomplicated group it would appear that the procedure is in actuality being performed for irritable bowel complaints. Reilly observes that the indications for the procedure's application seem to be diminishing.[103] He suggests that better medical treatment may be the reason.

In 1973, Hodgson proposed transverse teniamyotomy in the treatment of diverticular disease.[51] In a later article he and his co-workers reported four patients.[52] The two antimesenteric teniae are transversely incised at 2-cm intervals from the rectosigmoid junction proximally to the normal colon. These authors believe that the technique is simpler than Reilly's, but Reilly states that Hodgson's operation is less complete. More recently another report from Hodgson's group implied less enthusiasm for the technique.[76] However, decreased intraluminal pressure and decreased motility following natural and pharmacologic stimuli has been reported for transverse teniamyotomy.[65] Other modifications have been suggested with favorable functional results.[26]

Comment

I have had no experience with myotomy in the management of diverticular disease. However, I am of the opinion that careful and expeditious resection of acute inflammatory disease will prove to be the best operation with respect to morbidity, mortality, and long-term results.

The value of the technique for an irritable bowel, the "prediverticular state," and diverticulosis is perhaps less controversial and worthy of further investigation. Physiologic evaluation (motility and pressure studies) may permit identification of patients who will benefit from this approach.

COLONIC COMPLICATIONS OF TRANSPLANTATION

Patients who have undergone transplantation are prone to develop a variety of colonic complications, including prolonged ileus, intestinal obstruction, ischemic colitis, necrotizing enterocolitis, ulceration and hemorrhage, and perforated diverticulitis.[2, 16, 47, 57, 60, 82, 105, 109] Other causes of colonic perforation include overzealous use of exchange resin enemas and perforation of the colon by peritoneal dialysis trocars.[105]

A much higher percentage of renal transplant patients develop free perforations, as opposed to the more common mesenteric abscess or walled-off perforation in patients who have not undergone transplantation. The use of immunosuppressive agents and steroids are believed to be responsible. The complication can be of catastrophic consequence in this group of patients. Even when the patient does not manifest systemic signs and symptoms, surgical intervention should be performed early (Fig. 14-42). Because of diminished resistence in these patients, it is unlikely that a demonstrable perforation or abscess will resolve with conservative therapy.

GIANT COLONIC DIVERTICULUM

Giant colonic diverticulum is a rare clinical entity, although more than 50 cases have been reported in the past 30 years.[37, 49, 58, 73, 123] The condition was originally reported by Hughes and Greene and by Gabriel.[36, 55] The disease most frequently involves the sigmoid colon, but there are reports of solitary giant diverticula that have involved other areas of the bowel. All described cases originate from the antimesenteric border of the colon, with the lesion representing a pseudodiverticulum that becomes progressively enlarged.

Muhletaler and associates described the pathogenesis of giant diverticula.[84] They and others felt that the disease represents an unusual complication of diverticulitis. Theories include distention of a diverticulum from gas-forming organisms after the neck has been occluded, and a ball-valve mechanism causing gas trapping in the abscess cavity when the intraluminal pressure of the bowel increases. With few exceptions the reports have revealed that the diverticulum is not lined by mucosa or by muscularis mucosae. The wall of the cavity is usually composed of a colonic inflammatory reaction.

Patients may present with perforation, sepsis, intes-

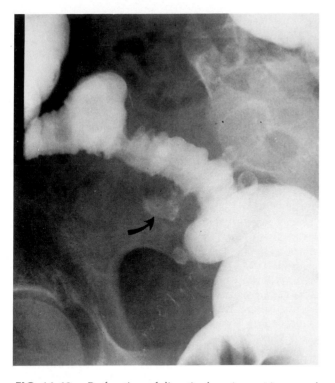

FIG. 14-42. Perforation of diverticulum *(arrow)* in a renal transplant patient. No symptoms were apparent except that the patient felt a mass.

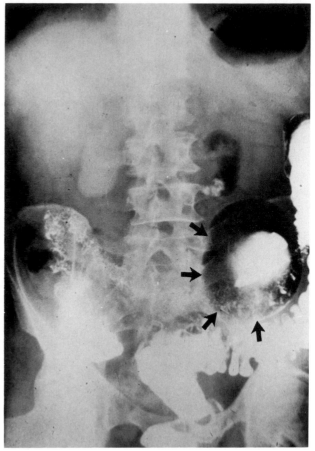

FIG. 14-43. Giant sigmoid diverticulum: barium fills part of the cavity; gas is also evident within the lumen *(arrow).*

tinal obstruction (due to compression by the mass), and rectal bleeding. Must complain of abdominal pain or the presence of an abdominal lump. A plain abdominal x-ray film may reveal a gas-filled mass of some considerable size. Differential diagnosis includes congenital duplication of the colon, colonic volvulus, emphysematous cholecystitis, infected pancreatic pseudocyst, pneumatosis cystoides intestinalis, giant duodenal diverticulum, intestinal obstruction, intra-abdominal lipoma, and intra-abdominal abscess.[37] Barium enema examination will usually confirm the diagnosis, because the diverticulum will fill approximately two thirds of the time (Fig. 14-43). Presumably, under some circumstances compression by the mass may preclude visualization. Fiberoptic colonoscopy perhaps should be able to identify the communication, but as of this writing no case has been reported employing this technique.

Treatment by means of resection of the diverticulum in continuity with the sigmoid colon is advised. There have been a few reports of diverticulectomy alone. This is not advised, however, because it is felt that it is important to remove the source of the complication,

namely, the sigmoid diverticular disease. The dissection is often quite difficult because of the inflammatory reaction induced by the mass.

DIVERTICULAR DISEASE OF THE RIGHT COLON

Diverticulitis of the cecum was first described by Potier in 1912.[98] Although the disease is not common, a number of reports and reviews have been published over the years.[6, 7, 38, 43, 61, 66, 72, 79, 117, 119] The type that involves the right colon may be solitary or multiple and should be distinguished from right-sided diverticula that exist concurrently with extensive diverticulosis throughout the colon. The former type of diverticula are thought to be congenital, and most are true diverticula, that is, they contain all layers of the intestine.

Murayama and co-workers measured the thickness of the right colon muscle in right-sided diverticular disease together with the counts of the number of haustrae in the right colon; they suggested that the etiology is the same as that of left-sided diverticular disease: abnormal thickening of the muscle in the wall of the colon.[85]

Right-sided diverticular disease is commoner in Japan than elsewhere. In support of the theory of a congenital origin, proponents have suggested that the condition tends to occur at a much earlier age than that of left-sided colitis. Characteristically, the solitary diverticulum has a shorter and wider neck than the multiple variety.[66]

Radiologic findings that are consistent with right-sided diverticulitis include the presence of a paracolic mass, a calcified fecalith, and a distended loop of small bowel near the mass.[14] However, these findings are found with acute appendicitis, so unless the patient has had the appendix previously removed, this triad of radiologic findings is not particulary helpful. On barium enema examination, an eccentric mural defect, a paracolic mass, or fistula are highly suspicious for the presence of cecal diverticulitis.[14]

The symptoms and signs of right-sided diverticulitis mimic appendicitis. Patients may complain of epigastric pain, nausea, and vomiting, with migration of the pain into the right iliac fossa. Depending on whether the process is localized or diffuse, low-grade fever, moderate tenderness, guarding, and rebound may be noted. The leukocyte count is usually elevated.

At the time of surgery it may be difficult to distinguish the condition from acute appendicitis or even from sigmoid diverticulitis. In the latter situation it is imperative to identify the source of the inflammation. Performing a transverse colostomy for acute cecal diverticulitis is unlikely to ameliorate the condition. The preoperative diagnosis is rarely correct, so a high index of suspicion must be maintained, particularly in patients who have undergone previous appendectomy or when rectal bleeding accompanies the abdominal signs and symptoms.

Ideally, surgical treatment should include excision of the involved diverticulum and closure. However, because the inflammatory mass usually involves a large portion of the cecum or right colon, a resective procedure is usually required. Resection is probably advisable in all cases when an inflammatory mass is present, because of the difficulty in distinguishing the lesion from a perforating carcinoma.

Kovalcik and Sustarsic reported 11 patients who underwent surgical procedures for cecal diverticulitis during a 10-year period.[61] The average age was 49 years, considerably less than the average age for patients with left-sided diverticulitis. Without benefit of preoperative barium enema, nine patients underwent resection, all but one of whom had a primary anastomosis. No deaths or anastomotic leaks were reported. Two patients who underwent elective resection underwent simple diverticulectomy. Gouge and co-workers reported 14 patients with diverticulitis of the ascending colon.[43] All patients at exploration had an inflammatory mass medial and posterior to the ascending colon. Eight were perforated with an abscess, but no free perforation or generalized peritonitis was noted. All patients underwent resection with ileocolic anastomosis. There were no deaths and no leaks. These authors also found a younger age for patients with right-sided diverticulitis (51 years as compared with 62 years); they also observed an equal sex distribution. McFee and associates reported 18 patients with right-sided diverticulitis; their average age was 46 years.[79] Barium enema examination was not helpful, and in only two patients was the preoperative diagnosis correct. All but one underwent resection with primary anastomosis. There were no deaths.

It appears, then, that the disease is rarely recognized preoperatively and that resection with primary anastomosis is the treatment of choice.

Reports of acute diverticulitis of the transverse colon are extremely rare. McClure and Welch identified 19 cases in the English-language literature and added three of their own.[78] All of their patients were found to have lesions in the right transverse colon, so these authors advocated right hemicolectomy. As with right colon diverticulitis, patients tend to be younger. The correct diagnosis is usually made at operation.

REFERENCES

1. Adams JT: The barium enema as treatment for massive diverticular bleeding. Dis Colon Rectum 1974; 17:439–441
2. Aguilo JJ, Zincke H, Woods JE et al: Intestinal perforation due to fecal impaction after renal transplantation. J Urol 1976; 116:153–155
3. Alexander-Williams J: Management of the acute complications of diverticular disease: The dangers of colostomy. Dis Colon Rectum 1976; 19:289–292
4. Alfidi RJ, Esselstyn CD, Tarar R et al: Recognition and angio-surgical detection of arteriovenous malformations of the bowel. Ann Surg 1971; 174:573–582
5. Almy TP, Howell DA: Diverticular disease of the colon. N Engl J Med 1980; 302:324–331
6. Anderson L: Acute diverticulitis of cecum: Study of 99 surgical cases. Surgery 1947; 22:479–488

7. Asch MJ, Markowitz AM: Cecal diverticulitis: Report of 16 cases and review of literature. Surgery 1969; 65:906–910

8. Auguste LJ, Wise L: Surgical management of perforated diverticulitis. Am J Surg 1981; 141:122–127

9. Baer JW: Pathogenesis of bleeding colonic diverticulosis: New concepts. CRC Critical Rev Diag Imaging 1978; 11:1–20

10. Baum S, Athanasoulis CA, Waltman AC: Angiographic diagnosis and control of large-bowel bleeding. Dis Colon Rectum 1974; 17:447–453

11. Baum S, Athanasoulis CA, Waltman AC et al: Angiodysplasia of the right colon: A cause of gastrointestinal bleeding. Am J Roentgenol 1977; 129:789–794

12. Baum S, Rösch J, Dotter CT et al: Selective mesenteric arterial infusions in the management of massive diverticular hemorrhage. N Engl J Med 1973; 288:1269–1272

13. Bell GA: Closure of colostomy following sigmoid colon resection for perforated diverticulitis. Surg Gynecol Obstet 1980; 150:85–89

14. Beranbaum SL: Diverticular disease of the right colon. From Greenbaum EI (ed):Radiographic Atlas of Colon Disease, pp 125-145. Chicago, Year Book Medical Publishers, 1980

15. Berman IR, Corman ML, Coller JA, Veidenheimer MC: Late onset Crohn's disease in patients with colonic diverticulitis. Dis Colon Rectum 1979; 22:524–529

16. Bernstein WC, Nivatvongs S, Tallent MB: Colonic and rectal complications of kidney transplantation in man. Dis Colon Rectum 1973; 16:255–263

17. Bloch O: Om extra-abdominal behandlung af cancer intestinalis (rectum, derfra, untaget) foretagne operationer og deref resultater. Nord Med Ark Stockh 1892; 2:1–36

18. Bokey EL, Chapuis PH, Pheils MT: Elective resection for diverticular disease and carcinoma: Comparison of postoperative morbidity and mortality. Dis Colon Rectum 1981; 24:181–182

19. Brodribb AJM: Treatment of symptomatic diverticular disease with a high-fibre diet. Lancet 1977; 1:664–666

20. Burkitt DP, Walker ARP, Painter NS: Effect of dietary fibre on stools and transit-times, and its role in the causation of disease. Lancet 1972; 2:1408–1412

21. Burkitt DP, Walker ARP, Painter NS: Dietary fibre and disease. JAMA 1974; 229:1068–1074

22. Chodak GW, Rangel DM, Passaro E Jr: Colonic diverticulitis in patients under age 40: Need for earlier diagnosis. Am J Surg 1981; 141:699–702

23. Classen JN, Bonardi R, O'Mara CS et al: Surgical treatment of acute diverticulitis by staged procedures. Ann Surg 1976; 184:582–586

24. Colcock BP, Stahmann FD: Fistulas complicating diverticular disease of the sigmoid colon. Ann Surg 1972; 175:838–846

25. Connell AM: Applied physiology of the colon: Factors relevant to diverticular disease. Clin Gastroenterol 1975; 4:23–36

26. Correnti FS, Pappalardo G, Mobarhan S et al: Follow-up results of a new colomyotomy in the treatment of diverticulosis. Surg Gynecol Obstet 1983; 156:181–186

27. Criado FJ, Wilson TH Jr: Technique for reestablishing continuity after the Hartmann operation. Am Surg 1981; 47:366–367

28. Dean ACB, Newell JP: Colonoscopy in the differential diagnosis of carcinoma from diverticulitis of the sigmoid colon. Br J Surg 1973; 60:633–635

29. Eastwood MA, Smith AN, Brydon WG, Pritchard J: Comparison of bran, ispaghula, and lactulose on colon function in diverticular disease. Gut 1978; 19:1144–1147

30. Eisenberg H, Laufer I, Skillman J: Arteriographic diagnosis and management of suspected colonic diverticular hemorrhage. Gastroenterology 1973; 64:1091–1100

31. Eng K, Rauson JHC, Localio SA: Resection of perforated segment: A significant advance in treatment of diverticulitis with free perforation or abscess. Am J Surg 1977; 133:67–72

32. Failes D, Killingback M, Stuart M, DeLuca C: Elective resection for diverticular disease. Aust NZ J Surg 1979; 49:66–72

33. Farkouh E, Hellou G, Allard M, Atlas H: Resection and primary anastomosis for diverticulitis with perforation and peritonitis. Can J Surg 1982; 25:314–316

34. Forde KA: Colonoscopy in complicated diverticular disease. Gastrointestinal Endosc 1977; 23:192–193

35. Forde KA: Colonoscopy in acute rectal bleeding. Gastrointest Endosc 1981; 27:219–220

36. Gabriel WB: Diverticulitis of the pelvic colon with large solitary diverticulum. Proc R Soc Med 1953: 46:416

37. Gallagher JJ, Welch JP: Giant diverticula of the sigmoid colon: A review of differential diagnosis and operative management. Arch Surg 1979; 114:1079–1083

38. Garner OP Jr, Bolin JA, LeSage MA, Nelson NC: Acute solitary cecal diverticulitis. Am Surg 1973; 39:700–705

39. Gear JSS, Ware A, Fursdon P et al: Symptomless

diverticular disease and intake of dietary fibre. Lancet 1979; 1:511–514

40. Gennaro AR, Rosemond GP: Colonic diverticula and hemorrhage. Dis Colon Rectum 1973; 16:409–415

41. Goldberger LE: Diverticular disease of the colon: Angiography in diverticular hemorrhage. In Greenbaum EI: Radiographic Atlas of Colon Disease, pp 113-124. Chicago, Year Book Medical Publishers, 1980

42. Goldberger LE, Bookstein JJ: Transcatheter embolization for treatment of diverticular hemorrhage. Radiology 1977; 122:613–617

43. Gouge TH, Coppa GF, Eng K et al: Management of diverticulitis of the ascending colon. Am J Surg 1983; 145:387–391

44. Greco RS, Kamath C, Nosher JL: Percutaneous drainage of peridiverticular abscess followed by primary sigmoidectomy. Dis Colon Rectum 1982; 25:53–55

45. Greif JM, Fried G, McSherry CK: Surgical treatment of perforated diverticulitis of the sigmoid colon. Dis Colon Rectum 1980; 23:483–487

46. Griffen WO Jr: Management of the acute complications of diverticular disease: Acute perforation of colonic diverticula. Dis Colon Rectum 1976; 19:293–295

47. Hadjiyannakis EJ, Evans DB, Smellie WAB, Calne RY: Gastrointestinal complications after renal transplantation. Lancet 1971; 2:781–785

48. Hartmann H: Nouveau procédé d'ablation des cancers de la partie terminale du colon pelvien. Congres Franc de Chir 1923; 30:411

49. Heimann T, Aufses AH Jr: Giant sigmoid diverticula. Dis Colon Rectum 1981; 24:468–470

50. Helbraun MA, Corman ML, Coller JA, Veidenheimer MC: Diverticular disease. Reported at the annual meeting of the American Society of Colon and Rectal Surgeons, San Diego, California, 1978

51. Hodgson WJB: Transverse taeniamyotomy for diverticular disease. Dis Colon Rectum 1973; 16:283–289

52. Hodgson WJB, Schauzer H, Bakare S, McElhinney AJ: Transverse taenia myotomy in localized acute diverticulitis. Am J Gastroenterol 1979; 71:61–67

53. Hool GJ, Bokey EL, Pheils MT: Diverticular coloenteric fistulae. Aust NZ J Surg 1981; 51:358–359

54. Howe HJ, Casali RE, Westbrook KC et al: Acute perforations of the sigmoid colon secondary to diverticulitis. Am J Surg 1979; 137:184–187

55. Hughes WL, Greene RC: Solitary air cyst of the peritoneal cavity. Arch Surg 1953; 67:931–936

56. Hyland JMP, Taylor I: Does a high fibre diet prevent the complications of diverticular disease? Br J Surg 1980; 67:77–79

57. Julien PJ, Goldberg HI, Margulis AR, Belzer FO: Gastrointestinal complications following renal transplantation. Radiology 1975; 117:37–43

58. Kempczinski RF, Ferrucci JT Jr: Giant sigmoid diverticula: A review. Ann Surg 1974; 180:864–867

59. Knoepp LF Jr, McCulloch JH: Colonoscopy in the diagnosis of unexplained rectal bleeding. Dis Colon Rectum 1978; 21:590–593

60. Koep LJ, Peters TG, Starzl TE: Major colonic complications of hepatic transplantation. Dis Colon Rectum 1979; 22:218–220

61. Kovalcik PJ, Sustarsic DL: Cecal diverticulitis. Am Surg 1981; 47:72–73

62. Kovalcik PJ, Veidenheimer MC, Corman ML, Coller JA: Colovesical fistula. Dis Colon Rectum 1976; 19:425–427

63. Labow SB, Salvati EP, Rubin RJ: The Hartmann procedure in the treatment of diverticular disease. Dis Colon Rectum 1973; 16:392–394

64. Laimon H: Hartmann resection for acute diverticulitis. Rev Surg 1974; 31:1–6

65. Landi E, Fianchini A, Landa L, Maniscalco L: Multiple transverse taeniamyotomy for diverticular disease. Surg Gynecol Obstet 1979; 148:221–226

66. Langdon A: Solitary diverticulitis of the right colon. Can J Surg 1982; 25:579–581

67. Lennard-Jones JE: Functional gastrointestinal disorders. N Engl J Med 1983; 308:431–435

68. Lubbers E-JC, de Boer HHM: Inherent complications of Hartmann's operation. Surg Gynecol Obstet 1982; 155:717–721

69. Madden JL: Treatment of perforated lesions of the colon by primary resection and anastomosis. Dis Colon Rectum 1966; 9:413–416

70. Madden JL, Tan PY: Primary resection and anastomosis in the treatment of perforated lesions of the colon, with abscess or diffusing peritonitis. Surg Gynecol Obstet 1961; 113:646–650

71. Madure JA, Fiore AC: Reanastomosis of a Hartmann rectal pouch. Am J Surg 1983; 145:279–280

72. Magness LJ, Sanfelippo PM, van Heerden JA, Judd ES: Diverticular disease of the right colon. Surg Gynecol Obstet 1975; 140:30–32

73. Maresca L, Maresca C, Erickson E: Giant sigmoid diverticulum: Report of a case. Dis Colon Rectum 1981; 24:191–195

74. Matolo NM, Link DP: Selective embolization for control of gastrointestinal hemorrhage. Am J Surg 1979; 138:840–844

75. Max MH, Knutson CO: Colonoscopy in patients

with inflammatory colonic strictures. Surgery 1978; 84:551–556

76. Mayefsky E, Sicular A, Hodgson WJB: Recurrent diverticulitis after conservative surgery. Mt Sinai J Med (NY) 1979; 46:556–558

77. Mayo WJ: Acquired diverticulitis of the large intestine. Surg Gynecol Obstet 1907; 5:8

78. McClure ET, Welch JP: Acute diverticulitis of the transverse colon with perforation. Arch Surg 1979; 114:1068–1071

79. McFee AS, Sutton PG, Ramos R: Diverticulitis of the right colon. Dis Colon Rectum 1982; 25:254–256

80. Von Mikulicz J: Chirurgische Erfahrung über das Darmcarcinom. Arch f Klin Chir 1903; 69:28–47

81. Miller MD, Johnsrude IS, Jackson DC: Improved technique for transcatheter embolization of arteries. Am J Roetgenol 1978; 130:183–184

82. Misra MK, Pinkus GS, Birtch AG, Wilson RE: Major colonic diseases complicating renal transplantation. Surgery 1973; 73:942–948

83. Morson BC: Diverticular disease of the colon. Acta Chir Belg 1979; 78:369–376

84. Muhletaler CA, Berger JL, Robinette CL Jr: Pathogenesis of giant colonic diverticula. Gastrointest Radiol 1981; 6:217–222

85. Murayama N, Baba S, Susumu K, Abe O: An aetiological study of diverticulosis of the right colon. Aust NZ J Surg 1981; 51:420–425

86. Noer R, Hamilton JE, Williams DJ, Broughton DS: Rectal hemorrhage: Moderate and severe. Ann Surg 1962; 155:794–805

87. Nunes GC, Robnett AH, Kremer RM, Ahlquist RE Jr: The Hartmann procedure for complications of diverticulitis. Arch Surg 1979; 114:425–429

88. Orebaugh JE, McCris JA, Lee JF: Surgical treatment of diverticular disease of the colon. Am Surg 1978; 44:712–715

89. Ouriel K, Schwartz SI: Diverticular disease in the young patient. Surg Gynecol Obstet 1983; 156:1–5

90. Painter NS: Diverticular disease of the colon: A disease of this century. Lancet 1969; 2:586–588

91. Painter NS: The treatment of uncomplicated diverticular disease of the colon with a high fibre diet. Acta Chir Belg 1979; 78:359–368

92. Painter NS: Diverticular disease of the colon: The first of the Western diseases shown to be due to a deficiency of dietary fibre. South Afr Med J 1982; 61:1016–1020

93. Painter NS, Burkitt DP: Diverticular disease of the colon: A deficiency disease of Western civilization. Br Med J 1971; 1:450–454

94. Parks TG: Natural history of diverticular disease of the colon. Clin Gastroenterol 1975; 4:53–69

95. Parks TG: The clinical significance of diverticular disease of the colon. Practitioner 1982; 226:643–654

96. Paul FT: Colectomy. Liverpool M Chir J 1895; 15:374

97. Pheils MT, Chapuis PH, Bokey EL, Hayward P: Diverticular disease: A retrospective study of surgical management— 1970–1980. Aust NZ J Surg 1982; 52:53–56

98. Potier F: Diverticulite et appendicite. Bull Mem Soc Anat (Paris) 1912; 87:29–31

99. Ramanath H, Hinshaw JR: Management and mismanagement of bleeding colonic diverticula. Arch Surg 1971; 103:311–314

100. Ramirez OM, Hernandez-Pombo J, Marupundi SR: New technique for anastomosis of the intestine after the Hartmann's procedure with the end-to-end anastomosis stapler. Surg Gynecol Obstet 1983; 156:366–368

101. Rankin FW, Brown PW: Diverticulitis of colon. Surg Gynecol Obstet 1930; 50:836–847

102. Reilly MCT: Sigmoid myotomy: A new operation. Proc R Soc Med 1964; 57:556–557

103. Reilly MCT: The place of sigmoid myotomy in diverticular disease. Acta Chir Belg 1979; 78:387–390

104. Rennie JA, Charnock MC, Wellwood JM et al: Results of resection for diverticular disease and its complications. Proc R Soc Med 1975; 68:575

105. Rice RP, Thompson WM: Colon complications following renal transplantation. In Greenbaum EI: Radiographic Atlas of Colon Disease, pp 89-93. Chicago, Year Book Medical Publishers 1980

106. Risholm L: Primary resection in perforating diverticulitis of the colon. World J Surg 1982; 6:490–491

107. Rösch J, Dotter CT, Brown MJ: Selective arterial embolization: A new method for control of acute gastrointestinal bleeding. Radiology 1972; 102:303–306

108. Sakai L, Daake J, Kaminski DL: Acute perforation of sigmoid diverticula. Am J Surg 1981; 142:712–715

109. Sawyerr OI, Garvin PJ, Codd JE et al: Colorectal complications of renal allograft transplantation. Arch Surg 1978; 113:84–86

110. Seldinger SI: Catheter replacement of needle in percutaneous arteriography; new technique. Acta Radiol (Stockh) 1953; 39:368–376

111. Smithwick RH: Experiences with surgical management of diverticulitis of the sigmoid. Ann Surg 1942; 115:969–985

112. Sniderman KW, Franklin J Jr, Sos T: Successful transcatheter Gelfoam embolization of a bleeding

cecal vascular ectasia. Am J Roentgenol 1978; 131:157–159

113. Staunton MD: Treatment of perforated diverticulitis coli. Br Med J 1962; 1:916–918

114. Swarbrick ET, Fevre DI, Hunt RH et al: Colonoscopy for unexplained rectal bleeding. Br Med J 1978; 2:1685–1687

115. Thompson HR: Diverticulosis and diverticulitis of the colon. In Maingot R (ed): Abdominal Operations, 7th ed, pp 1874-1875. New York, Appleton-Century-Crofts, 1980

116. Trowell HC, Burkitt DP: Diverticular disease in urban Kenyans. Br Med J 1979; 1:1795

117. Vaughn AM, Narsete EM: Diverticulitis of the cecum. Arch Surg 1952; 65:763–769

118. Veidenheimer MC, Corman ML, Coller JA: Colonic hemorrhage. Surg Clin North Am 1978; 58:581–590

119. Wagner DE, Zollinger RW: Diverticulitis of the cecum and ascending colon. Arch Surg 1961; 83:436–443

120. Wara P, Sørensen K, Berg V, Amdrup E: The outcome of staged management of complicated diverticular disease of the sigmoid colon. Acta Chir Scand 1981; 147:209–214

121. Watkins GL, Oliver GA: Management of perforative sigmoid diverticulitis with diffusing peritonitis. Arch Surg 1966; 92:928–933

122. Weckesser EC: Functional exteriorized colon for perforations due to diverticulitis. Am J Surg 1980; 139:298–300

123. Wetstein L, Camera A, Trillo RA, Zamora BO: Giant sigmoidal diverticulum: Report of a case and review of the literature. Dis Colon Rectum 1978; 21:110–112

124. Williams CB: Diverticular disease and strictures. In Hunt RH and Waye JD: Colonoscopy: Techniques, Clinical Practice and Colour Atlas, pp 363-381. London, Chapman and Hall, 1981

125. Williams RA, Wilson SE: Current management of massive lower gastrointestinal bleeding. Int Surg 1980; 2:157–163

126. Wolff BG, Ready RL, MacCarty RL et al: Effect of sigmoidal resection on progression of diverticulosis. Presented at Annual Meeting, American Society of Colon and Rectal Surgeons, 1983

CHAPTER 15

Nonspecific Inflammatory Bowel Disease

Nonspecific inflammatory bowel disease is an expression used to describe two conditions of unknown etiology: ulcerative colitis and Crohn's disease. The rationale for placing both diseases within the same chapter is that the two diagnoses are often confused. In many cases the symptomatology is similar; radiologic investigation may pose a problem in differentiation, and even pathologic evaluation may reveal an indeterminate colitis in as many as 15% of patients. The two conditions frequently affect young persons in their late teens and early twenties, and men and women in an approximately equal ratio; people living in Western countries are the most vulnerable. They are two of the most difficult and challenging diseases confronting the physician today.

HISTORICAL PERSPECTIVE

It is difficult to know if prior to the 19th century the disease ulcerative colitis was truly recognized as such. Infectious and noninfectious diarrheas have existed since antiquity, but most of the descriptions are of a clinical syndrome: diarrhea, rectal bleeding, the so-called "bloody-flux." Samuel Wilks is generally credited with coining the term *ulcerative colitis* at a court trial in a letter published in 1859 describing the appearance of the intestine.[274] Subsequently, the surgeon-general of the Union army after the Civil War referred to the disease *ulcerative colitis*, and included photomicrographs of the condition.[103] Other detailed descriptions followed,[275] and by the early 20th century over 300 cases of ulcerative colitis had been collected for presentation to the Royal Society of Medicine.[103]

Crohn's disease of the bowel was reported in 1932 by Crohn, Ginzburg, and Oppenheimer.[50] They described a transmural inflammatory disease of the terminal ileum. The authors allegedly listed their names in alphabetical order for the purpose of publication. It would appear that if one is at all concerned about eponymous immortality, it is helpful to have a name occurring early in the alphabet. Furthermore, many of the cases were based on the large clinical material of A. A. Berg.[178] Had Dr. Berg wished to include his name on the paper, the condition might be called Berg's disease today. A number of other papers followed from the experience of Crohn and his associates confirming the disease in the small bowel, but also noting that in a number of cases the colon was to some extent involved.

A recent review presented in the "Classics" section of the journal *Diseases of the Colon and Rectum* postulated that Moynihan was really describing Crohn's disease in 1907 when he presented lesions that mimicked a malignant bowel condition but that were benign.[196] In 1923, Moschowitz and Wilensky described four patients with a granulomatous disease of the intestine and the amelioration of the condition by intestinal bypass.[195]

In 1951, Marshak described the radiologic findings of what he felt was granulomatous disease of the colon as a distinct clinical entity separate from ulcerative colitis.[178] This view was not generally accepted until 1959 when Morson and Lockhart-Mummery described the characteristic pathologic features of granulomatous colitis.[193] Therefore, our concepts of Crohn's disease as confined to the colon are barely a quarter of a century old.

INCIDENCE AND EPIDEMIOLOGY

In a recent review, Kirsner and Shorter observed that nonspecific inflammatory bowel diseases, especially Crohn's disease, have become pervasive worldwide; the two conditions have emerged as one of the most important biomedical problems of our time.[148] Unfortunately, our knowledge of their pathogenesis continues to remain obscure.

In evaluating the epidemiology of the two conditions, our knowledge is frustrated by the plethora of diarrheal states throughout the world that may be infectious or parasitic in nature and that present with symptoms not unlike those of nonspecific inflammatory bowel disease. Furthermore, because of international inability to classify the two diseases as distinct from the numerous specific inflammatory bowel problems, our ability to obtain meaningful data is compromised. Most of the information, therefore, has been obtained from Western countries where the diseases are relatively prevalent. Ulcerative colitis and Crohn's disease in England, the United States, and Scandinavia are reported at incidence rates of four to six cases per 100,000 white adults per year, and prevalence rates between 40 and 100 per 100,000.[149] Most studies have demonstrated an increased incidence of Crohn's disease during the past 20 years.[22, 28, 73, 165, 184, 191, 207] The disease is more common in whites, among Jewish people, and among those of Western origin (especially northern Europe and the northern part of eastern Europe).[149] Other countries such as South American nations, the Soviet Union, and Japan have a much lower incidence and prevalence. As with carcinoma of the colon, the prevalence of inflammatory bowel disease in many industrialized countries, and the development of the conditions among those from low-risk populations who immigrate to higher-risk areas, suggest an environmental cause. Mendeloff believes that there is a marked deficiency in the investigation of these diseases because the mortality is low and the genetic determinants are multiple.[189] He suggests that for the future it will be necessary to develop better fundamental means of acquisition and recording of data, and that

at least for the immediate time a concerted effort should be made to identify those families in which multiple cases of inflammatory bowel disease exist and to investigate these people thoroughly; this would include genetic, psychological, and metabolic studies.

Investigative efforts to identify the etiologic agent responsible for inflammatory bowel disease have been unsuccessful. Inflammatory bowel disease that appears nonspecific in nature has been found in hamsters, horses, swine, and the canine population, but an experimental animal model for induction or transmission of the disease still eludes investigators. The two primary areas of investigation that continue to be actively pursued are immunology and infection.

The concept of circulating *antiepithelial antibodies* combining with antigens on the intestinal cell surface and damaging the cells seems a reasonable theory to explain the etiology of inflammatory bowel disease. This is the so-called *concept of autoimmunity.* However, in spite of the demonstration of anticolon antibodies in both blood and tissue of inflammatory bowel disease patients, current evidence would seem to militate against the likelihood that they play a primary pathogenetic role in the conditions.[228]

Immune complex mediation of inflammatory bowel disease has been felt by some to be a responsible factor, but more recent studies have failed to corroborate significantly increased frequency or concentration of these complexes regardless of disease activity.[228] Other immunologic mechanisms that have been investigated include abnormality and variability of circulating lymphocytes, lymphocyte cytotoxicity, defective cell-mediated immunity, immediate hypersensitivity, leukocyte chemotaxic impairment, and immunoregulatory cellular imbalance.[149, 228] A useful pathogenesis for inflammatory bowel disease may involve an interaction between host responses, immunologic genetic influences, and external agents, but no definitive proof has yet been forthcoming.

With respect to *infectious agents,* ulcerative colitis in particular has been attributed to bacterial causes for over 50 years. Crohn's disease had been confused with tuberculosis; Crohn, Ginzburg, and Oppenheimer suggested that the disease might be caused by a mycobacterial agent.[50] Subsequent studies have failed to demonstrate conclusively an association with an infective agent, and, in fact, the incidence of inflammatory bowel disease correlates inversely with that of the infectious dysenteries.[149] However, the concept of a microbial infection as the offending agent has been resurrected with the recognition of the new bacterial causes of enteritis and colitis (especially *Campylobacter jejuni* and *Clostridium difficile*).[26, 167, 200, 258] Although several studies suggest the possibility of these two organisms contributing to relapse of inflammatory bowel disease, Gurian and co-workers, in examination of stool specimens from 32 patients who had exacerbation of inflammatory bowel disease, revealed no *C. difficile* cytotoxin and negative cultures for *C. jejuni*.[111] Other bacteriologic agents (*Shigella, Salmonella, Streptococcus faecalis, Pseudomonas* variant, *Chlamydia, Mycobacteria,* and many others) have been suggested, but their roles have not been confirmed.

There has been considerable interest in a possible *viral etiology* of ulcerative colitis and Crohn's disease. Transmission of granulomatous lesions has been successfully carried out in experimental animals.[41, 65, 251] Tissue culture and electron microscopic investigation have also suggested that a viral agent is present in tissue from patients with inflammatory bowel disease.[7, 94, 273] However, there continues to remain considerable controversy over the specificity of these findings; whether indeed the evidence is convincing enough to accurately identify viral particles on electron microscopic examination of affected tissue remains unresolved.[228]

Dietary factors, especially cow's milk, have been implicated as possible causative agents for inflammatory bowel disease. Early studies seem to demonstrate an elevated milk-protein antibody level in ulcerative colitis patients, as compared with a control population. Subsequent reports wherein milk was excluded from the diet failed to achieve an improvement in the clinical response, and later studies concerning the implication of milk and milk products failed to demonstrate any correlation. Other factors that have been under investigation include chemical food additives, mercury ingestion, inadequate fiber, excess refined sugar intake, and even the increased consumption of corn flakes.[228] It is difficult for me to believe, however, that a dietary factor can be a major element in the etiology of inflammatory bowel disease, because this is often a disease of young people. If one is to use the analogy of the role of diet in diverticular disease and colorectal cancer, one must recognize that these conditions are primarily seen in the older age groups, people who have had many years of possible dietary "indiscretion."

Cigarette smoking has been found to have a negative correlation with ulcerative colitis.[35, 58, 118, 133] In some cases, complete remission of symptoms was obtained through the use of nicotine-laced chewing gum. In other patients, exacerbation of the disease was noted when the patient ceased smoking. Since the presented data is rather speculative, more substantial evidence by prospective clinical trials should resolve this issue.

Although ulcerative colitis and Crohn's disease are not classic *genetic disorders,* the occurrence of inflammatory bowel disease in family members born in widely separated areas or living apart for long periods, along with the increased incidence among Jews, and the predilection for familial aggregation of patients with ankylosing spondylitis in Crohn's disease, suggest a genetically mediated mechanism in the causation of the condtions.[75, 149] Numerous studies have demonstrated a familial association of inflammatory bowel disease.[5, 55, 75, 147, 150] Although the possibility of a common environment may contribute to the increased risk of inflammatory bowel disease, the shared genetic pool is much more likely to be the primary factor. A familial occurrence has been noted in 17.5% of over 600 patients with inflammatory bowel disease (IBD).[239] In a report from the Cleveland Clinic, Farmer and co-workers evaluated the family histories of over 800 patients with the onset of IBD before the age of 21.[75] Twenty-nine percent of those with ulcerative colitis had a positive history, and 35% of those with Crohn's had a positive family history for IBD. Although genetic counseling for families of patients with IBD has not been pursued, the relative frequency of familial occurrence is a reality to be considered by the physician and by the patient who plans to have children.

The *psychological aspects* and the possible psychosomatic factors contributing to the onset and exacerbations of inflammatory bowel disease, and of ulcerative colitis in particular, have been a subject of considerable debate since the original paper by Murray in 1930.[197] Karush and associates, in a book on psychotherapy in ulcerative colitis, state that the colitic patient develops susceptibility to the problem through "disruption and distortion of the relationship to the parents and to other significant persons as early as the second year of life."[139] The results are exaggerated emotional manifestations, egocentricity, dependency conflicts, and poor mechanisms for coping with the stresses of life. Frequent anxiety or depression, in the opinion of the authors, is also characteristic, and this predisposition, they felt, explains the relatively high incidence of schizophrenia in patients with ulcerative colitis. In their study of precipitating emotional factors, the authors reported that a well-defined event of powerful emotional impact preceded the onset of the disease by a few days or weeks. Subsequent recurrences were also heralded by such events. Although many papers have been published to support this susceptible personality description, opponents of the psychosomatic theory point out that the concept is based on either anecdotal or uncontrolled studies.[228] Bercovitz criticizes the reports as being retrospective, and notes that there are no long-term, prospective psychological studies available of any large group of people.[18]

The emotional stress of serious illness in a most vulnerable period of emotional development, the need for hospitalization, psychotropic medications (*e.g.,* corticosteroids), or the fear of surgery (especially the "mutilation'' of an ileostomy) may induce considerable stress. In fact, it would be the remarkable patient indeed who was not emotionally troubled by the consequences of his or her illness. The importance of providing emotional support to the patient cannot be overestimated. Psychotherapy has been demonstrated to be of value; an internist or a surgeon who understands the role of emotional conflicts and anxieties either as a cause or a result of the patient's illness can provide such support.

Age and Sex

Inflammatory bowel disease is a condition that occurs at any age, but most commonly becomes manifest before the age of 30 years. The incidence of ulcerative colitis and Crohn's disease is highest among teenagers.[149] There is a small secondary peak in the incidence of the two conditions late in the sixth decade. In most series both sexes are approximately equally affected. Farmer and colleagues reported 838 patients who were 20 years old or younger at the time of diagnosis at the Cleveland Clinic.[75] Thirteen percent of patients with ulcerative colitis and 5% of Crohn's disease patients were 10 years of age or younger. Approximately one third of each group were between the ages of 11 and 15. There were 316 patients with ulcerative colitis, with an almost 1:1 ratio of males to females, and 522 patients with Crohn's disease, 57% of whom were males. In Goligher's experience, approximately one half of the patients were between 20 and 39 years of age when the disease was diagnosed, with a 4-to-3 predominance of females over males.[100] With Crohn's disease, Goligher reported that in his own personal series females predominated in a 3-to-2 ratio.[102] There seemed to be a tendency for the disease to develop later than ulcerative colitis does, 70% of patients being between the ages of 20 and 49 years.

In our experience of 151 patients who underwent proctocolectomy, the mean age at surgery for both ulcerative colitis and Crohn's patients was 36 years.[46] Fifty-six percent of ulcerative colitis patients were men, while 57 percent who had Crohn's colitis were women.

DIFFERENTIAL DIAGNOSIS

Ulcerative colitis and Crohn's disease can usually be distinguished from each other on the basis of the patient's clinical course, the symptomatology, the manifestations, and the endoscopic findings. Ulcerative colitis is a disease characterized by exacerbations and remissions. In contrast, the patient with Crohn's disease has less clear-cut periods of flare-up and remission; the disease tends to run a more smoldering course. Frequently the patient is really not well and yet is not ill enough to warrant hospitalization.

Rectal bleeding is virtually a *sine qua non* for the diagnosis of ulcerative colitis. A physician might seriously question the diagnosis in the absence of rectal bleeding. Alternatively, bleeding is much less frequently seen in Crohn's colitis; in fact, 25% of patients with Crohn's disease never manifest bleeding. Since ulcerative colitis is an inflammatory disease of the mucosa, bleeding is a common complaint, whereas with the often-noted minimal involvement of the mucosa in Crohn's colitis, bleeding is frequently not observed.

Ulcerative colitis is a disease confined to the colon and rectum, whereas Crohn's disease can occur anywhere in the digestive tract, from the mouth to the anus. *Anorectal disease* in particular (fissures, abscesses, and fistulas) are more commonly noted in patients with Crohn's disease (at least 60%) than in patients with ulcerative colitis. A biopsy of a sinus tract or abscess cavity may demonstrate the granulomas characteristic of Crohn's colitis. The diagnosis may be suspected on examination of the perianal skin (Fig. 15-1).

Proctosigmoidoscopic examination is of value in differ-

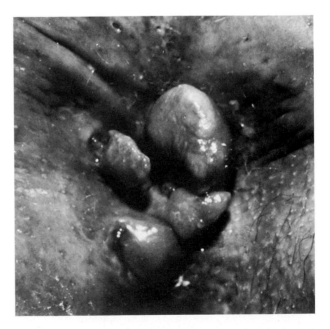

FIG. 15-1. Anal Crohn's disease. Note the thickened, edematous tags with furrowing and fissuring of the skin. (Corman ML, Veidenheimer MC, Nugent FW et al: Diseases of the Anus, Rectum and Colon. Part II: Non-specific inflammatory bowel disease. New York, Medcom, 1976)

entiating the two conditions. The rectum is always diseased during attacks of ulcerative colitis. Characteristic changes include contact bleeding, granularity, and ulceration. However, with Crohn's colitis, 40% of the patients have sparing of the rectum, irrespective of anal or perianal involvement. But when the rectum *is* involved by this condition, differentiation between the two diseases may be quite difficult.

Extracolonic manifestations were presumed to be noted only with ulcerative colitis, but now it is recognized that these can be observed in both conditions (see later).

Differential diagnosis may be difficult to establish by radiologic means and by clinical means; in approximately 10% of cases, differentiation cannot even be made pathologically, this group forming an indeterminate category.

Macroscopic Appearance

Ulcerative Colitis

Ulcerative colitis is a disease confined to the mucosa and submucosa of the bowel. The only exception to this is when transmural involvement produces the so-called *toxic megacolon* (see later). The bowel wall is not thickened, there are no granulomata, except foreign body giant cell reaction occasionally seen in an area of acute inflammation, and there are no skip areas. The rectum is always involved, and the disease extends proximally for varying distances, but always with continuity of involvement to the proximal extent of the disease (Fig. 15-2). Characteristically, the disease tends to involve the bowel more severely distally than proximally. Despite extensive inflammatory reaction, the bowel wall retains its normal thickness (see Fig. 15-2). The results of the confluence of numerous ulcers are the longitudinal furrows of denuded mucosa that alternate with islands of heaped-up mucosa, resulting in so-called pseudopolyps (Figs. 15-3, 15-4, and 15-5). Pseudopolyps are inflammatory polyps, not neoplastic lesions. These are seen during a quiescent phase of ulcerative colitis and are a later manifestation of this condition. They may be confused with familial polyposis (see Fig. 9-40), but the absence of normal mucosa between these polyps suggests the correct diagnosis. The entire colon including the cecum and appendix may be involved (Fig. 15-6). Characteristically, however, the disease does not affect the ileum. In fact, if the small bowel *is* involved for more than a few centimeters, the diagnosis is not ulcerative colitis. One exception to this is the so-called "backwash ileitis" seen occasionally when the entire colon is involved. This reversible condition, which may be demonstrated radiographically as edematous, thickened mucosal folds, is a nonspecific inflammatory reaction resulting from proximity of the ileum to the diseased colon.

The entire mucosa may be lost in patients with long-standing, chronic, ulcerative colitis (Fig. 15-7). Under these circumstances, the physician may be lulled into a false sense of security, since the patient's symptoms are often minimal. It is difficult to experience mucous discharge, diarrhea, or bleeding if there is no inflamed mucosa present. It is this type of patient who is predisposed to the development of carcinoma (see Relationship to Carcinoma).

Toxic megacolon is a condition in which acute inflammatory reaction extends through the entire thickness of the bowel wall to the serosa. Gangrene and perforation can result (Fig. 15-8). This is the only manifestation of ulcerative colitis that is not limited to the mucosa and submucosa. The term is a poor one, because it is not the colon that is toxic; it is the patient.

Crohn's Disease

Crohn's disease may have protean clinical and pathological manifestations. The condition can be confined to the colon alone or may involve only the anal canal. Fistulas, segmental involvement, rectal sparing, perianal disease, and abscess formation are all characteristic of granulomatous colitis.

Some of the earliest changes of the small intestine involved by Crohn's disease may be immediately recognizable in the serosal aspect if the patient is submitted to surgery. Subserosal extension of fat around the surface of the bowel ("fat wrapping") and the prominent vascular pattern in the serosa are very characteristic of the disease (Fig. 15-9). The serosal surface may be granular and bleed easily upon any intraoperative abrasion.

The disease frequently involves the bowel in a segmental fashion. This may produce extensive skip areas (Figs. 15-10 and 15-11), limited involvement of an area of the bowel (Fig. 15-12), or even a focal, isolated stricture (Fig. 15-13).

Classically, Crohn's colitis involves the intestine in an asymmetric fashion. Areas of the bowel may show involvement on the mucosal surface with sparing of adjacent sites, leaving islands of somewhat edematous but otherwise nonulcerated mucosa (Figs. 15-14, 15-15, and 15-16). Ulceration in an irregular fashion with large areas of uninvolved mucosa interspersed between broad, twisiting lesions is quite characteristic. The relative sparing between ulcers is not seen in ulcerative colitis. Another characteristic feature of the macroscopic appearance of Crohn's disease is the thickening of the bowel wall. Involvement through all the layers of the bowel, along with the cobblestone appearance of the mucosa, has been described as "stones in a running brook" (Fig. 15-17).

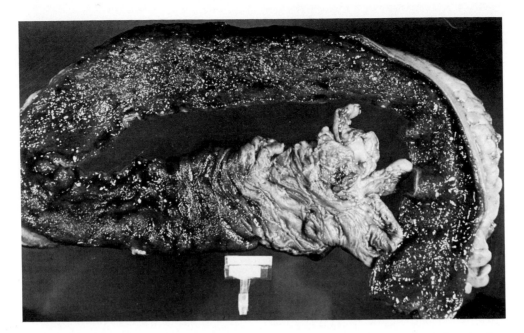

FIG. 15-2. Ulcerative colitis: a resected specimen (rectum removed separately) showing in-continuity involvement from the sigmoid to the mid-ascending colon. Loss of mucosa, deep ulceration, and extensive granularity are evident. (Corman ML, Veidenheimer MC, Nugent FW et al: Diseases of the Anus, Rectum and Colon. Part II: Non-specific inflammatory bowel disease. New York, Medcom, 1976)

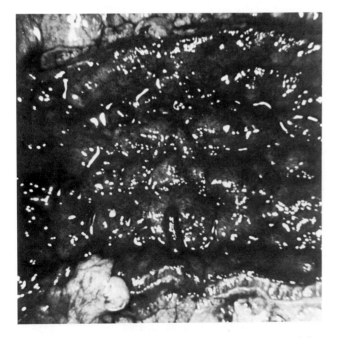

FIG. 15-3. Ulcerative colitis. Longitudinal furrows of denuded mucosa alternate with islands of heaped-up mucosa, demonstrating how loss of mucosal integrity contributes to fluid and electrolyte depletion. (Corman ML, Veidenheimer MC, Nugent FW et al: Diseases of the Anus, Rectum and Colon. Part II: Non-specific inflammatory bowel disease. New York, Medcom, 1976)

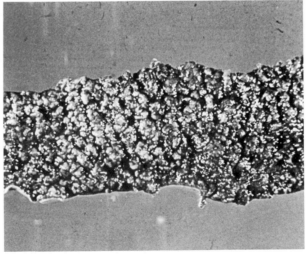

FIG. 15-4. Extensive pseudopolyps in active ulcerative colitis. Note the relative uniformity of the polyps as compared with the varied sizes seen in familial polyposis, Fig. 9-40. (Corman ML, Veidenheimer MC, Nugent FW et al: Diseases of the Anus, Rectum and Colon. Part II: Non-specific inflammatory bowel disease. New York, Medcom, 1976)

533

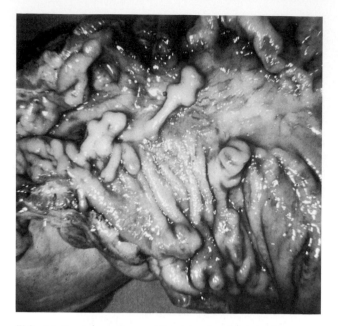

FIG. 15-5. Ulcerative colitis: islands of heaped-up mucosa and inflammatory polyps (pseudopolyps). (Corman ML, Veidenheimer MC, Nugent FW et al: Diseases of the Anus, Rectum and Colon. Part II: Non-specific inflammatory bowel disease. New York, Medcom, 1976)

Crohn's colitis frequently involves the colon and ileum in continuity. Cecal ulceration with involvement of the ileocecal valve can be seen with ileal disease (Fig. 15-18). Thickening of the bowel wall may produce narrowing sufficient to precipitate intestinal obstruction or to impede the passage of swallowed seeds or nuts (Fig. 15-19). Occasionally the ileal disease may terminate abruptly at the ileocecal valve, sparing the large bowel (Fig. 15-20).

One of the common manifestations of Crohn's disease is *fistula formation.* Fistulas may occur into any adjacent organ, such as the small or large bowel, bladder, vagina, uterus, ureter, or skin. Burrowing of the fissures deep into the bowel wall predisposes to fistula formation. Fistulas occur more commonly in the mesocolic aspect of the bowel than on the antimesocolic border (Fig. 15-21).

Occasionally, diffuse mucosal disease may produce a pseudopolypoid mucosal pattern similar to that of chronic ulcerative colitis. Giant pseudopolyps may actually mimic neoplasms clinically and radiographically. The condition is most likely the result of fusion of numerous finger-like pseudopolyps.[109] A number of reports and reviews of this manifestation have been published.[64, 109, 140] *(Text continues on p. 543)*

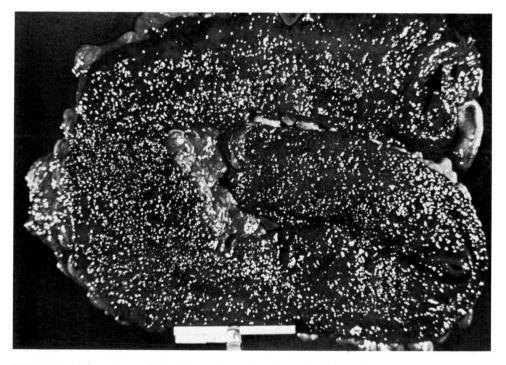

FIG. 15-6. Ulcerative colitis. The entire colon is involved by inflammatory change with sparing of the ileum *(arrow).* (Corman ML, Veidenheimer MC, Nugent FW et al: Diseases of the Anus, Rectum and Colon. Part II: Non-specific inflammatory bowel disease. New York, Medcom, 1976)

534

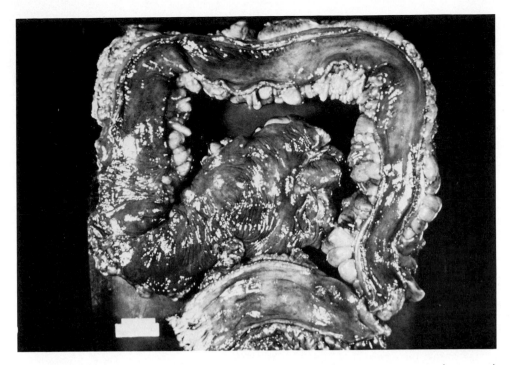

FIG. 15-7. Ulcerative colitis: complete desquamation of colonic mucosa. Note the normal bowel wall thickness. (Corman ML, Veidenheimer MC, Nugent FW et al: Diseases of the Anus, Rectum and Colon. Part II: Non-specific inflammatory bowel disease. New York, Medcom, 1976)

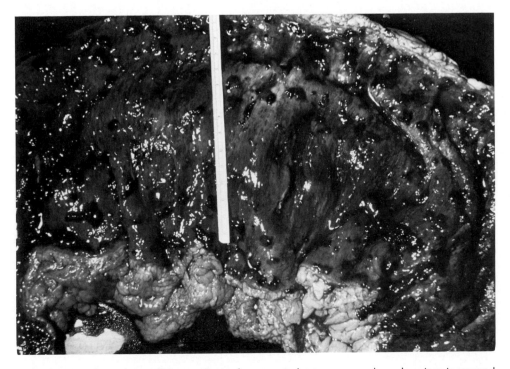

FIG. 15-8. Ulcerative colitis: portion of a resected transverse colon showing increased circumference of the bowel. There is practically no mucosa remaining, and in some areas circular muscle is exposed. (Corman ML, Veidenheimer MC, Nugent FW et al; Diseases of the Anus, Rectum and Colon. Part II: Non-specific inflammatory bowel disease. New York, Medcom, 1976)

535

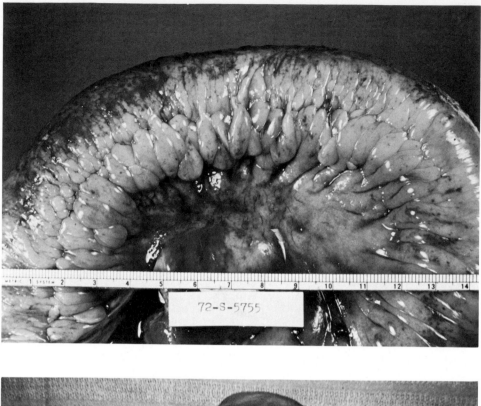

FIG. 15-9. Ileal Crohn's disease. Subserosal inflammation and "fat-wrapping" are evident. (Corman ML, Veidenheimer MC, Nugent FW et al: Diseases of the Anus, Rectum and Colon. Part II: Non-specific inflammatory bowel disease. New York, Medcom, 1976)

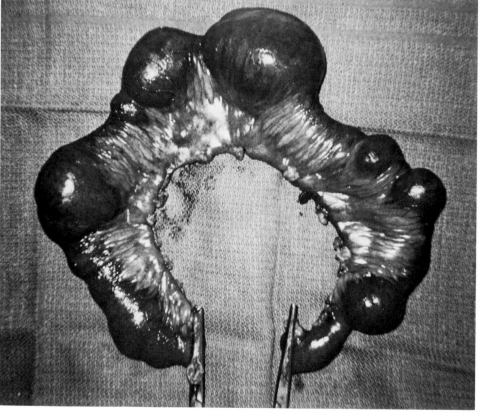

FIG. 15-10. Crohn's disease: segmental constrictions of small bowel with dilated bowel between each stenotic area. (Corman ML, Veidenheimer MC, Nugent NW et al: Diseases of the Anus, Rectum and Colon. Part II: Non-specific inflammatory bowel disease. New York, Medcom, 1976)

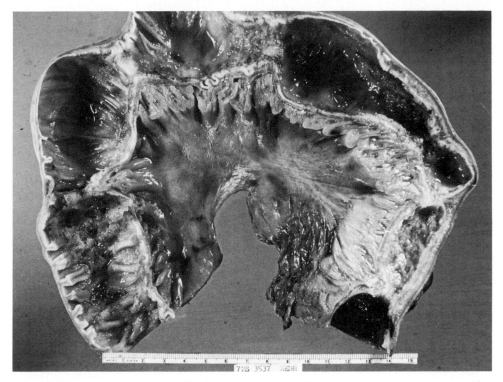

FIG. 15-11.   Crohn's disease. This opened specimen from the previous figure reveals the segmental nature of the disease. Thickening of the mesentery is a prominent feature. (Corman ML, Veidenheimer MC, Nugent FW et al: Diseases of the Anus, Rectum and Colon. Part II: Non-specific inflammatory bowel disease. New York, Medcom, 1976)

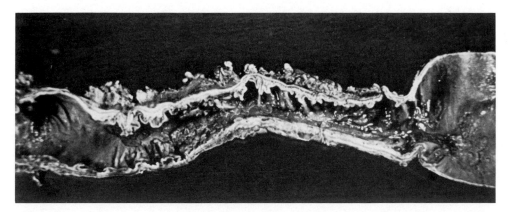

FIG. 15-12.   Crohn's colitis: segmental involvement of the sigmoid with marked narrowing of the midportion. Thickening of all layers of bowel is evident. At each end the bowel is less involved and more distensible. (Corman ML, Veidenheimer MC, Nugent FW et al: Diseases of the Anus, Rectum and Colon. Part II: Non-specific inflammatory bowel disease. New York, Medcom, 1976)

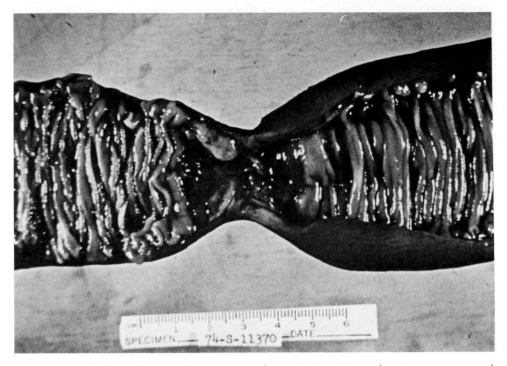

FIG. 15-13.   Crohn's disease: short segment of constriction. Note edematous mucosa and evidence of bowel dilatation on the right side, produced by partial obstruction. (Corman ML, Veidenheimer MC, Nugent FW et al: Diseases of the Anus, Rectum and Colon. Part II: Non-specific inflammatory bowel disease. New York, Medcom, 1976)

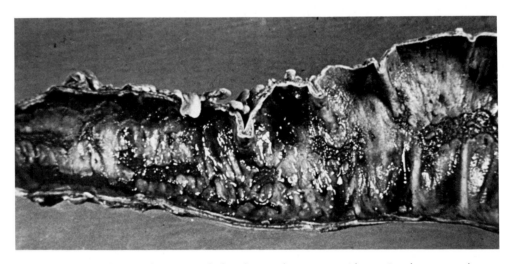

FIG. 15-14.   Crohn's colitis: irregularly ulcerated mucosa with sparing between ulcers. (Corman ML, Veidenheimer MC, Nugent FW et al: Diseases of the Anus, Rectum and Colon. Part II: Non-specific inflammatory bowel disease. New York, Medcom, 1976)

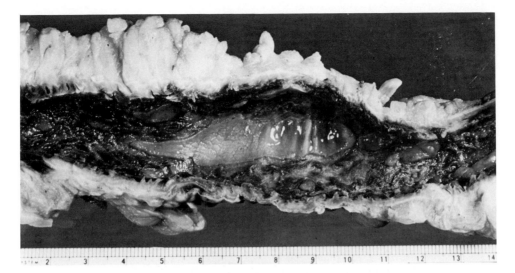

FIG. 15-15. Crohn's colitis. An island of normal mucosa lies in the middle of the specimen, with largely denuded, ulcerated mucosa on either side. (Corman ML, Veidenheimer MC, Nugent FW et al: Diseases of the Anus, Rectum and Colon. Part II: Non-specific inflammatory bowel disease. New York, Medcom, 1976)

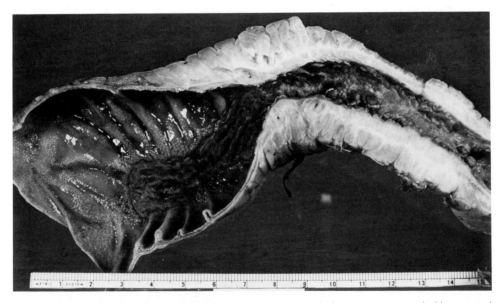

FIG. 15-16. Crohn's colitis: severe stenosis on the right and ulceration surrounded by normal mucosa on the left, a typical feature of this disease. (Corman ML, Veidenheimer MC, Nugent FW et al: Diseases of the Anus, Rectum and Colon. Part II: Non-specific inflammatory bowel disease. New York, Medcom, 1976)

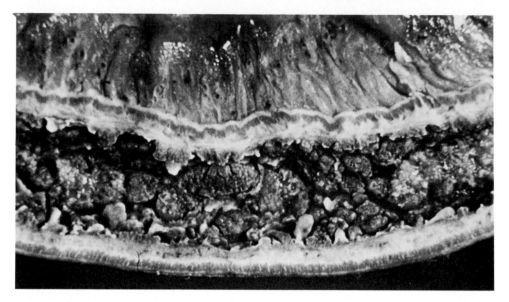

FIG. 15-17. Crohn's ileitis. The cobblestone appearance of the mucosa is produced by transverse and longitudinal intersecting ulcerations. Note the thickened bowel wall. (Corman ML, Veidenheimer MC, Nugent FW et al: Diseases of the Anus, Rectum and Colon. Part II: Non-specific inflammatory bowel disease. New York, Medcom. 1976)

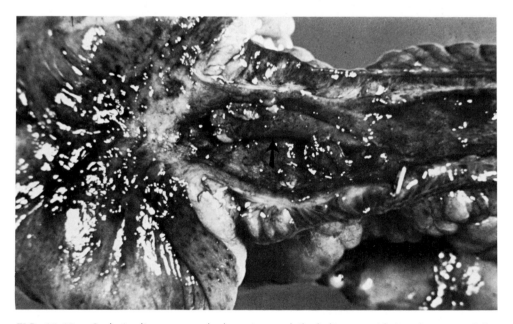

FIG. 15-18. Crohn's disease: cecal ulceration and ileal disease with involvement of the ileocecal valve. Note the large ileal mucosal tag *(arrow)*. (Corman ML, Veidenheimer MC, Nugent FW et al: Diseases of the Anus, Rectum and Colon. Part II: Non-specific inflammatory bowel disease. New York, Medcom, 1976)

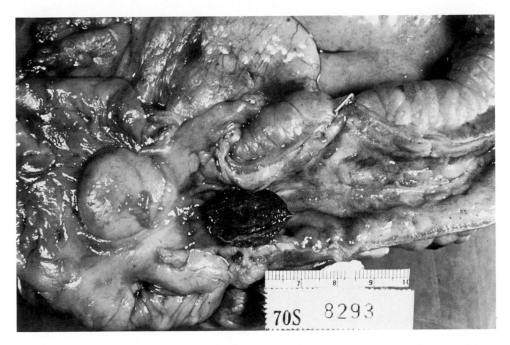

FIG. 15-19. Crohn's ileitis. This unusual specimen demonstrates a prune pit trapped in a narrowed segment of terminal ileum, precipitating intestinal obstruction. (Corman ML, Veidenheimer MC, Nugent FW et al: Diseases of the Anus, Rectum and Colon. Part II: Nonspecific inflammatory bowel disease. New York, Medcom, 1976)

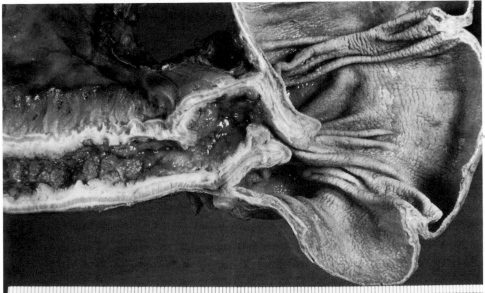

FIG. 15-20. Crohn's ileitis: ileal involvement with sparing of the large bowel. Note the abrupt cessation of the disease at the ileocecal valve. (Corman ML, Veidenheimer MC, Nugent FW et al: Diseases of the Anus, Rectum and Colon. Part II: Non-specific inflammatory bowel disease. New York, Medcom, 1976)

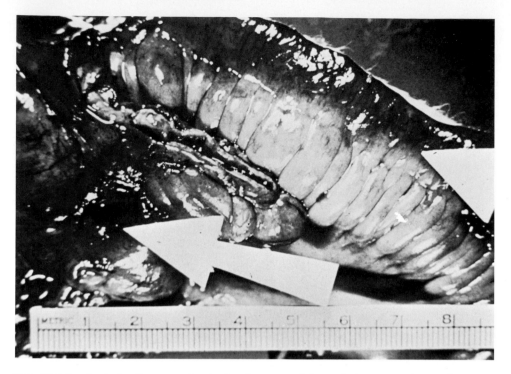

FIG. 15-21. Crohn's disease: a fistula that has passed through the mesocolon and into an adjacent structure at some distance from the point of origin in the bowel. One arrow points to the fistula; the other demonstrates the characteristic small bowel fat wrapping. (Corman ML, Veidenheimer MC, Nugent FW et al: Diseases of the Anus, Rectum and Colon. Part II: Non-specific inflammatory bowel disease. New York, Medcom, 1976)

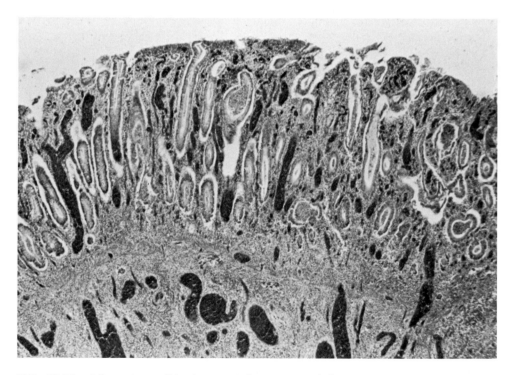

FIG. 15-22. Ulcerative colitis: intense inflammation of the mucosa with multiple crypt abscesses. (Original magnification × 80. Corman ML, Veidenheimer MC, Nugent FW et al: Diseases of the Anus, Rectum and Colon. Part II: Non-specific inflammatory bowel disease. New York, Medcom, 1976)

Histologic Appearance

Ulcerative Colitis

Ulcerative colitis is characterized histologically by an intense inflammation of the mucosa and submucosa, in addition to the presence of multiple crypt abscesses. Marked vascular engorgement accounts for the propensity toward rectal bleeding in patients with this condition (Fig. 15-22). There is an obvious decrease in mucus production by the crypt epithelial cells (Fig. 15-23). If the bowel is cut longitudinally it becomes apparent that there is sparing of the deeper parts of the

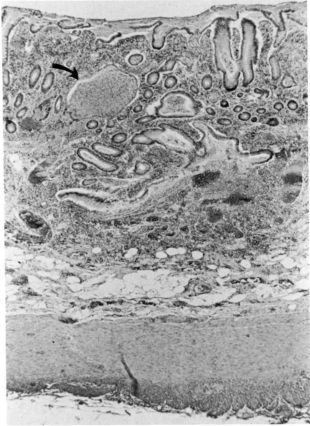

FIG. 15-24. Ulcerative colitis: marked inflammation of the mucosa and submucosa. Note the large crypt abscess *(arrow)* that has penetrated into the submucosa and has been lined partially by epithelial cells growing down into the abscess cavity. (Original magnification × 80. Corman ML, Veidenheimer MC, Nugent FW et al: Diseases of the Anus, Rectum and Colon. Part II: Non-specific inflammatory bowel disease. New York, Medcom, 1976)

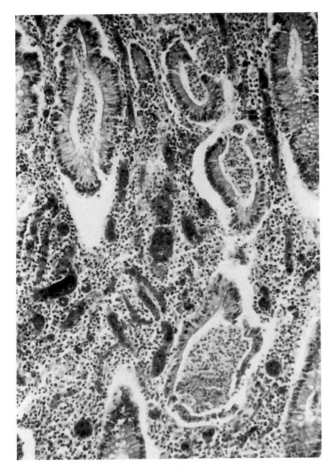

FIG. 15-23. Ulcerative colitis: crypt abscesses with degeneration of crypt epithelium and with communication between the crypt lumen and lamina propria. Note vascular engorgement and decrease in mucus production by crypt epithelial cells.(Original magnification × 280. Corman ML, Veidenheimer MC, Nugent FW et al: Diseases of the Anus, Rectum and Colon. Part II: Non-specific inflammatory bowel disease. New York, Medcom, 1976)

colonic wall; this is the most characteristic finding in ulcerative colitis (Fig. 15-24). Abscesses may enlarge to undermine the mucosa, which may then be shed into the bowel lumen, leaving an ulcer behind. When multiple ulcers form, the remaining nonulcerated mucosa extends above the muscularis as polypoid projections, resulting in the so-called pseudopolyps of ulcerative colitis (Figs. 15-25 and 15-26). If ulceration continues, the entire mucosa may become denuded, and broad areas of the submucosa may be exposed to the fecal stream. With toxic megacolon there is full-thickness involvement of the bowel, necrosis, and friability, the histologic manifestation of which is shown in Figure 15-27.

(Text continues on p. 547)

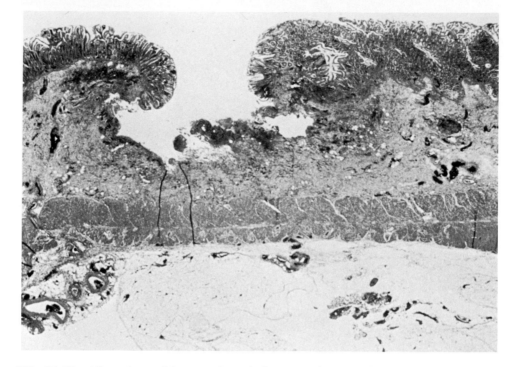

FIG. 15-25. Ulcerative colitis: an enlarged abscess undermines the mucosa to leave an ulcer. (Original magnification × 80. Corman ML, Veidenheimer MC, Nugent FW et al: Diseases of the Anus, Rectum and Colon. Part II: Non-specific inflammatory bowel disease. New York, Medcom, 1976)

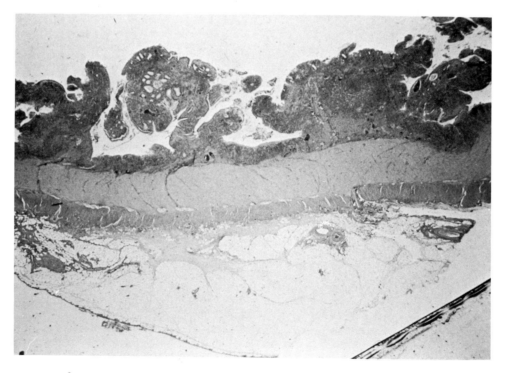

FIG. 15-26. Ulcerative colitis: confluence of ulcers results in pseudopolyps. (Original magnification × 80. Corman ML, Veidenheimer MC, Nugent FW et al: Diseases of the Anus, Rectum and Colon. Part II: Non-specific inflammatory bowel disease. New York, Medcom, 1976)

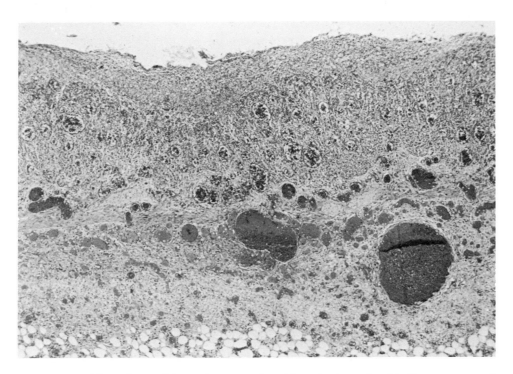

FIG. 15-27. Ulcerative colitis: toxic megacolon. Note the loss of epithelium, transmural necrosis, and hemorrhage. (Original magnification × 80. Corman, ML, Veidenheimer MC, Nugent FW et al: Diseases of the Anus, Rectum and Colon. Part II: Non-specific inflammatory bowel disease. New York, Medcom, 1976)

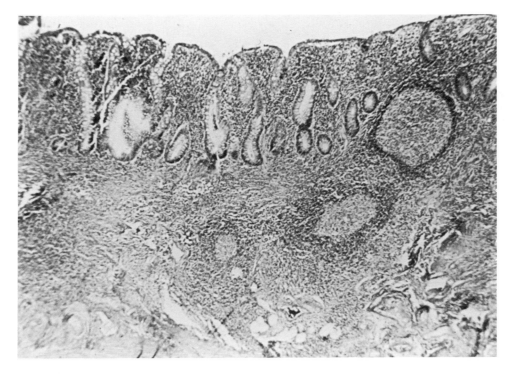

FIG. 15-28. Lymphoid hyperplasia. Although mucosal disease is relatively inactive, lymphoid hyperplasia is pronounced. (Original magnification × 80. Corman ML, Veidenheimer MC, Nugent FW et al: Diseases of the Anus, Rectum and Colon. Part II: Non-specific inflammatory bowel disease. New York, Medcom, 1976)

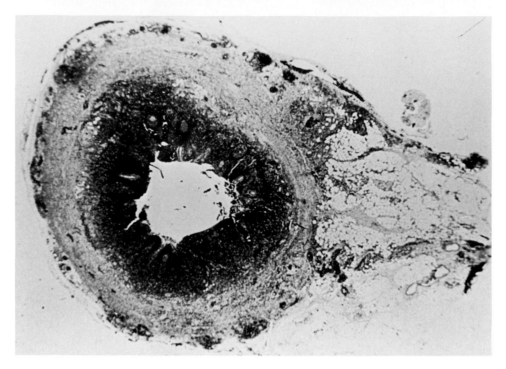

FIG. 15-29. Crohn's disease of the appendix. Cross section demonstrates inflammatory changes at all levels: mucosa, muscularis, and serosa. (Original magnification × 80. Corman ML, Veidenheimer MC, Nugent FW et al: Diseases of the Anus, Rectum and Colon. Part II: Non-specific inflammatory bowel disease. New York, Medcom, 1976)

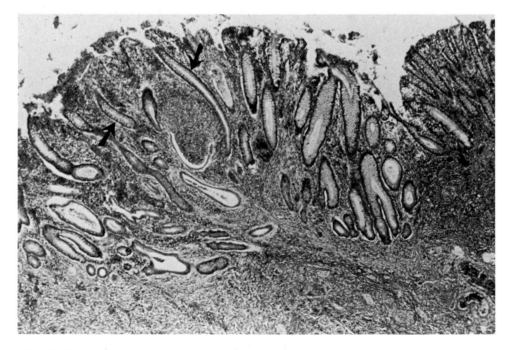

FIG. 15-30. Crohn's disease. Note the crypts (*arrows*) on either side of the crypt abscess contain an almost normal complement of goblet cells. (Original magnification × 80. Corman, ML, Veidenheimer MC, Nugent FW et al: Diseases of the Anus, Rectum and Colon. Part II: Non-specific inflammatory bowel disease. New York, Medcom, 1976)

Lymphoid hyperplasia involving the mucosa and submucosa occurs in up to 25% of patients with ulcerative colitis. This may be present beneath an area of relative inactivity (Fig. 15-28).

Crohn's Disease

The three primary pathologic findings in patients with Crohn's colitis are transmural inflammation and fibrosis, granulomas, and narrow, deeply penetrating ulcers or "fissures" (Fig. 15-29). The mucosal inflammation of Crohn's disease differs from that of ulcerative colitis in that typically there are fewer crypt abscesses, less congestion, and better preservation of the goblet cell population (Fig. 15-30).

Granulomas may occur in any part of the bowel wall and are usually identified in approximately two thirds of all patients with Crohn's colitis. If a biopsy is performed in an attempt to differentiate between the two inflammatory conditions, the material should be obtained if possible from a noninflamed area; a granuloma may be apparent with ulcerative colitis in the area of acute inflammation (Fig. 15-31). The microscopic appearance of the granuloma is not diagnostic, and the possibility of an infectious agent should always be considered (Fig. 15-32). Granulomas can also occur in the liver (Fig. 15-33) and in the omentum (Fig. 15-34).

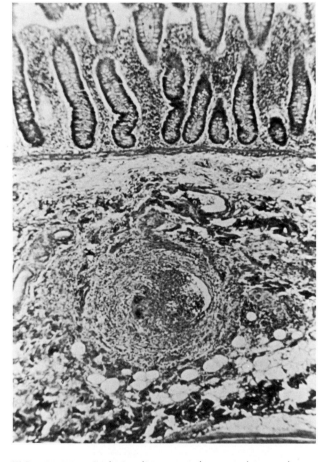

FIG. 15-31. Crohn's disease: submucosal granuloma. Note that the overlying mucosa has inflammatory cells in the lamina propria but no crypt abscess or ulceration. (Original magnification × 80. Corman ML, Veidenheimer MC, Nugent FW et al: Diseases of the Anus, Rectum and Colon. Part II: Non-specific inflammatory bowel disease. New York, Medcom, 1976)

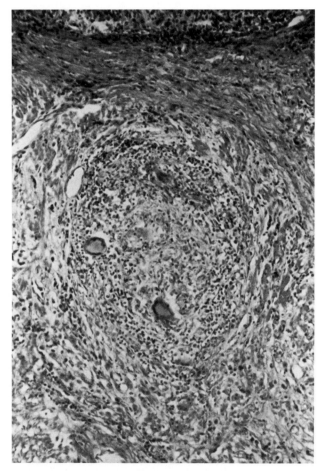

FIG. 15-32. Crohn's disease: granuloma within muscularis propria. (Original magnification × 280. Corman ML, Veidenheimer MC, Nugent FW et al: Diseases of the Anus, Rectum and Colon. Part II: Non-specific inflammatory bowel disease. New York, Medcom, 1976)

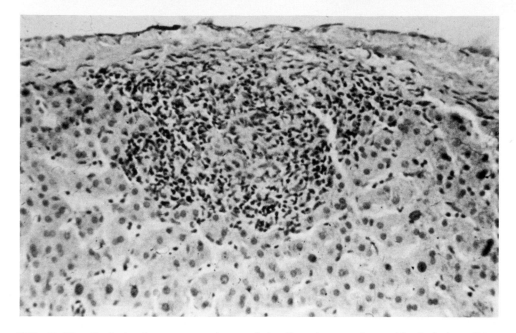

FIG. 15-33. Crohn's disease: granuloma of the liver in a patient with Crohn's colitis. (Original magnification × 260. Corman ML, Veidenheimer MC, Nugent FW et al: Diseases of the Anus, Rectum and Colon. Part II: Non-specific inflammatory bowel disease. New York, Medcom, 1976)

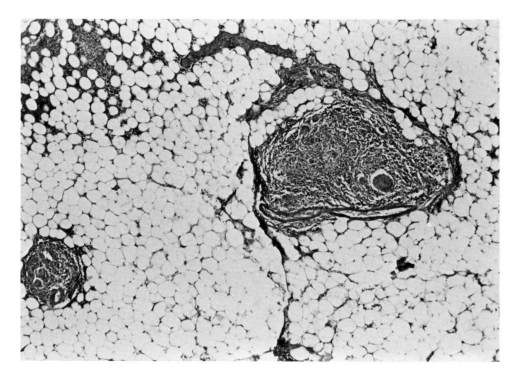

FIG. 15-34. Crohn's colitis. Two omental granulomas are seen in a patient with Crohn's colitis. (Original magnification × 80. Corman ML, Veidenheimer MC, Nugent FW et al: Diseases of the Anus, Rectum and Colon. Part II: Non-specific inflammatory bowel disease. New York, Medcom, 1976)

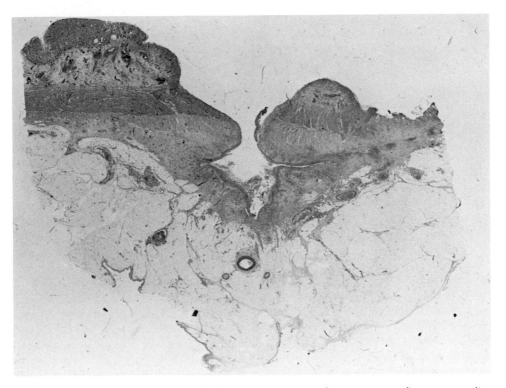

FIG. 15-35. Crohn's disease: a whole mount specimen demonstrates a fissure extending through the colon wall and into the pericolonic fat. This is the origin of a fistula. (Corman ML, Veidenheimer MC, Nugent FW et al: Diseases of the Anus, Rectum and Colon. Part II: Non-specific inflammatory bowel disease. New York, Medcom, 1976)

Narrow, deeply penetrating ulcers or "fissures" are the third characteristic feature of Crohn's disease. The fissures may penetrate through the inner circular layer of the muscularis and are visible on the radiographs after a barium enema as spicules (see later, under Radiographic Features). A sinus tract present in the fat adjacent to the bowel wall indicates that one of the fissures has penetrated through the wall (Fig. 15-35). When this occurs, a sinus may burrow into another organ to produce a fistula (Fig. 15-36).

Recent information about the pathology of inflammatory bowel disease has been gleaned from electron microscopy. Early epithelial changes in areas that appear to be uninvolved can be identified using this modality. These changes include necrosis of individual columnar epithelial cells; budding of the tips of microvilli; thickening, shortening, irregularity, and fusion of intestinal villi; numerous Paneth's cells; hyperplasia of goblet cells; and augmented mucous secretion.[148] Other studies such as tissue-enzyme analysis, jejunal-surface pH, and differences in sodium flux and mucosal potential imply that the disease often is far more extensive than is recognized by other more conventional means, and certainly much more extensive than is apparent at the time of surgery.

Another recent observation is the increased secretion of mucus by the bowel in Crohn's disease as compared with decreased colonic mucus in ulcerative colitis. This decrease may be explained by destruction of the epithelial cells.[148] A number of biochemical changes have also been observed.

Radiographic Features

Ulcerative Colitis

In any evaluation of a patient with inflammatory bowel disease, the importance of a plain film of the abdomen should not be underestimated. Without submitting the patient to the rigors of a barium enema examination, particularly when the patient may be acutely ill, the physician can obtain valuable information about the extent of disease (Fig. 15-37).

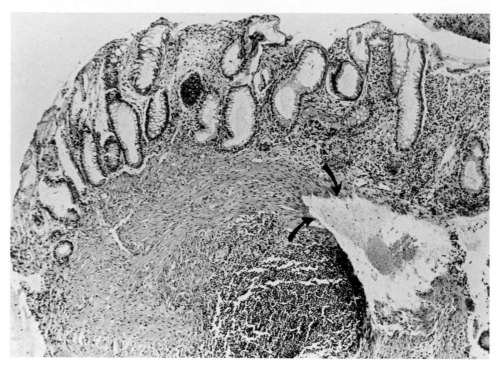

FIG. 15-36. Crohn's colitis with fistula: a sharply defined early fistula in the submucosa *(arrows)*. (Original magnification × 80. Courtesy of Rudolf Garret, M.D.)

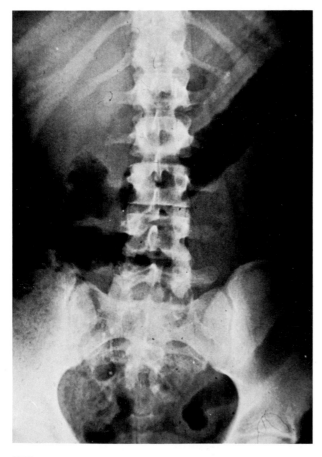

FIG. 15-37. Ulcerative colitis. This plain abdominal film of an acutely ill patient reveals some thickening of the colonic wall, especially in the region of the sigmoid where it overlies the iliac crest, and loss of haustral markings throughout the left colon and transverse colon to the region of the hepatic flexure. Subsequent barium enema demonstrated the disease to extend exactly to the point seen on the plain film. (Corman ML, Veidenheimer MC, Nugent FW et al: Diseases of the Anus, Rectum and Colon. Part II: Non-specific inflammatory bowel disease. New York, Medcom, 1976)

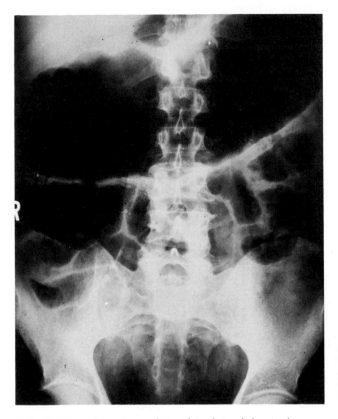

FIG. 15-38. Ulcerative colitis. This plain abdominal x-ray film reveals marked dilatation of the transverse colon (toxic megacolon). (Corman ML, Veidenheimer MC, Nugent FW et al: Diseases of the Anus, Rectum and Colon. Part II: Non-specific inflammatory bowel disease. New York, Medcom, 1976)

The importance of a plain film of the abdomen is further emphasized in patients who have toxic dilatation, a condition usually seen in the transverse colon (Figs. 15-38 and 15-39). When the radiographic appearance of toxic dilatation is noted, a barium enema examination is contraindicated, but serial abdominal films are diagnostically valuable. The effectiveness of medical therapy can be evaluated by determining the increase or decrease in the degree of dilatation. The abdominal examination should not be relied upon exclusively because the patient may frequently be confused or even obtunded. Furthermore, the high dose of steroids frequently used in the treatment of toxic megacolon may mask abdominal signs.

The radiologic findings during the acute phase of ulcerative colitis include edema, ulceration, and changes in colonic motility. Edema may be apparent even on the plain film of the abdomen such as in Figure 15-39. Initially, ulceration may be rather minimal and difficult to identify. As the disease becomes more fulminant, the ulceration becomes more obvious and may take on a collar-button appearance (Fig. 15-40). Edema and inflammation of the mucosa may result in the radiologic appearance that has been called "thumbprinting," a phenomenon which is characteristically observed in patients with ischemic colitis (Fig. 15-41).

When the disease enters a more chronic phase, other features become characteristic on barium enema examination. These include fibrosis, which results in shortening of the bowel, depression of the flexures, pseudopolyposis, and stricture formation. The bowel wall is less distensible, and the motility pattern is disturbed. Diffuse, confluent, symmetric disease beginning with the anorectal junction are the hallmarks of the radiological findings of chronic ulcerative colitis (Figs. 15-42 and 15-43). The presence of polypoid lesions throughout the entire colon may confuse the unini-

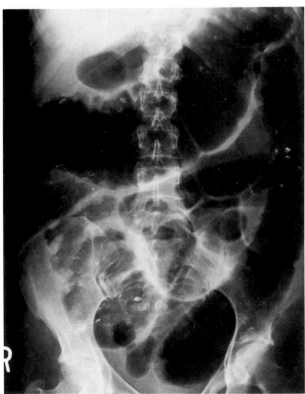

FIG. 15-39. Ulcerative colitis: toxic megacolon. Note the transverse colon dilatation, small bowel ileus, and fluid between the loops of the bowel.

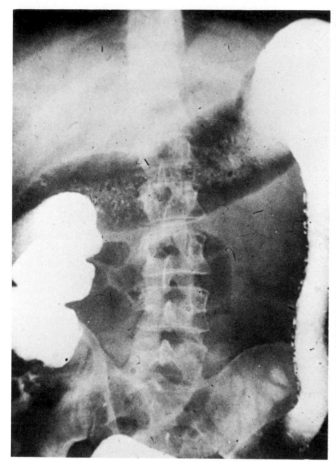

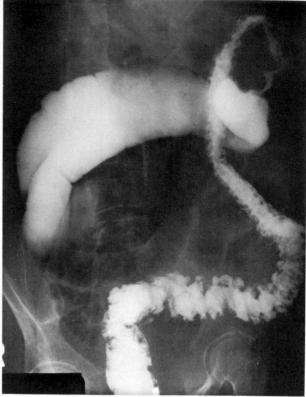

FIG. 15-41. Acute ulcerative colitis demonstrating edema of the bowel wall, flocculation of barium due to mucus (fuzzy appearance), and thumb-printing in the region of the splenic flexure.

FIG. 15-40. Acute ulcerative colitis. Note the loss of haustral markings up to and including the mid-ascending colon and numerous discrete ulcerations deep in the submucosa along the descending colon. (Corman ML, Veidenheimer MC, Nugent FW et al: Diseases of the Anus, Rectum and Colon. Part II: Non-specific inflammatory bowel disease. New York, Medcom, 1976)

tiated with the radiologic picture seen in familial polyposis. Both diseases commonly present with rectal bleeding and diarrhea (Fig. 15-44). In ulcerative colitis foreshortening of the bowel may be apparent, particularly in the flexures, and if the outline of the colon is carefully examined, numerous discrete ulcerations can usually be appreciated (Fig. 15-45).

Benign strictures are quite uncommon in ulcerative colitis. In fact, a stricture in this condition should be considered malignant until proved otherwise (see Relationship to Carcinoma). Radiologic examination will

usually reveal a smoothly outlined, concentric lumen with tapering margins (Fig. 15-46). Areas of spasm are frequently seen in ulcerative colitis and may be difficult to differentiate from stricture. The administration of propantheline (Pro-Banthine, 10 mg) intravenously may eliminate the stricture due to such spasm. If the lumen is concentric and the margins are smooth, the lesion may be benign; if the lumen is eccentric and the margins are irregular a carcinoma must be suspected.[179]

Another radiologic finding that is sometimes observed in patients with ulcerative colitis is the so-called backwash ileitis. This is a very poor term because it implies that the ulcerative colitis has somehow regurgitated through the ileocecal valve to cause the disease in the distal ileum. Marshak and Lindner were able to demonstrate the presence of this phenomenon in approximately 10% of patients with ulcerative colitis whom they had studied.[179] The changes may vary from

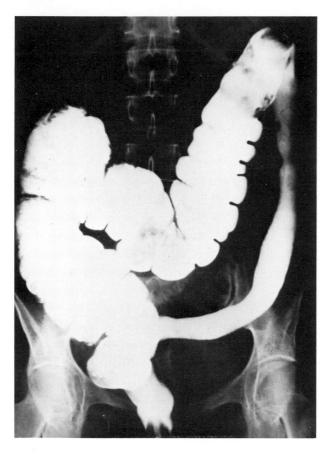

FIG. 15-42. Chronic ulcerative colitis. Typical changes of left-sided disease include loss of haustral pattern, shortening of the sigmoid, and narrowing of the entire descending and sigmoid colon. (Corman ML, Veidenheimer MC, Nugent FW et al: Diseases of the Anus, Rectum and Colon. Part II: Non-specific inflammatory bowel disease. New York, Medcom, 1976)

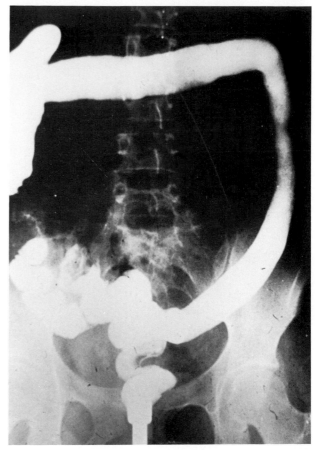

FIG. 15-43. Chronic ulcerative colitis: a classic example of diffuse, symmetric, confluent disease. Characteristically, the left side is more involved than the right. Note that there is more foreshortening of the splenic flexure than of the hepatic flexure, and there is suggestion of haustrae on the right but not on the left. (Corman ML, Veidenheimer MC, Nugent FW et al: Diseases of the Anus, Rectum and Colon. Part II: Non-specific inflammatory bowel disease. New York, Medcom, 1976)

simple lack of distensibility as the head of pressure is increased when the barium is inserted, to ileal dilatation, narrowing, rigidity, and changes that may mimic regional enteritis (Fig. 15-47).

Crohn's Disease

As previously mentioned, Crohn's disease can occur anywhere in the alimentary tract. The disease tends to be segmental and asymmetrical. Radiologic findings include skip lesions, contour defects, longitudinal ulcers, transverse fissures, eccentric involvement, pseu-

dodiverticula, narrowing or stricture formation, pseudopolypoid changes that may be cobblestone-like, sinus tracts, and fistulas.[179]

A plain film of the abdomen may be quite useful in the early stages of Crohn's colitis. Although toxic megacolon is much less common in Crohn's disease than it is in ulcerative colitis, acute toxic dilatation may occur before any firm cicatrix has formed in the bowel wall (Fig. 15-48).

(Text continues on p. 557)

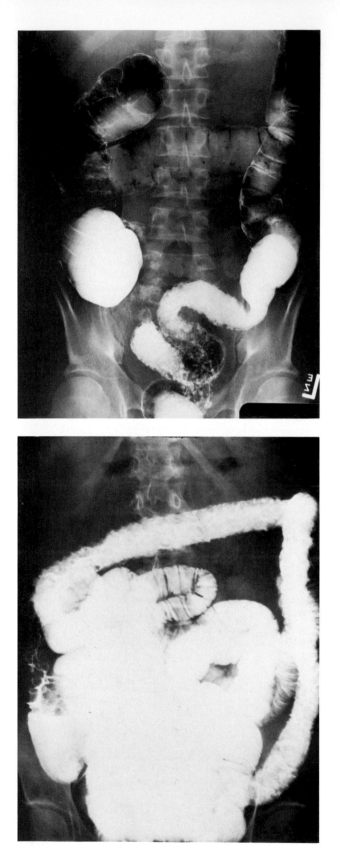

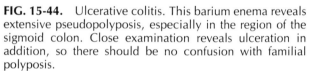

FIG. 15-44. Ulcerative colitis. This barium enema reveals extensive pseudopolyposis, especially in the region of the sigmoid colon. Close examination reveals ulceration in addition, so there should be no confusion with familial polyposis.

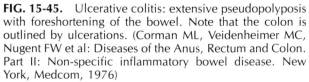

FIG. 15-45. Ulcerative colitis: extensive pseudopolyposis with foreshortening of the bowel. Note that the colon is outlined by ulcerations. (Corman ML, Veidenheimer MC, Nugent FW et al: Diseases of the Anus, Rectum and Colon. Part II: Non-specific inflammatory bowel disease. New York, Medcom, 1976)

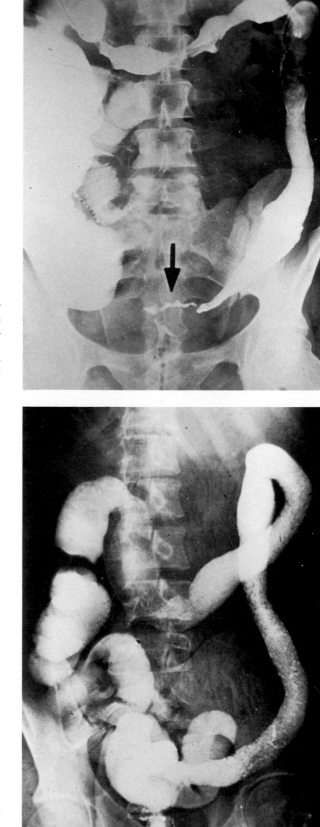

FIG. 15-46. Ulcerative colitis with stricture. Inflammatory changes are noted to the hepatic flexure with stricture in the distal sigmoid *(arrow)* . The patient subsequently underwent resection, and the lesion was found to be benign. (Corman ML, Veidenheimer MC, Nugent FW et al: Diseases of the Anus, Rectum and Colon. Part II: Non-specific inflammatory bowel disease. New York, Medcom, 1976)

FIG. 15-47. Extensive ulcerative colitis with loss of haustral markings and destruction of the normal mucosa throughout. Dilatation of the terminal ileum is evident, a characteristic observation in "backwash ileitis." (Corman ML, Veidenheimer MC, Nugent FW et al: Diseases of the Anus, Rectum and Colon. Part II: Non-specific inflammatory bowel disease. New York, Medcom, 1976)

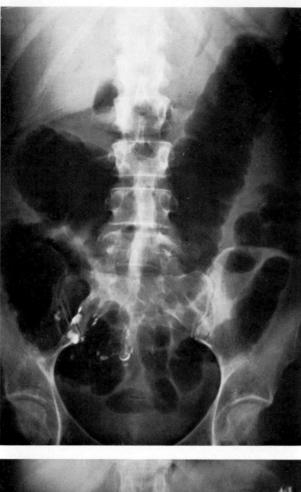

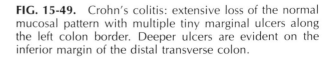

FIG. 15-48. Crohn's colitis. This plain abdominal film demonstrates marked colonic dilatation. Toxic megacolon may be recognized during the initial attack, before fibrosis and thickening develop. (Corman ML, Veidenheimer MC, Nugent FW et al: Diseases of the Anus, Rectum and Colon. Part II: Non-specific inflammatory bowel disease. New York, Medcom, 1976)

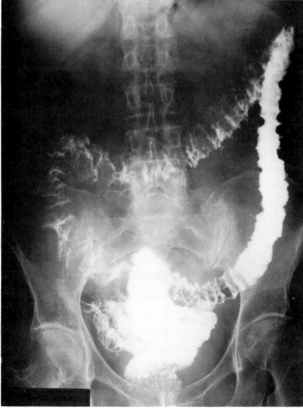

FIG. 15-49. Crohn's colitis: extensive loss of the normal mucosal pattern with multiple tiny marginal ulcers along the left colon border. Deeper ulcers are evident on the inferior margin of the distal transverse colon.

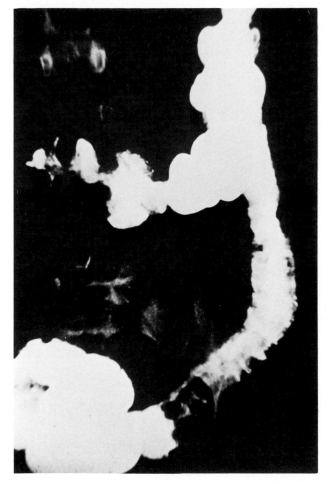

FIG. 15-50. Crohn's colitis. Extensive longitudinal and transverse ulcers are evident in the descending and sigmoid colon. (Corman ML, Veidenheimer MC, Nugent FW et al: Diseases of the Anus, Rectum and Colon. Part II: Non-specific inflammatory bowel disease. New York, Medcom, 1976)

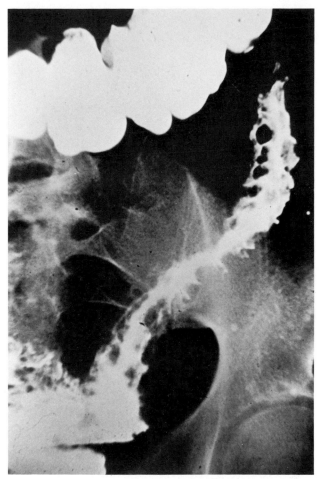

FIG. 15-51. Crohn's colitis: coarse cobblestoning of the left colon with intramural fistula traversing longitudinally along the bowel wall. (Corman ML, Veidenheimer MC, Nugent FW et al: Diseases of the Anus, Rectum and Colon. Part II: Non-specific inflammatory bowel disease. New York, Medcom, 1976)

The post-evacuation film is most useful in identifying numerous discrete ulcers (Fig. 15-49). Small ulcerations may combine to produce large, longitudinal ulcers (Fig. 15-50), and when the longitudinal ulcers combine with transverse fissures they produce the cobblestone appearance seen radiologically (Fig. 15-51). Intramural fistulas can result from the coalescing of the numerous longitudinal ulcers, which in turn may produce a double-lumen appearance (Fig. 15-52). Ulcerations may penetrate beyond the contour of the bowel and present as numerous, long spicules or as sinus tracts (Fig. 15-53). These deep fissures may be confused with diverticula, but with experience the physician

should readily differentiate them. If one examines the whole-mount specimen shown in Figure 15-35, one can readily perceive how such a radiologic picture can be achieved.

Figure 15-54 demonstrates a number of the classical changes that one may see in the radiographic appearance of Crohn's colitis. These include segmental distribution with sparing of the rectum, stenosis, thickening of the bowel wall, ulceration, and a suggestion of a double-lumen appearance.

Strictures are of variable length, and may be quite extensive indeed (Fig. 15-55). When a stricture occurs
(Text continues on p. 560)

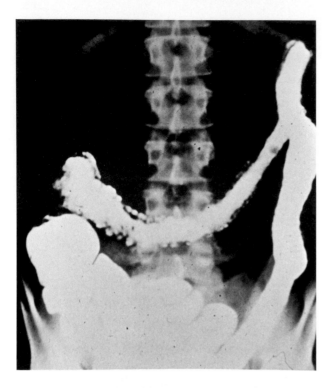

FIG. 15-52. Crohn's colitis. Longitudinal intramural fistulas are evident in the proximal transverse colon and splenic flexure. (Corman ML, Veidenheimer MC, Nugent FW et al: Diseases of the Anus, Rectum and Colon. Part II: Non-specific inflammatory bowel disease. New York, Medcom, 1976)

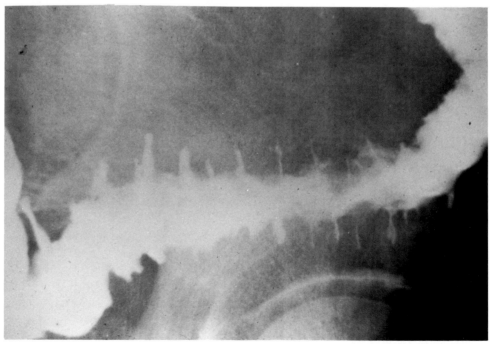

FIG. 15-53. Crohn's colitis: deep fissuring of the bowel wall in the sigmoid colon, giving a thornlike appearance. (Corman ML, Veidenheimer MC, Nugent FW et al: Diseases of the Anus, Rectum and Colon. Part II: Non-specific inflammatory bowel disease. New York, Medcom, 1976)

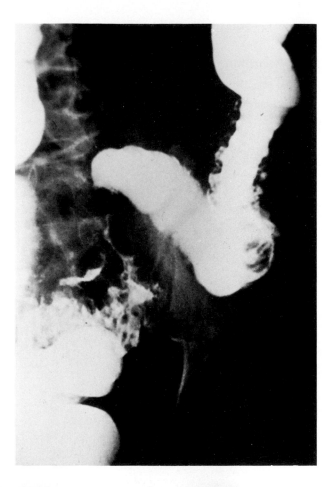

FIG. 15-54. Crohn's colitis: typical segmental involvement with a normal rectum, markedly stenotic lower sigmoid, relatively normal mid-sigmoid area, and then a further area of involvement of the upper sigmoid just distal to an uninvolved descending colon. Thickening of the bowel wall is seen in the upper sigmoid. (Corman ML, Veidenheimer MC, Nugent FW et al: Diseases of the Anus, Rectum and Colon. Part II: Non-specific inflammatory bowel disease. New York, Medcom, 1976)

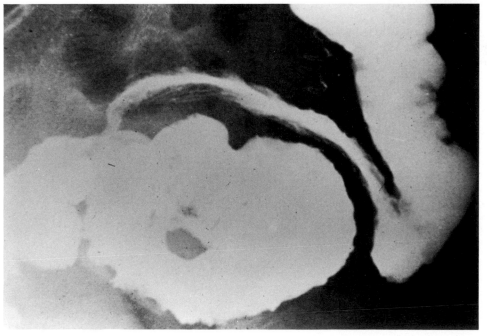

FIG. 15-55. Crohn's colitis: long sigmoid stricture with ulceration distally. (Corman ML, Veidenheimer MC, Nugent FW et al: Diseases of the Anus, Rectum and Colon. Part II: Non-specific inflammatory bowel disease. New York, Medcom, 1976)

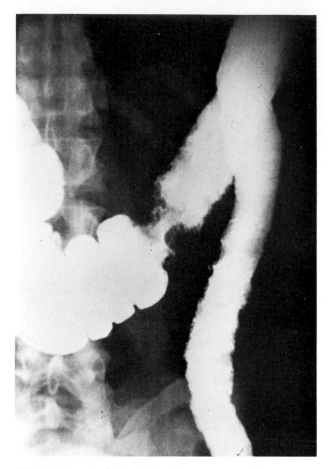

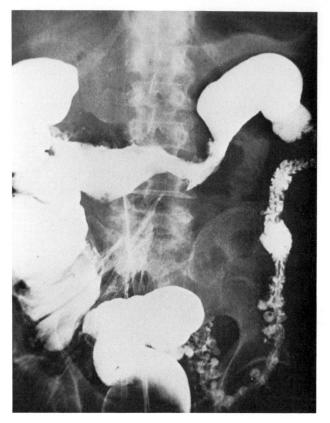

FIG. 15-57. Scirrhous carcinoma of the transverse colon. Contrast the absence of adjacent mucosal abnormality with the previous figure. (Corman ML, Veidenheimer MC, Nugent FW et al: Diseases of the Anus, Rectum and Colon. Part II: Non-specific inflammatory bowel disease. New York, Medcom, 1976)

FIG. 15-56. Crohn's colitis with transverse colon stricture, an ''apple core'' lesion suggestive of carcinoma. Note, however, that the distal bowel is ulcerated. (Corman ML, Veidenheimer MC, Nugent FW et al: Diseases of the Anus, Rectum and Colon. Part II: Non-specific inflammatory bowel disease. New York, Medcom, 1976)

in Crohn's disease it does not have the malignant association that a stricture assumes when it is seen in a patient with ulcerative colitis. However, patients with Crohn's disease have recently been shown to have an increased risk for the development of malignancy (see Relationship to Carcinoma). Differential diagnosis between a Crohn's stricture and that of a carcinoma should not be difficult. Close inspection will usually reveal that the bowel in an adjacent area is ulcerated (Fig. 15-56). Contrast this x-ray with Figure 15-57. Although a scirrhous carcinoma must always be considered in the differential diagnosis, the lack of associated ulceration or inflammatory changes elsewhere

in the colon usually clarifies the diagnosis. A most difficult differential diagnostic problem radiologically in patients with Crohn's disease is that of tuberculosis. When the condition is confined to the ileocecal region, it is virtually impossible to distinguish between the two diseases.

Crohn's disease of the terminal ileum has a characteristic appearance. Thickening of the bowel wall narrows the lumen, resulting in a degree of obstruction in some patients. This is the most frequent cause of abdominal pain in patients with Crohn's disease. The radiologic appearance of the terminal ileum has been described as a ''string sign'' (Fig. 15-58). Involvement of the terminal ileum may be seen as an isolated finding or may be associated with multiple diseased areas throughout the small intestine (Fig. 15-59).

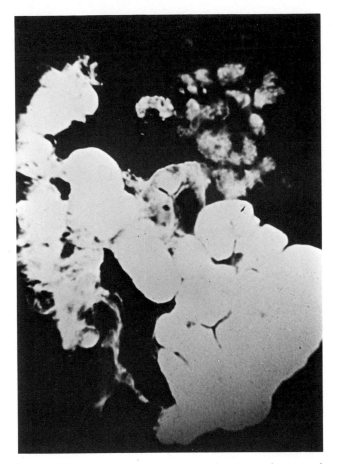

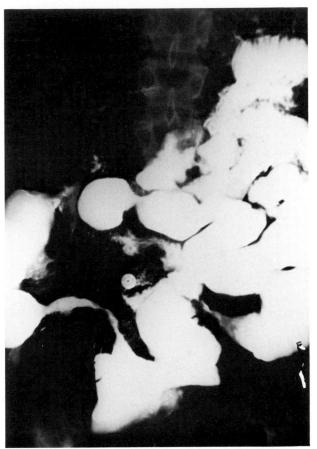

FIG. 15-58. Distal ileal Crohn's disease. Edema and thickening of the bowel wall produce the characteristic "string sign." (Corman ML, Veidenheimer MC, Nugent FW et al: Diseases of the Anus, Rectum and Colon. Part II: Non-specific inflammatory bowel disease. New York, Medcom, 1976)

FIG. 15-59. Small bowel Crohn's disease: terminal ileal disease in addition to multiple skip areas. (Corman ML, Veidenheimer MC, Nugent FW et al: Diseases of the Anus, Rectum and Colon. Part II: Non-specific inflammatory bowel disease. New York, Medcom, 1976)

Fistulous complications are frequently seen in patients with Crohn's disease. Communication between the ileum and colon is not uncommon (Fig. 15-60), but other types of fistulas have been reported, including coloduodenal (Fig. 15-61), and into the pelvic organs (Fig. 15-62).

SIGNS, SYMPTOMS, AND PRESENTATIONS

Patients with ulcerative colitis and Crohn's disease may present with very minimal symptoms and moderate complaints, or they may have fulminant manifestations. There is a considerable overlap in the symptomatology of the two conditions, but there are some differences in the presentation between the two. *Rectal bleeding* is always seen in patients with ulcerative colitis some time during the course of the illness. It can be safely said that if the patient does not bleed, the patient does not have ulcerative colitis. Patients with Crohn's disease also may bleed, but this is not as frequent a manifestation and may not be as severe. *Abdominal pain* may be mild or absent in patients with ulcerative colitis; it is rarely severe except in the condition of *toxic megacolon*. However, patients with Crohn's disease frequently have abdominal pain. This may be colicky in

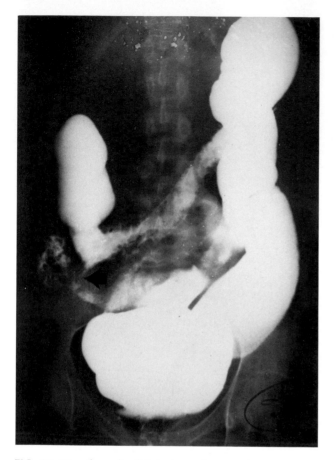

FIG. 15-60. Ileocolic fistula *(arrow)*: extensive transverse colon disease with communication to the ileum. (Corman ML, Veidenheimer MC, Nugent FW et al: Diseases of the Anus, Rectum and Colon. Part II: Non-specific inflammatory bowel disease. New York, Medcom, 1976)

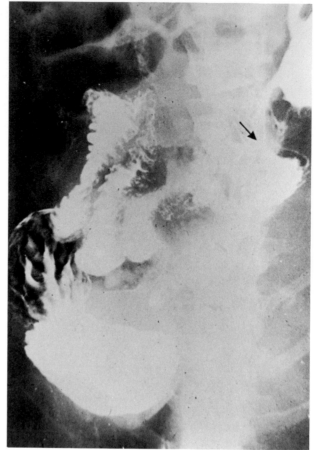

FIG. 15-61. Coloduodenal fistula. An upper gastrointestinal series demonstrates fistula *(arrow)* between the duodenum and the ascending colon. (Corman ML, Veidenheimer MC, Nugent FW et al: Diseases of the Anus, Rectum and Colon. Part II: Non-specific inflammatory bowel disease. New York, Medcom, 1976)

nature and be associated with intestinal obstruction, or it may be continual and related to the presence of a septic process within the abdomen. An abdominal mass is occasionally found on physical examination in a patient with Crohn's disease but is never seen in a patient with ulcerative colitis.

The presence of *diarrhea* and the *passage of mucus* are frequently observed in both conditions and do not serve as distinguishing characteristics.

Diarrhea may be manifested as two or three loose stools a day or may be as severe as twenty or more bowel movements within a 24 hour period. Often, patients with ulcerative colitis are more troubled by the frequency of the bowel movements than are patients with Crohn's disease, perhaps because the distal disease

tends to be associated with more urgency, and in some cases, *tenesmus*. Patients with Crohn's disease may have rectal sparing and are less likely to experience this urgency. However, *anal disease* is much more commonly seen in patients with Crohn's colitis. The presence of anal pain, swelling, and discharge may be a presenting feature of this condition and may be the only abnormality observed on examination and upon subsequent investigation.

Fever is usually not seen in patients with ulcerative colitis unless the person is acutely ill (toxic megacolon). However, in patients with Crohn's disease, a pyrexia is not uncommonly noted, and is usually due to the pres-

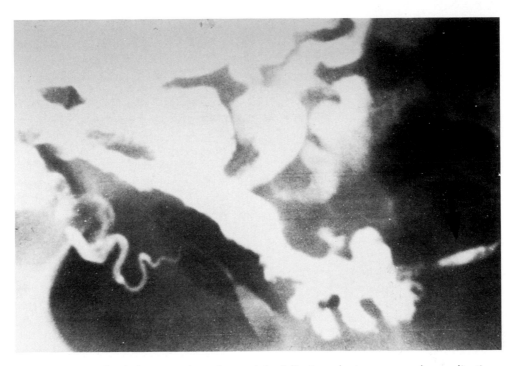

FIG. 15-62.   A fistula between the colon and the fallopian tube is an unusual complication of Crohn's colitis. Note that a second fistula passes into an abscess and out to the skin *(arrow)*. (Corman ML, Veidenheimer MC, Nugent FW et al: Diseases of the Anus, Rectum and Colon. Part II: Non-specific inflammatory bowel disease. New York, Medcom, 1976)

ence of an intra-abdominal abscess or undrained septic focus. *Nausea* and *vomiting* are not frequently seen in either condition unless there is evidence of intestinal obstruction. *Anorexia,* weight loss, anemia, and general debility are seen with relatively long-standing or fulminant disease.

The development of inflammatory bowel disease in *the elderly population* has been a source of some confusion. Many older patients who have signs and symptoms suggestive of inflammatory bowel disease are thought to have ischemic colitis. Conversely, patients thought to have inflammatory bowel disease subsequently may be proved to have ischemia as the cause of their symptoms. Brandt and co-workers reviewed 81 patients with colitis whose symptoms began after the age of 50 years.[30] In this retrospective review, one half of patients classified as having nonspecific inflammatory bowel disease were felt to really have had ischemic colitis. In older patients, ulcerative colitis may have a sudden and fulminating onset that may progress to a fatal outcome.

When the condition occurs in *children,* there may be a more rapid onset and progression than when the condition occurs in young adults. Symptoms are the same as for the adult disease, but toxic megacolon, bowel perforation, and massive hemorrhage are not uncommon sequellae. These youngsters often become chronically ill, have growth impairment and decreased mental acuity, and are less developed physically than their healthy peers (Fig. 15-63).[56, 57, 190, 255, 259]

Since inflammatory bowel disease is common in the child-bearing age, *pregnancy* is not infrequently an issue in the medical and surgical care of the patient. However, pregnancy developing in a patient who has inflammtory bowel disease is not that frequently seen. The reason probably is related to the fact that the patient may suffer any number of hormonal imbalances as a result of acute and chronic illness; a woman's ability to become pregnant is probably severely impaired. But ulcerative colitis and Crohn's disease do not adversely affect fertility, nor do they necessarily impede the progress of the pregnancy or the delivery of a normal, term infant. Pregnancy in association with a preexisting colitis or complicated by the development of inflammatory bowel disease is attended by the same prospect of a full-term delivery of a normal child as is

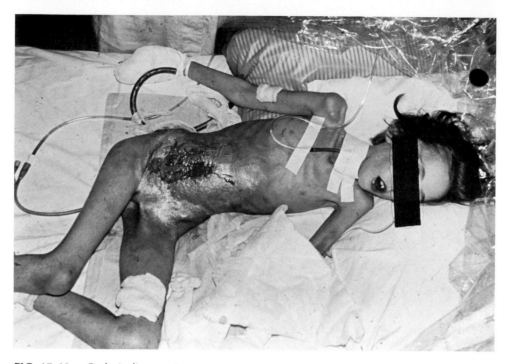

FIG. 15-63. Crohn's disease. Severe wasting in a 17-year-old girl, who looks much younger. Note the external abdominal wall fistula. (Corman ML, Veidenheimer MC, Nugent FW et al: Diseases of the Anus, Rectum and Colon. Part II: Non-specific inflammatory bowel disease. New York, Medcom, 1976)

pregnancy in the healthy woman.[285] Levy and associates reviewed 60 pregnancies in 31 ulcerative colitis patients in a retrospective fashion.[171] Twenty percent were improved, 18% deteriorated, and 62% demonstrated no change during the course of the pregnancy. Fourteen percent ended by spontaneous and two by artificial abortions. One premature birth was noted in 50 full-term deliveries. All of the births resulted in normal children. The authors concluded that pregnancy did not seem to aggravate the course of preexisting ulcerative colitis, nor did the colitis interfere with the outcome of the pregnancy.

Crohn and associates reported 74 pregnancies in 47 women whose colitis was inactive at the time of conception.[51] All subsequent therapeutic and spontaneous abortions (including one stillbirth) occurred in patients in whom the colitis became activated. There was no difference in the incidence of abortion in patients whose conception took place during an active phase of colitis when compared with those whose colitis was inactive at the time of conception. These observations have been confirmed by others.[61]

What happens to the colitis in patients who are pregnant? Zetzel reviewed a number of reported series

and found it helpful to group the pregnant patient into several categories.[285] Only 30% of patients in whom pregnancy developed in a quiescent phase of the colitis had an exacerbation of their disease, but 60% of patients developed an exacerbation when the pregnancy occurred during an active phase of the inflammatory bowel disease. In patients whose colitis developed initially during pregnancy or in the postpartum period, a particularly severe result was noted: over 60% had worsening of their symptoms.

In the management of a colitis patient who is contemplating pregnancy, there is no justification for suggesting that the patient avoid attempts at conception. As mentioned, patients who have a quiescent form of the disease are unlikely to experience problems with the subsequent pregnancy and delivery. Conversely, if the patient is experiencing an exacerbation of the colitis, the patient's own illness may preclude the possibility of becoming pregnant. If the disease is more than moderately active, Zetzel counsels a temporary waiting period and introduction of appropriate medical therapy to secure a remission.[285] However, even in this situation the chances of a normal pregnancy and delivery approximate 50%[285]; certainly, if the prospective parents wish to have a child, no benefit might be expected from a therapeutic abortion. Even in the severely ill pregnant woman there is no evidence to suggest that the pregnancy cannot be brought to a successful conclusion with a healthy baby.

If surgery becomes necessary during pregnancy, the method of treatment should be identical to that of a patient who is not pregnant. In other words, the drug management (steroids, Azulfidine) is not contraindicated. If surgery becomes necessary for fulminant disease, the operation should be performed as it is in the nonpregnant state. The exception to this would be the unusual situation in which the patient requires surgical intervention late in the course of the pregnancy. The enlarged uterus may preclude the possibility of performing a proctectomy, and a staged operation may be appropriate. It would not be advisable to perform an esoteric sphincter-saving operation in this type of patient.

A high fetal and maternal mortality has been reported if surgical intervention becomes necessary for fulminant colitis.[187, 214] Bohe and colleagues reported two cases of fulminant disease during pregnancy that required subtotal colectomy and ileostomy in one, and proctocolectomy in the other.[24] These operations were undertaken in the 32nd week and 33rd week of pregnancy, respectively. Pathologic report confirmed the diagnosis to be Crohn's disease. I have performed surgery in two patients during pregnancy: one, at 3 months, underwent a proctocolectomy, and the other, at 5 months, underwent a total abdominal colectomy and ileostomy; both patients proceeded to uneventful conclusions of their pregnancy and delivered normal, healthy infants. In my opinion it is not in the interest of the mother or of the fetus to delay surgery until the pregnancy can be terminated with a viable child. In other words, I do not advocate waiting until the 32nd week to perform a cesarean section while the mother is forced to postpone needed surgery.

If pregnancy develops following resection and ileostomy, the question arises of whether the prospective mother should undergo a cesarean section or deliver vaginally. This decision probably should be deferred to the obstetrician; my own feeling is that if the pregnant woman has an adequate pelvis for a normal vaginal delivery, this should be attempted. A cesarean section is not mandatory simply because the patient has an ileostomy. If an episiotomy is performed, there may be a delay in healing of the perineal wound, however.

PHYSICAL EXAMINATION

Physical examination is usually unrewarding in patients with ulcerative colitis unless the patient has ful-

minant disease. Abdominal tenderness is usually absent, as is abdominal distension. No masses are palpable. However, in the acutely ill person, abdominal distension associated with toxic megacolon may be noted. Diffuse tenderness may be apparent, and if perforation has ensued, all the usual signs and symptoms of an intra-abdominal catastrophe are noted.

On the other hand, Crohn's disease may demonstrate more obvious findings on physical examination. For example, mere inspection of the anal area will often demonstrate the characteristic edematous tags, fissures, or fistulas seen in this condition (see Fig. 15-1). Rectal examination will often reveal the anal canal to be stenotic, fibrotic, and thickened. If an anal fissure is apparent, severe pain is evident (Fig. 15-64). Pelvic examination in the woman may reveal a rectovaginal fistula, and bimanual examination the presence of a pelvic mass.

Abdominal findings are more common in patients with Crohn's disease than in those with ulcerative colitis. A mass may be associated with regional enteritis involving the small bowel when it is confined to the right iliac fossa. An enlarged mesenteric abscess can often be palpated. Crohn's colitis, however, usually does not demonstrate obvious abdominal physical findings. Extracolonic manifestations may be apparent, but these are seen in both conditions (see later).

ENDOSCOPIC EXAMINATION

Proctosigmoidoscopy, flexible fiberoptic sigmoidoscopy, and colonoscopy are important tools for evaluating the bowel and for confirming the presence or absence of inflammatory bowel disease. Proctosigmoidoscopic examination is particularly useful in differentiating Crohn's disease and ulcerative colitis; the rectum is always diseased during attacks of ulcerative colitis. The earliest apparent change is loss of vessel pattern due to edema of the bowel wall. The presence of contact bleeding, followed by granularity and ulceration, and more severe signs of inflammatory disease. In 40% of patients with Crohn's colitis, the rectum is spared, irrespective of anal or perianal involvement. However, when the rectum *is* involved by this condition, differentiation between the two diseases may be quite difficult.

In patient's with distal disease, that is, ulcerative proctitis or proctosigmoiditis, complete endoscopic examination by means of the colonoscope is unnecessary. The extent of disease can usually be determined with the rigid instrument or by the flexible fiberoptic sigmoidoscope. The presence of diffuse, confluent, symmetric disease from the dentate line cephalad to the limit of the inflammatory reaction is consistent with

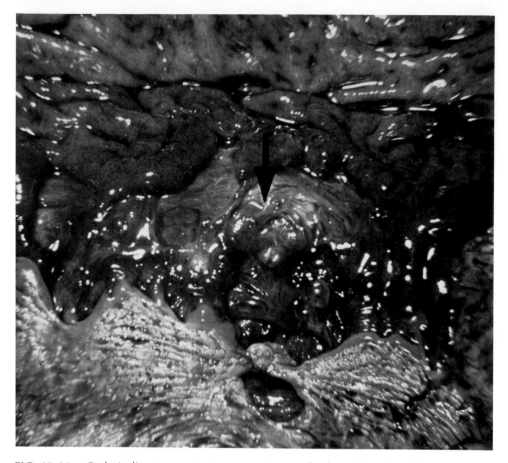

FIG. 15-64. Crohn's disease: proctectomy specimen with a broad-based anal fissure *(arrow)*. Just distal to the dentate line, an external opening of a fistula is evident. (Corman ML, Veidenheimer MC, Nugent FW et al: Diseases of the Anus, Rectum and Colon. Part II: Nonspecific inflammatory bowel disease. New York, Medcom, 1976)

ulcerative colitis or proctitis, depending on the extent of involvement. If the patient's symptoms are consistent with the endoscopic findings, appropriate treatment can be initiated without further contrast study or colonoscopy. Conversely, if the patient's disease extends beyond the limit of the endoscopic procedure performed, it is necessary to perform at some point total colonic evaluation. Colonoscopy should certainly supplement barium enema examination under these circumstances.

Generally, colonoscopy will identify inflammatory changes more proximal than what would be expected on the basis of the radiologic study. Furthermore, histologic examination of the biopsy specimen will often reveal more proximal disease that has been suspected by endoscopic examination.[72, 282] Das and associates reported 31 patients with idiopathic proctitis who were colonoscoped while they were asymptomatic.[54] Multiple biopsies were taken from throughout the colon and rectum. Although the obvious disease appeared limited to the distal 20 cm of the colon, microscopic abnormalities were seen commonly in more proximal locations. The authors postulated that the clinical course would be more consistent with distal disease if this indeed were confirmed by biopsy, whereas more proximal involvement usually implied that the patient would be refractory to conventional management (*e.g.*, topical steroids).

Ulcerative colitis and Crohn's disease are usually recognized by excluding other specific causes of inflammatory bowel disease such as amoebic colitis, ischemic colitis, pseudomembranous colitis, and so forth. The commonest differential diagnostic problem revolves around the numerous and varied infective colitides.

Other areas of concern in the differential include ischemic colitis, radiation changes, the so-called solitary ulcer syndrome, irritable bowel complaints (the diagnosis of exclusion), and, of course, the differentiation between the two nonspecific inflammatory bowel diseases, ulcerative colitis and Crohn's disease.[254] Biopsy may be helpful in one third of patients because histologic changes suggestive of Crohn's disease in particular may be apparent; up to 20% of such patients may exhibit granulomata (Fig. 15-65). In patients with ulcerative colitis, rectal biopsy is extremely important for recognizing dysplasia, especially in patients with long-standing disease (see Relationship to Carcinoma).

The place of colonoscopy in inflammatory bowel disease has been extensively reviewed by many authors. Teague and Waye recommend colonoscopy in inflammatory bowel disease for five indications: differential diagnosis, resolution of radiographic abnormalities (*e.g.*, filling defects and strictures), preoperative and postoperative evaluation in Crohn's disease, examination of stomas, and screening for premalignant and malignant changes.[254]

For the patient who has a history of inflammatory bowel disease, the preparation for colonoscopy includes a modified diet; clear liquids are suggested for 48 hours. Vigorous cleansing enemas, such as one would normally use in the evaluation of a noninflamed colon or in the performance of colonoscopy–polypectomy, are contraindicated. For the relatively active colitis patient, no laxative is suggested. If the colitis is minimal or relatively inactive, a reduced dose of a laxative is suggested (*e.g.*, magnesium citrate or one of the commercially available purgatives).

Waye describes a number of colonoscopic features in the differential diagnosis of inflammatory bowel disease.[269] He suggests that patients with ulcerative colitis have rectal involvement from the anal verge cephalad in continuity with whatever distal involvement is present. Erythema of the colonic wall is one of the early manifestations. More obvious changes include granularity, friability, bleeding, edema with interhaustral septal thickening and blunting, ulceration, mucosal bridging, the presence of pseudopolyps, and the superimposition of carcinoma (see Color Fig. 1-1).

With *granulomatous colitis* Waye describes the following major colonoscopic findings: a normal rectum (obviously this is not always the case), asymmetry or eccentricity of involvement, cobblestone appearance,

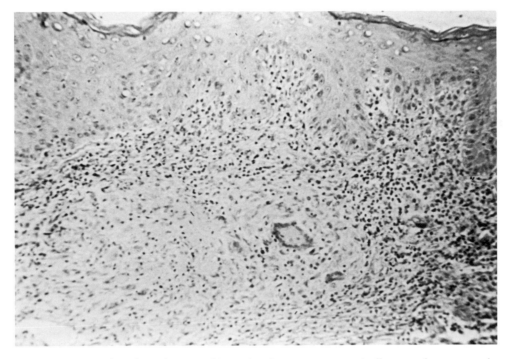

FIG. 15-65.   Anal Crohn's disease. This section from a macroscopically normal anus reveals submucosal granuloma. The patient subsequently proved to have Crohn's disease. (Original magnification × 80. Corman ML, Veidenheimer MC, Nugent FW et al: Diseases of the Anus, Rectum and Colon. Part II: Non-specific inflammatory bowel disease. New York, Medcom, 1976)

normal vasculature (since friability is not usually encountered except in advanced disease), edema of the bowel wall (as seen in ulcerative colitis), normal mucosa intervening between areas of ulceration, serpiginous ulcers (these may course for several centimeters), pseudopolyps (as in ulcerative colitis), and skip areas (lack of continuity of involvement).[269] He adds another observation, the presence of *amyloidosis* in the biopsy specimen.

There are, however, problems in the interpretation of the biopsies obtained by means of proctosigmoidoscopy or colonoscopy. In a prospective study, Geboes and Vantrappen performed over an 18 month period 71 colonoscopies on 59 patients with Crohn's disease.[90] In comparison with barium enema examination, the segmental nature of the involvement was more apparent with colonoscopy; microulceration was also more evident than by radiologic means. Radiographs yielded more information about the haustrae, especially in the right colon. Colonoscopy permitted a histologic diagnosis in 24% of patients, but granulomas were found in only 19 of 321 specimens. In over one quarter of the patients, the entire colon could not be examined, and no complications occurred. Hogan and colleagues observed that inconsistencies are often noted between macroscopic observations by the endoscopist and histologic interpretation of the biopsy specimen by the pathologist.[123] They felt that the reason for this problem is the overlapping of the histologic features of the two conditions. As discussed previously, the most useful lesion found on colonoscopic mucosal biopsy of patients with Crohn's disease is a granuloma. Changes in patients with ulcerative colitis are truly nonspecific, unless atypia or frank carcinoma supervenes.

Myren and co-workers performed routine and blind histologic evaluation by means of colonoscopy–biopsy in patients with and without inflammatory bowel disease.[199] In 110 patients, 278 biopsies were obtained at different levels of the colon. Clinical information including colonoscopic diagnosis was available to the pathologists at the initial routine examination. Later the sections were examined blindly and independently by two pathologists. Agreement between the pathologists was obtained in only two thirds of the patients. The authors concluded that a limiting factor in making reliable diagnoses is the small size of the tissue specimens available. Also, discrepancies may be due to the fact that biopsies are not always representative of the process in the colonic mucosa.

Myren and associates in another study performed colonoscopic evaluation in 40 patients and compared this with conventional barium enema.[198] Colonoscopic diagnosis and biopsy revealed complete agreement in 80% of the patients, whereas colonoscopic evaluation and radiologic survey revealed agreement in only 55% of patients. The only area where radiology seemed to have an advantage was the decreased haustration that seemed to be more apparent by x-ray techniques. Erosions, mucosal edema, vascular injection, and bleeding were not detected by barium enema. Others have confirmed the value of colonoscopy in evaluation of patients with nonspecific inflammatory bowel disease.[87, 252, 270, 276] However, it should be remembered that the procedure is contraindicated in patients with acute exacerbation of the colitis and certainly in patients who have toxic megacolon.

Farmer and co-workers reviewed 100 patients who underwent colonoscopy for *distal ulcerative colitis.*[75] They classified their patients in two groups: those whose disease was confined to the distal 25 cm, and those whose mucosal changes extended above that level, but not beyond the splenic flexure. Because flexible fiberoptic sigmoidoscopy or colonoscopy is not as accurate in defining disease in the rectum, whether it is inflammatory or neoplastic, there was a 5% disagreement about the presence of inflammation in that area of the bowel. Certainly, the rigid instrument is far more useful in evaluating the rectum than the flexible fiberoptic colonoscope. Biopsies were taken at multiple levels, and the retrospective review was performed over several years. It was determined that patients in whom the disease was limited to the rectum and sigmoid colon had a good prognosis for progression of the disease—only 10%. However, 25% of patients experienced recurrence. Prognosis was similar whether the disease was confined to the distal 25-cm level or was distal to the splenic flexure.

RADIOLOGIC INVESTIGATION

Although the standard barium enema examination has been routinely employed as the procedure of choice for evaluating inflammatory bowel disease, recent evidence suggests that the air-contrast technique is preferred. Radiologists have prided themselves in their ability to identify sometimes unusual radiographic features of inflammatory bowel disease; these include mucosal bridging and aphthoid ulcers.[21, 114, 231, 237] Although these findings are helpful in the evaluation of patients with inflammatory bowel disease, their ready documentation by means of colonoscopy would diminish the value of the radiologic observation.

Upper gastrointestinal and small bowel x-ray films are extremely useful for evaluating inflammatory bowel disease in this area of the alimentary tract. There is no adequate endoscopic examination of the small intestine, except possibly for the very distal ileum. Evaluation of the terminal ileum is best obtained by reflux on barium enema examination, but unfortunately as many as 20% of patients will not demonstrate this phenomenon. Alternatively, a small bowel follow-through study with good spot films is the preferred approach. The x-ray appearances of IBD are presented earlier in this chapter.

Ultrasound examination is of quite limited value in patients with inflammatory bowel disease because of the presence of considerable artifact associated with the loops of bowel. The presence of air or fluid in the intestine and adhesed loops of bowel may simulate a septic focus.

Sonnenberg and colleagues performed a prospective clinical trial comparing 51 patients with Crohn's disease with 124 controlled subjects by means of Grey scale ultrasound.[241] Diagnosis by ultrasound reflected primarily the thickening of the gastrointestinal wall itself, perceived with a characteristic "target" appearance. The study demonstrated that there were very few false-negative appearances. The occasional false-positive phenomenon was usually attributed to the presence of a gastrointestinal tumor.

Computed tomography (CT) has been able to demonstrate thickening of the colon, nodularity, adenopathy, and intra-abdominal abscess. Presence of a fistula, especially an enterocutaneous communication, has also been demonstrable by means of CT scan. In most cases, however, adequate evaluation of the intra-abdominal pathology can be obtained by means of endoscopic examination and standard contrast techniques.

EXTRACOLONIC MANIFESTATIONS

Increasing evidence supports the statement that inflammatory disease of the colon is a systemic problem rather than one localized to this organ. As previously discussed, many etiologic concepts have been considered, but regardless of the sequence of pathologic changes in the colon, there is little question about the presence of related events, at times profound, in distant areas of the body. The joints, skin, liver, kidneys, eyes, mouth, blood, nervous system, and, of course, other areas of the alimentary tract may be sites of lesions that, at least in the extraintestinal manifestations, seem dependent upon the presence of diseased bowel.

Esophageal Involvement

Patients with Crohn's disease of the esophagus will present with symptoms not unlike those associated with other lesions of that organ, such as carcinoma. Substernal discomfort, dysphagia, epigastric pain, weight loss, nausea, and vomiting are all part of the clinical spectrum. Other gastrointestinal manifestations are usually due to the presence of disease elsewhere in the alimentary tract.[70, 92, 120]

Physical examination is usually unrewarding except with manifestations outside of the upper gastrointestinal tract. Diagnosis is usually made by a high index of suspicion and radiologic investigation, which obviously would include an upper gastrointestinal series, a study that may reveal thickened mucosal folds, multiple ulcerations, or most commonly a stricture. This last radiologic finding makes differentiation from carcinoma quite difficult, except that the presence of disease elsewhere or the relatively young age of the patient would lead one to suspect an inflammatory process.

Endoscopic examination will usually reveal either an ulcerated mucosa or the presence of an inflammatory stricture. Biopsies usually show an inflammatory reaction, but the absence of granulomata does not exclude the diagnosis of Crohn's disease.[70]

Treatment usually consists of the standard medical management appropriate for Crohn's disease of the small or large bowel (see later). Resection is rarely indicated.

Gastroduodenal Crohn's Disease

Crohn's disease involving the stomach and duodenum may not be as rare as originally suspected. In 1981 Korelitz and co-workers performed random endoscopic biopsies of the stomach and duodenal mucosa in patients with Crohn's disease, frequently demonstrating the presence of microscopic alterations consistent with this inflammatory process in the upper gastrointestinal tract.[161] Clinically evident inflammatory bowel disease of the gastroduodenal area is believed to occur in approximately 2% or 3% of all patients with Crohn's disease. The condition can occur without evident involvement elsewhere in the gastrointestinal tract, but it is usually seen with disease elsewhere.

Patients usually present with epigastric abdominal symptoms exacerbated by eating, nausea, vomiting, and weight loss. Symptoms may not be dissimilar to those of ulcer disease. Obstruction, perforation, fistula, and hemorrhage can occur. Duodenocolic fistulas are a complication, but in evaluation of patients with this condition it is important to ascertain whether the fistula arose from inflammatory bowel disease in the intestinal tract outside of the duodenum (see Fig. 15-61).

Radiologic investigation may reveal the findings summarized by Cohen.[40] These include antral inflammation, contiguous disease in the duodenum, cobblestone mucosal appearance with thickened folds, reduced distensibility or stricture, and ulceration (Fig. 15-66). Barium enema examination is the preferred study to identify a fistula between the upper gastrointestinal tract and the colon. Endoscopic examination may reveal ulceration, cobblestoning, or stricture. As with

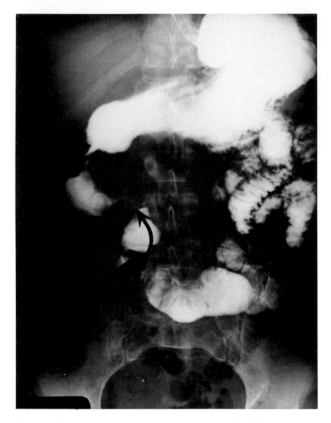

FIG. 15-66. Duodenal Crohn's disease. This film from an upper GI series demonstrates stricture of the second portion of the duodenum with a fistula from the third portion to the small bowel (arrow).

esophageal disease, the absence of granulomata does not necessarily mean that the patient does not have nonspecific IBD.

Treatment usually consists of antacids (ulcer regimen), steroids, Azulfidine, hyperalimentation, and possibly surgery. The primary indications for surgical intervention are the presence of a fistula and obstruction. In the latter situation, Nugent and co-workers reported 18 patients who were relieved of obstruction by means of gastrojejunostomy.[205] This is the treatment of choice for patients with duodenal disease. If hemorrhage is a complication, either resectional surgery or oversewing the bleeding point is the treatment of choice if the bleeding cannot be controlled by medical means. Usually, however, surgery for primary gastroduodenal Crohn's disease is not necessary. A number of cases and reviews have been published on the evaluation and management of Crohn's disease in this area.[42, 53, 74, 81, 227, 280] Ross and associates reviewed the long-term results of surgery for duodenal Crohn's disease that

had been initially reported by Farmer and co-workers.[74, 223] Of the 11 patients, 7 required a total of 10 further operations; the mean follow-up was approximately 14 years. Indications for subsequent surgery included marginal ulceration, recurrence producing obstruction at the enteroenterostomy, and duodenal fistula. Eight of the 11 patients also required surgery for Crohn's disease elsewhere in the intestinal tract. The authors concluded that bypass surgery alone was not satisfactory in the long term and suggested that vagotomy be added at the time of operation; functional results are felt to be better, particularly if reoperative surgery is done in an expeditious and timely manner.

Oral Manifestations

Basu and Asquith reviewed the oral manifestations of inflammatory bowel disease, describing a number of lesions.[14] These included recurrent aphthous ulcers, pyoderma gangrenosum, pyostomatitis vegetans, hemorrhagic ulceration, glossitis, macroglossia, and moniliasis. The authors reported that the incidence is not as uncommon as one might expect: up to 20% of patients have been described as having oral lesions.

Aphthous ulcers usually parallel the course or activity of the inflammatory bowel disease: the more active the disease, the more likely one is to develop this manifestation. Biopsy usually shows a chronic inflammatory reaction.

Pyostomatitis vegetans is an unusual manifestation of inflammatory bowel disease. Papillary projections of mucous membrane can be seen separated by small areas of ulceration (Fig. 15-67). Biopsy may reveal suprabasal separation of the oral epithelium and infiltration with eosinophils.

Rarely, the oral manifestations become evident before the intestinal disease is diagnosed. Scully and co-workers reported 19 patients with clinical evidence of oral Crohn's disease but no intestinal symptoms.[234] Over one third were demonstrated on either rectal biopsy or by contrast gastrointestinal x-ray films to have inflammatory bowel disease, even in the absence of symptoms.

Since the lesions are resistant to local therapy, general measures for soothing the oral discomfort are advised. Oral manifestations are ameliorated with appropriate treatment of the intestinal disease.

Cutaneous Manifestations

Pyoderma gangrenosum is a condition found exclusively in patients with inflammatory bowel disease but is fortunately uncommon, occurring in no more than 2% of

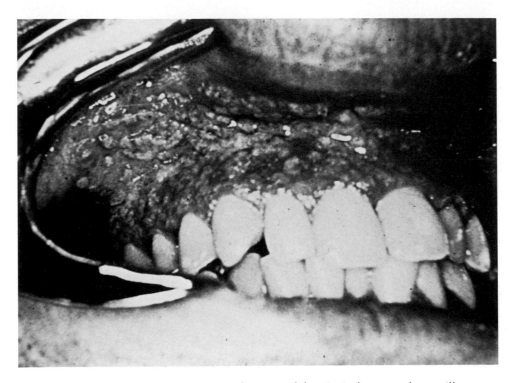

FIG. 15-67. Pyostomatitis vegetans: involvement of the gingival mucosa by papillary projections. (Corman ML, Veidenheimer MC, Nugent FW et al: Diseases of the Anus, Rectum and Colon. Part II: Non-specific inflammatory bowel disease. New York, Medcom, 1976)

patients. Schoetz and associates identified 8 patients out of 961 with Crohn's disease who had this condition (an incidence of 0.8%).[232] Clinically, the lesion appears as a spreading, undermining ulceration that has a characteristic violaceous border (Figs. 15-68 and 15-69).[14] The lesions are usually found on the extremities, the most common location being the anterior tibial area. However, the ulcers can occur on the trunk, buttocks, and other areas. Usually there are only one or two lesions, but these can be of considerable size.

Biopsy of the lesion shows no definite characteristics that would identify the ulcer as being specific for a complication associated with inflammatory bowel disease. A vasculitis has been suggested as a possible etiology.

Treatment consists of administration of systemic steroids and occasionally intralesional steroids, and, of course the management of the colitis. Topical measures also should include appropriate antibiotics if culture suggests the value of such treatment, or in the presence of lymphangitis or cellulitis. As with so many other extracolonic manifestations, the course of the pyoderma parallels the clinical course of the intestinal disease.

Rarely does the skin condition assume such significance that colectomy must be performed. I have experienced a situation in which a total colectomy with preservation of the rectum resulted in 90% healing, and the residual pyoderma failed to clear until proctectomy was subsequently performed (Fig. 15-70).

Polyarteritis nodosa is a rare cutaneous manifestation of Crohn's disease. Kahn and co-workers reviewed 11 cases in the literature and added one of their own.[138] The presence of erythematous, tender nodules in the extremities should lead one to suspect the diagnosis. Biopsy or excision may reveal an arteritis with lumenal narrowing by fibrinous thrombus.

The relationship of the cutaneous manifestation to systemic polyarteritis nodosa is controversial, but in the case reported by the authors, when subsequent resection of the bowel was carried out, there was no evidence of such an arteritis. The condition should be distinguished from other cutaneous manifestations, such as erythema nodosum.

Erythema nodosum is another cutaneous manifestation that is not uncommonly seen in association with inflammatory bowel disease. Generally, approximately 5% are afflicted.[134] The condition, however, is not ex-

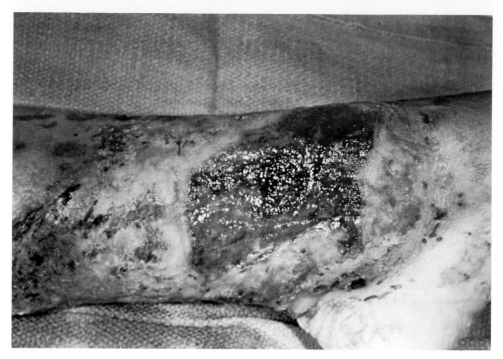

FIG. 15-68. Pyoderma gangrenosum: irregularly outlined, sharply defined ulceration with edematous edges and pyodermatous base in a patient with ulcerative colitis. (Courtesy of Rudolf Garret, M.D.)

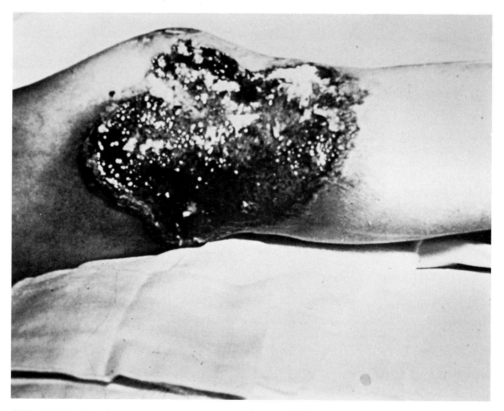

FIG. 15-69. Pyoderma gangrenosum: an undermined ulcer with a violaceous border. (Corman ML, Veidenheimer MC, Nugent FW et al: Diseases of the Anus, Rectum and Colon. Part II: Non-specific inflammatory bowel disease. New York, Medcom, 1976)

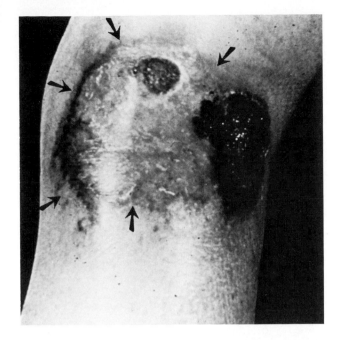

FIG. 15-70. Pyoderma gangrenosum. In this photograph taken 1 month following proctocolectomy, a much smaller ulcer is evident. Compare this with the original lesion outlined by arrows. (Corman ML, Veidenheimer MC, Nugent FW et al: Diseases of the Anus, Rectum and Colon. Part II: Non-specific inflammatory bowel disease. New York, Medcom, 1976)

clusively seen with ulcerative colitis and Crohn's disease but occurs in many other systemic diseases. Tender, subcutaneous nodules are usually seen on the pretibial aspects of the legs. As with other extracolonic manifestations, the clinical course usually parallels that of the intestinal disease.

Arthritis

Colitic arthritis is the commonest joint manifestation of inflammatory bowel disease, occurring in approximately 8% of patients. The large joints are involved primarily; they may be swollen, warm, and red (Fig. 15-71). Although any joint may be involved, small joints are less frequently affected (Fig. 15-72). The appearance may not be dissimilar to that of rheumatoid arthritis, but rheumatoid factor is absent from the blood.

Symptoms of the arthritis usually develop after the inflammatory bowel disease and are usually easily controlled by means of anti-inflammatory agents or by the use of steroids. The arthritis completely resolves after colectomy.

Other joint disorders that may be encountered are severe arthralgias and rheumatoid spondylitis.[1,131,186,287]

The incidence of *rheumatoid spondylitis* is considerably higher in patients with inflammatory bowel disease

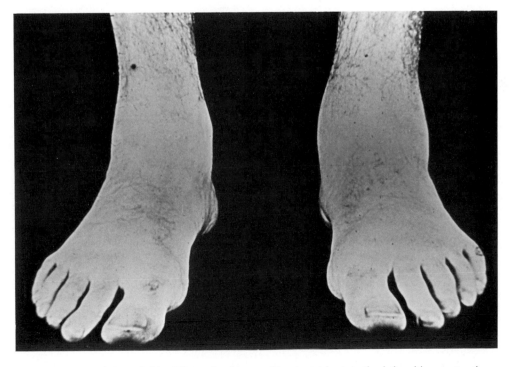

FIG. 15-71. Colitic arthritis. Bilateral ankle swelling is evident, in the left ankle greater than in the right, in a patient with ulcerative colitis. (Corman ML, Veidenheimer MC, Nugent FW et al: Diseases of the Anus, Rectum and Colon. Part II: Non-specific inflammatory bowel disease. New York, Medcom, 1967)

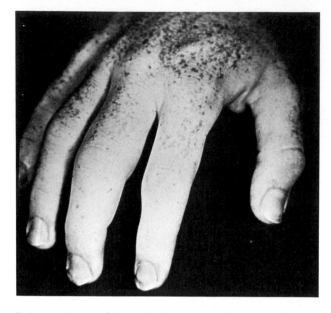

FIG. 15-72. Colitic arthritis: proximal interphalangeal joint involvement in a 20-year-old man with acute ulcerative colitis. (Corman ML, Veidenheimer MC, Nugent FW et al: Diseases of the Anus, Rectum and Colon. Part II: Non-specific inflammatory bowel disease. New York, Medcom, 1976)

than in the general population; estimates range in excess of 20 times. The well-known sex incidence (the ratio of men to women is 4 to 1) is reversed when rheumatoid spondylitis complicates inflammatory bowel disease. A genetic association between the two diseases has been demonstrated. In contradistinction to most other extracolonic manifestations, spondylitis does not parallel the activity of the bowel disease.

The patient initially develops pain in the lumbosacral region, but the discomfort may rapidly progress to involve the thoracic and cervical spine. As ankylosis develops the patient exhibits the characteristic dorsal kyphosis (Fig. 15-73).

Treatment consists of physiotherapy, anti-inflammatory agents, and steroids. As suggested, colectomy is not indicated simply for the treatment of the arthritic manifestations.

Ocular Manifestations

Ocular disease, including orbital congestion, uveitis, iritis, and keratitis are seen in approximately 5% of patients with inflammatory bowel disease. The most

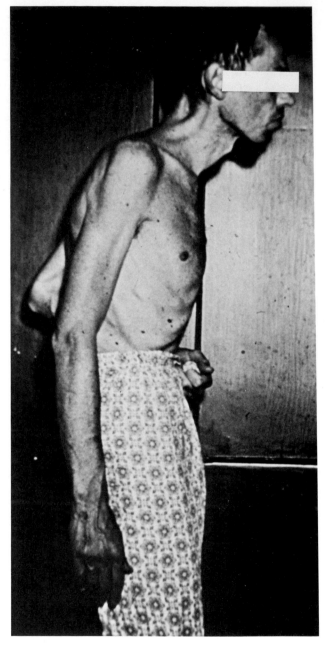

FIG. 15-73. Rheumatoid spondylitis. Note the kyphosis in this patient with chronic ulcerative colitis. (Corman ML, Veidenheimer MC, Nugent FW et al: Diseases of the Anus, Rectum and Colon. Part II: Non-specific inflammatory bowel disease. New York, Medcom, 1976)

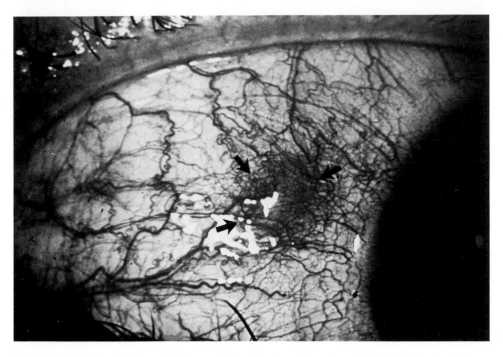

FIG. 15-74. Episcleritis: note the nodular, focal, erythematous lesion *(arrows)*. (Corman ML, Veidenheimer MC, Nugent FW et al: Diseases of the Anus, Rectum and Colon. Part II: Non-specific inflammatory bowel disease. New York, Medcom, 1976)

common ocular lesion is episcleritis, an inflammation overlying the sclera, under the conjunctiva. A thickened, deep red appearance is usually noted in one segment of the eye (Fig. 15-74). Burning, itching, and pain are the primary symptoms, but the patient often seeks medical attention because of the appearance. Steroids and anti-inflammatory agents are the treatments of choice. Because of the complications that may lead to a chorioretinitis, ophthalmologic consultation is advised.

Hepatobiliary Disease

Liver function studies and liver biopsy often show abnormal results in both ulcerative colitis and Crohn's disease patients. Cohen and associates performed a prospective study of liver function in 50 consecutive patients with regional enteritis.[39] Thirty percent had abnormal results of liver function tests, most commonly an elevation of the serum alkaline phosphatase, but none had significant liver disease. Fifteen patients of the 19 who underwent liver biopsy had evidence of chronic pericholangitis. The most significant finding

was the high incidence of gallstone disease (34%). Others reported an even higher associated incidence of liver abnormalities.[60, 67] *Fatty degeneration* is probably the most frequently encountered microscopic abnormality (Fig. 15-75); this may be due to the relatively poor nutritional state of many colitic patients. Occasionally a granuloma may be seen (see Fig. 15-33).

Another histologic manifestation of liver disease is *pericholangitis* (Fig. 15-76). The condition may present with jaundice, abdominal pain, fever, and pruritus. Many patients, however, are asymptomatic. Bacterial infection and an autoimmune process have been implicated as possible causative factors. Other hepatic abnormalities include chronic active hepatitis and, rarely, cirrhosis.

One of the most serious, albeit rare, consequences of inflammatory bowel disease that occurs as a complication of both ulcerative colitis and Crohn's disease is *primary sclerosing cholangitis*. In order to establish this diagnosis there must be no prior history of biliary surgery, no gallstones, and diffuse involvement of the extrahepatic biliary ducts.[267]

Symptoms include right upper quadrant abdominal pain, vomiting, jaundice, and pruritus. Laboratory studies reveal the usual changes suggestive of an ob-

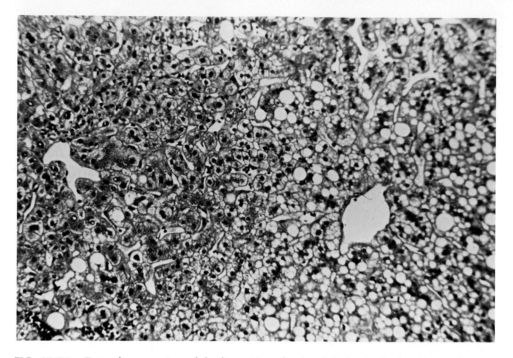

FIG. 15-75. Fatty degeneration of the liver. Note the fat globules in the liver parenchyma. (Original magnification × 260. Corman ML, Veidenheimer MC, Nugent FW et al: Diseases of the Anus, Rectum and Colon. Part II: Non-specific inflammatory bowel disease. New York, Medcom, 1967)

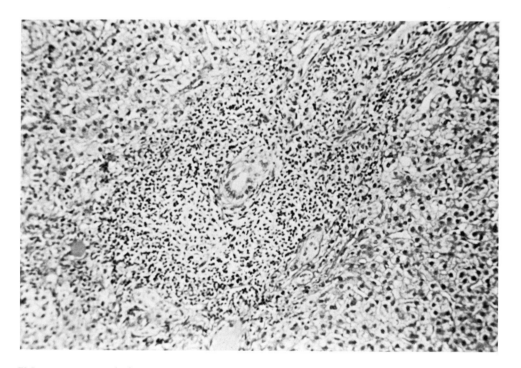

FIG. 15-76. Pericholangitis. An inflammatory infiltrate within the portal areas surrounds the bile ducts and may result in cirrhosis through a process of progressive fibrosis. (Original magnification × 260. Corman ML, Veidenheimer MC, Nugent FW et al: Diseases of the Anus, Rectum and Colon. Part II: Non-specific inflammatory bowel disease. New York, Medcom, 1967)

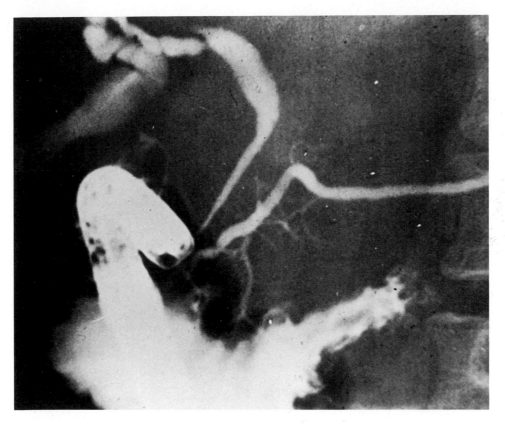

FIG. 15-77.   Sclerosing cholangitis. ERCP demonstrates narrowing of the distal common bile duct with complete obstruction at the level of the common hepatic duct. (Corman ML, Veidenheimer MC, Nugent FW et al: Diseases of the Anus, Rectum and Colon. Part II: Nonspecific inflammatory bowel disease. New York, Medcom, 1976)

structive jaundice. Cholangiogram reveals the strictured bile duct (Fig. 15-77).

When the sclerosing cholangitis has been established, removal of the inflammatory bowel disease does not reverse the condition. Because of the profoundly serious consequences of progressive cholangitis, a case may be made for "prophylactic" removal of the inflammatory bowel process if early changes in the biliary tract are observed, even when the gastrointestinal manifestations are felt to be quite minimal.

Bile Duct Carcinoma

Carcinoma of the bile duct arising in a patient with ulcerative colitis is a rare complication. The association was originally described by Parker and Kendall in 1954.[211] In 1974, Ritchie and colleagues identified 67 cases.[219] The condition is more common in men and is usually seen in patients who have had a prolonged history of colitis. Patients give a history of typical biliary obstruction with painless jaundice, weight loss, and pruritic symptoms. Diagnosis is usually confirmed by intravenous cholangiogram, ultrasound demonstration of dilated intrahepatic ducts, and endoscopic retrograde cholangiography. Prognosis is poor, with biliary diversion the usual surgical approach.[278]

Urologic Complications

Urologic complications are not uncommonly seen in association with inflammatory bowel disease. These include chronic interstitial nephritis, chronic pyelonephritis, acute tubular necrosis, urinary fistulas, ureteral obstruction, and nephrolithiasis.

Ureteral obstruction is much more frequently seen in association with Crohn's disease than with ulcerative

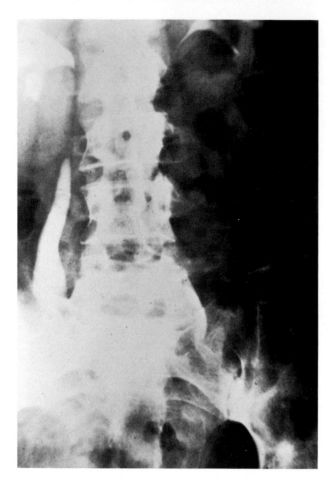

FIG. 15-78. Ureteral obstruction in a patient with distal ileitis and pelvic abscess. Note the dilated right collecting system and the right ureter. (Corman ML, Veidenheimer MC, Nugent FW et al: Diseases of the Anus, Rectum and Colon. Part II: Non-specific inflammatory bowel disease. New York, Medcom, 1976)

colitis (Fig. 15-78). The incidence has been reported to be as high as 50% in this group of patients. The inflammatory mass involving the terminal ileum and occasionally the sigmoid colon produces extrinsic compression of the distal ureters. The right is more frequently involved than the left. The result is hydroureter, hydronephrosis, and possible caliectasis. Symptoms related to the urinary tract may be minimal, and if present may actually be due to compression of the bladder by an inflammatory mass rather than from the obstruction of a ureter. Flank pain is suggestive of ureteral obstruction.

Treatment involves removal of the inflammatory mass that is causing the compression. Complete resolution may be expected, assuming that the obstruction has not produced irreversible renal damage. Preoperative identification of ureteral dilatation should warn the surgeon that a meticulous dissection may be required in order to avoid ureteral injury.

Nephrolithiasis and bladder calculi are seen in at least 5% of patients with inflammatory bowel disease. Following proctocolectomy and ileostomy, patients are still at a risk for the development of nephrolithiasis. Many factors contribute to the development of calculi in chronic inflammatory bowel disease: decreased urine volume, increased crystalloid concentration, urinary electrolyte and pH changes, and recurrent urinary tract infections. The more acid urine favors precipitation of urates, and, as a result, uric acid calculi are more common in patients with inflammatory bowel disease than in the "normal" population of stone formers. Intestinal absorption of oxylate is increased when ileal disease is present, and this is a further reason for formation of stones. Figure 15-79 demonstrates numerous bladder calculi that developed in a 60-year-old man who had extensive Crohn's disease of the small intestine for more than 20 years.

Bambach and associates reported that 10% of patients who underwent resection for inflammatory bowel disease gave a history of urinary stone formation after surgery.[13] Ileostomy patients were demonstrated to have a significantly lowered urinary pH and volume, and a higher concentration of calcium, oxylate, and uric acid. The authors advised close follow-up of patients with ileostomies, and with small bowel resections in particular, in order to assess fecal losses and urinary composition. Ideally, patients who are at increased risk for the formation of urinary stones could then be identified.

An adequate urinary volume should be maintained by encouraging the patient to consume sufficient water to increase urinary volume without increasing ileostomy output, alkalinization in selected patients, a diet low in oxylate and fat, and "slowing" medications to reduce the ileostomy volume.[13]

RELATIONSHIP TO CARCINOMA

Ulcerative Colitis

Carcinoma of the colon arising in a patient with ulcerative colitis was initially reported by Crohn and Rosenberg in 1925.[243] Since that time numerous cases have been reported, so that today there is a well-recognized association between chronic ulcerative colitis and the subsequent development of malignancy.

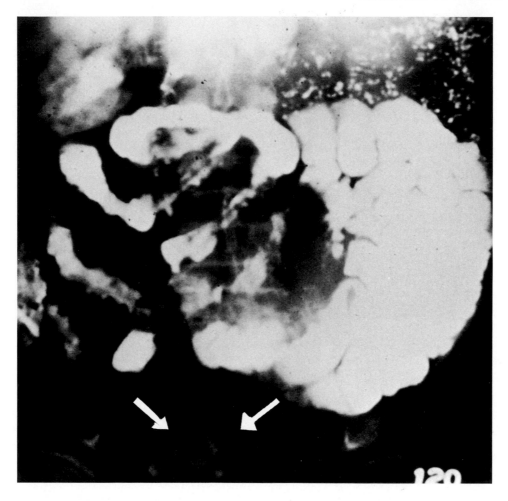

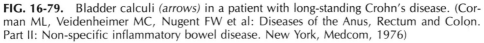

FIG. 16-79. Bladder calculi *(arrows)* in a patient with long-standing Crohn's disease. (Corman ML, Veidenheimer MC, Nugent FW et al: Diseases of the Anus, Rectum and Colon. Part II: Non-specific inflammatory bowel disease. New York, Medcom, 1976)

It appears that there are a number of factors that predispose a colitic patient to cancer. These include total colonic or pancolonic disease as opposed to distal or left-sided disease; prolonged duration of the illness (the earliest reported case was in a patient with the disease of 7 years' duration); age of onset of the disease (this is not really different from duration); continuous active disease as opposed to intermittent symptoms; and possibly the severity of the disease. The cumulative risk of cancer increases with the duration of the colitis, reaching 25% to 30% at 25 years' duration, 35% at 30 years, 45% at 35 years, and 65% at 40 years.[209] The overall incidence of carcinoma in patients with ulcerative colitis has been variously reported to be between 2% and 5%. Johnson and co-workers reported the

long-term findings in over 1400 patients with ulcerative colitis and noted that colorectal cancer developed in 63 (4.4%).[136] No statistically significant difference occurred in the probability of carcinoma of the colon and rectum developing following *proctitis* as compared with total colitis. Yet patients with left-sided disease seemed to fare considerably better with respect to the risk for the development of colorectal cancer. Greenstein reported that neoplasms developed in 11.2% of 267 patients with ulcerative colitis.[104] Thirteen percent of patients with universal colitis developed colorectal cancers and 5% of the patients with left-sided colitis developed malignant change. Patients with left-sided disease tended to develop cancer at least a decade later than patients with universal colitis. The median dura-

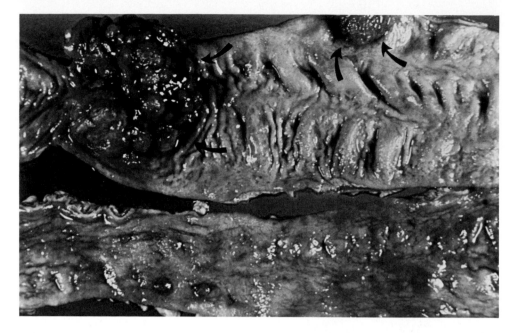

FIG. 15-80. Carcinomas in ulcerative colitis *(arrows)*. (Corman ML, Veidenheimer MC, Nugent FW et al: Diseases of the Anus, Rectum and Colon. Part II: Non-specific inflammatory bowel disease. New York, Medcom, 1976)

tion from onset of colitis to diagnosis of cancer was 20 years for those with universal colitis and 32 years for those with left-sided colitis.[104] No patient developed cancer with left-sided colitis before the 23rd year of disease.

In patients who undergo resective surgery for ulcerative colitis, the incidence of associated cancer is considerably higher. Van Heerden and Beart reported the Mayo Clinic experience with 726 patients who underwent surgical exploration for chronic ulcerative colitis between the years 1961 through 1975.[264] Seventy patients (9.6%) were found to have a carcinoma of the colon. These patients represented 1.4% of all patients who were diagnosed as having chronic ulcerative colitis during the period of study. Öhman reported the incidence to be 2.7% in the total series.[209]

Generally, the incidence of carcinoma is the same in both sexes, a not surprising statement in light of the fact that ulcerative colitis affects both sexes in approximately an equal ratio. Welch and Hedberg reported a bimodal distribution of the incidence—one peak was in the fourth decade and the other in the seventh decade.[272]

The distribution of tumors in patients with ulcerative colitis and carcinoma was reported by Öhman to demonstrate multicentricity much more commonly than in patients with colorectal cancer without IBD.[209] He also noted that 28% of patients had lesions of the transverse colon. Only 28% of lesions involved the rectum and rectosigmoid. The sigmoid colon comprised 17% of the series. Conversely, Riddell and colleagues reported that the rectum was the most common site of involvement, and that this was more noticeable in men than in women.[217] Over 40% of the cancers were found in the rectum in their study. Approximately 25% of patients had multiple tumors. It is certainly clear that multicentricity of the cancers is a frequently reported phenomenon (Fig. 15-80).

Another characteristic of colorectal cancer with ulcerative colitis is that very often the cancer tends to be infiltrative and scirrhous. Visible tumor involving the mucosa may not be observed even by careful endoscopic examination (Fig. 15-81). Although this is the most common clinical presentation of cancer in ulcerative colitis, it can also appear as a typical ulcerating or polypoid carcinoma (Fig. 15-82).

A fourth pathologic feature of carcinoma arising in ulcerative colitis is the tendency of the lesion to be highly aggressive and poorly differentiated. Over half of young ulcerative colitis patients with colorectal cancers have colloid carcinomas with histologically appearing mucous-secreting tumors of the signet-ring cell

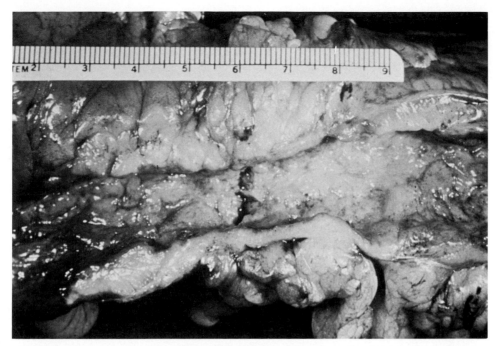

FIG. 15-81. Carcinoma of the sigmoid in ulcerative colitis. Note the characteristic infiltration of the bowel wall in an appearance that resembles the linitis plastica type of carcinoma seen in the stomach. (Corman ML, Veidenheimer MC, Nugent FW et al: Diseases of the Anus, Rectum and Colon. Part II: Non-specific inflammatory bowel disease. New York, Medcom, 1976)

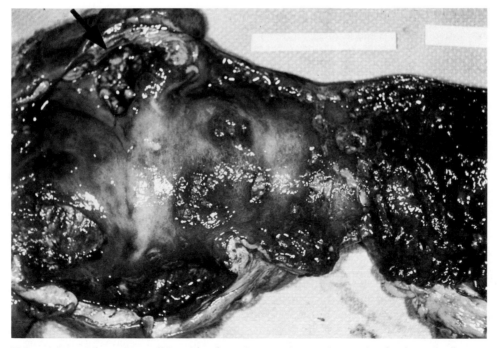

FIG. 15-82. Ulcerative colitis with ulcerating carcinoma *(arrow)* in the hepatic flexure. (Corman ML, Veidenheimer MC, Nugent FW et al: Diseases of the Anus, Rectum and Colon. Part II: Non-specific inflammatory bowel disease. New York, Medcom. 1976)

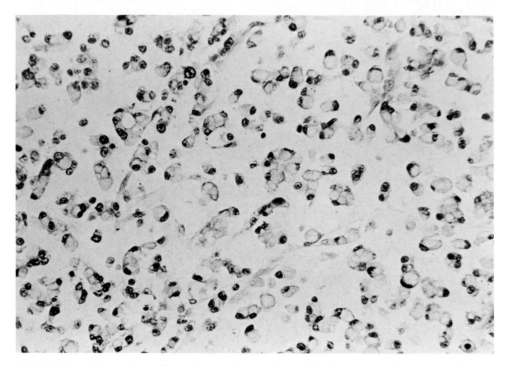

FIG. 15-83.   Signet-ring cell carcinoma in a patient with ulcerative colitis. (Original magnification × 600)

type (Fig. 15-83; see also Fig. 10-14).[243] The fact that the patient may be relatively asymptomatic or even completely without symptoms tends to lull the patient and the physician into a false sense of security. Witness the situation illustrated in Figure 15-7, in which the mucosa has been completely denuded. When there is no mucosa present, bleeding does not occur and mucous discharge is no longer apparent. This may cause the physician and the patient to believe that the medical measures that have been implemented are effectively controlling the disease. It is in just this kind of situation, a patient with long-standing ulcerative colitis, that a carcinoma can supervene. As suggested, physical examination, endoscopic examination, and even barium enema study may fail to identify the lesion. But when stricture occurs, the patient must be presumed to have a carcinoma until proved otherwise (Figs. 15-84 and 15-85). The presence of a stricture in a patient with ulcerative colitis is, in my opinion, an indication for surgery.

Ritchie and co-workers reviewed the St. Mark's Hospital experience of carcinoma complicating ulcerative colitis between the years 1947 and 1980; 67 patients with carcinoma were identified.[220] In comparison with those who underwent surgery for carcinoma of the colon and rectum in the same time period, it was felt that there was a higher proportion of inoperable and high-grade tumors in the colitic group, but the prognosis was found to be very similar in patients with and without colitis for the same stage of lesion. In the Mayo Clinic series, 40% of patients with carcinoma in chronic ulcerative colitis had a Dukes' A or B growth as compared with 63% in patients with carcinoma alone.[264] Conversely, 60% of the patients with carcinoma and ulcerative colitis were Dukes' C and D patients, as compared with 37% of patients with carcinoma alone. The mean age of their patients at the onset of the colitis was 26 years, with a duration of 17 years before the onset of malignancy. Twenty-three percent of these patients exhibited multicentric tumors. Those patients whose carcinoma was identified incidentally during prophylactic colectomy had a 72% 5-year survival, whereas those with clinical or radiographic evidence suggestive of cancer had a much poorer survival rate (35%).

The advanced nature of the cancerous change is attested to by the report of Johnson and co-workers.[136] Only 57% of their patients underwent curative resection. The overall survival rate for those operated on for cure was 61%. In Öhman's experience, two thirds of

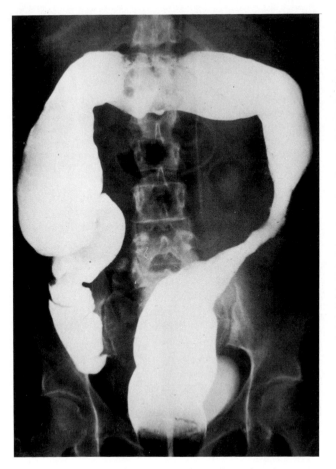

FIG. 15-84. Stricture in ulcerative colitis: foreshortening of the lower descending and sigmoid colon with stricture. Laparotomy revealed extensive carcinoma, hepatic metastases, and two additional unsuspected primary cancers in the resected specimen.(Corman ML, Veidenheimer MC, Nugent FW et al: Diseases of the Anus, Rectum and Colon. Part II: Non-specific inflammatory bowel disease. New York, Medcom, 1976)

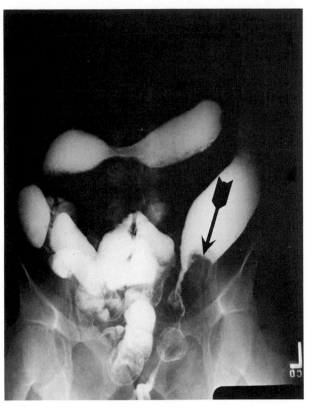

FIG. 15-85. Carcinoma in ulcerative colitis. Note the loss of haustrations, marked shortening, and sigmoid stricture. The tumor extends cephalad from the stricture to appear as a polypoid filling defect (arrow).

the patients operated upon for cure survived 5 years, as compared with a 69% rate in noncolitic patients.[209] All patients with Dukes' A lesions survived 5 years. Lavery and associates reviewed the Cleveland Clinic experience of 79 patients from 1950 through 1979 found to have carcinoma arising in ulcerative colitis.[168] In comparing their survival statistics with noncolitic cancer patients, they, too, noted no statistically significant difference in survival rates for the same stage of invasion. The poorer results were due to the fact that a higher percentage of patients presented with more advanced or incurable disease at the time of surgery.

Dysplasia

In 1967 Morson and Pang described a phenomenon which they called *dysplasia,* a frequent and widespread histologic change that extended to the rectum in patients with carcinoma complicating ulcerative colitis.[194] They suggested that biopsy of the rectum could detect this premalignant situation and possibly dictate the requirement for surgical intervention.

This is a singular advance in the management of patients with long-standing chronic ulcerative colitis. Prior to the concept of dysplasia, in order to protect the patient from the development of malignancy, particularly since the cancer may be far advanced and still asymptomatic when discovered, "prophylactic" proctocolectomy was advocated. Many patients having little or no complaint referable to the gastrointestinal tract were submitted to this procedure, purely on the basis of the premalignant potential of the colon.

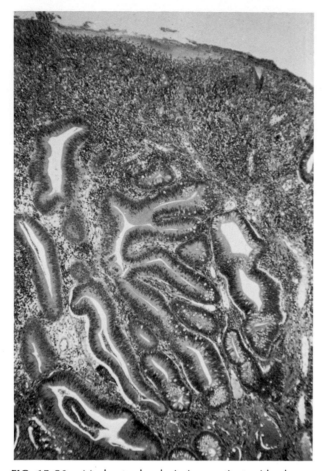

FIG. 15-86. Moderate dysplasia in a patient with ulcerative colitis. Note the loss of polarity and decreased mucus production. (Original magnification × 80. Courtesy of Rudolf Garret, M.D.)

The problem is to identify those patients who upon biopsy and histologic examination are found to have the dysplastic phenomenon. There are mild degrees of dysplasia, moderate degrees, and severe degrees; the correct interpretation of the biopsies rests on the talent and the experience of the pathologist. It is imperative, therefore, to have available someone who is not only competent but also interested in this particular aspect of colon pathology.

The criteria for diagnosing dysplasia are problematic and vary from institution to institution. Dysplasia includes adenomatous and villous changes in the mucosa, irregular budding tubules beneath the muscularis mucosae, and cellular alterations consisting of fewer goblet cells, hyperchromatic nuclei, stratified nucleoli, and course chromatin (Figs. 15-86, 15-87, and 15-88).[148] The following criteria have been proposed by Nugent and colleagues[204]:

Mild dysplasia
Crypt architecture preserved
Stratified nuclei but not reaching the lumenal surface
Crowding and hyperchromasia of nuclei
Mitoses in upper portion of crypt
Goblet cell mucin usually moderately diminished
Moderate dysplasia
Distortion of crypt architecture with branching and lateral buds
Nuclear abnormalities as in mild dysplasia, but stratification reaching lumenal surface
Goblet cell mucin usually depleted
Marked dysplasia
Distortion of crypt architecture more marked, frequently with villous configuration of surface epithelium
Nuclear abnormalities as in moderate dysplasia but with loss of polarity frequently present
"Back-to-back" glands frequently present.

The last category includes all abnormalities short of invasive carcinoma and encompasses what some might designate "carcinoma in situ."

Nugent and co-workers reviewed the clinical and histologic data in a retrospective fashion in 23 patients with known colon carcinoma and chronic ulcerative colitis.[204] All but one of these patients were found to have dysplasia at a remote site from the cancer. On the basis of this experience the authors continued a prospective study in 36 patients with chronic ulcerative colitis. Colonoscopy was performed in those who had a pancolitis of more than 5 years' duration. The number of biopsy specimens taken ranged from three to ten; eight were demonstrated to exhibit dysplasia. One patient with mild dysplasia underwent a colectomy for intractable disease and was found to have a Dukes' A carcinoma. Five patients with severe dysplasia were submitted to resection, and one was found to have a Dukes' C carcinoma. The study now includes 17 patients who have been identified as harboring dysplasia. Ten of these have been submitted to operation, and four patients have been found to have an unsuspected carcinoma. As of this writing seven patients are still unoperated.

Dickinson and associates surveyed 43 patients with long-standing ulcerative colitis in which the disease extended proximal to the splenic flexure.[62] Dysplasia was found in nine patients in one or more biopsies (severe in two, moderate in one, and mild in six). The two patients with severe dysplasia were subsequently found to harbor a carcinoma.

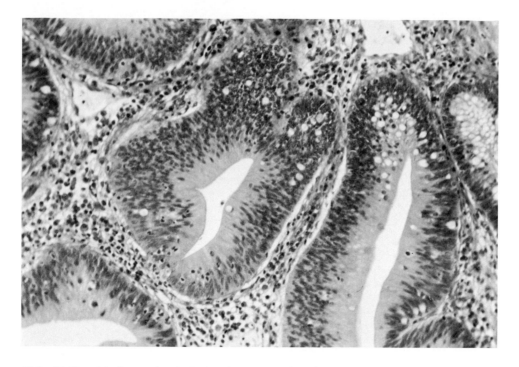

FIG. 15-87. Moderate dysplasia in ulcerative colitis: loss of polarity and proliferation of epithelial cells. (Original magnification × 260. Courtesy of Rudolf Garret, M.D.)

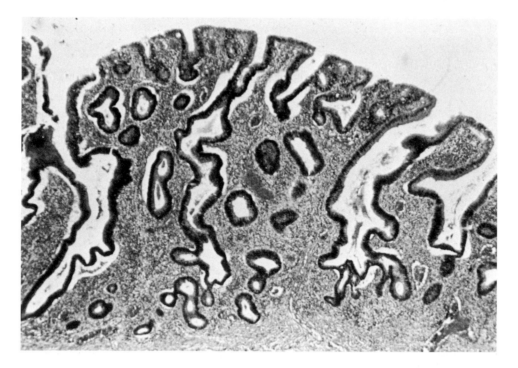

FIG. 15-88. Severe dysplasia: atypical hyperplasia with irregularly shaped crypts lined by crowded cells with hyperchromatic nuclei. (Original magnification × 80. Corman ML, Veidenheimer MC, Nugent FW et al: Diseases of the Anus, Rectum and Colon. Part II: Non-specific inflammatory bowel disease. New York, Medcom, 1976)

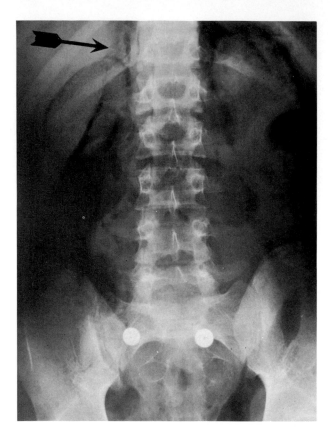

FIG. 15-89. Retroperitoneal gas from a colon perforated during colonoscopy–biopsy for dysplasia in a 19-year-old patient with ulcerative colitis. The renal outlines are clearly evident, as is the right adrenal gland (*arrow*).

Blackstone and co-workers performed colonoscopy on 112 patients with long-standing ulcerative colitis over a 4-year period.[23] In 12 patients a polypoid mass was identified which on biopsy revealed dysplasia. Seven of these patients were subsequently found to have invasive carcinoma. Twenty-seven patients were found to have dysplasia in the absence of a polypoid excrescence (*i.e.*, a flat mucosa), and only one carcinoma was found subsequently. The authors felt that the presence of a single polypoid mass was highly significant for the possible presence of concurrent invasive cancer. This was strong evidence to support the need for colectomy.

For many years it has been known that endoscopic examination, either proctosigmoidoscopy or colonoscopy, was not consistently effective in the identification of even far advanced carcinoma arising in ulcerative colitis and less effective in early disease.[52] With the advent of the dysplastic phenomenon surveillance is advised for those patients who have had a minimum of 7 years of total or subtotal colonic disease. These patients are then submitted to total colonoscopy with biopsy of any demonstrable lesion. As mentioned, the biopsy of a specific, elevated lesion will yield a much higher incidence of dysplasia. Multiple random biopsies should be taken throughout the colon (ten are suggested). This should be performed every other year, or more often if dysplasia is identified. It must be remembered, however, that colonoscopy in ulcerative colitis is not necessarily a benign procedure; performing multiple biopsies may be quite hazardous (Fig. 15-89). As with patients who are bleeding, I believe the examiner who is to perform colonoscopy and multiple biopsies on a patient with chronic ulcerative colitis should be a highly experienced endoscopist. Histologic findings should be an indication for colectomy only if dysplasia is severe, is consistent in more than one biopsy obtained at different sites, or is found in sequential biopsies taken from an endoscopic lesion. Preferably, biopsies should be obtained in areas free from inflammatory reaction.[216]

Barium enema examination is useful only to demonstrate the macroscopic anatomy of the colon: the loss of haustrations, shortening, and possible stricture. It is unlikely that a barium enema will reveal a carcinoma earlier than will endoscopic examination. Proctosigmoidoscopy or flexible fiberoptic sigmoidoscopy is recommended on alternate years.

Treatment of Carcinoma

If a carcinoma is identified in a patient with ulcerative colitis, proctocolectomy is the treatment of choice. No attempt should be made to preserve the rectal mucosa. Alternative operations may, however, include the continent ileostomy (Kock), and the ileoanal anastomosis with intervening pouch (see later, under Surgical Management).

In the absence of a known carcinoma, surgeons have on occasion attempted to preserve the rectum in the hope that some day reestablishment of intestinal continuity might be possible. The rectum is either oversewn or brought out as a mucous fistula. Another alternative operation is the ileorectal anastomosis, maintaining intestinal continuity, but preserving potentially malignant rectal mucosa.

Aylett reported the largest experience with ileorectal anastomosis in patients with ulcerative colitis.[8–10] Over 400 patients underwent this operation, only 8% of whom had to undergo conversion to an ileostomy. Twelve patients underwent proctectomy because of carcinoma in the retained rectum.

Johnson and co-workers reported their experience with rectal preservation in patients with ulcerative colitis.[135] Of the 172 patients who underwent subtotal colectomy and mucous fistula, over half subsequently required rectal excision. In 27% the rectum remained as a mucous fistula. An additional 101 patients underwent an initial primary ileorectal anastomosis. Of the 273 patients at risk for the development of rectal cancer, 10 (3.6%) subsequently developed a malignant lesion. The authors estimated that the cumulative probability of developing a cancer in the rectum following subtotal colectomy was 17% at 27 years from the onset of the disease. Unfortunately, more than half of the patients had disseminated disease at the time of rectal removal, and there were no Dukes' A lesions. Although the experience of the authors was reasonably favorable, the fact that when cancer developed it was relatively far advanced in most cases indicates that careful follow-up evaluation is a requisite.

Grundfest and colleagues reviewed the Cleveland Clinic experience of total abdominal colectomy and ileorectal anastomosis for ulcerative colitis.[108] This retrospective study involved 89 patients between the years 1957 and 1977. Twenty-one percent of the patients required subsequent proctectomy, with the overall incidence of carcinoma being 4.8%. The cumulative risk of developing a rectal cancer was 12.9% ($\pm$ 8.3%) after 25 years, considerably less than when the colon is left intact. The authors caution that preexisting colonic cancer with severe colonic dysplasia is a relative contraindication to rectal preservation. They also strongly recommend frequent proctosigmoidoscopy and rectal biopsy to look for dysplasia.

Khubchandani and associates performed a prospective study to evaluate dysplasia in 34 patients who had previously undergone colectomy and ileorectal anastomosis for inflammatory bowel disease.[145] One patient with a history of 23 years' duration of disease demonstrated severe dysplasia. Subsequent proctectomy revealed carcinoma in situ. The authors recommended multiple biopsy examinations of the rectum, ideally from relatively free areas, every 6 months. If a biopsy demonstrates severe dysplasia, a repeat examination is suggested 3 months later. If sequential biopsy demonstrates severe dysplasia, excision of the rectum is recommended.

Evaluation of the rectum by means of proctosigmoidoscopy or flexible fiberoptic sigmoidoscopy can usually be performed relatively easily in a patient whose rectum is in continuity with the intestinal tract. However, if a patient has a mucous fistula or an oversewn rectal stump, after a time it may be impossible to pass an instrument in the disused rectum. In my experience these are the patients who are at the greatest risk for the development of malignancy. If continuity has not been reestablished within 2 years following colectomy, the rectum should be removed. Sphincter

impairment would probably be of sufficient magnitude that subsequent anastomosis would produce an unsatisfactory functional result.

Others have also expressed their concern about the retained rectum after colectomy for ulcerative colitis.[158, 163, 169, 185]

Crohn's Disease

For many years it was felt that there was no increased risk for the development of carcinoma in patients who had Crohn's disease. There have been a number of recent case reports, however, with the authors suggesting that there *is* an increased incidence. In 1980, Zinkin and Brandwein identified 43 patients with adenocarcinoma arising in a segment of Crohn's colitis and added one of their own.[286] Hawker and associates reviewed the literature on Crohn's disease of the *small intestine* and identified 61 cases, including their own experience.[119] There were 41 tumors of the ileum, 18 of the jejunum, 1 in the duodenum and ileum, and 1 in the ileum and colon. Eighteen occurred in bypassed intestinal loops.

Most people now accept the thesis that there is an increased risk for cancer in patients with Crohn's disease, but there is no question that it is not comparable to that associated with chronic ulcerative colitis. It is very difficult to assess the true incidence of Crohn's disease and carcinoma in the small bowel because small bowel carcinoma is such a rare condition. Greenstein calculated that the increased risk for the development of malignancy in Crohn's disease approximated that found in universal colitis by a factor of at least one third.[104] Even in large clinical series, the number of cancers of the small bowel is so small that one rarely reads reports of more than two or three cases. However, the association appears genuine and is based on several observations.

There is a different distribution of small bowel cancer in Crohn's disease when compared with cancer of the small intestine that occurs in the absence of the inflammatory condition. In Crohn's disease, two thirds of the small bowel cancers occur in the ileum, whereas no more than 30% occur in this area in the absence of Crohn's.[119] In the large intestine, Crohn's disease with cancer is usually found on the right side of the colon, as compared with the usual distal bowel involvement in the general population. In a study from Birmingham, England, Gyde and colleagues demonstrated a significant excess of tumors in both the upper and lower gastrointestinal tract in patients with Crohn's disease.[112] Their study further demonstrated that the whole tract may be at an increased risk and that this risk is not merely confined to areas of obvious inflammatory involvement.

The likelihood of the development of carcinoma is greatly enhanced in patients who have undergone bypass intestinal surgery.[106, 119] This is particularly true when chronic inflammatory disease persists for many years. Lavery and Jagelman identified two cases of carcinoma that developed in the out-of-circuit rectum after subtotal colectomy and ileostomy for Crohn's disease.[169] The mortality rate from patients who develop cancer in excluded loops is extremely high (greater than 80%), probably because recognition is very late in the progression of the disease.[104] The observation of new signs and symptoms after a prolonged period of quiescence, particularly in long-standing disease, especially if the patient had previously undergone an exclusion or bypass procedure, should be vigorously evaluated for the possible presence of a malignancy.

The age at which colonic carcinoma develops in patients with Crohn's disease is quite young and is also associated with long duration of the process. More than half the patients who developed colonic cancer were under the age of 40 years.[240]

Additional features of carcinoma in Crohn's disease include multifocal lesions and metachronous intestinal and extra-intestinal cancers.

As with carcinoma in ulcerative colitis, radiologic diagnosis of malignant change in patients with Crohn's disease is virtually impossible. Endoscopic examination likewise is of very little benefit in establishing the diagnosis. However, dysplasia probably is as significant a finding as it is with ulcerative colitis, and this method deserves further study. Unfortunately, the small intestine does not lend itself very well to investigation by means of biopsy, particularly in an excluded segment. It is probably a reasonable precaution to recall all patients who have undergone a bypass or exclusion procedure for Crohn's disease to evaluate the candidacy of that patient for a resection.

MEDICAL MANAGEMENT

Ulcerative Proctitis and Proctosigmoiditis

The primary treatment of ulcerative proctitis is a short course of a hydrocortisone retention enema given once or twice daily. Enema kits containing 100 mg of hydrocortisone (Cortenema) or 40 mg of methylprednisolone acetate (Medrol Enpak) are convenient and effective for treating disease confined to the lower bowel. I have found the latter medication is occasionally more effective, but this may be due to the equivalent corti-

sone dose being double that contained in Cortenema. The packaging of the former product permits easier administration.

Very often, retention enemas containing cortisone administered over 2 weeks will resolve the patient's complaints. The rapidity of the clinical response and the lack of complications usually encountered with systemic steroid therapy are the primary advantages of this method of treatment. The rectal installation of steroids has the advantage of a medication applied directly to the involved mucosa, although it should be remembered that with persistent and frequent use the patient ultimately may develop side-effects associated with hyperadrenalcorticism. If this occurs, the medication should be reduced to alternate days so that within 2 or 3 weeks it can be discontinued. Some patients require longer treatment, and others have difficulty retaining the enema because of tenesmus or diarrhea.[242]

Additional medical measures include dietary restrictions. This involves the omission of all foods that tend to produce frequency of bowel movements (*e.g.*, fruits, milk products [especially if the patient has a lactose intolerance], and fiber). However, there can be no hard-and-fast rule about complete restriction of these products for every patient. Some patients may be more tolerant than others.

The addition of a bulk agent, such as one of the psyllium-containing products, may be of benefit in producing some form to the stool. The addition of "slowing" medications may also be helpful for the patient having frequent bowel movements out of proportion to the degree of inflammatory involvement of the rectum. Products such as diphenoxylate (Lomotil), loperamide (Imodium), codeine, and deodorized tincture of opium individually or in combination may be quite ameliorative for this patient.

Sulfasalazine (Azulfidine) has for many years been the standard drug of choice to prevent exacerbations of inflammatory bowel disease. The efficacy of the drug may be due to the fact that it is broken down by bacteria in the bowel to produce a sulfapyridine, an antibiotic. Another effect of the breakdown product of the drug is to decrease the amount of prostaglandins in the stool, one of the effects of the cortisones. The dosage is usually begun at 2 g per day, up to a maximum of 4 g a day. Increasing the dose further causes unpleasant side-effects. Spiro recommends that the medication be continued at a dose of 2 g a day for at least 1 year in order to prevent exacerbation.[242] This is the only drug proved to have prophylactic benefits in the treatment of ulcerative colitis.

Side-effects of sulfasalazine include skin rash, bone marrow depression, nausea, headache, and malaise. Folic acid deficiency is very frequently unrecognized; folic acid supplements taken daily are recommended. Other side-effects of greater consequence include hemolysis in patients with glucose 6-phosphate dehydrogenase deficiency, exfoliative skin disorders, and temporary infertility in men.

Oral steroids should be considered in patients who fail to respond to the above measures. The medication should, however, not be used for the treatment of diarrhea, but rather for patients who continue to bleed. A beginning dose of prednisone, 20 mg, is suggested on a daily basis, which is then reduced by 5 mg after 1 week; ideally, the medication is completely withdrawn in a period of 4 to 6 weeks. Higher doses of steroids may be used transiently on an outpatient basis, but are not recommended for prolonged use. Every attempt should be made to taper the dosage in a reasonable, nonprecipitous way.

One of the important aspects of educating the patient is to have him recognize that he may have a relatively chronic condition that is subject to exacerbations and remissions. In some patients, bleeding persists for many months or a year. All too often the patient will, either on his own initiative or upon the advice of the physician, increase the dose of prednisone to the point where steroid complications are evident.

The value of *psychiatric counseling* was discussed earlier. Although the disease may not be of psychogenic origin, there is sufficient evidence to suggest that emotions do play a role in the exacerbation or remission of the condition. In addition to the medication and dietary measures presented, it is often helpful to supplement these with psychotherapy.

Ulcerative Colitis Versus Crohn's Disease: Difference in Approach

Although it is true that the primary drugs for the treatment of both ulcerative colitis and Crohn's disease are identical, the approach to therapy for the two conditions is quite different. For example, since ulcerative colitis is a disease subject to exacerbations and remissions, the physician endeavors to remove steroids from the medical management as soon as the patient's condition permits. Crohn's disease, however, tends to pursue a more smoldering course, with less clear-cut exacerbations and remissions—hence, the often required continuous low-dose steroid therapy.

Because the therapy for both conditions depends on the patient's symptoms, treatment must be individualized; the physician endeavors to control the disease rather than to cure.[151] Factors that contribute to the medical decision making with respect to *ulcerative colitis* include the extent of involvement of the inflammatory disease, the duration of the illness, and the status of the disease (exacerbated or remitted). Patients with ulcerative colitis tend to have the most severe manifestations early in the course of the illness, with the pos-

sibility of cancer development being the primary concern later in the course of the disease. However, patients with *Crohn's disease* have a poorer prognosis the longer the disease persists.[156]

The primary drugs available for the treatment of ulcerative colitis and Crohn's disease are sulfasalazine and steroids. The outpatient management with these drugs is the same with more diffuse involvement as it is with the limited distal disease previously mentioned. However, if the patient is ill enough to require hospitalization, intravenous administration of a steroid is recommended (Fig. 15-90).

Acute medical management includes dietary restriction, intravenous fluids, protein replacement, blood transfusions, and the steroid therapy of choice. There is some controversy over the relative merits of adrenocorticotropic hormone (ACTH) and hydrocortisone or methylprednisolone. Some physicians believe that ACTH is more effective in controlling the acutely ill patient. The initial dose recommended is 40 units in

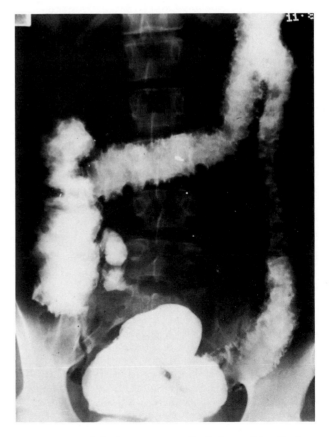

FIG. 15-90. Fulminant acute Crohn's colitis. Barium enema reveals total colonic ulceration and bowel wall edema.

1000 ml, over 8 hours. Therefore, a total of 120 units are given during a 24-hour period. If the physician prefers, the equivalent of 300 mg of hydrocortisone (approximately 60 mg of Prednisone) is recommended. Intravenous hydrocortisone, however, requires either continuous administration, or intravenous bolus injections no less frequently than every 4 hours. After this period of time, the blood level falls to inadequate therapeutic levels. If cortisone acetate is given intramuscularly, however, the effective therapeutic level can be maintained for a longer period of time. This, of course, is quite inconvenient and uncomfortable for the patient.

With a good response, the medication can be reduced at the rate of 5 mg (Prednisone) every 4 or 5 days, or it may be reduced more rapidly.[156] In a patient with acute Crohn's disease, a dramatic response is often observed with intravenous steroid administration; an abdominal mass may rapidly disappear, or a patient's acute abdominal symptoms may resolve.

Although there is no definitive study available on the efficacy of sulfasalazine in preventing exacerbations of Crohn's disease, most physicians recommend that this drug be used. Even when the patient is recovering from resective surgery, with no evidence for continued abdominal disease, sulfasalazine is recommended. Korelitz believes that sulfasalazine is more effective in preventing recurrences in Crohn's disease than it is with ulcerative colitis.[156] He further observes that in the natural course of the disease, the inflammatory process may tend to extend distally, but rarely proximally. However, once the patient undergoes surgery, proximal involvement is more likely to develop, usually at and just above the anastomosis.

Metronidazole (Flagyl) was initially introduced for the treatment of *Trichomonas vaginalis* infections but was subsequently demonstrated to be a very effective antibiotic against anaerobic organisms. It was also found to have effective activity against gram-positive and gram-negative bacteria. Metronidazole is a substituted imidazole that is rapidly absorbed orally and rectally; it can also be given intravenously in the acutely ill patient.

Recently, a controlled clinical trial from Sweden compared the efficacy of metronidazole with sulfasalazine in the treatment of patients with active Crohn's disease.[222, 262] Seventy-eight patients participated in the study during two 4-month periods. Metronidazole was demonstrated to be slightly more effective than sulfasalazine. The drug has been suggested to be particularly useful in the management of anal and perianal complications (see Surgical Management, Indications). A number of theories suggesting the mechanism of its action have been proposed: immunosuppression, an effect on wound healing, stimulation of leukocyte chemotaxis, and, of course, its antimicrobial effect.

Because of the supposition that inflammatory bowel disease is an autoimmune condition, the treatment with *immunosuppressive drugs* has been recommended.[159, 216, 256, 279] The two drugs that have been used are 6-mercaptopurine and its analogue, azathioprine. Korelitz uses immunosuppressive drugs when other treatment modalities fail and when there is no indication for operative intervention, and as an option offered to the patient prior to surgery.[157] Present and co-workers performed a double-blind study on 83 patients and noted a 67% response with 6-mercaptopurine as compared with only an 8% improvement with a placebo.[216] Most studies have demonstrated efficacy in approximately two thirds of patients. The drugs are felt not to be effective in the treatment of fulminating disease but should be used in those patients who can tolerate the relatively slow response to treatment. The drugs have also been recommended for the treatment of perianal disease and small bowel obstruction (when surgery is contraindicated), and in the treatment of children; prophylaxis after two surgical resections is another possible indication.

Complications include bone marrow suppression, liver abnormalities (including liver necrosis), pancreatitis, and hair loss. The initial concern about the possible induction of cancer does not seem to be justified on the basis of over a decade of experience. Theodor and associates in a retrospective study of 35 patients in whom Imuran (azathioprine) was employed, reported a "clearly superior response when compared with non-treatment or steroid therapy."[256] However, two patients died of fatal septicemia on Imuran therapy, and seven patients were subsequently submitted to colectomy.

Although immunosuppressive drugs have been shown to be effective in both ulcerative colitis and Crohn's disease, and with few exceptions the complications have been reversible, there is a fear on the part of most physicians to employ this modality in the management of their patients with inflammatory bowel disease.

Hyperalimentation, either parenteral or oral, has been recommended in a supportive role for patients with inflammatory bowel disease. Increasing evidence suggests that patients frequently are hospitalized with varying states of malnutrition. It has been demonstrated, furthermore, that patients who have lost greater than 20% of their usual weight before undergoing abdominal surgery have a higher morbidity and mortality than those who have not exhibited weight loss. There is currently an extensive literature on how to interpret nutritional data and when to use intravenous hyperalimentation. With inflammatory bowel disease, the theory for implementing intravenous hyperalimentation is that the bowel is "put to rest." If this were attempted without supplementary intravenous caloric intake, the patient's nutritional status would rapidly deteriorate. Intravenous hyperalimentation, therefore, permits the patient with IBD to be managed with bowel rest while simultaneously providing adequate amino acids and calories for anabolism.[63]

Fazio and colleagues reported the Cleveland Clinic's experience of 81 courses of total parenteral nutrition in the treatment of Crohn's disease.[79] Two groups of patients were treated, one as definitive therapy, and a second for adjunctive treatment. Indications in the former group included diffuse small intestinal disease, short bowel syndrome, acute ileitis or colitis (in which there was inadequate response to alternative medical treatment), poor nutrition, and enteric fistulas. A subsequent report revealed 23 patients in the primary therapy group.[116] A remission occurred in approximately two thirds of the patients; the remaining 8 patients required operation during the hospitalization.

In the adjunctive group, 58 patients were treated, of whom almost one quarter underwent remission, obviating the need for surgical intervention during that hospitalization. These patients, in fact, satisfied the criteria for primary therapy, although this was not the design in that group of patients. The course of treatment ranged from 10 to 264 days. The average treatment course was almost 3 weeks.

Of the 21 patients with Crohn's disease who were treated with total parenteral nutrition as primary therapy, there were only four (19%) who did not eventually require surgery. Three of the five patients with ulcerative colitis who were so treated responded well enough to medical therapy to have deferred surgery for an average of 2 years. The authors concluded that there appeared to be no lasting benefit for hyperalimentation as a primary method of therapy for patients with inflammatory bowel disease, particularly for Crohn's. But if the purpose of the treatment is to defer surgical intervention so that it can be pursued on an elective basis, hyperalimentation should be considered.

Shiloni and Freund studied the effect of total parenteral nutrition on 19 patients suffering from active Crohn's disease.[235] Although only approximately one third did not require surgery during the follow-up (up to 3 years), the authors felt that the treatment was highly effective as supportive therapy, enabling a patient to undergo uneventful major surgery. Others have recommended preoperative total parenteral nutrition for at least 5 days in patients with inflammatory bowel disease who have severe protein depletion.[221]

My own attitude is to use total parenteral nutrition only in those patients for whom surgery should be avoided, or whose nutritional status is so poor that one may anticipate a very high morbidity and mortality. The concept of short-term intravenous hyperalimentation in preparation for bowel surgery may have certain theoretical advantages, but expeditiously performed surgery should allow the patient to commence oral intake earlier, a much preferred method of administrating calories. One cannot dispute the facts that intravenous hyperalimentation is costly and is not without morbidity.

One other application of hyperalimentation is for the patient who has a short bowel syndrome secondary to multiple resections for Crohn's disease.[107, 170, 246] There are approximately 1000 such patients who have been discharged on home parenteral nutrition since the institution of a registry in 1981. It should be noted that most would not have been able to survive outside of a hospital without this technique. Almost all patients who require rehospitalization do so because of problems with the catheter, and in the experience of the Cleveland Clinic, mortality is usually due to the underlying disease process rather than to the therapy.[246] In my own experience, while this therapeutic modality may be quite cumbersome for the patient, it does permit a relatively normal life-style.

Toxic Megacolon

Patients with toxic megacolon may present with very minimal symptoms or may be critically ill. High fever, tachycardia, and abdominal pain are frequently noted. The most important aspect of the management of a patient with acute toxic dilatation is the assessment through the use of plain abdominal x-ray films. Clinical signs and symptoms may be masked by the patient's medications, especially by steroids. The usual signs of peritonitis may be absent or minimal.

My own philosophy is to adopt the attitude that toxic megacolon requires urgent surgical intervention, not emergency surgical management. The patient should be given the opportunity to recover from the acute attack. The usual supportive measures of intravenous fluid replacement and blood, colloid, and steroid therapy should be supplemented with broad-spectrum antibiotic coverage. With serial abdominal films, the effectiveness of the medical management can be assessed. If the dilatation decreases one may be reasonably assured that surgery can be deferred. Conversely, if colonic dilatation progresses during the period of maximum therapy, surgical intervention is advised.

Any medications that "slow" the gastrointestinal activity, such as anticholinergics or opiates, are discontinued. A nasogastric tube is advised. Some physicians have suggested a long (Miller-Abbott) tube in an attempt to decompress the colon, but I do not advise it. Placing the patient on the abdomen for a few minutes every 2 or 3 hours may help to distribute the gas, moving it into the rectum. Rectal tubes have also been advocated, but these are potentially dangerous and can lead to perforation of the sigmoid colon. Barium enema examination and colonoscopy are contraindicated; in fact, occasionally barium enema examination has been reported to precipitate toxic megacolon.

SURGICAL MANAGEMENT

Indications

The surgical indications in *ulcerative colitis* include toxic megacolon, perforation, hemorrhage, and the possibility of malignant degeneration. Proctocolectomy for ulcerative colitis in the absence of carcinoma is curative. Operative treatment in *Crohn's disease* is advised primarily for complications (abscess, fistula, obstruction), or for severe inanition (see Fig. 15-63); surgical intervention may not cure the patient.

Surgery is almost always required for *toxic megacolon*. In the series reported by Fazio from the Cleveland Clinic, only 7 of 115 patients (6%) were successfully managed medically, and 5 of these 7 came to colectomy in later years.[77] However, a period of observation to permit an opportunity for medical resolution is encouraged in order to avoid an emergency procedure.

Surgical intervention is advised if there is not a rapid response to intensive medical therapy.

Perforation usually occurs in the patient who exhibits toxic dilatation of the colon. Diagnosis can usually be made quite readily on the basis of physical examination and a decubitus film of the abdomen. A walled-off perforation may become evident at the time of laparotomy, and may be converted to a free perforation as the bowel is mobilized. Both ulcerative colitis and Crohn's disease can produce perforation, the latter early in the course of the illness.

Hemorrhage is rarely an indication for surgery in ulcerative colitis, and is virtually unheard of as an indication for surgery in granulomatous colitis (Fig. 15-91). Usually even massive hemorrhage can be controlled by medical means. It should be remembered, however, that a subtotal or total colectomy without proctectomy may not succeed in stopping the bleeding. Whatever the predisposing factors, it may be necessary to perform a proctectomy in order to establish hemostasis.

Internal and external *fistulas* associated with Crohn's disease are indications for surgical intervention.[95, 96, 130, 164] Although total parenteral nutrition may succeed in effecting temporary closure of the fistula, patients

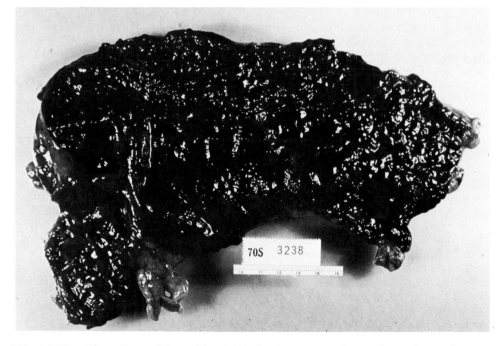

FIG. 15-91. Ulcerative colitis: a blood clot in the cecum of a patient who underwent emergency proctocolectomy for hemorrhage. (Corman ML, Veidenheimer MC, Nugent FW et al: Diseases of the Anus, Rectum, and Colon. Part II: Non-specific inflammatory bowel disease. New York, Medcom, 1976)

almost invariably develop symptoms severe enough to justify surgical intervention. The presence of a fistula virtually excludes the diagnosis of ulcerative colitis.

Abscess formation is usually a consequence of fistula in Crohn's disease.[105, 248] Greenstein and co-workers reported that 20% of 230 patients with Crohn's colitis and ileocolitis underwent surgery for intra-abdominal abscess.[105] The most frequent site of origin was the terminal ileum, with the abscess located in the right lower quadrant.

Operation for *presumed appendicitis* occasionally becomes an indication for surgery in Crohn's disease. Considerable controversy exists over the appropriate treatment when Crohn's disease is recognized at the time of operation.[162, 181, 238] Simonowitz and associates reviewed the records of 20 patients who underwent incidental appendectomy and made the following recommendations: if the patient has abdominal pain for less than 1 week, appendectomy is followed by minimal complications.[238] For patients who have symptoms longer than this period of time, incidental appendectomy is followed by an 83% incidence of fistula or sinus tract arising not from the appendiceal stump but from the terminal ileum. My own attitude is to perform an appendectomy if I am convinced on clinical grounds that the cecum is free of disease.

Crohn's disease confined to the appendix is a very rare entity. Lindhagen and associates identified 50 cases and added 12 of their own.[172] The indications for surgery were appendicitis in eight cases, appendiceal abscess in two, suspected pyosalpinx in one, and ovarian cyst in one. All but two of the eight appendicitis patients underwent appendectomy; the other patients underwent a more extensive resection. There was no incident of subsequent fecal fistula. With a median follow-up of almost 14 years, and with no further manifestation of the disease, the authors concluded that when Crohn's disease is confined to the appendix the prognosis is very favorable.

Anorectal disease, in the absence of other complications of inflammatory bowel disease, is rarely an indication for surgical intervention outside of the anal area. However, in those patients where loss of sphincter creates fecal incontinence, or in the presence of a rectovaginal or anovaginal fistula, radical surgery may be indicated for these complications alone. Usually a permanent ileostomy is required, but a diversionary procedure on a temporary basis may permit the surgeon to perform a reconstruction on selected patients.

In our reported experience with anal complications in patients with Crohn's disease, 22% of 1098 were so afflicted.[277] Crohn's colitis was much more frequently associated with an anal lesion than Crohn's disease of the small bowel (52% versus 14%). In our experience,

when an anal lesion became manifest, Crohn's disease ultimately developed elsewhere in the intestinal tract. Within 1 year following the anal manifestation, Crohn's disease presented elsewhere in 59% of patients. All of the remaining patients developed gastrointestinal disease within 5 years.

Definitive surgery has been recommended and has been successfully performed in patients with anal fistulas in Crohn's disease.[4, 80, 122, 177] The success that these authors have had is, I am certain, due to careful patient selection. One must make a distinction between anal Crohn's disease and a fistula in ano in the patient who has Crohn's disease without anal involvement. In this latter group, definitive anal surgery may be safely undertaken with reasonable expectation of healing. This is particularly true if the involved segment in the bowel either has been resected or is quiescent. Conversely, healing of wounds in a patient with anal Crohn's disease or in a patient with active disease elsewhere in the gastrointestinal tract will often lead to chronic, draining, indolent, painful ulcers, which create more problems in management than did the original pathology (see Fig. 4-32). With anal Crohn's disease the optimal form of therapy is medical management and simple drainage of the abscess when it occurs.

Metronidazole has been successfully employed in the treatment of perineal Crohn's disease.[20, 29, 71] Bernstein and associates demonstrated that drainage, erythema, and induration diminished dramatically in all 21 patients so treated, with complete healing obtained in more than half of those that were maintained on therapy.[20] Eisenberg compared surgery alone in the management of complicated anal Crohn's disease with surgery plus metronidazole.[71] The patients were randomly allocated, but it was not a double-blind study. An intravenous loading dose of 15 mg/kg (usually 1 g) was given, with maintenance therapy of 500 mg intravenously every 6 hours for 5 days. Outpatient treatment was continued at the dosage of 250 mg, three times daily, for 4 weeks or until complete healing occurred. Twelve of 14 patients (86%) receiving metronidazole treatment had a satisfactory response with complete healing of anorectal–perineal Crohn's disease without relapse during a follow-up period of from 1 to 5 years. In the control group, 11 of 17 patients (65%) treated by surgery alone had satisfactory healing.

In a follow-up study of long-term administration of metronidazole, Brandt and colleagues evaluated whether the drug could be reduced or stopped in these patients without creating an exacerbation.[29] They reported that dosage reduction was associated with recurrent disease activity in all patients, but that healing occurred promptly when the full dosage of metronidazole was reinstituted.

It appears, then, that definitive anal surgery can be undertaken even in the presence of anal Crohn's disease with some reasonable expectation of success if supplementary metronidazole therapy is administered.

Preparation of the Patient

In elective surgery, preparation of the patient is not significantly different for patients undergoing resection for inflammatory bowel disease than for patients who undergo surgery for cancer. However, it is a wise idea to limit the amount of laxative administered. In fact, if a patient is troubled by diarrhea, a preoperative cathartic should be avoided. On the morning of surgery an enema should be given until the returns are clear; this is the only mechanical bowel preparation advised under these circumstances. Patients who are to undergo small bowel resection do not require a mechanical preparation unless the possibility of colonic resection also exists. The antibiotic preparation should be the same as that described in Chapter 10.

Since most patients undergoing surgery for inflammatory bowel disease have been on *steroids* for varying periods of time, it is imperative that adequate "coverage" be maintained to prevent adrenal insufficiency caused by the stress of surgery. Unless the patient had been on short-term cortisone therapy many months prior to the operation, steroid protection should be afforded even if corticosteroids had been withdrawn up to 2 years previously. The following protocol is recommended:

1. 9:00 P.M., night before surgery: cortisone acetate, intramuscularly, 100 mg
2. 6:00 A.M., day of surgery: cortisone acetate, 100 mg intramuscularly
3. Postoperatively, day of surgery: cortisone acetate, 100 mg intramuscularly, three times daily
4. First postoperative day: cortisone acetate, 100 mg, three times daily, intramuscularly (A tapering schedule is advised after the third postoperative day, depending on the condition of the patient.)

Intravenous hydrocortisone is not advised because of the requirement for continuous infusion or the need to administer it every 4 hours. Uniform blood levels are more difficult to maintain by the intravenous method.

In the emergency situation it is obviously not possible to prepare the bowel adequately, particularly for toxic megacolon. Preoperative preparation includes the correction of any fluid and electrolyte abnormalities, blood replacement as necessary, the placement of a nasogastric tube, the insertion of a Foley catheter (adequate urine output must be clearly established before surgery is undertaken), and possibly the insertion of a hyperalimentation catheter.

An *intravenous pyelogram* should be performed routinely on any patient who is to undergo elective bowel resection. It is of particular value in patients with inflammatory bowel disease, especially Crohn's disease, because of the high likelihood of associated urinary tract abnormalities (see Figs. 15-78 and 15-79).

Preoperative stoma marking should be considered for all patients who are to undergo surgery for inflammatory bowel disease, and it is imperative if an ileostomy is contemplated. Although preoperative marking is strongly advised for patients who are to undergo abdominoperineal resection for cancer, the consequences of a poorly placed stoma are not as profound as they would be in those patients who are to have an *ileostomy.* It must be remembered that to the patient the stoma is the most important feature of the operation. An improperly located stoma that does not permit convenient management may cause a patient to become significantly disabled and reclusive. The surgeon should make as much effort to create a satisfactory stoma both in terms of the preoperative location and in the technique of construction as he does to secure adequate hemostasis. The techniques of stomal construction are discussed in the following chapter, as are the complications of ileostomy and colostomy.

The optimal site is selected for the sitting, supine, and standing positions. It should be away from any bony promontories, scars, or umbilicus. Often two sites are selected in the hypogastrium, one on each side; should it not be possible to create the stoma in one position, an alternative is available. The ileostomy should always be brought through the split thickness of the rectus muscle (Fig. 15-92). In the elective situation it may be helpful to have the patient wear the appliance for a day to be certain that the location is satisfactory (*e.g.,* not interfering with the belt line).

In the emergency situation, it may not be possible to adequately mark the site preoperatively, particularly if a perforation precipitates the need for surgical intervention. Even under these circumstances, however, an effort should be made to mark the site preoperatively. Attempts to do this during the operation, with the abdominal wall open, will often result in the stoma being in a less-than-satisfactory location. On the operating table a site may be selected with some degree of assurance; a metal flange can be used that corresponds to the diameter of the face plate of an appliance (Fig. 15-93). Although the patient can be examined only in the supine position under these circumstances, it is a better alternative than a mere guess. The flange can be autoclaved so that a patient whose requirement for an ileostomy was unsuspected at the time of laparotomy can still benefit from an intelligent effort in establishing the appropriate site.

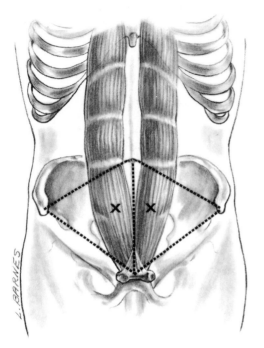

FIG. 15-92. When choosing a site for ileostomy location, scars, bony prominences, and the umbilicus must be avoided.

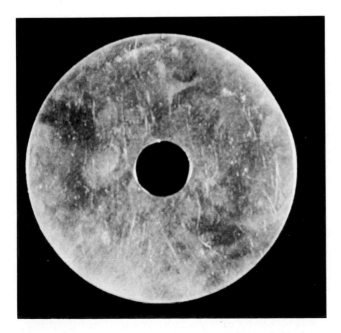

FIG. 15-93. A metal flange corresponding to the face plate diameter can be sterilized to use as a template for stoma site marking on the operating table.

Choice of Operation

There are basically five operations currently available for the surgical treatment of *ulcerative colitis:* proctocolectomy and ileostomy; total or subtotal colectomy with rectal preservation (ileorectal anastomosis, mucous fistula of rectum, closure of rectal stump); total abdominal proctocolectomy with ileoanal anastomosis; proctocolectomy with reservoir ileostomy (Kock); and total abdominal proctocolectomy with ileoanal anastomosis and intervening pouch (Parks). In patients with toxic megacolon, a sixth option is a diverting loop ileostomy with decompressive skin-level ("blowhole") colostomy.

For patients with *Crohn's disease* involving the colon and rectum, proctocolectomy with ileostomy is considered the only appropriate operation, although preservation of the rectum may be contemplated if this area is relatively spared. When Crohn's disease involves other segments of the gastrointestinal tract, the choice of operation will depend on the location and extent of disease. The Parks procedure and the Kock operation are contraindicated in patients with granulomatous colitis.

The *incision* for all colon resections, including surgery for inflammatory bowel disease, should always be through the midline. The reasons for this were discussed previously, and include rapid and facile entry into the peritoneal cavity, good exposure of all areas within the abdomen, and, most important, accessibility of both sides of the abdomen for possible stomal placement. If a paramedian incision is used, that side of the abdomen is excluded as a possible location for an ileostomy. This may not seem very important at the time of the procedure, particularly if the surgeon contemplates locating the stoma on the opposite side, but if the ileostomy ever requires relocation, unless the scar is flat, it may be extremely difficult to find a satisfactory site for the stoma. The alternative of placing the stoma in a pararectus location is unsatisfactory (see Chap. 16). If a total abdominal colectomy or proctocolectomy is contemplated, the incision is usually from xyphoid to pubis. In patients with long-standing ulcerative colitis, however, when foreshortening of the bowel may be present, one should begin the incision in the hypogastrium, ascertain the height of the flexures, and extend the incision cephalad if further exposure is required. When operating for toxic megacolon it is imperative to have adequate exposure in order to avoid possible injury to the colon or to the spleen.

Exploration of the abdomen will usually reveal the extent of pathology in patients with Crohn's disease, since this is a transmural inflammatory process, and the serosa is virtually always involved. However, in patients with ulcerative colitis one may be singularly unimpressed with the amount of disease as it appears from the serosal aspect. One may appreciate only tortuosity of the vessels, a pallor on the serosal aspect, and, of course, in the case of long-standing, chronic ulcerative colitis, bowel shortening.

When operating for *ulcerative colitis* one should have a preconceived plan of the surgery to be performed. That is to say, almost irrespective of the operative findings, the entire colon should be removed. Whether one wishes to contemplate a more esoteric operation is a decision that should be made *preoperatively*. One must depend on the preoperative evaluation, history, endoscopy, and radiologic studies, not on the operative findings, to determine the extent of resection for ulcerative colitis. Conversely, in patients with *Crohn's disease,* it is not uncommon to discover that involvement is more extensive than could be appreciated by preoperative evaluation. In both conditions one must inspect the entire small bowel for the possibility of other lesions. The bowel should be carefully examined even in patients with presumed ulcerative colitis, because occasionally one may discover a lesion in the proximal bowel consistent with Crohn's disease. Obviously, this might impel the surgeon to perform an alternative operation.

Proctocolectomy and Ileostomy

Proctocolectomy and ileostomy has become the conventional operative approach to the treatment of ulcerative colitis and for most patients with granulomatous colitis in which the rectum or anus is involved. However, it is interesting to note that in the past 10 years there have been very few reports on the management of inflammatory bowel disease by this operation. A great deal of interest, as manifested by the voluminous literature on the subject, has arisen in the treatment of ulcerative colitis; particular attention has been given to various sphincter-saving approaches and to the continent, reservoir ileostomy. But proctocolectomy and conventional ileostomy should be considered the benchmark procedure against which all other operations should be compared. It has become established as a safe, curative approach that permits the patient to live a virtually normal life-style.

The operation has evolved in a sequential way, beginning initially with appendicostomy as a decompressive procedure, then ileostomy, and then staged operations to effect removal of the colon and rectum.[33, 37, 38, 44, 166, 175, 188] During the era of staged procedures, which included staged thyroidectomy, esophageal diverticulectomy, abdominoperineal resection, and pancreatectomy, it was considered perfectly reasonable to perform four operations before completely extirpating the bowel for ulcerative colitis (ileostomy, right hemicolectomy, left hemicolectomy, abdominoperineal resection). With advances in anesthesia, blood transfusion, and antibiotics, and better surgical techniques, the staged procedures were reduced to two operations (total abdominal colectomy followed by proctectomy), and finally to proctocolectomy in one stage.[32, 49, 89, 97]

The technique of proctocolectomy essentially combines the operations previously discussed in Chapters 10 and 11: total abdominal colectomy with proctectomy, ideally in the perineolithotomy position (synchronous combined). There are some minor differences, however, which are important to consider. First, this is not a cancer operation; hence, it is not necessary to remove a large area of mesentery containing the lymphatic structures. The presence of large lymph nodes is of no clinical significance. Some surgeons had thought it prudent to remove these nodes in patients with Crohn's disease, believing that their presence predisposed the patient to recurrence. There is no evidence to suggest that this is the case, and the surgeon is not advised to pursue a more radical excision in an effort to eliminate this tissue. Furthermore, it is not necessary to excise areas of parietal peritoneum as one often does for carcinoma of the colon. The peritoneal cut may be made directly on the bowel wall, expediting the dissection.

In patients with Crohn's disease, retroperitoneal inflammation may pose some risk for ureteral injury during mobilization of the right colon or the rectosigmoid. Great care should be taken during this maneuver to identify the ureter and to keep it out of harm's way. Likewise, duodenal injury is possible, particularly if transmural involvement by Crohn's disease creates fixation of the bowel to the second and third portions of the duodenum. Careful dissection between these structures must be performed, dropping the duodenum posteriorly until it is well out of the area of dissection. Foreshortening and thickening of the mesentery of the right colon and proximal transverse colon also predisposes the duodenum to possible injury. By clamping the blood vessels on one side only, dividing the mesentery on the bowel side, one is less likely to incorporate the side of the duodenum. Back-bleeding can then be addressed with the bowel delivered away from the area of potential injury. This maneuver is analogous to that which one performs to divide the lateral ligaments of the rectum (see Figs. 11-14 and 11-15).

Another difference in surgical technique when removing the colon and rectum for inflammatory bowel disease compared with removing it for cancer is in the rectal mobilization. Because of potential injury to sympathetic and parasympathetic nerves, it has been suggested that the rectal dissection posteriorly be performed between the rectum and the mesorectum. This maneuver is more likely to avoid injury to the presacral nerves, the sympathetic innervation to the pelvic viscera. However, the dissection is tedious and often quite hemorrhagic. Furthermore, the technique fails to protect the parasympathetic innervation, which is usually of greater concern, particularly in men. Erection is a parasympathetic-mediated response, which is transmitted through the nervi erigentes, arising from the second, third, and fourth sacral nerves. Parasympathetic nerve injury results in impotence; injury to the presacral sympathetic nerves impedes ejaculation. The presacral nerves originate from the thoracic and lumbar segments of the spinal cord and usually are readily identified if the surgeon makes a modicum of effort to do so. Since there is a ready plane of dissection between the mesentery of the rectum and the sacrum, I prefer to directly visualize the presacral nerves, displace them posteriorly, and proceed in this plane as I do with proctectomy for carcinoma. In order to accomplish this safely, it is important to begin the dissection into the hollow of the sacrum sharply with a scissors rather than to initiate mobilization of the rectum bluntly from the promontory of the sacrum by means of the hand only. After the dissection has proceeded well below the sacral promontory, it is possible to complete the mobilization by placing the hand into the presacral space.

An organized approach to the operation minimizes morbidity and mortality. Having ascertained the extent of the pathology, mobilization of the sigmoid colon and rectum proceed, and the perineal surgeon commences his portion of the operation. After completion of the proctectomy the rectum is delivered to the abdominal operator, wrapped in a towel, and the rest of the colectomy is completed while the perineal surgeon closes the bottom end wound. Alternatively, the abdominal surgeon may elect to perform a total colectomy initially, calling the perineal surgeon in at the appropriate stage of the operation to complete the proctectomy.

If two teams are not available, the patient is placed in the supine position on the operating table, and the total abdominal colectomy is completed. The rectum is divided and secured in a rubber glove (see Fig. 11-19), the abdomen closed, the ileostomy created, and the perineal dissection undertaken with the patient either in the left lateral position or in the lithotomy position as described for the one-team approach for carcinoma of the rectum.

In contradistinction from proctectomy for carcinoma, the floor of the pelvis is not reconstituted. This is because there is a tendency for delayed perineal wound healing in inflammatory bowel disease. If one closes the perineal floor with parietal peritoneum, a diaphragm-like effect is created, resulting in a large dead space that has the propensity of not healing. One must endeavor to create the pelvic floor as low as possible. Since it is not necessary to excise the levator muscle widely as is done for cancer, it is always possible to reapproximate this muscular structure. It is the levatores, then, that form the floor of the pelvis in patients who undergo proctectomy for inflammatory bowel disease.

The perineal dissection is undertaken in a manner somewhat different from that for carcinoma. The technique that I prefer is the intersphincteric dissection advocated by Lyttle and Parks (Fig. 15-94).[174] This permits a much smaller perineal wound. In fact, the diameter of the incision is such that it is impossible to insert a Lace retractor, the preferred retractor to facilitate the perineal portion of the dissection for cancer of the rectum (see Fig. 11-28). The dissection is carried out in the intersphincteric plane, between the internal and external anal sphincters. When the levator ani muscle is encountered, it is divided close to the rectum and the dissection completed anteriorly and posteriorly in a manner identical to that for carcinoma of the rectum. A Jackson-Pratt drain is placed into the pelvis and brought out through a stab wound in the buttock (see Fig. 15-94, *D*). Levator ani muscle is then approximated and the skin closed. The drain is usually removed at 72 hours, depending on the amount of drainage.

In creating the ileostomy in patients with ulcerative colitis, I prefer an *extraperitoneal approach*. This technique permits total obliteration of the paraileostomy gutter, thereby avoiding the potential for herniation. It also facilitates subsequent entrance into the abdominal cavity without the risk of injuring the mesentery to the small bowel and stoma. Kocher clamps are placed on the cut edge of the parietal peritoneum. The peritoneum is then gently stripped off the inner aspect of the abdominal wall to the point where the ileostomy site is located. An abdominal wall opening is then created (see Fig. 11-16), and the end of the ileum is delivered through the opening (Fig. 15-95, *A*). The cut edge of the mesentery is then secured to the peritoneum that has been mobilized (Fig. 15-95, *B*). Following closure of the abdomen the ileostomy is matured (see Figs. 16-38, 16-39, and 16-40).

An *intraperitoneal ileostomy* is recommended in patients who undergo proctocolectomy for granulomatous colitis, in patients who have already had a portion of the terminal ileum removed, and in those patients for whom an adequate "stripping" of the parietal peritoneum is not technically possible. As suggested, the primary disadvantages of this technique are the technical difficulties associated with complete obliteration of the right lateral gutter; the inferior aspect does not lend itself to closure in a satisfactory fashion, and to all intents and purposes it effectively impedes entrance into the abdominal cavity from the right upper quad-

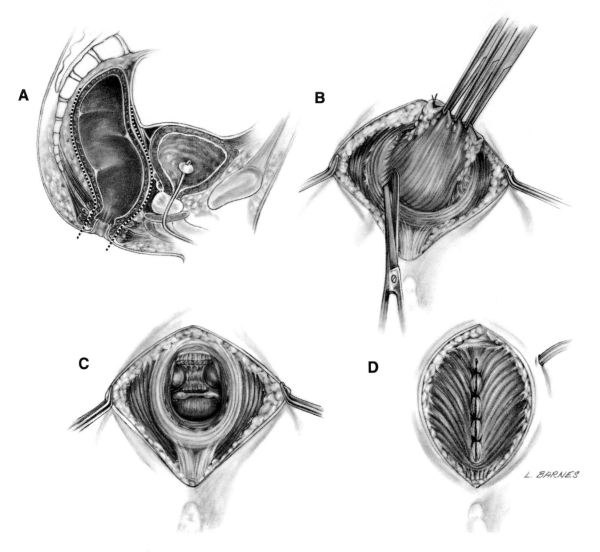

FIG. 15-94. Technique of intersphincteric proctectomy. **A.** Outline of the area removed. **B.** Dissection proceeds in the intersphincteric plane. **C.** Intact external sphincter and levators following rectal removal. **D.** Closure of levators with drainage.

rant. The surgeon must be wary of performing an abdominal operation particularly in this area. This cautionary note is best exemplified by the example of a patient who underwent a cholecystectomy several years following intraperitoneal obliteration of the lateral gutter. The surgeon elected a subcostal incision to avoid the ileostomy, but in entering the peritoneal cavity the mesentery to the small intestine was inadvertently divided, which resulted in necrosis of the stoma. The technique for creating an intraperitoneal ileostomy

and obliteration of the lateral space is illustrated in Figure 15-96.

If the surgeon prefers, the lateral gutter may be left completely open. As with sigmoid colostomy, it is better to have a very large opening than a small one. But some form of tethering still is required in order to avoid torsion of the distal ileum on itself. A few anchoring sutures placed from the serosa of the ileum and its mesentery to the parietal peritoneum will usually prevent this complication (Fig. 15-97).

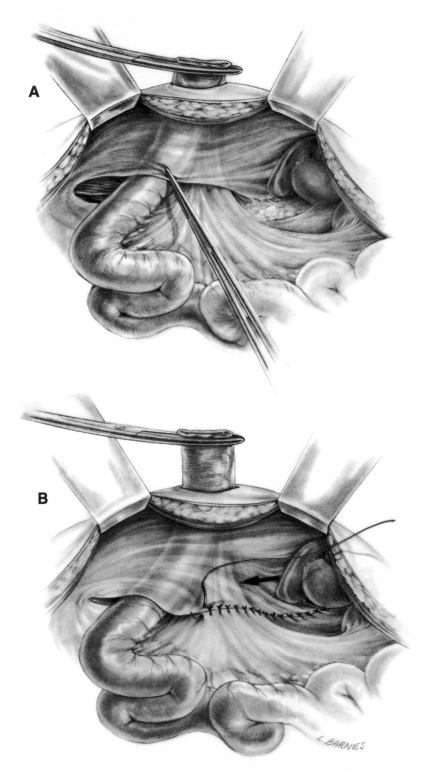

FIG. 15-95. Extraperitoneal ileostomy. **A.** Mobilized peritoneum on the abdominal wall with the terminal ileum delivered through the ileostomy site, and closure of the mesenteric defect. **B.** The peritoneum overlies the cut edge of the mesentery *(arrow).*

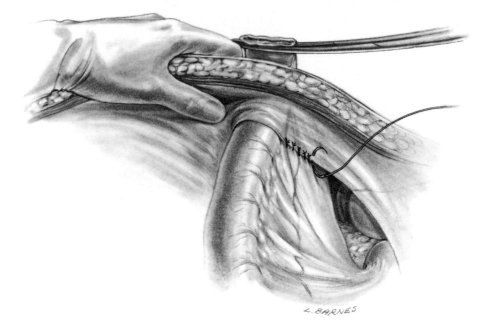

L. BARNES

FIG. 15-96. Intraperitoneal fixation. The falciform ligament is the cephalad limit of closure. The cut edge of the mesentery is sutured to the parietal peritoneum.

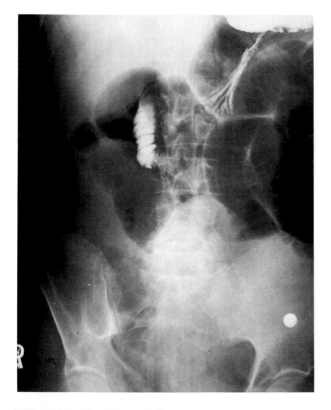

FIG. 15-97. Small bowel obstruction secondary to torsion of the ileum on its mesentery. Barium study reveals complete obstruction proximal to the ileostomy.

Complications

Most complications following proctocolectomy are not unique to the operation: wound infection, intra-abdominal sepsis, wound dehiscence, ureteral and splenic injury, and urinary, pulmonary, and cardiovascular problems. These are discussed in Chapter 10. Complications attributed more specifically to this operation include ileostomy problems, sexual dysfunction, and perineal wound difficulties.

Stomal Problems. Most stomal complications and their management are discussed in the following chapter. A special problem is recurrence in the ileum or in the ileostomy following proctocolectomy for Crohn's disease (Fig. 15-98). Although proctocolectomy is usually curative when granulomatous colitis is confined to the colon, rectum, and anus, between 10% and 15% of patients will develop a recurrence proximally, usually at the site of the ileostomy. A paraileostomy abscess in a patient who underwent resection for Crohn's disease implies recurrence until proved otherwise. Evaluation may include endoscopic examination of the ileostomy, radiologic investigation by means of a barium enema through the stoma, or both.

Treatment almost always requires resection of the involved ileum and ileostomy with relocation of the stoma to another site. In the acute situation it may be possible to drain the abscess by inserting a clamp at

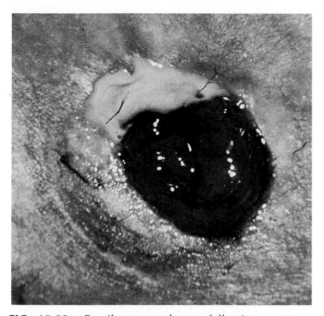

FIG. 15-98. Paraileostomy abscess following proctocolectomy and ileostomy for Crohn's disease. The patient was demonstrated to have terminal ileal recurrence.

the mucocutaneous junction and liberating the pus. This, then, can be incorporated in the ileostomy appliance with a drain left in the cavity. Alternatively, if the abscess "points" at some distance from the ileostomy, drainage should be effected outside of the face plate of the appliance. Every attempt should be made to avoid draining the abscess directly under the face plate; such a maneuver will cause it to be impossible to manage the ileostomy effluent.

Recurrent Crohn's Disease. Recurrent Crohn's disease can develop any time following resection for the condition, even as early as a few days postoperatively. On two occasions I have had to reoperate on patients who underwent proctocolectomy and ileostomy whose entire small bowel was felt to be normal at the time of resection. Because of acute peritoneal signs, the patients were submitted to reexploration within 1 week of the surgery and found to have fulminant inflammatory bowel disease involving extensive areas of the ileum and jejunum.

Intestinal Obstruction. In patients who develop intestinal obstruction following ileostomy, consideration must be given to a paraileostomy hernia as the cause of the problem. Initial conservative management includes nasogastric intubation and possibly an attempt to relieve the obstruction by irrigating the ileostomy. Occasionally the obstruction may be due to inspissated

fecal material or undigested food. As long as the patient is passing flatus it is usually possible to delay surgical intervention. However, if a complete intestinal obstruction is present, early surgical intervention becomes necessary. Occasionally the etiology of the problem is a simple adhesion, but if a paraileostomy hernia with entrapment of the small intestine is the cause, the small bowel must be reduced and the defect closed.

A nonviable distal ileum usually is due to torsion. Obviously, if the stoma itself is necrotic the preoperative diagnosis is self-evident, and resection of the stoma and nonviable bowel is necessary. However, if the blood supply to the ileostomy is preserved, the surgeon may be tempted to resect the nonviable bowel and perform an anastomosis a few inches from the end of the ileostomy. Such a resection is a dangerous undertaking. Unless the area of nonviability is at least 25 cm from the ileostomy, no anastomotic attempt should be made. The stoma should be resected in continuity with the nonviable bowel and a new ileostomy created, usually in the left lower quadrant. Even though this means sacrificing further intestine, the risk of anastomotic leak is so great that preservation of this small segment is not justified.

Sexual Dysfunction. Sexual dysfunction has been mentioned as an unfortunate sequela of proctectomy. It is this complication that makes many surgeons reluctant to remove the rectum at the time of the initial procedure, preferring to perform proctectomy at a later date when it is hoped that the patient will have achieved all procreative ambitions. I am not convinced, however, that a young man in his thirties, with perhaps sufficient children, is particularly grateful for impotence at that age any more than he might have been 10 years previously.

To delay operation, however, is not without problems. The patient must contend with another major operation, with its implications of loss of work, of family hardship, and of changes in life-style. Many patients who feel well are reluctant to submit to an operation that will make them, at least for a time, unwell. Some are lost to follow-up, and some refuse operation. Finally, the risk of malignancy developing in ulcerative colitis and perhaps also in Crohn's colitis has been discussed, and is a very real concern. Many surgeons have experienced the tragedy of incurable carcinoma arising in the long-forgotten, retained rectum.

Impotence after abdominoperineal resection for carcinoma of the rectum is not an uncommon problem, but one questions whether preservation of the rectum and deferment of proctectomy in men is justified solely because of the possibility of subsequent impotence.

We reviewed our experience with 76 postpubescent males who underwent proctocolectomy between the years 1964 and 1973.[45] All patients were interviewed

Table 15-1. Impotence after Proctectomy for Inflammatory Bowel Disease

Reference	Number of patients	Impotence Number	Percent
Bacon and co-workers[11]	39	1	2.8
Burnham et al[36]	118	6	5.1
Donovan and O'Hara[66]	21	1	4.8
May[183]	47	3	6.4
Stahlgren and Ferguson[244]	25	0	0.0
Van Prohaska and Siderius[265]	79	0	0.0
Watts et al[268]	41	7	17.1
Corman et al[45]	76	0	0.0
Total reported series	446	18	4.0

(Corman ML, Veidenheimer MC, Coller JA: Impotence after proctectomy for inflammatory disease of the bowel. Dis Colon Rectum 1978; 21:418–419)

by telephone or reexamined. The mean age of patients at proctectomy was 36 years (range 14 to 71 years). One patient was found to have transient impairment of the ability to achieve an erection, but normal sexual function subsequently developed; after 6 years of follow-up, his function in this area was normal.

Table 15-1 summarizes the reports of other series on impotence following proctectomy for inflammatory bowel disease. While the report of Watts and associates found a high incidence of impotence, patients in their series were older than those in most others.[268] In fact, five of seven patients with impotence were in their late 50s and 60s. When this series is excluded from the overall figures, the rate of impotence is 2.7%. The vast majority of patients in all series who are impotent are in the older age groups.

In my opinion, impotence appears to be less the result of the type of operative approach than of the age of the patient. It seems difficult to believe that careful attention to dissection close to the bowel wall is the reason for a low incidence of impotence whereas the "radical" operation for cancer produces a high incidence. Although one cannot gainsay meticulous surgical technique, preoperative libido is probably a more important factor. The recent report from the Mayo Clinic Group seems to concur with this opinion.[283]

Other concerns about sexual dysfunction are related primarily to the concept of an ileostomy itself, or the need for an external appliance and its impact on sexuality and the body image. These aspects are discussed in the following chapter.

Persistent Perineal Sinus. Persistent perineal sinus is one of the most troubling sequelae of proctectomy for inflammatory bowel disease. The failure of

perineal wounds to heal readily has stimulated considerable discussion and has served as an impetus for the development of a number of operative approaches to deal with the problem (Figs. 15-99 and 15-100).[6, 31, 128, 176, 218, 226, 229, 236] We reviewed our experience with 160 patients who underwent proctectomy for the treatment of inflammatory bowel disease.[46] The mean ages of the patients were the same in both conditions (36 years). The sex incidence for the combined diseases was also the same, but more men than women were diagnosed as having ulcerative colitis and more women than men as having Crohn's colitis. The perineal wounds in 75% of patients with ulcerative colitis were healed by the end of the follow-up period without reoperation, whereas only 52% of wounds in the patients with Crohn's colitis were healed. By the end of the follow-up study, only 11% of patients with ulcerative colitis were not healed, but

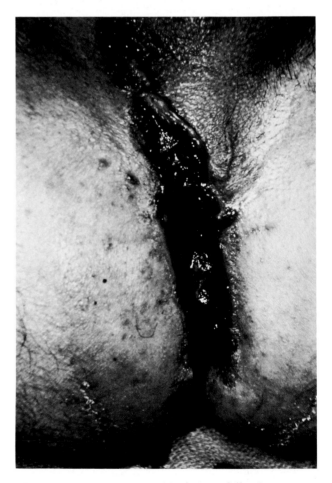

FIG. 15-99. Persistent perineal sinus following proctectomy for inflammatory bowel disease. A chronic, indolent draining wound.

over one third of the patients with Crohn's colitis had not healed.

A number of factors besides the diagnosis seem to be contributing to delayed healing. *Youth* was felt to be a contributing factor, based on our study. All patients more than 50 years of age with ulcerative colitis and all patients more than 60 years old with Crohn's colitis had healed perineal wounds. With respect to *sex*, women with ulcerative colitis (97.5%) were more likely to heal the perineal wound *per primum*, whereas only 82% of men achieved such healing. However, no statistically significant difference in healing was seen when comparing sex distributions in patients with Crohn's disease.

Evaluation of the presence or absence of a *stoma* before proctectomy revealed that in patients with ulcerative colitis, diversion implied an excellent chance for healing. Interestingly, the opposite was true for patients with Crohn's colitis.

Perineal disease, specifically fistula in ano (present at the time of proctectomy), was not a statistically significant factor in nonhealing, although the numbers were small. The rates of nonhealing were almost the same in patients with ulcerative colitis and in patients with Crohn's colitis when a fistula was present. However, in the absence of a perianal fistula, a patient with Crohn's colitis did not heal as well as a patient with ulcerative colitis. These factors are summarized in Table 15-2.

The number of prior operations, extent of disease,

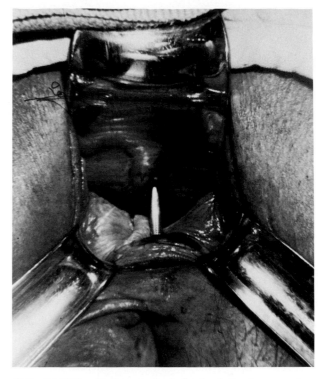

FIG. 15-100. Perineovaginal fistula following proctectomy. Treatment requires fistulotomy. Pregnancy is unlikely to occur in this situation.

Table 15-2.   Healing After Proctectomy

	Ulcerative colitis			Crohn's colitis		
	Healed	Not healed	Percent healed	Healed	Not healed	Percent healed
Age, years						
<20	10	4	71.4	0	2	0.0
20–29	17	2	89.5	14	7	66.7
30–39	21	2	91.3	9	5	64.3
40–49	15	2	88.2	8	5	61.6
50–59	9	0	100.0	6	2	75.0
60–69	7	0	100.0	2	0	100.0
>69	1	0	100.0	1	0	100.0
Sex						
Men	41	9	82.0	17	9	65.4
Women	39	1	97.5	23	12	65.7
Stoma						
Yes	50	1	98.0	25	18	58.1
No	30	9	76.9	15	3	83.3
Fistula						
Yes	4	2	66.7	25	16	61.0
No	76	8	90.5	15	5	75.0

(Corman ML, Veidenheimer MC, Coller JA, Ross VH: Perineal wound healing after proctectomy for inflammatory bowel disease. Dis Colon Rectum 1978; 21:155–159)

Table 15-3. Perineal Wound Healing: Summary of Literature

Author, Year	Diagnosis	Healed, months	Number healed	Number not healed	Percent healed
Hughes, 1965[125]	Ulcerative colitis	Not stated	58	13	81.7
Watts and co-workers, 1966[268]	Ulcerative colitis	6	70	23	75.3
Jalan and co-workers, 1969[132]	Ulcerative colitis Crohn's colitis	6 12	48 67	58 39	45.3 63.2
Roy and co-workers, 1970[225]	Ulcerative colitis Crohn's colitis	3 3	Not stated Not stated	Not stated Not stated	81.6 76.3
Oates and Williams, 1970[208]	Both	Not stated	41	12	77.4
de Dombal and co-workers, 1971[59]	Crohn's colitis	6	39	29	57.4
Ritchie, 1971[218]	Ulcerative colitis Crohn's colitis	6 6	121 4	101 15	54.5 21.1
Broader and co-workers, 1974[31]	Ulcerative colitis Crohn's colitis	6 12	33 11	8 2	80.5 84.6
Irvin and Goligher, 1975,[129]	Ulcerative colitis Crohn's colitis	6 6	23 12	10 7	69.7 63.2
Corman and co-workers, 1978[46]	Crohn's colitis Ulcerative colitis	6 6	17 40	44 50	27.9 44.4

(Corman ML, Veidenheimer MC, Coller JA, Ross VH: Perineal wound healing after proctectomy for inflammatory bowel disease. Dis Colon Rectum 1978; 21:155–159)

emergent, urgent, or elective nature of the surgical procedure, contamination of the wound, presence or absence and duration of steroid therapy, level of serum albumin, and nutritional state of the patient were all analyzed as factors and found to have no significant role in the delay in perineal wound healing.

A number of studies have been summarized in Table 15-3, which serves to indicate the magnitude of the problem.

Many treatments have been advocated to avoid a delay in perineal wound healing. Some authors have demonstrated that packing of the perineal wound is associated with delayed healing.[132, 225] I concur, and have advocated the primary closure method as described in Figure 15-94

Once a perineal sinus has developed, vigorous curettage, creating a pyramidal defect, should be undertaken at 6-month intervals until healing is achieved. Alternative methods include the gracilis myocutaneous

flap,[12] the use of an omental graft,[226] skin grafting,[6] and the use of a fibrin adhesive.[146]

Results

Primary proctocolectomy and ileostomy today can be carried out with very low morbidity and mortality. In a personal experience of 134 operations performed in one stage, I have experienced one death (0.7%). Mavroudis and Schrock reported an operative mortality of 2% in 100 patients who underwent total abdominal colectomy, proctectomy, or both.[182] In the experience of Goligher, 10 operative deaths were noted in 113 patients who underwent proctocolectomy and ileostomy for Crohn's disease, a rate of 9%.[98] In his personal experience in the management of 504 patients with ulcerative colitis, there were 34 operative deaths, an operative mortality of 6.7%.[101] He broke down the mortality among elective, urgent, and emergency surgery, showing the rate in the first category to be under 3%, in the second, 10.7%, and in emergency cases, almost 25%. Other reports suggest that the overall operative mortality for proctocolectomy and ileostomy is between 7% and 10%.

Late mortality due to carcinoma arising in the retained rectum is not a source of concern in patients who undergo proctocolectomy. However, this is certainly a problem that needs to be considered if a sphincter-saving approach is undertaken.

Recurrence following proctocolectomy for Crohn's disease, when the disease is confined to the colon, has been reported to be between 10% and 15%.[98, 160, 247] The prognosis appears to be particularly salutary if total proctocolectomy is performed as compared with a restorative operation.[206] The recurrence rate following restorative surgery in the small and large bowel is discussed later.

Turnbull reported that 6% of 261 patients who underwent proctocolectomy and ileostomy for ulcerative colitis developed small bowel *obstruction* relieved by laparotomy.[260] The complication usually developed within 5 years of the original operation. Sources for the obstruction included an adhesion (most common), ileal torsion, and paraileostomy hernia.

Ileostomy–Colostomy (Treatment of Toxic Megacolon)

Because of the high mortality rate associated with the surgical treatment of toxic megacolon by colectomy (in some series, in excess of 30%), Turnbull and colleagues in 1971 advocated a lesser procedure.[261] This consisted of a diversionary loop ileostomy and two decompressive colostomies, one in the transverse colon and the other in the sigmoid. The colostomies were created at the skin level and were designed to vent the dilated colon as a "blowhole." The major impetus for suggesting this operative approach was to avoid inadvertent gross fecal soiling of the peritoneal cavity when a walled-off perforation had been liberated by mobilization of the bowel. This usually occurs in the region of the splenic flexure, an area that is predisposed to bowel wall necrosis. Considerable contamination can result when the dilated colon is decompressed through this inadvertent orifice. It is the opinion of the Cleveland Clinic group that diversion and decompression will avoid this very serious consequence.

The technique consists of making a small midline incision and identifying a loop of distal ileum. This is brought out through a previously marked site in the right lower quadrant, usually over a small rod (Fig. 15-

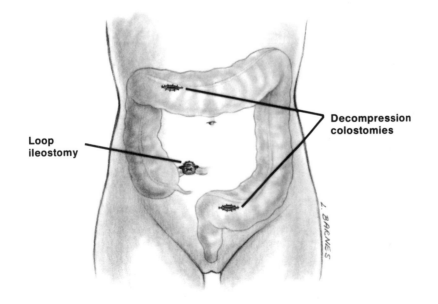

Loop ileostomy

Decompression colostomies

FIG. 15-101. Diverting ileostomy and decompression colostomies for toxic megacolon. (After Turnbull RB Jr, Hawk WA, Weakley FL: Surgical treatment of toxic megacolon: Ileostomy and colostomy to prepare patients for colectomy. Am J Surg 1971; 122:325–331)

101). Ideally, the proximal limb is placed inferiorly and the distal limb superiorly so that subsequent colon resection will not necessitate a change in the fixation of the distal ileum. Exploration of the right upper quadrant of the abdomen identifies the maximum point of dilatation of the transverse colon, and a small incision is made in the skin, fascia, and rectus muscle. If the sigmoid colon is dilated, it, too, can be decompressed by making a small incision in the left iliac fossa, permitting the bowel to bulge into the incision. In more recent reports from the Cleveland Clinic, however, this second blowhole has been felt to be rarely necessary. The abdomen is then closed, and the loop ileostomy is matured, emphasizing the proximal limb (see Figs. 16-55, 16-56, and 16-57).

Attention is then turned to the dilated transverse colon. Seromuscular sutures are placed into the colon and to the peritoneum and rectus fascia with interrupted fine catgut sutures. A second row of seromuscular sutures is placed between the bowel and the subcutaneous fat. The bowel is then opened and the contents liberated. With successful decompression, sutures may now be placed between the cut edge of the bowel and the skin. The same procedure can be used for the sigmoid colon if an opening is necessary in this area.

Although also an advocate of this particular approach, Fazio points out several potential disadvantages.[77] These include the necessity for further major abdominal surgery and possible continued bleeding if hemorrhage was a presenting problem (approximately one quarter of these patients will continue to bleed postoperatively); in addition, if a septic focus persists, earlier surgical intervention may be required.

The Cleveland Clinic group points out that the procedure should not be performed in cases of free perforation, but only when obvious acute colonic dilatation exists *without peritonitis*.

Results

Fazio reported the Cleveland Clinic experience of 115 patients seen from 1961 to 1967 with toxic megacolon; only seven were discharged following medical management.[77] Of interest is the fact that five of the seven required colectomy subsequently. Subtotal colectomy with ileostomy was performed in 26 patients and decompression/diversion in the remaining 83. The mortality rate following subtotal colectomy was 11.5%. Three patients died after decompression/diversion, a mortality rate of 3.6%. However, two additional patients succumbed following elective colectomy, bringing the overall mortality to 6% for the decompression/diversion group. Of the 17 patients found to have free perforations, there were 5 deaths, a mortality rate of almost 30%.

Fazio is reluctant to draw dogmatic conclusions about the value of diversion and decompression. Certainly the mortality appears lower when patients are treated by this technique, but the series is uncontrolled, and it appears that many of the patients who were treated initially by colectomy actually had free perforations, a much higher-risk group.

Zelas and Jagelman reported loop ileostomy as the sole initial procedure in patients who were severely debilitated with Crohn's colitis.[284] This technique was employed in 79 patients, 91% of whom improved. Definitive resection was then undertaken at a later stage without an operative death. They recommended loop ileostomy in certain severely ill patients with this disease. Likewise, Harper and associates discussed the value of ileostomy for IBD. In 102 patients with Crohn's colitis, there was an immediate clinical improvement in 95, with sustained remission of symptoms for considerable lengths of time.[117] In a number of patients who might otherwise have been treated by proctocolectomy, it was possible subsequently to restore intestinal continuity.

Comment

I am able to restrain my enthusiasm for the decompression/diversion technique in the treatment of toxic megacolon primarily for the reasons that were alluded to by Fazio. It is troublesome as a concept to commit the patient to at least one other operation when the procedure can be accomplished in one stage, removing the source of sepsis, and liberating the patient from contending with at least two abdominal orifices. Draining upper and lower abdominal wounds may be a justified, albeit unaesthetic experience, if one is convinced that it is the only life-saving measure available, but I believe that expeditious, well-conceived resection can accomplish the optimal goal. To free a sealed perforation, I suggest that the transverse colon might possibly be decompressed by simple needle aspiration before "attacking" the splenic flexure. Another alternative would be to mobilize the sigmoid and descending colon and the transverse colon, dividing the bowel at the point of planned resection and exteriorizing the bowel so that minimal contamination will result should a sealed perforation be encountered. Finally, there is a certain impracticality in the advice on the technique for creating the colon decompression. In my experience, attempting to suture a profoundly dilated, possibly necrotic transverse colon is more than a frustrating experience, it is impossible. Passing a suture into the bowel itself is likely to cause perforation; the procedure is analogous to trying to suture wet toilet paper. In an admittedly small personal experience of 17 patients with toxic megacolon, I have applied resection as the modality of therapy, with no deaths.

Ileorectal Anastomosis

Total abdominal colectomy with ileorectal or ileosigmoid anastomosis for ulcerative colitis has been advocated by a number of authors, but particularly by Aylett.[8–10] The subject has been addressed earlier with respect to the risk of the subsequent development of malignancy in the rectal segment. The technical aspect of total colectomy is identical to the surgical approach described in Chapter 10.

Farnell and colleagues reported the Mayo Clinic experience with rectal preservation in nonspecific inflammatory bowel disease.[76] Sixty-three patients with ulcerative colitis and 80 patients with Crohn's disease underwent colectomy and ileorectal or ileosigmoid anastomosis. Follow-up was a minimum of 5 years up to a maximum of 17 years. During this interval, no patient developed carcinoma in the residual rectum. The requirement for subsequent proctectomy was quite similar in both ulcerative colitis patients and Crohn's disease patients (24% versus 29%, respectively). The quality of life was felt to be satisfactory in over half of the patients with ulcerative colitis, but only approximately one third of the patients with Crohn's disease were satisfied. Early age of onset of ulcerative colitis was demonstrated to be a poor prognostic factor for subsequent rectal preservation. Patients who developed the disease later in life were more likely to avoid subsequent proctectomy. Preoperative proctoscopic examination revealed a normal rectum in slightly over half of the patients with ulcerative colitis, whereas the rectum was felt to be uninvolved in 70% of patients with Crohn's disease. Moderate disease was present in 38% of the former and 19% of the latter. Interestingly enough, the presence of moderate rectal mucosal disease did not increase the likelihood of subsequent proctectomy.

Buchmann and co-workers reported 105 patients treated with colectomy and ileorectal anastomosis for Crohn's disease.[34] The mean follow-up was approximately 7½ years. The presence or absence of ileal disease or perianal disease at the time of the anastomosis did not affect the prognosis, but patients with sigmoidoscopic evidence of inflammatory disease in the rectum appeared to do less well. The risk of reoperation for recurrence after this anastomosis was calculated actuarially to be 50% after 16 to 20 years. The authors felt that the anastomotic procedure as described was a reasonable alternative for most patients with Crohn's colitis who do not have severe involvement of the rectum.

From the same unit, Keighley and associates performed balloon distention of the rectum and barium enema examination to assess rectal capacity.[142] They determined that a severely contracted rectum was associated with the need for a stoma in 6 of 7 patients, compared with only 2 of 13 patients who did not have radiologic signs of narrowing. Others have also been relatively enthusiastic in recommending ileorectal anastomosis for selected patients with inflammatory bowel disease.[126, 137]

Comment

In my opinion, ileorectal anastomosis for Crohn's colitis is the procedure of choice when the rectum is relatively spared and when the patient does not have significant anal disease. With the passage of time, the likelihood of symptoms that warrant either proctectomy or diversion is probably on the order of one third of the patients. But even those individuals who must undergo a second procedure can still be relatively well served by temporarily avoiding an ileostomy. The problem, of course, is to select the appropriate patients, an exceedingly difficult task. One is often surprised at the degree of inflammatory reaction that a patient may harbor in the rectum or indeed in the anal region and still have a relatively salutary result following a restorative operation. However, patients who demonstrate pelvic sepsis, an intra-abdominal abscess, or a fistula to the rectum should probably undergo a temporary diverting loop ileostomy to protect the anastomosis. This is obviously a surgical judgment decision, and each patient must be treated on an individual basis.

Those who are troubled by frequent bowel movements can often be helped by the addition of a bulk agent containing psyllium and "slowing" medications such as codeine, deodorized tincture of opium, and Lomotil or Imodium.

With ileorectal anastomosis for ulcerative colitis, I reiterate what I stated previously, that the possibility of carcinoma arising in the residual rectum is a source of great concern. If the patient truly understands this risk and is willing to submit to frequent (6-month) follow-up examinations, I believe that ileorectal anastomosis should be considered in those in whom the rectum is not severely involved by inflammatory disease. However, if concern for possible development of carcinoma is great enough, and conventional proctocolectomy is an unacceptable option, consideration should be given to one of the newer operative approaches (see later).

Other Restorative Operations

Alternative operations for *ulcerative colitis* to restore intestinal continuity besides ileorectal anastomosis are contraindicated. Segmental resection of the sigmoid colon, right colon, and so forth will result in a uniform 100% recurrence rate that will necessitate further resection. The only exception to this admonition is the patient who has severe proctitis or proctosigmoiditis with profound urgency and tenesmus. An abdominoperineal resection might be performed without the patient developing recurrent disease.

With *Crohn's disease,* restoration of intestinal continuity is certainly a viable option under many circumstances, depending on the location and the extent of disease. Because Crohn's disease can occur anywhere in the gastrointestinal tract, it is difficult to discuss the operative choices as they pertain solely to the colon and rectum.

Management of Small Bowel Crohn's Disease

As mentioned earlier, the indications for surgery for regional enteritis include inanition, intra-abdominal sepsis, intestinal obstruction, fistulas, urologic complications, and extra-intestinal manifestations. The choice of operative procedure depends on the intra-abdominal findings.

Occasionally a patient is submitted to laparotomy with a presumed diagnosis of acute appendicitis. An inflamed, erythematous, edematous, *acute distal ileitis* may be identified. The appendix may be safely removed if there is no evidence of cecal disease. Conversely, if the ileum and cecum appear to be involved by a chronic inflammatory process, appendectomy may result in a fecal fistula. Laparotomy alone may lead to a fistula through handling of the diseased bowel, presumably from disrupting microperforations of the distal ileum.[78] No resection of the ileal involvement is advised. In an extensive review of the incidence of progression of regional enteritis involving only the distal ileum, Gump and associates reported that less than 10% of patients developed subsequent identifiable ileitis.[110]

When surgery is indicated for other than acute ileitis, resection of the involved segment is performed. Types of operations include limited small bowel resection, multiple small bowel resections, resection of distal ileum in continuity with cecum or right colon, right hemicolectomy, subtotal colectomy, total colectomy, and, of course, proctocolectomy.

When an enteroenteric fistula is identified, it is important to try to ascertain whether the bowel was involved primarily by Crohn's disease or secondarily. For example, in the latter situation, resection of the segment of bowel that is not involved in the Crohn's process can be avoided. A not-infrequent circumstance is when the involved terminal ileum creates an ileosigmoid fistula. Resection of the ileum is undertaken with division of the fistulous communication to the sigmoid colon. Whether a resection of the sigmoid is appropriate depends on the degree of inflammatory reaction. Usually, if the opening can simply be sutured, no resection is advised.

Partial resections of the involved colon (transverse colectomy, left partial colectomy, sigmoid resection), are usually not advised because of the high rate of recurrence. Wide lymphadenectomy is also not indicated, because there has been no evidence to suggest that enlarged residual lymph nodes contribute to subsequent recurrence.

The resection is usually undertaken with a margin of a minimum of 10 cm. If multiple "skip" areas are present it is sometimes necessary to leave behind residual disease in order to avoid serious nutritional problems. Under these circumstances one endeavors only to remove or bypass the most constricting portions that may be causing the symptoms. If two segments are involved in relative proximity (less than 30 cm), it is probably safer to perform an en bloc resection of both segments rather than to perform two anastomoses.

A bypass or exclusion procedure has been advocated for distal ileal and cecal Crohn's disease. These operations are to be condemned because of the high incidence of persistent septic problems and the association with subsequent development of carcinoma. The only patients for whom bypass surgery is not contraindicated are those with duodenal lesions and those who have multiple "skip" areas throughout the small bowel.

Results. Trnka and co-workers reviewed 113 patients with Crohn's disease whose initial procedure involved an anastomosis.[257] The recurrence rate was 29% at 5 years, 52% at 10 years, and 84% at 25 years. There was no relationship between the incidence of recurrence and the age of the patient, the sex, the duration of disease, the presence or absence of granulomas, the length of the resected specimen, and the presence or absence of disease at the proximal resection margin. Patients with colon disease who underwent an anastomosis had a much higher incidence of recurrence than those patients who had small bowel involvement. Frikker and Segall also reported that patients with small bowel disease had a better prognosis than did patients with ileocolic involvement.[86]

Wolff and associates reported the Mayo Clinic experience of over 700 patients who underwent surgery for Crohn's disease with an anastomosis.[281] Those patients who were demonstrated to have microscopic involvement of the resection margin were found to have a recurrence rate of approximately 90% within the follow-up period of 8 years. Those patients who did not have such involvement had a 55% incidence of recurrence at 10 years. The authors concluded that clear margins should be obtained in resections for Crohn's disease if this is at all possible. Most surgeons feel that visual impression is as accurate as frozen section histologic examination.

Lock and co-workers reported the Cleveland Clinic experience of 127 patients with Crohn's disease of the *large bowel* who underwent excisional surgery.[173] Initial involvement of the terminal ileum in addition to the large bowel was associated with a statistically significant higher incidence of overall recurrence and earlier postoperative recurrence when compared with patients who had ileal sparing.

Homan and Dineen compared the results of resection, bypass, and exclusion for ileocecal Crohn's disease.[124] In a total of 161 patients, resection was performed in 115, bypass with exclusion in 25, and bypass alone in 21. Recurrence rates were 25% for resection, 63% for bypass with exclusion, and 75% for bypass alone. With 15 years of follow-up, bypass was seen to be associated with a 94% recurrence rate. The authors concluded that resection can be performed with a morbidity and mortality equivalent to either of the bypass procedures and that the recurrence rate following resection is significantly lower than either bypass or exclusion.

In our reported experience with the long-term fol-low-up of small intestinal Crohn's disease, the commonest indication for surgical treatment was chronic obstruction (35%), followed by internal fistulas (30%), intractability (22%), and abscess formation (11%).[250] Eighty-five percent of the patients had a resection of the terminal ileum and cecum with an anastomosis performed between the distal ileum and the ascending colon. The average length of small bowel removed at the initial resection was 57 cm. No frozen-section biopsies of the proximal margin were performed; subsequent histologic examination revealed two instances (3%) in which the surgeon did not suspect involvement.

Recurrent Crohn's disease developed after the initial bowel resection in 51 patients (69%). Of these patients, 28 (55%) required a second operation. Of these, 18 had further recurrence of the disease, but in none did further operative intervention prevent subsequent recurrence. Some patients even required a third and fourth procedure because of disease-related complications. In other words, no patient was cured if he or she required a third operation (Fig. 15-102).

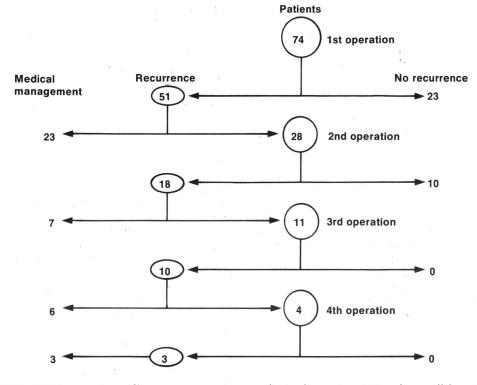

FIG. 15-102. Pattern of recurrence in patients who underwent resection for small bowel Crohn's disease. (Based on data from Stone W, Veidenheimer MC, Corman ML, Coller JA: The dilemma of Crohn's disease: Long-term follow-up of Crohn's disease of the small intestine. Dis Colon Rectum 1977; 20:372–376)

As mentioned previously, patients who require re-resection after an initial procedure for sigmoid diverticulitis should be presumed to have Crohn's colitis until proved otherwise. In our experience with 25 patients resected for "diverticulitis" a second time, all were found to have Crohn's disease in the specimen.[19] The illness is characterized by the requirement for multiple operations, failure of diversionary procedures to control the distal disease, presence of anorectal disease, rectal bleeding, and fistulas.

Comment. The results of surgery for Crohn's disease are less than satisfactory. The idea that repeated resections will ultimately cure the patient is completely erroneous. Unless one is to extirpate the entire gastrointestinal tract, one can never be truly assured that recurrent disease will not develop. It is evident from our study and from the research of others that the more resections that are required, the less the likelihood of cure. No patient was cured in our series who required more than two operations for the treatment of the disease.

One must, therefore, limit surgical intervention to those patients who have complications severe enough to justify an operation. Long-standing disease is not a surgical indication as it classically has been for ulcerative colitis. Since it is too soon to make a determination of the appropriateness of dysplasia in patients with Crohn's disease, and since the incidence of malignant change is so low, this in itself is not an indication for surgical intervention. Bypass procedures and exclusion operations should not be performed except in the critically ill patient. Under these circumstances definitive resection should be undertaken at the earliest possible time.

Total Abdominal Colectomy (Mucosal Proctectomy) and Ileoanal Anastomosis

In 1977, Martin and colleagues described a procedure in children whereby the entire colon was removed in the usual manner, but the mucosa was stripped from the rectal muscular sleeve and an anastomosis effected between the ileum and the anal canal.[180] By this means intestinal continuity was reestablished and all of the potential disease-bearing area was extirpated. The procedure is theoretically suitable for patients with ulcerative colitis and those with familial polyposis. However, patients who have Crohn's disease, particularly with anal manifestations, should not be submitted to this operation. Although the procedure is not a new one (with the exception of the denuded muscular cuff), it had fallen into disrepute because of complications associated with the anastomosis and the poor functional results.

Operative Technique. The total abdominal colectomy is undertaken in the usual manner and the bowel resected as low as possible in the rectum. Initially, the mucosal stripping was undertaken commencing at the level of the sacral promontory in order to preserve a long muscular sleeve (Fig. 15-103). Utsunomiya and co-workers advocate a balloon catheter as a rectal internal stent to facilitate the mucosal stripping (Fig. 15-103, C).[263] The procedure is performed by infiltrating the submucosa with a dilute epinephrine solution. The initial advantage of preserving this muscular sleeve was theoretical; it was felt that it protected the anastomosis. However, complications such as "sleeve abscess" developed, and the tedious dissection required to create the sleeve caused most surgeons to abandon this particular approach. In current practice, one endeavors to amputate the rectum as low as is possible, removing the residual mucosa (if any) by way of the perineal dissection.

Tension on the ileal mesentery is a potential problem, because the ileum must be brought virtually to the perianal skin. Complete mobilization of the ileal mesentery up to the level of the duodenum is usually required. The ileal artery may be divided to further elongate the mesentery, and the parietal peritoneum of the distal ileum may be incised.

The anastomosis is effected at the level of the dentate line using paired Gelpi or Parks' retractors for exposure. Interrupted 000 long-term absorbable sutures are suggested between the edge of the ileum and the anal canal and underlying internal sphincter (Fig. 15-104). A protecting loop ileostomy should be performed in all cases (see Figs. 16-55, 16-56, and 16-57).

Results. Utsunomiya and associates reported a few patients who underwent the above operation, but in the same paper described a technique with an intervening pouch (see later).[263] It is difficult to interpret the results because of the multiplicity of techniques used. Beart and co-workers reported the Mayo Clinic experience with 50 patients who underwent total abdominal colectomy, excision of the rectal mucosa, and ileoanal anastomosis.[17] Forty-one patients were operated on for chronic ulcerative colitis; familial polyposis was the diagnosis in seven patients, and Crohn's disease in two. The authors emphasized the importance of meticulous hemostasis, preservation of the anoderm, careful stripping of all the rectal mucosa, and avoidance of tension on the suture line. A number of these patients had an intervening "reservoir."

Forty-two patients had reestablishment of intestinal continuity by closure of the ileostomy; no deaths occurred in the series. Two had anastomotic strictures requiring conversion to an ileostomy, and nine additional patients were dissatisfied because of stool fre-

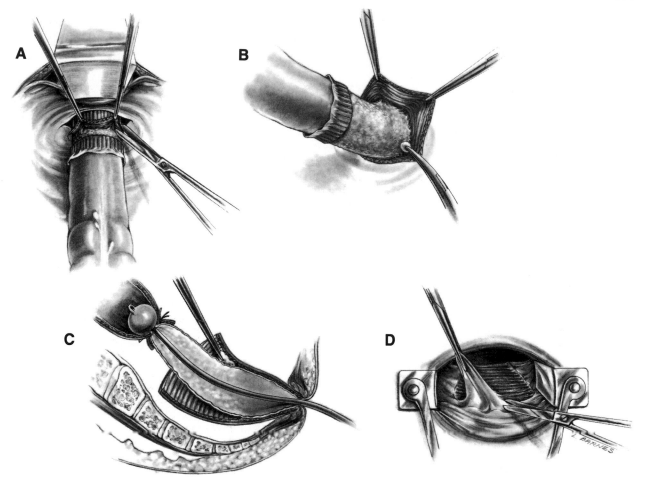

FIG. 15-103. Rectal mucosal stripping. **A.** Commencing at the top of the rectum. **B.** Completed from above. **C.** Facilitated by internal stent. **D.** By perineal route.

quency and were converted to either a Kock pouch (see later) or a conventional ileostomy. In the remaining 30 patients, stool frequency averaged eight per day, but most required "slowing" medications. Heppell and colleagues reviewed 12 of these patients at least 4 months after the procedure by means of physiologic studies.[121] Anal sphincter resting pressure and squeeze pressure of patients who underwent the procedure were similar to those of healthy controls, although the rectal inhibitory reflex was absent. The greater the capacity of the new rectum, the fewer the number of bowel movements. Although the procedure did indeed preserve the anal sphincter, the usual decreased capacity and compliance of the distal bowel impaired continence.

Coran reported the procedure on 36 children and adults with ulcerative colitis and familial polyposis.[43] Four patients were converted to an ileostomy subsequently. The median stool frequency was seven per 24 hours. This was interpreted by the author to be an encouraging result.

Comment.   The ileoanal anastomosis successfully reestablishes intestinal continuity but with the distinct disadvantage of frequent bowel movements. It requires great motivation indeed on the part of the patient to avoid an ileostomy and willingness to accept seven or more bowel movements per day. One wonders how many bowel movements the patient had preoperatively; I suspect no more, and probably fewer. In any

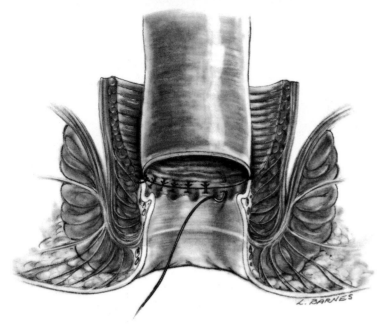

FIG. 15-104. Endoanal anastomotic technique. Paired Gelpi retractors are suggested.

event, the discussion appears moot. Witness the Mayo Clinic's experience and their concern about the decreased reservoir function of the rectum; they have abandoned this procedure in favor of the ileoanal anastomosis with intervening pouch.

Total Proctocolectomy and Ileoanal Anastomosis with Intervening Pouch (Parks)

As mentioned, total abdominal proctocolectomy with ileoanal anastomosis is associated with frequent bowel movements, urgency, and fecal incontinence in a high percentage of cases. With the success of the ileal reservoir as described by Kock (see later), Parks and Nicholls described an operation that combines an ileal pouch that eliminates propulsive activity and acts as a storage organ, with the preservation of the entire sphincter mechanism.[212]

Technique. The patient is placed in the perineolithotomy position as if for an abdominoperineal resection. Following completion of the colectomy and excision of the rectum as far distally as is possible, an ileal reservoir is created. The two types of reservoir or pouch are the S-type (Fig. 15-105, and the J-type (Fig. 15-106). The former is that which was originally described by Parks, but the latter is simpler and is the preferred procedure according to Utsunomiya and coworkers.[263] In the S-pouch, the terminal 50 cm of

ileum are measured and folded twice to give three segments of bowel, the proximal two of which are 15 cm long, and the distal segment, 20 cm long. A 5-cm length of ileum projects beyond the pouch, which is the area to be used for the anastomosis. The ileum is opened on its antimesenteric border (see Fig. 15-105, *B*), and the adjacent loops are sutured (see Fig. 15-105, *C*). An interrupted technique may be used, but a continuous suture of 000 long-term absorbable material is more expeditious. The two outer edges are then folded across to complete the pouch, with the closure effected using the same suture material (see Fig. 15-105, *D*).

The anastomosis is performed by the transanal approach using a Parks retractor or paired Gelpi retractors placed at right angles. As mentioned previously, no attempt is made to preserve a muscular sleeve. Any small amount of residual rectal mucosa is removed by the anal route. A dilute solution of epinephrine injected under the submucosa facilitates the dissection. The full thickness of the ileum is sutured to the anal canal at the level of the dentate line, incorporating the underlying internal anal sphincter muscle.

FIG. 15-105. S-type (Parks) ileal reservoir. **A.** The bowel is aligned. **B.** The antimesenteric aspect is opened after serosal apposition. **C.** Suturing of the adjacent walls. **D.** The reservoir is completed with an ileoanal anastomosis. ▶

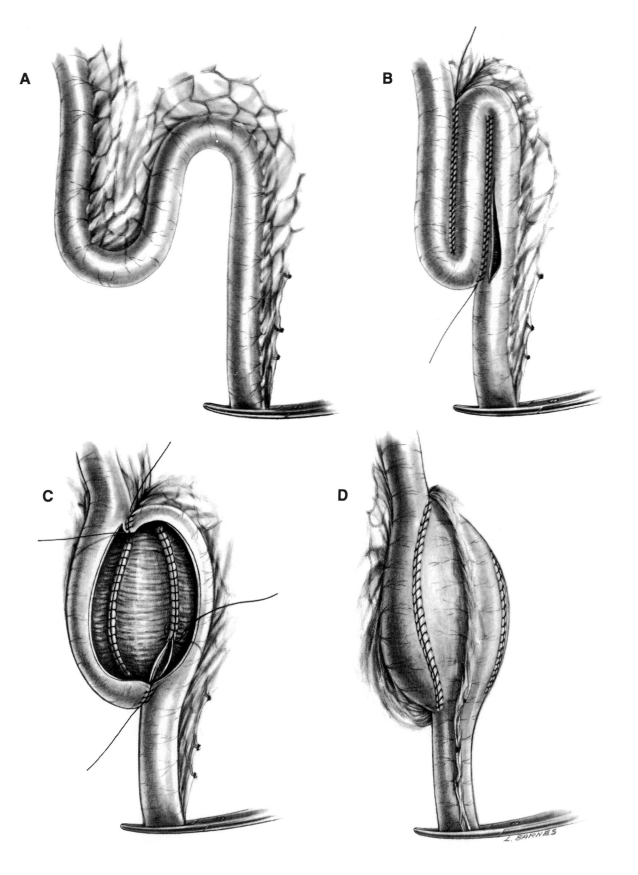

Parks and associates advised draining the pelvis through the intersphincteric plane, but some surgeons prefer either no drainage or a suprapubic suction drain.[213] An alternative would be to drain the pelvis through the levators and the buttocks with a suction drain. A loop ileostomy is *always performed* to protect the anastomosis.

The J-pouch is prepared by selecting the point at which the ileal loop reaches the lowest level of the pelvis, usually about 25 cm from the end of the ileum. Apposition of the loop is performed using a continuous seromuscular suture, and a long side-to-side anastomosis is created. The authors suggest using a GIA stapling device to create the reservoir.[263] The length of the pouch is approximately 20 cm. An anastomosis is effected between the side of the pouch and the anal canal in the manner described above (see Fig. 15-106, *C*). Again, a loop ileostomy is always performed.

Results. Parks and colleagues reported 21 patients, 17 with ulcerative colitis and 4 with polyposis.[213] There was no mortality and no disturbance of urinary or sexual function. All patients were observed to be continent of feces completely during the day, but one patient was incontinent at night. The average frequency of bowel evacuation was approximately 4 times in 24 hours. Approximately half of the patients required a catheter to facilitate defecation. Two patients required medications to reduce the frequency of bowel actions.

Pescatori and associates reviewed 34 patients who underwent this operation, studying them by "evacuation pouchography."[215] The purpose of the study was to determine why some patients could evacuate spontaneously and others had to insert a catheter several times a day to empty the pouch. The 50% who were able to have a spontaneous evacuation had a signifi-

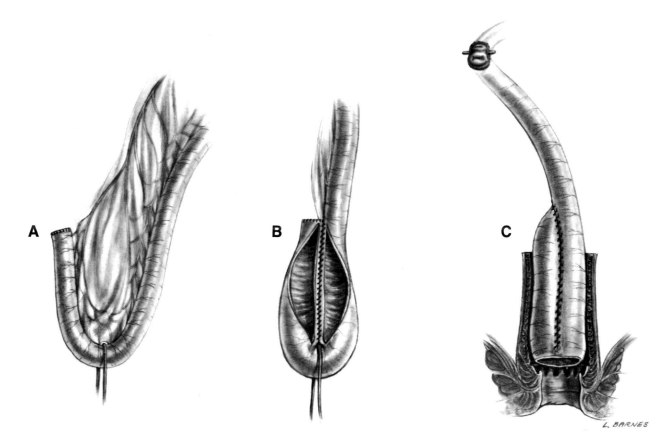

FIG. 15-106. J-type (Utsunomiya) ileal reservoir. **A.** The bowel is aligned. **B.** The antimesenteric aspect is opened and the adjacent walls are sutured. **C.** The reservoir is completed with a side-to-end ileoanal anastomosis.

cantly shorter distal segment (mean 8 ± 3 cm), as compared with those who had to use a catheter to empty the pouch, in whom the distal segment was longer (mean 11 ± 4 cm). The authors felt that the longer the distal segment, the more likely it was to be angulated. Short segments were demonstrated to fill on straining as compared with the longer segments, which often failed to fill while the patient strained.

Rothenberger and co-workers reported their experience in 29 patients with this operation.[224] Operative time averaged 5½ hours, and the average hospital stay following surgery averaged 10 days. The length of time from the completion of the restorative procedure to closure of the loop ileostomy averaged 3 months. Complications included skin excoriation, strictured anastomosis, "pouchitis," partial incontinence, and peritonitis. The length of follow-up of 24 patients whose ileostomy was closed averaged 4.5 months. Fourteen emptied their pouches spontaneously by straining. Eight patients occasionally used the catheter to empty the pouch, whereas only two patients found it necessary to always empty the pouch by means of the catheter. Four patients reported minimal leakage during the day or at night; mucus discharge was common. All patients reported total continence for gas and often found it difficult to eliminate flatus. The mean number of bowel movements in a 24-hour period was six (range: 2 to 11). All but six patients required some medication to control the consistency or frequency of bowel action. The authors felt that the functional results were indeed promising and that the patient satisfaction was quite high. Others also reported a gratifying experience with this operative approach.[115]

Utsunomiya and co-workers reported their experience with the J-pouch.[263] They felt that the J-pouch was superior because the reservoir is located in the lowest part of the pelvic area, similar to the normal rectal ampulla. This is a theoretic advantage over the Parks procedure. They also believed that their method has the potential advantage of posing less risk of mesenteric injury.

Taylor and colleagues reported the initial Mayo Clinic experience with 74 patients who underwent the ileal-pouch anal anastomosis using a J-reservoir.[253] In comparing their patients with those who underwent a straight ileoanal anastomosis, the authors noted that stool frequency with the pouch was less (mean, 7 stools per 24 hours, as opposed to 11 stools in 24 hours in the straight ileoanal group). Major nocturnal incontinence was also less in the pouch group (0% versus 20%).

As of this writing, the updated report by Beart of the Mayo Clinic included 118 patients who underwent the J-pouch, ileoanal anastomosis. There were no operative or postoperative deaths. An average follow-up of 8 months following ileostomy closure revealed that all patients could defecate spontaneously; the mean stool frequency was approximately 7 in 24 hours. During the day, 83% had complete fecal continence, 12% had minor staining, and 5% had fecal leakage. At night, two thirds were completely continent, 31% noted minor staining, and 3% had fecal leakage. Only two patients were considered failures. Since each patient served as his own control, the only patients who were dissatisfied when comparing their operation to the prior ileostomy were the two reported failures. Beart concludes that "although no available alternative will establish normal stooling patterns, the procedure does seem to offer a very acceptable quality of life when compared with the other alternatives available."

Fonkalsrud reported his experience with a modified pouch procedure in which he created a "lateral" ileal reservoir.[83–85] This was accomplished by performing an ileoanal anastomosis, dividing and oversewing the proximal end approximately 25 to 30 cm above the peritoneal reflection. A temporary end ileostomy is then used for diversion (Fig. 15-107, *A*). A lateral reservoir is constructed over the entire length of the original segment on a subsequent operation (Fig. 15-107, *B*).

The author reported his experience with 21 patients (mean age approximately 17 years) with ulcerative colitis and polyposis. The author felt that the procedure was superior to the results obtained by an S-shaped reservoir. A mean of four continent bowel movements per 24 hours was achieved within 4 weeks in patients with lateral reservoirs. There was no mortality and a relatively low morbidity, sepsis being the most frequently observed problem.

Comment. The ileal reservoir with endoanal anastomosis in the treatment of patients with ulcerative colitis must still be considered an experimental operation, in my opinion. There is no question that many patients seem quite pleased with the results and do serve as their own controls (since each has a protecting ileostomy for a time), but in most surgeons' experience, the procedure has a high morbidity. Mortality is low primarily because an ileostomy is a requisite until the ileoanal anastomosis has healed.

Before the surgeon offers this procedure as an alternative to conventional ileostomy or reservoir ileostomy, the patient should be highly motivated to accept the consequences: frequent bowel movements and possible soilage. If the patient has such an incentive, I believe that the procedure can be reasonably offered knowing that the long-term follow-up evaluation is still lacking. Because of the risk of recurrence, the operation is contraindicated in patients with Crohn's disease.

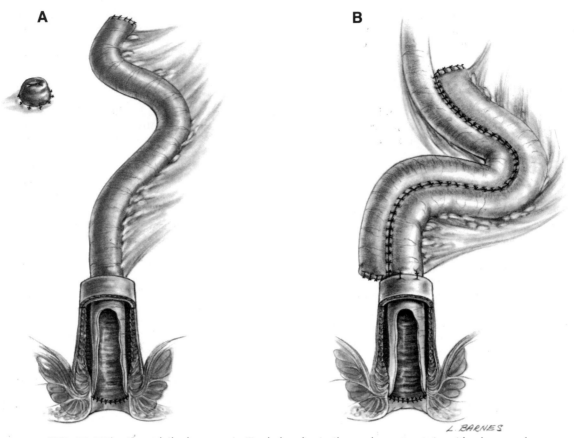

FIG. 15-107. Lateral ileal reservoir (Fonkalsrud). **A.** Ileoanal anastomosis with closure of the proximal ileum and ileostomy. **B.** Lateral reservoir, created after takedown of the end ileostomy.

Continent Ileostomy (Kock)

Because of the not-uncommon problems associated with conventional ileostomy, including skin irritation, appliance management difficulties, and the psychological disability associated with wearing an appliance, Kock devised a method of creating a reservoir from the terminal ileum, and subsequently modified it to create an intestinal obstruction by means of an intussuscepted portion of distal ileum, the so-called nipple valve.[152–154] However, in spite of some considerable success, problems arose in maintaining the position of the nipple. Extrusion not uncommonly developed, usually within 3 months of surgery. A number of modifications have been proposed to address this complication, including implantation of Mersilene mesh to reinforce the nipple,[15] magnetic closure using the Maclet closure device[230] (see Chap. 16), stripping the serosa, and even a protecting loop ileostomy created above the reservoir.[127] Bokey and Fazio suggest the use of a fascial sling threaded through the mesentery to prevent reduction of the nipple.[25] Gerber and co-workers recommend encircling the ileal outlet with a 1-cm strip of Marlex mesh passed through the mesentery of the reservoir and outlet.[93]

Technique. There are two basic reservoir techniques that may be employed. One is the S-shaped reservoir such as was described for the Parks procedure (see Fig. 15-105). This technique requires approximately 10 cm for each segment (three segments in all to create the pouch). An additional 18 to 20 cm are required to make the nipple valve and the conduit.

The Kock technique involves preparation of approximately a 50-cm segment of terminal ileum. Thirty centimeters are used to create the pouch and the remainder to make the valve and the external conduit. Figures 15-108 through 15-116 illustrate the procedure of creating the continent (reservoir) ileostomy.

(Text continues on p. 620)

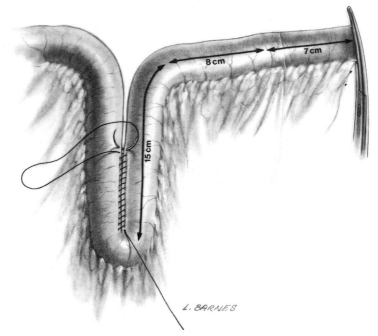

FIG. 15-108. Continent ileostomy: apposition of the bowel.

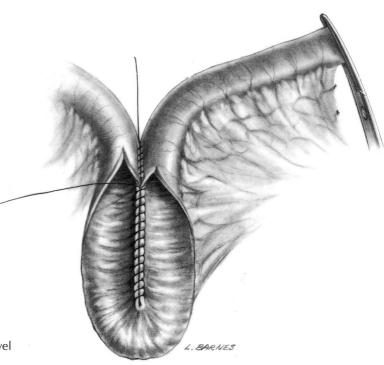

FIG. 15-109. Continent ileostomy: bowel opened and posterior row completed.

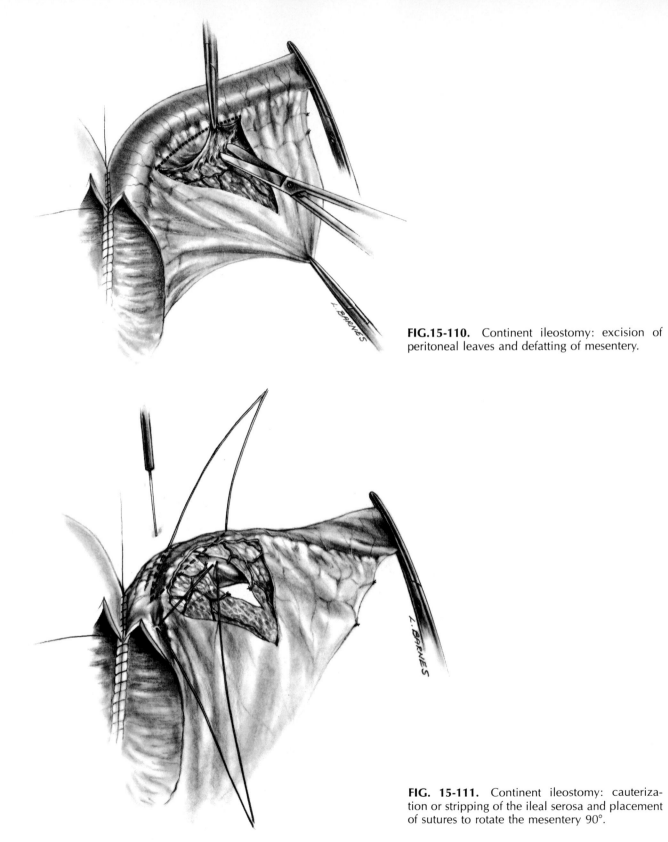

FIG.15-110. Continent ileostomy: excision of peritoneal leaves and defatting of mesentery.

FIG. 15-111. Continent ileostomy: cauterization or stripping of the ileal serosa and placement of sutures to rotate the mesentery 90°.

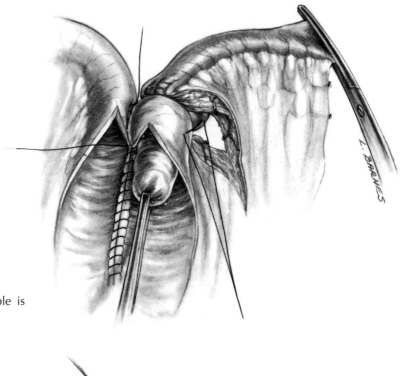

FIG. 15-112. Continent ileostomy: a nipple is created and sutures are secured.

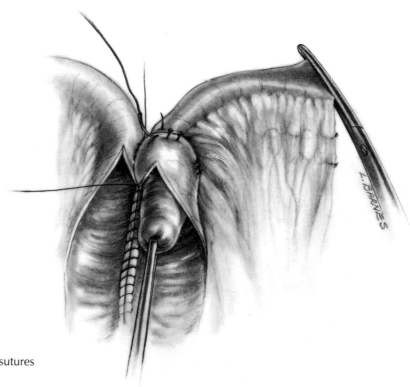

FIG. 15-113. Continent ileostomy: silk sutures placed from conduit to reservoir.

Before the ileostomy is "matured," the competence of the nipple valve should be tested by means of clamping the afferent limb with a rubber-shod clamp. A catheter is then inserted through the nipple valve into the reservoir and inflated with air. If the air fails to escape after the catheter has been removed, one may assume that the valve is competent. The catheter is then re-

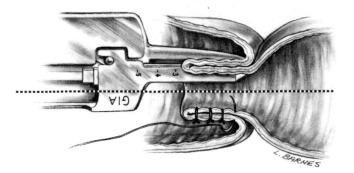

FIG. 15-114. Continent ileostomy: Application of SGIA-50 stapler to nipple valve in three aspects. Alternatively, sutures may be used.

placed into the reservoir, and the air should escape. The completed reservoir is shown in Figure 15-117.

The stoma can be made quite low on the abdominal wall and flush with the skin.

Postoperative Care.   Prior to leaving the operating room, the surgeon places a heavy silk suture around a silastic catheter which has been inserted into the pouch. The suture is secured to the skin and a dressing applied in such a manner that the catheter exits upwards and gently curves into a drainage tube, and from thence into a drainable bag. The straight exit of the catheter minimizes the risk of necrosis of the conduit should the catheter be under tension on one side. Initially, I was inclined to look at the ileostomy every 24 hours to ascertain viability, but more recently I have left the dressing in place for 72 hours before examining the stoma. An alternative is to use a Marlen continent ileostomy drainage system (Fig. 15-118).

Usually there will be only serosanguineous drainage for the first several days; eventually this becomes bile-stained and then feculent. The patient is then begun on a progressive intake, but a low-residue diet is suggested to avoid plugging of the catheter. The catheter

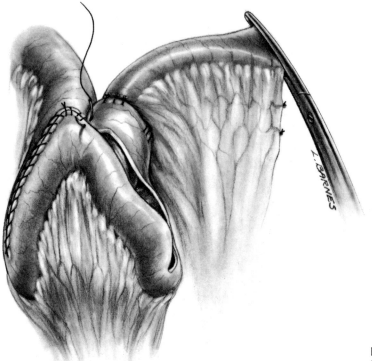

FIG. 15-115. Continent ileostomy: the reservoir is closed by folding over.

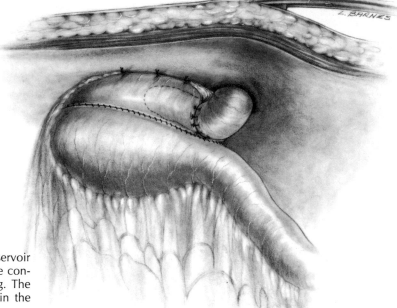

FIG. 15-116. Continent ileostomy. The reservoir is anchored to the abdominal wall after the conduit has been brought through the opening. The ileostomy opening is usually placed low in the abdomen.

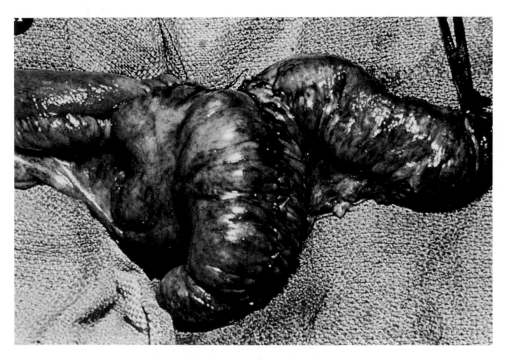

FIG. 15-117. Continent ileostomy: completed reservoir and nipple.

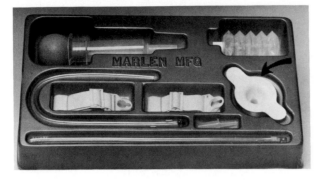

FIG. 15-118. The continent ostomy set includes catheters, lubricant, belts, irrigating syringe, and a device for immediate postoperative support of the catheter *(arrow)*. (Courtesy of Marlen Manufacturing and Development Co.)

remains in place for 3 weeks, after which the patient is advised to clamp it for 10 or 15 minutes every 3 or 4 hours. During the night it is left to drain continuously.

After 1 month the patient is instructed on intermittent catheterization, initially every 3 or 4 hours and usually once during the night. After approximately 1 week of this regimen, nightly intubations are omitted and the interval for catheterization during the day is extended. Ultimately the patient develops a time frequency based on his convenience and the feeling of fullness that impels a requirement for drainage. Various continent ileostomy catheters are shown in Figure 15-119. Occasionally, formed fecal material and high-residue items (such as popcorn, mushrooms, *etc.*) require irrigation by means of a syringe, but this is usually unnecessary. A simple dressing is placed over the flush stoma, or one of the commercially available security pouches may be used.

Complications. The greatest concern in the postoperative period is the possibility of *leakage* from one of the reservoir suture lines. Obviously, this can be of catastrophic consequence, requiring emergency surgical intervention. Initially the complication was reported much more commonly than it is today. This is

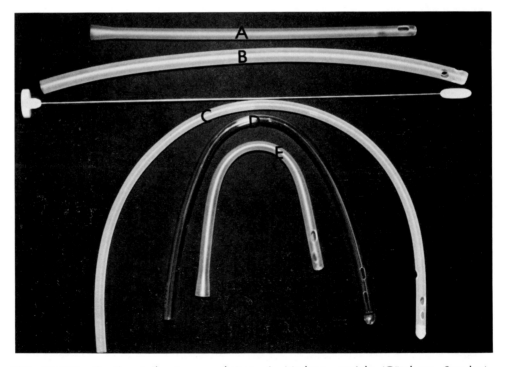

FIG. 15-119. Continent ileostomy catheters. **A.** Medena, straight (Göteborg, Sweden). **B.** Heyer-Schulte, with introducer (Goleta, California). **C.** Waters (Rochester, Minnesota). **D.** Marlen (Bedford, Ohio). **E.** Medena (curved).

due to the improved techniques of reservoir construction and the careful selection of patients who undergo this procedure. Cranley reviewed the development of the procedure and reported that anastomotic leak occurred in 8.8% of cases.[48] In the experience of Goligher with 62 reservoir operations, leakage occurred in seven cases with the development of diffuse peritonitis in three and of a localized abscess in four.[101] An additional two patients required a proximal loop ileostomy for presumed leakage, although no defect in the reservoir could be identified at the time of surgery. Goligher commented that his complications seemed to be more frequently observed than those of other surgeons.

The report by Kock and associates in 1981 revealed seven deaths in 314 patients (2.2%).[155] All of the operative deaths occurred before 1975, with no deaths recorded in the succeeding 152 patients. Twenty-four percent of patients operated on between 1967 and 1974 and 7% of patients in the latter period developed early complications. Anastomotic leak or fistula occurred in 19 patients in the earlier group, but only in one from the latter.

Palmu and Sivula reported an experience of 51 patients; there were two perforations of the reservoir (one death), four fecal fistulas, and eight intestinal obstructions.[210] Gelernt and colleagues reported their experience on 54 patients and noted a fecal fistula in 6, with hemorrhage from the ileal reservoir noted in 5 patients.[91] In a report by Halvorsen and associates, of the 36 patients who underwent a reservoir ileostomy three died from septic complications.[113] Of the 150 patients reported from the Mayo Clinic, 16 patients required excision of the pouch, but only 1 because of a fistula.[16]

If surgical intervention becomes necessary in the immediate postoperative period because of presumed suture line leakage, every attempt should be made to preserve the ileal reservoir. This can usually be accomplished by a diversionary proximal loop ileostomy and appropriate surgical drainage with or without closure of the leak. Subsequent radiologic investigation may reveal that the fistula spontaneously closed even without repair.

If it appears, however, that the reservoir is beyond salvation, it must be resected and a neoileostomy created. If the patient had undergone a procedure for what subsequently proved to be Crohn's disease, a suture line leak has an ominous prognosis indeed. Under such circumstances it is probably the wiser course to remove the pouch and create a new ileostomy.

Late complications of the continent ileostomy procedure are myriad and include incontinence due to reduction of the nipple valve, ileitis (pouchitis), recurrent Crohn's disease, catheter perforation, detachment of the pouch from the abdominal wall, volvulus of the reservoir, urolithiasis, obstruction from inspissated material, stomal stenosis, and intestinal obstruction from a lost catheter.

Obviously, the complication associated with reduction of the nipple valve with resultant *incontinence* is the most troublesome and the most frequently observed late management problem. If this complication does develop, it is often difficult for the patient to intubate the reservoir. The kinking of the intra-abdominal portion of the distal ileum may in itself create a partial small bowel obstruction. Usually, however, the patient is incontinent and *not* obstructed.

Reconstruction of the nipple may be accomplished by performing an enterotomy in the reservoir, reintussuscepting the distal ileum, and resecuring it. However, it may not be possible to accomplish this maneuver because of necrosis of the ileum, inadequate length of the conduit, or bowel injury during the process of mobilization. Under these circumstances a new nipple may be created without sacrificing the reservoir. This is accomplished by using the afferent limb, oversewing the old efferent conduit opening, and performing an anastomosis of the proximal ileum to another part of the reservoir (Fig. 15-120). This is the method usually required to convert the reservoir ileoanal anastomosis (Parks) to the continent ileostomy (Kock). Usually there is insufficient length of terminal ileum remaining (that had been anastomosed to the anal canal) to create a nipple valve and conduit. By oversewing the efferent end and using the proximal bowel to create a new nipple and conduit, the reservoir from that operation can be preserved.

Schrock reported a 15% incidence of immediate postoperative complications in 39 patients.[233] Late complications developed in 46% of these patients. Factors that contributed to the complications included older age (greater than 40 years), obesity, and the presence of Crohn's disease. By far the most common complication was spontaneous reduction of the nipple valve, usually occurring within 3 months. This complication was noted by the author in one third of his patients. A much higher incidence of nipple valve failure was noted in patients who underwent a secondary operation rather than a primary procedure, that is, proctocolectomy and continent ileostomy at the same time. Forty-six percent of secondarily operated patients had nipple failure as compared with 13% of primary surgery patients. Increased weight gain may be a contributing factor, since the patients were generally well and had a much more fatty mesentery when operated upon the second time.

Dozois and colleagues reported the factors that affected the revision rate in the Mayo Clinic experience.[69] Among the almost 300 patients who underwent continent ileostomy and who were followed for at least 1 year, revision was required less often in women, in

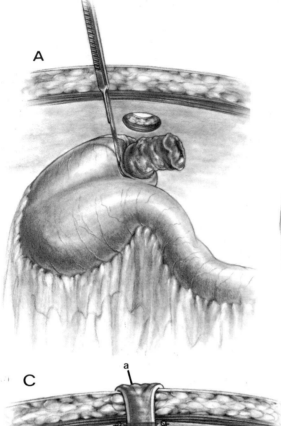

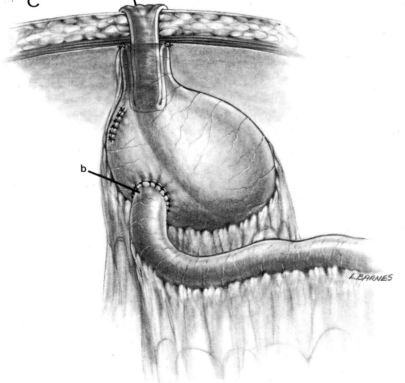

FIG. 15-120. Construction of a new nipple valve. **A.** Resection of the old conduit. **B.** Division of the proximal (afferent) limb for the creation of a new nipple. **C.** Final position of reservoir and conduit.

younger patients, and in patients who underwent primary proctocolectomy and continent ileostomy; this was the same experience that Schrock reported. The authors advised that if a malfunctioning valve develops, it ideally should be revised rather than a new one created; revision was felt to be technically simpler and the long-term results were comparable.

Gerber and associates reported a 19% incidence of nipple valve slippage in their first 48 patients; in the next 48, the incidence of nipple valve slippage was only 4%.[93] The authors attributed their success to stapling the nipple valve rather than suturing and the placement of a Marlex mesh sleeve around the conduit. The authors reported success in patients with *Crohn's colitis,* but their experience with *ileocolitis,* even with removal of the entire diseased bowel, was associated with a prohibitively high incidence of postoperative complications.

Flake and co-workers reported their initial experience on 11 patients. Three quarters required further surgery.[82] Four patients required a completely new Kock ileostomy, two required stomal revision, and two underwent revision of the valve with removal of the reservoir. Subsequently, two patients underwent conversion to a conventional ileostomy.

In the Mayo Clinic experience the results from the first 149 patients were compared with those from the last 150 patients.[68] There were no operative deaths. Fifteen pouches were excised in the early group, as opposed to only five in the later group. Furthermore, the need for revision of the valve by 1 year was 43% in the early group but 22% in the later group. Long-term follow-up demonstrated complete continence in 60% of the patients in the early group and 75% in the later group. The initial experience of Kock and associates revealed a 50% incidence of nipple valve complications necessitating revisional surgery.[155] With the newer modifications, their more recent experience demonstrated a malfunction rate of 6%.

Approximately one third of the patients of Palmu and Sivula required revision for nipple insufficiency, but Gelernt and associates, in an experience of 54 patients, stated that no nipple revision had ever been required.[91, 210] Only three patients reported some degree of incontinence. Halvorsen and colleagues reported disinvagination of the nipple in over one third of their patients.[113] Telander and co-workers reported a 20% requirement for revision of the nipple valve in patients under 19 years of age who underwent this procedure.[255]

The diagnosis of nipple valve slippage can usually be made clinically. However, it is valuable to confirm the position of the nipple radiographically. This can be done by a barium enema study through the stoma or by an upper gastrointestinal x-ray study (Fig. 15-121).

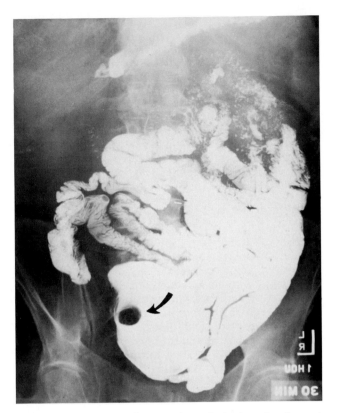

FIG. 15-121. Normal reservoir and nipple valve *(arrow)* demonstrated on a film from an upper gastrointestinal series.

The radiographic feature of a normal continent ileostomy on a plain abdominal film is the presence of a lobulated, gas-filled structure in the middle or right lower abdomen. With contrast material, the terminal, invaginated ileal segment resembles an inverted nipple protruding into the pouch.[192, 245] Barium enema examination can reveal the size of the reservoir; the effluent can be measured and the adequacy of the emptying confirmed. Other complications of continent ileostomy may also be confirmed radiographically, such as small bowel obstruction, anastomotic leakage, intra-abdominal abscess, fistula formation, failure of the reservoir to dilate, and the presence of recurrent Crohn's disease.[192]

Obstruction at the level of the reservoir is usually due to reduction of the nipple valve and kinking of the conduit. This will require revision to relieve the problem. The purpose of the operation, of course, is to create an intestinal obstruction. One of the distinct disadvantages is the need to have a catheter readily available. If a patient loses the catheter and is unable to conveniently obtain one (*e.g.,* on a camping trip or overboard on a boat), a serious problem ensues. The patient will not be able to relieve the obstruction until the proper equipment is available. Patients who enjoy outings away from civilization are well advised to secure the catheter on their person with great care.

Other unusual complications of the reservoir and the nipple valve have been reported. These include the development of an enormous ileal reservoir, the result of chronic outlet obstruction due to volvulus of the reservoir,[266] and volvulus with obstruction leading to perforation.[2]

Hemorrhage from the nipple valve or reservoir has also been reported. This may be due to trauma from insertion of the catheter (perforation of the pouch can actually occur) but is usually associated with a nonspecific inflammation of the mucosa, the so-called pouchitis. Bonello and co-workers estimate that the incidence of mucosal enteritis occurs in 13% to 43% of patients who have undergone a continent ileostomy.[27] Although the etiology is unknown, most authors believe that the manifestations are due to a change in the flora of the pouch, particularly with an overgrowth of anaerobic bacteria. Patients usually manifest increased ileostomy outputs that require more frequent intubation. Abdominal pain, bleeding, nausea, vomiting, and pyrexia may be observed.[27] Barium enema study is usually not helpful, although thickening of the mucosal folds may be apparent. Endoscopic examination will reveal an erythematous, ulcerated mucosa. Contact bleeding and friability are evident. Bonello and associates advocate oral metronidazole (Flagyl) as the treatment of choice.[27] Continuous drainage of the reservoir may have an ameliorative effect, and in the rare situation, removal of the pouch may be necessary.

Detachment of the continent ileostomy from the anterior abdominal wall has been reported to produce angulation of the efferent limb and difficulty intubating the pouch.[271] Operative correction is required.

Urolithiasis is a well-known associated complication in patients who have undergone conventional ileostomy. Stern and co-workers evaluated the problem in patients who underwent Kock ileostomies and compared them with nine matched patients who had undergone the conventional operation.[249] Both ileostomy groups demonstrated reduced urinary volume, with the Kock procedure having the lower volume. There was no significant reduction in urinary pH or elevation in urine uric acid concentration in the continent ileostomy group. The results seemed to suggest that there was no added risk of uric acid stone formation in pouch patients.

Malabsorption has been suggested as a possible concern because of intestinal stasis and bacterial overgrowth. Kelly and associates compared the nature and frequency of malabsorption in 42 pouch patients with 19 patients who underwent conventional ileostomy.[143] Almost one third with the reservoir were found to have excess fecal volumes accompanied by increased fecal losses of electrolytes, nitrogen, and fat, and by decreased vitamin B_{12} uptake. The remaining patients had fecal and urinary outputs similar to those of patients with conventional ileostomies. Gadacz and colleagues performed absorptive studies and motor function analysis of the pouch in 8 patients.[88] The pouch absorbed vitamin B_{12} that was instilled together with intrinsic factor. Other studies on patients who had documented malabsorption or symptoms of a malfunctioning pouch revealed that the number of jejunal and ileal anaerobic bacteria decreased in patients during treatment with metronidazole, implicating overgrowth of anaerobic bacterial flora in the pathogenesis of the syndrome.[144]

Kay and associates determined bile acid and neutral steroid excretion in 15 patients, 5 with conventional ileostomy, 5 with continent ileostomy, and 5 with continent ileostomy and an ileal resection.[141] Bile acid excretion rates were significantly increased in patients with a continent ileostomy and an ileal resection. Also, continent ileostomy was associated with a significant increased percentage of water content and a reduction in the pH of the ileal effluent. We have observed multiple calcium salt stones in the pouch of one patient (Fig. 15-122).

Physiologic studies of the nipple valve and pouch reveal that electrical and motor patterns of the undistended ileum are similar with both types of ileostomy, but the anatomic and motor properties of the pouch allow it to accept far larger intraluminal volumes both during fasting and after feeding.[3] Pressure studies on the pouch, the nipple valve, and the outlet demonstrate the presence of a high pressure zone in the nipple valve relative to the pouch.[203] Distention of the pouch with air causes a tonic contraction that travels from the pouch, along the intestinal layers of the intussuscepted nipple valve and the outlet.[203] It is postulated that this is the mechanism for desusception of the nipple valve, a complication that the authors suggest may be avoided by frequent intubation of the pouch. Other studies have demonstrated the functions of the mucosa and smooth muscle of the continent ileal pouch to be similar to those of normal ileum.[88]

Nilsson and colleagues performed morphologic and histochemical studies on the continent ileostomy reservoir up to 10 years after its construction.[202] No alarming changes in terms of dysplasia, fibrosis, or progressive atrophy were found. Histochemical investigation of the mucosa revealed largely unchanged, strong enzymatic activity involved both in oxidative metabolism and secretory functions.[202]

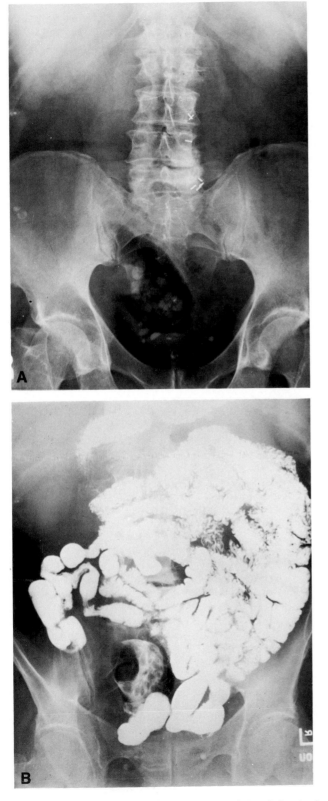

Comment.   Most observers experienced with the continent ileostomy believe that the operation offers a reasonably satisfactory alternative to the conventional procedure.[16, 99, 201] The encumbrance of an appliance, the occasional "accidents" with appliance management, the unaesthetic proboscis on the abdominal wall, the sexual inhibition, and the psychological embarrassment have stimulated many patients to seek an alternative procedure. But unfortunately, the operation is no panacea. In spite of the many improvements in surgical technique, the procedure is still fraught with numerous complications. The Kock pouch is also not for everyone; it is contraindicated in patients with Crohn's disease, and the results in older people and people who are somewhat obese are quite poor. The patient should *request* this operation; it must not be "sold" by the surgeon.

However, after a decade of experience I do not believe that we should consider this procedure experimental. The quality of life for patients who have elected the continent ileostomy is unquestionably improved in the vast majority of cases. With the passage of time I expect that more patients will embrace this alternative, and that ultimately the conventional ileostomy will probably be used virtually exclusively for patients with Crohn's disease.

The admonition to the surgeon, "Be not the first to abandon the old or the last to adopt the new," should be well heeded. I believe that now we have reached the point with the Kock ileostomy that it deserves complete legitimacy in our surgical armamentarium. My only concern is that because of the complexity of the operation, it should probably be performed only by those surgeons with patient volume adequate enough to gain sufficient experience with the technique.

REFERENCES

1. Acheson ED: An association between ulcerative colitis, regional enteritis, and ankylosing spondylitis. Q J Med 1960; 29:489–499
2. Agrez MV, Dozois RR, Beahrs OH: Volvulus of the Kock pouch with obstruction and perforation: A case report. Aust NZ J Surg 1981; 51:311–313
3. Akwari OE, Kelly KA, Phillips SF: Myoelectric and motor patterns of continent pouch and conventional ileostomy. Surg Gynecol Obstet 1980; 150:363–371
4. Alexander-Williams J: Perianal Crohn's disease. World J Surg 1980; 4:203–208
5. Almy TP, Sherlock P: Genetic aspects of ulcerative colitis and regional enteritis. Gastroenterology 1966; 51:757–763

FIG. 15-122.   Continent ileostomy. **A.** Plain abdominal film reveals radiopaque objects in the reservoir (note air shadow). **B.** A small bowel series confirms "stones" in the pouch.

6. Anderson R, Turnbull RB Jr: Grafting the un-healed perineal wound after coloproctectomy for Crohn's disease. Arch Surg 1976; 111:335–338

7. Aronson MD, Phillips CA, Beeken WL, Forsyth BR: Isolation and characterization of a viral agent from intestinal tissue of patients with Crohn's disease and other intestinal disorders. Prog Med Virol 1975; 21:165–176

8. Aylett SO: Diffuse ulcerative colitis and its treatment by ileorectal anastomosis. Ann R Coll Surg Engl 1960; 27:260–284

9. Aylett SO: Three hundred cases of diffuse ulcerative colitis treated by total colectomy and ileo-rectal anastomosis. Br Med J 1966; 1:1001–1005

10. Aylett SO: Rectal conservation in the surgical treatment of ulcerative colitis. Arch Mal App Dig 1974; 63:585–587

11. Bacon HE, Bralow SP, Berkley JL: Rehabilitation and long-term survival after colectomy for ulcerative colitis. JAMA 1960; 172:324–328

12. Baek S-M, Greenstein A, McElhinney AJ, Aufses AH Jr: The gracilis myocutaneous flap for persistent perineal sinus after proctocolectomy. Surg Gynecol Obstet 1981; 153:713–716

13. Bambach CP, Robertson WG, Peacock M, Hill GL: Effect of intestinal surgery on the risk of urinary stone formation. Gut 1981; 22:257–263

14. Basu MK, Asquith P: Oral manifestations of inflammatory bowel disease. Clin Gastroenterol 1980; 9:307–321

15. Bayer I, Feller N, Chaimoff Ch: A new approach to the nipple in Kock's reservoir ileostomy using mersilene mesh. Dis Colon Rectum 1981; 24:428–431

16. Beart RW Jr, Beahrs OH, Kelly KA et al: Continent ileostomy: A viable alternative. Mayo Clin Proc 1979; 54:643–645

17. Beart RW Jr, Dozois RR, Kelly KA: Ileoanal anastomosis in the adult. Surg Gynecol Obstet. 1982; 154:826–828

18. Bercovitz ZT: Etiology and pathogenesis. In Bercovitz ZT, Kirsner JB, Lindner AE et al (eds): Ulcerative and Granulomatous Colitis, pp 180-181. Springfield, Charles C Thomas, 1973

19. Berman IR, Corman ML, Coller JA, Veidenheimer MC: Late onset Crohn's disease in patients with colonic diverticulitis. Dis Colon Rectum 1979; 22:524–529

20. Bernstein LH, Frank MS, Brandt LJ, Boley SJ: Healing of perineal Crohn's disease with metronidazole. Gastroenterology 1980; 79:357–365

21. Beubige EJ, Bagless TM, Milligan FD: Mucosal bridging in Crohn's disease of the colon. Gastrointest Endosc 1975;21:189

22. Binder V, Both H, Hansen PK et al: Incidence and prevalence of ulcerative colitis and Crohn's disease in the county of Copenhagen, 1962 to 1978. Gastroenterology 1982; 83:563–568

23. Blackstone MO, Riddell RH, Rogers BHG, Levin B: Dysplasia-associated lesion or mass (DALM) detected by colonoscopy in long-standing ulcerative colitis: An indication for colectomy. Gastroenterology 1981; 80:366–374

24. Bohe MG, Ekelund GR, Genell SN et al: Surgery for fulminating colitis during pregnancy. Dis Colon Rectum 1983; 26:119–122

25. Bokey LE, Fazio VW: The mesenteric sling technique: A new method of constructing an intestinal nipple valve for the continent ileostomy. Cleve Clin Q 1978; 45:231–236

26. Bolton RP, Sherrif RJ, Read AE: *Clostridium difficile* associated diarrhoea: a role in inflammatory bowel disease? Lancet 1980; 1:383–384

27. Bonello JC, Thow GB, Manson RR: Mucosal enteritis: A complication of the continent ileostomy. Dis Colon Rectum 1981; 24:37–41

28. Brahme F: Crohn's disease in a defined population. Gastroenterology 1975; 69:342–351

29. Brandt LJ, Bernstein LH, Boley SJ, Frank MS: Metronidazole therapy for perineal Crohn's disease: A follow-up study. Gastroenterology 1982; 83:383–387

30. Brandt L, Boley S, Goldberg L et al: Colitis in the elderly. Am J Gastroenterol 1981; 76:239–245

31. Broader JH, Masselink BA, Oates GD et al: Management of the pelvic space after proctectomy. Br J Surg 1974; 61:94–97

32. Brooke BN: The outcome of surgery for ulcerative colitis. Lancet 1956; 2:532–536

33. Brown JY: Value of complete physiological rest of large bowel in ulcerative and obstructive lesions. Surg Gynecol Obstet 1913; 16:610

34. Buchmann P, Weterman IT, Keighley MRB et al: The prognosis of ileorectal anastomosis in Crohn's disease. Br J Surg 1981; 68:7–10

35. Bureš J, Fixa B, Komárková O, Fingerland A: Non-smoking: a feature of ulcerative colitis. Br Med J 1982; 285–440

36. Burnham WR, Lennard-Jones JE, Brooke BN: The incidence and nature of sexual problems among married ileostomists (abstr). Gut 1976; 17:391

37. Cattell RB: The surgical treatment of ulcerative colitis. JAMA 1935; 104:104–109

38. Cave HW: The surgical management of chronic intractable ulcerative colitis. Am J Surg 1939; 46:79–82

39. Cohen S, Kaplan M, Gottlieb L, Patterson J: Liver disease and gallstones in regional enteritis. Gastroenterology 1971; 60:237–245

40. Cohen WN: Gastric involvement in Crohn's disease. Amer J Roentgen 1967; 101:425–430

41. Cohen Z, Cook MG, Festenstein H: The transmission of human Crohn's disease in inbred strains of mice (abstr). Ann R Coll Physicians Surg Canada 1978; 2:51

42. Comfort MW, Weber HM, Baggenstoss AH et al: Non-specific granulomatous inflammation of the stomach and duodenum: Its relation to regional enteritis. Am J Med Sci 1950; 220:616–632

43. Coran AG: The ileal endorectal pull-through procedure. Surgical Rounds 1982; November:40–50

44. Corbett RS: Discussion on the surgical treatment of idiopathic ulcerative colitis and its surgical sequelae. Proc R Soc Med 1940; 33:647

45. Corman ML, Veidenheimer MC, Coller JA: Impotence after proctectomy for inflammatory disease of the bowel. Dis Colon Rectum 1978; 21:418–419

46. Corman ML, Veidenheimer MC, Coller JA, Ross VH: Perineal wound healing after proctectomy for inflammatory bowel disease. Dis Colon Rectum 1978; 21:155–159

47. Corman ML, Veidenheimer MC, Nugent FW et al: Diseases of the Anus, Rectum and Colon. Part II: Non-specific inflammatory bowel disease. New York, Medcom, 1976

48. Cranley B: The Kock reservoir ileostomy: A review of its development, problems and role in modern surgical practice. Br J Surg 1983; 70:94–99

49. Crile G Jr, Thomas CY Jr: Treatment of acute toxic ulcerative colitis by ileostomy and simultaneous colectomy. Gastroenterology 1951; 19:58–68

50. Crohn BB, Ginzburg L, Oppenheimer GD: Regional ileitis: A pathologic and clinical entity. JAMA 1932; 99:1323–1329

51. Crohn BB, Yarnis H, Walter RI et al: Ulcerative colitis as affected by pregnancy. NY State J Med 1956; 56:2651–2657

52. Crowson TD, Ferrante WF, Gathright JB Jr: Colonoscopy: Inefficacy for early carcinoma detection in patients with ulcerative colitis. JAMA 1976; 236:2651–2652

53. Danzi JT, Farmer RG, Sullivan BH Jr et al: Endoscopic features of gastroduodenal Crohn's disease. Gastroenterology 1976; 70:9–13

54. Das KM, Morecki R, Nair P, Berkowitz JM: Idiopathic proctitis: I. The morphology of proximal colonic mucosa and its clinical significance. Am J Dig Dis 1977; 22:524–528

55. Dassei PM: A familial pattern in inflammatory disease of the bowel (Crohn's disease and ulcerative colitis). Dis Colon Rectum 1977; 20:669–671

56. Daum F, Alperstein G: Inflammatory bowel disease in children and adolescents. Ped Gastroenterol 1982; 6:26–30

57. Davidson M: Juvenile ulcerative colitis. N Engl J Med 1967; 277:1408–1410

58. de Castella H: Non-smoking: A feature of ulcerative colitis. Br Med J 1982; 284:1706

59. de Dombal FT, Burton I, Goligher JC: The early and late results of surgical treatment for Crohn's disease. Br J Surg 1971; 58:805–816

60. de Dombal FT, Goldie W, Watts J et al: Hepatic histological changes in ulcerative colitis: A series of 58 consecutive operative liver biopsies. Scand J Gastroenterol 1966; 1:220–227

61. de Dombal FT, Watts JM, Watkinson G, Goligher JC: Ulcerative colitis and pregnancy. Lancet 1965; 2:599–601

62. Dickinson RJ, Dixon MF, Axon ATR: Colonoscopy and the detection of dysplasia in patients with longstanding ulcerative colitis. Lancet 1980; 2:620–622

63. Diehl JT, Steiger E, Hooley R: The role of intravenous hyperalimentation in intestinal diseases. Surg Clin North Am 1983; 63:11–25

64. Di Febo G, Gizzi G, Cappelo IP: Unusual case of colonic sub-obstruction by giant pseudopolyposis in Crohn's colitis. Endoscopy 1981; 13:90–92

65. Donnelly BJ, Delaney PV, Healy TM: Evidence for a transmissable factor in Crohn's disease. Gut 1977; 18:360–363

66. Donovan MJ, O'Hara ET: Sexual function following surgery for ulcerative colitis. N Engl J Med 1960; 262:719–720

67. Dordal E, Glagov S, Kirsner JB: Hepatic lesions in chronic inflammatory bowel disease. Gastroenterology 1967; 52:239–253

68. Dozois RR, Kelly KA, Beart RW Jr, Beahrs OH: Improved results with continent ileostomy. Ann Surg 1980; 192:319–324

69. Dozois RR, Kelly KA, Ilstrup D et al: Factors affecting revision rate after continent ileostomy. Arch Surg 1981; 116:610–613

70. Dyer NH, Cook PL, Kemp-Harper RA: Oesophageal stricture associated with Crohn's disease. Gut 1969; 10:549–554

71. Eisenberg HW: Combined metronidazole and surgery in the management of complicated Crohn's disease. Cont Surg 1982; 21:95–102

72. Emmanouilidis A, Manoussos O, Nicolaou A et al: Colonoscopy in ulcerative colitis. Am J Proctol Gastroenterol Colon and Rectal Surg 1983; 34:5–8

73. Evans JG, Acheson ED: An epidemological study of ulcerative colitis and regional enteritis in the Oxford area. Gut 1965; 6:311–324

74. Farmer RG, Hawk WA, Turnbull RB Jr: Crohn's disease of the duodenum (transmural duodenitis): Clinical manifestations: Report of 11 cases. Am J Dig Dis 1972; 17:191–198

75. Farmer RG, Michener WM, Mortimer EA: Studies of family history among patients with inflammatory bowel disease. Clin Gastroenterol 1980; 9:271–278

76. Farnell MB, Van Heerden JA, Beart RW Jr, Weiland LH: Rectal preservation in nonspecific inflammatory disease of the colon. Ann Surg 1980; 192:249–253

77. Fazio VW: Toxic megacolon in ulcerative colitis and Crohn's colitis. Clin Gastroenterol 1980; 9:389–407

78. Fazio VW: Regional enteritis (Crohn's disease): Indications for surgery and operative strategy. Surg Clin North Am 1983; 63:27–48

79. Fazio VW, Kodner I, Jagelman DG et al: Inflammatory disease of the bowel: Parenteral nutrition as primary or adjunctive treatment (symposium). Dis Colon Rectum 1976; 19:574–578

80. Fielding JF: Perianal lesions in Crohn's disease. J R Coll Surg Edinb 1972; 17:32–37

81. Fitzgibbons TJ, Green G, Silberman H et al: Management of Crohn's disease involving the duodenum, including duodenal cutaneous fistula. Arch Surg 1980; 115:1022–1028

82. Flake WK, Altman MS, Cartmill AM, Gilsdorf RB: Problems encountered with the Kock ileostomy. Am J Surg 1979; 138:851–855

83. Fonkalsrud EW: Total colectomy and endorectal ileal pull-through with internal ileal reservoir for ulcerative colitis. Surg Gynecol Obstet 1980; 150:1–8

84. Fonkalsrud EW: Endorectal ileal pullthrough with lateral ileal reservoir for benign colorectal disease. Ann Surg 1981; 194:761–766

85. Fonkalsrud EW: Endorectal pullthrough with ileal reservoir for ulcerative colitis and polyposis. Am J Surg 1982; 144:81–87

86. Frikker MJ, Segall MM: The resectional reoperation rate for Crohn's disease in a general community hospital. Dis Colon Rectum 1983; 26:305–309

87. Frühmorgen P: Diagnosis of inflammatory disease of the colon by colonoscopy. Acta Gastroenterol 1974; 37:154–158

88. Gadacz TR, Kelly KA, Phillips SF: The continent ileal pouch: Absorptive and motor features. Gastroenterology 1977; 72:1287–1291

89. Gardner C, Miller GG: Total colectomy for ulcerative colitis. Arch Surg 1951; 63:370–372

90. Geboes K, Vantrappen G: The value of colonoscopy in the diagnosis of Crohn's disease. Gastrointest Endosc 1975; 22:18–23

91. Gelernt IM, Bauer JJ, Kreel I: The reservoir ileostomy: Early experience with 54 patients. Ann Surg 1977; 185:179–184

92. Gelfand MD, Krone CL: Dysphagia and esophageal ulceration in Crohn's disease. Gastroenterology 1968; 55:510–514

93. Gerber A, Apt MK, Craig PH: The Kock continent ileostomy. Surg Gynecol Obstet 1983; 156:345–350

94. Gitnick GL, Rosen VJ, Arthur MH, Hertweck SA: Evidence for the isolation of a new virus from ulcerative proctitis patients: Comparison with virus derived from Crohn's disease. Dig Dis Sci 1979; 24:609–619

95. Givel J-C, Hawker P, Allan RN, Alexander-Williams J: Enterovaginal fistulas associated with Crohn's disease. Surg Gynecol Obstet 1982; 155:494–496

96. Goldwasser B, Mazor A, Wiznitzer T: Enteroduodenal fistulas in Crohn's disease. Dis Colon Rectum 1981; 24:485–486

97. Goligher JC: Primary excisional surgery in treatment of ulcerative colitis. Ann R Coll Surg Engl 1954; 15:316–325

98. Goligher JC: Inflammatory disease of the bowel (symposium): results of resection for Crohn's disease. Dis Colon Rectum 1976; 19:584–587

99. Goligher JC: Continent ileostomy: Commentary. World J Surg 1980; 4:147–148

100. Goligher JC: Surgery of the Anus, Rectum and Colon, 4th ed, p 689. London, Ballière Tindall, 1980

101. Goligher JC: Surgery of the Anus, Rectum and Colon, 4th ed, pp 793–814. London, Ballière Tindall, 1980

102. Goligher JC: Surgery of the Anus, Rectum and Colon, 4th ed, p 828. London, Ballière Tindall, 1980

103. Goligher JC, de Dombal FT, Watts J McK, Watkinson G: Ulcerative Colitis, p 2. London, Ballière, Tindall and Cassell, 1968

104. Greenstein A: Cancer in inflammatory bowel disease. Surgical Rounds 1982; October: 44–56

105. Greenstein AJ, Sachar DB, Greenstein RJ et al: Intraabdominal abscess in Crohn's (ileo) colitis. Am J Surg 1982; 143:727–730

106. Greenstein AJ, Sachar D, Pucillo A et al: Cancer in Crohn's disease after diversionary surgery: A report of seven carcinomas occurring in excluded bowel. Am J Surg 1978; 135:86–90

107. Grundfest S, Steiger E: Home parenteral nutrition. JAMA 1980; 244:1701–1703

108. Grundfest SF, Fazio V, Weiss RA et al: The risk of cancer following colectomy and ileorectal anastomosis for extensive mucosal ulcerative colitis. Ann Surg 1981; 193:9–14

109. Grüner OPN, Refsum S, Fausa O, Hognestad J: Giant pseudopolyposis causing colonic obstruction: Report of a case seemingly associated with Crohn's disease of the colon. Scand J Gastroenterol 1978; 13:65–69

110. Gump FE, Lepore M, Barker HG: A revised concept of acute regional enteritis. Ann Surg 1967; 166:942–946

111. Gurian L, Klein K, Ward TT: Role of *Clostridium difficile* and *Campylobacter jejuni* in relapses of inflammatory bowel disease. West J Med 1983; 138:359–360

112. Gyde SN, Prior P, Macartney JC et al: Malignancy in Crohn's disease. Gut 1980; 21:1024–1029

113. Halvorsen JF, Heimann P, Hoel R, Nygaard K: The continent reservoir ileostomy: Review of a collective series of thirty-six patients from three surgical departments. Surgery 1978; 83:252–258

114. Hammerman AM, Shatz BA, Susman N: Radiographic characteristics of colonic "mucosal bridges:" Sequelae of inflammatory bowel disease. Radiology 1978; 47:611–614

115. Handelsman JC, Fishbein RH, Hoover HC Jr et al: Endorectal pull-through operation in adults after colectomy and excision of rectal mucosa. Surgery 1983; 93:247–253

116. Harford FJ Jr, Fazio VW: Total parenteral nutrition as primary therapy for inflammatory disease of the bowel. Dis Colon Rectum 1978; 21:555–557

117. Harper PH, Truelove SC, Lee ECG et al: Split ileostomy and ileocolostomy for Crohn's disease of the colon and ulcerative colitis: A 20 year survey. Gut 1983; 24:106–113

118. Harries AD, Baird A, Rhodes J: Non-smoking: A feature of ulcerative colitis. Br Med J 1982; 284:706

119. Hawker PC, Gyde SN, Thompson H, Allan RN: Adenocarcinoma of the small intestine complicating Crohn's disease. Gut 1982; 23:188–193

120. Heffernon EW, Kepkay PH: Segmental esophagitis gastritis and enteritis. Gastroenterology 1954; 26:83–88

121. Heppell J, Kelly KA, Phillips SF et al: Physiologic aspects of continence after colectomy, mucosal proctectomy, and endorectal ileo-anal anastomosis. Ann Surg 1982; 195:435–443

122. Hobbis JH, Schofield PF: Management of perianal Crohn's disease. J R Soc Med 1982; 75:414–417

123. Hogan WJ, Hensley GT, Geenen JE: Endoscopic evaluation of inflammatory bowel disease. Med Clin North Am 1980; 64:1083–1102

124. Homan WP, Dineen P: Comparison of the results of resection, bypass, and bypass with exclusion for ileocecal Crohn's disease. Ann Surg 1978; 187:530–535

125. Hughes ESR: The treatment of ulcerative colitis. Ann R Coll Surg Engl 1965; 37:191–206

126. Hughes ESR, McDermott FT, Masterton JP: Ileorectal anastomosis for inflammatory bowel disease: 15-year follow-up. Dis Colon Rectum 1979; 22:399–400

127. Hultén L, Fasth S: Loop ileostomy for protection of the newly constructed ileostomy reservoir. Br J Surg 1981; 68:11–13

128. Hultén L, Kewenter J, Knutsson U et al: Primary closure of perineal wound after proctocolectomy or rectal excision. Acta Chir Scand 1971; 137:467–469

129. Irvin TT, Goligher JC: A controlled clinical trial of three different methods of perineal wound management following excision of the rectum. Br J Surg 1975; 62:287–291

130. Irving M: Assessment and management of external fistulas in Crohn's disease. Br J Surg 1983; 70:233–236

131. Jalan KN, Prescott RJ, Walker RJ et al: Arthropathy, ankylosing spondylitis, and clubbing of fingers in ulcerative colitis. Gut 1970; 11:748–754

132. Jalan KN, Smith AN, Ruckley CV et al: Perineal wound healing in ulcerative colitis. Br J Surg 1969; 56:749–753

133. Jick H, Walker AM: Cigarette smoking and ulcerative colitis. N Engl J Med 1983; 308:261–263

134. Johnson ML, Wilson HT: Skin lesions in ulcerative colitis. Gut 1969; 10:255–263

135. Johnson WR, McDermott FT, Hughes ESR et al: The risk of rectal carcinoma following colectomy in ulcerative colitis. Dis Colon Rectum 1983; 26:44–46

136. Johnson WR, McDermott FT, Hughes ESR et al: Carcinoma of the colon and rectum in inflammatory disease of the intestine. Surg Gynecol Obstet 1983; 156:193–197

137. Jones PF, Bevan PG, Hawley PR: Ileostomy or ileorectal anastomosis for ulcerative colitis. Br Med J 1978; 1:1459–1463

138. Kahn EI, Daum F, Aiges HW, Silverberg M: Cutaneous polyarteritis nodosa associated with Crohn's disease. Dis Colon Rectum 1980; 23:258–262

139. Karush A, Daniels GE, Flood C, O'Conner JF: Psychotherapy in Chronic Ulcerative Colitis, p 148. Philadelphia, WB Saunders

140. Katz S, Rosenberg RF, Katzka I: Giant pseudopolyps in Crohn's colitis. Am J Gastroenterol 1981; 76:267–271

141. Kay RM, Cohen Z, Siu KP et al: Ileal excretion and bacterial modification of bile acids and cholesterol in patients with continent ileostomy. Gut 1979; 21:128–132

142. Keighley MRB, Buchmann P, Lee JR: Assessment of anorectal function in selection of patients for ileorectal anastomosis in Crohn's colitis. Gut 1982; 23:102–107

143. Kelly DG, Branon ME, Phillips SF, Kelly KA: Diarrhea after continent ileostomy. Gut 1980; 21:711–716

144. Kelly DG, Phillips SF, Kelly KA et al: Dysfunction of the continent ileostomy: Clinical features and bacteriology. Gut 1983; 24:193–201

145. Khubchandani IT, Stasik JJ Jr, Nedwich A: Prospective surveillance by rectal biopsy following ileorectal anastomosis for inflammatory disease. Dis Colon Rectum 1982; 25:343–347

146. Kirkegaard P, Madsen PV: Perineal sinus after removal of the rectum: Occlusion with fibrin adhesive. Am J Surg 1983; 145:791–794

147. Kirsner JB: Genetic aspects of inflammatory bowel disease. Clin Gastroenterol 1973; 2:557–575

148. Kirsner JB, Shorter RG: Recent developments in "nonspecific" inflammatory bowel disease, Part I. N Engl J Med 1982; 306:775–785

149. Kirsner JB, Shorter RG: Recent developments in nonspecific inflammatory bowel disease, Part II. N Engl J Med 1982; 306:837–848

150. Kirsner JB, Spencer JA: Family occurrences of ulcerative colitis, regional enteritis, and ileocolitis. Ann Intern Med 1963; 59:133–144

151. Kirsner JB, Wall AJ: The medical treatment of ulcerative colitis and Crohn's disease of the colon. In Kirsner JB, Shorter RG: Inflammatory Bowel Disease, pp 279–293. Philadelphia, Lea & Febiger, 1975

152. Kock NG: Intra-abdominal "reservoir" in patients with permanent ileostomy: Preliminary observations on a procedure resulting in fecal "continence" in five ileostomy patients. Arch Surg 1969; 99:223–231

153. Kock NG, Darle N, Hultén L et al: Ileostomy. Curr Probl Surg 1977; 14:1–52

154. Kock NG, Darle N, Kewenter J et al: The quality of life after proctocolectomy and ileostomy: A study of patients with conventional ileostomies converted to continent ileostomies. Dis Colon Rectum 1974; 17:287–292

155. Kock NG, Myrvold HE, Nilsson LO, Philipson BM: Continent ileostomy: An account of 314 patients. Acta Chir Scand 1981; 147:67–72

156. Korelitz BI: Therapy of inflammatory bowel disease, including use of immunosuppressive agents. Clin Gastroenterol 1980; 9:331–349

157. Korelitz BI: The treatment of ulcerative colitis with "immunosuppressive" drugs. Am J Gastroenterol 1981; 76:297–298

158. Korelitz BI, Dyck WP, Klion FM: Fate of the rectum and distal colon after subtotal colectomy for ulcerative colitis. Gut 1969; 10:198–201

159. Korelitz BI, Glass JL, Wisch N: Long-term immunosuppressive therapy of ulcerative colitis. Am J Dig Dis 1973; 18:317–322

160. Korelitz BI, Present DH, Alpert LI et al: Recurrent regional ileitis after ileostomy and colectomy for granulomatous colitis. N Engl J Med 1972; 287:110–115

161. Korelitz BI, Waye JD, Kreuning J et al: Crohn's disease in endoscopic biopsies of the gastric antrum and duodenum. Am J Gastroenterol 1981; 76:103–109

162. Kovalcik P, Simstein L, Weiss M, Mullen J: The dilemma of Crohn's disease: Crohn's disease and appendectomy. Dis Colon Rectum 1977; 20:377–380

163. Kurtz LM, Flint GW, Platt N, Wise L: Carcinoma in the retained rectum after colectomy for ulcerative colitis. Dis Colon Rectum 1980; 23:346–350

164. Kurtz RS, Heimann TM, Aufses AH: The management of intestinal fistulas. Am J Gastroenterol 1981; 76:377–380

165. Kyle J: An epidemiological study of Crohn's disease in northeast Scotland. Gastroenterol 1971; 61:826–833

166. Lahey FH: Ulcerative colitis. NY St J Med 1941; 41:475–481

167. La Mont JT, Trnka YM: Therapeutic implications of *Clostridium difficile* toxin during relapse of chronic inflammatory bowel disease. Lancet 1980; 1:381–383

168. Lavery IC, Chiulli RA, Jagelman DG et al: Survival with carcinoma arising in mucosal ulcerative colitis. Ann Surg 1982; 195:508–512

169. Lavery IC, Jagelman DG: Cancer in the excluded rectum following surgery for inflammatory bowel disease. Dis Colon Rectum 1982; 25:522–524

170. Lees CD, Steiger E, Hooley RA et al: Home parenteral nutrition. Acta Chir Scand (Suppl) 1981; 507:113–120

171. Levy N, Roisman I, Teodor I: Ulcerative colitis in pregnancy in Israel. Dis Colon Rectum 1981; 24:351–354

172. Lindhagen T, Ekelund G, Leandoer L et al: Crohn's disease confined to the appendix. Dis Colon Rectum 1982; 25:805–808

173. Lock MR, Fazio VW, Farmer RG et al: Proximal recurrence and the fate of the rectum following excisional surgery for Crohn's disease of the large bowel. Ann Surg 1981; 194:754–760

174. Lyttle JA, Parks AG: Intersphincteric excision of the rectum. Br J Surg 1977; 64:413–416

175. Maingot R: Terminal ileostomy in ulcerative colitis. Lancet 1942; 2:121–124

176. Manjoney DL, Koplewitz MJ, Abrams JS: Factors influencing perineal wound healing. Am J Surg 1983; 145:183–189

177. Marks CG, Ritchie JK, Lockhart-Mummery HE: Anal fistulas in Crohn's disease. Br J Surg 1981; 68:525–527

178. Marshak RH, Lindner AE: Chronic inflammatory disease of the colon: Historical perspective. In Bercovitz ZT, Kirsner JB Lindner AE et al (eds): Ulcerative and Granulomatous Colitis, pp xvii–xx. Springfield, Charles C Thomas, 1973

179. Marshak RH, Lindner AE: Radiologic diagnosis of chronic ulcerative colitis and Crohn's disease of the colon. In Kirsner JB, Shorter RG (ed): Inflammatory Bowel Disease, pp 241–276. Philadelphia, Lea & Febiger, 1975

180. Martin LW, LeCoultre C, Schubert WK: Total colectomy and mucosal proctectomy with preservation of continence in ulcerative colitis. Ann Surg 1977; 186:477–480

181. Marx FW Jr: Incidental appendectomy with regional enteritis. Arch Surg 1964; 88:546–551

182. Mavroudis C, Schrock TR: The dilemma of preservation of the rectum: Retention of the rectum in colectomy for inflammatory disease of the bowel. Dis Colon Rectum 1977; 20:644–648

183. May RE: Sexual dysfunction following rectal excision for ulcerative colitis. Br J Surg 1966; 53:29–30

184. Mayberry J, Rhodes J, Hughes LE: Incidence of Crohn's disease in Cardiff between 1934 and 1977. Gut 1979; 20:602–608

185. Mayo CW, Fly OA Jr, Connelly ME: Fate of the remaining segment after subtotal colectomy for ulcerative colitis. Ann Surg 1956; 144:753–757

186. McEwen C, Di Tata D, Lingg C et al: Ankylosing spondylitis and spondylitis accompanying ulcerative colitis, regional enteritis, psoriasis and Reiter's disease: A comparative study. Arthritis Rheum 1971; 14:291–318

187. McEwan HP: Ulcerative Colitis in pregnancy. Proc R Soc Med 1972; 65:279–281

188. McKittrick LS, Miller RH: Idiopathic ulcerative colitis: a review of 149 cases with particular reference to the value of, and indications for surgical treatment. Ann Surg 1935; 102:656–673

189. Mendeloff AL: The epidemiology of idiopathic inflammatory bowel disease. In Kirsner JB, Shorter RG (eds): Inflammatory Bowel Disease pp 3-19. Philadelphia, Lea & Febiger, 1975

190. Michener WM: Ulcerative colitis in children. Pediatr Clin North Am 1967; 94:159–173

191. Miller DS, Keighley AC, Langman MJS: Changing patterns in epidemiology of Crohn's disease. Lancet 1974; 2:691–693

192. Montagne J-P, Kressel HY, Moss AA, Schrock TR: Radiologic evaluation of the continent (Kock) ileostomy. Radiology 1978; 127:325–329

193. Morson BC, Lockhart-Mummery HE: Crohn's disease of the colon. Gastroenterologia 1959; 92:168–173

194. Morson BC, Pang LSC: Rectal biopsy as an aid to cancer control in ulcerative colitis. Gut 1967; 8:423–434

195. Moschowitz E, Wilensky AO: Non-specific granulomata of the intestine. Am J Med Sci 1923; 166:48–66

196. Moynihan B: The mimicry of malignant disease in the large intestine. Edinburgh Med J 1907; 21:228–236. Reproduced and discussed in "Classics of Colon and Rectal Surgery." Dis Colon Rectum 1981; 24:133–139

197. Murray CB: Psychogenic factors in the etiology of ulcerative colitis and bloody diarrhea. Am J Med Sci 1930; 180:239–248

198. Myren J, Eie H, Serck-Hanssen A: The diagnosis of colitis by colonoscopy with biopsy and x-ray examination. A blind comparative study. Scand J Gastroenterol 1976; 11:141–144

199. Myren J, Serck-Hanssen A, Solberg L: Routine and blind histological diagnoses on colonoscopic biopsies compared to clinical-colonoscopic observations in patients without and with colitis. Scand J Gastroenterol 1976; 11:135–140

200. Newman A, Lambert JR: (Letter) *Campylobacter jejuni* causing flare-up in inflammatory bowel disease. Lancet 1980; 2:919

201. Nilsson LO, Kock NG, Kylberg F et al: Sexual adjustment in ileostomy patients before and after conversion to continent ileostomy. Dis Colon Rectum 1981; 24:287–290

202. Nilsson LO, Kock NG, Lindgren I et al: Morphological and histochemical changes in the mucosa of the continent ileostomy reservoir 6-10 years after its construction. Scand J Gastroenterol 1980; 15:737–747

203. Nordgren S, Cohen Z, Greig PD, Diamant NE: Pressure studies on the continent reservoir ileostomy. Surg Gynecol Obstet 1982; 155:646–652

204. Nugent FW, Haggitt RC, Colcher H, Kutteruf GC: Malignant potential of chronic ulcerative colitis. Gastroenterology 1979; 76:1–5

205. Nugent FW, Richmond M, Park SK: Crohn's disease of the duodenum. Gut 1977; 18:115–120

206. Nugent FW, Veidenheimer MC, Meissner WA, Haggitt RC: Prognosis after colonic resection for Crohn's disease of the colon. Gastroenterology 1973; 65:398–402

207. Nunes GC, Ahlquist RE: Increasing incidence of Crohn's disease. Am J Surg 1983; 145:587–580

208. Oates GD, Williams JA: Primary closure of the perineal wound in excision of the rectum. Proc R Soc Med 1970; (Suppl) 63:128

209. Öhman U: Colorectal carcinoma in patients with ulcerative colitis. Am J Surg 1982; 344–349

210. Palmu A, Sivula A: Kock's continent ileostomy: Results of 51 operations and experiences with correction of nipple-valve insufficiency. Br J Surg 1978; 65:645–648

211. Parker RGF, Kendall EJC: Liver in ulcerative colitis. Br Med J 1954; 2:1030–1032

212. Parks AG, Nicholls RJ: Proctocolectomy without ileostomy for ulcerative colitis. Br Med J 1978; 2:85–88

213. Parks AG, Nicholls RJ, Belliveau P: Proctocolectomy with ileal reservoir and anal anastomosis. Br J Surg 1980; 67:533–538

214. Patterson M, Eytinge EJ: Chronic ulcerative colitis and pregnancy. N Engl J Med 1952; 246:691–694

215. Pescatori M, Manhire A, Bartram CI: Evacuation pouchography in the evaluation of ileoanal reservoir function. Dis Colon Rectum 1983; 26:365–368

216. Present DH, Korelitz BI, Wisch N et al: Treatment of Crohn's disease with 6-Mercaptopurine: A long-term randomized, double-blind study. N Engl J Med 1980; 302:981–987

217. Riddell RH, Shove DC, Ritchie JK et al: Precancer in ulcerative colitis. In Morson BC (ed): The Pathogenesis of Colorectal Cancer, pp 95–118. Philadelphia, WB Saunders, 1978

218. Ritchie JK: Ileostomy and excisional surgery for chronic inflammatory disease of the colon: A survey of one hospital region. Gut 1971; 12:528–540

219. Ritchie JK, Allan RN, Macartney J et al: Biliary tract carcinoma associated with ulcerative colitis. Q J Med 1974; 43:263–279

220. Ritchie JK, Hawley PR, Lennard-Jones JE: Prognosis of carcinoma in ulcerative colitis. Gut 1981; 22:752–755

221. Rombeau JL, Barot LR, Williamson CE, Mullen JL: Preoperative total parenteral nutrition and surgical outcome in patients with inflammatory bowel disease. Am J Surg 1982; 143:139–143

222. Rosén A, Ursing B, Alm T et al: A comparative study of metronidazole and sulfasalazine for active Crohn's disease: The cooperative Crohn's disease study in Sweden. I. Design and methodologic considerations. Gastroenterology 1982; 83:541–549

223. Ross TM, Fazio VW, Farmer RG: Long-term results of surgical treatment for Crohn's disease of the duodenum. Ann Surg 1983; 197:399–406

224. Rothenberger DA, Vermeulen FD, Christenson CE et al: Restorative proctocolectomy with ileal reservoir and ileoanal anastomosis. Am J Surg 1983; 145:82–88

225. Roy PH, Sauer WG, Beahrs OH, Farrow GM: Experience with ileostomies: Evaluation of long-term rehabilitation in 497 patients. Am J Surg 1970; 119:77–86

226. Ruckley CV, Smith AN, Balfour TW: Perineal closure by omental graft. Surg Gynecol Obstet 1970; 131:300–302

227. Rutgeerts P, Onette E, Vantrappen G et al: Crohn's disease of the stomach and duodenum: A clinical study with emphasis on the value of endoscopy and endoscopic biopsies. Endoscopy 1980; 12:288–294

228. Sachar DB, Auslander MO, Walfish JS: Aetiological theories of inflammatory bowel disease. Clin Gastroenterol 1980; 9:231–257

229. Saha SK, Robinson AF: A study of perineal wound healing after abdominoperineal resection. Br J Surg 1976; 63:555–558

230. Salmon R, Bloch P, Loygue J: Magnetic closure of a reservoir ileostomy. Dis Colon Rectum 1980; 23:242–243

231. Samach M, Train J: Demonstration of mucosal bridging in Crohn's colitis. Am J Gastroenterol 1980; 74:50–54

232. Schoetz DJ Jr, Coller JA, Veidenheimer MC: Pyoderma gangrenosum and Crohn's disease: Eight cases and a review of the literature. Dis Colon Rectum 1983; 26:155–158

233. Schrock TR: Complications of continent ileostomy. Am J Surg 1979; 138:162–169

234. Scully C, Cochran KM, Russell RI et al: Crohn's disease of the mouth: An indicator of intestinal involvement. Gut 1982; 23:198–201

235. Shiloni E, Freund HR: Total parenteral nutrition in Crohn's disease: Is it a primary or supportive mode of therapy? Dis Colon Rectum 1983; 26:275–278

236. Silen W, Glotzer DJ: The prevention and treatment of the persistent perineal sinus. Surgery 1974; 75:535–542

237. Simkins KC: Aphthoid ulcers in Crohn's colitis. Clin Radiol 1977; 28:601–608

238. Simonowitz DA, Rusch VW, Stevenson JK: Natural history of incidental appendectomy in patients with Crohn's disease who required subsequent bowel resection. Am J Surg 1982; 143:171–173

239. Singer HC, Anderson JGD, Frischer H et al: Fam-

ilial aspects of inflammatory bowel disease. Gastroenterology 1971; 61:423–430

240. Smith TR, Conradi H, Bernstein R, Greweldinger J: Adenocarcinoma arising in Crohn's disease: Report of two cases. Dis Colon Rectum 1980; 23:498–503

241. Sonnenberg A, Erckenbrecht J, Peter P, Niederau C: Detection of Crohn's disease by ultrasound. Gastroenterology 1982; 83:430–434

242. Spiro HM: Office management of ulcerative colitis and proctitis. Med Times 1982; April:44–48

243. Stahl D, Tyler G, Fischer JE: Inflammatory bowel disease—relationship to carcinoma. In Current Problems in Cancer, pp 5-71. Chicago, Year Book Medical Publishers, 1981

244. Stahlgren LH, Ferguson LK: Effects of abdominoperineal resection on sexual function in sixty patients with ulcerative colitis. Arch Surg 1959; 78:604–610

245. Standertskjöld-Nordenstam C-G, Palmu A, Sivula A: Radiologic assessment of nipple-valve insufficiency in Kock's continent reservoir ileostomy. Br J Surg 1979; 66:269–272

246. Steiger E, Srp F: Morbidity and mortality related to home parenteral nutrition in patients with gut failure. Am J Surg 1983; 145:102–105

247. Steinberg DM, Allan RN, Thompson H et al: Excisional surgery with ileostomy for Crohn's colitis with particular reference to factors affecting recurrence. Gut 1974; 15:845–851

248. Steinberg DM, Cooke WT, Alexander-Williams J: Abscess and fistulae in Crohn's disease. Gut 1973; 14:865–869

249. Stern H, Cohen Z, Wilson DR, Mickle DAG: Urolithiasis risk factors in continent reservoir ileostomy patients. Dis Colon Rectum 1980; 23:556–558

250. Stone W, Veidenheimer MC, Corman ML, Coller JA: The dilemma of Crohn's disease: Long-term follow-up of Crohn's disease of the small intestine. Dis Colon Rectum 1977; 20:372–376

251. Taub RN, Sachar D, Janowitz HD, Siltzbach LE: Induction of granulomas in mice by inoculation of tissue homogenates from patients with inflammatory bowel disease and sarcoidosis. Ann NY Acad Sci 1976; 278:560–564

252. Tawile NT, Priest RJ, Schuman BM: Colonoscopy in inflammatory bowel disease. Gastrointest Endosc 1975; 22:11–13

253. Taylor BM, Beart RW Jr, Dozois RR et al: Straight ileoanal anastomosis v ileal pouch-anal anastomosis after colectomy and mucosal proctectomy. Arch Surg 1983; 118:696–701

254. Teague RH, Waye JD: Inflammatory bowel disease. In Hunt RH, Waye JD (eds): Colonoscopy:

Techniques, Clinical Practice, and Colour Atlas, pp 343-362. London, Chapman & Hall, 1981

255. Telander RL, Smith SL, Marcinek HM et al: Surgical treatment of ulcerative colitis in children. Surgery 1981; 90:787–794

256. Theodor E, Niv Y, Bat L: Imuran in the treatment of ulcerative colitis. Am J Gastroenterol 1981; 76:262–266

257. Trnka YM, Glotzer DJ, Kasdon EJ et al: The long-term outcome of restorative operation in Crohn's disease: Influence of location, prognostic factors and surgical guidelines. Ann Surg 1982; 196:345–353

258. Trnka YM, LaMont JT: Association of *Clostridium difficile* toxin with symptomatic relapse of chronic inflammatory bowel disease. Gastroenterology 1981; 80:693–698

259. Tumen HJ, Valdes-Dapena A, Haddad H: Indications for surgical intervention in ulcerative colitis in children. Am J Dis Child 1968; 116:641–651

260. Turnbull RB Jr: The surgical approach to the treatment of inflammatory bowel disease (IBD): A personal view of techniques and prognosis. In Kirsner JB, Shorter RG (ed): Inflammatory Bowel Disease, pp 338-385. Philadelphia, Lea & Febiger, 1975

261. Turnbull RB Jr, Hawk WA, Weakley FL: Surgical treatment of toxic megacolon: Ileostomy and colostomy to prepare patients for colectomy. Am J Surg 1971; 122:325–331

262. Ursing B, Alm T, Bárány F et al: A comparative study of metronidazole and sulfasalazine for active Crohn's disease: The cooperative Crohn's disease study in Sweden. II. Result. Gastroenterology 1982; 83:550–562

263. Utsunomiya J, Iwama T, Imajo M et al: Total colectomy, mucosal proctectomy, and ileoanal anastomosis. Dis Colon Rectum 1980; 23:459–466

264. Van Heerden JA, Beart RW Jr: Carcinoma of the colon and rectum complicating chronic ulcerative colitis. Dis Colon Rectum 1980; 23:155–159

265. Van Prohaska J, Siderius NJ: The surgical rehabilitation of patients with chronic ulcerative colitis. Am J Surg 1962; 103:42–46

266. Wapnick S, Grosberg S, Farman J et al: Volvulus of the Kock reservoir. Dis Colon Rectum 1979; 22:55–57

267. Warren KW, Athanassiades S, Monge JI: Primary sclerosing cholangitis. Am J Surg 1966; 3:23–28

268. Watts JM, de Dombal FT, Goligher JC: Long-term complications and prognosis following major surgery for ulcerative colitis. Br J Surg 1966; 53:1014–1023

269. Waye JD: The role of colonoscopy in the differential diagnosis of inflammatory bowel disease. Gastrointest Endosc 1977; 23:150–154

270. Waye JD: Endoscopy in inflammatory bowel disease. Clin Gastroenterol 1980; 9:279–296

271. Weinstein M, Rubin RJ, Salvati EP: Detachment of the continent ileostomy pouch from the anterior abdominal wall: Report of two unusual cases. Dis Colon Rectum 1976; 19:705–706

272. Welch CE, Hedberg SE: Colonic cancer in ulcerative colitis and idiopathic colonic cancer. JAMA 1965; 191:815–818

273. Whorwell PJ, Phillips CA, Beeken WL et al: Isolation of reovirus-like agents from patients with Crohn's disease. Lancet 1977; 1:1169–1171

274. Wilks S: The morbid appearance of the intestine of Miss Banks. Medical Times and Gazette 1859; 2:264

275. Wilks S, Moxon W: Lectures on Pathological Anatomy, 2nd ed, pp 408; 672. London, J & A Churchill, 1875

276. Williams CB, Waye JD: Colonoscopy in inflammatory bowel disease. Clin Gastroenterol 1978; 7:701–717

277. Williams DR, Coller JA, Corman ML et al: Anal complications in Crohn's disease. Dis Colon Rectum 1981; 24:22–24

278. Williams SM, Harned RK: Bile duct carcinoma associated with chronic ulcerative colitis. Dis Colon Rectum 1981; 24:42–44

279. Wisch N, Korelitz BI: Immunosuppressive therapy for ulcerative colitis, ileitis, and granulomatous colitis. Surg Clin North Am 1972; 52:961–969

280. Wise, L, Kyriakos M, McCown A, Ballinger WF: Crohn's disease of the duodenum: A report and analysis of eleven new cases. Am J Surg 1971; 121:184–193

281. Wolff BG, Beart RW Jr, Frydenberg HB el al: The importance of disease-free margins in resection for Crohn's disease. Dis Colon Rectum 1983; 26:239–243

282. Wolff WI, Shinya H, Geffen A et al: Comparison of colonoscopy and the contrast enema in five hundred patients with colorectal disease. Am J Surg 1975; 129:181–186

283. Yeager ES, Van Heerden JA: Sexual dysfunction following proctocolectomy and abdominoperineal resection. Ann Surg 1980; 191:169–170

284. Zelas P, Jagelman DG: Loop ileostomy in the management of Crohn's colitis in the debilitated patient. Ann Surg 1980; 191:164–168

285. Zetzel L: Fertility, pregnancy, and idiopathic inflammatory bowel disease. In Kirsner JB, Shorter RG (eds): Inflammatory Bowel Disease, pp 146-153. Philadelphia, Lea & Febiger, 1975

286. Zinkin LD, Brandwein C: Adenocarcinoma in Crohn's colitis. Dis Colon Rectum 1980; 23:115–117

287. Zvaifler NJ, Martel W: Spondylitis in chronic ulcerative colitis. Arthritis Rheum 1960; 3:76–87

CHAPTER 16

Intestinal Stomas

The applications of colostomy and ileostomy have been discussed in detail in Chapters 11 and 15. The purposes of this chapter are to amplify upon the methods of creating a satisfactory stoma, the methods of closure, the results with these procedures, the complications and their management, and enterostomal therapy.

GENERAL PRINCIPLES

Unfortunately, many patients who have undergone ostomy surgery are unsure of whether they have a colostomy or an ileostomy when they leave the hospital. In addition, some patients have had unpleasant associations with ostomies through family and friends; myths and misunderstandings further prejudice the patient's attitude. The surgeon must confront the patient's fears of the disease itself, the potential for complications, and, indeed, the possible mortality; these issues must be addressed as part of a comprehensive rehabilitative program.

The location of the stoma has a direct bearing on subsequent ostomy management. Establishment of the stoma site before surgery is usually the responsibility of the surgeon, but in many instances may be delegated to a trained enterostomal therapist. Proper location of the stoma can prevent complications such as prolapse, hernia, and skin problems.

The groin, the waistline, the costal margins, the umbilicus, skin folds, and scars frequently interfere with appliance management. It is advisable to leave a 5-cm margin of smooth skin around the stoma. The stoma should always be placed at the summit of the infra-umbilical bulge and within the rectus muscle. When the site is being marked, it is helpful to have the patient lie in the supine position and tense the abdominal muscles. This allows one to feel the lateral border of the rectus muscle. A triangle is formed by drawing an imaginary line from the umbilicus to the pubis, one from the umbilicus to the anterosuperior iliac spine, and another from the pubis to the anterosuperior iliac spine (the inguinal ligament; see Fig. 15-92). The stoma should be in the center. The face plate should be taped over the site and the patient should stand, sit, and bend with the face-plate in place. Slight adjustments may be required because of interference from skin creases and from adiposity.

If a site is not selected until the patient is in the operating room, what is perceived to be an ideal location may subsequently present a difficult management problem. The outer margin of the face plate may appear at the waistline or in the groin, or the stoma may be found on the undersurface of the infraumbilical bulge, making it impossible for the patient to fit the skin barrier properly and to center the pouch. Another factor to consider is the patient's preference for clothing style, especially where the belt is worn, because stomas must be placed below the waist and preferably below the belt line. Should the patient require a second stoma, the new opening must be placed either above or below the existing one. Occasionally, it may be necessary to keep a face plate in place for 24 hours to ensure the patient's subsequent comfort and ease of movement.

This is especially true when the abdomen contains multiple scars. The proper location is marked permanently by wiping the skin with alcohol, placing a drop of India ink on the spot, and pricking with a fine hypodermic needle. An alternative method is to scratch a mark onto the proposed location.

The above considerations are applicable to all intestinal stomas—ileostomy, sigmoid colostomy, transverse colostomy, and urinary conduit.

SIGMOID COLOSTOMY

The most common indication for performing a permanent sigmoid colostomy is carcinoma of the rectum. Other possible indications for either a permanent or temporary stoma in this area include diverticulitis, Crohn's disease, congenital anomalies, anal incontinence, and colorectal trauma.

The technique for creating a satisfactory end sigmoid colostomy has been described previously as it pertains to the abdominoperineal resection for carcinoma of the rectum (see Figs. 11-16 to 11-18). It is important that the colon be brought through the split rectus muscle and sutured to the skin without tension. Ideally, redundant colon should be excised in order to permit a satisfactory irrigation should the patient elect to do so. Many surgeons perform a paramedian incision and then must create the stoma either in a pararectus location or bring the colostomy through the wound. Neither of these methods is in my opinion acceptable. A pararectus colostomy predisposes to peristomal hernia (see later). A "flush" colostomy can be reasonably safely performed because the colostomy effluent is noncorrosive, but this technique is not advised. With the patient's possible weight gain, the stoma tends to retract. This makes appliance managment more difficult. Hence, the stoma should be permitted to pout slightly, but not to the extent of a conventional ileostomy.

When the colostomy has been created, a simple, transparent drainable bag is placed before the patient leaves the operating room (see Fig. 16-58). This permits visualization of the stoma during the immediate postoperative course; the viability of the bowel can be determined on a continual basis. Usually, when the colostomy begins to function (after 4 or 5 days), the bag is removed and the stoma and skin carefully inspected.

Results

Whittaker and Goligher reviewed their experience with colostomy following abdominoperineal resection of the rectum in 251 patients who survived for at least 2 years.[98] Upon comparison of extraperitoneal and intraperitoneal colostomy, it appeared that the complication rate was higher with the latter technique; the difference, however, was not statistically significant. Table 16-1 demonstrates the results of this study. It can be appreciated that colostomy construction is associated with a high incidence of complications. Almost 50% of the patients in this series (patients who survived for at least 2 years) developed a stomal problem. One can only conjecture that had the series been followed for a longer period of time, the complication rate would be higher. Furthermore, the study failed to include those patients who had no specific stomal problem; it included only those with difficulties in appliance management.

Marks and Ritchie reviewed their experience with complications following abdominoperineal resection for carcinoma of the rectum during the period 1968 through 1972, at the St. Mark's Hospital.[54] Of the 227 patients who formed the basis of this study, three died in the postoperative period. By far the commonest stomal problem encountered was hernia, which occurred in 23 patients, approximately 10%. It was felt that the cumulative risk of developing a pericolostomy hernia in the sixth postoperative year was approximately 33%. The authors believed that extraperitoneal colostomy seemed to offer some protection against herniation. The other reported complications included retraction, stenosis, abscess, and prolapse. The cumulative incidence

Table 16-1. Complications of Terminal Colostomy (251 Patients)

Complication	Number of cases	Percent of series
Infection	34	14
Mucocutaneous separation	24	10
Pericolostomy hernia	36	14
Prolapse	12	5
Recession (retraction)	1	0.4
Stenosis	9	4
Fistula	1	0.4

(Modified from Whittaker M, Goligher JC: A comparison of the results of extraperitoneal and intraperitoneal techniques for construction of terminal iliac colostomies. Dis Colon Rectum 1976; 19:342–344)

of all these stomal complications was approximately 7%. This report and others confirm that most colostomy hernias seem to develop in the first few years.[52]

Complications

Most colostomy complications are preventable. The principles of stomal construction have already been outlined. The bowel must be drawn through the abdominal wall without tension; it must be brought through the split rectus muscle; it must be sutured primarily to the skin; and the viability of the end of the colon must be clearly demonstrated.[93] Although no method guarantees that subsequent complications will be avoided, attention to the above principles will minimize the risk.

Ischemia and Stomal Necrosis

Ischemia and stomal necrosis are obviously due to inadequate blood supply. This is more likely to develop if the ascending branch of the left colic artery is not preserved, a consequence of high ligation of the inferior mesenteric artery (on the aorta). Another possible source for compromise of the blood supply occurs if the meandering artery has been divided or if collateral circulation from the middle colic vessels is inadequate.

Recognition of stomal ischemia should not be difficult. If the mucosa looks blue it probably is ischemic. Occasionally, after a difficult abdominoperineal resection, one may be less compulsive in creating the colostomy or perhaps somewhat less concerned about the possible nonviability of the stoma. It is better to reopen the abdomen to free a further length in order to effect a satisfactory stoma at the time of the resection than to have to return the patient to the operating room several days or weeks later. The philosophy expressed by the statement, ''It looks a bit dark, but it will probably be all right,'' is delusional. If the stoma is nonviable, the bowel may retract into the peritoneal cavity, causing peritonitis and necessitating emergency surgical intervention. Less critical, but almost as unpleasant a consequence, is the situation illustrated in Figure 16-1. The sigmoid colostomy has retracted and the

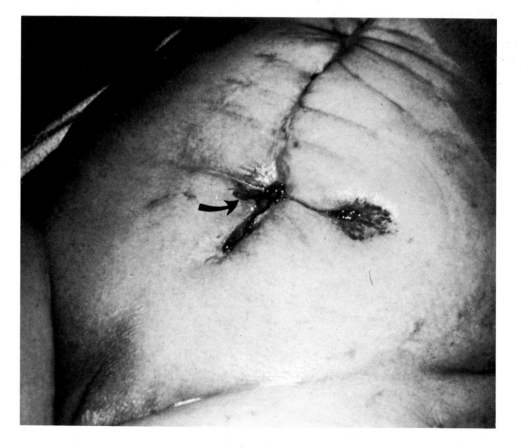

FIG. 16-1. Sigmoid colostomy: retraction with feces draining entirely from the abdominal wound *(arrow).*

stool presents in the lower portion of the abdominal incision, tracking subcutaneously from the original opening in the rectus fascia. In a less ominous consequence, the stoma may merely separate from the skin at the area of nonviability with a resultant stricture (Fig. 16-2).

If the patient cannot cope with the retraction or stenosis, revision is required. This may or may not be possible without a laparotomy. An attempt is made to circumcise the colostomy, free up sufficient bowel, and resuture it (Fig. 16-3). The patient should be prepared preoperatively for the possibility of a laparotomy if there is insufficient length of bowel available to create an adequate stoma by this method. Dilatation alone of skin-level stenoses is not recommended. The trauma from manipulation may cause hemorrhage and further inflammatory reaction, and may actually worsen the condition.

Rarely, the stenosis occurs at the fascial level. This is usually due to an inadequate opening in the fascia itself. Treatment will require mobilization of the bowel, enlargement of the opening in the fascia, and resuture of the colon.

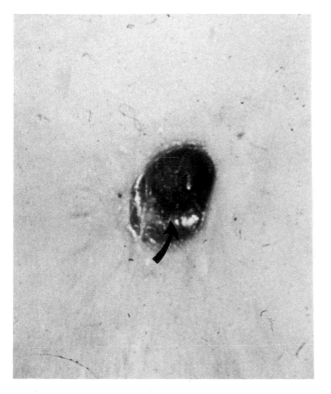

FIG. 16-2. Sigmoid colostomy. Separation on the inferior aspect *(arrow)* resulted in subsequent stenosis and requirement for a revision.

Paracolostomy Abscess

Paracolostomy abscess is an unusual postoperative complication. It should be particularly rare if the stoma is not placed in the abdominal incision. The problem is more likely to be seen with an ileostomy, if sutures are placed too deeply and penetrate the bowel lumen during the process of eversion. Another possible cause of a parastomal abscess in a patient who has undergone an ileostomy is recurrent Crohn's disease. If the colostomy retracts and there is fecal contamination in the subcutaneous tissue, an abscess can result. But by far the most common reason for paracolostomy abscess is incorrect irrigation technique; either the irrigating fluid or the device used for insertion into the stoma perforates the bowel. Symptoms include an unrewarding irrigation associated with immediate pain.[44] Predisposing factors include alcoholism, psychological disturbances, and the presence of a pericolostomy hernia. Usually a phlegmon of the abdominal wall develops. If the process dissects into the peritoneal cavity or starts within the abdomen, it can lead to generalized peritonitis.

Treatment usually requires laparotomy and relocation of the colostomy, but Reynolds and co-workers reported satisfactory management by means of adequate surgical drainage and intravenous hyperalimentation or an elemental diet.[66] No proximal diversion was undertaken. However, in my limited experience with this complication, usually with patients who developed a bowel perforation secondary to irrigation, this was a major septic problem requiring urgent surgery and extensive debridement, drainage, stomal relocation, and, in some cases, proximal colostomy.

Isa and Quan reviewed the Memorial Hospital experience with colostomy perforation.[44] This was observed 10 times in a 10-year period ending in 1975. In nine cases the cause of the perforation was irrigation of the colostomy, and in one case a barium enema examination. Barium enema complication can usually be avoided by the use of a cone tip (see Fig. 1-22, *B*) or by other devices.[77] The Memorial Hospital group strongly condemns the use of catheters with intraluminal balloons.

Hemorrhage

Colostomal hemorrhage is extremely unusual in the immediate postoperative period. However, because of underlying portal hypertension, the mucosa of the exposed bowel is predisposed to the possibility of considerable bleeding. Goldstein and co-workers concluded in their review that control of major stomal hemorrhage by local measures is often ineffective and that portasystemic shunting may be required to control the bleeding.[34] Finemore reported varices associated with

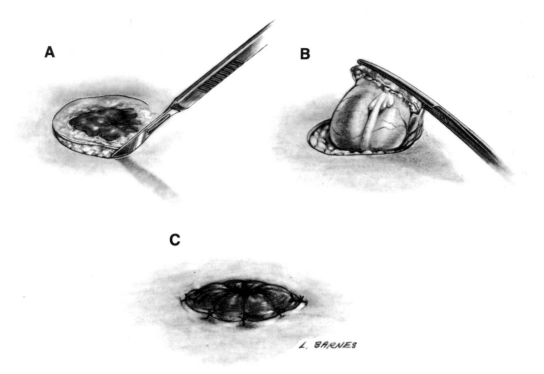

FIG. 16-3. Revision of retracted or stenotic colostomy. **A.** Skin is incised. **B.** Bowel is mobilized. **C.** New stoma is matured.

hepatic metastatic carcinoma.[27] A characteristic bluish skin around the stoma may be appreciated. This also can be seen in a patient with an ileostomy (see Fig. 16-53).

Prolapse

Colostomy prolapse is an uncommon complication following abdominoperineal resection. Chandler and Evans identified only 2 patients with this complication in 217 who underwent the procedure (less than 1%).[16] The complication occurs much more frequently in patients who have undergone a loop colostomy (see later) than in those with an end colostomy. The etiology of the problem may be an oversized opening in the abdominal wall, a redundant sigmoid loop leading to the stoma, sudden increased abdominal pressure (*e.g.,* straining or coughing), or a rigid appliance worn with a tight belt.[51] The condition is frequently associated with a pericolostomy hernia. Adequate fixation of the mesentery and bowel to the peritoneum has been suggested as a means for preventing this complication, but I do not agree with this view. In my experience, patients who develop colostomy prolapse usually have a

stoma that was initially created somewhat too long. This situation, in combination with the presence of a redundant loop of sigmoid colon, especially in a thin patient, particularly if that individual has chronic lung disease, tends to predispose to the problem (Figs. 16-4 and 16-5).

In the absence of an associated hernia, treatment of a prolapse usually does not require a laparotomy. The colostomy is incised and the bowel liberated, resected, and resutured (Fig. 16-6). If the prolapse occurs several months after the initial operation, the incision should be made into the mucosa rather than into the skin. The blood supply from the adjacent skin will be sufficient to maintain viability of the stoma, and an anastomosis is in actuality effected between the new end of the colon and the mucosa. This is an important point to remember, because if the skin is incised, too large an opening will be created when the stoma is subsequently matured (Fig. 16-7). It is important to liberate as much intra-abdominal colon as is possible and to resect it in order to avoid recurrent prolapse. With a particularly mobile colon, one may actually create an end transverse colostomy in the left iliac fossa.

Rarely, sigmoid colostomy prolapse may produce

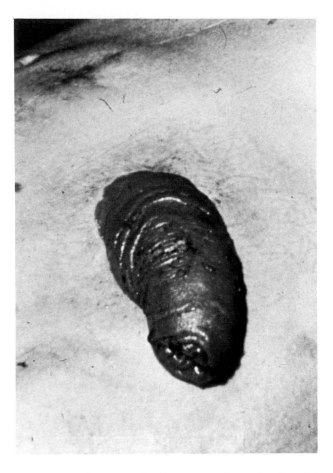

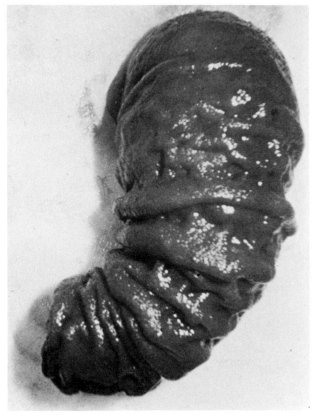

FIG. 16-5. This sigmoid colostomy prolapse developed 6 months following the procedure; the patient was lifting a heavy object.

FIG. 16-4. This sigmoid colostomy prolapse developed 1 month following operation after a bout of coughing. Considerable redundant sigmoid colon had been permitted to remain.

compromise of the blood supply to the bowel and gangrene of the stoma (Fig. 16-8). Depending on the level of involvement, resection of the necrotic bowel may be accomplished without a laparotomy, or a full laparotomy may be required. If a prolapse is associated with a pericolostomy hernia, relocation of the stoma may be necessary.

Peristomal Hernia

Peristomal hernia is the commonest late complication of abdominoperineal resection. As mentioned, the usual reason for this complication is the placement of the stoma in a pararectus location. Other possibilities include placement of the stoma into the incision, itself, and the creation of too large an opening in the abdominal wall (Figs. 16-9 through 16-11).

The choice of operative approach to the repair of peristomal hernias is usually dependent on the size of the defect. Relatively small openings can be repaired by direct suture, circumcising the colostomy, repairing the defect, and rematuring the stoma (Fig. 16-12). This technique is only possible for small hernias and is suggested when the colostomy had been created in the proper location, that is, through the split rectus muscle. If a small hernia is present in conjunction with an improperly located stoma, the colostomy should be relocated. This can usually be accomplished by a simple intraperitoneal tunnel method, repairing the defect at the original site by primary suture (Fig. 16-13).

Repair of larger defects usually requires the addition of a synthetic material, such as Marlex.[1, 64, 72, 84] My own preference is to attempt a direct repair whenever possible using the patient's normal tissue; however, in the huge hernias illustrated in Figures 16-9 through 16-11, such a procedure would be technically impossible. Relocation in my opinion is always advisable in

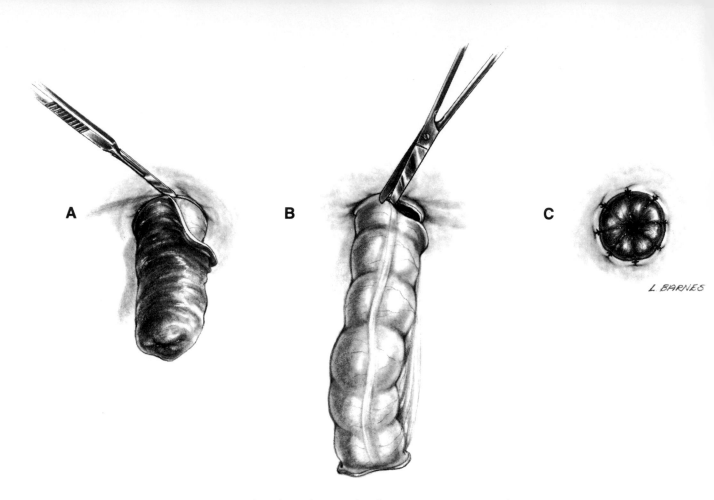

FIG. 16-6. Revision of prolapsed sigmoid colostomy. **A.** Incision at the mucocutaneous junction. **B.** Delivery and resection of redundant bowel. **C.** Colostomy matured.

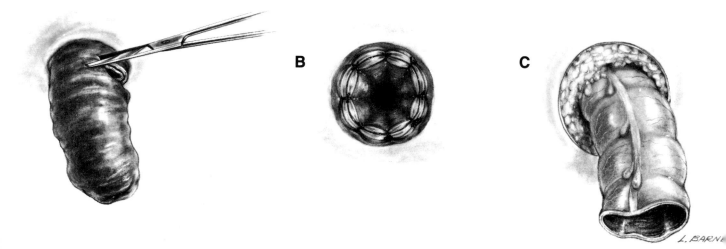

FIG. 16-7. Revision of prolapsed sigmoid colostomy (after several months). **A.** Incision into mucosa. **B.** Final maturation. **C.** Incorrect incision in the skin creates a large opening.

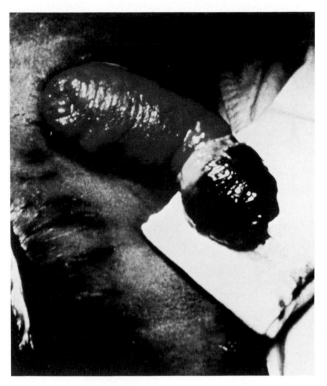

FIG. 16-8. Gangrene at the end of a prolapsed colostomy.

these situations. If the split rectus muscle is still available, I prefer this location, but all too often the entire left side of the abdomen is incorporated by hernia. One has essentially two recourses: using the right side of the abdomen or placing the stoma at the umbilicus. My own preference is for the latter location. The use of the umbilical site is not a unique concept, however; some surgeons prefer to create the colostomy in the umbilicus initially. Raza and colleagues evaluated 101 patients in whom they performed an umbilical colostomy.[65] They strongly supported the concept of this stoma because of their low incidence of complications: only four patients required reoperation. There were no peristomal hernias and no prolapses in their experience. If an umbilical colostomy is created, the technique of construction is essentially the same, but it is important to remove all of the skin that tends to turn inward.

In the repair of the hernia, some surgeons prefer to keep the stoma at the original location, using the mesh around the colostomy. Others actually bring the bowel through the middle of the Marlex. As stated, my own preference is to use mesh if necessary to effect the repair and relocate the stoma elsewhere. Unfortunately, many of these patients are elderly or represent a high risk for a major abdominal operation, and this is indeed a major procedure. There may be no recourse for some patients except to use some form of abdominal support.

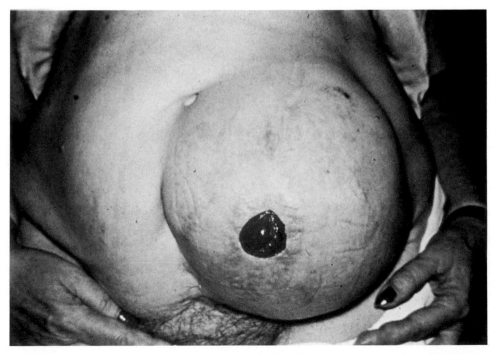

FIG. 16-9. Massive pericolostomy hernia. Note that the stoma has been brought through the left paramedian incision.

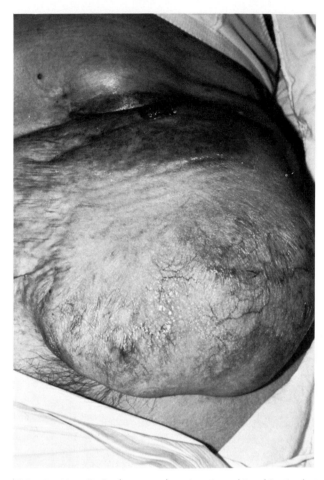

FIG. 16-10. Pericolostomy hernia. Atrophic skin is the only covering of the abdominal cavity. The stoma is at the apex of the defect.

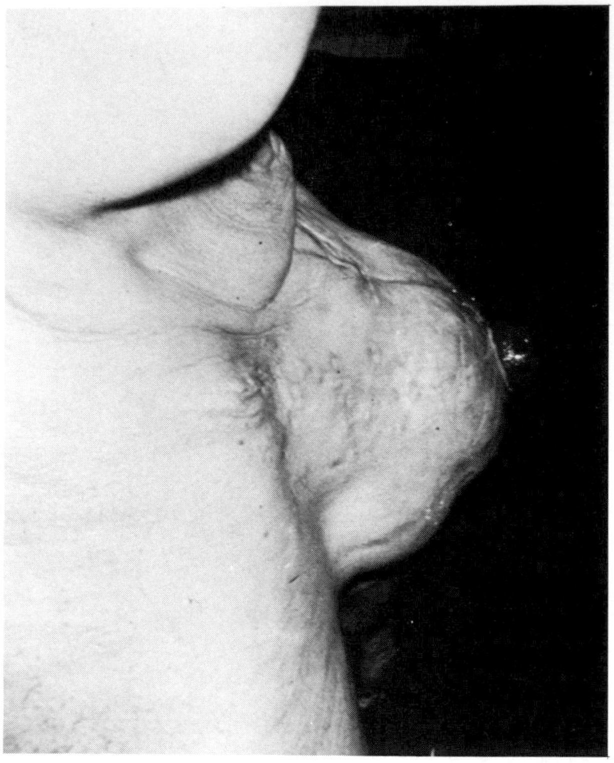

Fig. 16-11. Typical pericolostomy hernia with the stoma at the center of the defect.

Recurrent Disease

Recurrent disease may develop at the site of the stoma. This is usually seen in patients who have undergone abdominoperineal resection or a diversionary colostomy for inflammatory bowel disease (ulcerative colitis or Crohn's disease). The mucosa appears edematous and friable, bleeds easily, and may be granular or ulcerated. Medical management of the underlying disease process may resolve the inflammation and ameliorate the patient's complaints. However, because of diarrhea and the inability to maintain an appliance satisfactorily, a more extensive bowel resection and possible ileostomy may be required.

Recurrent malignancy may also occur at the site of the colostomy (Fig. 16-14). This may be due to tumor implantation at the time of the resection or inadequate

margin of resection, or it may actually represent a second primary. Probably the most likely explanation is tumor implantation. This is a rare and potentially fatal complication. Radical resection of the involved area including part of the abdominal wall with relocation of the stoma is the recommended treatment.

Alternative Techniques

In addition to the conventional maturation technique for sigmoid colostomy, the circular stapling device has been advocated for performing end colostomies.[50] The method has been used only on dogs, but it does have a certain potential appeal. Instead of a disk of skin being excised from the abdominal wall, a small opening is created just large enough to pass the center rod without the anvil. A pursestring is created of the distal colon in the usual manner and the anvil inserted into the bowel. The cartridge and anvil are approximated, and the instrument is fired. One donut consists of the skin, and the other is made up of the bowel. In effect, it is a colocutaneous anastomosis by means of the circular stapling device. Although the procedure does

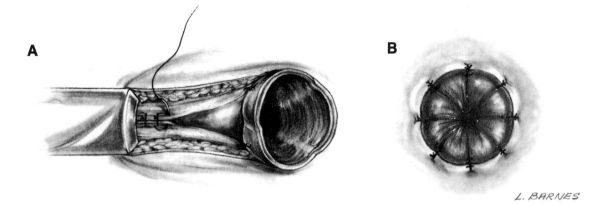

L. BARNES

FIG. 16-12. Pericolostomy hernia repair for a small defect at the correctly located site. **A.** Direct repair (note serosa to fascia sutures). **B.** Closure.

have theoretical appeal, it would certainly make the subcutaneous dissection and rectus splitting much more tedious. Furthermore, it is more likely that the inferior epigastric vessels will be injured during the course of the preliminary dissection. Hopefully, one may anticipate reports on the clinical experience with this technique.

The search for continence in a colostomy has stimulated many attempts to control bowel movements by means of prosthetic devices. Tenney and co-workers reviewed the various approaches that have been attempted or proposed that address this concept.[88] The authors considered the concepts in accordance with four categories: external devices, surgical technique alone, surgical technique with passive implanted devices, and surgical technique with active implanted devices.

In the first category, a simple inflatable cuff has been attempted by the Mayo Clinic group, using the cuff end of a tracheostomy tube. The procedure was performed initially in animals and then in patients who had failed nipple valves following a Kock continent ileostomy. It was also considered in patients with conventional ileostomies who had not undergone a reservoir procedure. Kock and associates proposed a technique, analogous to the continent ileostomy, of using the descending colon to create a nipple valve.[48] Because the procedure has been performed only in dogs, its application in humans has not as yet been determined.

Szinicz described an implantable hydraulic sphincter prosthesis that consists of a compressible driving and control system together with a sleeve that is implanted around the bowel.[86] The sleeve is connected to the compliance chamber by means of a connecting tube. The author reported his experience in animal experi-

ments and in seven patients. Heiblum and Cordoba implanted an inflatable plastic balloon in the subcutaneous tissue around the stoma in order to achieve fecal continence.[39] The connecting tube from the balloon was tunneled subcutaneously and brought out through a small wound at some distance from the stoma. The authors reported their experience in six patients, all but one of whom underwent the prosthesis insertion secondarily. Complete continence to feces and gas was obtained. One device had to be removed because it eroded the skin; subcutaneous infection was a problem in three patients.

Intestinal smooth muscle has been used to construct a continent colostomy.[78] Freely transplanted large intestinal muscle (usually the sigmoid), devoid of mucosa and mesenteric fat, is prepared in a 10- to 15-cm-long segment. The seromuscular sleeve is incised longitudinally through one of the tenia, soaked in an antibiotic solution, and sutured to the serosa of the bowel approximately 2 or 3 cm proximal to the site for the creation of the stoma. Sutures are placed so that the transplant becomes accordionated. This creates a length of approximately 6 cm, which in effect increases the muscular mass. The author emphasizes that, after securing one edge of the graft, the muscle must be stretched maximally, and the graft wrapped around the bowel and secured. The mesenteric vessels are incorporated by the graft.

Schmidt reported his experience with this technique in over 500 patients, 231 of whom underwent surgery in his own unit.[78] Approximately 80% of the patients did not require an appliance, there was no mortality, and only five required removal of the surgical implant. Apparently the transplants are nourished by means of a secondary vascularization. An irrigation technique

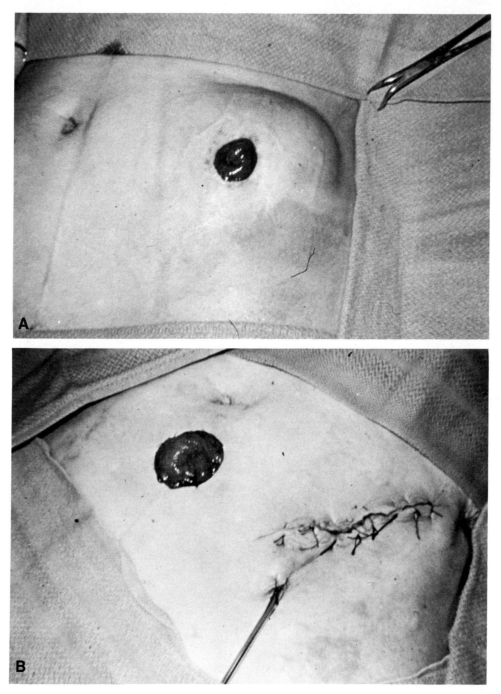

FIG. 16-13. Pericolostomy hernia repair for small defects in the pararectus location, **A.** The stoma has been relocated after intraperitoneal tunneling, and the defect repaired, **B.** The wound should be closed secondarily, not by the primary closure and drainage method which is shown.

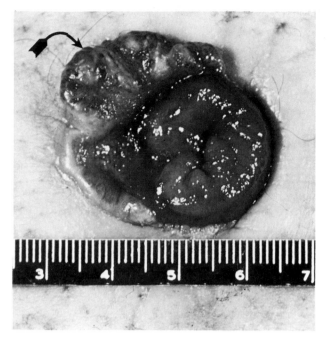

FIG. 16-14. Recurrent carcinoma adjacent to the stoma *(arrow)*. (Courtesy of Rudolf Garret, M.D.)

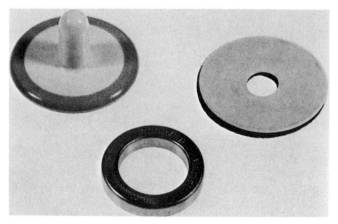

FIG. 16-15. Magnetic ring, cap, and disposable charcoal filter. (Khubchandani IT, Trimpi HD, Sheets JA, Stasik JJ Jr, Balcavage CA: The magnetic stoma device: A continent colostomy. Dis Colon Rectum 1981; 24:344)

facilitates defecation. In most patients who underwent the procedure secondarily, "nearly all viewed their postoperative situation as markedly improved."

In 1975, Feustel and Hennig of Erlangen, Germany, described a device to create continence in patients who underwent conventional sigmoid colostomy: a magnetic ring implant (Fig. 16-15).[26] A ring of samarium cobalt encased in a plastic is buried in the subcutaneous tissue around the colon. The colostomy is matured in the usual manner and when the wound has completely healed (usually several weeks later), an external cap containing a ring magnet in the top and a core magnet in the center pin is inserted to create a plug. Khubchandani and co-workers recommend that the site for creating the colostomy should be higher than that usually employed if the magnetic stoma device is to be implanted.[47] They recommend penetrating the full thickness of the abdominal wall with a needle and injection of methylene blue in order to help orient the surgeon with the subsequent dissection.

It is extremely important for the bowel to come through the abdominal wall at a right angle to the skin so that the cap will sit exactly in the center of the ring. Failure to effect this may result in necrosis of the bowel wall. A 2.5-cm disk of skin is excised from the previously marked site; no attempt is made to remove subcutaneous tissue. A cruciate incision is made in the fascia in the usual manner, and the rectus muscle is

split. The peritoneal cavity is entered and by blunt dissection a plane is created between the abdominal wall and the stoma site. The ring is then passed into the pocket and secured in place with interrupted 3-0 monofilament nylon sutures (Fig. 16-16). The space where the tunnel was created at the abdominal wound is closed. Scarpa's fascia is secured to the edge of the rectus fascia, completely excluding the ring (Fig. 16-16, *C*). The bowel is then brought through the ring and the colostomy matured in the usual manner. The cap is inserted 4 to 6 weeks later, the patient managing the stoma in a conventional manner up until that time. Patients may elect to use the cap only on special occasions or may wear it all the time except in preparation for evacuation. Evacuation may be facilitated by an irrigation. Alternatively, a colostomy bag may be used during the hours of sleep until the bowel evacuates. This is ideal if the patient is fortunate enough to have a regular bowel regimen.

An alternative technique involves the implantation of the device from the outside. This is the preferred method for the patient who has the procedure performed secondarily. If the ring is implanted from the outside, a larger disk of skin must be excised than if it is tunneled from the abdominal wall. The subcutaneous tissue is bluntly dissected off the fascia, and the ring is inserted using traction on the skin (Fig. 16-17, *A*). The ring is then secured and Scarpa's fascia sutured to obliterate the entire surface, as has been previously described. If the colostomy has been created several months previously, it is possible to simply circumcise the colostomy approximately 1 cm from the mucocutaneous junction, seat the ring, obliterate the space, and resuture the skin (Fig. 16-17, *B* and *C*). Necrosis

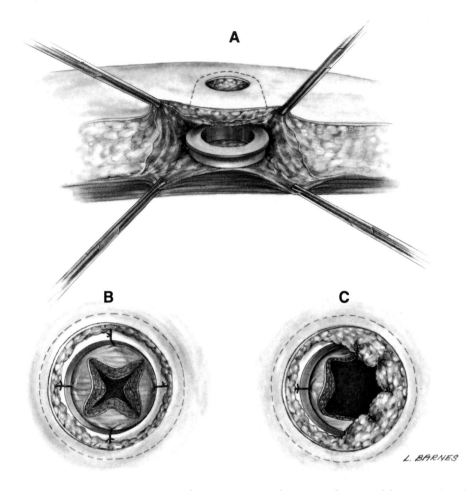

FIG. 16-16. Magnetic continent colostomy. **A.** Development of a tunnel between the abdominal wound and the stomal site. **B.** Securing of the ring to the fascia. **C.** Obliteration of the ring surface by suturing Scarpa's fascia to the anterior rectus fascia. Care must be taken to avoid dimpling of skin.

of the skin between the incision and the mucosa should not occur because collateral circulation should be adequate this long following the initial creation of the colostomy.

Results of the continent colostomy device were initially quite favorable, although subsequent results have been less optimistic.[35] Khubchandani and associates reported their experience in 14 patients; one half had good results.[47] There was no morbidity attributable to insertion of the ring, and there was no incident of wound infection. The authors emphasize that meticulous attention must be given to avoiding wound contamination; the colostomy must be constructed in a strictly perpendicular manner, and mucosal eversion must be minimal, or, ideally, nonexistent. Patients who

are relatively obese are poor candidates; the authors believe that subcutaneous adipose tissue in excess of 5 cm contraindicates the operation. If the abdominal wall is not flat enough to bear the disk, this is also a contraindication. Patients who are too thin (subcutaneous tissue less than 1 cm) should also not undergo the operation. Other problems include triggering security monitors at airports, disturbances of television reception if one is sitting close, malfunctioning of a wrist watch, and adherence of patient to anything metallic (*e.g.*, a kitchen sink).[47] The authors further emphasize that the patient must be physically and mentally able to cope with the magnetic device.

Alexander-Williams and associates reviewed their experience with 61 patients, 55 primary and 6 secon-

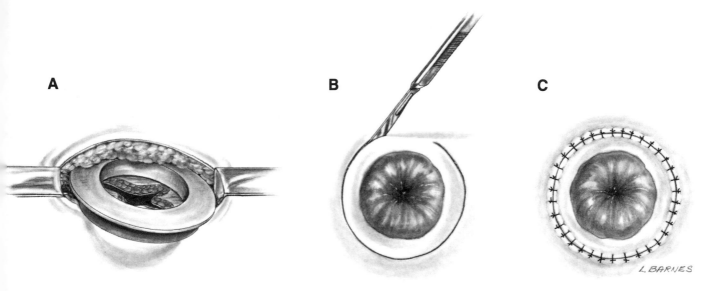

FIG. 16-17. Magnetic continent colostomy (external placement). **A.** The ring is inserted after mobilization of the fat off the rectus fascia. **B.** Incision for late ring insertion. **C.** Closure.

dary implants.[5] One patient died, possibly as the result of sepsis at the site of the implant. Twelve (20%) required removal of the ring because of failure of healing or late skin necrosis. Approximately half of the remaining patients were not using the magentic cap at all at the time of the review. The reason for this failure was the fact that the device did not afford complete continence. Of the 21 patients that used the cap regularly, 15 were continent. In these authors' experience, therefore, only one quarter of the patients who underwent the operation were completely continent. Kewenter reported 21 patients who underwent magnetic colostomy, all but three of whom had the procedure performed at the time of the primary resection.[46] Three patients died soon after operation (unrelated to the surgery). Eight of the patients were considered a success in that the cap was used under all circumstances, and two patients were considered partial successes. If one groups these two categories together, excluding the patients who expired, the rate of success with the procedure in Kewenter's experience was 44%.

It appears from the foregoing that implantation of the magnetic stoma device is not a very forgiving technique. It requires meticulous dissection and careful patient selection. Complete control is effected in no more than 50% of patients. For these reasons I have not been willing to consider the operation or to recommend it for my patients who have undergone sigmoid colostomy. I believe a technique recently developed by my colleague Elliot Prager holds greater promise.

In 1983, Prager described a device for control of feces following abdominoperineal resection and sigmoid colostomy.[63] It is composed of two parts, a silicone ring, which is produced in three different internal diameters with a flange on the upper surface reinforced with dacron mesh, and a silicone balloon, which is made in varying lengths. The balloon is inflated and deflated by means of a 30-ml syringe. The ring is implanted within the peritoneal cavity and sewn onto the undersurface of the abdominal wall where the opening has been made for the stoma to be delivered (Fig. 16-18). The ring can be positioned directly under the abdominal wall defect and held in place by an obdurator while the sutures are placed. The obdurator is also calibrated on the handle to determine the thickness of the abdominal wall; this will determine the length of plug that is subsequently employed. When the bowel is brought through the ring, it should be delivered in a gentle arc to avoid angulation and possible obstruction (Fig. 16-19). The abdominal incision is then closed and the colostomy matured in the usual manner. Beginning approximately 1 week after the operation, the patient begins to use the plug (Fig. 16-20). It may be used on the first day for an hour at a time, with half-hour intervals between insertions. On the second day, this is increased to two-hour intervals. With each subsequent day the plug is used for a more extended period of time. As of this writing, preliminary experience with 17 patients revealed no incident of infection and no evidence of injury to the stoma. Colostomy manage-

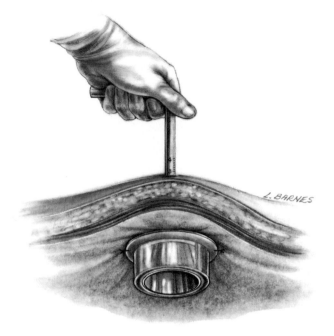

FIG. 16-18. Continent colostomy (Prager): implantation of a ring using an obturator to hold position and to facilitate suture placement. Note the calibration for determination of plug length. Rings are available in several diameters for different bowel circumferences.

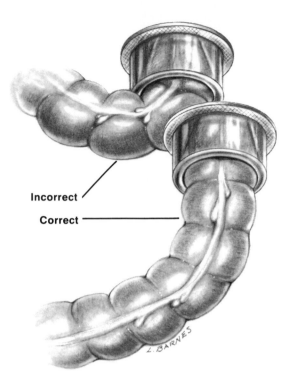

FIG. 16-19. Continent colostomy (Prager). Note that the angulation of the bowel relative to the ring must be virtually nonexistent.

ment proceeds with or without irrigation in the usual way. Although the experience is still limited and the follow-up period is short, the procedure in my opinion has promise, particularly since there are no absolute restrictions on the type of patient who is a candidate for the procedure, and thus far, side-effects are nonexistent.

TRANSVERSE COLOSTOMY

Transverse colostomy is a procedure usually employed on a temporary basis for obstructing and perforating lesions of the colon, for trauma, because of anastomotic disruption, and in order to protect an anastomosis. With the advent of improved anastomotic techniques, the procedure is now used primarily in emergency situations.

Technique

A properly constructed loop transverse colostomy is a fully diverting stoma. Unless the proximal limb retracts, it is impossible for the stool to pass into the distal limb.

Numerous modifications have been proposed to simplify the technique, to facilitate appliance management, and to expedite closure with presumed lower morbidity.[7, 14, 25, 41, 53, 69, 70, 74, 85] However, intra-abdominal or skin-level colostomies without a rod or tube colostomy may vent the colon adequately but are not truly diverting.[25, 85] The problem can be obviated by "stapling" the distal end,[61, 74] or by dividing the colon, creating an end transverse colostomy and performing a side-to-side colon anastomosis of the distal segment.[53] This last method, an alternative to the concept of a "double-barrel" colostomy, is time consuming to create and requires a full laparotomy to close.

Most surgeons are confident with a loop colostomy, because the technique is simple and, if the stoma is properly constructed, it completely diverts the fecal stream. Rombeau and co-workers performed a barium enema in 25 patients following loop transverse colostomy.[70] Follow-up films were obtained up to 4 days later; barium was not visible in the distal colon in any of the patients. This same study performed 4 weeks following diverting colostomy failed to show barium in the distal colon segment.

Suggested alternatives to the use of a cumbersome

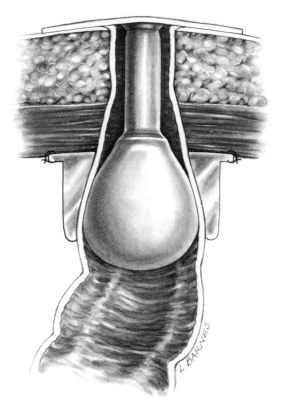

FIG. 16-20. Continent colostomy (Prager): plug in position.

rod have included a deep retention suture with retained polyethylene sleeve as a bridge,[14] the use of the skin as a rod,[7] and suturing of the fascia between the leaves of the mesentery.[69] One may elect to simply use a No. 14 French red rubber catheter to support the spur of the loop, using the cut ends of a No. 22 French catheter sewn into each end. Alternatively, one may employ the system prepared commercially by Hollister (Fig. 16-21) or by Convatec (Fig. 16-22).

For many years the ritual of "unveiling the stoma" had been a standard part of the postoperative management of patients who underwent a temporary diverting colostomy. A large plastic or glass rod was placed beneath the bowel and a rubber hose was attached to both ends to keep it from slipping out of place. A bulky dressing was then applied. Approximately 48 hours later the dressing was removed, and at the bedside, a cautery or soldering iron was employed to open the colon. The bloody, feculent scene that resulted might be reminiscent of the Battle of Sebastopol: assistants rushing to find hemostats, and feces on the floor, on the bedclothes, and on the walls. Ultimately, a temporary appliance was draped around the large rod and changed frequently because the apparatus was certain to leak. Not uncommonly, additional problems included ischemia or gangrene of the stoma when hidden from view by the dressing, and retraction of the colostomy into the peritoneal cavity if the rod slipped out.

Today there is no excuse for such unpleasantness. There are three important reasons for opening the colostomy at the time of operation: (1) for patients with obstruction it affords an immediate opportunity to decompress the bowel; (2) it obviates the necessity of a subsequent tedious bedside procedure; and (3) it provides the physician and the nursing staff with an opportunity to inspect the viability of the stoma at frequent intervals. A dressing tends to dissuade anyone from examining the site and precludes any possibility of identifying nonviable bowel.[18]

As has been suggested in Chapter 14, if a transverse colostomy is performed in an emergency situation, it should still be accompanied by a full exploratory laparotomy, identifying the nature of the pathology. Ideally, the colostomy should be created as distally as is possible, and if it is performed in the transverse colon should be accomplished on the left side. This is an important point, because if a transverse colostomy is present for a sufficient time, the distal limb will tend to prolapse. By placing it in the left transverse colon, the splenic flexure tends to tether the bowel and prevent the prolapse. Another reason for performing the colostomy in the distal transverse colon is that the stool is theoretically somewhat more formed than it would be in a more proximal location. There is simply no practical or theoretical advantage for using the right transverse colon as the stomal site.

As with sigmoid colostomy and ileostomy, the transverse colostomy should be brought through the split rectus muscle (Fig. 16-23). The omentum is freed from the colon for a sufficient distance to permit exteriorization without tension. A Penrose drain is passed through the leaves of the mesentery and the bowel delivered through the abdominal wound. A rod is passed through the same plane as the drain (Figs. 16-24 and 16-25). The colostomy is then "matured" by opening it longitudinally and suturing the bowel edge to the skin (Fig. 16-26). An appliance is then used (Fig. 16-27). A properly constructed loop transverse colostomy should be fully diverting, relatively easy to manage, and not offensive (Fig. 16-28). The bridge or rod can be removed as soon as sufficient edema is present to maintain exteriorization of the colon. It is not necessary to leave the rod in place for a week, as has been sometimes advised, because very often the rod itself will cause an element of obstruction that impedes the progress of the patient. Conversely, if the colostomy

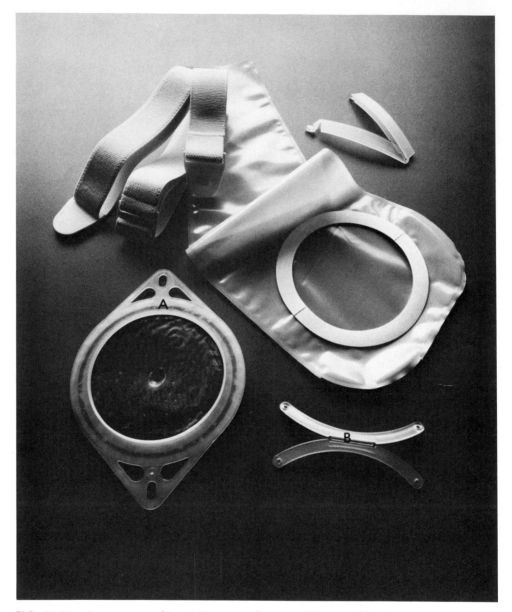

FIG. 16-21. Loop ostomy kit. **A.** Karaya gasket assembly. **B.** Folding loop ostomy bridge. (Courtesy of Hollister, Inc.)

seems to be functioning well even with the rod in place, and very little edema is evident, the bridge may be maintained for a longer period of time.

In an obese patient it sometimes is impossible to deliver the transverse colon out as a loop. Under this circumstance the bowel must be divided and the distal end oversewn. The colostomy is then created using the end of the transverse colon, maturing it in a similar manner to that of a conventional sigmoid colostomy.

Results

My associates and I reviewed our experience with complications of colostomy construction and closure.[58] In 162 patients who underwent a loop colostomy, 12 (7.4%) developed a *prolapse,* 6 (3.7%) were noted to have *retracted stomas,* and 4 (2.5%) were noted to have an *abscess.* In the series, almost 14% of patients developed a complication related to the colostomy construction alone. This does not, of course, take into consideration the morbidity associated with closure of a colostomy (see Colostomy Closure).

Embarking upon a transverse colostomy should not be taken lightly. As has been discussed in Chapter 11, one must justify that the procedure is indicated, and is not done simply because it makes the surgeon "feel better." The overall complication rate in 248 patients who underwent colostomy reported by Abrams and co-workers was 41%.[3] A hospital death rate of 24% was also noted. However, many of the patients had other serious illnesses, and one cannot blame the colostomy exclusively for the high morbidity and mortality. Wara and co-workers reviewed 250 patients who underwent transverse colostomy for proximal fecal diversion; the morbidity rate was 28%.[95] The two most important factors affecting the morbidity rate were

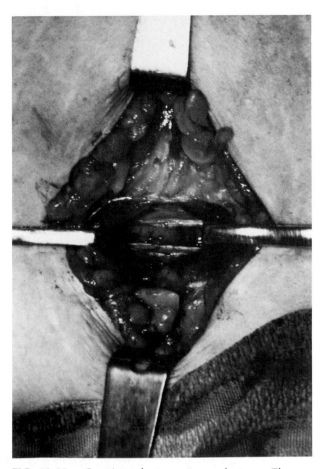

FIG. 16-23. Creation of a transverse colostomy. The rectus muscle is split.

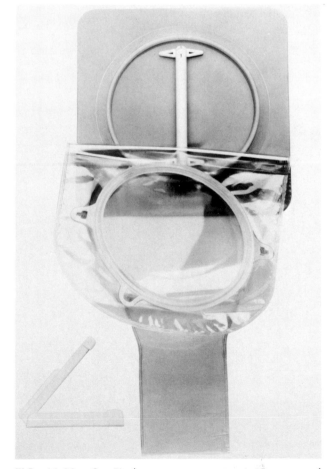

FIG. 16-22. Sur-Fit loop ostomy system. (Courtesy of Convatec, a division of E.R. Squibb and Sons, Inc.)

emergency colostomies and colostomies in infants. The overall incidence of specific colostomy complications was 26.4% in adults and 50% in children. Excluding infection, the commonest complication was prolapse, followed by retraction, peristomal hernia, and stomal necrosis. Miles and Greene noted a complication rate related to stomal construction of 11% in almost 200 patients, and Smit and Walt reported almost a 10% incidence of complications related to creation of the stoma.[57, 82]

The methods for preventing complications of transverse colostomy are quite similar to those of sigmoid colostomy. The size of the opening must be adequate in order to avoid edema, stricture, and obstruction. The appropriate site must be selected ideally before the operation, but this is not always possible if the transverse colostomy construction was unanticipated. If the colostomy is created with the bowel under tension, it is

(Text continues on p 658)

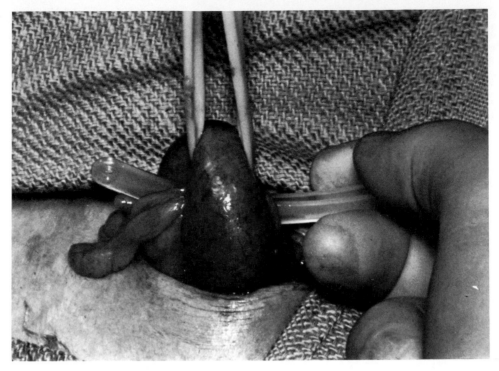

FIG. 16-24. Creation of a transverse colostomy. The bridge is passed through the mesentery. Traction on the Penrose drain delivers the bowel.

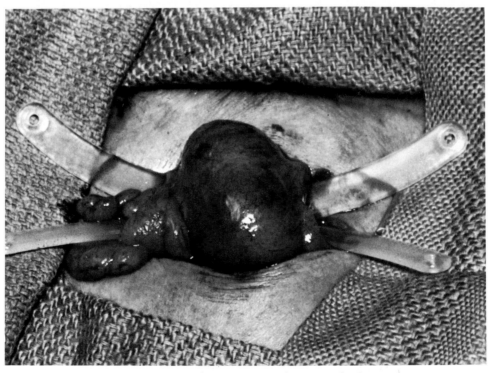

FIG. 16-25. Creation of a transverse colosotomy: bridge in place.

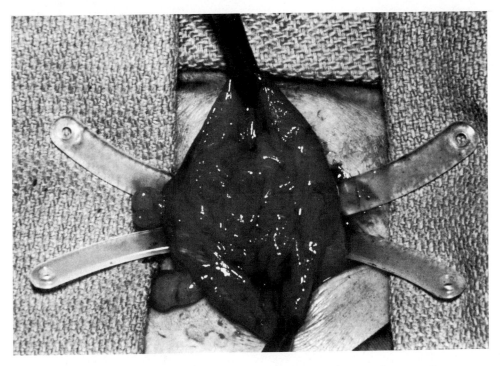

FIG. 16-26. Creation of a transverse colostomy: colostomy is matured.

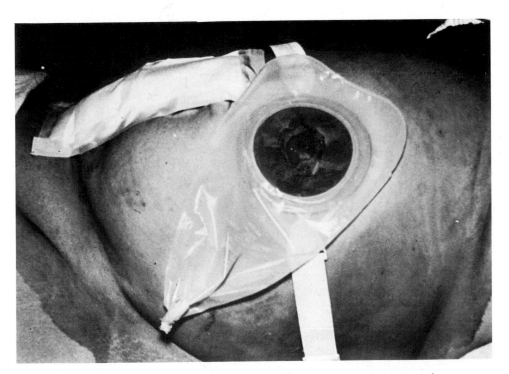

FIG. 16-27. Creation of a transverse colostomy: appliance is secured.

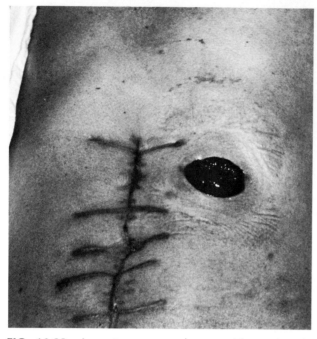

FIG. 16-28. Loop transverse colostomy. The patient is shown 1 month following perforated diverticulitis with fecal peritonitis.

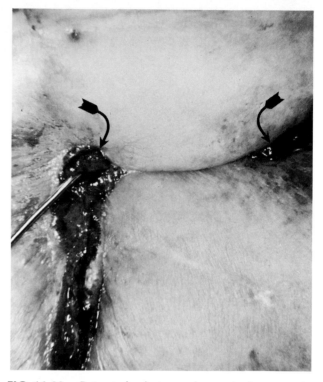

FIG. 16-29. Retracted colostomy, the result of mesenteric tension in an obese patient. Only two fecal fistulas remain *(arrows)*.

likely to retract or necrose (Fig. 16-29). A more common complication is colostomy prolapse, usually of the efferent limb (Fig. 16-30). If a colostomy is brought through the abdominal incision, it will always prolapse (Fig. 16-31). Winkler and Volpe advised that loop transverse colostomy is a holdover from the past, and that it is all too often permanent rather then temporary; they suggest that all colostomies should be created as end stomas.[101] Although their suggestion emphasizes the magnitude of the problem, I prefer a loop stoma because of the relative ease of subsequent closure.

Chandler and Evans reported that 40% of adult loop colostomies involving the right side of the transverse colon prolapsed, a statistically significant increase exceeding the rate for loop colostomies in more distal sites.[16] They further observed that obstruction at the time the colostomy was created seemed to predispose to an increased incidence of prolapse. Thirty-eight percent of all stomas originally made for obstruction prolapsed, compared with only 7% of those placed in unobstructed bowel. These authors proposed that the mechanism for this appeared to be a disproportion between the size of the fascial defect and the smaller diameter of the bowel following decompression.

Schofield and co-workers recommend rotating the colostomy 90° so that the proximal end is in a depen-

dent position.[79] These authors contend that stool is less likely to flow into the distal loop. In addition, they suggest that this method avoids colostomy prolapse and hernia. It is difficult for me to understand why that would be so, since the predisposing factors remain. Furthermore, with a properly constructed standard loop colostomy, overflow into the distal limb should not occur.

A number of techniques have been devised to treat colostomy prolapse. Zinkin and Rosin modified the technique originally described by Mayo and have adapted it to an office procedure.[55, 103] A smooth-backed button is placed on the abdominal wall, and a nonabsorbable suture is passed through the button-hole, skin, fascia, and intestine. A finger in the lumen of the intestine helps to reduce the prolapse and to direct the entrance of the needle through the bowel. The result is to fix the reduced intestine firmly against the anterior abdominal wall, preventing further intussusception. Krasna uses a pursestring suture to narrow the colostomy orifice, whereas Colmer and Foxx describe an external prolapse control device that consists of attaching the base of a Gellhorn pessary to the face plate of a colostomy appliance.[17, 49] The device is held

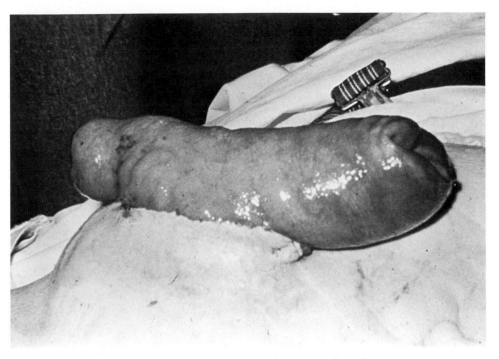

FIG. 16-30.   Loop transverse colostomy with prolapse.

in place by a colostomy bag belt. Since the "cork" is not completely obstructing, the stool passes around it, but the prolapse remains reduced.

Fortunately, most patients who have undergone a transverse colostomy are inconvenienced for a relatively short period of time. When the colostomy is performed for terminal disease, however, patients sometimes live long enough to develop severe management problems with the stoma. This is particularly true when abdominal distension as a result of liver enlargement or ascites produces a peristomal hernia or an irreducible prolapse. In fact, the problems associated with stomal management may be a source of greater disability than all other aspects of the care of the terminally ill patient. Therefore, one should endeavor to avoid if at all possible a permanent loop transverse colostomy.

Occasionally, a so-called temporary colostomy may become permanent. This is usually because a distal anastomosis has failed to heal or the patient has developed other serious medical problems that preclude further surgical intervention. If a problem arises, the surgeon might consider one of the methods described to control prolapse of the efferent limb. Another possibility, which can be accomplished with a local anesthetic, is to circumcise the distal limb, divide the bowel, oversew it, and resuture the end colostomy stoma (Fig. 16-32).

COLOSTOMY CLOSURE

It is the high morbidity associated with colostomy closure that has stimulated a voluminous literature that addresses the factors that predispose to the complications. Attempts are made to proselytize colleagues in an effort to convince the skeptics of the optimal method for reestablishing intestinal continuity. Controversy still exists over the relative merits of intra-abdominal versus extra-abdominal closure, closure with resection versus closure without resection, or primary wound closure versus delayed.

Yajko and co-workers reported a 28% incidence of complications associated with colostomy closure in 100 patients.[102] Wound infection was noted in 10% and fecal fistula in 4%. These authors advocate an open, two-layer anastomosis with delayed wound closure.

Beck and Conklin analyzed the records of 77 Vietnam war casualties who underwent loop colostomy closure.[8] The total postoperative complication rate was 9% with simple loop closure as compared with 24% with resection and anastomosis. These authors felt that closure without resection was technically easier and associated with a lower morbidity than resection of the stoma with reanastomosis.

Wara and associates noted a morbidity rate of 57% (a leakage rate of 10%) and a mortality rate of 1.7% in 105 patients.[95] They noted a significantly increased

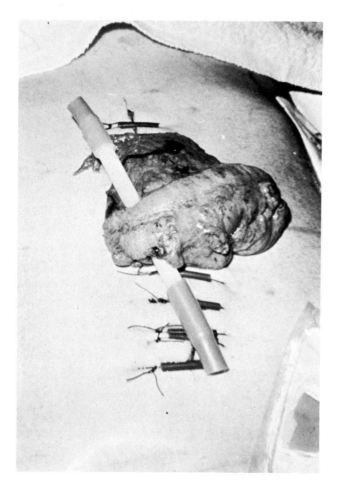

FIG. 16-31. Prolapsed loop colostomy created at the time of surgery with the colon brought through the abdominal incision.

incidence of fecal fistula and incisional hernia when closure was performed as a single procedure subsequent to a definitive resection; they believe that the difference might be explained by better accessibility when the colostomy was performed at the same time as the definitive resection.

Smit and Walt reported a complication rate of 30% in 167 patients who underwent colostomy closure.[82] Wound infection was seen in over 17% of the patients. These authors felt that the optimal period for closure was from 2 to 3 months after colostomy construction. They further noted that there was a higher incidence of complications in patients who did not undergo a full bowel preparation or who were not on antibiotics. They therefore suggested the use of antibiotics with complete bowel preparation as if for colon resection in all patients who are to undergo colostomy closure.

Todd and colleagues reviewed their experience in a retrospective fashion of 206 colostomy closures.[91] These authors found that the method employed did not significantly influence the postoperative morbidity or mortality, and that there was no evidence that the timing of the colostomy closure was a critical factor in the subsequent anastomotic complications. Varnell and Pemberton found that the time interval between colostomy creation and closure did not affect morbidity, nor did intraoperative wound management, the use of systemic antibiotics alone, and the location of the loop colostomy.[94] Their morbidity rate was 44 percent. Conversely, Freund and co-workers felt that the two major factors determining subsequent complications were timing and technique of closure.[28] Simple closure was associated with fewer complications than resection, and colostomies closed sooner than 12 weeks after their construction had twice the incidence of complications than those which were closed after that time.

Oluwole and associates concurred that colostomy closure 3 months following construction is preferred.[62] Other factors associated with a lower incidence of complications in their experience included mechanical and antibiotic bowel preparation, intraperitoneal closure, resection of the anastomosis, and delayed (secondary) skin closure. Rosen and Friedman, however, noted that the incidence of wound infection was not significantly improved by the use of systemic or nonabsorbable intestinal antibiotics.[71] Furthermore, intraperitoneal drainage alone or in combination with subcutaneous drainage resulted in the highest rate of wound infection in their experience.

Rickwood and co-workers reported a study of 100 consecutive colostomy closures in infants and children; they used a resection technique with intraperitoneal closure.[67] Wound infection was noted in 43 patients, a fecal fistula in 5, and other major complications in 8 instances. The overall morbidity, therefore, was in excess of 50%.

Besides the studies already referred to, I have selected nine recent reports from the literature on the results of colostomy closure.[6, 11, 23, 29, 40, 42, 59, 76, 97] The mean morbidity rate was 24% (range: 14% to 38%).

We reviewed our experience with colostomy closure from 1963 to 1974.[58] The combined early and late morbidity was 49%; wound infections were found in approximately 25% of the patients. A fecal fistula occurred in 9.3% of patients. Closure of the colostomy without resection was associated with the lowest incidence of complications (6.8%) when compared with other types of closure. Superficial subcutaneous drains did not prevent wound infections, and patients with intra-abdominal drains had an even higher incidence. Analysis of the intervals between creation and closure

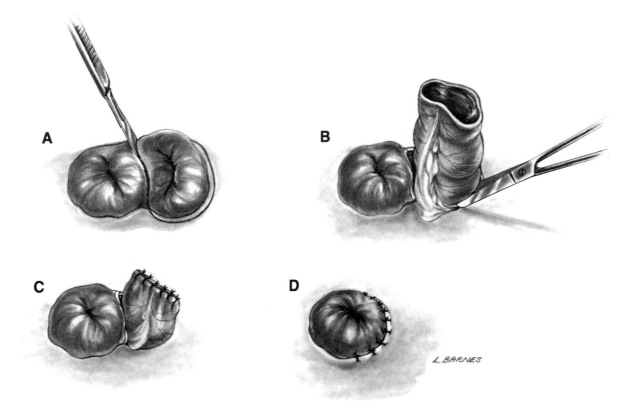

FIG. 16-32. Surgical treatment of loop colostomy prolapse. **A.** The mucosal rim is circumcised. **B.** The bowel is divided. **C.** The bowel is oversewn or stapled. **D.** Final maturation as an end stoma.

of the colostomies demonstrated that patients whose stomas were closed within 3 months after creation had a morbidity rate in excess of 50% (see Table 16-2). This rate decreased to approximately 34% for closure after a 4-month to 1-year interval.

Late complications occurred in 28 patients, incisional hernia, suture sinus, and intestinal obstruction being the most frequently seen (Table 16-3). With a complication rate such has been reported in most series, particularly with respect to closure of the colostomy, the surgeon should be circumspect in the initial selection of patients for a diversionary procedure.

Two recent reports, however, note a remarkably low incidence of problems associated with colostomy closure. Salley and co-workers reported a complication rate of 7.8 percent in 166 patients operated on from 1974 to 1981.[75] The sepsis rate was extremely low, only 2.4 percent. The authors attributed their low incidence of complications to a vigorous mechanical bowel preparation and the use of luminal and parenteral antibiotics. With respect to operative technique,

the bowel was sutured both by resection and by simple closure, and the wounds were closed by four different methods. Garnjobst and associates reviewed their experience of 125 consecutive colostomy closures, noting a complication rate of 5.6 percent in the early phase, and a later complication rate of 4 percent (primarily due to incisional hernia).[30] The authors attribute their low morbidity to simple closure rather than resection of the bowel (no local complications in 63 patients), meticulous surgical technique, antibiotic wound irrigation, and primary wound closure.

If, after reading the above outlined review, the surgeon is not confused about the optimal means of avoiding complications following colostomy closure, I would be greatly surprised. If one can extract a thread of consistency from the data, it is that early closure of the colostomy is associated with a high morbidity and that resection of the bowel in the experience of most surgeons is more hazardous than simple closure. Wound infection is by far the commonest complication; its avoidance, therefore, should be possible by delayed

Table 16-2. Interval Between Colostomy and Closure

Interval (Months)	Number of patients	Number with complications	Percent with complications
0–3	41	21	51.2
4–6	35	12	34.3
7–12	26	9	34.6
>12	16	3	18.8
	118	45	

(Mirelman D, Corman ML, Veidenheimer MC, Coller JA: Colostomies: Indications and contraindications: Lahey Clinic experience, 1963–1974. Dis Colon Rectum 1978; 21:172–176)

Table 16-3. Late Complications of Colostomy Closure

Complication	Number of patients	Percent of series
Incisional hernia	19	16.4
Suture sinus	3	2.6
Intestinal obstruction	2	1.7
More than one above	4	3.7
	28	24.4

(Mirelman D, Corman ML, Veidenheimer MC, Coller JA: Colostomies: Indications and contraindications: Lahey Clinic experience, 1963–1974. Dis Colon Rectum 1978; 21:172–176)

wound closure. The following technique is the procedure that I have adopted, which is associated with a morbidity rate of less than 5%.

Technique

The patient is placed on a full bowel preparation as if for colon resection. Irrigation of both limbs of the colostomy and of the rectum is performed the morning of surgery until the returns are clear. A broad-spectrum intravenous antibiotic is administered on call to the operating room; the patient is given another dose during surgery, and the antibiotics are continued for 48 hours following the operation. The colostomy is circumcised by means of a diathermy cautery, leaving a cuff of skin (Fig. 16-33, A). Four Kocher clamps are placed on the skin around the colostomy, and four triple hooks (Lahey) are placed on the surrounding skin to act as rectractors (Fig. 16-33, B). The Kocher clamps are held by the surgeon and serve as a handle while the assistant uses the hooks as retractors. The peritoneal cavity is entered, a clamp is placed on the fascia, and the bowel is freed (Fig. 16-33, C).

With the colostomy now separated from the abdominal wall, the skin and any remaining fibrous tissue is excised (Fig. 16-34, A). Closure of the anterior wall of the bowel is then effected in a transverse fashion (Fig. 16-34, B). Alternatively, if considerable edema and fi-

brosis prevent safe closure, the bowel is resected and an anastomosis performed as if for any colon resection. The fascia is then approximated with interrupted long-term absorbable sutures (Fig. 16-34, C).

Because of the high incidence of wound infection I prefer to leave the wound open for closure secondarily. This is accomplished by placing the skin sutures in loosely and securing them on a tongue depressor (Fig. 16-35, A). The wound is packed either with iodoform gauze or a Betadine-soaked gauze, and the wound is secondarily closed 4 or 5 days later (Fig. 16-35, B). The wound is closed completely by pulling on the tongue depressor and the assistant merely cuts each suture in turn while the surgeon ties it. With this technique no anesthetic is required, and the tension produced by individualy pulling and tying the sutures is avoided.

Postoperatively the patient is maintained on intravenous fluids until either good bowel sounds are established or the patient has passed flatus. No nasogastric tube is advised.

CECOSTOMY

The procedure of cecostomy could be removed from our surgical armamentarium with very little consequence to health care delivery. In fact, because the operation is used for the wrong indications, it probably is responsible for adverse results more often than it

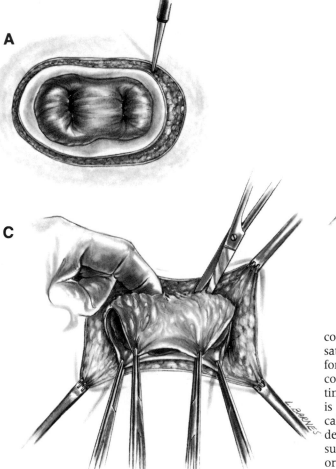

FIG. 16-33. Technique of loop colostomy closure. **A.** The colostomy is circumcised. **B.** Kocher clamps on the skin around the stoma serve as a handle, and triple hooks are used as retractors. **C.** The peritoneal cavity is entered and the colostomy is dissected from the abdominal incision.

ameliorites a condition. The procedure has been advocated to "protect" a left-sided anastomosis, in the treatment of large bowel obstruction, for cecal perforation, and in the treatment of cecal volvulus.[90] In my opinion the only indication for cecostomy is in the patient with Ogilvie's syndrome (see Chap. 17). Ileus on a nonsurgical basis that produces profound cecal dilatation and the risk of possible perforation may be treated by cecostomy. The point is that cecostomy is a decompressive maneuver; it is a vent. It does not divert the fecal stream. If diversion is required, a loop ileostomy should be considered (see later) if the transverse colon is not suitable. A loop ileostomy is an eminently satisfactory procedure not only for diversion, but also for permitting reasonable appliance management. Cecostomy virtually always commits the patient to continued hospitalization until such time as the opening is surgically closed. An exception to this is if the so-called tube cecostomy is employed, a technique that definitely should be stricken from the list of approved surgical procedures. The tube may become obstructed or the cecum may become detached from the abdominal wall, leading to generalized fecal peritonitis. Furthermore, sepsis can develop around the tube, and ultimately the fistula may still require surgical closure.

With the limited indication that I mentioned, cecostomy should be performed by the exteriorization technique. If it is to be performed as a "blind" procedure for acute cecal dilatation, a small incision is made in the right lower quadrant in a similar manner to the approach used for appendectomy. However, instead of splitting the muscle, the external and internal oblique and transversus abdominis are divided. The peritoneum is exposed and carefully incised. The cecum will tend to pout into the open wound, but if it is so distended that it cannot be delivered through the incision, it can be decompressed by needle or trocar aspiration. The seromuscular surface of the cecum is sutured to the abdominal wall with the interrupted long-term absorbable sutures (Fig. 16-36). After walling off the peritoneal cavity in this manner, the cecum is opened and the cut edge of the bowel is sutured to the full thickness of the skin in a similar manner to the maturation of an ordinary colostomy.

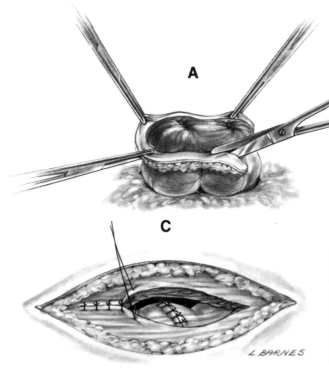

FIG. 16-34. Technique of loop colostomy closure. **A.** Excision of the skin and eschar. **B.** The anterior wall is closed transversely. **C.** The fascia is closed.

Even using this technique, appliance management is extremely difficult. The effluent is corrosive and liquid. But since the cecostomy does not truly divert, drainage may actually be quite minimal. It may consist mostly of gas, hence its primary benefit for decompressing an acutely dilated cecum. At least with the technique mentioned, the cecum is unlikely to become detached or to retract into the peritoneal cavity, leading to a possible life-threatening situation.

The paucity of recent literature on the subject is a testament to its lack of applicability and to its replacement by alternative diversionary procedures.

ILEOSTOMY

An ileostomy is usually advised for inflammatory bowel disease (ulcerative colitis or Crohn's disease). Other indications include familial polyposis, carcinomatosis, trauma, and congenital anomalies. Ideally, the patient should be well informed about the need for an ileostomy long before the operation is required. It is usually of great benefit to acquaint the patient with someone of comparable age, sex, and socioeconomic status who has an ileostomy and is well adjusted to it,

so that the patient can be assured that a normal lifestyle is possible. Unfortunately, some patients do not receive adequate preoperative counseling, either because the physician fails to mention the possibility of an ileostomy during the course of treatment of the condition or because the patient requires urgent surgical intervention, such as may be necessary for hemorrhage, toxic megacolon, perforation, or sepsis. Under these circumstances, the patient may always believe that the operation was performed too precipitously, and that perhaps with more vigorous medical management, surgery might have been avoided or at least deferred until a later time.

As has been previously discussed, preoperative consideration of the placement of the stoma is mandatory. The patient may actually wear the appliance before operation and note areas where subsequent appliance management may become difficult: skin folds, the waist line, and the usual position of pants or belt. One should not delay the determination of the site of the stoma until the time of the operation, because abdominal skin folds may not be apparent when the patient is lying down.

Prior to the early 1950s, for a patient to be confronted with an ileostomy was a traumatic event indeed. Before the advent of satisfactory appliance adhesives and the eversion techniques currently used, skin was actually grafted onto the end of the ileum in order for the corrosive effluent to be able to pass into some kind of appliance (Fig. 16-37). A signal advance was made for ileostomy construction by Brooke's publication, which stated rather undramatically, "A more simple device is to evaginate the ileal end at the time of the operation and suture the mucosa to the skin; no complications have accrued from this."[12] This author further observed that the ileostomy did not retract, but stood out in conical form; furthermore, prolapse was not encountered.

At about the same time, Turnbull suggested that so-called ileostomy dysfunction could be prevented by

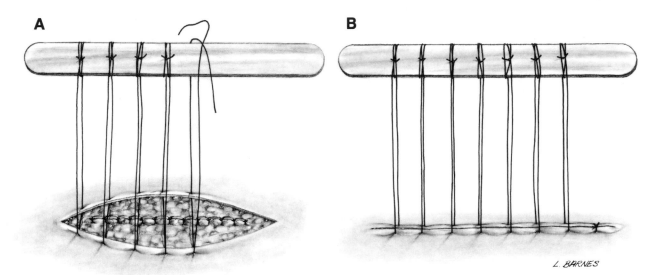

FIG. 16-35. Delayed wound closure. **A.** Sutures are placed and taped onto a tongue depressor. **B.** The wound is pulled closed and the sutures tied.

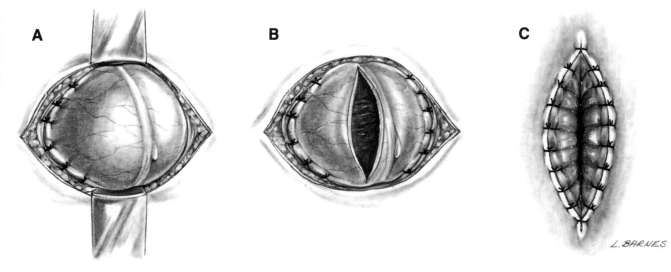

FIG. 16-36. Technique of cecostomy. **A.** Obliteration of the peritoneal opening by suture of the bowel wall to the fascia. **B.** Opening of the cecum. **C.** Primary maturation to the skin.

covering the serosa of the newly constructed ileostomy with mucosa.[92] He advised a technique whereby the seromuscular coat of the distal half of the exteriorized ileostomy was removed and the residual mucosal tube was pulled down over the ileostomy as a viable sliding graft. Subsequently, Crile and Turnbull explained the concept of ileostomy dysfunction on the basis of a violation of the basic surgical principle in exposing an

unprotected surface.[21] This exposure leads to serositis with fibrinopurulent exudate by the third or fourth postoperative day. These authors stated that this, in reality, is a peritonitis of the protruding segment. What results is an ileus and a functional obstruction of the ileostomy, with small bowel dilatation and diarrhea leading to excess loss of fluids and electrolytes. It was on the basis of the writings of Brooke and of Crile and

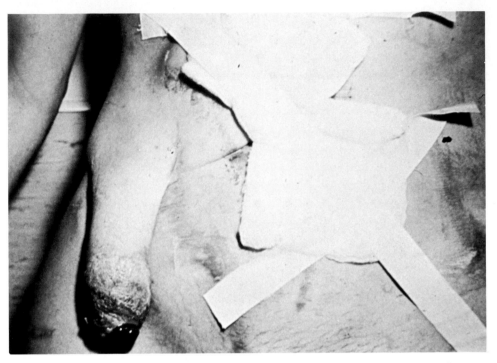

FIG. 16-37.   Skin-grafted ileostomy created before the development of effective adhesives and the current maturation technique. (Corman ML, Veidenheimer MC, Coller JA: Ileostomy complications: Prevention and treatment. Contemp Surg 1976; 8:36–41)

Turnbull that our current concepts of primary ileostomy maturation developed.

Despite the advances in operative technique, the creation of a satisfactory ileal stoma and the proper management of ileostomy complications are often unachieved ideals. This is not difficult to comprehend, for four reasons.

First, most busy general surgeons perform perhaps only two or three ileostomies in a given year. Second, when the procedure is performed on an emergency basis, the surgeon's main concern is with saving the patient's life, and sufficient care may not be given to creating the stoma. For example, during a colectomy and ileostomy for toxic megacolon, the colon must be removed as expeditiously as possible. In addition, the patient's cardiac, renal, and pulmonary functions may be severely compromised. With these pressing concerns, the surgeon may not be as meticulous as he should be in performing the ileostomy.

The third reason for difficulties after ileostomy may be the surgeon's lack of familiarity with techniques for properly locating and maturing the stoma. The fourth is in the area of postoperative care. Unfortunately, a mystique surrounds stomal management; surgeons who can successfully treat gangrene of the abdominal wall are confounded by a peristomal dermatitis. In the past, patients, themselves, had to search for answers in a morass of ignorance and superstition. It was because of this that the ostomy associations were formed. Even today patients with stoma problems are most often referred to these groups. Enterostomal therapy is designed to meet the needs of such patients, but the person's own physician can assist greatly by learning how to use simple principles. Besides problems with the appliance itself, the primary causes of difficulty after ileostomy are improper placement and incorrect construction of the stoma.

Technique

A disk of skin is excised from a previously marked site on the abdominal wall. Because subcuticular sutures are used instead of sutures through full-thickness skin, I find it easier to cut the skin obliquely such as is illustrated in Figure 11-16, *A*. This emphasizes the subcuticular aspect for easy suturing. The ileostomy is brought through the split rectus muscle and protrudes for approximately 4 or 5 cm. There is no reason to create a stoma that when everted is longer than 2 cm; the appliances that we now have available are so satisfactory that a penile-type stoma is truly unnecessary. Following extraperitoneal or intraperitoneal fixation (see Figs. 15-95 and 15-96), the mesentery to the distal ileum is trimmed (Fig. 16-38). Turnbull and Weakley advise passing an absorbable suture around the mesentery at skin level and excising the mesenteric fat from the ileostomy to overcome the bowing effect.[93] It is

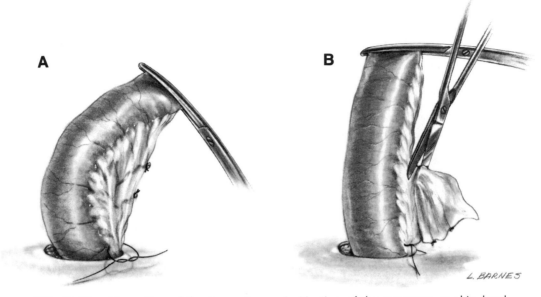

FIG. 16-38. Maturation of ileostomy stoma. **A.** Ligation of the mesentery at skin level. **B.** Trimming of the mesentery to remove "chordee." (After Turnbull RB, Weakley FI · Atlas of Intestinal Stomas. St. Louis, CV Mosby, 1967)

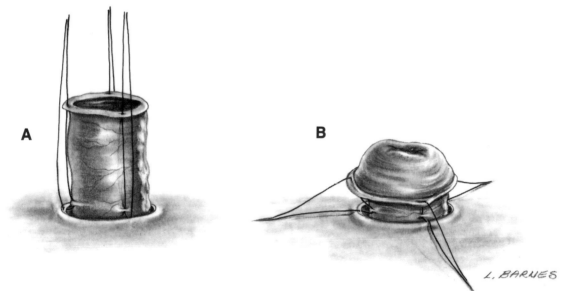

FIG. 16-39. Maturation of ileostomy stoma. **A.** Three sutures are placed incorporating the seromuscular layer to facilitate eversion. **B.** The sutures are secured, everting the bowel.

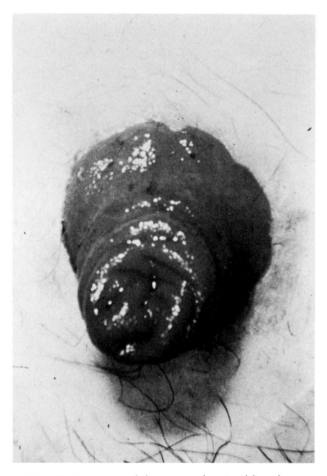

FIG. 16-40. Normal ileostomy of optimal length.

their feeling that the submucosal vascular supply can nourish at least 6 cm of ileum after the mesentery has been divided. I believe that this is always a safe maneuver in patients with ulcerative colitis. However, patients with Crohn's disease, who have a thickened mesentery or in whom the bowel is partially obstructed, often do not tolerate mesenteric stripping for this distance. One should exercise caution in carrying out this maneuver when such a problem is recognized.

At this point any redundant ileum should be amputated; the final length of the ileostomy should be approximately 2 cm. Three sutures are then placed through the full thickness of the end of the bowel, the seromuscular aspect of the ileum (at the skin level), and the subcuticular skin. One suture is placed on the antimesenteric aspect and one each on either side of the mesentery (Fig. 16-39). A seromuscular bite aids in the subsequent eversion of the bowel. Some sur-

geons criticize this technique because of the risk of possible fistula should the suture be placed too deeply. Obviously, care is required if one is to perform the technique properly and avoid this complication. The bowel is then everted and primarily matured (Fig. 16-40). A Babcock clamp placed within the bowel lumen may aid in the eversion. Interrupted sutures of 4-0 chromic catgut complete the construction.

Results

As recently as 30 years ago, the complication rate for ileostomy alone approached 100%. More recently, Morowitz and Kirsner reported their experience using a questionnaire of almost 2000 patients who had undergone ileostomy for ulcerative colitis.[60] Patient satisfaction with the ileostomy was certainly great in comparison with the preoperative status. This was substantiated by the dramatic decrease in the number of colitis patients under the care of a physician after the operation. Furthermore, the ileostomy seemed to have an ameliorative effect on marital status, and there appeared to be no significant effect on child-bearing. The authors, however, comment that, on the negative side, at least one fourth of the patients required ileostomy revision. Reoperation for bowel obstruction was performed in over 10%, and diarrhea and nephrolithiasis were frequent problems. Medication was required in 20%. There was a relatively low number of unemployed persons in the study. Conversely, Halevy and colleagues reported a survey from the Israel Ostomy Association and noted a low rate of rehabilitation as measured by return to previous occupation and problems with sexual and social adjustment.[37]

We have reported that ileostomy complications requiring revision are more frequently noted in patients who have Crohn's disease as compared with patients with ulcerative colitis.[33] Roy and co-workers reported that 9.7% of their patients with ulcerative colitis needed revision, as compared with 26.5% of patients with Crohn's disease.[73] Steinberg and colleagues found a similar incidence.[83]

Advanced age does not appear to be a contraindication to ileostomy. We reviewed our experience with ileostomy in the elderly, that is, patients over 60 years of age.[2] The median age was 64 at the time of surgery; there was no mortality. All of the patients accepted and managed their ileostomy stoma in much the same manner as younger people; no specialized nursing care was necessary. Four of ten patients required ileostomy revision; although this is a small series, this incidence is not significantly greater than in younger patients.

My colleagues and I reviewed our experience with ileostomy complications requiring revision during a 10-

year period ending in 1973.[33] Eighty-four revisions were performed on 50 patients. The reasons for revision are summarized in Table 16-4. Thirty-one patients underwent only one revision; subsequent stomal operations were required in 19 patients. Nine of these patients underwent a third revision, four a fourth, and two a fifth.

Complications: Prevention and Treatment

Complications following an ileostomy may be due to technical error on the part of the surgeon, such as improper location or faulty maturation technique. Second, recurrent disease may be a cause for subsequent stomal problems. Third, the patient, either through inadequate education, neglect, or misuse, can cause stomal problems that might actually necessitate surgical intervention.

Stenosis and Retraction

Stenosis and retraction are the commonest indications for revision in our experience.[33] Thirty percent of revisions were performed for these indications. The primary causes of stenosis and retraction are inadequate initial stomal length and inadequate skin excision (Fig. 16-41). Retraction can also be due to one of these factors (Fig. 16-42), but may also be caused by weight gain after the operation (Fig. 16-43). I have on occasion noted a patient to triple his weight within a period of 1 year following the operation.

Table 16-4.   Reasons for Ileostomy Revision

Complication	Number	Percent
Stenosis	20	23.8
Fistula	12	14.2
Prolapse	10	11.9
Retraction	10	11.9
Recurrent disease	8	9.5
Small-bowel obstruction	8	9.5
Poor placement	5	6.0
Stomal bleeding	3	3.6
Dermatitis	2	2.4
Necrosis	2	2.4
Stomal pain	2	2.4
Paraileostomy hernia	1	1.2
Paraileostomy abscess	1	1.2
Total	84	100.0

(Goldblatt MS, Corman ML, Haggitt RC et al: Ileostomy complications requiring revision: Lahey Clinic experience, 1964–1973. Dis Colon Rectum 1977; 20:209–214)

Vascular compromise with resulting ischemia and necrosis may also lead to retraction. The attitude that the stoma may be a little purple or perhaps a bit blue but will probably be all right is usually an unfulfilled prophesy as mentioned previously. It is far preferable to reopen the abdomen and create an adequate length of viable bowel, prolonging the operation for whatever time is necessary, than to return on a subsequent occasion or to relegate the patient to disability because of his difficulty in managing the appliance.

Handelsman and Fishbein recommend that retraction or prolapse of the ileostomy can be prevented by placing a ribbon of fascia obtained from the abdominal wall through the mesentery adjacent to the bowel between the vessels.[38] It is neither wrapped around the bowel nor sutured to it. The authors believe that this technique will secure the position of the ileostomy without risking a possible fistula from suturing the bowel wall.

Correction of the retraction or stenosis requires excision of sufficient skin to create a proper-sized opening and mobilizing the bowel as far as is required in order to create a stoma of adequate length. Intraperitoneal mobilization of the ileum is carried out as far as possible, and the stoma is matured in the usual manner. Unfortunately, retraction is a complication that may necessitate a laparotomy in order to obtain the desired length of ileum. I prefer to warn the patient that this eventuality may be necessary should I be unable to obtain sufficient length by means of a more limited approach.

Prolapse

Prolapse may be of two types, *fixed* (irreducible) and *sliding*. In my experience the fixed type always occurs without any prior history of stomal revision. Conversely, the sliding type is always seen with the second or later revision. This implies inadequate abdominal fixation and indicates that mobilizing an ileostomy when performing a revision predisposes to subsequent problems with the sliding type of prolapse (Fig. 16-44). Prolapse is usually not associated with skin problems if it is of the fixed type, but if it retracts and becomes flush, leakage can occur. Too long a stoma is prone to trauma from contact with the appliance and may lead to psychological problems as well.

If the patient's prolapse is not really a prolapse, but simply an ileostomy that was created too long initially, treatment is relatively simple. The ileal mucosa is incised, preserving a rim, and the stoma is inverted. This maneuver is identical to that shown earlier for colostomy prolapse (see Figs. 16-6 and 16-7). Redundant ileum is resected, and the stoma is matured in the usual manner. One should not attempt to perform any intra-

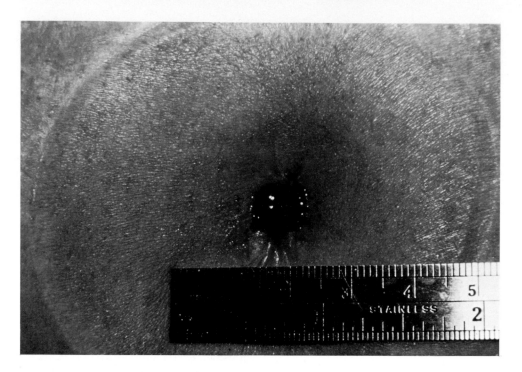

FIG. 16-41. Stenotic ileostomy due to inadequate skin excision and necrosis of the end of the ileum.

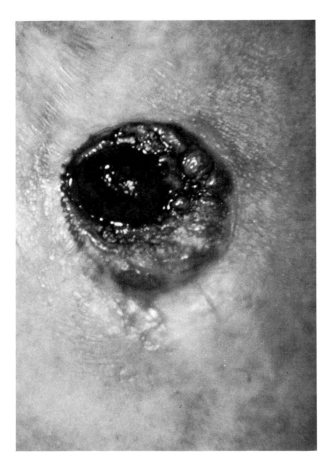

FIG. 16-42. Retracted ileostomy with stricture due to inadequate length of the initially created stoma. (Corman ML, Veidenheimer MC, Coller JA: Ileostomy complications: Prevention and treatment. Contemp Surg 1976; 8:36–41)

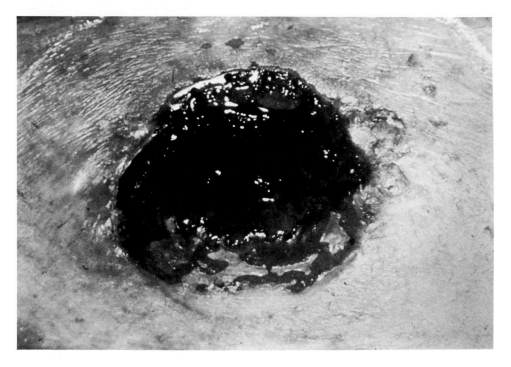

FIG. 16-43. Retracted ileostomy with severe dermatitis secondary to weight gain. (Corman ML, Veidenheimer MC, Coller JA: Ileostomy complications: Prevention and treatment. Contemp Surg 1976; 8:36–41)

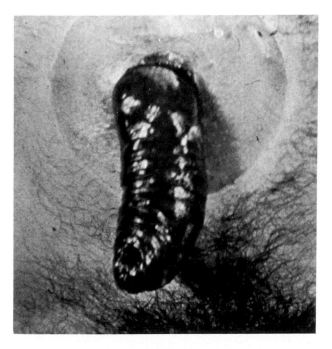

FIG. 16-44. Ileostomy "Prolapse" in this patient was due to creating too long a stoma initially.

abdominal dissection in order to avoid disrupting intraperitoneal fixation. Occasionally, with a sliding type of prolapse so much small bowel is delivered that some form of intraperitoneal fixation is required. Reduction of the ileum is usually technically difficult to accomplish and may result in recurrence of the prolapse, but resection of a long segment of ileum is not justified. Intraperitoneal fixation may be required by means of a full laparotomy to treat the complication adequately.

Fistula

Fistula is not an uncommon reason for ileostomy revision; approximately 15% of revisions are done for this reason. The most frequent cause of fistula is recurrent Crohn's disease (see Fig. 15-98). Erosion of the stoma by a rigid face plate of an appliance or from deep placement of a suture (Fig. 16-45) are other possible reasons for the development of a fistula. This complication presents a much more difficult management problem than does prolapse. Closure of the fistula may be attempted if no inflammatory disease is present, but subsequent breakdown is quite likely. If the fistula is resected, laparotomy may be required in order to obtain sufficient length of ileum for adequate maturation.

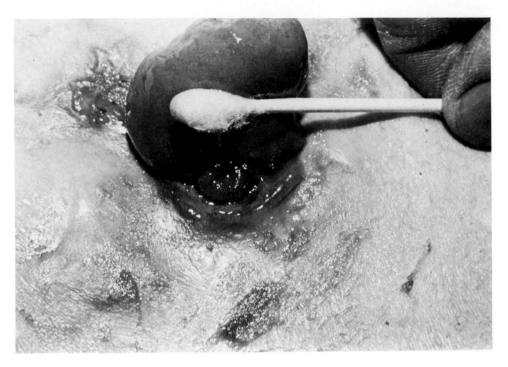

FIG. 16-45. Ileostomy fistula presumed secondary to a deeply placed seromuscular anchoring suture. (Corman ML, Veidenheimer MC, Coller JA: Ileostomy complications: Prevention and treatment. Contemp Surg 1976; 8:36–41)

Greenstein and co-workers identified 15 of 214 patients with an ileostomy constructed for Crohn's disease who developed a paraileostomy fistula.[36] In every case this was due to recurrent disease. All patients required resection and reconstruction of the stoma. If the skin at the original stomal site has been injured by the ileal effluent or if sufficient additional small bowel must be resected, the stoma should be created in an alternate site, usually the left lower quadrant.

Seeding

Seeding of viable ileal mucosa can develop along the suture line if subcuticular sutures for maturation are not employed (Fig. 16-46). Such seeding can lead to persistent secretion, and consequently to problems in fitting the appliance (Fig. 16-47).

For what apparently seems a rather trivial problem, treatment is quite extensive. Attempts at cauterizing of the ectopically located mucosa are fruitless. The only effective treatment is excision, and even with this procedure the viable ileal mucosal cells may grow again to the surface from a deeply implanted location. A plastic surgical procedure, rotating a skin flap to cover the defect, may be attempted successfully, but all too often relocation of the stoma may be required. This is

a totally preventable complication if one uses a subcuticular suturing technique.

Complications of Improper Placement

The above complications are due to errors in ileostomy maturation technique. Another cause of difficulty after stomal construction is the initial improper placement of the stoma. As discussed previously, the site chosen should be free of eschar, especially if the eschar is irregular rather than flat. The stoma should not be near any bony promontory, such as the iliac crest (Fig. 16-48) or the rib margin (Fig. 16-49), and should be placed in such a way that the intestine can be pulled through the split rectus muscle. Failure to do this often results in peristomal herniation (Fig. 16-50). Bringing the stoma through the incision is contraindicated with an ileostomy, not only because of the risk of hernia, but also because of the difficulty in maintaining an appliance and the delay in wound healing created by spilling of the effluent on the skin (Fig. 16-51). The stoma should be placed in an area where the patient can care for it properly and maintain an appliance with confidence and without leakage (Fig. 16-52).

If the stoma is improperly located and the appliance management is unsatisfactory, relocation is necessary.
(Text continues on p 676)

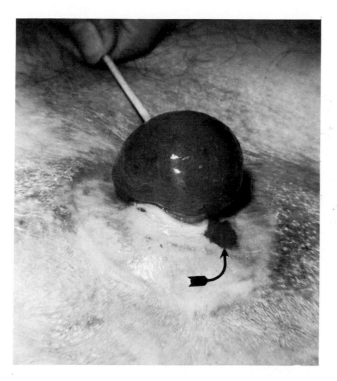

FIG. 16-46. Mucosal "seeding" *(arrow)* due to improper suturing of the ileum to the subcuticular skin.

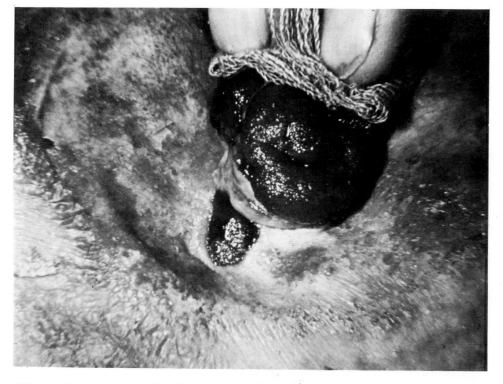

FIG. 16-47. Mucosal seeding leading to inability to maintain the appliance. Note the severe skin changes. (Corman ML, Veidenheimer MC, Coller JA: Ileostomy complications: Prevention and treatment. Contemp Surg 1976; 8:36–41)

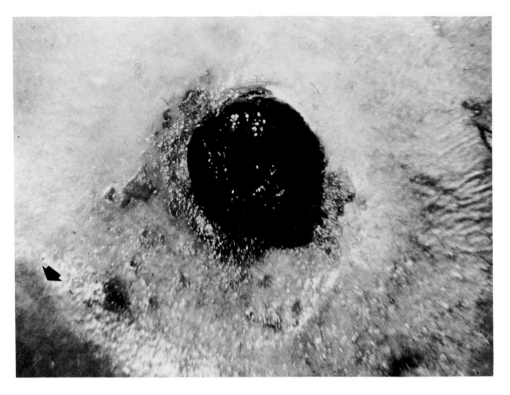

FIG. 16-48. Positioning the stoma too close to the iliac crest causes an inability to maintain the appliance. Note the parastomal dermatitis. The arrow indicates the anterior superior iliac spine. (Corman ML, Veidenheimer MC, Coller JA: Ileostomy complications: Prevention and treatment. Contemp Surg 1976; 8:36–41)

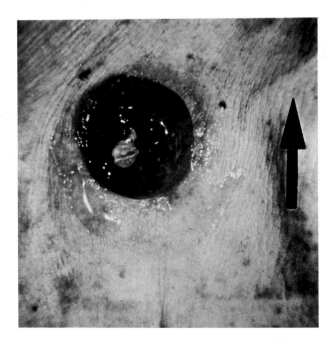

FIG. 16-49. Ileostomy too close to the rib margin *(arrow)*. (Corman ML, Veidenheimer MC, Coller JA: Ileostomy complications: Prevention and treatment. Contemp Surg 1976; 8:36–41)

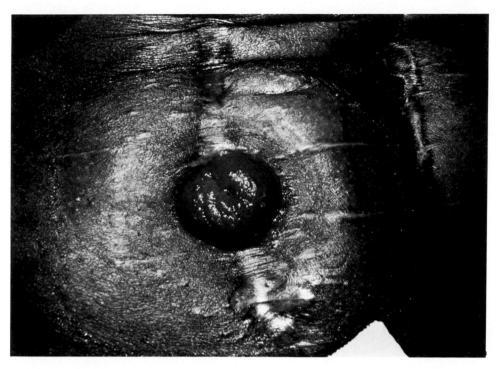

FIG. 16-50. Ileostomy through an abdominal incision creates difficulty in appliance management. Note hernia.

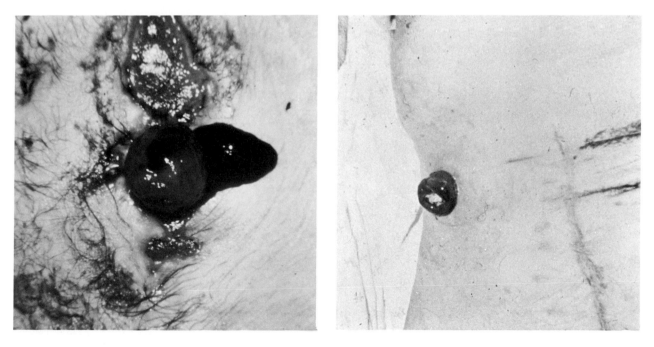

FIG. 16-51. Open, indolent incision due to bringing the ileostomy through the wound.

FIG. 16-52. Appliance management is a challange when the stoma is placed on the hip. (Corman ML, Veidenheimer MC, Coller JA: Ileostomy complications: Prevention and treatment. Contemp Surg 1976; 8:36–41)

This usually involves a full laparotomy with its attendant morbidity and mortality. Taylor and associates suggest that it is possible to perform a revision and relocation of the stoma without a complete abdominal exploration.[87] As usual, the site selection is carefully determined preoperatively. The ileal stoma is mobilized by a circumstomal incision into the peritoneal cavity. The diseased segment is delivered if possible and resected. The bowel is returned to the peritoneal cavity after closure of the distal end. Long sutures are left outside the abdomen should retrieval be necessary. By blunt dissection from the old abdominal wall opening, an adequate space is created to tunnel the distal ileum to the new site. A disk of skin is excised, the rectus is split, and the peritoneal cavity is entered at the new site. The ileum is pulled through by means of the long sutures that had been left attached, and the new stoma is constructed. Although by this technique one can avoid a larger incision, I do not believe that it is a quantum advance in the treatment of ileostomy complications requiring revision. The fact of the matter is that stomal placement errors are completely preventable complications.

Other Complications

Patients who have chronic ulcerative colitis coexisting with liver disease and portal hypertension may suffer hemorrhagic parastomal varices following proctocolectomy and ileostomy (Fig. 16-53). Adson and Fulton identified 19 cirrhotic patients who bled repeatedly from the mucocutaneous junction of the ileal or colonic stomas and added three patients of their own.[4] These were treated by portasystemic shunting with no evidence of recurrent bleeding. These authors advise a trial of stomal revision to control hemorrhage, but when stomal and esophageal varix bleeding coexist, a portasystemic shunt procedure is justified.

Trauma to the ileostomy can be accidental or deliberate (Fig. 16-54). Wilkinson and Humphreys reported a patient who suffered a laceration of the ileostomy as a result of a seat belt injury.[99] Following satisfactory repair, the patient was admitted to another hospital at a later time with total avulsion of his stoma as a result of direct trauma during a brawl. Although these types of injuries are not necessarily preventable, one should create the stoma of sufficient prominence to satisfactorily maintain an appliance; any further length not only is unsightly but also increases susceptibility to trauma.

Stomal ulceration is usually due to trauma from the appliance. However, the condition may also be secondary to recurrent Crohn's disease or to a specific bacterial infection. *Campylobacter jejuni* has been reported to cause profound ulceration of the stoma in association with an acute ileitis.[56] This case report emphasizes the importance of obtaining a stool culture in the evaluation of a patient with suspected recurrent inflammatory bowel disease.

Carcinoma of an ileostomy has been reported, presumably due to seeding of viable tumor cells at the time of the original procedure.[9, 22, 45, 81] Although this is not a totally preventable complication, particular attention should be given to appropriate cancer technique; if the tumor appears to have seeded the abdomen or has breached the seromuscular surface of the bowel wall, perhaps at least a change of gloves is in order at the time of the maturation of the ileostomy.

Loop Ileostomy

Loop ileostomy was originally described by Turnbull and Weakley as a procedure to divert the fecal stream primarily in the treatment of toxic megacolon (see Chap. 15).[93] It is also a technique that is effective for the treatment of colonic obstruction (much preferred to a cecostomy), and to protect an ileorectal anastomosis, especially when performed for inflammatory bowel disease.

An indication for loop ileostomy that is not generally appreciated is in the situation in which an end ileal stoma is technically difficult to create. Such a problem arises with obese patients in whom the mesentery may be shortened and thickened, and it can also be encountered when the small intestine has been resected.[20] In this last situation the blood supply often enters radially, with little collateral circulation between the arcade vessels. Every surgeon has been confronted with the problem of a bowel length that precludes creation of an adequate stoma. This necessitates trimming the mesentery, which in turn may result in the loss of viability of the distal end of the stoma. When the devitalized bowel is excised, sufficient length is unavailable, and the mesenteric vessels are again divided with the same resultant viability problem. Finally, the surgeon may compromise and accept a less-than-optimal stomal length or construct an ileostomy of sufficient protrusion but of questionable viability. These problems can be avoided by using the loop ileostomy. The technique is illustrated in Figures 16-55 and 16-56 as the alternative to an end stoma, but it is also applicable to the in-continuity creation of an ileostomy.

After the colectomy has been performed the distal end of the small intestine is oversewn. A disk of skin where the stoma is to be placed is excised in the same manner and at the same location as if for a conventional ileostomy. A point is selected 10 cm proximal to the closed ileum (a more proximal site is chosen in a severely obese patient), and a Penrose drain is placed

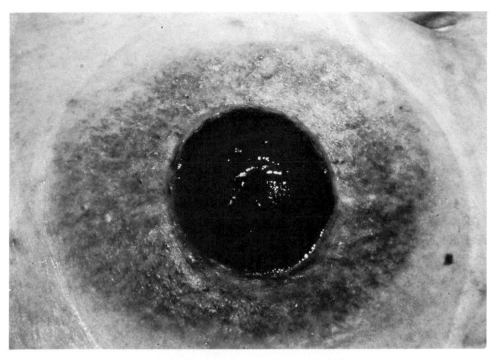

FIG. 16-53.   Peristomal varices in a patient with portal hypertension.

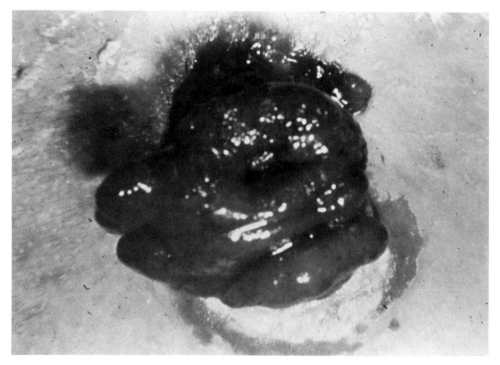

FIG. 16-54.   Macerated ileostomy with multiple fistulas in a psychotic patient who attempted to "destroy" the stoma.

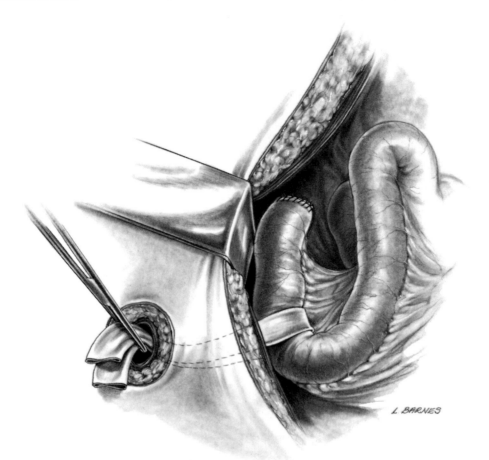

L. BARNES

FIG. 16-55. Loop ileostomy. The distal ileum is closed and the loop prepared for exteriorization.

around the intestine. The loop of small intestine is brought through the split rectus muscle (see Fig. 16-55). A rod supports the loop, and the bowel is opened at the level of the skin on the distal, nonfunctioning side. The stoma is created by eversion with interrupted mucosubcuticular sutures of fine catgut (see Fig. 16-56). Eversion may be facilitated by means of a Babcock clamp.

The rod is usually removed in 3 to 7 days, and in time, the distal end completely retracts. The general appearance and the functional results are identical to those obtained by conventional end ileostomy (Fig. 16-57).

Closure of a loop ileostomy usually requires resection. The procedure can be undertaken without a full laparotomy, circumcising the ileostomy as if for a revision. The proximal and distal bowel are immobilized and the bowel resected on the abdominal wall. A conventional single-layer, interrupted anastomosis is performed and the bowel returned to the peritoneal cavity.

Postoperative Care*

Preserving the integrity of the skin is the greatest concern in the immediate postoperative period. Moist, weeping, oily, eroded skin will lead to leakage, odor, and in the case of an ileostomy, loss of face plate adhesion. Meticulous attention to skin care must begin in the operating or recovery room with the first application of the skin barrier and placement of the pouch.

A *skin barrier* is a porous material that adheres directly to the skin to afford protection from the contents of the colon or ileum. The pouch is put on top of the barrier. In contrast to a skin barrier, a *skin protective agent,* such as Skin Prep or Skin Gel, provides a clear dressing that coats the skin. This is to be used only

*In part from Hunt N, Corman ML: Enterostomal therapy. Contemporary Education 1982; April: 79–92

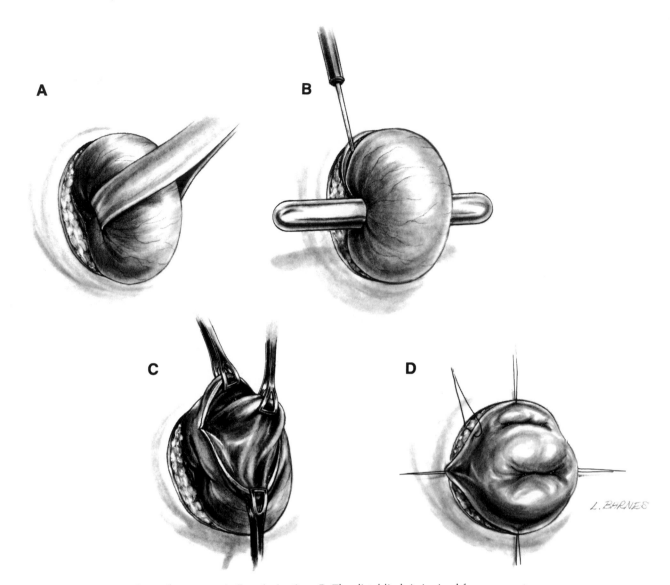

FIG. 16-56. Loop ileostomy. **A.** Exteriorization. **B.** The distal limb is incised from mesentery to mesentery at skin level. Care must be taken to make certain which side is proximal. **C.** Eversion. **D.** Maturation.

under tapes or adhesive coverings of cement or double-faced disks. Generally, protective agents are used when tape-like products contact the skin, to protect the epidermis from irritation. These protective agents are available as sprays, wipes, paint-on solutions, or pastes. Distinction must be made between a skin barrier and a protecting agent; patients with ileostomies should *never* use a protective agent in place of a skin barrier.

A comprehensive listing of ostomy suppliers and products is provided on pp 681–683. The most commonly employed skin barriers are discussed below.

Karaya Products

Karaya is a resin that forms a protective base when combined with glycerin, thus inhibiting the corrosive effects of ileal contents. It is refined and marketed in different forms, including powders, washers, wafers, and blankets, and mixed with natural clays. It is also manufactured in paste form, which provides an excellent means for filling in crevices created by abdominal folds near the stoma.

Karaya is nonallergenic, although the ingredients in

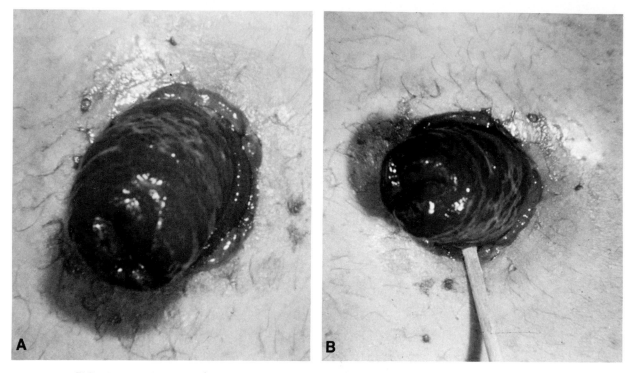

FIG. 16-57. **A.** Loop ileostomy simulates on inspection an end stoma. **B.** A cotton-tip applicator disappears into the distal limb.

some products may cause sensitivity. Under these circumstances all that is required is a change to a karaya product manufactured by another company. Karaya stretches, and when it is used as a washer around a stoma, it should measure about one-quarter inch smaller than the base of the stoma in order to fit it snugly.

One disadvantage of karaya products is early breakdown in the presence of urine. Therefore, they should never be used with urinary diversions. An exception to this admonition is Colly-Seel, which is effective because of its plasticized nature. Karaya is hygroscopic and melts easily in heat or even when the patient has an elevated temperature. Thus, for ostomates who live in hot climates, a different skin barrier should be used (*e.g.*, Stomahesive or Hollihesive).

Colly-Seel

Colly-Seel is another, more solid form of karaya. Natural clays have been added, which cause it to be less vulnerable to heat; thus, it is a suitable barrier for both urinary and ileostomy effluents. Colly-Seel is available in varying thicknesses as well as in washer, wafer, and sheet form. It does not stretch, and when measured, the inner diameter should be cut approxi-

mately the same or $\frac{1}{16}$ inch larger than the diameter of the stomal base. It must be moistened slightly before application. Colly-Seel is recommended for patients with soft or flabby abdomens or when considerable scarring is present. It should be placed on the abdomen while it is still sticky. This is the one exception when the use of Skin Prep or Skin Gel may be helpful in establishing good adhesion.

Stomahesive

Stomahesive is composed of gelatin, pectin, carboxymethylcellulose sodium, and polyisobutylene. It is nonallergenic and looks like a piece of American cheese. Its shiny surface is affixed to the appliance, and the sticky side is secured to the skin. It should be cut to fit snugly around the stoma and may be used as a washer or as a whole wafer. The product is also available in a powder or a paste. Stomahesive is excellent for use directly on excoriated skin.

A skin barrier such as Stomahesive is appropriate for intestinal as well as urinary tract diversions and should be placed on the skin immediately after the operation. The inner diameter should be cut relatively snugly around the base of the stoma; the outer

Ostomy Manufacturers and Products

Company	Products
Atlantic Surgical Co., Inc. 5200 N.E. 12th Avenue Fort Lauderdale, FL 33334 (305) 772-3493	Appliances Adhesive foam pads Karaya powder Stoma paper guide strips
Bard/Coloplast Home Health Division C.R. Bard, Inc. Berkeley Heights, NJ 07922	Disposable pouches ReliaSeal
Blanchard Ostomy Products 2216 Chevy Oaks Circle Glendale, CA 91206 (213) 242-6789	Karaya washers
Byron Products 19738 Greenside Terrace Gaithersburg, MD 20879	Ostomy support belts (Reliabelt)
Convatec/E.R. Squibb and Sons, Inc. P.O. Box 4000 Princeton, NJ 08540	Appliances Stomahesive wafers Stomahesive powder Stomahesive paste Duoderm Kenalog Spray Mycostatin powder
Dansac Inc. 2020 Wolff St. Racine, WI 53404 (414) 632-5665	Disposable pouches
D'Odor P.O. Box 1211 Leesburg, Florida 32949 (904) 326-5292	Deodorant Pectin-off Night drainage unit
Foxy Enterprises 4594 Edgemont Avenue Brookhaven, PA 19015 (215) 876-3314	Ostomy pouch covers
John F. Greer Co. 530 E. 12th Street Oakland, CA 94606 (415) 465-4162	Appliances Irrigation equipment Adhesive disks Stomapaper guidestrips Derma Benz
Hollister, Inc. 2000 Hollister Drive Libertyville, IL 60048	Disposable appliances Karaya washers Karaya paste Skin gel Hollihesive Premium Paste Fecal and urinary incontinence devices Appliance belts, clamps

Ostomy Manufacturers and Products (Continued)

Company	Products
Hudson Ostomy Center P.O. Box 1146 Fort Lee, NJ 07024 (201) 854-3461	Appliances
Marlen Manufacturing and Development Co. 5150 Richmond Road Bedford, OH 44146 (216) 292-7060	Appliances Stoma paper guidestrips Karaya powder
Mason Laboratories, Inc. 119 Horsham Road P.O. Box 334 Horsham, PA 19044 (800) 523-2302	Colly Seels Colly-Seel Appliances
A B Medena S-43400 Kungsbacka, Sweden	Kock pouch catheters
3M Medical Products Division 3M Center St. Paul, MN 55101 (602) 733-5454	Double-faced adhesive Adhesive foam pads Micropore paper tape
Nu-Hope Labs, Inc. 2900 Rowene Ave. Los Angeles, CA 90039 (213) 666-5249	Appliances Adhesive foam pads Skin protectant Nu-Gard Electrolytes plus Support belts Appliance covers Adhesive tape strips
The Parthenon Co., Inc. 3311 West 2400 South Salt Lake City, UT 84119	Deodorant tablets Devrom oral deodorant (bismuth subgallate)
The Perma-Type Co., Inc. P.O. Box 448 Farmington, CT 06032-0448 (800) 243-4234	Appliances Karaya powder Fresh tabs
H.W. Rutzen and Son 345 West Irving Park Road Chicago, IL 60618 (312) 267-4344	Appliances
Rystan Co. Dept. OQ 470 Mamaroneck Ave. White Plains, NY 10605 (914) 761-0044	Derifil deodorant and tablets
Torbot Co. 1185 Jefferson Blvd. Warwick, RI 02886 (401) 739-2241	Appliances

Ostomy Manufacturers and Products (Continued)

Company	Products
United, Division of Howmedica, Inc. P.O. Box 1970 Largo, FL 33540 (813) 392-1261	Appliances Adhesive foam pads Stoma paper guide strips Bismuth subgallate Banish Skin Prep Uri-Kleen Uni-Solve Uni-Wash Uni-Salve Uni-Derm
Waters Instruments, Inc. P.O. Box 6117 Rochester, MN 55903-6117 (507) 288-7777	Kock pouch catheters

aspect should be rounded and made slightly smaller than the adhesive portion of a soft-backed disposable clear pouch. The skin must be completely dry before applying Stomahesive or any other skin barrier.

Hollihesive

Hollihesive is similar to Stomahesive, except that it is a bit more flexible and stickier to the touch. It, too, is available as a paste.

Reliaseal

Reliaseal is similar in composition to Stomahesive. It comes as a round or oval disk with precut inner diameter sizes at one-eighth-inch intervals. It has two adhesive sides, one covered with white paper and the other with blue. The white paper is peeled off and that side is placed directly on the skin. Then the blue paper covering is removed, and that side is placed directly on the face plate of the pouch. "Blue to the sky" is a helpful memory device to teach patients how to use this barrier. Reliaseal is also an effective washer for an ileal conduit. When using Stomahesive or Reliaseal, many patients choose to add a small karaya or Stomahesive washer before applying the barrier for an added peristomal seal.

Crixiline

Crixiline is an extremely sticky silicone-like barrier that comes in rings and sheets. This barrier also is available attached to a disposal, soft-backed, open- or closed-ended pouch called Stomaplast-plus with a micropore tape backing. This product is very useful around drains. For good adhesion the skin must be dry.

APPLIANCE MANAGEMENT

Following establishment of an ostomy, the appliance selected is usually a transparent, odorproof, drainable bag (Figs. 16-58 and 16-59). This permits ready visualization of the color and integrity of the stoma and allows the contents to be emptied without the need for frequent change of the appliance.

Procedure for Application of Disposable Appliance

1. Empty the contents and remove the appliance.
2. Cleanse the skin with warm water and dry the area.
3. Measure the stoma and either cut out a disk or select an appliance with an appropriate-sized opening approximately $1/8$ inch larger than the stoma.
4. Apply a skin protective agent around the stoma and allow it to dry.
5. Place the bag on the skin by centering the opening around the stoma. During the immediate postoperative period, when the patient is not ambulatory, place the bag diagonally for ease of drainage. Pull the skin taut, and place the adhesive surface firmly against the skin to avoid wrinkles.
6. Insert a deodorant into the bag (optional).
7. Close the opened end of the bag, and secure with a clamp or rubber band. "Picture frame" the edges of the bag with micropore tape.

    In patients with an ileostomy, the pouch should be changed on the first postoperative day. This enables inspection of the base of the stoma, cleansing of the peristomal skin, and use of a larger opening if the stoma is edematous. Appliance changes should continue every other day or three times a week until the patient leaves the hospital. The major difference between an

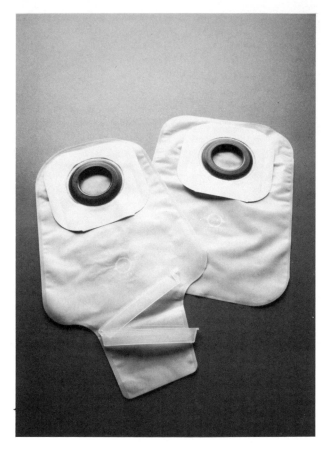

FIG. 16-58. Drainable and closed pouches with karaya seal and adhesive. (Courtesy of Hollister, Inc.)

month, or until their first visit, and have access to at least one supply source from which they can obtain all of their equipment. If necessary, arrangements are made for a visiting nurse. Written instructions should also be given as part of the discharge planning.

At the postoperative visits, it is important to examine and remeasure the stoma, and to ensure that the patient is using the appropriate appliance. The peristomal skin should also be examined for any irritation or lesion. Obviously, questions about ostomy management must also be addressed.

The following factors are essential to a properly fitting appliance:

It must permit 3 to 7 days of wear.
It must not leak contents or cause odor.
It must not cause skin or stomal irritation.
It must be comfortable for all levels of activity.
It must not require a wardrobe change.
It must be unobtrusive.

Both disposable and reusable pouches are available. Some disposal pouches come with an adhesive or microporous tape backing and, in some instances, with a soft plastic face plate and belt tabs (see Figs. 16-58 and 16-59). A number of such commonly used products include the Hollister, Sur-Fit (Convatec), United Surgical, Marlen, ColoPlast-Bard, and Nu-Hope pouches. They are lightweight, easy to apply, and very effective choices for the firm abdomen not requiring a more rigid face plate for peristomal support. In addition, no assembly is required.

The disadvantages of the disposable system include shorter wearing time, increased cost, and limitation to certain body configurations. A face plate with a firm base provides better peristomal support, particularly in a patient with a "flabby" abdomen. A disposal pouch *always* requires a skin barrier to enhance the wearing time and to provide adequate skin protection for a patient with an ileostomy.

Reusable or "permanent" appliances are available in one or two pieces, depending on whether the face plate is detachable (Figs. 16-60 and 16-61). A face plate for any appliance must always have a means of attachment to the body regardless of the type of skin barrier used. Attachment is usually accomplished through the use of precut double-faced adhesive seals. The inner diameter of an adhesive disk must equal exactly the inner diameter of the face plate.

A one-piece appliance may be preferred by patients with arthritis affecting the hands, those who have poor eyesight or who are blind, active youngsters who need a secure pouch construction with ease of application, patients with a neurologic deficit, and those with flush stomas. The choice of the one-piece appliance may also be simply personal preference.

ileostomy and a colostomy appliance is that some form of protective ring *must* be used around the ileostomy stoma because of the corrosive nature of the effluent. During the first 6 to 8 days after surgery, a disposable, soft-backed pouch will be required in addition to an appropriate skin barrier. By the seventh or eighth day, the stoma should be remeasured, because the edema will usually have resolved, although it usually takes from 4 to 6 weeks for the stoma to shrink to its smallest size. Therefore, several face plate changes will be required during this initial period. Once the appropriate equipment has been selected and obtained, the patient should remain in the hospital for 3 more days for training. It is often advantageous at this time to have a member of the family or a close friend present so that a second person may learn the procedure.

Patients may be taught to remeasure their stoma to accommodate for shrinkage before the first postoperative visit. They are given sufficient supplies to last 1

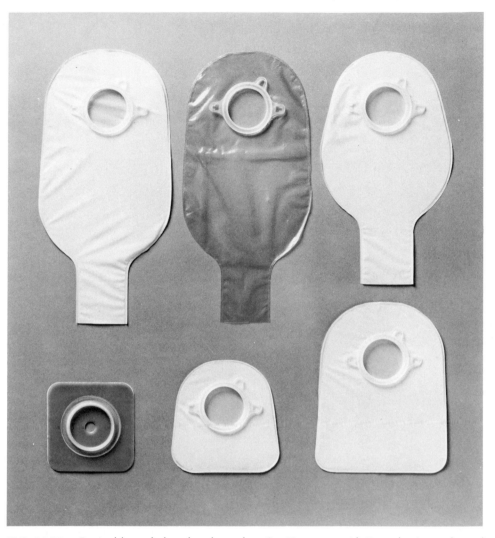

FIG. 16-59. Drainable and closed-end pouches: Sur-Fit system with Stomahesive wafer and flange. (Courtesy of Convatec, a division of E.R. Squibb & Sons, Inc.)

The main advantages of the two-piece system are cost effectiveness and durability. An elastic ring around the neck of the pouch holds the appliance to the face plate. The attachment of a double-faced adhesive disk to the back of the face plate is the same as that with the one-piece appliance. Generally, the firmer the abdomen, the softer and flatter the face plate. For example, a pregnant woman will require a soft, flat face plate, but a corpulent person will need a firm, convex face plate to lend sufficient peristomal support to prevent undermining of the seal. Most patients, with the exception of those who are very slender or who have firm abdomens, will need a slightly convex face plate. Face plates can be obtained from any manufacturer of reusable appliances. In addition to the reusable system, many patients have a supply of disposable pouches available for an emergency, for rapid change, or for camping and traveling. Figure 16-62 outlines the procedure for application of a conventional reusable appliance. With a well-positioned stoma of adequate length, a properly applied reusable pouch should remain in place without leakage and without skin injury for 4 to 7 days. One may also shower or bathe with the pouch in place. Although it is important for patients

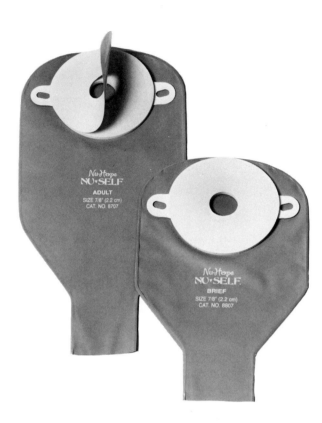

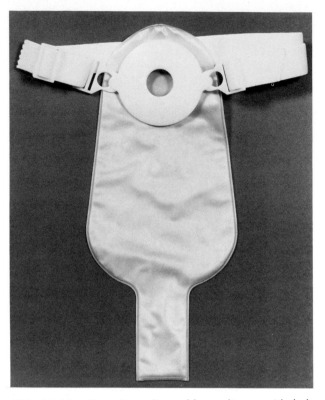

FIG. 16-61. Two-piece disposable appliance with belt. (Courtesy of Marlen Manufacturing and Development Co.)

FIG. 16-60. Semi-disposable one-piece vinyl pouch with foam pad coated with adhesive. (Courtesy of Nu-Hope Laboratories)

to be aware of the availability of both systems, more and more of my patients seem to select a disposable appliance.

When removing the pouch, if a protective skin shield was used, the appliance may be pulled directly away from the skin. However, if an adhesive cement was employed, it is necessary to drip a solvent with a pipette between the skin and the face plate as it is lifted off. All of the solvent should then be washed off the skin.

With knowledge of a few basic principles, a satisfactory management protocol can be developed. What may seem complex in the beginning will be routine in a brief time as these patients gain confidence that the system will not leak and will enable them to return to productive activity.

ADHESIVE PRODUCTS FOR APPLIANCES

Double-Faced Adhesive Disk

The most popular way of adhering a reusable appliance is by a double-faced adhesive cloth disk. This must measure exactly the inner diameter of the face plate. Before a new disk is applied, the face plate should be cleansed of any residual adhesive.

Cement

Patients who have had their stomas for a number of years have learned to work with a special appliance cement as the adhesive agent. This is an acceptable method, although more time-consuming. Today, cement is occasionally recommended for a patient with a difficult abdominal contour or in whom a satisfactory seal cannot be established by other means.

Cement is applied as a thin coat beyond the area covered by the face plate; it is then permitted to dry, and the procedure is repeated. Failure to allow the cement to adequately dry can result in severe skin irritation. A thin coat of cement is applied to the face plate and also permitted to dry, and this step is repeated. A washer is placed around the stoma, and the face plate with the attached pouch is secured. To remove the appliance from the skin, ostomy cement remover should be used, and then the appliance can be gently lifted off the skin.

Belt and Tape

Many patients feel secure when wearing a belt. The belt, however, is not meant to hold an appliance in place; it is intended merely to support the weight of the pouch. Belts may ride up on the hip and cause detachment of the appliance, which may then lead to stomal laceration. Some patients wear the belt too tightly and cause deep indentation marks on the skin. With few exceptions (*i.e.,* active children), the use of belts should be discouraged.

When possible, an alternative to the belt, such as framing the face plate or adhesive area with paper tape, should be considered. When the patient swims or bathes, many types of waterproof tapes are available.

PREVENTION AND TREATMENT OF SKIN IRRITATION

The ostomate is subjected to skin problems in spite of fastidious care and a proper-fitting appliance. To pre-

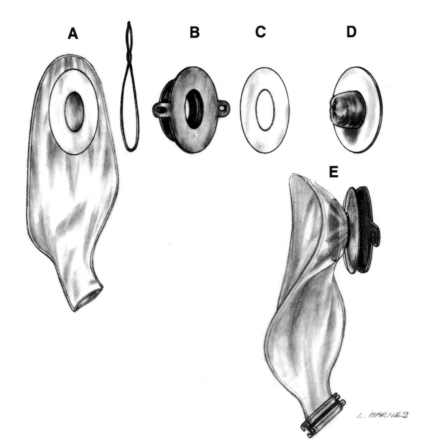

FIG. 16-62. Application of a reusable appliance. **A, B.** Mount the face plate on the pouch (if using a two-piece appliance) and apply the elastic O-ring. **C.** Apply the double-faced adhesive disk to the back of the face plate. **D.** After the skin is prepared, place the skin protector around the stoma. **E.** After exposure of the other side of the adhesive disk, the appliance is seated with the aid of a guidestrip.

vent complications from developing, it is important for the patient to return annually for a stomal inspection. This provides the physician (or enterostomal therapist) with an opportunity to remeasure the stoma and to evaluate the integrity of the peristomal skin. In addition, the patient can be informed about any new developments in equipment.

Weight gain or loss has major implications for stomal management (Fig. 16-63). Face plate size and convexity may require a change (Fig. 16-64). Skin sensitivity to products may develop even after many years of use (Figs. 16-65 and 16-66). Even mild skin irritation must be treated promptly to prevent serious consequences. Mild or moderate dermatitis may be treated by gently washing of the peristomal skin with warm water; soap should not be used. The area should be permitted to dry thoroughly. A hair dryer held approximately 1 foot away from the skin can be used to dry the surface. Karaya powder should be dusted on the area, and the excess brushed off. After a skin protective agent is applied and permitted to dry, a skin barrier is used with a clean appliance.

Severe irritation may be caused by improper fitting of the face plate, leakage, allergy to the adhesive product, or yeast infection (Figs. 16-67, 16-68, and 16-69). Cleansing the area with an antacid usually relieves irritation. This is done by decanting the antacid (*e.g.,* Amphojel, Maalox, Milk of Magnesia) and spreading it thinly over the skin. After drying, a skin protective agent is applied, followed by a skin barrier and a clean pouch. Occasionally, a small piece of Telfa may be placed over a draining area to prevent undermining of the skin barrier, and to allow drainage to take place. This appliance must be changed daily.

Problems with yeast or fungal infections often occur during warm weather or whenever moisture accumulates under the appliance. The area should be cleansed and dried gently, and a small amount of Kenalog should be sprayed on the affected area. After the excess is wiped off, the area should be dusted lightly with Mycostatin powder; the skin barrier should follow, and then the pouch. Depending on the severity of the infection, this unit may be left in place for 48 hours and the process repeated once or twice more if necessary.

Hirsute patients should remove excess hair around the stoma for a radius of approximately 10 cm, with scissors or an electric razor. A hand razor or depilatory should not be used.

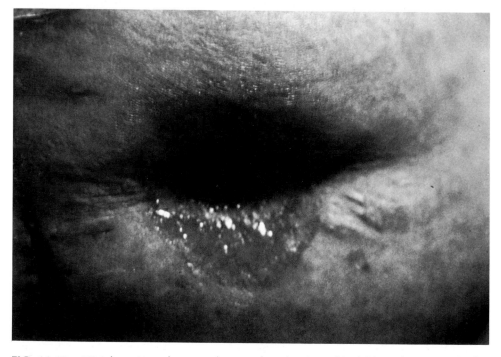

FIG. 16-63.   Weight gain and poor colostomy location in a skin fold result in a stoma that cannot be managed by conventional means. Note dermatitis inferior to the retracted ostomy opening.

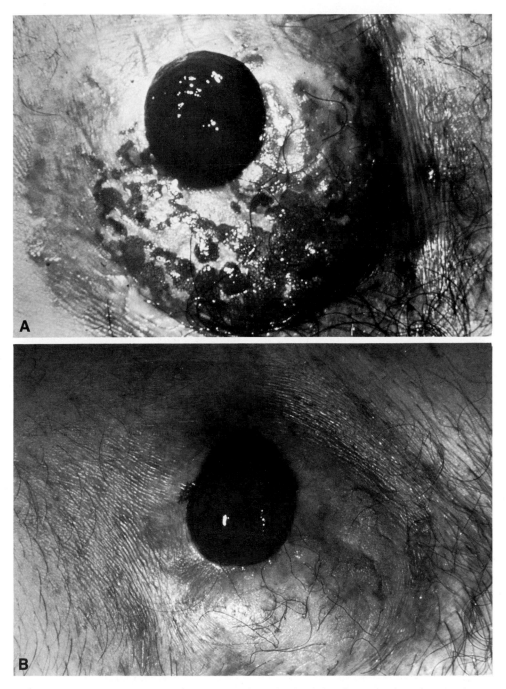

FIG. 16-64. **A.** Severe peristomal dermatitis from the face plate being too large. **B.** Resolution following use of a proper-fitting appliance. (Corman ML, Veidenheimer MC, Coller JA: Ileostomy complications: Prevention and treatment. Contemp Surg 1976; 8:36–41)

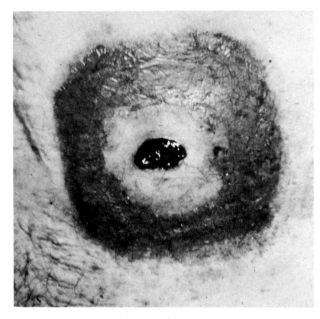

FIG. 16-65. Pericolostomy dermatitis from an allergy to adhesive. Note the halo of protected skin around the stoma from the Karaya ring.

ODOR CONTROL

Diet and personal hygiene probably are the most effective means of decreasing odor.[10] Gazzard and associates studied 50 ileostomy patients and 50 colostomy patients in an attempt to ascertain which foods upset stomal function.[31] Only a small variety of foodstuffs produced symptoms in a significant number of patients. Patients with colostomies found flatulence more of a problem than odor, particularly after eating vegetables or fruit. Items in this study that tended to be associated with an increased odor were different for ileostomy patients as compared with those who had a colostomy. Fish, eggs, cheese, and onions, in that order, were a greater problem for ileostomy patients, and green vegetables were the primary agent in patients with a colostomy. Yogurt, buttermilk, and parsley have been said to decrease odor in colostomy patients.[10]

A number of products are available that help to reduce odor. Liquid deodorants are generally more successful than tablets for use in pouches, because tablets do not dissolve quickly enough. Recommended products include Banish, Greer Guard, and Nil-Odor. Approximately 6 drops are placed inside the pouch after each emptying. If this is not adequate for control of odor, several other oral preparations are very effective. Derifil (chlorophyllin), one to three tablets daily taken orally, has been demonstrated to be an effective agent

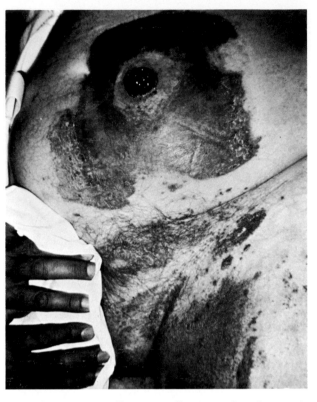

FIG.16-66. Severe allergy to adhesive and to the pouch itself. The bag hung in the groin, hence the inflammation in that area. Skin testing with a piece of pouch plastic yielded a positive response.

for eliminating or reducing odors of fecal and urinary drainage. Devrom (bismuth subgallate), a chewable tablet taken ½ hour before meals, two or three times daily, is also an effective odor reduction agent. It also tends to thicken and darken the stool.

COLOSTOMY IRRIGATION

Colostomy irrigation is a method of bowel control offered to selected patients with sigmoid or descending colon colostomies. Much depends on personal interest, bowel habits before surgery, manual dexterity, available toilet facilities, and life-style. Irrigation techniques are usually taught on the fifth or sixth postoperative day, and for some, a few months following the operation.

Most patients tend to return to the bowel habits they had before operation, usually within 6 to 12 weeks. In other words, if a patient defecated every morning after breakfast the colostomy will probably continue to function on that schedule. Under these

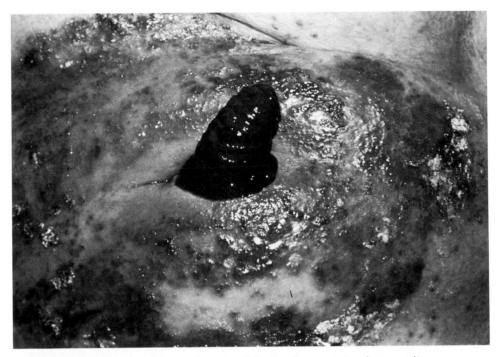

FIG. 16-67. Severe dermatitis with a yeast infection in a patient whose appliance management was poor, with frequent leakage.

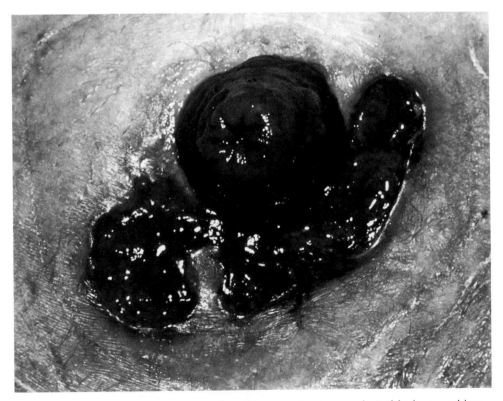

FIG. 16-68. Ulcerating areas around an ileostomy due to a neglected leakage problem.

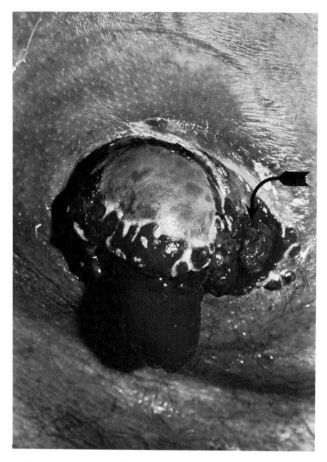

FIG. 16-69. Fecal fistula *(arrow)* secondary to erosion from an improperly fitted appliance.

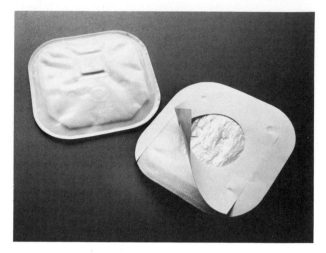

FIG. 16-70. Stoma cap: a soft patch of odor-barrier material that absorbs mucus. (Courtesy of Hollister, Inc.)

circumstances, irrigating may be unnecessary, and such patients can frequently avoid an appliance for the rest of the day or merely use a small dressing or Stomacap (Fig. 16-70). A closed-ended "security pouch" can also be used.

Conversely, if a patient had irregular bowel function preoperatively, the colostomy will probably act irregularly postoperatively. These patients are often more content by irrigating. However, under no circumstances should the patient be directed to irrigate the stoma. It is advisable to learn the technique, but the decision of whether to use irrigation should be left to the individual.

A nipple, cone, or catheter is inserted into the stoma. The cone tip is now being used more frequently for colostomy irrigations than the catheter, not only because there is less chance of perforating the bowel, but also because it provides a dam to prevent backflow. If a catheter is selected it should be inserted no more than 3 inches. A rubber nipple with a hole enlarged to accommodate the catheter tip acts as a flange and temporary dam while fluid is running in. Many companies manufacture irrigation kits (Fig. 16-71). The colon does not need to be washed out; the bowel is merely stimulated with the irrigant to produce evacuation. Tepid water (1500 ml) may ultimately be instilled; the first 500 ml are allowed to enter and are evacuated, clearing the distal bowel. The remaining 250 to 1000 ml is permitted to flow in gradually over a period of 7 to 10 minutes. The bottom of the bag for irrigation should be at shoulder height when the patient is seated. Most of the returns are usually collected within 15 minutes. The collecting sleeve can be closed while the patient tends to other activities. After approximately 45 minutes the irrigant usually will have been expelled. Over a period of time the patient may require irrigations only every 48 hours or even every 72 hours. Some patients may never be able to irrigate completely and may require a pouch all of the time. Under these circumstances it is difficult to justify the time and effort expended to perform this task. An alternative technique has been suggested by Schwemmle and co-workers; a specially constructed basin is used at stoma level when the patient is standing.[80] Obviously, this requires a special plumbing arrangement in the patient's bathroom.

Watt categorized those patients who probably are not candidates for controlling bowel elimination by irrigation as follows: those with an irritable bowel syndrome; patients who underwent irradiation therapy and sustained radiation enteritis; and the terminally ill. Stomal management problems such as hernia and ste-

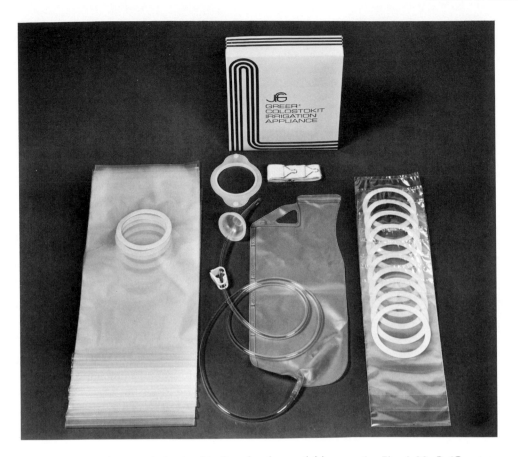

FIG. 16-71. Colostomy irrigating kit. See also the available cone tip, Fig. 1-22, *B*. (Courtesy of John F. Greer Co.)

nosis, poor eyesight, impaired dexterity, fear of the irrigation procedure, and resentment of the time necessary also militate against irrigation.[96]

Terranova and co-workers evaluated irrigation and compared the technique with natural evacuation in 340 patients.[89] They concluded that because of the feeling of security gained by relative continence, cleanliness, and the avoidance of an appliance, the vast majority of patients preferred irrigating. Williams and Johnston performed a prospective randomized study using colostomy irrigation and natural evacuation in 30 selected patients.[100] The mean time spent managing the stoma was 45 minutes per day in the spontaneous group versus 53 minutes when irrigation was performed. Because of reduction of odor and flatus, the lack of requirement for medication, and the ability of many to avoid an appliance, irrigation seemed to offer an improved life-style. Doran and Hardcastle performed a controlled trial of colostomy management by natural evacuation, by irrigation, and by means of a foam enema.[24] By evaluating 20 patients who used each technique for 2 months, the authors concluded that almost all felt that irrigation or the foam enema improved their quality of life. Furthermore, the patients opted to continue with irrigation on completion of the study.

SEXUAL FUNCTION

Many studies have been published that address the psychological and sexual aspects of patients who have undergone an operation resulting in an ileostomy or colostomy.[13, 15, 32, 68] Problems expressed include impotence, dyspareunia, decreased physical attractiveness, concern for odor, fear of injuring the stoma, and fear of rejection by the sexual partner. The studies uniformly indicate that patients believe that the surgeon should discuss these factors prior to performing permanent ostomy surgery. Brouillette and colleagues observed that many of the problems were resolved by the patients themselves, but the authors strongly advocate that an understanding surgeon as well as knowledgeable enterostomal therapist and site visitor can create a climate in which the patient can feel at ease in asking for guidance in sexual matters.[13]

ADDITIONAL CONSIDERATIONS

Insurance coverage is an important consideration. In the United States, patients with Medicare are afforded protection, which is included under ''prosthetic devices.'' This will provide coverage for much of the appliance expense. The usual cost for equipment is between $300 and $600 a year.

As part of a comprehensive rehabilitative planning program it is helpful to provide other resources for information. The local chapter of the American Cancer Society or the United Ostomy Association will make available a number of booklets or brochures, which the patient will usually find quite helpful (see the list below).

Additional Resources for Information

Local chapter of the American Cancer Society

United Ostomy Association (UOA)
2001 West Beverly Blvd.
Los Angeles, CA 90057

Suggested pamphlets published by the UOA:

Ileostomy: A Guide
Urinary Ostomies— A Guide for Patients
Colostomies: A Guide
Sex, Pregnancy and the Female Ostomate
Sex, Courtship and the Single Ostomate
Sex and the Male Ostomate
All About Jimmy and His Friend (an ostomy coloring storybook)

International Association for Enterostomal Therapy
505 North Tustin Avenue, Suite 282
Santa Ana, CA 93705
(714) 972-1720

Other publications:
Jeter KF: These Special Children. Palo Alto, Bull Publishing Co., 1982
Mullen BD, McGinn KA: The Ostomy Book (Living Comfortably with Colostomies, Ileostomies, and Urostomies). Palo Alto, Bull Publishing Co., 1980
Cox BG, Wentworth AE: The Ileal Pouch Procedure. Rochester, Minnesota, Mayo Comprehensive Cancer Center, 1977

REFERENCES

1. Abdu RA: Repair of paracolostomy hernias with Marlex mesh. Dis Colon Rectum 1982; 25:529–531
2. Abrams AV, Corman ML, Veidenheimer MC: Ileostomy in the elderly. Dis Colon Rectum 1975; 18:115–117
3. Abrams BL, Alsikafi FH, Waterman NG: Colostomy: A new look at morbidity and mortality. Am Surg 1979; 45:462–464
4. Adson MA, Fulton RE: The ileal stoma and portal hypertension: An uncommon site of variceal bleeding. Arch Surg 1977; 112:501–504
5. Alexander-Williams J, Amery AH, Devlin HB et al: Magnetic continent colostomy device. Br Med J 1977; 1:1269–1270
6. Anderson E, Carey LC, Cooperman M: Colostomy Closure: A simple procedure? Dis Colon Rectum 1979; 22:466–468
7. Baker FS: The ''rodless'' loop colostomy. Dis Colon Rectum 1975; 18:528
8. Beck PH, Conklin HB: Closure of colostomy. Ann Surg 1975; 181:795–798
9. Blake DP, Scheithauer BW, van Heerden JA: Metastasis to a Brooke ileostomy: An unusual cause of stomal dysfunction. Dis Colon Rectum 1981; 24:644–646
10. Boston A, Litman L, Rush A et al: Controlling colostomy odor. Am J Nurs 1977; 77:444
11. Bozzetti F, Nava M, Bufalino R et al: Early local complications following colostomy closure in cancer patients. Dis Colon Rectum 1983; 26:25–29
12. Brooke BN: The management of an ileostomy including its complications. Lancet 1952; 2:102–104
13. Brouillette JN, Pryor E, Fox TA Jr: Evaluation of sexual dysfunction in the female following rectal resection and intestinal stoma. Dis Colon Rectum 1981; 24:96–102
14. Browning GGP, Parks AG: A method and the results of loop colostomy. Dis Colon Rectum 1983; 26:223–226
15. Burnham WR, Lennard-Jones JE, Brooke BN: Sexual problems among married ileostomists: Survey conducted by the ileostomy association of Great Britain and Ireland. Gut 1977; 18:673–677
16. Chandler JG, Evans BP: Colostomy prolapse. Surgery 1978; 84:577–582
17. Colmer ML, Foxx MJ: A device for the control of colostomy prolapse. Surg Gynecol Obstet 1981; 152:827–828
18. Corman ML, Veidenheimer MC, Coller JA: An appliance for management of the diverting loop colostomy. Arch Surg 1974; 108:742–743

19. Corman ML, Veidenheimer MC, Coller JA: Ileostomy complications: Prevention and treatment. Contemp Surg 1976; 8:36–41

20. Corman ML, Veidenheimer MC, Coller JA: Loop ileostomy as an alternative to end stoma. Surg Gynecol Obstet 1979; 149:585–586

21. Crile G Jr, Turnbull RB Jr: The mechanism and prevention of ileostomy dysfunction. Ann Surg 1954; 140:459–465

22. Cuesta MA, Donner R: Adenocarcinoma arising at an ileostomy site: Report of a case. Cancer 1976; 37:949–952

23. Dolan PA, Caldwell FT, Thompson CH, Westbrook KC: Problems of colostomy closure. Am J Surg 1979; 137:188–191

24. Doran J, Hardcastle JD: A controlled trial of colostomy management by natural evacuation, irrigation, and foam enema. Br J Surg 1981; 68:731–733

25. Eng K, Localio A: Simplified complementary transverse colostomy for low colorectal anastomosis. Surg Gynecol Obstet 1981; 153:734–735

26. Feustel H, Hennig G: Kontinent kolostomi durch magnetverschluss. Dtsch Med Wochenschr 1975; 100:1063–1064

27. Finemore RG: Repeated haemorrhage from a terminal colostomy due to mucocutaneous varices with coexisting hepatic metastatic rectal adenocarcinoma: A case report. Br J Surg 1979; 66:806

28. Freund HR, Raniel J, Muggia-Sulam M: Factors affecting the morbidity of colostomy closure: A retrospective study. Dis Colon Rectum 1982; 25:712–715

29. Garber HI, Morris DM, Eisenstat TE et al: Factors influencing the morbidity of colostomy closure. Dis Colon Rectum 1982, 25:464–470

30. Garnjobst W, Leaverton GH, Sullivan ES: Safety of colostomy closure. Am J Surg 1978; 136:85–89

31. Gazzard BG, Saunders B, Dawson AM: Diets and stoma function. Br J Surg 1978; 65:642–644

32. Gloeckner MR, Starling JR: Providing sexual information to ostomy patients. Dis Colon Rectum 1982; 25:575–579

33. Goldblatt MS, Corman ML, Haggitt RC et al: Ileostomy complications requiring revision: Lahey Clinic experience, 1964–1973. Dis Colon Rectum 1977; 20:209–214

34. Goldstein WZ, Edoga J, Crystal R: Management of colostomal hemorrhage resulting from portal hypertension. Dis Colon Rectum 1980; 23:86–90

35. Goligher JC, Lee PWR, McMahon MJ, Pollard M: The Erlangen magnetic colostomy control device: Technique of use and results in 22 patients. Br J Surg 1977; 64:501–507

36. Greenstein AJ, Dicker A, Meyers S, Aufses AH Jr: Peri-ileostomy fistulae in Crohn's disease. Ann Surg 1983; 197:179–182

37. Halevy A, Adam Y, Eshchar J: Ileostomates in Israel. Dis Colon Rectum 1977; 20:482–486

38. Handelsman JC, Fishbein RH: Stabilization of ileostomy position with fascia. Surgery 1983; 93:88–90

39. Heiblum M, Cordoba A: An artificial sphincter: A preliminary report. Dis Colon Rectum 1978; 21:562–566

40. Henry MM, Everett WG: Loop colostomy closure. Br J Surg 1979; 66:275–277

41. Hines JR: A method of transverse loop colostomy. Surg Gynecol Obstet 1975; 141:426–428

42. Hines JR, Harris GD: Colostomy and colostomy closure. Surg Clin North Am 1983; 57:1379–1382

43. Hunt N, Corman ML: Enterostomal therapy. Contemporary Education 1982; April:79–92

44. Isa S, Quan SHQ: Colostomy perforation. Dis Colon Rectum 1978; 21:92–93

45. Johnson WR, McDermott FT, Pihl E, Hughes ESR: Adenocarcinoma of an ileostomy in a patient with ulcerative colitis. Dis Colon Rectum 1980; 23:351–352

46. Kewenter J: Continent colostomy with the aid of a magnetic closing system: A preliminary report. Dis Colon Rectum 1978; 21:46–51

47. Khubchandani IT, Trimpi HD, Sheets JA et al: The magnetic stoma device: A continent colostomy. Dis Colon Rectum 1981; 24:344–350

48. Kock NG, Geroulantos S, Hahnloser P et al: Continent colostomy: An experimental study in dogs. Dis Colon Rectum 1974; 17:727–734

49. Krasna IH: A simple purse string suture technique for treatment of colostomy prolapse and intussusception. J Pediatr Surg 1979; 14:801–802

50. Krause R, Freund HR, Fischer JE: A new technique for performing end enterostomies using a stapling device. Am J Surg 1979; 138:461–462

51. Kretschmer KP: The Intestinal Stomas: Indications, Operative Methods, Care, Rehabilitation, 128 pp. Philadelphia, WB Saunders, 1978

52. Kronborg O, Kramhöft J, Backer O, Sprechler M: Late complications following operations for cancer of the rectum and anus. Dis Colon Rectum 1974; 17:750–753

53. Lau JTK: Proximal end transverse colostomy in children: A method to avoid colostomy prolapse in Hirschsprung's disease. Dis Colon Rectum 1983; 26:221–222

54. Marks CG, Ritchie JK: The complications of synchronous combined excision for adenocarcinoma of the rectum at St. Mark's Hospital. Br J Surg 1975; 62:901–905

55. Mayo CW: Button colopexy for prolapse of colon

through colonic stoma. Mayo Clin Proc 1939; 14:439–441

56. Meuwissen SGM, Bakker PJM, Rietra PJGM: Acute ulceration of ileal stoma due to *Campylobacter fetus* subspecies *jejuni*. Br Med J 1981; 282:1362

57. Miles RM, Greene RS: Review of colostomy in a community hospital. Am Surg 1983; 49:182–186

58. Mirelman D, Corman ML, Veidenheimer MC, Coller JA: Colostomies: Indications and contraindications: Lahey Clinic experience, 1963–1974. Dis Colon Rectum 1978; 21:172–176

59. Mitchell WH, Kovalcik PJ, Cross GH: Complications of colostomy closure. Dis Colon Rectum 1978; 21:180–182

60. Morowitz DA, Kirsner JB: Ileostomy in ulcerative colitis: A questionnaire study of 1803 patients. Am J Surg 1981; 141:370–375

61. Moseson MD, Labow SB, Hoexter B: Technique for totally diverting loop transverse colostomy. Dis Colon Rectum 1983; 26:195

62. Oluwole SF, Freeham HP, Davis K: Morbidity of closure of colostomy. Dis Colon Rectum 1982; 25:422–426

63. Prager E: The continent colostomy. Dis Colon Rectum (in press)

64. Prian GW, Sawyer RB, Sawyer KC: Repair of peristomal colostomy hernias. Am J Surg 1975; 130:694–696

65. Raza SD, Portin BA, Bernhoft WH: Umbilical colostomy: A better intestinal stoma. Dis Colon Rectum 1977; 20:223–230

66. Reynolds HM Jr, Frazier TG, Copeland EM III: Treatment of paracolostomy abscess without proximal diverting colostomy: Report of two cases. Dis Colon Rectum 1976; 19:458–459

67. Rickwood AMK, Hemalatha V, Brooman P: Closure of colostomy in infants and children. Br J Surg 1979; 66:273–274

68. Rolstad BS, Wilson W, Rothenberger DA: Sexual concerns in the patient with an ileostomy. Dis Colon Rectum 1983; 26:170–171

69. Rombeau JL, Turnbull RB Jr: Hidden-loop colostomy. Dis Colon Rectum 1978; 21:177–179

70. Rombeau JL, Wilk PJ, Turnbull RB Jr, Fazio VW: Total fecal diversion by the temporary skin-level loop transverse colostomy. Dis Colon Rectum 1978; 21:223–226

71. Rosen L, Friedman IH: Morbidity and mortality following intraperitoneal closure of transverse loop colostomy. Dis Colon Rectum 1980; 23:508–512

72. Rosin JD, Bonardi RA: Paracolostomy hernia repair with Marlex mesh: A new technique. Dis Colon Rectum 1977; 20:299–302

73. Roy PH, Saver WG, Beahrs OH, Farrow GM: Experience with ileostomies: Evaluation of long-term rehabilitation in 497 patients. Am J Surg 1970; 119:77–86

74. Sachatello CR, Maull KI: Rapid totally diverting loop sigmoid colostomy with noncontaminating rectal irrigation. Am J Surg 1977; 134:300

75. Salley RK, Bucher RM, Rodning CB: Colostomy closure: Morbidity reduction employing a semi-standardized protocol. Dis Colon Rectum 1983; 26:319–322

76. Samhouri F, Grodsinsky C: The morbidity and mortality of colostomy closure. Dis Colon Rectum 1979; 22:312–314

77. Sarashina H, Ozaki A, Fukao K et al: A new device for barium-enema examination following colostomy. Radiology 1979; 133:241–242

78. Schmidt E: The continent colostomy. World J Surg 1982; 6:805–809

79. Schofield PF, Cade D, Lambert M: Dependent proximal loop colostomy: Does it defunction the distal colon? Br J Surg 1980; 67:201–202

80. Schwemmle K, Kunze H-H, Padberg W: Management of the colostomy. World J Surg 1982; 6:554–559

81. Sigler L, Jedd FL: Adenocarcinoma of the ileostomy occurring after colectomy for ulcerative colitis: Report of a case. Dis Colon Rectum 1969; 12:45–48

82. Smit R, Walt AJ: The morbidity and cost of the temporary colostomy. Dis Colon Rectum 1978; 21:558–561

83. Steinberg DM, Allan RN, Brooke BN et al: Sequelae of colectomy and ileostomy: Comparison between Crohn's colitis and ulcerative colitis. Gastroenterology 1975; 68:33–39

84. Sugarbaker PH: Prosthetic mesh repair of large hernias at the site of colonic stomas. Surg Gynecol Obstet 1980; 150:577–578

85. Sykes FR: Transcutaneous defunctioning colostomy. Br J Surg 1979; 66:505–506

86. Szinicz G: A new implantable sphincter prosthesis for artificial anus. Int J Artif Organs 1980; 3:358–362

87. Taylor RL, Rombeau JL, Turnbull RB Jr: Transperitoneal relocation of the ileal stoma without formal laparotomy. Surg Gynecol Obstet 1978; 146:953–958

88. Tenney JB, Eng M, Graney MJ: The quest for continence: A morphologic survey of approaches to a continent colostomy. Dis Colon Rectum 1978; 21:522–533

89. Terranova O, Sandei F, Rebuffat C et al: Irrigation vs natural evacuation of left colostomy: A comparative study of 340 patients. Dis Colon Rectum 1979; 22:31–34

90. Thomson JPS: Caecostomy and colostomy. Part

I: Surgical procedures and complications. Clin Gastroenterol 1982; 11:285–296

91. Todd GJ, Kutcher LM, Markowitz AM: Factors influencing the complications of colostomy closure. Am J Surg 1979; 137:749–751

92. Turnbull RB Jr: Management of ileostomy. Am J Surg 1953; 86:617–624

93. Turnbull RB, Weakley FL: Atlas of Intestinal Stomas, 207 pp. St Louis, CV Mosby, 1967

94. Varnell J, Pemberton LB: Risk factors in colostomy closure. Surgery 1981; 89:683–686

95. Wara P, Sørensen K, Berg V: Proximal fecal diversion: Review of ten years' experience. Dis Colon Rectum 1981; 24:114–119

96. Watt RC: Colostomy irrigation: Yes or no? Am J Nurs 1977; 77:442–444

97. Wheeler MH, Barker J: Closure of colostomy: A safe procedure? Dis Colon Rectum 1977; 20:29–32

98. Whittaker M, Goligher JC: A comparison of the results of extraperitoneal and intraperitoneal techniques for construction of terminal iliac colostomies. Dis Colon Rectum 1976; 19:342–344

99. Wilkinson AJ, Humphreys WG: Seat-belt injury to ileostomy. Br Med J 1978; 1:1249–1250

100. Williams NS, Johnston D: Prospective controlled trial comparing colostomy irrigation with "spontaneous-action" method. Br Med J 1980; 281: 107–109

101. Winkler MJ, Volpe PA: Loop transverse colostomy: The case against. Dis Colon Rectum 1982; 25:321–326

102. Yajko RD, Norton LW, Bioemendal L, Eiseman B: Morbidity of colostomy closure. Am J Surg 1976; 132:304–306

103. Zinkin LD, Rosin JD: Button colopexy for colostomy prolapse. Surg Gynecol Obstet 1981; 152: 89–90

CHAPTER 17

Miscellaneous Colon and Rectal Conditions

This chapter is devoted to a potpourri of colon and rectal conditions, which are incorporated here for the sake of convenience.

RADIATION ENTERITIS

Radiation injuries to the gastrointestinal tract are among the most difficult management problems facing the surgeon. It is not uncommon for the patient to suffer the deleterious effects of ionizing radiation long after the primary disease process for which the radiation was employed had been cured. Radiation is indeed a two-edged sword. Because of the serious consequences and the late complications (which are sometimes lethal), many surgeons are reluctant to employ this modality if another alternative is felt to be reasonably efficacious.

Radiation damage is cumulative and progressive. A finite amount of radiation is tolerable, beyond which additional radiotherapy at any time following the initial treatment may precipitate complications. Certain conditions, such as diabetes mellitus, hypertension, and previous abdominal surgery are believed to predispose the bowel to radiation injury.[9] Other factors that increase the risk include infection, single portal therapy, overlapping portals of therapy, poorly calibrated or uncalibrated dosimeters, inadequate vaginal packing during implants, and overlooking signals of distress or masking them by overmedication.[159]

Cervical cancer is the most commonly radiated le-sion, and thus is associated with the most radiation complications. Other primary diseases for which radiation therapy subsequently may produce problems include carcinoma of the endometrium, carcinoma of the bladder, carcinoma of the rectum or rectosigmoid, prostatic cancer, ovarian cancer, and carcinoma of the anal canal.

Marks and Mohiudden reported that the most common area of injury was the ileum, followed by the rectum, rectosigmoid, cecum, sigmoid colon, and jejunum.[120] Others have reported that although the small bowel is more sensitive to irradiation, the most common site of injury is the rectum, owing to its fixity in the pelvis.[9] The commonest lesion noted in the Cleveland Clinic report was proctitis; other complications included ulceration, stricture, and fistula to the vagina, bladder, or both.[108] Schmitz and colleagues reported that the original diseases in their 37 patients with radiation injuries were cervical carcinoma in 29 and endometrial carcinoma in 8.[169]

Since radiotherapy has been only recently advocated either for primary or adjunctive therapy for carcinoma of the rectum, it is too early to determine what the frequency of complications will be from its use. Hopefully, there will not be the incidence that has been seen hitherto for the treatment of carcinoma of the cervix and endometrium, primarily because of improved techniques of radiation administration. Most studies report that radiation injury develops in the bowel in approximately 5% of patients receiving pelvic or abdominal radiotherapy.[43, 135] Patients receiving more than 5000 R are most likely to develop this complication. Radiation dosages less than 5000 R are much less likely to be associated with the subsequent development of complications. All patients are not equally susceptible to intestinal radiation injury, however. For example, children are more likely to have complications associated with radiation enteritis,[48] and people with light complexions are more sensitive than those with dark.[169]

Early onset of symptoms such as cramping or diarrhea and an objective confirmation of radiation changes on endoscopy or biopsy should alert the physician to consider modification of the treatment plan by reducing the dose, increasing fractionation over longer periods of time, or temporarily interrupting the therapy.[135]

Symptoms

The symptoms of radiation injury depend on whether one is dealing with the acute process, usually occurring during the course of the treatment, or the result of therapy, weeks, months, or even years later. Nausea, vomiting, diarrhea, and cramping abdominal pain are seen in 75% of patients who undergo radiotherapy.[9] Proctoscopic examination may reveal loss of vessel pattern, edema, contact bleeding, and telangiectasis. Ulceration and granularity may be noted. Later changes may include thickening of the rectal wall with stricture and a fistula into the vagina or to the bladder. Because of complications of radiation to the small intestine, malabsorption, partial intestinal obstruction, and severe diarrhea may lead to malnutrition and fluid and electrolyte imbalance.

Investigative Studies

Proctosigmoidoscopy has been employed as the primary tool for evaluating radiation injury to the lower bowel. More recently, colonoscopy has been used for studying patients with presumed radiation colitis, particularly for bleeding and for inspection of a colonic stricture.[154] Endoscopic evidence of injury includes pallor of the mucosa, prominent submucosal telangiectatic vessels, friability, erythema, and granularity.

Radiologic study performed during the course of therapy will usually not be helpful in identifying specific radiation changes. Increased irritability and motility of the small bowel is usually noted, and there may be some associated spasticity in the colon.[159] However, months or years after the treatment, profound radiologic changes may be apparent on contrast study of the intestinal tract. Commonly involved areas include the sigmoid colon, rectum, and terminal ileum (Fig. 17-1).

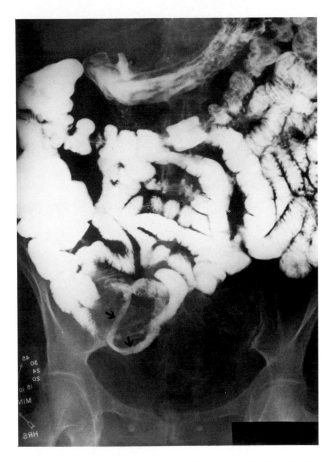

FIG. 17-1. Radiation enteritis. Terminal ileal radiation changes include rigidity and edema of the bowel wall, apparent mass between loops, and destruction of the mucosal pattern.

Angiographic studies may reveal arterial and venous irregularity, beading and focal obstruction of the bowel wall vasculature, and crowding of vessels because of foreshortening of the intestine.[159]

Pathology

Three phases of radiation effects have been identified: (1) acute, primarily affecting the mucosa; (2) subacute, with predominant effect in the submucosa; and (3) chronic, generally affecting all layers of the bowel wall.[120] Depending on the phase, the changes may vary from a colitis with capillary dilatation, hemorrhage, edema, and inflammatory cell infiltration in the acute situation, to an ischemia from an obliterative endarteritis and fibrosis in the chronic (Figs. 17-2, 17-3, and

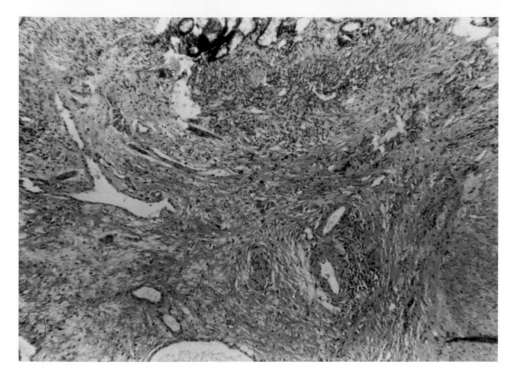

FIG. 17-2. Radiation colitis. Subacute changes include fibrosis of the submucosa, sclerosis of blood vessels, and perivascular mononuclear cell infiltrate. (Original magnification × 240. Courtesy of Rudolf Garret, M.D.)

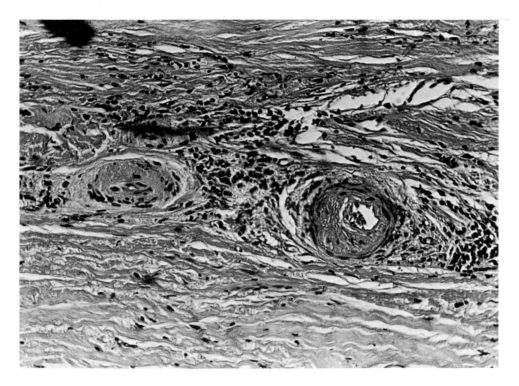

FIG. 17-3. Radiation colitis. Chronic changes reveal fibrosis, dilatation of the lymphatics, and virtual obliteration of the blood vessels. (Original magnification × 280. Courtesy of Rudolf Garret, M.D.)

17-4). The normal submucosal space may be altered by the deposition of dense hyaline material lacking the normal fibrillar structure of collagen.[95]

Treatment

The most frequent indication for surgical intervention in a patient with radiation injury is the presence of a fistula, frequently to the vagina or to the bladder, but also to the skin and other areas of the intestinal tract. Obstructive symptoms may also require surgical treatment.

Prior to operation it is important to evaluate the entire intestinal tract for the presence of associated radiation-induced abnormalities and for the possibility of recurrent primary disease. Upper gastrointestinal x-ray, barium enema, and complete endoscopic examination are indicated. Evaluation of the urinary tract is particularly important because of the high incidence of associated damage to the outflow tracts. Ureteral obstruction necessitates cystoscopy and retrograde pyelography. In addition, if a resection is attempted it is helpful to have ureteral catheters inserted at the time of operation. The presence of ureteral catheters does not guarantee that injury will not occur, but by palpating the indwelling catheter, possible trauma may be avoided.

The patient is placed on a bowel preparation (see Chap. 10). Perioperative antibiotics are strongly recommended.

The choice of surgical procedure will depend on the level of the injury, the patient's prognosis, and the extent of radiation damage as determined at the time of exploration. An elderly woman with a rectovaginal fistula who has severe radiation changes is probably optimally treated by a diversionary procedure, a sigmoid colostomy. Conversely, a patient with an obstructing lesion of the distal ileum may be treated by resection or possibly a bypass procedure. If an associated rectal or rectosigmoid lesion is found, a concomitant colostomy or an additional colon resection may be necessary. Obviously, this is a judgment that must be made at the time of laparotomy. Characteristically, there is a tendency to underestimate the amount of damage produced by the radiation when examination of the serosal surface of the intestine is performed. If one is to anticipate a favorable result of the operation, all radiation-injured tissue must be adequately excised and an anastomosis effected in relatively normal bowel.

Marks has been an advocate of combined abdominotranssacral reconstruction for the radiation-injured rectum (see Fig. 11-79).[119] He emphasizes also the importance of excising all radiation-injured tissue, per-

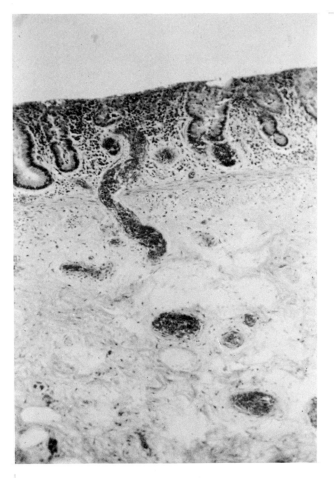

FIG. 17-4. Radiation proctitis: atrophy of the mucosa with fibrosis and telangiectasis of the submucosa. (Original magnification × 170)

forming an anastomosis in normal bowel, mobilizing the splenic flexure, use of ureteral catheters, and the obligatory implementation of a diversionary procedure. With abdominal wall radiation one should consider avoiding retention sutures if at all possible, and instead use delayed primary wound closure or permit the wound to heal by second intention.

Lopez and co-workers used a segment of nonirradiated colon for repair of post-irradiation rectal stricture.[110] The normal proximal bowel was turned down and anastomosed to the side of the rectum below the site of the injury, creating an end-to-side anastomosis. A proximal anastomosis was effected between the upper colon and the apex of the U of the distally rotated bowel. The authors reported successful application of this technique in one patient.

Home parenteral nutrition has been advocated for the treatment of patients with severe radiation enteritis.[108] Five patients have been reported from the Cleveland Clinic who would have been unable to survive their severe state of malnutrition without this treatment. They were not considered candidates for surgical intervention because of extensive disease and their poor nutritional state. One patient died of recurrent carcinoma after 14 months, and another died as a result of a pharmaceutical error after 30 months. The other three remained free of morbidity relating to the parenteral nutrition at the time of the follow-up report.

Treatment of Proctitis

Ulcerative proctitis secondary to radiation-induced injury produces symptoms of rectal bleeding, abdominal pain, diarrhea, passage of mucus, rectal pain, and tenesmus. It is a troublesome condition to treat. Proctosigmoidoscopic examination may reveal edema of the mucosa, granularity, ulceration, or contact bleeding. Narrowing may or may not be evident.

Management is usually directed to dietary measures, the addition of "slowing" medications, bulk agents, and antispasmotics. Retention enemas containing hydrocortisone have been recommended, but I have not found them particularly helpful. Many patients simply need to be reassured that they are not harboring a recurrent tumor. Periodic examinations are advised.

Results

Cram and associates reviewed their experience with 89 patients with radiation injury to the bowel of whom 31 required surgical intervention.[43] These authors tended to perform a resection or a bypass for small bowel disease, and a colostomy for large bowel involvement. Although they conceded that the conservative approach to large bowel radiation injury is not universally accepted, they felt that the high morbidity and mortality associated with resection and the requirement for possibly multiple procedures impelled them to adopt this particular approach.

Anseline and co-workers reported the Cleveland Clinic experience of 104 patients with radiation injury to the rectum as a result of therapy for gynecologic or urologic malignancy.[9] Fifty patients were treated surgically, and 54 were treated conservatively. The authors concluded that diversion was the safest form of treatment for rectovaginal fistula, rectal stricture, and proctitis that was unresponsive to medical measures. A high morbidity and mortality was recorded in patients who underwent resection.

Wellwood and Jackson reported their experience of 38 patients with intestinal complications after radiotherapy, noting a mortality rate of 37%.[213] These authors advised formation of a combined surgical–radiotherapy clinic in order to monitor and investigate patients who were at risk. They also suggested that prompt radiologic investigation of the intestinal tract be performed if symptoms suggestive of radiation damage are elicited; tests for malabsorption should also be performed.

Morgenstern and co-workers reported 50 patients with radiation enteropathy; the most frequent indication for surgical intervention was intestinal obstruction.[135] They advocate fixation of the intestinal loops outside of the pelvis, or the tacking of omentum to obliterate the pelvic cavity. These authors emphasized that because of the seriousness of the complication, investigative efforts should be undertaken to identify an indicator for intestinal mucosal damage in order to predict which patients are at risk.

Cooke and deMoor reported 37 patients with radiation damage to the rectum, 28 of whom had rectovaginal fistulas.[41] Treatment involved resection with restoration of continuity by means of coloanal anastomosis. They reported technical success in all but two patients with no mortality. Although some patients had impairment of fecal continence, the overwhelming results were favorable.

Schmitt and Symmonds reported 93 patients with small bowel radiation enteritis.[168] Over two thirds underwent intestinal resection, and 20 underwent bypass procedures; adhesions were lysed in 8 patients. Factors used to select the appropriate operative procedure included the age and general medical condition of the patient, the location, extent, and degree of the radiation changes, and whether the procedure was carried out on an elective or an emergency basis. Anastomotic dehiscence occurred in 10 patients; there were six operative deaths.

Comment

Intestinal complications of radiation therapy present difficult management problems. My own attitude is to attempt resection for patients who are symptomatic when the disease involves primarily the small intestine. Conversely, because of my lack of success with restorative operations for patients who have radiation changes in the rectum, particularly with stricture or fistula, I prefer a proximal diversionary procedure. My tendency is to limit resective sphincter-saving operations to those patients whose prognosis for long-term survival is good and in whom the disease is no lower than the mid-rectum.

VASCULAR DISEASES

Mesenteric Occlusion

Major occlusive disease is usually caused by mesenteric vascular obstruction by atheroma, thrombus, or embolus. However, many patients who develop ischemic changes of the small and large bowel do not have a demonstrably significant vascular lesion.

Acute mesenteric ischemia usually occurs in patients over 50 years of age, particularly in those with arteriosclerotic heart disease or valvular involvement. Other factors that predispose to the complication include long-standing congestive heart failure, cardiac arrhythmias, recent myocardial infarction, hypovolemia, hypotension, and gastrointestinal hemorrhage.[27]

The most frequent symptoms of mesenteric occlusion are abdominal pain and rectal bleeding. The pain is often out of proportion to the physical findings. A metabolic acidosis also is characteristic. Signs and symptoms of peritonitis rapidly ensue in the presence of intestinal infarction. In patients with so-called abdominal angina, abdominal pain is also evident, usually developing 15 to 20 minutes following the ingestion of food.[64] Pain is characteristically epigastric or periumbilical; weight loss and malnutrition may ensue.

Boley and his colleagues have proposed an aggressive algorithmic approach to the diagnosis and therapy of mesenteric occlusive and nonocclusive disease.[27, 30] The protocol advocates initial treatment directed at correction of the predisposing or precipitating causes of the ischemia. Vasopressors and digitalis are discontinued if at all possible. After the initial supportive measures have been completed, radiologic studies are undertaken. A plain film of the abdomen is obtained to be certain that there is no other obvious cause for the abdominal signs and symptoms, such as a perforation or intestinal obstruction. Angiography is then performed. Following a flush aortogram, selective angiography is undertaken to detect emboli, thrombosis, or mesenteric vasoconstriction in the superior mesenteric artery or its branches (Fig. 17-5).[30] Based upon the angiographic findings and the presence or absence of peritoneal signs, the patient is then treated according to a protocol that these authors devised.

If the angiogram is normal, and no peritoneal signs are found, observation is the treatment of choice. With a normal angiogram and the presence of peritoneal signs, exploratory laparotomy is undertaken. If an angiogram demonstrates a major embolus, with or without peritoneal signs, preoperative papaverine infusion is begun, and an embolectomy is performed with or without a bowel resection. If a minor occlusion or

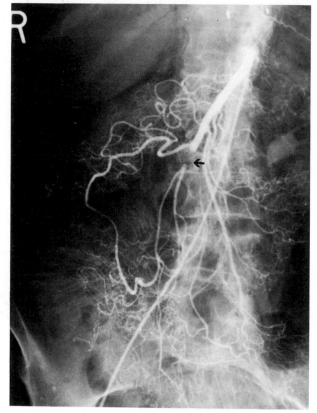

FIG. 17-5. Superior mesenteric artery embolism *(arrow)*. Note the collateral circulation through the meandering vessel.

embolus is noted, in the absence of peritoneal signs, papaverine may be considered and the patient observed. With peritoneal signs, preoperative papaverine is infused and a laparotomy and limited resection performed if indicated.

With a major nonembolic occlusion and peritoneal signs, papaverine may be infused and arterial reconstruction performed with or without a resection if necessary. A second-look procedure may be considered subsequently depending on the nature of the original pathology. If a major occlusion is not associated with peritoneal signs, and there is good collateral blood supply identified by angiogram, observation is the treatment of choice. In the absence of collaterals, and in the presence of splanchnic vasoconstriction, papaverine is infused; a laparotomy with arterial reconstruction and possible resection is undertaken. In this case, also, a second-look procedure may be indicated later.

If the angiogram fails to demonstrate an occlusion (splanchnic vasoconstriction only), in the absence of

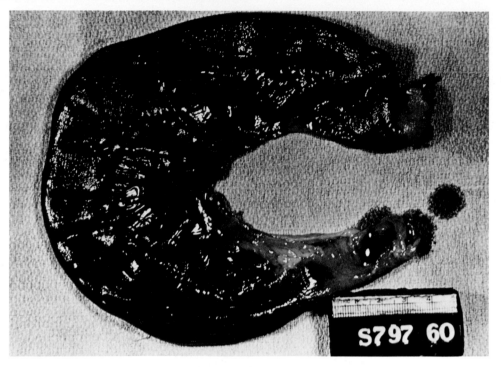

FIG. 17-6. A resected segment of small bowel showing infarction from prolonged hypotension due to nonocclusive vascular disease. (Courtesy of Rudolf Garret, M.D.)

peritoneal signs papaverine is infused. The patient is observed and the angiogram subsequently repeated. If peritoneal signs exist, preoperative papaverine is infused, and an exploratory laparotomy is performed. A resection is undertaken if indicated (Fig. 17-6). A repeat angiogram and possibly a second-look operation should be considered.

Boley and co-workers reported their experience with 47 patients with intestinal ischemia from superior mesenteric artery emboli.[27] The overall mortality was 66%. Patients with infarction of more than 50% of the small intestine did especially poorly (17 of 19 such patients died). A survival rate of 55% was obtained in patients managed according to the above protocol, whereas only 20% of those treated by traditional methods survived. The best results were obtained in those patients who were diagnosed within 24 hours of the onset of pain.

Ischemic Colitis

Ischemic colitis is a term coined by Marston and associates to describe a syndrome due to occlusive or nonocclusive vascular disease as it affects the large bowel.[121] It is a disease that usually is found in the aging population, with an increased incidence in women.[146] These authors classified the condition into three categories: gangrenous, strictured, and transient or reversible.

In the first category, the ischemia may lead to fulminant signs and symptoms. The patient may complain of severe abdominal pain, nausea, and vomiting. Bowel movements may be absent, or bloody diarrhea may be noted. Physical examination may reveal evidence of peritonitis if the bowel is involved by transmural disease, and certainly if there is a perforation. Plain abdominal x-ray may demonstrate free gas under the diaphragm. In a patient who has a suspected bowel infarction, barium enema is contraindicated (Fig. 17-7).

The development of an *ischemic stricture* probably is a sequela of more extensive inflammatory disease initially, but not to the point of bowel perforation. Patients may have minimal symptoms, or nausea, vomiting, and abdominal distention may develop. Barium enema often reveals a lesion difficult to distinguish from carcinoma.

In patients who have reversible or transient ischemic disease, rectal bleeding may be the only complaint.

Abdominal pain and tenderness on the left side is usually minimal or may not be evident. Proctosigmoidoscopic examination almost always will reveal rectal sparing, with inflammatory changes commencing usually at a level of approximately 15 cm. It is very difficult to distinguish the condition from nonspecific inflammatory bowel disease, except that the age of the patient and the history are often helpful. The rectum is rarely involved in the ischemic process because of its abundant collateral blood supply.[139] In fact, if the rectum *is* involved, serious consideration should be given to another cause (*e.g.*, ulcerative colitis, antibiotic-associated colitis, or any of the number of infectious colitides that are discussed later in this chapter). Other endoscopic changes include pallor of the mucosa and hemorrhagic areas. The latter are more likely to be appreciated early in the evolution of the inflammatory reaction.

The plain film of the abdomen may reveal characteristic thumb-printing, usually in the region of the splenic flexure. The vascular supply to this area is the most vulnerable, because of inadequate circulation through the marginal artery of Drummond. Barium enema examination shows thumb-printing, edema of the bowel wall, and narrowing primarily in the areas of the splenic flexure, the distal transverse colon, and the descending colon (Fig. 17-8).

Ischemic colitis may develop following resection of an abdominal aortic aneurysm.[59, 80, 93, 107] The changes may be reversible or, as with ischemic colitis not associated with aneurysmectomy, may subsequently lead to stricture, gangrene, or perforation. The combination of intra-abdominal sepsis with a prosthetic vascular graft is potentially catastrophic.

Rectal bleeding within the first 72 hours following aneurysmectomy is a characteristic symptom that requires investigation. Forde and co-workers suggest that colonoscopy is a particularly useful technique for establishing the diagnosis of ischemic colitis in the postoperative period.[59] The findings are as those previously described; the rectum and distal sigmoid colon are of-

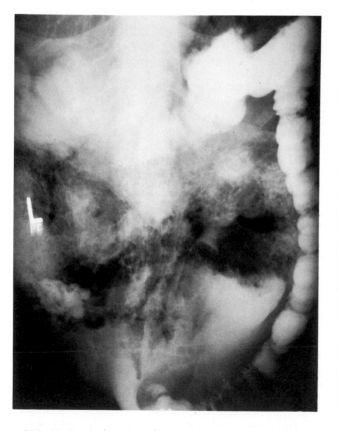

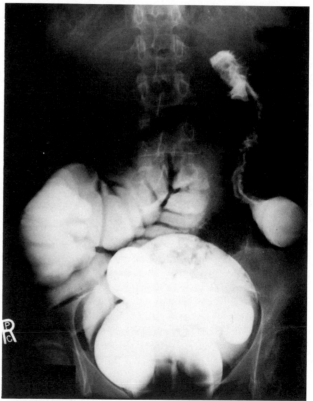

FIG. 17-7. Ischemic colitis: transverse colon perforation. Note the extravasation of barium into the peritoneal cavity (the marker is on the wrong side.)

FIG. 17-8. Ischemic colitis. Barium enema reveals thumb-printing of the splenic flexure, and edema and spasm of the descending colon. Note the preservation of mucosa.

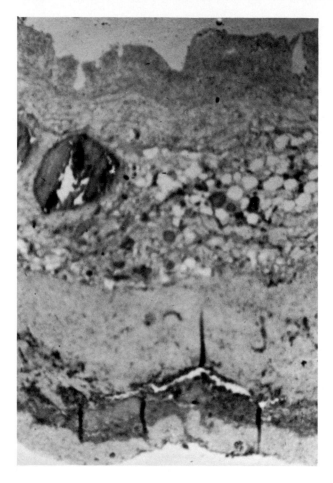

FIG. 17-9. Ischemic colitis: necrotic mucosa, serosal hemorrhage, and transmural involvement. (Original magnification × 120. Courtesy of Rudolf Garret, M.D.)

ten spared, with more proximal mucosal ulceration apparent. Dark blue or black nodular areas are suggestive of possible gangrene. Ernst and associates performed a prospective study on 50 patients to determine the incidence of this complication.[52] Colonoscopic examination was performed within 4 days of operation; three patients had evidence of ischemia (6%). Arteriographic evaluation of collateral circulation by the superior mesenteric artery revealed that colon ischemia did not develop when the collateral blood supply was identified. These authors suggest that despite the relative rarity of clinically significant colitis following aortic reconstruction, colonoscopy may be of value for early detection of possible ischemic changes so that therapy might, if necessary, be initiated sooner.

Pathologic changes of the colon may reveal disease limited to the mucosa and submucosa, or, in the situation when perforation has developed, transmural involvement may be evident (Fig. 17-9).

Management

Medical management includes intravenous fluid replacement, nasogastric suction, broad-spectrum antibiotic therapy, and the usual supportive measures. Surgical intervention is indicated for signs and symptoms of peritonitis and for obstruction.

The intraoperative diagnosis of the degree of colonic ischemia is often difficult to determine. Care must be taken at the time of resection to ensure adequacy of the blood supply to the anastomosis. Subtotal or total colectomy may be the safer approach.

Results

In the experience of West and co-workers with 27 patients who had colonic ischemia, 12 had reversible or transient colitis and 13 developed a stricture or gangrene that required surgery.[214] In the experience of these authors, the sigmoid colon was the most frequent area of symptomatic stricture presentation. Kim and co-workers analyzed the risk factors for the development of ischemia of the colon following abdominal aortic resection for aneurysm.[93] Prolonged cross-clamp time, hypoxemia, rupture of the aneurysm, hypotension, and arrhythmia occurred with significantly greater frequency among the patients with ischemia than among control subjects. In a study of postoperative colonoscopy following abdominal aortic reconstruction, Hagihara and colleagues determined that 11 of 163 patients who underwent reconstruction of the abdominal aorta demonstrated ischemic changes (7%).[80] These authors implied that the incidence might have been even higher if all patients surviving resection of ruptured abdominal aneurysms had undergone colonoscopy.

Abel and Russell reported their experience in the management of 18 patients with ischemic colitis.[1] They excluded all patients who developed ischemic symptoms following abdominal aortic surgery. Approximately 60% were 70 years of age or older; there were 14 women. Abdominal pain was the most common presenting symptom (72%). Diarrhea was noted in two thirds, and nausea and vomiting were frequent complaints. Laboratory tests were not found to be helpful.

Nine patients were submitted to surgery because of signs and symptoms that implied transmural involvement; four were noted to have gangrenous bowel, and two expired. Of the five patients who underwent exploratory laparotomy without resection, three died. Of the nine patients managed medically, four died.

It is evident that ischemic colitis is a disease associated with a very high mortality rate, probably because of the fact that many are elderly and have multisystem diseases.

Angiodysplasia

As is discussed in Chapter 14, unexplained massive lower intestinal bleeding, even in the presence of known diverticulosis, must be presumed to be due to angiodysplasia. The symptoms, diagnosis, and treatment for this condition are outlined in that chapter. The etiology of the condition remains somewhat problematic. Boley and associates suggested that the vascular lesions are degenerative, the results of the aging process.[28] They propose that muscular contraction or increased intraluminal pressure produces obstruction of the perforating veins. These submucosal structures become dilated and tortuous, with an associated arte-

riovenous (A–V) communication. Others suggest a congenital etiology, but this only serves to cause confusion. I think it would be simpler to accept the concept that angiodysplasia is an acquired condition and should be distinguished from the blood vessel tumor, hemangioma. A rare cause of lower gastrointestinal hemorrhage is variceal bleeding. This may be due to a congenital vascular abnormality, portal hypertension, obstruction of mesenteric venous circulation, splenic vein thrombosis, or a cardiac anomaly.[212]

Pathologically, the lesions appear to be ectasias, or dilatations of vascular structures. They represent collections of thin-walled dilated vessels (either capillaries or veins) lying usually in the submucosa (Figs. 17-10 and 17-11). Rarely, the condition may be associated

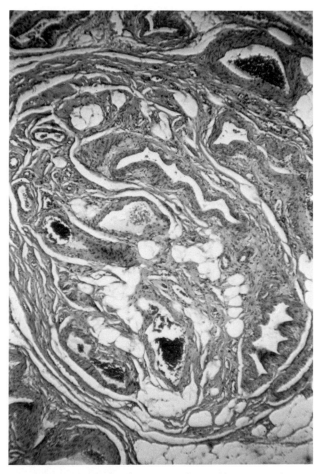

FIG. 17-11. Angiodysplasia: vascular malformation showing thick-walled veins and arteries in an irregular distribution. (Original magnification × 250. Courtesy of Rudolf Garret, M.D.)

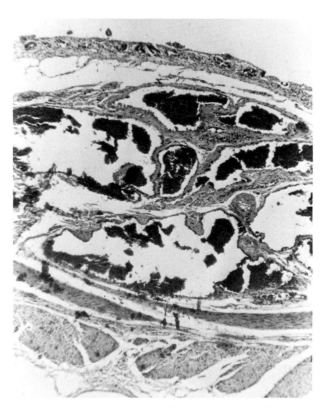

FIG. 17-10. Angiodysplasia of the cecum. Note the irregular veins and arteries. (Original magnification × 120. Courtesy of Rudolf Garret, M.D.)

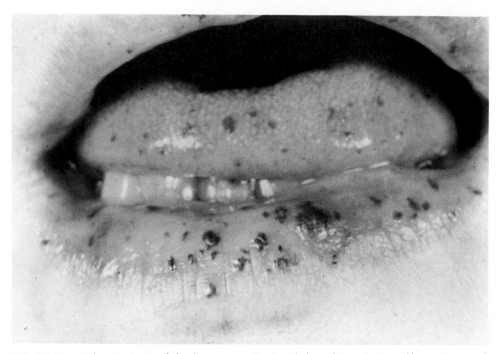

FIG. 17-12.   Telangiectasis of the lips in a patient with hereditary A–V malformations and gastrointestinal hemorrhage. (Courtesy of Rudolf Garret, M.D.)

with vascular malformations elsewhere in the gastrointestinal tract (*e.g.,* Osler-Weber-Rendu disease, Fig. 17-12).

The diagnosis is usually made by selective mesenteric arteriography. The cecal branch of the ileocolic artery usually is the most likely site for the malformation (see Figs. 14-30 through 14-32). The characteristic angiographic signs of angiodysplasia were described by Boley and co-workers and include a dense, slowly emptying vein (92%), a vascular tuft (68%), and an early filling vein (56%).[29] Extravasation of the contrast material is the least frequently observed finding (8%). Injection of the major blood vessel in the resected specimen may reveal a vascular tuft (Fig. 17-13).

Although most of the literature advocates angiography to establish the diagnosis, more recently colonoscopy has been used. Max and associates identified a lesion in 14 of 26 patients, confirming arteriographic findings in many.[124] Of interest is the fact that it was the only modality able to establish the diagnosis in three patients. Tedesco and co-workers, using colonoscopy, noted that in 11% of 46 patients with recurrent episodes of melena, vascular malformations were the cause.[190] Skibba and associates employed colonoscopy to establish the diagnosis of angiodysplasia of the cecum in a patient with gastrointestinal bleeding of unknown origin.[177] Thanik has also successfully used colonoscopy in the evaluation of hemorrhage from this condition.[191] Recently, bleeding from hereditary hemorrhagic telangiectasis, an autosomal dominant disease, has been evaluated successfully by means of colonoscopy.[178]

Localizing the site of acute gastrointestinal hemorrhage has been attempted using technetium sulfur colloid scintigraphy.[174] The imaging agent used for conventional liver scans is injected into the venous circulation, and with the abdomen of the patient under the gamma camera, a radionuclide angiogram is obtained. The principle of the study is that the labeled colloid is rapidly cleared from the bloodstream by the reticuloendothelial system, but an active site of bleeding appears as a "hot spot," since the extravasated isotope is no longer recirculating and cannot be cleared by the system.[174] Simpson and Previti, and Alavi and co-workers, have successfully used this approach to identify the site of bleeding.[3, 174] Baum suggests that as radionuclide scans are more widely employed, angiography will eventually be performed only in those patients with positive scans.[19]

Numerous studies have been published on the diagnosis and treatment of vascular malformations of the intestine. Richardson and associates reported 39 pa-

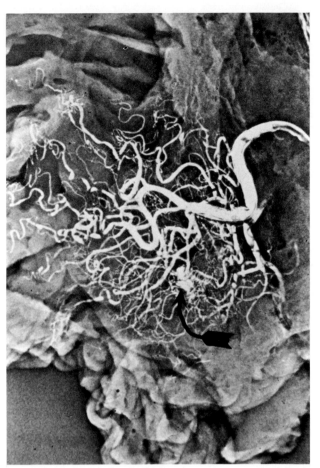

FIG. 17-13. Angiodysplastic lesion *(arrow)* in an injected specimen following resection for cecal arteriovenous malformation.

tients with bleeding due to this cause.[155] There appeared to be a bimodal age distribution, with younger patients having no associated disease, whereas older people often had an associated cardiac lesion (especially aortic stenosis and severe atherosclerotic disease). The commonest site of bleeding was the cecum, with resection controlling the hemorrhage in the vast majority of patients.

Love clarified the syndrome of calcific aortic stenosis and gastrointestinal bleeding, and suggested treatment of the bleeding by aortic valve replacement.[113] More recently, Shbeeb and co-workers reviewed Love's experience and confirmed the association of calcific aortic stenosis and obscure gastrointestinal bleeding in the elderly.[173] These authors suggest that this operation will not only correct the cardiac hemodynamic instability

but will also stop the gastrointestinal hemorrhage. They believe that an awareness of the association will lead to early diagnosis, and thus spare these patients from multiple hospitalizations and transfusions. A mechanism for this association and the ameliorative response of cardiac surgery is not clear. It may be a consumption phenomenon or qualitative alteration of platelet function produced by the roughened stenotic valve in the area of greatest pressure and velocity of the bloodstream.[113] This subtle coagulation defect combined with a thin-walled vascular lesion may tend to promote the hemorrhage.

Comment

The numerous reports in the literature reinforce the fact that an algorithmic approach to the treatment of gastrointestinal hemorrhage, such as is presented in Figure 14-29, is the most effective way to diagnose and treat the condition.[12, 75, 79, 134, 184, 187]

VOLVULUS

Sigmoid Volvulus

Sigmoid volvulus is a relatively rare condition that has been recognized since antiquity. Ballantyne stated that the authors of the papyrus Ebers from ancient Egypt wrote that either the volvulus spontaneously reduced or the sigmoid colon rotted.[14] Detorsion was recognized even then as the requirement for ameliorating the condition. Whether this is to be accomplished by medical or surgical means has been the subject of a considerable volume of literature, especially in the past 200 years.

In the United States sigmoid volvulus is a rare cause of intestinal obstruction, whereas in other areas of the world it is the single most common etiology for this presentation. Ballantyne reported that 30% of intestinal obstructions were caused by sigmoid volvulus in Pakistan, 25% in Brazil, 20% in India, 17% in Poland, and 16% in Russia.[15] In the United States, the incidence is only approximately 3%. The overall distribution of volvulus at various sites indicated that the sigmoid colon is by far the most commonly involved site (1400 cases) as compared with the cecum (400 cases), the transverse colon (35 cases), and the splenic flexure (4 cases).[15]

In Ballantyne's report, two different age patterns appeared.[15] In countries where sigmoid volvulus was relatively prevalent, the disease was usually seen in middle-aged men. However, in English-speaking countries (including the United States) the average age was considerably older, and the condition was as likely to occur in either sex.

Pathogenesis

The pathogenesis of sigmoid volvulus is obscure. The majority of patients are elderly and have a high incidence of associated medical or psychiatric problems.[6] In the few patients whom I have treated, most seem to come from either psychiatric institutions or nursing homes.

The condition is associated with an extremely redundant colon, a finding that may be seen in a number of illnesses, such as Chagas' disease, Parkinson's disease, paralytic conditions, ischemic colitis, ulcer disease, and many others.[15] Neurologic conditions in particular are frequently seen in association with volvulus. In fact, the high incidence of the condition in institutionalized patients may be more a reflection of the associated neurological disease than the fact that the patient happens to reside in such a facility.

An interesting fact is that sigmoid volvulus is the commonest cause of intestinal obstruction in pregnant women, presumably because a redundant colon is predisposed to torsion and twisting as the uterus rises out of the pelvis.[15] The condition also may be associated with aganglionic megacolon. In addition, mobilization of the colon coincident with other surgical procedures can predispose to volvulus. For example, this may occur following a Teflon sling procedure for rectal prolapse in a patient who often has a considerably redundant colon.

Signs and Symptoms

Patients with sigmoid volvulus usually present with the characteristic signs and symptoms of colonic obstruction. These include absence of bowel movements, failure to pass flatus, crampy abdominal pain, nausea, and vomiting. Physical examination may reveal a distended abdomen; minimal to mild tenderness may be noted. Peritoneal irritation is usually absent unless viability of the bowel is compromised. Rectal examination usually demonstrates an empty ampulla.

Investigations

The plain abdominal x-ray will usually reveal a markedly dilated sigmoid colon and proximal bowel, with relatively minimal gas noted in the rectum (Fig. 17-14). Agrez and Cameron reviewed the radiologic findings in 20 patients diagnosed as having a sigmoid volvulus.[2] Radiographic features included a distended

ahaustral sigmoid loop, the bent inner-tube appearance. In analyzing the plain films of 18 patients found to have sigmoid volvulus, an enlarged ahaustral loop was seen in 11 of them. In the remaining patients it was not possible to differentiate the distended loop from that of the transverse colon.

Barium enema examination may demonstrate complete retrograde obstruction to the flow of barium at the level of the torsion or may reveal an area of narrowing with proximal dilatation if the obstruction is incomplete or recently reduced (Fig. 17-15). In the experience of Agrez and Cameron, ten patients were submitted to barium enema study.[2] In three, there was a probable torsion point; four were definitely diagnostic (*e.g.*, bird's beak sign or mucosal spiral pattern), and three had markedly redundant sigmoid loops. None of the barium enema examinations relieved the volvulus.

Treatment

Ballantyne reviewed the evolution of nonoperative and operative treatment of sigmoid volvulus since the original description from Egyptian antiquity.[14] Suppositories, clysters, enemas, reduction by external manipulation, and the use of a rectal tube have all had their advocates. It was not until the 20th century that laparotomy was employed for the treatment of this condition.

Initial treatment depends on whether the surgeon believes that the bowel is viable or nonviable. In the former circumstance, attempt at reduction should be made by means of proctosigmoidoscopy and insertion of a rectal tube. If the volvulus can be reduced, an explosive discharge of gas and feces will be immediately recognized. The rectal tube should be left in place for approximately 48 hours in order to avoid the possibility of immediate recurrence. Colonoscopy has also been successfully employed in the therapy of sigmoid volvulus.[68, 167, 183] An attempt at colonoscopic reduction should be considered if proctosigmoidoscopic reduction has been unsuccessful.

If necrotic bowel is observed at the time of endoscopic examination, the surgeon should prepare the patient for an exploratory laparotomy. Proctosigmoidoscopic examination should be undertaken even if the patient has signs and symptoms of nonviable bowel in order to attempt to confirm the extent of involvement and if possible to establish the diagnosis with certainty. The procedure should be performed, however, with great care in order to avoid perforating the bowel.

In reviewing almost 600 patients, Ballantyne found that proctosigmoidoscopy and rectal tube insertion were successful in reducing the sigmoid volvulus in 40% of cases, proctosigmoidoscopy alone in 19%, barium enema in 5.4%, and other modalities in approxi-

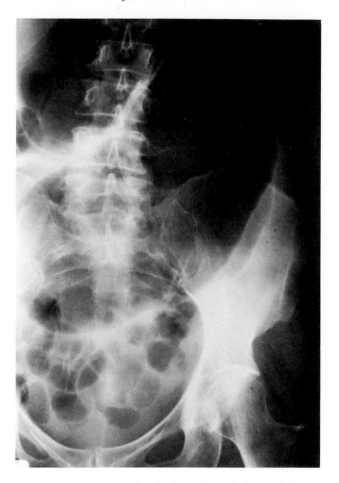

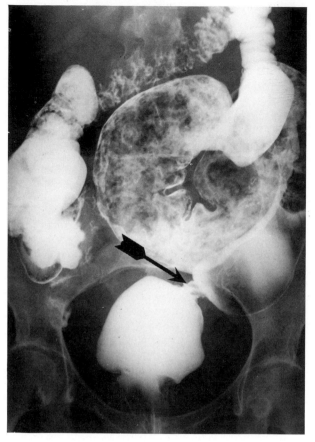

FIG. 17-14. Sigmoid volvulus. Plain abdominal film reveals a massive dilatation of the sigmoid and the so-called bent tire appearance. (Courtesy of Hector P. Rodriguez, M.D.)

FIG. 17-15. Sigmoid volvulus. Barium enema reveals a dilated sigmoid loop with a "corkscrew" appearance of the narrowed segment at the rectosigmoid junction indicated by the arrow. (Courtesy of Hector P. Rodriguez, M.D.)

mately 6%.[14] Seventy percent of patients were successfully reduced by some means in the 19 series reviewed by this author.

Although nonsurgical reduction of the volvulus allows one to avoid emergency surgical intervention, the recurrence rate is very high; in a combined series of 149 patients who were followed after successful reduction, 43% developed a recurrence.[14] There was a mortality rate in excess of 10% in this group. If the patient can possibly undergo an elective operation, this optimally should be performed during the same hospitalization after the bowel has been adequately prepared.

If one has been unsuccessful in reducing the volvulus, laparotomy is indicated. The choice of procedure depends on whether the viability of the bowel is com-

promised. Possible surgical alternatives include resection and anastomosis (with or without a proximal colostomy), Hartmann resection, exteriorization resection, detorsion, and detorsion with colopexy.

Obviously, if the colon is demonstrated to be nonviable, a resection is indicated. This is undertaken for the same reason and in the same manner that one would perform a resection of a perforated colon for any other condition (diverticulitis, carcinoma). The object is to remove the focus of sepsis. Whether to perform an anastomosis, a Hartmann procedure, or one of the other surgical options available is a judgement that each individual surgeon must make. The pros and cons of the different operative approaches are discussed in Chapter 14.

Irrespective of the viability of the bowel, my own preference is to resect the segment containing the volvulus.

Results

Ballantyne reviewed the experience of 25 American series that included over 600 patients.[14] Delayed elective resection with primary anastomosis was associated with the lowest mortality rate (8%). Operative mortality, however, in patients who underwent resection on an emergency basis was extremely high irrespective of the method of treatment (at least 25%). When one combines the American experience with that of other countries, it becomes clear that the prognosis of patients with sigmoid volvulus falls into two groups: viability or nonviability of the colon is the primary variable. Patients with viable bowel had an overall 12.3% operative mortality as compared with an operative mortality of 52.9% in patients with nonviable bowel.[14]

Ballantyne reported his personal experience of 12 patients with sigmoid volvulus.[13] There were 7 men and 5 women, with a mean age of approximately 69 years. Two thirds had neuropsychiatric disorders. The two patients who underwent emergency resection both expired, whereas mortality following elective resection was 25%.

Ryan reported 66 patients with sigmoid volvulus.[163] Emergency operation was required in almost half and was associated with a 22% operative mortality rate. The mortality rate with viable colon was twice as high when resection was carried out as when detorsion alone was performed. Because of this observation, Ryan recommends performing only detorsion unless gangrene or perforation require resection.

Anderson and Lee reported 134 patients with sigmoid volvulus.[6] Rectal decompression was effective in 85% of the patients. The best results in patients who had a nonviable colon were obtained with a Hartmann resection, although the number in this group was small. Because of the general success of a resective procedure when viable bowel was found, these authors do not advise detorsion alone. However, they had an extremely limited experience with this approach.

As stated, my own attitude is to perform resection with or without a primary anastomosis depending on the patient's condition and whether the operation is undertaken on an elective or an emergency basis.

Cecal Volvulus

Cecal volvulus is less common than volvulus of the sigmoid colon, representing approximately 25% to 30% of patients with this condition. The *sine qua non* for developing this type of volvulus is a failure of fusion of the parietal peritoneum to the cecum and ascending colon. This resultant mobility predisposes the bowel to twist on its axis, to rotate and twist, or to fold upwards. Volvulus of the cecum occurs in younger patients on average than volvulus in the sigmoid. Precipitating causes are said to include distal obstruction, meteorism occurring in unpressurized air travel, pregnancy, and adynamic ileus.[55]

Signs and Symptoms

Abdominal pain is the predominant complaint; the pain may be relatively low grade and colicky in nature. Abdominal distension is frequently present and may be asymmetrical, with a mass in the hypogastrium or on the right side. Bowel sounds are usually obstructive in nature.

Radiologic investigation usually reveals characteristic findings. The cecum and ascending colon can be found in any part of the abdomen, but the most common displacement is into the epigastrium and left upper quadrant.[55] An obliquely oriented cecum and ascending colon may be identified extending across the abdominal cavity (Fig. 17-16). Usually no gas can be seen distal to the point of obstruction. Multiple gas–fluid levels may be noted in the small intestine. Barium enema may reveal the classic bird-beak deformity due to obstruction in the region of the cecum (Fig. 17-17).

Colonoscopy has been successfully employed to reduce volvulus of the right colon, although it is important to recognize that unless the procedure is initiated early, persistent efforts are very likely to be more harmful than helpful.[8]

Choice of Operation

Choices of surgical procedure for cecal volvulus without perforation or gangrene include appendectomy, cecopexy, cecostomy, and resection. Obviously, if the viability of the bowel is compromised or if perforation is present, resection is required.

Results

O'Mara and colleagues reported 50 patients who underwent surgery for cecal volvulus.[142] Nine had a gangrenous cecum at the time of surgery; of these, there were three operative deaths (33%). A variety of operations were performed in the 41 patients who had no evidence of gangrenous bowel at the time. Four underwent tube cecostomy, with one death; seven patients underwent resection and primary anastomosis,

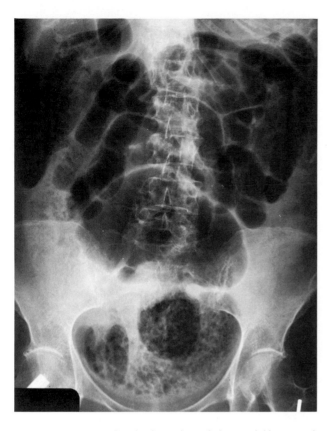

FIG. 17-16.   Cecal volvulus. Plain abdominal film reveals extensive small bowel gas with a large gas-filled shadow in the hypogastrium.

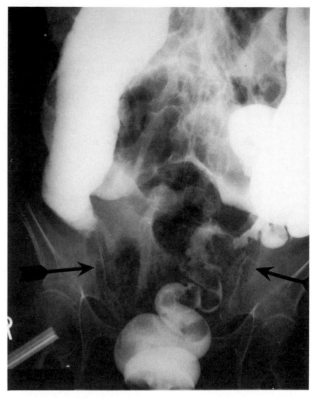

FIG. 17-17.   Cecal volvulus. Barium enema demonstrates obstruction in the region of the cecum; the cecal tip and terminal ileum are not visualized. The dilated cecum is outlined by arrows.

with no deaths; and twelve underwent detorsion alone, with two operative deaths. Cecopexy was performed on 18 patients, with no deaths. Howard and Catto reported 16 patients with cecal volvulus, 14 of whom underwent a nonresectional procedure.[84] In a follow-up averaging 5.6 years, no recurrence was demonstrable. These authors concluded that a resectional operation for viable bowel is unnecessary. Conversely, Todd and Forde, in a review of a number of series, noted that the recurrence rate for cecopexy was approximately 28%.[202] They advised that the operation of choice should be a tube cecostomy. With no recurrence following that procedure, as well as no recurrence following resection in their search of the literature, these authors advocate tube cecostomy as the treatment of choice because this procedure is less hazardous.

Anderson and Lee reported 41 cases of acute cecal volvulus.[5] They emphasize that prompt surgery is imperative. As with other series, the mortality rate approached 55% if the patient harbored necrotic bowel.

Cecopexy was associated with a 25% recurrence rate, but cecopexy with cecostomy was effective in preventing recurrence of symptoms.

Transverse Colon Volvulus

The transverse colon is probably the area of the colon in which volvulus least frequently occurs. Volvulus in this area may be associated with distal obstructing lesions, chronic constipation, prior abdominal surgery, or pregnancy. Anderson and co-workers identified 59 cases in the literature and added 7 of their own.[7] The condition is usually not diagnosed preoperatively. The radiologic findings are not really characteristic, except for the demonstration of obvious colonic dilatation. Gangrene in the reported series was found in approximately 16% of patients. In reviewing the literature,

Anderson and associates noted that simple colopexy was followed by a high incidence of recurrence.[7] They therefore suggested that at the very least the transverse colon should be resected. This is usually accomplished by means of an extended right hemicolectomy. Successful decompression by means of the colonoscope has been recently described.[88]

PNEUMATOSIS CYSTOIDES INTESTINALIS (PNEUMATOSIS COLI)

Pneumatosis cystoides intestinalis (pneumatosis coli, when the condition is confined to the colon) is a relatively uncommon disease of unknown etiology. It is characterized by the presence of gas-filled cysts within the wall of portions of the gastrointestinal tract. Koss reported an extensive review of the condition and noted that it most commonly occurs in the jejunum and ileum, with only 6% of cases being seen in the colon.[101] The disease is noted usually in the older age groups, but it can occur at any age. Its association with other conditions has been well documented. The most frequently associated diseases are pulmonary (*e.g.,* chronic obstructive lung disease), but it can also be seen with peptic ulcer, collagen disease, acute gastroenteritis, nontropical sprue, intestinal obstruction, mesenteric occlusion, ischemic colitis, inflammatory bowel disease, following abdominal trauma, as a result of endoscopic maneuvers (especially colonoscopy), with steroid therapy, following organ transplantation, and after surgical procedures on the bowel.[67, 77, 98, 129, 130]

The reasons for the occurrence in association with such diverse entities are not clear. One possibility is that increased intraluminal pressure may force the gas into the wall of the bowel. This may account for its association with certain primary diseases of the gastrointestinal tract. However, on close inspection of the bowel in such patients, it does not appear that the integrity of the mucosa is breached. The theory for the condition occurring in association with chronic obstructive pulmonary disease is that a pulmonary bleb ruptures and dissects retroperitoneally along the vessels, reaching the bowel wall. In support of this postulate is the fact that segmental distribution of the blebs usually is observed (Fig. 17-18). A third theory, which may be more relevant in infants with severe gastroenteritis, speculates that gas-forming bacteria account for the formation of the cysts.[76]

Many patients who harbor this condition do so without symptoms. The lesions may be noted on radiographic examination or at the time of endoscopy. When symptoms are present, they may be very vague, or they may include abdominal pain, diarrhea, and the passage of mucus and blood in the stool. Physical examination is usually not revealing. Rarely is there abdominal tenderness or distension. Digital examination of the rectum may reveal the presence of an extramucosal mass if the cysts indeed extend into that area. Barium enema examination may reveal well-demarcated, lucent wall defects of varying size, usually grouped in clusters with an intact overlying mucosa (Fig. 17-19).[25] The condition may be confused with inflammatory bowel disease, multiple polyposis, or carcinoma. Differential diagnosis has been established by means of colonoscopy; some have advocated its use as

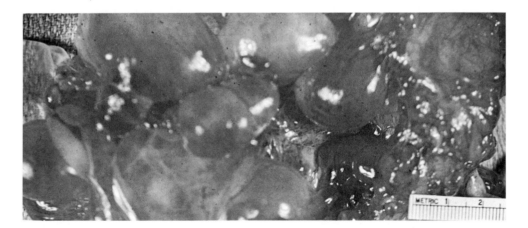

FIG. 17-18. Pneumatosis coli: cysts filled with gas, measuring up to 3 cm in diameter. (Courtesy of Rudolf Garret, M.D.)

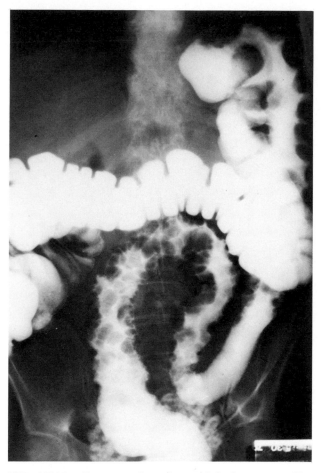

FIG. 17-19. Pneumatosis coli: multiple lucent cyst-like defects throughout the left colon.

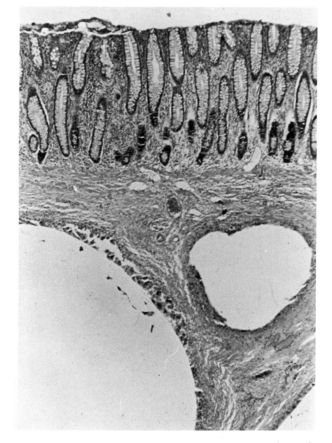

FIG. 17-20. Pneumatosis coli. Cystic spaces occupy the submucosa. (Original magnification × 120. Corman ML, Veidenheimer MC, Swinton NW: Diseases of the Anus, Rectum and Colon. Part I: Neoplasms. New York, Medcom, 1972)

the primary diagnostic tool for confirming the presence of the benign cysts.[47, 60]

Histologic examination of the biopsy specimen may reveal a normal mucosa beneath which cystic spaces are seen to be lined by endothelium.[71] There may be mild inflammatory infiltrate, and multinucleated giant cells are noticed frequently (Figs. 17-20 and 17-21).

It is important to recognize this entity and differentiate it from neoplasm. Treatment is nonsurgical.

In 1973 Forgacs and co-workers proposed replacement of the gas (which consists mainly of nitrogen) with oxygen.[61] By administering oxygen at relatively high concentration, resorption of the gas in the cysts should occur. Although there is no consistent recommendation about its administration, most authors believe that it is necessary to reach an arterial Po_2 in

excess of 300 mm Hg to achieve the desired results. A concentration of oxygen between 55% and 75% is generally used in the inhaled gas.[133] A minimum of 48 hours of therapy is recommended up to 5 days. Holt and co-workers suggest a standardized regimen of intermittent high-flow oxygen therapy.[83] One must be concerned, however, about the possibility of oxygen toxicity, and in fact my own attitude is to treat only those patients who have symptoms. In my experience I have been pleased with the ameliorative effect of oxygen therapy, and have found it necessary to employ the treatment for only 2 days.

Pneumoperitoneum can supervene in a patient with pneumatosis. If the patient has been known to harbor cysts, a trial of conservative therapy is advocated. Ab-

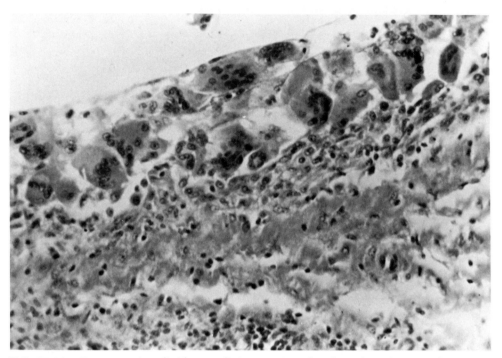

FIG. 17-21. Pneumatosis coli. The cyst lining consists of multinucleated giant cells, which probably represent a reaction to the gaseous material trapped within the cyst. (Corman ML, Veidenheimer MC, Swinton NW: Diseases of the Anus, Rectum and Colon. Part I: Neoplasms. New York, Medcom, 1972)

dominal signs and symptoms are usually absent. Usually no communication with the gastrointestinal tract exists; therefore, one should not treat the radiographic finding. Expectant management will usually be followed by gradual disappearance of the free gas. If one mistakenly embarks on an exploratory laparotomy for this presentation, it is probably better to close the abdomen, rather than to undertake a resection. In the rare situation in which the disease continues to cause symptoms and the cysts are localized to a limited segment of the bowel, resection might be contemplated.

COLORECTAL TRAUMA

Trauma to the colon or rectum may be due to blunt or penetrating injury of the abdomen or perineum, which may affect the blood supply to the bowel and the intraperitoneal or extraperitoneal intestine. The colon is injured in from 15% to 39% of penetrating abdominal injuries.[143] If the injury is to the rectum or perineum, associated trauma to the sphincter mechanism may be seen as well as damage to adjacent organs, the bladder,

urethra, and vagina. The therapy designed for the treatment of colon and rectal injuries depends on a number of factors, including the nature of the trauma (blunt or sharp), whether it is a high velocity injury from a bullet, or whether it is due to a knife or other form of impalement. The duration of time between the onset of the injury and the commencement of the medical care may also determine the type of therapy that is appropriate.

Colon Injury

Prior to the antibiotic era, especially with the experience gained from World War I, a conservative approach to colon injury was recommended. This usually consisted of exteriorization of the affected bowel, followed by a delayed resection and anastomosis. With the experience gained by World War II, it was felt that initial resection could be safely performed, but that colostomy was mandatory for such injuries. In recent years, there has been a greater tendency for the surgeon to perform primary resection and anastomosis, or even to attempt closure of the defect, depending on the nature of the trauma, the extent of the injury, the presence of associated injuries, the amount of spillage, and the length of delay in initiating therapy. It is not my purpose to discuss the total management of the acute abdominal or perineal injury. Obviously the appropriate resuscitative procedures must be initiated: intravenous fluid replacement, blood transfusion, and broad-spectrum antibiotics. Investigative studies may include endoscopy, cystoscopy, intravenous pyelography, Gastrografin enema, and possibly CT scan. Perforation due to endoscopic or radiologic investigation has been discussed in Chapter 1.[138, 176, 219] What I have elected to do in this discussion is to present to the reader a number of recent studies on the management and the results of treatment of perforating injury of the colon.

Stone and Fabian performed a randomized controlled study of primary closure versus exteriorization in patients with perforating colon trauma.[185] During a 44-month period, 268 patients with colon wounds were entered into the study. Excluded were those with profound preoperative shock, patients with blood loss in excess of 20% of estimated normal volume, patients with more than two intra-abdominal organ systems injured, those with significant fecal contamination, and patients in whom the surgery was begun more than 8 hours following the injury. Approximately one half had to be excluded because they did not meet these criteria. The authors determined that morbidity for the patients who were randomized to have a colostomy was 10 times as great as those who underwent a primary closure. The average postoperative stay was 6 days longer if a colostomy had been created, exclusive of the need for subsequent hospitalization for colostomy closure. The immediate mortality rate was identical, although one late death occurred following colostomy closure. The authors concluded that primary suture of colon wounds could be safely performed in selected patients if they met the criteria outlined.

Parks reported 106 patients who sustained colon injury as a consequence of the civil disturbances in Northern Ireland.[147] As would be expected, those patients who sustained multiple organ injuries had a much higher mortality rate. There were no deaths among patients who had isolated colonic or rectal injuries. Unfortunately, large bowel trauma tends to occur more often in association with injuries to other organs than it does in isolation. The author felt that primary closure of the wound should be considered if the injury is limited, of less than 4 hours' duration, with minimal peritoneal contamination and blood loss, and little or no associated injury.

There is a controversy about whether penetrating injuries of the right colon should be treated differently from those in the left. This is because it has been generally felt that right colon trauma is usually associated with a more favorable result than when the distal bowel is injured. Thompson and co-workers compared their experience in patients who sustained injury to the right colon with those who had a left colon injury.[198] Both groups of patients were similar with respect to the mechanism of injury, the presence of shock at admission, the degree of fecal contamination, the severity of the trauma, and the frequency of associated intra-abdominal problems. The number of patients managed by primary repair, resection, resection with exteriorization, and colostomy were comparable in right and left injuries, but it is to be remembered that these are historical controls. The treatment of right colon injuries resulted in a morbidity rate of 32% and a 2% mortality rate; left-sided injuries were found to have a 33% morbidity rate and a 4% mortality rate. Because of the comparable results, the authors concluded that penetrating trauma to the right and left colon should be managed similarly for the same degree of trauma, contamination, and so forth.

Wiener and associates at the University of Texas in Galveston reported their experience of 181 patients who sustained traumatic injury of the colon.[215] The authors emphasized that it is important to distinguish the treatment of colon injuries in civilian practice from the method of therapy commonly employed for war injuries. Treatment, according to the authors, must be individualized, with primary repair possible (debridement and suture or resection and anastomosis) in selected cases. In their experience, primary closure or resection resulted in a shorter hospital stay and a lower morbidity. Alternatively, exteriorization with a proximal colostomy was felt to be a reasonable alternative but one that should be reserved for the more severely injured patient. Criteria for exteriorization in these authors' experience included extensive damage to the bowel wall, questionable viability of the bowel, difficult or insecure repair, severe associated injury, and an easily mobile injured segment. Lou and associates reported a successful experience of 50 patients treated by an exteriorization repair method.[112] There was no mortality and a relatively low complication rate (18%). These authors felt that this method should be employed for those patients who cannot be treated by another approach. Likewise, Dang and associates reported a successful experience with an exteriorization repair technique in 82 patients who suffered colonic injury.[46] Although the study was uncontrolled, the overall mortality rate was 2.4%, as compared with no mortality in the patients who underwent an exteriorization repair. These authors concluded that this type of repair with early "drop-back" is safe and economical for most patients with moderate risk injury and even for some selected patients who may be at greater risk.

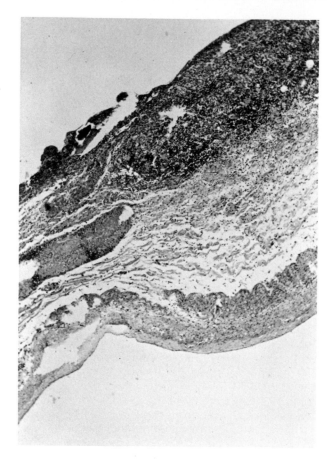

FIG. 17-22. Stercoral ulcer, the floor of which is lined by inflammatory exudate. (Original magnification × 120. Courtesy of Rudolf Garret, M.D.)

Kirkpatrick and Rajpal reported their experience in 165 patients with colonic injuries.[96] Their results demonstrated that primary closure with exteriorization was a safe and reliable method of management if the patients were selected from a rigid protocol. They recommended that the procedure be performed in all patients with lesions above 18 cm in which one suture line is required and in which the additional operating time of 20 minutes did not compromise the management of other injuries. These authors felt that if the patient could not fulfill these criteria, a colostomy should be performed. In their experience it was possible to reduce the need for colostomy to approximately one half of those who sustained colonic injury.

Flint and colleagues reviewed their experience with colonic injury in order to ascertain whether an intraoperative classification could permit assessment of pa-tients and a determination of the appropriate choice of operative procedure.[58] Grade 1 injuries were characterized by minimal contamination and the absence of other organ involvement. These wounds were managed by primary closure, that is, suture closure of the perforation. Grade 2 injuries implied through-and-through perforation with moderate contamination, and Grade 3 injury indicated severe tissue loss, devascularization, and heavy contamination. The authors advocated either exteriorization with or without subsequent colostomy or resection with colostomy. There was one death in 25 patients classified according to Grade 1; there were no complications in this group of patients. In 116 patients with a Grade 2 injury, the mortality rate was 2% and the complication rate 20%. With a Grade 3 injury (16 patients), there were 4 deaths (25%) and a complication rate of 31%.

Weil reported 66 patients who sustained retroperitoneal injury of the colon and rectum.[211] These injuries usually affected the intraperitoneal anterior and retroperitoneal posterior walls. The authors emphasize that the retroperitoneum must be inspected when an intraperitoneal hole is found or whenever the wound is in the flank or the back. In my opinion, colostomy is virtually always required for such injuries.

Blunt trauma to the abdomen is not usually associated with colonic injury, occurring in less than 5% of these cases. Mobile colon segments (transverse and sigmoid) are more susceptible to injury, although other areas of the bowel can be involved. Bubenik and colleagues describe three patients who sustained colonic injury following such trauma.[34] A characteristic scenario seemed to evolve. Perforation was discovered 7 to 10 days following injury and was indicated by signs of sepsis. A particularly prominent sign for occult infection was the syndrome of post-traumatic pulmonary insufficiency.

Obviously, if bowel injury is recognized in association with injury to other organs, the same principles already outlined should be applied. Unfortunately, some patients present many days following the initial injury, and are found on exploratory laparotomy to have considerable contamination and infection. Resection or exteriorization in addition to a diversionary procedure are indicated.

An uncommon cause of perforation of the colon is the so-called stercoral ulcer. A hard, scybalous fecal mass may produce an ulcerating lesion in the colon or rectum which can then lead to a perforation (Fig. 17-22). Bauer and co-workers described 4 patients who developed a perforation of the colon secondary to a hard mass of feces.[18] Treatment depends on the degree of contamination, the condition of the patient, and the other factors previously discussed. As with perforation of the colon irrespective of etiology, removing the nidus of sepsis from the peritoneal cavity is essential. A resection of the involved bowel is undertaken, and the decision of whether an anastomosis should be performed must rest with the judgment of the individual surgeon.

Rectal Trauma

Injuries to the anus and rectum may be the result of trauma from various surgical procedures (including obstetric, gynecologic, and urologic), following proctosigmoidoscopy, from ingested foreign bodies (Fig. 17-23), and from blunt and penetrating injuries to the perineum (Figs. 17-24 and 17-25). Trauma to the anorectal area may be secondary to gunshot wound, impalement, pneumatic injury, sexual assault, or insertion of enema nozzles and thermometers.

Usually the diagnosis of rectal injury is not difficult to establish; the history of trauma is usually self-evident. Occasionally, a high index of suspicion must be maintained if one is to establish the nature of the patient's complete injury and to initiate proper therapy. This is particularly true for avulsion injuries of the perineum and gunshot wounds of the abdomen. The mortality rate can approach 100% if an unsuspected rectal injury continues to provide a source for sepsis. Maxwell lists five factors that can determine the outcome of rectal injury: the extent of soft tissue trauma, the presence of associated injury, the delay in the onset of treatment, the general health and age of the patient, and the amount of fecal contamination.[125]

Haas and Fox describe a wide variety of injuries and procedures used in treating the various types of anorectal trauma.[78] They classify the types of injury into intraperitoneal perforations, retroperitoneal perforations, subperitoneal perforations, incomplete perforations, and perineal injuries. Sixty-two cases of rectal trauma between the sacral promontory and the anus were reviewed. The choice of therapy is dictated by the anatomic location, the pathology, and the etiology; the authors emphasize that there is no "best treatment" for anorectal injury.

If rectal injury is suspected, broad-spectrum antibiotic therapy should be initiated within as short a period of time as possible, hopefully not longer than 6 hours after injury. It has been demonstrated that the results of surgical treatment are improved if antibiotics are given very early after the onset of the injury. In *unsuspected* rectal trauma, the usual complaint is rectal pain. This may be delayed for several hours following the initial injury up to several days later. Abdominal

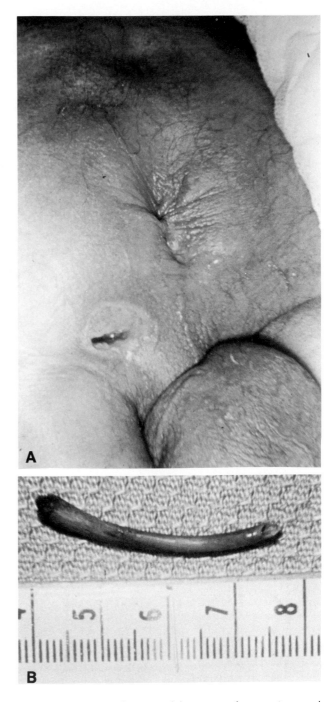

FIG. 17-23. **A.** Perforation of the rectum from an ingested foreign body, which produced an ischiorectal abscess. **B.** A chicken bone was the source of the perforation. (Courtesy of Daniel Rosenthal, M.D.)

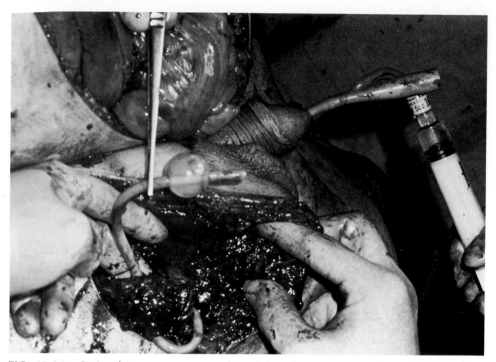

FIG. 17-24. Perineal trauma: severe avulsion injury from a motorcycle accident with lacerated urethra and rectum. (Courtesy of Imad Shbeeb, M.D.)

pain is an ominous sign implying peritonitis. Obviously, rectal bleeding with a history of trauma suggests at least a mucosal tear.

Physical examination should include digital rectal examination and careful palpation of the perineal area. Asking the patient to "tighten up" may help in evaluating the efficacy of the contractile mechanism. Anoscopic and proctosigmoidoscopic examination should be performed, although care must be taken to avoid exacerbating the injury. Barium enema examination is contraindicated if rectal injury is suspected; Gastrografin should be employed. Obviously the presence of intraperitoneal gas implies a perforated viscus.

The combination of blunt pelvic and perineal injury is associated with a very high morbidity and mortality. Kusminsky and associates emphasize the importance of performing a colostomy and washing out the distal rectum in order to avoid continued fecal contamination.[103] The authors reported their experience of 14 patients with this type of injury and noted a mortality rate of 42%. Obviously, such a high rate is due to extensive associated injuries.

Minor to moderate injuries of the anus below the level of the levator ani muscle may be treated by debridement, suture, drainage, antibiotic therapy, tetanus prophylaxis, and close observation. Intravenous fluid replacement and restriction of oral intake is advised. One might also consider the implementation of an elemental diet for several days until the patient's condition is felt to have become stabilized.

Injuries above the levatores usually require a colostomy at the minimum. Drainage, debridement, and distal washout of the rectum should be performed. I do not believe that one can be critical of the surgeon who errs on the side of conservatism in the management of rectal trauma by performing a colostomy; conversely, the treatment of a rectal injury without a diversionary procedure is usually inconsistent with optimal care.

Robertson and co-workers describe the Ochsner Clinic experience with 36 patients who underwent treatment for rectal trauma.[157] The authors caution that peritoneal lavage may be a valuable diagnostic study in the evaluation of blunt abdominal trauma, but may give false-negative results in patients who have undergone isolated rectal perforation or retroperitoneal or rectosigmoid perforation.[157] In choosing the therapy, the location, the cause, the length of time since the injury, and the association with other organ system involvement dictate the appropriate treatment.

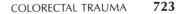

useful for a hollow body such as a jar.[54, 85] Drilling a hole in the bottom of a bottle or jar and inserting a Foley catheter is another means to remove such an item if the open end is directed cephalad. Garber and colleagues suggest using the more rigid endotracheal tube to remove such objects.[66] Berci and Morgenstern describe an operating proctoscope and tenaculum for extraction of foreign bodies.[21]

Eftaiha and associates reported their experience with the removal of 31 objects from the rectum.[50] They employ the principles of biplane abdominal roentgenograms to identify the location, type, and number of foreign materials, and they emphasize the necessity of an anesthetic. This is an important point; when one has established the presence of the foreign body it should always be removed under an anesthetic in order to avoid possible further injury. This is particularly true if the object is glass. Whenever possible transanal extraction should be accomplished, and laparotomy is undertaken only as a last resort. Proctosigmoidoscopic

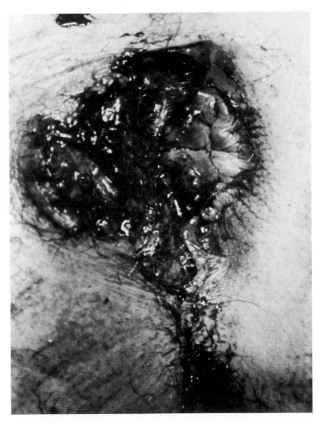

FIG. 17-25. Anorectal impalement injury. The anus is displaced to the right side. (Courtesy of Daniel Rosenthal, M.D.)

Foreign Body

The presence of a foreign body in the colon or rectum poses a particular problem in management. The ingestion of foreign objects may occur accidentally (*e.g.,* a swallowed dental bridge, nail, or screw, Fig. 17-26) or may be intentional, such as may be appreciated in treating the psychiatric population.

Extracting foreign bodies from the rectum has become virtually an epidemic problem in the last decade. Colonic foreign bodies may be removed by means of the colonoscope or, if symptoms of peritoneal irritation develop, may necessitate laparotomy and colotomy in order to effect extraction.[180] The list of objects that have been removed from the rectum is legion: lightbulbs, catheters, pens and pencils, glass tubes, candles, vibrators, bottles, and jars, to name a few (Figs. 17-27 and 17-28). A number of techniques have been suggested to remove these objects. A Foley catheter is particularly

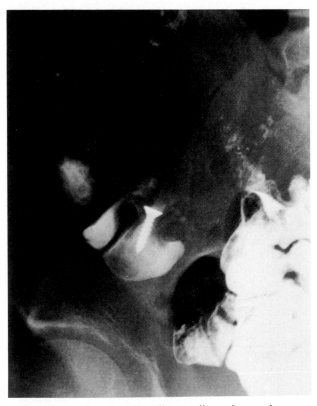

FIG. 17-26. An accidentally swallowed wood screw lodged in the cecum. Because of peritoneal signs, a laparotomy was undertaken. (Courtesy of Albert Medwid, M.D.)

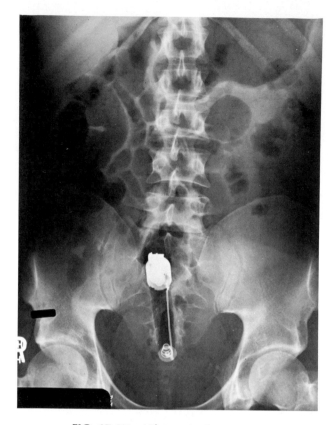

FIG. 17-27.   Vibrator in the rectum.

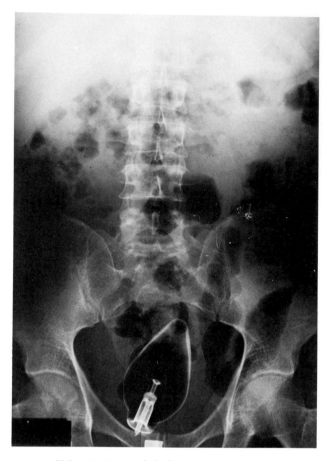

FIG. 17-28.   Lightbulb in the rectum.

examination should be performed after removal of the foreign body in order to be certain that no injury to the bowel has been sustained. It is also advisable to keep the patient in the hospital until a bowel movement has been achieved and the surgeon is convinced that sepsis or a perforation is unlikely.

If a laparotomy is required, an attempt should be made to "milk" the foreign body down into the field of vision of the perineal operator; hence, the perineolithotomy position should be used. Obviously, if injury to the rectum has occurred, the principles such as have been previously discussed apply. If the object cannot be removed transanally, a colotomy should be undertaken. In the controlled situation, without fecal contamination, no colostomy is performed.

SOLITARY RECTAL ULCER

Solitary ulcer of the rectum is an unusual condition initially described by Madigan and subsequently by Madigan and Morson; they collected a series of 68 cases.[115, 116] Unfortunately the term is rather confusing since the condition does not necessarily have to be solitary, does not have to be confined to the rectum, and may actually be polypoid rather than ulcerating. The condition is confused with inflammatory bowel disease, villous adenoma, colitis cystica profunda, and other inflammatory and neoplastic diseases affecting the colon and rectum.

The etiology is uncertain, but chronic constipation and fecal impaction may play a role. Some believe that the victims are often "unusual personalities."[200] Manual disimpaction may result in secondary inflammatory reaction, ulceration, and fibrosis, and autoeroticism may be involved. Turnbull, in fact, suggested that the treatment of the condition should be bilateral long-arm casts.[203] Some authors have observed a characteristic electromyographic finding in patients with solitary rectal ulcers.[105] Straining at stool in these patients is presumed to fail to inhibit the puborectalis muscle, which results in a repeated desire to defecate. Others have postulated that solitary rectal ulcer represents a stage prior to prolapse of the rectum. Duff and Wright reported 21 patients with benign ulcers of the rectum.[49] They felt that rectal prolapse, either complete or incomplete, was the condition most commonly associated with the disease.

Symptoms usually constitute varying bowel complaints: constipation, diarrhea, passage of mucus, tenesmus, rectal bleeding, and proctalgia fugax (see later). Martin and co-workers reviewed 51 patients with the syndrome and noted that 98% presented with rectal bleeding, 96% with the passage of mucus, and 93% with tenesmus.[123] About half of the patients were constipated. Bleeding was severe enough to require transfusion in three patients.

In the St. Mark's Hospital experience of 119 patients, the condition occurred equally in men and women. Classically, physical examination reveals an ulcer with hyperemic edges and surrounding induration. Alternatively, exophytic lesions may be seen. In my own experience, a combination of ulcerating and polypoid lesions is often noted on the posterior rectal wall, usually at a level of 6 to 8 cm. In the experience of Thomson and co-workers with six patients, the lesions were not necessarily solitary or ulcerated.[199]

There are characteristic features that permit the pathologist to distinguish solitary rectal ulcer from other inflammatory lesions on the basis of a rectal biopsy. Inflammatory changes may consist of replacement of the normal lamina propria by fibroblasts arranged at right angles to the muscularis mucosae (Figs. 17-29 and 17-30).[162] The microscopic appearance, however, is quite variable. Changes described include loss of nor-

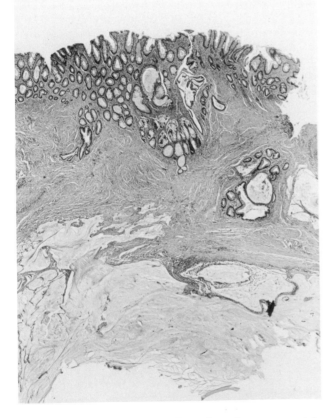

FIG. 17-29. Solitary rectal ulcer. The submucosa contains a large mucous lake *(bottom)* and a group of glands in the submucosa between the lake and the overlying mucosa. (Original magnification × 20. Courtesy of Rodger C. Haggitt, M.D.)

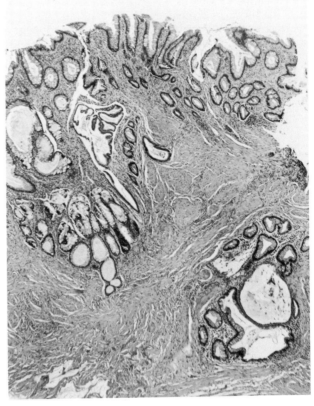

FIG. 17-30. Solitary rectal ulcer. Markedly hyperplastic muscularis mucosa separates a group of glands in the submucosa *(lower right)* from the overlying mucosa. Fibers of muscularis mucosa extend into and obliterate the lamina propria between crypts. (Original magnification × 40. Courtesy of Rodger C. Haggitt, M.D.)

mal polarity of the glandular epithelial cells, shortening of the crypts, mucin depletion, mucosal thickening, and inflammatory reaction in the submucosa. Many of the changes are those which have been previously described for patients with inflammatory bowel disease.

Franzin and associates reported a follow-up study of 27 patients with solitary ulcer of the rectum.[63] The authors noted a striking change in the evolution of the histologic pattern. Although there might have been an improvement in the patient's symptoms, the histologic appearance seemed to suggest chronic ischemia and an evolution to a transitional mucosa.

Treatment of the condition is rather problematical. I have been sorely tempted on occasion to consider Turnbull's admonition. A number of these patients are obviously psychologically disturbed. However, when the histologic-appearing lesion is proximal to the rectum, every one of the patients in my experience were subsequently proved to have inflammatory bowel disease, particularly Crohn's. With the lesion confined to the rectum, one might consider a trial of hydrocortisone enemas, although I have not been impressed with any ameliorative effect. Psychological counseling should augment medical management. Rarely, a colostomy may be indicated for the treatment of massive rectal bleeding.

SOLITARY CECAL ULCER

Solitary cecal ulcer is a condition of uncertain etiology. A number of theories have been postulated to explain its occurrence, including drugs (especially corticosteroids), stasis with stercoral ulceration, diverticulitis, arteriovenous malformation, and ischemia.[26] In the recent literature, solitary cecal ulcer seems to be quite frequently associated with end-stage renal disease.[106, 131]

Patients may present with signs and symptoms suggestive of acute appendicitis. Massive hemorrhage is not an uncommon consequence. The diagnosis may occasionally be made preoperatively by means of colonoscopy.

The surgical treatment for perforation requires a resection of the involved segment. In patients with hemorrhage, the protocol used in Chapter 14 would apply. However, since the lesion may actually be due to ischemia, Last and Lavery suggest that the use of intra-arterial vasopressin may precipitate a perforation.[106] Although conservative therapy should be considered, the differential diagnosis of a possible ulcerating carcinoma implies that at least a biopsy should be obtained.

LATE-ONSET HIRSCHSPRUNG'S DISEASE AND MEGACOLON

Hirschsprung's disease occurs once in 5000 births; it is seen more commonly in boys than in girls, in a ratio of 4 to 1. A physiologic intestinal obstruction is caused by lack of peristalsis in the aganglionic segment. Because of the failure to pass meconium in the first 24 to 48 hours, diagnosis is usually established within a relatively short time following birth. Depending on the level of the aganglionic segment the infant may be reasonably adequately treated by rectal examination, laxatives, and enemas for varying periods of time. If the aganglionic segment is long, medical management is not possible, and a colostomy is performed proximal to the aganglionic segment. When the child achieves a weight of approximately 20 pounds, definitive surgery is undertaken in the form of an abdomino-anal pull-through procedure or endoanal anastomosis (Swenson, Duhamel, Soave).

Occasionally a child may reach several years of age or even adulthood with a mild form of Hirschsprung's disease, that is, short-segment involvement. This manifestation may be limited to 3 or 4 cm of distal rectum and cause symptoms of severe constipation or absence of defecation except by means of rectal stimulation and enemas.

Udassin and associates reported 39 children who underwent treatment for a mild form of Hirschsprung's disease.[205] The diagnosis was based on clinical, radiographic, manometric, and histologic studies. The authors distinguished the mild from the severe cases on clinical grounds. In the former situation were classified patients who were constipated, who had abdominal distension, and who exhibited soiling with stool in the rectum. The onset of symptoms tended to be late. In the severe form, the rectal ampulla was empty, soiling did not occur, and the onset of symptoms was usually within the first month of life.

When a barium enema study is performed for short-segment involvement, it does not show the decompressed rectum seen with a classical Hirschsprung's lesion. On the contrary, the rectum may be quite dilated down to the level of the aganglionic segment (Fig. 17-31). The absence of ganglion cells on rectal biopsy has been felt to be diagnostic of Hirschsprung's disease (Fig. 17-32). However, in recent years, some authors have felt that in the short-segment form of the condition, biopsy is superfluous. The diagnosis can be made on clinical grounds supplemented by barium enema and pressure studies.

One of the problems with obtaining a biopsy for distal disease is that it is possible for ganglion cells to be absent normally at a very distal location. Furthermore, it is important to include the muscularis propria in order to obtain an adequate specimen for interpretation. As suggested, manometric studies are also useful in establishing the diagnosis of short-segment Hirschsprung's disease. With inflation of the proximal (rectal) balloon there is failure of the internal sphincter relaxation response.[206] This physiologic finding is pathognomonic for Hirschsprung's disease.

The treatment for short-segment disease is anorectal myectomy. A number of reports have been published demonstrating that the technique can be safely and simply used in children, not only as a primary procedure for short-segment involvement, but also as a secondary operation after a failed low anterior resection or pull-through. The procedure is essentially an extensive internal anal sphincterotomy. The internal anal sphincter is divided (or ideally partially excised) from the level of the dentate line, incorporating the muscularis of the bowel wall for a distance of approximately 8 cm.

Udassin and colleagues reported 39 children treated by a modification of this technique.[205] Four subsequently had to undergo a Duhamel operation because of failure. The mean age of the patients at diagnosis was approximately 6 years. Over two thirds were, as expected, boys. Long-term follow-up results revealed that 27 patients were essentially without symptoms; seven had good results, and in one, the result was equivocal. Nissan and co-workers reported their experience of 35 patients with biopsy-proven Hirschsprung's disease, 11 of whom were treated by anorectal myectomy.[140] The eldest was 14 years and the youngest, 7 months. The authors advised incising the mucosa transversely about 1 cm proximal to the mucocutaneous junction on the posterior wall of the anal canal. My own preference is to perform the procedure laterally. Elevation of the mucosa is performed and a strip of muscularis, including the internal sphincter, is excised as proximally as possible, including both muscle layers. The authors estimated the length of muscle removed to be from 6 to 10 cm. Thomas and co-workers reported 11 patients with chronic constipation but without evidence of a long aganglionic segment on barium enema x-ray.[196] They performed a sphincterotomy and rectomyotomy through a posterior approach. Four patients had previously undergone a Swenson procedure. The results were mixed and greatly depended on the length of the aganglionic segment, that is, the shorter the segment of involvement, the more successful myotomy was in achieving a satisfactory result.

Lynn and Van Heerden reported the Mayo Clinic experience of 37 patients who underwent rectal myectomy for this condition.[114] Lynn had described this procedure previously. Of the 28 patients in whom rectal myectomy was the definitive procedure and who had

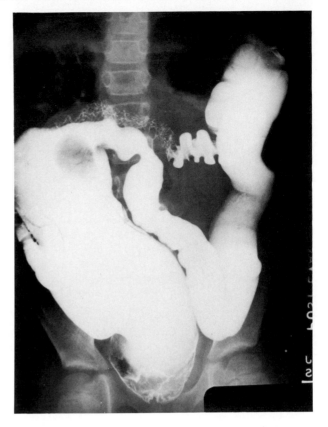

FIG. 17-31. Short-segment Hirschsprung's disease: markedly enlarged rectum with retained stool. No distal narrowing is noted because of the short length of involvement.

adequate follow-up, 20 had excellent results, 6 were improved, and 2 were relatively unchanged. Of the 4 patients who underwent the procedure following a previous operation, 3 had excellent results and 1 was improved.

Adult Hirschsprung's disease is a rather nebulous clinical entity. Speaking personally, I do not know whether it truly exists, except perhaps as the untreated short-segment form. Patients with severe chronic constipation, defecating once every 2 weeks, may be felt to have this disease. But in the absence of demonstrable objective evidence (manometric studies, absence of ganglion cells) the condition may be due to any of a number of causes. The matter, however, may be somewhat academic. Once the colon becomes markedly dilated, even if the patient developed the problem initially as a result of short-segment Hirschsprung's disease, anorectal myectomy will probably not significantly ameliorate the symptoms. It is this type of patient who will usually require a much more aggressive surgical approach, if surgery is to be considered at all.

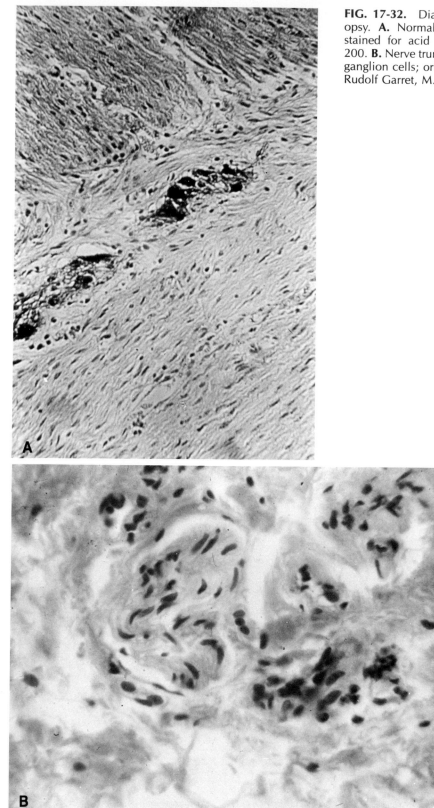

FIG. 17-32. Diagnosis of Hirschsprung's disease by biopsy. **A.** Normal ganglion cells in the submucosa are stained for acid phosphatase; original magnification × 200. **B.** Nerve trunk in the submucosa of the bowel without ganglion cells; original magnification × 600. (Courtesy of Rudolf Garret, M.D.)

Poisson and Devroede reviewed the problem of chronic constipation from a surgical perspective.[149] In those patients not found to have Hirschsprung's disease, manometric studies demonstrated a decreased amplitude of the rectoanal inhibitory reflex, a hypertonic anal canal that relaxes much more than is normal when rectal distension is performed, and a markedly unstable pressure in the upper anal canal. The authors emphasized that it is very important to ask about the onset of constipation. Those with a congenital type of constipation have problems from birth. In my experience, the adult patient with megacolon usually states that the problems of defecation began in early childhood.

Of course, an accurate history must be obtained, a complete physical examination must be performed, and appropriate diagnostic studies must be undertaken. One needs to ascertain whether the patient is taking any of the host of drugs that may produce constipation. The chronic constipation and colonic dilatation as seen on barium enema examination may be completely reversible after the medication has been discontinued.[37] Numerous medical diseases can be associated with chronic constipation and even megacolon. Included are various neurologic abnormalities, (*e.g.,* multiple sclerosis), diabetes mellitus, and connective tissue disorders, such as scleroderma.[69, 118, 165, 172] Radiologic study will often reveal a huge colon with considerable fecal residue (Fig. 17-33). Transit time studies using radiopaque markers may be useful.

Taylor and co-workers studied anorectal motility in the management of patients with adult megacolon.[188] Measurements were performed on 19 patients with the condition, and the results were compared with those of 12 normal subjects. Adult Hirschsprung's disease was recognized by the absence of anal canal inhibition on rectal distension. Those patients with non-Hirschsprung's megacolon had an elevated anal canal pressure and were treated by repeated anal dilatation. Those patients with normal anal canal pressures were treated with enemas and suppositories with little improvement. The authors concluded that anorectal motility studies were useful in the evaluation and subsequent management of patients with adult megacolon.

Many studies have been generated from Devroede's unit in Sherbrooke, Canada.[122, 149] By using anorectal manometry as well as radiopaque markers, the authors attempted to identify those patients who would respond to a particular surgical procedure. Patients who failed to improve following myectomy seemed to suffer essentially from colorectal inertia. This the authors found to be particularly true when markers were present in the right colon after a week or more following ingestion. The authors further caution that histologic examination is of limited value in the selection of pa-

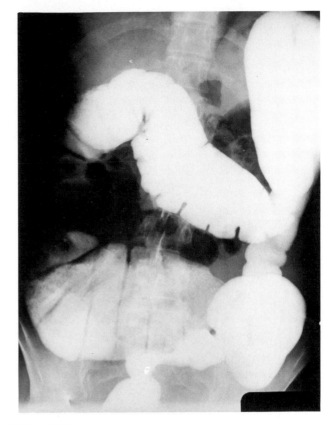

FIG. 17-33. Adult megacolon. Barium enema demonstrates a large-caliber bowel, especially in the proximal right colon. The patient moved her bowels once in 2 weeks.

tients with constipation for surgery. This is emphasized by the observation that absence of ganglion cells does not necessarily predict the efficacy of surgical treatment.

Belliveau and colleagues reported 48 patients treated for chronic, incapacitating constipation by resection.[20] Over 80% were women; most underwent subtotal colectomy. The authors reported an overall success rate of approximately 80% with a mean follow-up period of 5 years. McCready and Beart reported their experience of surgery on 50 adult patients with so-called Hirschsprung's disease.[126] A number of operations were employed, including the Swenson procedure, rectal myectomy, and a variety of bowel resections. Eight of 13 patients were improved or cured by rectal myectomy. Because of the diverse treatments, it is difficult to interpret the results of this study. Although the morbidity rate was low, there was a rather high failure rate.

My own approach to treating the adult patient with

megacolon is to perform a subtotal or total abdominal colectomy. I assume that the person would not have achieved adulthood without prior surgical intervention had there been an extensive aganglionic segment. Also, in my experience, the majority of patients who develop megacolon as adults have an associated medical problem, most commonly diabetes mellitus. I do not believe that colonic dilatation can resolve nor colon function be restored to normal in these patients by a limited anorectal procedure. However, if the person is a high risk for a major abdominal operation, anorectal myectomy might be considered.

COLONIC ILEUS (OGILVIE'S SYNDROME)

Intestinal pseudo-obstruction (colonic ileus, or Ogilvie's syndrome) was described initially in 1948 by the

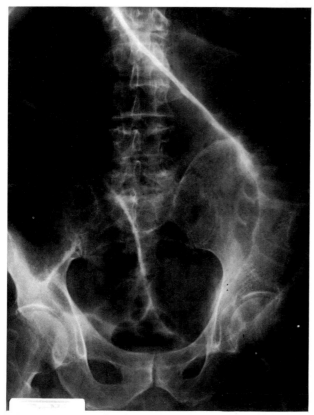

FIG. 17-34. Pseudo-obstruction of the colon (Ogilvie's syndrome): a massively dilated colon in an uncontrolled diabetic.

man who ultimately achieved eponymous recognition.[141] The patient exhibits signs and symptoms of colonic obstruction, but there is no evidence of an intrinsic or extrinsic lesion present. This condition is often seen in association with other diseases, and occasionally complicates the postoperative course of a patient who has undergone many types of operations, particularly abdominal surgery. Differential diagnosis includes Hirschsprung's disease (especially short-segment involvement; see above), toxic megacolon (ulcerative colitis, Crohn's disease), and a distal obstructing lesion. Predisposing illnesses and associated conditions are scleroderma, dermatomyositis, systemic lupus erythematosus, periarteritis nodosa, Chagas' disease, myotonic dystrophy, multiple sclerosis, familial dysautonomia, psychotic disorders, hypothyroidism, diabetes mellitus, hypoparathyroidism, renal failure, porphyria, congestive heart failure, lead poisoning, electrolyte imbalance, cesarean section, radiotherapy, and many others.[10, 16, 70, 111, 128, 137, 152]

The etiology of the condition is somewhat problematical. Probably many factors, including the underlying disease, are associated with the development of the dilatation. Impairment of electrical activity to the intestine as well as a defect in intestinal motility may be precipitated by numerous intrinsic and extrinsic agents such as secretin, glucagon, epinephrine, anticholinergics, and prostaglandins. Ogilvie suggested that distention of the colon was due to an interference with the sympathetic nerve supply.[141] Ravo and associates believe that the involvement of the sacral parasympathetic nerve supply to the colon may be the explanation for the syndrome, on the basis of their experience with the condition in pregnant women.[152]

The syndrome is characterized by massive colonic dilatation suggesting an obstructive etiology. The cecum is particularly dilated, a potentially dangerous consequence that can on occasion lead to perforation. Plain abdominal x-ray films will reveal marked dilatation typically localized to the large intestine. It is usually out of proportion to any distended loops of small bowel.[128] Meyers observed that the massive cecal distension may be horizontally oriented, a characteristic radiographic presentation (Fig. 17-34).[128] Close observation by means of serial plain abdominal x-ray films is required, similar to that performed for evaluation of toxic dilatation in a patient with acute inflammatory bowel disease. Barium enema examination is not required to establish the diagnosis and may be relatively contraindicated. If one is to undertake the procedure to rule out the presence of colon pathology, serious consideration should be given to performing the study with Gastrografin.

Colonic decompression has been advocated as an effective therapeutic modality in selected patients with nonobstructive colonic dilatation.[158, 186] Strodel and co-workers reviewed 44 patients who underwent 52 colonoscopic examinations for colonic ileus.[186] Approximately one quarter developed the condition while convalescing from recent surgery, whereas two thirds had major systemic disorders. The mean cecal diameter prior to colonoscopy was approximately 13 cm. On the basis of radiographic or clinical criteria, 38 patients (86%) were successfully decompressed on the initial colonoscopic examination; perforation of the cecum occurred in one patient. The authors advocate at least an attempt at colonoscopic decompression before performing cecostomy.

Another possible therapeutic modality is the use of ceruletide, a synthetically produced decapeptide that has been demonstrated to stimulate intestinal motility. Madsen and colleagues performed a double-blind clinical trial involving 18 patients and demonstrated a statistically significant effect on restoration of peristalsis in patients who had intestinal paralysis following abdominal surgery.[117] An intramuscular injection of 0.3 μg per kg body weight was given every 8 hours until passage of flatus or feces occurred or until three injections were administered.

Initial conservative management should include restriction of oral intake, nasogastric intubation, and correction of any fluid or electrolyte abnormalities. I believe it is important to distinguish the condition from other causes of megacolon that have been previously described. The easiest way that I find to distinguish these conditions is that the patient with so-called Ogilvie's syndrome usually develops the manifestation while in the hospital for another problem (usually post-surgical). There may or may not be an antecedent history of colonic ileus. In the patient with intestinal pseudo-obstruction, surgical intervention should not be performed unless there is a genuine fear of impending cecal perforation. As stated in Chapter 16, this is the only indication for performing a cecostomy in my opinion (see Fig. 16-36).

INTUSSUSCEPTION

Intussusception in the adult is always a surgical disease. This is in contradistinction to children, in whom medical management (*e.g.*, reduction by barium enema) may result in cure. Patients present with signs and symptoms of intestinal obstruction.

Nagorney and associates reviewed the Mayo Clinic experience with 144 cases of adult intussusception treated at that institution since 1910.[136] Almost nine out of ten were associated with a definitive pathologic process (malignant neoplasm, benign tumor, metastatic lesion, Meckel's diverticulum). Two thirds of the colonic intussusceptions were associated with primary carcinoma of the colon, whereas only one third of the intussusceptions of the small intestine were associated with an underlying malignancy; most of the latter were metastatic. The authors advocate resection of intussusception of the colon without any attempt at surgical reduction in order to minimize operative manipulation of the possible underlying malignancy.

COLONIC DUPLICATION

Colonic duplication is an uncommon congenital anomaly that usually occurs during infancy or early childhood.[17] However, occasional cases can present in the older age groups. Obstruction and the presence of an abdominal mass are usually the signs and symptoms apparent in infancy. Progressive abdominal pain, bleeding, and rarely perforation are characteristic of childhood or adult onset.[164]

True intestinal duplications must be distinguished from enteric cysts, whose characteristics include intimate attachment to some part of the alimentary tract, a smooth muscle coat, and a mucosal lining similar to that of the stomach, small bowel, or colon.[17] Four subtypes have been described: (1) a tubular duplication branching into the mesenteric leaves; (2) a double-barreled, communicating structure; (3) a free-lying, cystic duplication connected to the alimentary tract by a thin mesenteric stalk; and (4) a cystic duplication attached to the bowel by a common wall.[164]

Plain abdominal x-ray films may demonstrate a soft tissue mass, evidence of small or large bowel obstruction, and the presence of a gas-filled structure with air–fluid level on the erect film.[17] Barium enema examination may demonstrate displacement of the bowel, compression by the mass, or, in the case of a communicating lesion, an irregular double lumen. The condition is not uncommonly associated with other congenital anomalies such as malrotation, Meckel's diverticulum, lumbosacral spine anomalies, and genitourinary problems. An intravenous pyelogram should be part of the evaluation.

Treatment may involve excision of the mass with preservation of the normal colon (a communication is usually not demonstrable). Alternatively, an *en bloc* resection with anastomosis may be required when there is a double-barreled, communicating lesion.

MELANOSIS COLI

Melanosis coli is a condition that is commonly seen in patients who consistently use laxatives of the anthracene type (senna, cascara). The pigment produces no

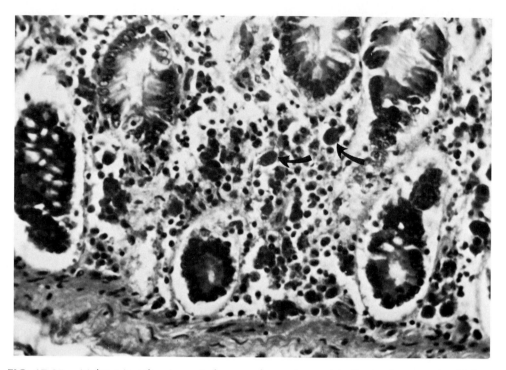

FIG. 17-35. Melanosis coli: pigmented macrophages *(arrows)* in the lamina propria. (Original magnification × 600. Corman ML, Veidenheimer MC, Swinton NW: Diseases of the Anus, Rectum and Colon. Part I: Neoplasms. New York, Medcom, 1972)

symptom. Proctosigmoidoscopic examination reveals the mucosa to be brown, deep purple, or black (Color Fig. 17-1). However, on careful inspection, the mucosa, although smooth, takes on a rather cobblestone appearance.

The condition usually occurs in the older age groups. Apparently, it takes years of laxative use or abuse to cause the color change. Biopsy of the rectum will reveal the presence of pigment-laden macrophages in the lamina propria giving the mucosa the characteristic color (Fig. 17-35). The cells do not contain true melanin, and the lesion should not be confused with malignant melanoma. There is no increased association with colorectal cancer.

Wittoesch and associates reviewed 887 patients with this condition. The overall incidence on routine proctosigmoidoscopic examination was approximately 1%.[217] The greatest incidence was in the fifth, sixth and seventh decades. The youngest patient was 20 years old. Approximately three fourths were women. Virtually all patients were habitual users of laxatives.

When the patient stops taking the anthracene laxative the pigment often disappears within 3 to 6 months.[181]

AMYLOIDOSIS

Amyloidosis not uncommonly affects the colon in association with a number of systemic diseases, particularly pulmonary, renal, hematologic, and arthritic. The value of rectal biopsy to establish the diagnosis of systemic amyloid has been a matter of controversy. Biopsies of the liver, spleen, and oral tissue (particularly gingiva) have been employed as alternatives.[170] Von Dinges and co-workers performed an autopsy study of 100 cases and took biopsy specimens of the rectum and gingiva.[208] In this unselected study there was a higher incidence of amyloid detected in the gingival and buccal mucosa than in the rectal mucosa; three fourths of the biopsies taken from the mouth yielded positive results, as compared with one third of the rectal mucosal specimens. The authors concluded that in view of the frequently found extensive amyloid deposits present in the mouth, biopsy should be obtained from the rectal mucosa. The theory behind this recommendation is that amyloid found on gingival biopsy is of less significance than if it were found on rectal biopsy.

Gafni and Sohar performed rectal biopsy on 30 cases of known amyloidosis; a positive result was found in

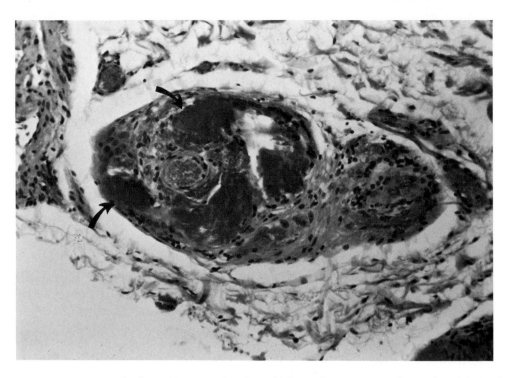

FIG. 17-36. Amyloidosis. Congo red stain, which produces green color under polarized light, reveals homogeneous material *(arrows)* within the wall of an artery in the submucosa of the rectum (Original magnification × 280)

26.[65] In a study by Kyle and co-workers, 17 of 20 patients with primary systemic amyloidosis were found to have positive rectal biopsies for amyloid.[104] In two of the three remaining patients the specimen did not contain submucosal tissue.

This is an important point; it is imperative that adequate submucosal tissue be obtained in order to establish the diagnosis. Although some authors have advocated a suction biopsy forceps, my own preference is to employ the ordinary rectal biopsy instrument. Since one is not taking a sample of tissue from an exophytic lesion, the biopsy should be obtained from the valve of Houston or from the posterior rectal wall. If bleeding is encountered, slight pressure with an epinephrine-soaked cotton swab is advised. Electrocoagulation should be used sparingly because of the risk of perforating the bowel.

Special stains are important for identification of amyloid. A homogeneous eosinophilic material can be identified by means of Congo red stain; this material may be overlooked with the standard H & E technique (Fig. 17-36).

Another use of rectal biopsy is in the assessment of different modalities of treatment for the systemic disease. Bacon and co-workers evaluated repeat rectal biopsies in a group of patients who underwent penicillamine therapy.[11] Improvement could be observed by means of repeat histologic examination.

Rarely, amyloidosis of the colon may produce a mass lesion or obstructive symptoms.[89, 102]

PROCTALGIA FUGAX (LEVATOR SPASM)

Proctalgia fugax (fleeting rectal pain) or levator spasm is a frequently heard complaint. Most physicians, unfortunately, fail to recognize this entity, and often classify the patient as a hysteric, prescribing various sedatives or tranquilizers as treatment.

The condition occurs predominantly in women. Characteristically, the patient complains of severe, episodic, often agonizing pain deep within the rectum. The location of the pain distinguishes the condition from that of thrombosed hemorrhoids or anal fissure; the symptoms for these conditions are often anal or perianal. The pain is often on the left side, may awaken the patient from sleep, and is usually unrelated to bowel activity (occasionally it may be exacerbated by defecation). It usually lasts for just a few seconds but occasionally may persist for several hours.

Physical examination is usually unrewarding, but sometimes a tender, spastic puborectalis muscle may be felt, particularly on the left side. The characteristic discomfort may be duplicated when the physician presses on the sensitive area.

Proctalgia fugax is analogous to a charley horse of the hamstring muscle; in this instance, it is a spasm of the levatores. It often occurs in patients who spend a great deal of time on the toilet: straining, with diarrhea, or reading the newspaper.

Treatment consists of instructions on bowel management and removing the library from the toilet. Sitz baths may offer some relief, but often the pain has ceased before the bath water can be drawn. Grant and colleagues believe that the syndrome is optimally treated in almost two thirds of patients by levator massage.[74] I, personally, believe that this treatment is contraindicated and prefer perineal strengthening exercises (see Chap. 5). With a vigorous exercise program and assurance that the person is not neurotic, the symptoms usually abate within a few weeks. In the intractable situation, muscle relaxants may be useful, but pain medication should not be given because of the risk of habituation. The teaching of self-hypnosis has been of benefit in some patients.

Recently Sohn and co-workers reported the use of electrogalvanic stimulation by means of a specially designed rectal probe.[179] The authors theorize that the technique may overstimulate and overcontract the levator muscle to fatigue it. They reported their results with 80 patients: excellent, 69%; good, 21%; and poor, 10%. I have had no experience with this technique.

Coccygodynia

Coccygodynia was originally described by Simpson in 1859 [175]; comprehensive reviews have been published by Thiele.[192–195] The condition is another manifestation of proctalgia fugax, but the pain is directed to the coccyx. Classically, the pain is characterized by exacerbation when the person rises from a sitting position.

In order to initiate proper therapy it is important to recognize the clinical syndrome and the characteristic pain. Some authors advocate levator massage, but I prefer to use perineal strengthening exercises and appropriate bowel management if the patient has difficulty in defecation.

Coccygectomy has been performed, but in my opinion it should be condemned for the treatment of this condition unless the coccyx has been injured or is dislocated. Even under these circumstances, coccygectomy rarely alleviates the pain. Johnson suggests that injection of a local anesthetic and cortisone may be beneficial.[90] He cautions, however, that the relief is usually only temporary. Albrektsson evaluated the long-term effect of sacral rhizotomy in 24 patients with coccygodynia.[4] Only six responded well to the procedure; serious complications occurred in 25%. I find it difficult to justify a surgical procedure of any kind in a patient with coccygodynia.

SARCOIDOSIS

Sarcoidosis is a generalized granulomatous disease with protean manifestations. The condition usually creates restrictive lung disease but can occasionally involve the gastrointestinal tract. In the limited number of cases reported, patients usually do not have symptoms referable to the bowel.[99, 201] Proctosigmoidoscopic examination may reveal mild inflammatory changes or a submucosal rectal nodule.

The characteristic noncaseating granuloma of sarcoidosis may be seen on biopsy or excision of a nodule (Fig. 17-37). Histologic examination may confirm a granuloma composed primarily of histiocytes; there is no evidence of caseous necrosis.

Differential diagnosis must include Crohn's disease, but the presence of a lesion in the lung will usually clarify any problem.

INFECTIOUS COLITIDES

Infections of the gastrointestinal tract may be caused by bacteria, fungi, or a host of parasitic organisms. The upper intestine tends to be attacked by organisms that produce toxins (*e.g.,* *Vibrio cholerae*), whereas in general colon infection is often associated with organisms that produce dysentery (*e.g.,* *Shigella*). In the former situation infection tends to leave the mucosa uninvolved, whereas in the latter, the intestinal mucosa is often ulcerated or destroyed. Upper intestinal organisms tend to produce diarrhea with severe dehydration; however, usually there is no septicemia. Those that affect the large bowel often produce severe abdominal pain, tenesmus, and signs and symptoms of generalized infection (*e.g.,* malaise, pyrexia). A rapid onset is often due to the presence of a toxin produced by a bacterium rather than to the bacterium itself; this type of syndrome is occasionally associated with certain restaurant

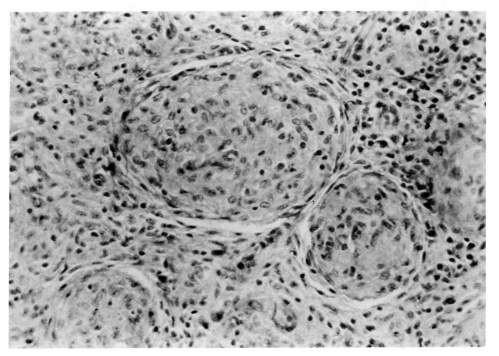

FIG. 17-37. Sarcoidosis: granuloma without caseous necrosis. Note the characteristic epithelioid cells. (Original magnification × 360. Corman ML, Veidenheimer MC, Swinton NW: Diseases of the Anus, Rectum and Colon. Part I: Neoplasms. New York, Medcom, 1972)

foods. Gorbach states that the incubation period from a toxin is so brief that the symptoms occur either when one is paying the check or when on the way to the parking lot.[73]

In this final section the various infectious diarrheas are discussed: presentation, diagnosis, and therapy.

Bacterial Infections

Pseudomembranous Colitis

Pseudomembranous enterocolitis is an uncommon infectious disease, but it can produce a potentially lethal illness. The condition has also been called antibiotic-associated diarrhea. Virtually all antibiotics have been reported to cause this syndrome (*e.g.*, tetracycline, chloramphenicol, clindamycin, lincomycin, ampicillin). Bloody diarrhea associated with abdominal pain may commence within 48 hours after the administration of the antibiotic. Any patient who develops diarrhea while on antibiotic therapy must be considered at risk for the development of this complication, although

the colitis may be unassociated with antibiotic therapy.[51] The condition can occur up to 6 weeks after discontinuance of the antibiotic. Toxic megacolon is a recognized complication.[40]

The condition has been reported as a complication of sulfasalazine therapy in a patient with inflammatory bowel disease.[150] The occurrence of this particular complication poses a considerable challenge in the differential diagnosis because the symptoms of the two diseases are so similar.

Recent evidence suggests that the colitis is caused by a change in the flora of the colon and overgrowth of toxin-producing strains of *Clostridium difficile* (Fig. 17-38). The organism is a spore-forming gram-positive anaerobic bacillus that is the component of the normal intestinal flora in about 3% of individuals.[53] It is difficult to isolate. Tests for the presence of the cytotoxin are performed by demonstrating the effect after incubation with viable cells. Clinically, the released toxin causes disruption of the endothelial cell membrane. Fluorescent antibody techniques are currently under development.

Proctosigmoidoscopic examination may reveal diffuse edema, multiple ulceration, and the presence of

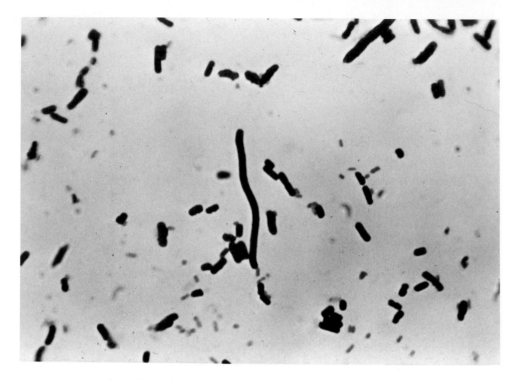

FIG. 17-38. *Clostridium difficile.* Gram stain of stool reveals gram-positive rods. (Original magnification × 800)

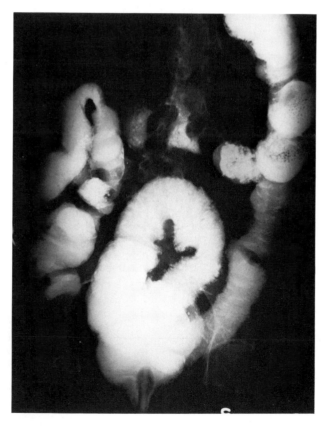

FIG. 17-39. Pseudomembranous colitis. Barium enema demonstrates extensive ulceration. Note the collar-button appearance of the ulcers extending into the bowel wall.

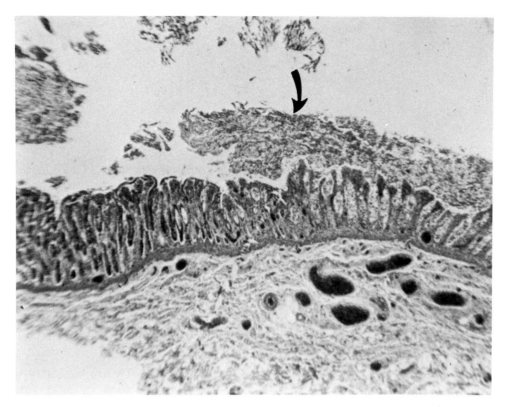

FIG. 17-40.   Pseudomembranous colitis. Superficial necrosis *(arrow)* with acute inflammatory mucosal exudate. (Original magnification × 80)

the adherent so-called pseudomembrane. Seppälä and associates stressed the importance of colonoscopy in the diagnosis of the condition.[171] (See Color Fig. 1-2). In a review of 16 patients with histologically proved antibiotic-associated pseudomembranous colitis, only 31% were confirmed by sigmoidoscopy, as compared with 85% in whom colonoscopy was performed. Others have reported the importance of total colonoscopy as the means for establishing the diagnosis, particularly since there is not uncommonly right-sided involvement with a relatively normal distal bowel.[35, 161, 166, 189] Tedesco demonstrated that five of six patients with tissue-culture evidence of a clostridial toxin in the stool had either a normal or merely an edematous rectal mucosa distally.[189] Thus, proctosigmoidoscopy would have failed to identify the abnormality.

Barium enema examination may demonstrate "thumb-printing" due to edema of the bowel wall. In more advanced stages severe ulceration may be present (Fig. 17-39). The procedure, however, is relatively contraindicated in the acutely ill patient because of the risk of precipitating toxic megacolon or a perforation.[53]

Biopsy of the lesion is not mandatory for confirming the diagnosis. However, if there is any question of the etiology of the inflammatory change, biopsy should be performed (Figs. 17-40 and 17-41). The most frequent indication for surgery is perforation, although pseudomembranous colitis may be a terminal complication in someone with a malignancy. Figures 17-42 and 17-43 demonstrate the appearance of the mucosa in such patients. Rarely does a patient survive who requires surgery.

Treatment, as stated, requires the discontinuation of the antibiotic, and fluid and electrolyte replacement. Depending on the severity of the manifestation, it may not be necessary to use an alternative antibiotic. Medications that slow peristalsis should be avoided, since elimination of the toxin is inhibited.[53] Those patients with a pyrexia, abdominal signs and symptoms, or leukocytosis, or who are elderly or debilitated, should be treated with vancomycin. The drug may be given orally in a dosage of 125 mg ever 6 hours for 5 days.[53] Improvement in symptoms usually occurs within 48 hours, but the diarrhea may not disappear for a week or more. Although treatment should be continued for at least 5 days, treatment for more than 10 days is

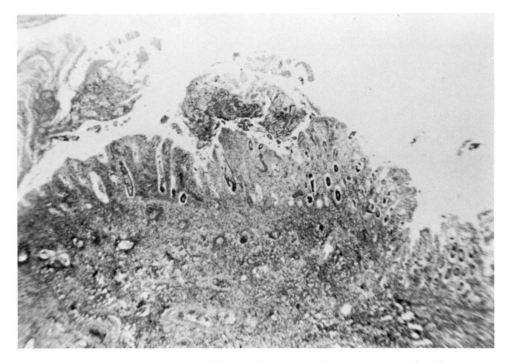

FIG. 17-41. Pseudomembranous colitis: total necrosis of the mucosa with inflammatory exudate in the submucosa. (Original magnification × 80)

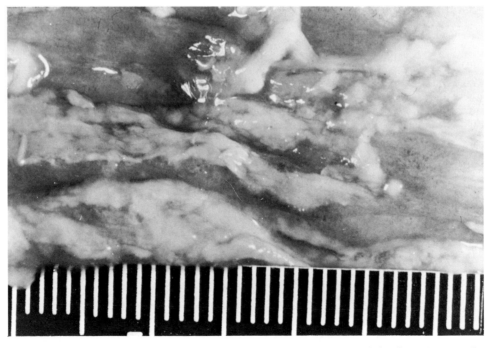

FIG. 17-42. Pseudomembranous colitis: postmortem appearance of the bowel. Note the mucosal exudate.

rarely necessary. Unfortunately, the drug currently is quite expensive. Milder cases may be treated with bacitracin, or metronidazole. Cholestyramine has also been shown to be effective.

Walters and co-workers recently reported relapse of antibiotic-associated colitis while the patient was maintained on vancomycin therapy.[209] Eight of fifteen patients so treated demonstrated a clinical relapse after therapy was discontinued. The results suggested to the authors that stool cultures should be done during and after treatment to dictate whether the antibiotic therapy should be maintained or reinstituted, or alternative therapeutic approaches considered.

Campylobacter Enteritis

Campylobacter jejuni has become one of the major causes of infectious diarrhea in the United States today and is an important cause of diarrhea throughout the world. The organism is a curved or spiral gram-negative rod. Transmission occurs by way of the fecal–oral route through contaminated fruit and water or by direct contact with infected animals or persons.[24] The organism is not uncommonly isolated from patients in the hospital who have diarrhea.

Symptoms and findings may be difficult to differentiate from those of other diseases affecting the intestinal tract, particularly inflammatory bowel disease. In fact, *Campylobacter* enteritis must be considered in the differential diagnosis of any patient who presents with rectal bleeding and diarrhea. Abdominal pain, fever, nausea, and vomiting may be associated. As suggested, rectal bleeding is quite common.

Proctosigmoidoscopic examination usually reveals edematous, inflamed mucosa. A high index of suspicion needs to be maintained if one is to establish the diagnosis and to initiate therapy promptly. Examination of the fecal specimen within 2 hours of passage by dark-field or phase-contrast microscopy may identify the organism.[24] The presence of polymorphonuclear leukocytes in the fecal stream is not uncommon but is not pathognomic for the condition.

Usually the infection is self-limited, but relapses are not uncommon. In severe cases, hospitalization and fluid and electrolyte replacement may be necessary. Erythromycin is the drug of choice, although tetracycline, doxycycline, and clindamycin may be used. Appropriate stool precautions (particularly in a hospitalized patient) are indicated, with proper disposal of contaminated linens and washing of hands.

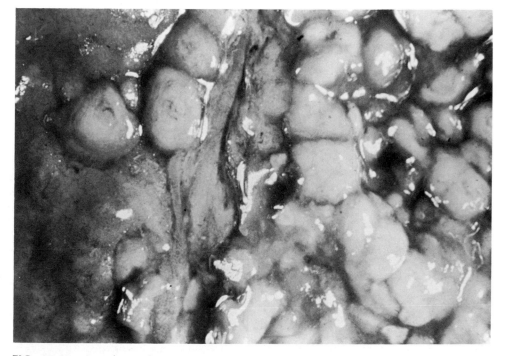

FIG. 17-43. Pseudomembranous colitis. Whitish plaques of pseudomembrane cannot be wiped off. The patient expired of acute leukemia.

Yersinia Enterocolitis

Yersinia enterocolitica is a relatively recently recognized cause of enteric infection. *Yersinia* enterocolitis is of particular interest to the surgeon because of its prevalence and because of its occasional confusion with regional enteritis. A former name for the causal organism was *Pasteurella pseudotuberculosis,* again implying confusion of the condition with another bacterial infection that tends to involve the ileocecal region. The disease is caused by a gram-negative rod resembling non-lactose fermenting *Escherichia coli.*[207] Epidemics due to contamination of food have been reported.[23]

The organism may produce signs and symptoms of an acute gastroenteritis; diarrhea is frequently observed in addition to abdominal pain. A syndrome simulating appendicitis is seen in 40% of the patients.[207] The condition may produce generalized septicemia and metastatic abscess in other organs. The disease may pursue a chronic course for many weeks, particularly if not treated with the appropriate antibiotics.

Results of radiologic examination were evaluated in a review by Vantrappen and colleagues.[207] A coarse, irregular, nodular mucosal pattern was seen in the terminal ileum. Ulcerations were also noted. In contrast to Crohn's disease, the infection of the terminal ileum is usually confined to the mucosa and submucosa; the characteristic "string-sign" is absent. Endoscopic examination demonstrates signs of inflammatory disease in approximately one half of the patients. The diagnosis is established by isolation of the bacteria from the stool. Treatment is with tetracycline or chloramphenicol.

Typhoid Fever

Typhoid fever is caused by the bacillus *Salmonella typhi.* These bacteria produce extensive epithelial invasion along the small bowel and colon without extensive destruction of the intestinal mucosa.[31] The epithelial lining is not appreciably disturbed. The bacteria breaches the mucosa and submucosa in areas of an inflammatory reaction. An endotoxin is produced upon autolysis of the bacterial cell. The condition is endemic in many underdeveloped countries.

If the organism enters the bloodstream, severe septicemia can result. Of surgical interest is the fact that acute cholecystitis may occur; this may progress to gangrene and perforation. Intestinal perforation can occur as well, and on rare occasion massive lower gastrointestinal hemorrhage can develop.[216] Bowel resection may be necessary under these circumstances.

Diagnosis is usually established when the symptoms occur in an endemic area. However, in Western countries it is unlikely to be considered in the initial differential diagnosis.

Abdominal examination may reveal mild tenderness or generalized peritonitis if a perforation has ensued. A maculopapular rash and splenomegaly are not uncommon. Stool culture may reveal the organism or, in the case of typhoid sepsis, blood culture may identify *Salmonella.*

Medical management includes the use of either chloramphenicol or ampicillin.

Tuberculosis

Tuberculosis involving the intestinal tract may be due to either *Mycobacterium tuberculosis* or *Mycobacterium bovis.* In the former situation, the disease is primary in the lungs and is carried to the intestinal tract by swallowing the sputum. The latter organism produces the infection in association with swallowing nonpasteurized milk. Although the condition is extremely unusual in most Western countries today (since pasteurization of milk is standardized), when the disease does affect the intestinal tract it is usually due to the pulmonary strain. Thus, in Western countries, infection of the bowel is almost always associated with primary disease in the lungs.

When tuberculosis affects the intestinal tract it usually localizes in the ileocecal region. The possible reasons for this are believed to be the presence of abundant lymphoid tissue in the area, an increased physiologic stasis, and an increased rate of absorption in the proximal bowel.[92] Although the condition is most commonly seen in the proximal colon and ileum, segmental colonic involvement has occasionally been observed.[33]

The commonest presenting complaint is abdominal pain. This is usually confined to the hypogastrium and is most frequently localized to the right lower quadrant. Other complaints include anorexia, fever, and weight loss.

Physical examination may reveal the presence of a mass, usually in the right lower quadrant. In the rare situation when tuberculosis involves the rectum or anus, a stricture may be apparent. Depending on whether the lesion produces ulceration or stricture, it can mimic carcinoma. In fact, in the absence of a pulmonary lesion, it would not be at all unlikely for the surgeon to perform a cancer operation for this disease.[94]

The diagnosis requires a high index of suspicion. Obviously, when a pulmonary lesion is present, intestinal tuberculosis should be considered. The acid-fast bacilli will only rarely be identified in the stool. Although a positive tuberculin test may be useful, it does not confirm the diagnosis with any certainty.

Radiologic investigation is helpful but not necessarily diagnostic of the condition. A plain abdominal x-ray film in a patient with intestinal obstruction secon-

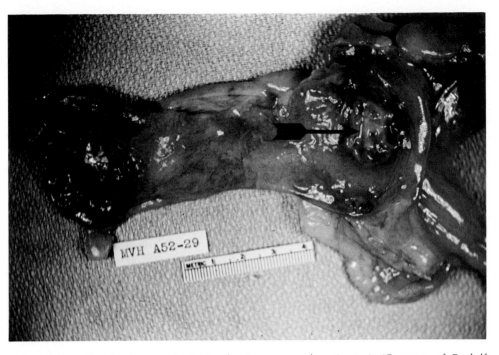

FIG. 17-44. Cecal tuberculosis. Note the transverse ulcer *(arrow)*. (Courtesy of Rudolf Garret, M.D.)

dary to a stricture or mass may reveal the absence of gas shadows in the right iliac fossa or distortion of the cecum and ascending colon by a mass.[39] Free perforation with pneumoperitoneum is extremely rare. Barium enema study may reveal retrograde obstruction, stricture, or a "conical cecum." The terminal ileum may be normal, dilated, ulcerated, or strictured. The distinction between tuberculosis and Crohn's disease may not be possible radiologically or endoscopically, although colonoscopy and biopsy have been useful diagnostic modalities.[33, 62, 82, 100]

Examination of the resected specimen may reveal thickening of the bowel wall, mucosal ulceration, localized segmental disease, or skip lesions. The mucosal appearance may demonstrate characteristic transverse ulcers (Fig. 17-44). The classical histologic criteria include the presence of submucosal or serosal Langhans' giant cells and the presence of caseous necrosis (Fig. 17-45). The organism may be demonstrated in the specimen or may be grown by guinea pig culture.

Surgical treatment is limited to those patients with symptomatic, localized disease. Conventional antituberculous agents should be used in the uncomplicated case. Approximately half of the patients with colonic or ileocolonic tuberculosis may be adequately treated with medical therapy alone.[45] Possible regimens include a combination of isoniazid with ethambutol or rifampin. Patients with ulcerating lesions are more likely to respond to medical management than are those with the hypertrophic form of the disease. Obviously, if the distinction cannot be made between tuberculosis and carcinoma by endoscopic or radiographic means, surgical treatment is indicated.

Gonococcal Proctitis

Gonorrhea is a common, sexually transmitted, acute infectious disease of the mucous membranes affecting the urethra, vagina, and cervix, but rectal gonorrhea has been recognized only relatively recently. Most physicians, in fact, did not appreciate the concept of rectal coitus in men prior to Kinsey's report in 1948, which discussed the widespread incidence of male homosexuality.[144]

The disease is caused by the bacterium *Neisseria gonorrhoeae* (the gonococcus), a gram-negative coccus occurring in pairs or clumps. Characteristically, the organism appears on smears as intracellular gram-negative diplococci (Fig. 17-46). In order to confirm the presence of the organism by culture, rectal swabs are inoculated on a selective chocolate agar (Thayer Martin) and sent to the laboratory without delay,

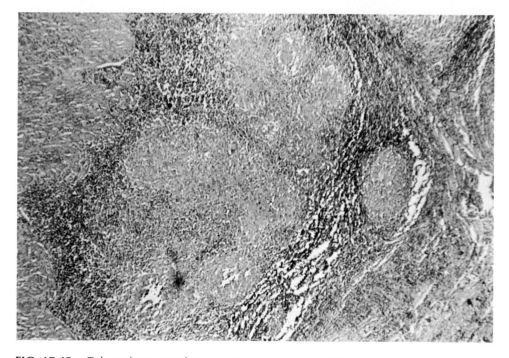

FIG. 17-45. Tuberculous granulomas (note caseous necrosis) in a mesenteric lymph node. (Original magnification × 180. Courtesy of Rudolf Garret, M.D.)

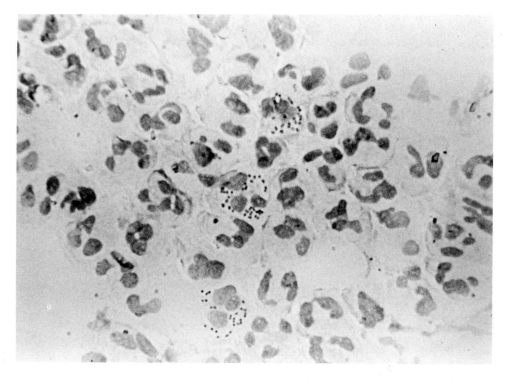

FIG. 17-46. Gonorrhea. Smear reveals gram-negative intracellular diplococci in the cytoplasm of polymorphonuclear cells. (Original magnification × 1000)

where they are placed in a carbon dioxide jar and incubated.

In men, the disease is most commonly associated with the homosexual population and is due to anal intercourse. However, in women the disease is usually transferred to the rectum by discharge from the vagina, presumably when the rectal mucosa is everted during defecation.[38] Usually only the lower rectum is involved.

Eradication of the disease is particularly difficult because the patient may report no symptoms. If symptoms are evident, they may include pruritus, mucous discharge, rectal bleeding, diarrhea, and complaints referable to either gonorrhea or syphilis in other sites. Disseminated disease may occur (septicemia), as well as pericarditis, endocarditis, meningitis, perihepatitis, and gonococcal arthritis. Characteristically the arthritis produces an acute purulent effusion of a single joint.[38]

Proctosigmoidoscopic examination will usually reveal edematous, friable mucosa with occasional areas of ulceration. Biopsy may show degeneration of the epithelium, capillary engorgement, and infiltration with inflammatory cells.[144] However, in many persons no identifiable lesion will be seen.

Quinn and co-workers reviewed their experience of anorectal infections in 52 homosexual men.[151] They reported that the gram stain of the rectal exudate was insensitive for the diagnosis of rectal gonorrhea, with up to 50% of culture-positive cases being missed. The authors further observed that because of the reported high prevalence of asymptomatic anorectal gonorrhea and the frequency of mixed infections, the isolation of the organism from a homosexual man with anorectal symptoms did not prove that the gonococcus was responsible for the symptoms. Lebedeff and Hochman, in a study of 1262 patients who had rectal symptoms, a gonorrhea contact, or a previously positive rectal culture for the organism, showed that 554 had culture-proven rectal gonorrhea.[109] Of the patients who demonstrated organisms, 82% had symptoms, one quarter had a history of contact, and 10% had a history of a prior positive culture. Of those that reported symptoms, 71% complained of mucus in the stool and 62% reported rectal discomfort.

Janda and associates studied the prevalence and pathogenicity of *Neisseria* in 815 homosexual men.[87] Interestingly, *Neisseria meningitidis* was isolated from more patients than *N. gonorrheae*. When the organism occurred in the rectum it was not usually associated with clinical illness.

Stansfield evaluated anorectal gonorrhea in women.[182] In a retrospective assessment of 159 patients who had undergone proctosigmoidoscopy, 127 (80%) had known contacts with patients with the disease. One half of these individuals harbored the organism. Of these, the vast majority had the organism in the rectum as well as in the urethra and cervix; only four (6.3%) had the organism confined to the rectum. Gram-stain smears demonstrated positive results in less than half of the patients with rectal gonorrhea.

Treatment of rectal gonorrhea has been a particular problem, because of the greater difficulty in eradicating the organism from this area than from the genitourinary tract.[38] Alternative regimens include the use of procaine penicillin, 4.8 million units, in two equally divided simultaneous intramuscular injections, with 1 g of probenecid given orally prior to or at the time of penicillin injection; or 1.5 g of tetracycline in an initial oral dose, followed by 500 mg 4 times a day for 4 days; or spectinomycin, 2 g by intramuscular injection.[144] Other antibiotics suggested include kanamycin intramuscularly, 2 g, or cotrimoxazole orally, three tablets, twice daily for 3 days.[38] Fiumara reported 80 patients with gonorrheal proctitis treated with the penicillin regimen followed by ampicillin, 500 mg orally four times daily for 4 days.[57] Of these, 78 patients returned for post-treatment culture. In addition, spectinomycin, 4 g intramuscularly, was given to 22 patients; all were cured at subsequent examination.

The importance of close follow-up examination with culture in order to assess the adequacy of the therapy cannot be overestimated.

Shigellosis

Shigellosis, also known as bacillary dysentery, is caused by the *Shigella* organism, a gram-negative, non-spore-forming rod. The condition may present acutely, with fever, diarrhea, and severe dehydration. The patient may actually seek emergency care.[81] This is another condition that is virtually epidemic in the gay population. In Heller's experience the clinical presentation may be one of subacute or chronic abdominal distress without fever or without diarrhea; alternatively, the organism may persist in the stool of untreated patients for prolonged periods in a "carrier state."[81] Obviously, this presents an epidemiologic problem. The author states that unlike the heterosexual population in which the need for antibiotic therapy may not be indicated, all homosexual men with *Shigella* cultures should be treated.

The hallmark of the inflammatory reaction is invasion and destruction of the intestinal mucosa.[31] Watery diarrhea is succeeded by severe abdominal pain, tenesmus, and rectal bleeding. The small bowel phase of the symptoms may be determined by an enterotoxin, whereas the invasive phase is typical of the large bowel.[31]

Sigmoidoscopic examination may reveal the typical changes of a proctitis, with edema, friability, and ulceration. The appearance may not be distinguishable from that of nonspecific inflammatory bowel disease. The most satisfactory means for establishing the diagnosis is culture obtained by swabbing any ulcerating lesion during endoscopy; alternatively, mucus or fecal material may be used for culture.[45]

As suggested, because of the usually self-limited aspect of the condition, supportive measures may be the only treatments required, although some people believe that all patients should be treated irrespective of the severity of symptoms.

Ampicillin is the drug of choice; alternatively, trimethoprim–sulfamethoxazole (Bactrim, Septra) may be used in patients who are sensitive to ampicillin or who have a resistant organism.[45] As with other infectious colitides, it is important to reevaluate the stool for the elimination of the bacterium.

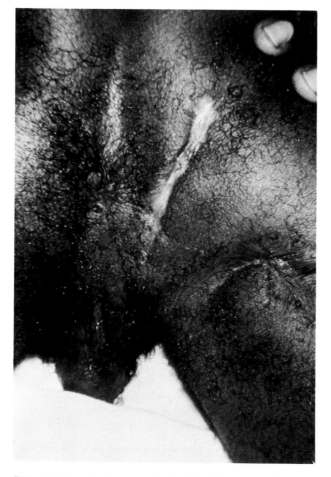

FIG. 17-47. Actinomycotic fistula. (Courtesy of Daniel Rosenthal, M.D.)

Actinomycosis

Actinomycosis is a suppurative, granulomatous disease that tends to form draining sinus tracts, discharging granules (see Fig. 8-18). The organism, *Actinomyces israelii*, an anaerobic, gram-positive bacterium, is a normal inhabitant of the mouth, lungs, and intestinal tract.[197] When the disease involves the colon or rectum, it usually presents with an abdominal mass, a fistula, or a sinus (Fig. 17-47). Differential diagnosis from neoplasm may be quite difficult.

Weese and Smith reviewed their experience of 57 patients who were subsequently proved to have this condition.[210] In only 4 was the disease correctly diagnosed on admission. Udagawa and associates reported 2 patients with primary actinomycotic infections involving the colon and rectum.[204] The diagnosis was established by histologic examination and by bacteriologic culture. In 1 patient, the presence of an abdominal mass was noted by the patient herself. Back pain, weight loss, and night sweats were also prominent complaints. Barium enema examination revealed segmental involvement of the descending colon by a stricture, and resection was undertaken. In the second patient proctologic examination revealed a mass in the perianal area. This is a much more frequent finding in patients who present with actinomycosis and is more likely to lead one to suspect the diagnosis. Others have pointed out that the lesion usually masquerades as an abdominal neoplasm.[197] Hence, unless material is available for histologic study, the disease is usually not diagnosed until resection has been performed.

For actinomycosis confined to the colon, resection is the treatment of choice in addition to antibiotic therapy (penicillin). Large doses are recommended over a prolonged period of time.

Viral Infection: Herpes Simplex Proctitis

Herpes simplex proctitis has been stated to be the most common cause of nongonoccocal proctitis in sexually active male homosexuals.[151] In a report by Goodell and associates the virus was detected in approximately 20% of 102 male homosexuals who presented with anorectal pain, discharge, tenesmus, or rectal bleeding, as compared with 3 of 75 homosexual men without intestinal symptoms.[72] The likelihood of having proctitis due to the herpes virus is greater if the patient has tenesmus, anorectal pain, constipation, and perianal ulceration. Difficulty in urinating, sacral paresthesias, and diffuse ulceration of the distal rectal mucosa also suggest the etiology of the condition.

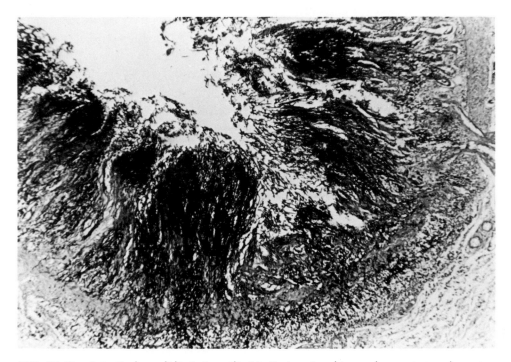

FIG. 17-48.   Intestinal candidiasis (moniliasis). Postmortem biopsy demonstrates characteristic pseudohyphae replacing mucosa. (Original magnification × 180. Courtesy of Rudolf Garret, M.D.)

The diagnosis is established by immunoassay of the antibody to the virus. In addition, herpes simplex virus may be isolated from rectal swabs or biopsy specimens. The natural history of recurrence of the proctitis after the initial episode and the possible beneficial treatment with antiviral agents has yet to be determined.[72]

Fungal Infection: Candidiasis (Moniliasis)

Fungal infections of the gastrointestinal tract are extremely rare in the healthy person. Candidiasis usually occurs in immunosuppressed patients, those with severe debilitating disease, and those who are taking steroids; it also may develop following prolonged administration of broad-spectrum antibiotics. Diffuse fungal infections are common causes of death in patients with terminal cancer.

Infection of the skin of the perianal area is discussed in Chapter 8. When the fungus affects the gastrointestinal tract it usually produces diarrhea and occasionally abdominal pain. Internal fistulas may develop. The diagnosis of the condition is established by demonstrating the yeast, spores, or pseudomycelia by means of microscopic examination. Biopsy may demonstrate the characteristic pseudohyphae (Fig. 17-48). Nystatin, 500,000 to 1,000,000 units orally, three times daily, is the usual treatment for intestinal candidiasis.

Parasitic Infection

Amebiasis

Amebiasis is a worldwide disease that is most commonly found in the tropics. It is caused by the protozoan *Entamoeba histolytica*. It is an uncommon although frequently diagnosed cause of traveller's diarrhea. A patient will often report to the physician that he has "amebiasis" based on a travel experience or contact with persons who are known to harbor the organism. However, Gorbach believes that even in the tropics, amebiasis is the "refuge of the diagnostically destitute," and that, in fact, the patient's symptoms are rarely due to this cause.[73]

Entamoeba histolytica exists in the colon as either a trophozoite (Fig. 17-49) or as a cyst. The cytoplasm of

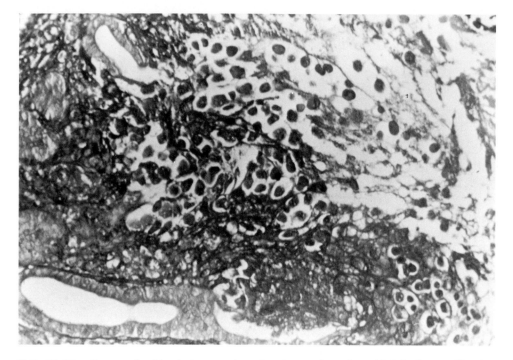

FIG. 17-49. *Entamoeba histolytica:* trophozoites in a colon ulcer. (Original magnification × 280. Courtesy of Rudolf Garret, M.D.)

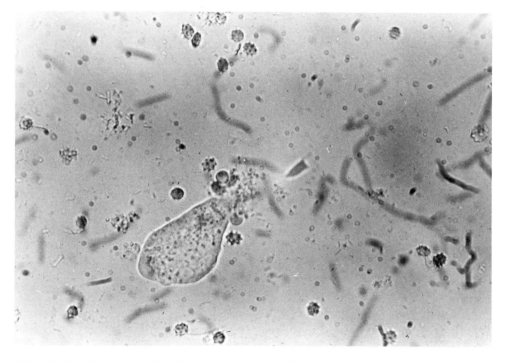

FIG. 17-50. *Entamoeba histolytica* ingesting red blood cells. (Wet preparation; original magnification × 360. Courtesy of Rudolf Garret, M.D.)

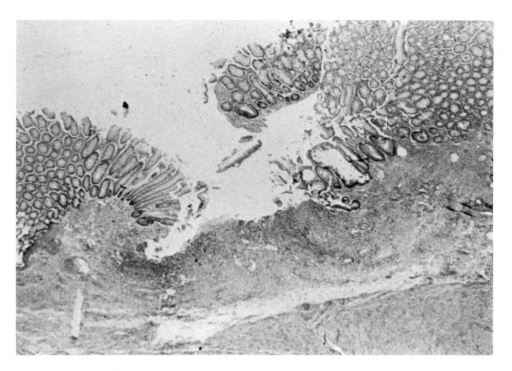

FIG. 17-51. Amebic ulcer. Note the characteristic flask shape. (Original magnification × 80)

the organism usually is quite granular owing to ingestion of many bacteria and other cellular debris (Fig. 17-50).

Transmission occurs either through water or food contaminated by carriers of the cysts. An outbreak of amebiasis occurred in a chiropractic clinic in patients who received colonic irrigation therapy.[86] *Entamoeba histolytica* infection has also been found in homosexuals.[36] The swallowed cysts pass into the small intestine where the trophozoites are released. These burrow into the mucosa and result in the characteristic flask-shaped ulcer (Fig. 17-51). Ulcers are usually identified in the cecum and ascending colon, but the process may be diffuse throughout the bowel; it is rare for the small intestine to be involved. Although the histologic appearance is usually indistinguishable from nonspecific inflammatory bowel disease, the overhanging mucosa, undermining margins, or flask shape, along with the appropriate history, suggest amoebic colitis (Fig. 17-52). Occasionally a granulomatous reaction may lead to the formation of a mass, the so-called ameboma. When this clinical picture is present, it may be difficult to distinguish the ameboma from that of granulomatous colitis or carcinoma.

Symptoms of amebiasis may be minimal, or the disease may be acute and fulminant. The commonest complaint is diarrhea, which may be bloody and contain mucus. Bowel movements can be frequent, in excess of 10 per day. Abdominal pain and tenesmus are associated complaints.

Physical examination may reveal abdominal tenderness, most marked in the hypogastrium. The liver may be enlarged, but hepatomegaly does not necessarily indicate the presence of a liver abscess. Toxic dilatation of the colon may develop in the fulminant condition, a clinical and radiologic manifestation which is not dissimilar to that of the complication when it occurs in ulcerative colitis. Perforation can supervene with generalized peritonitis.

The diagnosis is established by microscopic examination of fresh stool specimens for the trophozoites. Ninety percent of patients with symptomatic amebiasis will demonstrate this finding.[45] The trophozoites may be seen to contain ingested red cells (see Fig. 17-50). It is important that stool examination be undertaken before any barium investigation; the use of mineral oil and broad-spectrum antibiotics also impedes the ability to identify the protozoan.[45] In addition to stool culture and at least three stool examinations for ova and parasites, amebic titer by indirect hemagglutination technique may establish the diagnosis. An amebic titer by this means should be obtained if examination reveals colonic inflammation, and if the results of stool examination and cultures are negative.[127]

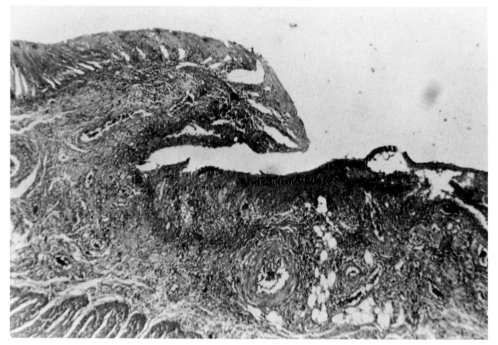

FIG. 17-52. Amebic ulcer. Note the undermined margin. (Original magnification × 180. Courtesy of Rudolf Garret, M.D.)

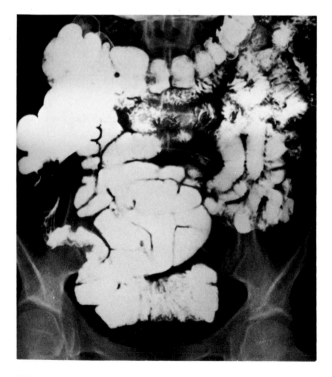

FIG. 17-53. Cecal ameboma. Barium enema demonstrates extrinsic compression of the cecum and terminal ileum with marked narrowing. The mucosa appears intact.

Sigmoidoscopic examination is a valuable method for diagnosis; ulcerations are usually visible in the rectum in up to 85% of the cases.[91] However, because the disease occurs more frequently in a proximal location than it does distally, a negative proctosigmoidoscopic examination does not rule out the diagnosis. Colonoscopy has been felt to be a useful technique for this reason. Crowson and Hines reported the diagnosis of the disease by means of colonoscopy in a patient in whom sigmoidoscopy was normal.[44] In the two patients of Rozen and co-workers, the symptom of rectal bleeding caused the authors to perform multiple colonoscopic biopsies which identified the etiology of the disease.[160]

Barium enema examination may reveal a multitude of changes in the patient with amebic colitis. As mentioned, toxic dilatation can occur, a contraindication to the performance of the study. Characteristic changes include the so-called collar-button ulcer, a cobblestone appearance, thumb-printing, and the signs of nonspecific inflammatory bowel disease. Amebiasis is almost always multifocal, so that a careful search throughout the length of the colon for other areas of infection is an important aspect of differential diagnosis.[145] The presence of a stricture or tumor-like ameboma may confuse the interpretation (Fig. 17-53); an ameboma can also involve the rectum.[158] Extra-intestinal amebiasis can lead to hepatitis, amoebic abscess of the liver, pulmonary disease, and involvement of the pericardium, brain, and skin (see Chap. 8).

The drug of choice for the treatment of asymptomatic patients with intestinal amebiasis is diiodohydroxyquin (Diodoquin).[45, 91] Other drugs that have been demonstrated to be efficacious include emetine hydrocholoride, dehydroemetine, and paromomycin (Humatin). For severe intestinal disease, metronidazole (Flagyl), 750 mg, three times daily for 5 to 10 days has also been recommended.[45]

If the patient requires surgical intervention for perforation, resection of the involved bowel must be performed. Total abdominal colectomy may be required if multiple areas of perforation are identified.

Balantidiasis

Balantidiasis is caused by a protozoan, *Balantidium coli*, a ciliate that is the only known member of the subphylum Ciliophora known to affect humans.[45] The trophozoite is quite large and may occasionally be seen with the naked eye (Fig. 17-54). Locomotion is by means of longitudinal rows of cilia that cover the body and propel it forward with a spiral motion.[97] A cyst develops when the organism is passed in the feces, and is the source for dissemination of the disease. Balantidiasis is found where poor sanitation is a problem.

After the cyst is ingested, the organism passes into the small intestine where it excysts, and the trophozoite then passes into the colon where it penetrates the intestinal epithelium.[45] Ulcerations are produced, not dissimilar to those seen with amebic colitis. In fact, the two conditions not uncommonly may coexist.

The usual symptoms are abdominal discomfort, distension, flatulence, and a loose, offensive, pale stool.[97] Mucus and blood may accompany the loose bowel movements.

Proctosigmoidoscopic examination may reveal the same changes seen in amebiasis. The diagnosis is made by examination of a fresh stool specimen. Patients with frequent bowel movements may pass only the trophozoites, however. An additional method is to obtain the trophozoites by duodenal aspiration or by the use of a recoverable nylon yarn swallowed in a weighted capsule.[97]

A number of drugs are effective in the treatment of balantidiasis. Some authors advocate tetracycline either alone or in combination with diiodohydroxyquin (Diodoquin)[45] or mepacrine.[97] Other alternatives include carbasone, ampicillin, metronidazole (Flagyl), and furazolidone (Furoxone). Treatment should be directed toward the asymptomatic carrier as well as the patient with acute or chronic illness in order to eliminate the organism and prevent its spread.[45]

Giardiasis

Giardiasis is also a disease caused by a protozoan, *Giardia lamblia*. It is a worldwide condition, with the vast majority of patients being asymptomatic. So-called traveler's diarrhea is commonly attributed to this protozoan. Contaminated water is believed to be the source of the infection in most cases. There is an increased incidence in the homosexual population.

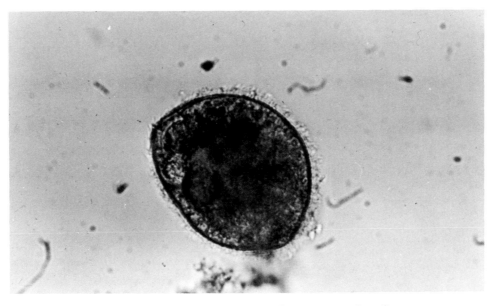

FIG. 17-54. *Balantidium coli*, trophozoite. Note the cilia.

As with balantidiasis, the protozoan exists both as a cyst and as a trophozoite. Infection results from ingestion of the cyst, which excysts in the small intestine.

If the patient is symptomatic, the most common complaint is diarrhea, but symptoms not unlike those of amebiasis may be reported. Rarely, the disease can pursue a fulminating course.

Proctosigmoidoscopic examination may reveal changes impossible to differentiate from those of amebiasis. The diagnosis is made by examination of scrapings of the base of the ulcer for the trophozoites.[45] Rectal biopsy may also be helpful in identifying the organism. Loose stool contains only the trophozoites; in formed stool there may be cysts and trophozoites.[97]

The drug of choice for the treatment of the condition is tetracycline. Alternatives include paromomycin, carbasone, ampicillin, and possibly metronidazole. Treatment of the asymptomatic carrier is somewhat controversial, but prudence would seem to dictate that both the asymptomatic person and the acute or chronically ill patient should undergo therapy in order to prevent spread of the disease.

Trypanosomiasis (Chagas' Disease)

It had been thought that trypanosomiasis was a condition confined to Central and South America, but more recent evidence suggests that the disease is present in the United States, particularly Texas.[32] Chagas' disease is caused by *Trypanosoma cruzi*, which is transmitted by a reduviid bug. The trypanosomes are deposited from the feces of the bug when it is taking a blood meal. Phagocytosis of the invading organisms is performed by histiocytes in the skin, fat, and muscle; this is the so-called leishmanial form of the disease. Involvement of the myocardium and central nervous system can occur.

Rupture of the cell causes escape of a large number of the trypanosomal forms into the circulation. In the gastrointestinal tract the disease is most likely to affect the esophagus, but the colon is also occasionally involved. In the intestine, the release of the toxin destroys the submucosal and myenteric plexus, which may result in colonic dilatation. The patient may be severely constipated as the bowel becomes progressively dilated because of the neurologic abnormality and the presence of inspissated feces. Volvulus is a potential complication.

Radiologic examination may reveal an enormously dilated and elongated colon. In contradistinction to other forms of megacolon, the distribution may be segmental.[145]

Patients with achalasia caused by the disease may undergo treatment with pneumatic dilatation of the esophagus or possibly esophagomyotomy.[45] Resection of the aperistaltic esophagus or colon may be necessary if symptoms warrant.

Schistosomiasis (Bilharziosis)

Schistosomiasis is a worldwide condition affecting perhaps 200 million people. The disease is caused by a trematode, a blood fluke which is seen in three forms: *Schistosoma mansoni, S. japonicum,* and *S. haematobium.* A snail host is required to complete the life cycle. The disease is frequently seen in tropical and subtropical climates.

The life cycle of the organism is of some interest. The infection is acquired by exposure to contaminated water containing the cercarial form of the organism (Fig. 17-55).[45] The cercaria invades the skin, loses its tail, and enters the host's subcutaneous veins. From there it spreads to the heart and lungs, and may produce a transient pneumonitis. Ultimately reaching the portal circulation, it grows, feeds, and differentiates into a male or a female form (Fig. 17-56). Following fertilization, the worms migrate together into the terminal mesenteric venules. There, the female deposits the fertilized eggs. The egg secretes a lytic substance that permits it to migrate through the surrounding tissue, into the intestinal lumen, and into the stool.[45]

The three forms of the infestation are differentiated on the basis of the appearance of the schistosoma ova (Figs. 17-57 and 17-58). The *S. mansoni* ovum has a prominent lateral spine, the *S. haematobium* has a projecting terminal spine, and the *S. japonicum* has no definite spine. *S. japonicum* preferentially invades the superior mesenteric veins, thus involving the small intestine and ascending colon; *S. mansoni* usually invades the inferior mesenteric veins, perforating through the descending colon; and *S. haematobium* tends to invade the bladder vessels, thus producing symptoms in the bladder, pelvic organs, and rectum.[45]

Symptoms initially are referable to the skin (see Chap. 8). If migration through the bowel wall occurs, patients develop severe lower abdominal pain, diarrhea, rectal bleeding, and the passage of mucus. Other symptoms include fever, urticaria, and facial swelling.[45] Bessa and associates reported 40 patients with colonic schistosomiasis due to *S. mansoni,* a common health problem in Egypt.[22] The primary complaint was severe diarrhea; three patients developed intestinal obstruction due to rectal or sigmoid stricture. Three quarters of the patients had a palpable mass.

Children are particularly susceptible to acute dysentery.[45] Fibrosis and thickening may result, and polyp formation may also occur. Other complications include intussusception and rectal prolapse. Portal involvement may produce granulomas, hepatosplenomegaly, and portal hypertension. Central nervous system complications can develop. *(Text continues on p 754)*

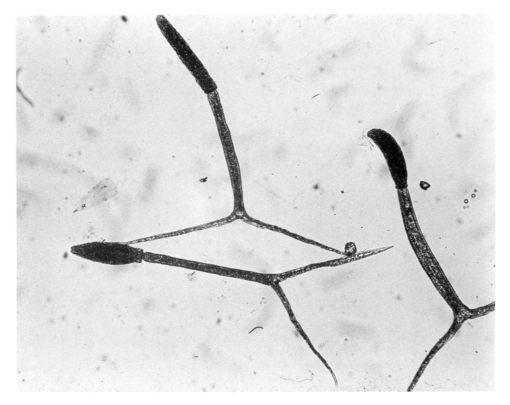

FIG. 17-55. Schistosoma: fork-tailed cercaria. (Courtesy of Rudolf Garret, M.D.)

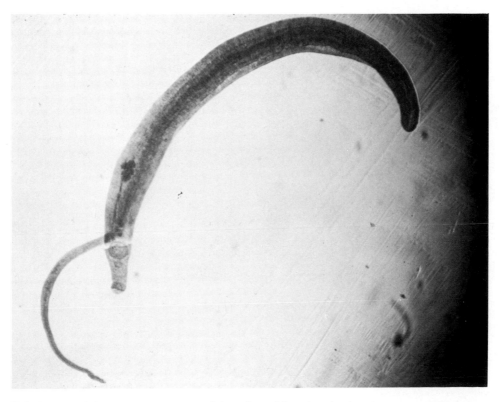

FIG. 17-56. *Schistosoma mansoni,* adult male and female. The female occupies the male's genital groove. (Courtesy of Rudolf Garret, M.D.)

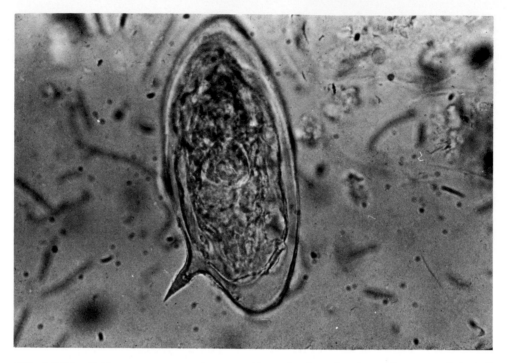

FIG. 17-57. *Schistosoma mansoni* ovum. Note the lateral spine. (Courtesy of Rudolf Garret, M.D.)

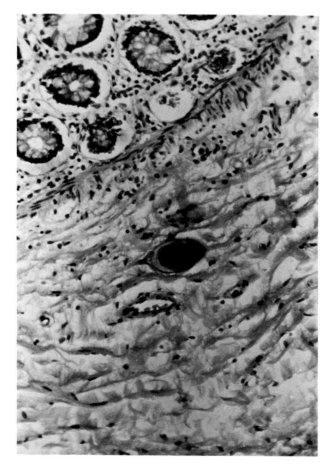

FIG. 17-58. *Schistosoma haematobium* ovum in the rectal wall. Note the terminal spine. (Original magnification × 180. Courtesy of Rudolf Garret, M.D.)

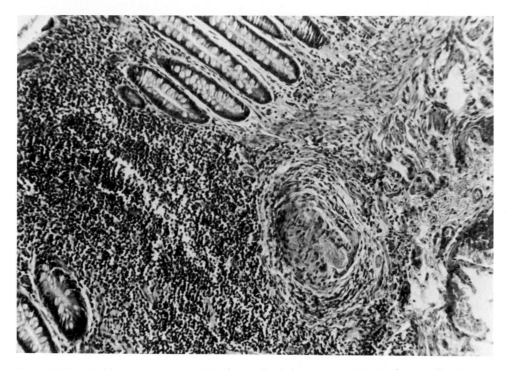

FIG. 17-59. *Schistosoma mansoni* in the wall of the rectum. (Original magnification × 250. Courtesy of Rudolf Garret, M.D.)

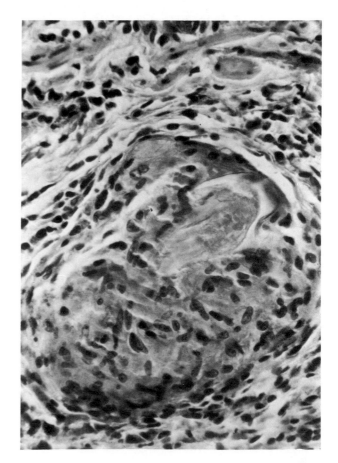

FIG. 17-60. *Schistosoma mansoni* in the wall of the rectum surrounded by epithelioid cells. (Original magnification × 600. Courtesy of Rudolf Garret, M.D.)

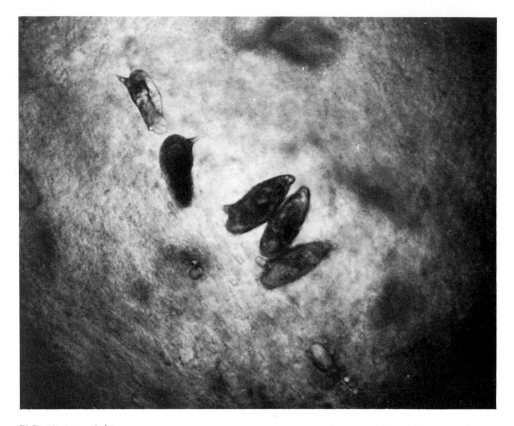

FIG. 17-61. *Schistosoma mansoni* ova, wet preparation. (Courtesy of Rudolf Garret, M.D.)

The diagnosis is usually made by identification of the ova in fresh stool specimens. Rectal biopsy frequently reveals the presence of the eggs in the mucosa or submucosa (Figs. 17-59 and 17-60). The diagnosis may also be made by means of a wet preparation; the biopsy specimen is compressed between two cover slips and examined for the ova (Fig. 17-61). A skin test and numerous serologic tests are also available for the diagnosis; the complement fixation test and indirect hemagglutination test may be valuable.[45]

The medical management of schistosomiasis is not without risk. Drugs employed vary, depending on which species is involved. A number of chemotherapeutic agents are variously effective; they include sodium antimony dimercaptosuccinate (Astiban), antimony potassium tartrate (Tartar emetic), stibophen (Fuadin), and niridazole. The reader is referred to a current drug resource reference for specific dosages.

Treatment of the complications of the colon involve a variety of resective and diversionary procedures. Anastomosis without a colostomy appears to be associated with a prohibitively high incidence of leakage.[22]

Patients with long-standing schistosomal colitis are at an increased risk for the development of carcinoma. Ming-Chai and co-workers reported a retrospective study of 60 patients with schistosomal granulomatous disease of the large intestine without obvious evidence of carcinoma and noted that 36 had mild to severe dysplasia.[132] The authors regarded the changes as presumptive evidence for the premalignant potential of schistosomal colitis, and felt that the findings were analogous to those observed in patients with long-standing chronic ulcerative colitis. Although as of this writing there are no published studies of the use of colonoscopy in the diagnosis of premalignant change and the performance of prophylactic colectomy on the basis of such change, it may be anticipated that such a protocol will appear.

Cirrhosis with portal hypertension may produce massive hemorrhage from varices that requires portacaval shunting. However, because of the high risk of this procedure, a new approach has been considered that involves cannulation of the portal vein, followed by trapping of the adult worms in a filter system (Fig.

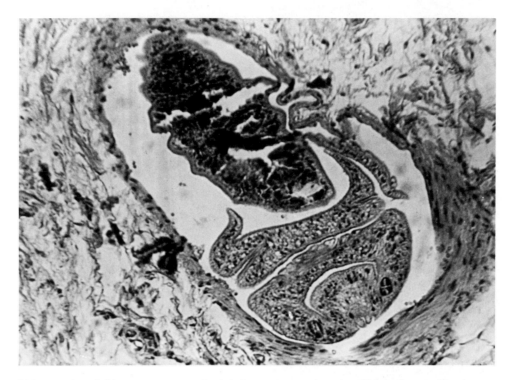

FIG. 17-62. *Schistosoma mansoni* adult in a mesenteric vein. (Original magnification × 120. Courtesy of Rudolf Garret, M.D.)

17-62).[45] Administration of antimony potassium tartrate has been demonstrated to increase the yield of the worms removed by stimulating migration into the portal circulation.

Ascariasis

Ascariasis is caused by a large round worm, *Ascaris lumbricoides* (Fig. 17-63). The disease is a worldwide problem; it is estimated that approximately 25% of the world's people are affected.[148] The condition is endemic in tropical and subtropical areas, but epidemics have been reported in Europe and even in small, focal areas of the United States. Infection occurs from ingestion of the eggs in contaminated food and drink (Fig. 17-64). Following ingestion, the larvae emerge from the ovum and migrate through the wall of the small intestine into the portal venous system, passing through the liver and into the lungs.[32] Ultimately the larvae migrate through the capillaries, into the alveoli and the bronchioles, and are coughed up and swallowed. In the small intestine they develop into the adult worm.

Intestinal ascariasis usually produces cramping abdominal pain. If the parasitic load is small, there may be very minimal symptoms. However, due to the large size of the adult worm, a number of complications referable to the gastrointestinal tract can ensue. Intestinal obstruction may result from blockage by a bolus of worms, particularly in the distal ileum, although it has been suggested that a major cause for obstruction may be spasm produced by irritation of the mucosal sensory receptors.[148] Allergic reaction (asthma, urticaria, and conjunctivitis) may be the result of absorption of toxins from the worm.[32]

Physical examination may reveal minimal signs, but obviously in the presence of intestinal obstruction, abdominal distension and diffuse tenderness may be noted. Occasionally perforation can ensue, and the patient will present with signs of peritonitis.

The diagnosis of ascariasis is made by finding the eggs, larvae, or adult worms. It usually takes approximately 2 months from the time of infection before the eggs will appear in the stool. The worms may also be recovered from the sputum, and occasionally from emesis.[32] Laboratory studies are usually of no value, since the only significant abnormality is the presence of an eosinophilia.

Small bowel x-ray films may reveal the presence of the worms in the distal ileum. Characteristically, the

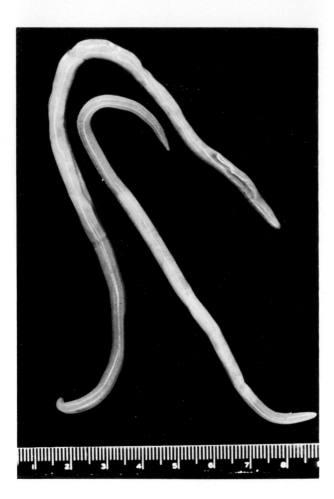

FIG. 17-63. *Ascaris lumbricoides,* adult worms. (Courtesy of Rudolf Garret, M.D.)

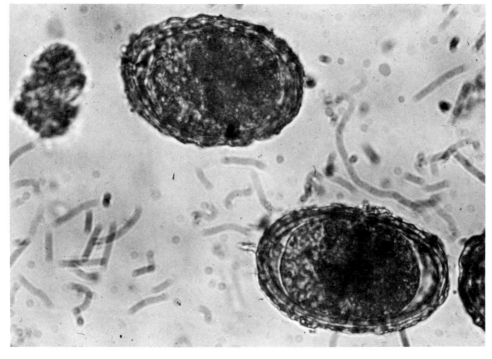

FIG. 17-64. *Ascaris lumbricoides,* ova. (Courtesy of Rudolf Garret, M.D.)

756

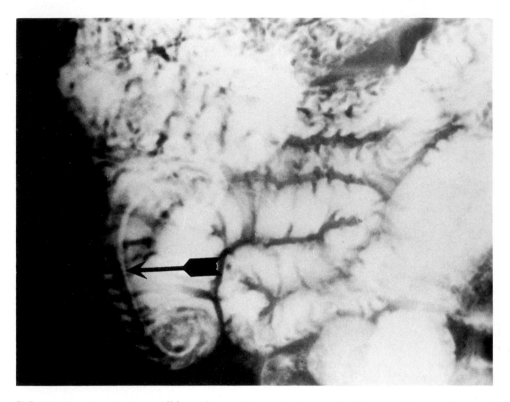

FIG. 17-65. Ascariasis: small bowel x-ray demonstrates ascaris. The gastrointestinal tract of the worm can be identified *(arrow)*.

gastrointestinal tract of the worm may be identified because it is filled with the contrast material (Fig. 17-65).

Treatment with piperazine derivatives has been advocated, but is associated with potentially serious side-effects. Other recommended drugs include levamisole, thiabendazole, and fenbendazole.

In a patient with intestinal obstruction, in the absence of an acute surgical problem, nasogastric intubation is recommended. Consideration should be given to placement of piperazine through the nasogastric tube.[148] If surgery is required and perforation has not occurred, it is best to attempt manipulation of the worms through the ileum into the cecum rather than to open the bowel. Resection is advised if required, as opposed to enterotomy and extraction of the worms.

Strongyloidiasis

Strongyloidiasis is a parasitic disease often seen in tropical climates and caused by another roundworm, *Strongyloides stercoralis*. The condition usually occurs in the small bowel, but the colon may occasionally be the site of involvement. Not too dissimilar to hookworm, the larvae penetrate the skin and are carried by way of the circulation to the lungs. They then rupture into the alveola and develop into adolescent worms.[32] The swallowed female invades the small intestinal mucosa where it remains, depositing eggs (Fig. 17-66).

Symptoms referable to the intestinal tract may be minimal, or the patient may complain of diarrhea, nausea, vomiting, and abdominal pain. Rectal pain and tenesmus have been reported in association with involvement in that area, and a proctitis may be present on sigmoidoscopy.[153]

The diagnosis is established by examination of duodenal secretions; suction biopsy of the duodenum is a poor way of finding the parasite.[32] Additionally, strongyloidiasis can be diagnosed by finding the larvae in the feces; this is the only intestinal nematode from which larvae rather than eggs are identified in the stool.[56]

In the severe form of the disease, mortality is usually due to dehydration and electrolyte imbalance, the result of vomiting and diarrhea.[56] The drug of choice for the treatment of the condition is thiabendazole (Mintezol).

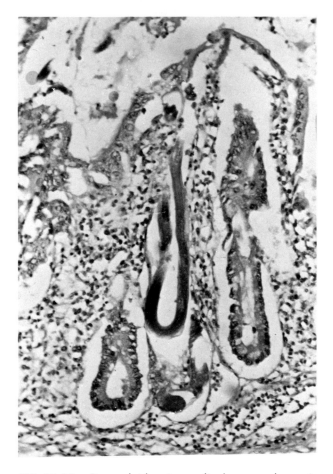

FIG. 17-66. *Strongyloides stercoralis:* larvae and eggs in intestinal mucosa. (Original magnification × 280. Courtesy of Rudolf Garret, M.D.)

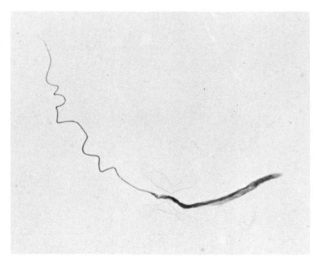

FIG. 17-67. Adult *Trichuris trichiura*. Note the slender neck, which gives the worm its common name, whipworm. (Courtesy of Rudolf Garret, M.D.)

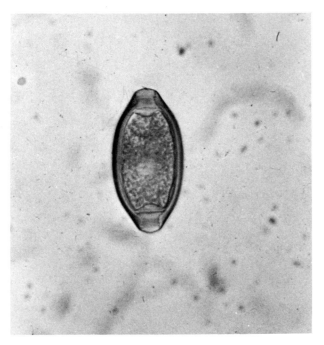

FIG. 17-68. *Trichuris trichiura* ovum. Note the characteristic barrel shape with a ''plug'' at either end. (Courtesy of Rudolf Garret, M.D.)

Trichuriasis

Trichuriasis is caused by the roundworm *Trichuris trichiura,* the so-called whipworm. Its common name is misleading because the whip or tail is actually its head (Fig. 17-67). In some areas of the world up to 90% of the population is infected; it may be the most commonly recognized intestinal helminth in people returning from tropical areas.[218]

The egg has a characteristic barrel shape with a nonstaining prominence at each end (Fig. 17-68). Ingestion of food or water containing the eggs is the method of contamination. In the intestinal tract the eggs are digested, releasing larvae into the small intestine. The larvae reside in the mucosa for several days, and then relocate to the cecal area where they mature (Fig. 17-69).[32]

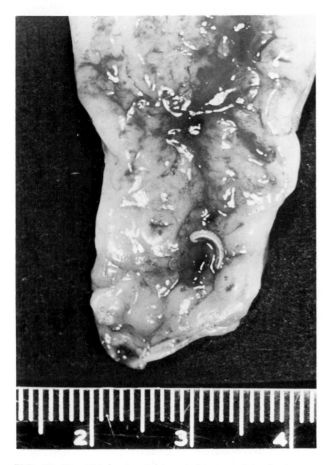

FIG. 17-69. *Trichuris trichiura* (whipworm) in the lumen of the appendix. (Courtesy of Rudolf Garret, M.D.)

Patients may be virtually asymptomatic or have moderate or severe infective symptoms, depending on the extent of involvement. Lower abdominal pain, diarrhea, and rectal bleeding may be reported. Nausea, vomiting, flatulence, abdominal distension, headache, and weight loss may be noted.[218] Appendicitis and rectal prolapse may be a consequence of whipworm infection.[32] Rectal prolapse is thought to result from straining at defecation due to a massive number of worms in the rectum.[218] A number of worms together, creating blockage of the appendiceal lumen, accounts for the signs and symptoms of appendicitis.

The worm has been demonstrated to suck blood from the colon, and it is estimated that 0.005 ml may be lost per day per worm.[218] Hence, severe infestation may cause anemia. However, significant blood loss in the adult has only rarely been recognized.

The diagnosis is made by the identification of the characteristic eggs in the stool. Egg counts are useful in determining the degree of infection and for evaluating the efficacy of treatment.[218] Barium enema examination may reveal evidence of the worms on air-contrast study.

Treatment with mebendazole (Vermox) has been found to be highly effective against *Trichuris* and other worms.[32]

REFERENCES

1. Abel ME, Russell TR: Ischemic colitis: Comparison of surgical and nonoperative management. Dis Colon Rectum 1983; 26:113–115
2. Agrez M, Cameron D: Radiology of sigmoid volvulus. Dis Colon Rectum 1981; 24:510–514
3. Alavi A, Dann RW, Baum S, Biery DN: Scintigraphic detection of acute gastrointestinal bleeding. Radiology 1977; 124:753–756
4. Albrektsson B: Sacral rhizotomy in cases of anococcygeal pain: A follow-up of 24 cases. Acta Orthop Scand 1981; 52:187–190
5. Anderson JR, Lee D: Acute caecal volvulus. Br J Surg 1980; 67:39–41
6. Anderson JR, Lee D: The management of acute sigmoid volvulus. Br J Surg 1981; 68:117–120
7. Anderson JR, Lee D, Taylor TV, McLean Ross AH: Volvulus of the transverse colon. Br J Surg 1981; 68:179–181
8. Anderson MJ Sr, Okike N, Spencer RJ: The colonoscope in cecal volvulus: Report of three cases. Dis Colon Rectum 1978; 21:71–74
9. Anseline PF, Lavery IC, Fazio VW et al: Radiation injury of the rectum: Evaluation of surgical treatment. Ann Surg 1981; 194:716–724
10. Attiyeh FF, Knapper WH: Pseudo-obstruction of the colon (Ogilvie's syndrome). Dis Colon Rectum 1980; 23:106–107
11. Bacon PA, Tribe CR, Harrison P, Mackenzie JC: Rheumatoid disease, amyloidosis, and its treatment with penicillamine (abst) Arthritis Rheum 1981; 44:454
12. Baer JW: Vascular ectasias. In Greenbaum EI (ed): Radiographic Atlas of Colon Disease, pp 623–630. Chicago, Year Book Medical Publishers, 1980
13. Ballantyne GH: Sigmoid volvulus: High mortality in county hospital patients. Dis Colon Rectum 1981; 24:515–520
14. Ballantyne GH: Review of sigmoid volvulus: History and results of treatment. Dis Colon Rectum 1982; 25:494–501

15. Ballantyne GH: Review of sigmoid volvulus: Clinical patterns and pathogenesis. Dis Colon Rectum 1982; 25:823–830

16. Bardsley D: Pseudo-obstruction of the large bowel. Br J Surg 1974; 61:963–969

17. Bass EM: Duplication of the colon. In Greenbaum EI (ed): Radiographic Atlas of Colon Disease, pp 153–158. Chicago, Year Book Medical Publishers, 1980

18. Bauer JJ, Weiss M, Dreiling DA: Stercoraceous perforation of the colon. Surg Clin North Am 1972; 52:1047–1053

19. Baum S: Angiography and the gastrointestinal bleeder. Radiology 1982; 143:569–572

20. Belliveau P, Goldberg SM, Rothenberger DA, Nivatvongs S: Idiopathic acquired megacolon: The value of subtotal colectomy. Dis Colon Rectum 1982; 25:118–121

21. Berci G, Morgenstern L: An operative proctoscope for foreign-body extraction. Dis Colon Rectum 1983; 26:193–194

22. Bessa SM, Helmy I, Mekky F, Hamam SM: Colorectal schistosomiasis: Clinicopathologic study and management. Dis Colon Rectum 1979; 22:390–395

23. Black RE, Jackson RJ, Tsai T et al: Epidemic *Yersinia enterocolitica* infection due to contaminated chocolate milk. N Engl J Med 1978; 298:76–79

24. Blaser MJ, Reller LB: *Campylobacter* enteritis. N Engl J Med 1981; 305:1444–1452

25. Bloch C: The natural history of pneumatosis coli. Radiology 1977; 123:311–314

26. Blundell CR, Earnest DL: Idiopathic cecal ulcer: Diagnosis by colonoscopy followed by nonoperative management. Dig Dis Sci 1980; 25:494–503

27. Boley SJ, Feinstein FR, Sammartano R et al: New concepts in the management of emboli of the superior mesenteric artery. Surg Gynecol Obstet 1981; 153:561–569

28. Boley SJ, Sammartano R, Adams A et al: On the nature and etiology of vascular ectasias of the colon. Gastroenterology 1977; 72:650–660

29. Boley SJ, Sprayregen S, Sammartano RJ et al: The pathophysiologic basis for the angiographic signs of vascular ectasias of the colon. Radiology 1974; 125:615–621

30. Boley SJ, Sprayregen S, Siegelman SS, Veith FJ: Initial results from an aggressive roentgenological and surgical approach to acute mesenteric ischemia. Surgery 1977; 82:848–855

31. Bottone EJ, Keush GT: Bacterial agents of diarrheal diseases. API Species 1981; 5:29–38

32. Brandborg LL: Parasitic diseases. In Sleisenger MH, Fordtran JS (eds): Gastrointestinal Disease, 2nd ed, pp 1154–1181. Philadelphia, WB Saunders, 1978

33. Breiter JR, Hajjar J-J: Segmental tuberculosis of the colon diagnosed by colonoscopy. Am J Gastroenterol 1981; 76:369–373

34. Bubenik O, Meakins JL, McLean APH: Delayed perforation of the colon in blunt abdominal trauma. Can J Surg 1980; 23:473–475

35. Burbige EJ, Radigan JJ: Antibiotic-associated colitis with normal appearing rectum. Dis Colon Rectum 1981; 24:198–200

36. Burnham WR, Reeve RS, Finch RG: *Entamoeba histolytica* infection in male homosexuals. Gut 1980; 21:1097–1099

37. Campbell WL: Cathartic colon: Reversibility of roentgen changes. Dis Colon Rectum 1983; 26:445–448

38. Catterall RD: Sexually transmitted diseases of the anus and rectum. Clin Gastroenterol 1975; 4:659–669

39. Chawla S: Tuberculosis of the colon. In Greenbaum EI (ed): Radiographic Atlas of Colon Disease, pp 557–575. Chicago, Year Book Medical Publishers, 1980

40. Cone JB, Wetzel W: Toxic megacolon secondary to pseudomembranous colitis. Dis Colon Rectum 1982; 25:478–482

41. Cooke SAR, deMoor NG: The surgical treatment of the radiation-damaged rectum. Br J Surg 1981; 68:488–492

42. Corman ML, Veidenheimer MC, Swinton NW: Diseases of the Anus, Rectum, and Colon. Part I: Neoplasms. New York, Medcom, 1972

43. Cram AE, Pearlman NW, Jochimsen PR: Surgical management of complications of radiation-injured gut. Am J Surg 1977; 133:551–553

44. Crowson TD, Hines C Jr: Amebiasis diagnosed by colonoscopy. Gastrointest Endosc 1978; 24:254–255

45. Curtis KJ, Sleisenger MH: Infectious and parasitic diseases. In Sleisenger MH, Fordtran JS: Gastrointestinal Disease, 2nd ed, pp 1679–1715. Philadelphia, WB Saunders, 1978

46. Dang CV, Peter ET, Parks SN, Ellyson JH: Trauma of the colon: Early drop-back of exteriorized repair. Arch Surg 1982; 117:652–656

47. Desbaillets LG, Mangla JC: Pneumatosis cystoides intestinalis diagnosed by colonoscopy. Gastrointest Endosc 1974; 20:126–127

48. Donaldson SS, Jundt S, Ricour C et al: Radiation enteritis in children. Cancer 1975; 35:1167–1178

49. Duff TH, Wright FF: Acute and chronic ulcers of the rectum. Surg Gynecol Obstet 1981; 153:398–400

50. Eftaiha M, Hambrick E, Abcarian H: Principles of management of colorectal foreign bodies. Dis Colon Rectum 1977; 112:691–695

51. Ellis ME, Watson BM, Milewski PJ, Jones G: *Clostridium difficile* colitis unassociated with antibiotic therapy. Br J Surg 1983; 70:242–243

52. Ernst CB, Hagihara PF, Daugherty ME et al: Ischemic colitis incidence following abdominal aortic reconstruction: A prospective study. Surgery 1976; 80:417–421

53. Fekety R, Quintiliani R: Current approach to the treatment of antibiotic-associated diarrhea. Infections in Surgery 1982; September: 13–24

54. Ferguson EF: The Foley catheter in colon-rectal surgery. Contemp Surg 1983; 22:43–48

55. Figiel LS, Figiel SJ: Volvulus of the cecum and right colon. In Greenbaum EI (ed): Radiographic Atlas of Colon Disease, pp 637–645. Chicago, Year Book Medical Publishers, 1980

56. Filho EC: Strongyloidiasis. Clin Gastroenterol 1978; 7:179–200

57. Fiumara NJ: Treating gonorrhea. Am Fam Physician 1981; 23:123–126

58. Flint LM, Vitale GC, Richardson JD, Polk HC Jr: The injured colon: Relationships of management to complications. Ann Surg 1981; 193:619–623

59. Forde KA, Lebwohl O, Wolff M, Voorhees AB: The endoscopy corner: Reversible ischemic colitis: Correlation of colonoscopic and pathologic changes. Am J Gastroenterol 1979; 72:182–185

60. Forde KA, Whitlock RT, Seaman WB: The endoscopy corner: Pneumatosis and cystoides intestinalis: Report of a case and colonoscopic findings of inflammatory bowel disease. Am J Gastroenterol 1977; 68:188–190

61. Forgacs P, Wright PH, Wyatt AP: Treatment of intestinal gas cysts by oxygen breathing. Lancet 1973; 1:579–582

62. Franklin GO, Mohapatra M, Perrillo RP: Colonic tuberculosis diagnosed by colonoscopic biopsy. Gastroenterology 1979; 76:362–364

63. Franzin G, Dina R, Scarpa A, Fratton A: The evolution of the solitary ulcer of the rectum: An endoscopic and histopathological study. Endoscopy 1982; 14:131–134

64. Friedman G, Sloan WC: Ischemic enteropathy. Surg Clin North Am 1972; 52:1001–1012

65. Gafni J, Sohar E: Rectal biopsy for the diagnosis of amyloidosis. Am J Med Sci 1960; 240:332–336

66. Garber HI, Rubin RJ, Eisenstat TE: Removal of a glass foreign body from the rectum. Dis Colon Rectum 1981; 24:323

67. Gefter WB, Evers KA, Malet PF et al: Nontropi-cal sprue with pneumatosis coli. AJR 1981; 137:624–625

68. Ghazi A, Shinya H, Wolff WI: Treatment of volvulus of the colon by colonoscopy. Ann Surg 1976; 183:263–265

69. Glick ME, Meshkinpour H, Haldeman S et al: Colonic dysfunction in multiple sclerosis. Gastroenterology 1982; 83:1002–1007

70. Golladay ES, Byrne WJ: Intestinal pseudoobstruction. Surg Gynecol Obstet 1981; 153:257–273

71. Goodall RJK: Pneumatosis coli: Report of two cases. Dis Colon Rectum 1978; 21:61–65

72. Goodell SE, Quinn TC, Mkrtichian E et al: Herpes simplex virus proctitis in homosexual men. N Engl J Med 1983; 201:868–871

73. Gorbach SL: Infectious diarrheas. Presented at Annual Meeting, American Society of Colon and Rectal Surgeons. Boston, Massachusetts, 1983

74. Grant SR, Salvati EP, Rubin RJ: Levator syndrome: An analysis of 316 cases. Dis Colon Rectum 1975; 18:161–163

75. Groff WL: Angiodysplasia of the colon. Dis Colon Rectum 1983; 26:64–67

76. Gruenberg JC, Batra SK, Priest RJ: Treatment of pneumatosis cystoides intestinalis with oxygen. Arch Surg 1977; 112:62–64

77. Gruenberg JC, Grodsinsky C, Ponka JL: Pneumatosis intestinalis: A clinical classification. Dis Colon Rectum 1979; 22:5–9

78. Haas PA, Fox TA Jr: Civilian injuries of the rectum and anus. Dis Colon Rectum 1979; 22:17–23

79. Hagihara PF, Chuang VP, Griffen WO: Arteriovenous malformations of the colon. Am J Surg 1977; 133:681–687

80. Hagihara PF, Ernst CB, Griffen WO Jr: Incidence of ischemic colitis following abdominal aortic reconstruction. Surg Gynecol Obstet 1979; 149:571–573

81. Heller M: The gay bowel syndrome: A common problem of homosexual patients in the emergency department. Ann Emerg Med 1980; 9:487–493

82. Hiatt GA: Miliary tuberculosis with ileocecal involvement diagnosed by colonoscopy. JAMA 1978; 240:561–562

83. Holt S, Gilmour HM, Buist TAS et al: High-flow oxygen therapy for pneumatosis coli. Gut 1979; 20:493–498

84. Howard RS, Catto J: Cecal volvulus: A case for nonresectional therapy. Arch Surg 1980; 115:273–277

85. Hughes JP: Foreign body of the rectum removal. Am J Proctol Gastroenterol Colon Rectal Surg 1983; 34:16

86. Istre GR, Kreiss K, Hopkins RS et al: An outbreak of amebiasis spread by colonic irrigation at a chiropractic clinic. N Engl J Med 1982; 307:339–342

87. Janda WM, Bohnhoff M, Morello JA, Lerner SA: Prevalence and site-pathogen studies of Neisseria meningitidis and N gonorrhoeae in homosexual men. JAMA 1980; 244:2060–2064

88. Joergensen K, Kronborg O: The colonoscope in volvulus of the transverse colon. Dis Colon Rectum 1980; 23:357–358

89. Johnson DH, Guthrie TH, Tedesco FJ et al: Amyloidosis masquerading as inflammatory bowel disease with a mass lesion simulating malignancy. Am J Gastroenterol 1982; 77:141–145

90. Johnson PH: Coccygodynia. J Arkansas Med Soc 1981; 77:421–424

91. Juniper K: Amoebiasis. Clin Gastroenterol 1978; 7:3–29

92. Kasulke RJ, Anderson WJ, Gupta SK, Gliedman ML: Primary tuberculous enterocolitis: Report of three cases and review of the literature. Arch Surg 1981; 116:110–113

93. Kim MW, Hundahl SA, Dang CR et al: Ischemic colitis after aortic aneurysmectomy. Am J Surg 1983; 145:392–394

94. King HC, Voss EC Jr: Tuberculosis of the cecum simulating carcinoma. Dis Colon Rectum 1980; 23:49–53

95. Kinsella TJ, Bloomer WD: Tolerance of the intestine to radiation therapy. Surg Gynecol Obstet 1980; 151:273–284

96. Kirkpatrick JR, Rajpal SG: The injured colon: Therapeutic considerations. Am J Surg 1975; 129:187–191

97. Knight R: Giardiasis, isosporiasis, and balantidiasis. Clin Gastroenterol 1978; 7:31–47

98. Koep LJ, Peters TG, Starzl TE: Major colonic complications of hepatic transplantation. Dis Colon Rectum 1979; 22:218–220

99. Konda J, Ruth M, Sassaris M, Hunter FM: Sarcoidosis of the stomach and rectum. Am J Gastroenterol 1980; 73:516–518

100. Koo J, Ho J, Ong GB: The value of colonoscopy in the diagnosis of ileocecal tuberculosis. Endoscopy 1982; 14:48–50

101. Koss LG: Abdominal gas cysts (pneumatosis cystoides intestinorum hominis): An analysis with a report of a case and a critical review of the literature. Arch Pathol 1952; 53:523–549

102. Kumar SS, Appavu SS, Abcarian H, Barreta T: Amyloidosis of the colon: Report of a case and review of the literature. Dis Colon Rectum 1983; 26:541–544

103. Kusminsky RE, Shbeeb I, Makos G, Boland JP: Blunt pelviperineal injuries: An expanded role for the diverting colostomy. Dis Colon Rectum 1982; 25:787–790

104. Kyle RA, Spence RJ, Dahlin DC: Value of rectal biopsy in the diagnosis of primary systemic amyloidosis. Am J Med Sci 1966; 251:501–506

105. Lane RH: Clinical application of anorectal physiology. Proc R Soc Med 1975; 68:28–30

106. Last MD, Lavery IC: Major hemorrhage and perforation due to a solitary cecal ulcer in a patient with end-stage renal failure. Dis Colon Rectum 1983; 26:495–498

107. Launer DP, Miscall BG, Beil AR Jr: Colorectal infarction following resection of abdominal aortic aneurysms. Dis Colon Rectum 1978; 21:613–617

108. Lavery IC, Steiger E, Fazio VW: Home parenteral nutrition in management of patients with severe radiation enteritis. Dis Colon Rectum 1980; 23:91–93

109. Lebedeff DA, Hochman EB: Rectal gonorrhea in men: Diagnosis and treatment. Ann Intern Med 1980; 92:463–466

110. Lopez MJ, Kraybill WG, Johnston WD, Bricker EM: Postirradiation reconstruction of the rectum in a male. Surg Gynecol Obstet 1982; 155:67–71

111. Lopez MJ, Memula N, Doss LL, Johnston WD: Pseudo/Obstruction of the Colon During Pelvic Radiotherapy. Dis Colon Rectum 1981; 24:201–204

112. Lou MA, Johnson AP, Atik M et al: Exteriorized repair in the management of colon injuries. Arch Surg 1981; 116:926–929

113. Love JW: The syndrome of calcific aortic stenosis and gastrointestinal bleeding. J Thorac Cardiovasc Surg 1982; 83:779–783

114. Lynn HB, Van Heerden JA: Rectal myectomy in Hirschsprung's disease: A decade of experience. Arch Surg 1975; 110:991–994

115. Madigan MR: Solitary ulcer of the rectum. Proc R Soc Med 1964; 57:403

116. Madigan MR, Morson BC: Solitary ulcer of the rectum. Gut 1969; 10:871–881

117. Madsen PV, Nielsen-Lykkegaard M, Nielsen OV: Ceruletide reduces postoperative intestinal paralysis: A double-blind, placebo-controlled trial. Dis Colon Rectum 1983; 26:159–160

118. Mapp E: Colonic manifestations of the connective tissue disorders. Am J Gastroenterol 1981; 75:386–393

119. Marks G: Combined abdominotranssacral reconstruction of the radiation-injured rectum. Am J Surg 1976; 131:54–59

120. Marks G, Mohiudden M: The surgical management of the radiation-injured intestine. Surg Clin North Am 1983; 63:81–96

121. Marston A, Pheils MT, Thomas ML et al: Isch-aemic colitis. Gut 1966; 7:1–15

122. Martelli H, Devroede G, Arhan P, Duguay C: Mechanisms of idiopathic constipation: Outlet obstruction. Gastroenterology 1978; 75:623–631

123. Martin CJ, Parks TG, Biggart JD: Solitary rectal ulcer syndrome in Northern Ireland, 1971–1980. Br J Surg 1981; 68:744–747

124. Max MH, Richardson JD, Flint LM Jr et al: Co-lonoscopic diagnosis of angiodysplasias of the gastrointestinal tract. Surg Gynecol Obstet 1981; 152:195–199

125. Maxwell TM: Rectal injuries. Can J Surg 1978; 21:524

126. McCready RA, Beart RW Jr: Adult Hirsch-sprung's disease: Results of surgical treatment at the Mayo Clinic. Dis Colon Rectum 1980; 23:401–407

127. Merritt RJ, Coughlin E, Thomas DW et al: Spec-trum of amebiasis in children. Am J Dis Child 1982; 136:785–789

128. Meyers MA: Colonic ileus. In Greenbaum EI (ed): Radiographic Atlas of Colon Disease, pp 95–98. Chicago, Year Book Medical Publishers, 1980

129. Meyers MA, Ghahremani GG: Pneumatosis coli. In Greenbaum EI (ed): Radiographic Atlas of Co-lon Disease, pp 389–399. Chicago, Year Book Medical Publishers, 1980

130. Miercort RD, Merrill FG: Pneumatosis and pseudo-obstruction in scleroderma. Radiology 1969; 92:359–362

131. Mills B, Zuckerman G, Sicard G: Discrete colon ulcers as a cause of lower gastrointestinal bleed-ing and perforation in end-stage renal disease. Surgery 1981; 89:548–552

132. Ming-Chai C, Chi-Yuan C, Fu-Pan W et al: Co-lorectal cancer and schistosomiasis. Lancet 1981; 1:971–973

133. Miralbés M, Hinojosa J, Alonso J, Berenguer J: Oxygen therapy in pneumatosis coli: What is the minimum oxygen requirement? Dis Colon Rec-tum 1983; 26:458–460

134. Moore JD, Thompson NW, Appleman HD, Foley D: Arteriovenous malformations of the gastroin-testinal tract. Arch Surg 1976; 111:381–389

135. Morgenstern L, Thompson R, Friedman NB: The modern enigma of radiation enteropathy: Seque-lae and solutions. Am J Surg 1977; 134:166–172

136. Nagorney DM, Sarr MG, McIlrath DC: Surgical management of intussusception in the adult. Ann Surg 1981; 193:230–236

137. Nanni G, Garbini A, Luchetti P et al: Ogilvie's syndrome (acute colonic pseudo-obstruction): Review of the literature (October 1948 to March 1980) and report of four additional cases. Dis Colon Rectum 1982; 25:157–166

138. Nelson RL, Abcarian H, Prasad ML: Iatrogenic perforation of the colon and rectum. Dis Colon Rectum 1982; 25:305–308

139. Nelson RL, Schuler JJ: Ischemic proctitis. Surg Gynecol Obstet 1982; 154:27–33

140. Nissan S, Bar-Maor JA, Levy E: Anorectal myomectomy in the treatment of short segment Hirschsprung's disease. Ann Surg 1969; 170:969–977

141. Ogilvie H: Large-intestine colic due to sympa-thetic deprivation: New clinical syndromes. Br Med J 1948; 2:671–673

142. O'Mara CS, Wilson TH Jr, Stonesifer GL, Cam-eron JL: Cecal volvulus: Analysis of 50 patients with long-term follow-up. Ann Surg 1979; 189:724–731

143. Oreskovich MR, Carrico CJ, Baker LW: Compli-cations of penetrating colon injury. Infections in Surgery 1983; 2:101–105

144. Owen RL: Rectal gonorrhea. In Sleisenger MH, Fordtran JS (eds): Gastrointestinal Disease, 2nd ed, pp 1692–1693. Philadelphia, WB Saunders, 1978

145. Palmer PES: Amebiasis and tropical diseases of the colon. In Greenbaum EI: Radiographic Atlas of Colon Disease, pp 9–29. Chicago, Year Book Medical Publishers, 1980

146. Parks TG: Ischaemic disease of the colon. Colo-proctology 1980; 4:213–218

147. Parks TG: Surgical management of injuries of the large intestine. Br J Surg 1981; 68:725–728

148. Pawłowski ZS: Ascariasis. Clin Gastroenterol 1978; 7:157–178

149. Poisson J, Devroede G: Severe chronic constipa-tion as a surgical problem. Surg Clin North Am 1983; 63:193–217

150. Pokorney BH, Nichols TW Jr: Pseudomembran-ous colitis: A complication of sulfasalazine ther-apy in a patient with Crohn's colitis. Am J Gas-troenterol 1981; 76:374–376

151. Quinn TC, Corey L, Chaffee RG et al: The etiology of anorectal infections in homosexual men. Am J Med 1981; 71:395–406

152. Ravo B, Pollane M, Ger R: Pseudo-obstruction of the colon following Caesarean section: A review. Dis Colon Rectum 1983; 26:440–444

153. Reddy KR, Thomas E: Proctitis: An unusual pre-sentation of *Strongyloides stercoralis* infestation. Am J Proctol Gastroenterol Colon Rectal Surg 1983; 34:11–13

154. Reichelderfer M, Morrissey JF: Colonoscopy in radiation colitis. Gastrointest Endosc 1980; 26:41–43

155. Richardson JD, Mas MH, Flint LM Jr et al: Bleeding vascular malformations of the intestine. Surgery 1978; 84:430–436

156. Robbins RD, Schoen R, Sohn N, Weinstein MA: Colonic decompression of massive cecal dilatation (Ogilvie's syndrome) secondary to Caesarean section. Am J Gastroenterol 1982; 77:231–232

157. Robertson HD, Ray JE, Ferrari BT, Gathright JB Jr: Management of rectal trauma. Surg Gynecol Obstet 1982; 154:161–164

158. Rominger JM, Shah AN: Ameboma of the rectum. Gastrointest Endosc 1979; 25:71–73

159. Roswit B: Radiation injury of the colon and rectum. In Greenbaum EI (ed): Radiographic Atlas of Colon Disease, pp 461–472. Chicago, Year Book Medical Publishers, 1980

160. Rozen P, Baratz M, Rattan J: Rectal bleeding due to amebic colitis diagnosed by multiple endoscopic biopsies: Report of two cases. Dis Colon Rectum 1981; 24:127–129

161. Russo A, Cirino E, Sanfilippo G et al: Ampicillin-associated colitis. Endoscopy 1980; 12:97–99

162. Rutter KRP, Riddell RH: The solitary ulcer syndrome of the rectum. Clin Gastroenterol 1975; 4:505–529

163. Ryan P: Sigmoid volvulus with and without megacolon. Dis Colon Rectum 1982; 25:673–679

164. Ryckman FC, Glenn JD, Moazam F: Spontaneous perforation of a colonic duplication. Dis Colon Rectum 1983; 26:287–289

165. Sacher P, Buchmann P, Burger H: Stenosis of the large intestine complicating scleroderma and mimicking a sigmoid carcinoma. Dis Colon Rectum 1983; 26:347–348

166. Sakurai Y, Tsuchiya H, Ikegama F et al: Acute right-sided hemorrhagic colitis associated with oral administration of ampicillin. Dig Dis Sci 1979; 24:910–915

167. Sanner CJ, Saltzman DA: Detorsion of sigmoid volvulus by colonoscopy. Gastrointest Endosc 1977; 23:212–213

168. Schmitt EH, Symmonds RE: Surgical treatment of radiation induced injuries of the intestine. Surg Gynecol Obstet 1981; 153:896–900

169. Schmitz RL, Chao J-H, Bartolome JS Jr: Intestinal injuries incidental to irradiation of carcinoma of the cervix of the uterus. Surg Gynecol Obstet 1974; 138:29–32

170. Selikoff IJ, Robitzek EH: Gingival biopsy for the diagnosis of generalized amyloidosis. Am J Pathol 1947; 23:1099–1111

171. Seppälä K, Hjelt L, Sipponen P: Colonoscopy in the diagnosis of antibiotic-associated colitis: A prospective study. Scand J Gastroenterol 1981; 16:465–468

172. Shamberger RC, Crawford JL, Kirkham SE: Progressive systemic sclerosis resulting in megacolon: A case report. JAMA 1983; 250:1063–1065

173. Shbeeb I, Prager E, Love J: The aortic valve—colonic axis. Dis Colon Rectum (in press)

174. Simpson AJ, Previti FW: Technetium sulfur colloid scintigraphy in the detection of lower gastrointestinal tract bleeding. Surg Gynecol Obstet 1982; 155:33–36

175. Simpson JY: Clinical lectures on the diseases of women. Lecture XVII. On coccygodynia, and the diseases and deformities of the coccyx. Med Times and Gaz 1859; 40:1–7

176. Sjogren RW, Heit HA, Johnson LF et al: Serosal laceration: A complication of intra-operative colonoscopy explained by transmural pressure gradients. Gastrointest Endosc 1978; 24:239–242

177. Skibba RM, Hartong WA, Mantz FA et al: Angiodysplasia of the cecum: Colonoscopic diagnosis. Gastrointest Endosc 1976; 22:177–179

178. Sogge MR, Dale JA, Butler ML: Detection of typical lesions of hereditary hemorrhagic telangiectasia by colonoscopy. Gastrointest Endosc 1980; 26:52–53

179. Sohn N, Weinstein MA, Robbins RD: The levator syndrome and its treatment with high-voltage electrogalvanic stimulation. Am J Surg 1982; 144:580–582

180. Sorenson RM, Bond JH Jr: Colonoscopic removal of a foreign body from the cecum. Gastrointest Endosc 1975; 21:134–135

181. Spiro HM: Clinical Gastroenterology, 3rd ed, pp 729–730. New York, Macmillan, 1983

182. Stansfield VA: Diagnosis and management of anorectal gonorrhoea in women. Br J Vener Dis 1980; 56:319–321

183. Starling JR: Initial treatment of sigmoid volvulus by colonoscopy. Ann Surg 1979; 190:36–39

184. Stewart WB, Gathright JB Jr, Ray JE: Vascular ectasias of the colon. Surg Gynecol Obstet 1979; 148:670–674

185. Stone HH, Fabian TC: Management of perforating abdominal trauma: Randomization between primary closure and exteriorization. Ann Surg 1979; 190:430–436

186. Strodel WE, Nostrant TT, Eckhauser FE, Dent TL: Therapeutic and diagnostic colonoscopy in nonobstructive colonic dilatation. Ann Surg 1983; 197:416–421

187. Talman EA, Dixon DS, Gutierrez FE: Role of arteriography in rectal hemorrhage due to arteriovenous malformations and diverticulosis. Ann Surg 1979; 190:203–213

188. Taylor I, Hammond P, Darby C: An assessment of anorectal motility in the management of adult megacolon. Br J Surg 1980; 67:754–756

189. Tedesco FJ: Antibiotic associated pseudomembranous colitis with negative proctosigmoidoscopy examination. Gastroenterology 1979; 77:295–297

190. Tedesco FJ, Pickens CA, Griffin JW Jr et al: Role of colonoscopy in patients with unexplained melena: Analysis of 53 patients. Gastrointest Endosc 1981; 27:221–223

191. Thanik KD, Chey WY, Abbott J: Vascular dysplasia of the cecum as a repeated source of hemorrhage: Role of colonoscopy in diagnosis. Gastrointest Endosc 1977; 23:167–169

192. Thiele GH: Tonic spasm of the levator ani, coccygeus and piriformis muscles: Its relationship to coccygodynia and pain in the region of the hip and down the leg. Trans Am Proc Soc 1936; 37:145–155

193. Thiele GH: Coccygodynia and pain in the superior gluteal region and down the back of the thigh: Causation by muscles and relief by massage of these muscles. JAMA 1937; 109:1271–1275

194. Thiele GH: Coccygodynia: The mechanism of its production and its relationship to anorectal disease. Am J Surg 1950; 79:110–116

195. Thiele GH: Coccygodynia: Cause and treatment. Dis Colon Rectum 1963; 6:422–434

196. Thomas CG Jr, Bream CA, De Connick P: Posterior sphincterotomy and rectal myotomy in the management of Hirschsprung's disease. Ann Surg 1970; 171:796–810

197. Thompson JR, Watts R Jr, Thompson WC: Actinomycetoma masquerading as an abdominal neoplasm. Dis Colon Rectum 1982; 25:368–370

198. Thompson JS, Moore EE, Moore JB: Comparison of penetrating injuries of the right and left colon. Ann Surg 1981; 193:414–418

199. Thomson G, Clark A, Handyside J, Gillespie G: Solitary ulcer of the rectum—or is it? A report of 6 cases. Br J Surg 1981; 68:21–24

200. Thomson H, Hill D: Solitary rectal ulcer: Always a self-induced condition? Br J Surg 1980; 67:784–785

201. Tobi M, Kobrin I, Ariel I: Rectal involvement in sarcoidosis. Dis Colon Rectum 1982; 25:491–493

202. Todd GJ, Forde KA: Volvulus of the cecum: Choice of operation. Am J Surg 1979; 138:632–634

203. Turnbull RB Jr: Personal communication

204. Udagawa SM, Portin BA, Bernhoft WH: Actinomycosis of the colon and rectum: Report of two cases. Dis Colon Rectum 1974; 17:687–695

205. Udassin R, Nissan S, Lernau O, Hod G: The mild form of Hirschsprung's disease (short segment). Ann Surg 1981; 194:767–770

206. Ustach TJ, Tobon F, Schuster MM: Simplified method for diagnosis of Hirschsprung's disease. Arch Dis Child 1969; 44:964–967

207. Vantrappen G, Agg HO, Ponette E et al: Yersinia enteritis and enterocolitis: Gastroenterological aspects. Gastroenterology 1977; 72:220–227

208. Von Dinges HP, Werner R, Watzek G: The incidence and significance of amyloid deposits in gingival, buccal and rectal mucous membranes. Wien Klin Wochensch 1978; 90:431–435

209. Walters BAJ, Roberts R, Stafford R, Seneviratne E: Relapse of antibiotic associated colitis: endogenous persistence of *Clostridium difficile* during vancomycin therapy. Gut 1983; 24:206–212

210. Weese WC, Smith IM: A study of 57 cases of actinomycosis over a 36-year period: A diagnostic "failure" with good prognosis after treatment. Arch Intern Med 1975; 135:1562–1568

211. Weil PH: Injuries of the retroperitoneal portions of the colon and rectum. Dis Colon Rectum 1983; 26:19–21

212. Weingart J, Höchter W, Ottenjann R: Varices of the entire colon—an unusual cause of recurrent intestinal bleeding. Endoscopy 1982; 14:69–70

213. Wellwood JM, Jackson BT: The intestinal complications of radiotherapy. Br J Surg 1973; 60:814–818

214. West BR, Ray JE, Gathright JB Jr: Comparison of transient ischemic colitis with that requiring treatment. Surg Gynecol Obstet 1980; 151:366–368

215. Wiener I, Rojas P, Wolma FJ: Traumatic colonic perforations: Review of 16 years' experience. Am J Surg 1981; 142:717–720

216. Wig JD, Malik AK, Khanna SK et al: Massive lower gastrointestinal bleeding in patients with typhoid fever. Am J Gastroenterol 1981; 75:445–448

217. Wittoesch JH, Jackman RJ, McDonald JR: Melanosis coli: General review and a study of 887 cases. Dis Colon Rectum 1958; 1:172–180

218. Wolfe MS: Oxyuris, trichostrongylus and trichuris. Clin Gastroenterol 1978; 7:201–217

219. Wu TK: Occult injuries during colonoscopy: Measurement of forces required to injure the colon and report of cases. Gastrointest Endosc 1978; 24:236–238

Index

767

Page numbers followed by the letter *f* indicate illustrations; those followed by the letter *t* indicate tables.